Ditch the scales

The only way to create a beautiful body and a healthy life

BY DONNA STILL

Book Cover Design and Type Setting by **Neil Coe**
(neil@cartadesign.co.uk)

About the Author photography by **Ricky Hutton**

Set in Myriad Roman 11pt on 14pt

First published in 2008 by;

Ecademy Press
6 Woodland Rise, Penryn,
Cornwall UK TR10 8QD
info@ecademy-press.com
www.ecademy-press.com

Printed and Bound by;
Lightning Source in the UK and USA

Printed on acid-free paper from managed forests. This book is printed on
demand, so no copies will be remaindered or pulped.

ISBN 978-1-905823-37-6

Disclaimer:
Information is for educational purposes only. The contents do not constitute health advice
in any way. You should consult your medical practitioner before embarking on any drastic
lifestyle changes.

Whatever you can do or dream you can do, begin it. Boldness has genius, power and magic in it.

Goethe

Acknowledgments

My sincere thanks and heartfelt love goes to all those who have supported me with unconditional love and guidance throughout the development process of ditch the scales. I have the deepest gratitude to two people who are, in my opinion, two of the greatest mentors a person could have: Tony Robbins and Joseph McIlendon III. Over a weekend, they unleashed a power within me that is so strong, so resourceful it enabled me to step up and take on my own challenges, breaking through fears and limitations in a way that I would never have imagined. I honour both for the outstanding way in which they touch and change lives forever!

I'd also especially like to thank all the people who have been involved in the research, development and completion of this book; without their help and input it would not have been possible. I offer special thanks to the following: Alan, Joe, Rachael, Daniel and Holly Still, Denise Rollison, Jo Adams, Di Gilder, Lucia Cinnery, Lynn Jones, Karina Cordon, Marie Mc Creedy, Susan Savery, John Cassidy-Rice, Hazel Dudley, Francesca Flinn, Errol Denton, Pummi Mathu, Anita Bhardway, Jo Bell, Richard Love, Ruth Crone, My coaches, Shyanne Smith, Sandy Warr and vitally editor and publisher Mindy Gibbins-Klein for her time, friendship and unquestionable belief in my ability to develop my initial thoughts and ideas onto paper and finally into print.

I feel totally honoured and blessed to have worked with you all.

I dedicate this book to my husband Alan and children, Joe, Su, Rachael, Daniel and Holly for their support and showing me how to love unconditionally.

With much love
XOX

CONTENTS

About the Author

Donna Still is a life strategies & success coach who works with individuals and business' to develop sensible strategies for change and change management. Having read thousands of books attended hundreds of hours of personal development programmes and trained as a professional, personal performance coach, a Master NLP practitioner & Trainer, Donna is the proprietor of **Ultimate Life** Personal development and consultancy.

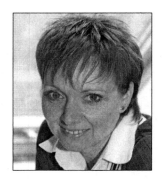

Donna has a straight talking no nonsense approach to life and living and believes that it is in the challenging times that we grow the most. These are the times when we are tested to our limits, the times when we discover our true inner strengths, the times when we find out who we really are. Donna has always been interested in education and personal development and since 2001 has followed a path to help others develop to their true and fullest potential. Working with people from all areas of society, assisting them to develop strategies to live a successful life full of confidence and a true sense of purpose.

Donna realised many years ago that the diet industry is set up to ensure you keep going back and spending your hard earned pounds on yet another product that gives you promises that might not necessarily work for you. Asking what is the difference that makes the difference between all the programmes available. She set about extensive research into diet and weightloss methods. What made some programmes work for some people? What would it take to create a healthy balanced lifestyle? How could it be implemented easily for everyone taking into consideration that we are all different? Donna noticed that the one overriding factor is of course the individual, It was the individual who created success through their belief and value system. She then asked, how could I help those who needed it develop a support system that was individualised. What was needed was a new dynamic approach to health that dealt with what was happening within and this is precisely why Donna developed the *Ditch the Scales* coaching programme and then wrote this book ditch the scales, to make the principles and techniques more widely available to all.

Donna launched her Ditch the Scales coaching and support programme in March 2007. Designed for those who are serious about making a change in their life and gaining full control of their health once and for all. Ditch the scales is also beneficial to anyone who has ever suffered health problems as a result of being overweight or obese, or those who suffer low confidence and self-esteem because of their life time struggles with weight. It is equally beneficial to anyone who has ever entertained the thought that they might like to lose weight, what ever there age or gender.

Donna now spends most of her time encouraging and supporting individuals to create their Ultimate Life strategies and make it their reality through her ditch the scales and coaching programmes and is regularly invited to share her experiences and life/health strategies by occupational health therapists, GP's etc. During 2008 ditch the scales will be available as a series of workshops. To find out more about workshop dates and to register your interest in the ditch the scales workshops please visit the website at: www.ditchthescales.com

"Life is a gift, capture the magic moments, cherish yourself, live with passion"

– Tony Robbins

Birthday Suit

You already know that even the most expensive designer outfit in the world cannot change how you feel inside. If you don't like or love yourself, then how can you expect anyone else to? If you are not comfortable in your own skin, then no amount of expensive clothing or cosmetic surgery will change a thing. That's why I have written this book and developed the ditch the scales coaching and lifestyle programme to support you on your quest for a confident, slimmer, healthier you.

I too spent many years struggling with diets and failed miserably. Until, that is, I discovered the key to unlock my own success. The true reason why I had always previously failed every diet I tried and never become what I'd always dreamed of, slim and healthy, I never realised at the time, but I grew up with expectations of being fat. It wasn't uncommon for my sister and me to be referred to as, 'fatty and skinny,' no prizes for guessing which one I was!

I know the challenges you will face every day and wish to support you, to encourage you, to help you make that decision to make a lasting change that will impact your life in ways that you may never have imagined. I have already helped numerous clients take those incredible, tentative first steps to make positive decisions for lasting change not only in the way they view themselves but also their relationship with food, banishing forever the necessity of the old habits of binge eating, over eating and comfort eating.

By participating and engaging fully with each of the exercises contained within these pages you will gain benefits that will far exceed your expectations, benefits that will permeate into every area of your life. You will find that you will become more confident as your self esteem grows, as a result of working through the issues and challenges that you face on a daily basis to uncover the truths about who you really are. You may even find a few surprises here and there! If I were to ask you 'Who are you?', how would you reply? Have your weight and the issues surrounding it become part of your identity? We shall see. Do you find yourself often saying, 'It's just the way I am and I've never been any different'? You know already who you are at your core. Can you imagine how it would feel to be able to express those thoughts and feelings both verbally and physically? To really express your true self! I know already that you have the ability to be a beautifully confident, healthy person; it's just that your life's traumas' and challenges have allowed you to forget your true self.

Contained within these covers is the formula for your success, the key ingredients for you to become healthy and slim and create the body image/shape you have always desired but previously thought was unachievable. Because you have tried all the diets, joined all the clubs and always sabotaged your best efforts and failed miserably. Or maybe you have reached your target then found yourself slipping back into old habits.

You may have gathered by now this book is not about faddy diets or following regimes; it's about you, who you are and what you want to become. It's about working out real strategies that will help you live a full and exciting life. Have you ever given yourself the opportunity to dream? What is your dream body size? What is the vision you hold in your mind's eye of the ideal you? You may never have dared to create a vision of yourself as your ideal shape and size. You may even still be harbouring old emotions and feelings from events so long ago that you can no longer remember them, but buried deep somewhere in the back of your mind is a little voice from the past that pops up now and again, that stops or blocks you from achieving your desired vision. Working through the exercises will enable you to look at your past experiences and make new decisions and choices about how they will affect you from today.

The strategies you will develop will work equally well in virtually any other area of your life where you must make changes. Make a commitment today to yourself to make the changes necessary. You are halfway there; all you need to do now is continue reading through the book answering the questions as honestly as you can, then **act** on the outcomes and findings. You have already shown the intention that you are ready to take action, to create the massive changes necessary to achieve the body of your dreams, grow your confidence and obtain the best physical health you can.

I have written this book to help you kick-start your own successful achievement of attaining a healthy balanced life and to be comfortable in your own skin, to be full of confidence to achieve your dreams and aspirations. Ditch the scales is a pulling together of all the experiences, strategies and exercises I've found useful and developed during my own mission to become healthy and that of helping others to achieve the same results; writing about it has been a truly cathartic experience. Included of course are my own personal experiences and a small sample of those who have been coached to make dramatic and lasting changes in their lives as a result of the 'Ditch the scales coaching programme,' showing you that losing weight can be effortless and fun when you have the right mindset. Once you've **decided** and made a firm **commitment** to yourself, you too can enjoy the experience.

My Journey

The incredible things I've discovered and learned for myself during my journey of education have been so powerful that I've used them to change my own body and self-image. I'll take you through how I transformed myself from a large size 16/18 to a petite size 8/10 in just 6 months. I lost the first 2 stone in the first two months; it just dropped off so fast it was beyond my wildest dreams. The more I looked in the mirror, the better I felt, the more the weight dropped off, it was effortless!

I now have the body shape that I had always dreamed of, the body I always knew I had lurking deep inside the layers of previously bulging fat. I now eat more than I have ever eaten. I never feel hungry. I never get cravings. I have more energy than ever before and I wake up in the mornings feeling alive and full of energy. This is very different to how I felt previously. I was sluggish in the morning, my joints ached so much that I had to lie in bed and exercise them just so that I could stand up; it was agony just to walk to the bathroom. I would always feel fuzzy headed, like my head was clothed in cotton wool; it would take at least two cups of coffee before I would feel conscious in the morning. Now, I don't even need an alarm clock.

It is achievable for you also and it can last a lifetime. Because I have more energy than ever before I sleep less so I have more time to do the things I love. I feel and look amazing and as a result my self-confidence has blossomed. As I was losing the weight the more I congratulated myself the easier it became. My confidence soared. I was and still am walking taller. I'm prepared to put myself forward which was something that I would never have previously done. I'd always preferred to be a bystander. I am also regaining my feminine personal power, the power to make my own decisions, the power to decide what I want, no longer a passive voice but a strong voice that will be heard and it feels great.

You too can and will achieve this for yourself.

For most of my adult life I'd had a love-hate relationship with food. I had tried many diet plans, slimming pills and food replacement programmes, which of course worked in the short term; however there was never any lasting, long-term change. Sure I'd lose weight only to put it all back on again and more when I stopped following the plan. The slimming club scenario wasn't for me either, each week I'd turn up for the weigh-in after having felt like I'd starved and deprived myself all week only to find that I'd put on yet a couple more pounds. The resulting dwindling self-confidence compounded my low self-esteem and feelings of guilt and denial that were keeping me locked in a constant cycle of yo-yo dieting. Of course it was going to take more than just changing my eating habits.

February 9th 2006 was the date I committed to myself that I would become the healthy person I am today.

I decided,

> NEVER again would I suffer the agony of the tops of my legs chafing together until they were a mass of sores and bleeding during the summer.

> NEVER again would I suffer the embarrassment of being breathless after climbing just one flight of stairs.

> NEVER again would I tolerate the pain of aching joints.

> NEVER again was I going to settle for being anything more than a healthy for me size 10.

I wasn't even sure if it was possible at this stage, but I was sure as hell going to do everything I could to get there! I started by setting myself the goal of becoming HEALTHY, which is what I needed to do in order to be able to complete the BELA (basic expedition leader) training in my role as a civilian instructor in the air cadets. For me this was a major turning point. I had a really powerful motivating goal, a reason why I must change my habits **NOW**. I knew that I was going to have to walk almost 20 miles carrying all my equipment over two days to gain the award and I had already previously struggled with the five-mile walk, which took me a full two hours longer than the rest of the group, and left me unable to walk for three days afterwards. A massive shift was required if I was going to successfully complete the BELA training programme.

I quickly began to realise through educating myself by attending personal development seminars and reading books that the reason I was so fat and unfit was because I wasn't really taking any notice of what I was putting into my body. The fat was actually doing me a favour. It was preventing me from being poisoned to death from all the toxins I was consistently stuffing into my long-suffering, obese body. I realised I was just eating or starving, constantly bouncing between the two.

Due to my now stable personal relationship I found that the past fifteen years I'd learned to really enjoy my food and drink, maybe a little too much at times and I had been very creative in the kitchen. I loved to bake and create new dishes. So in my daily round of rushed activities of running the home, working full time and raising four children, I just cooked meals and baked loads of cakes without much thought to the nutritional balance, other than we were having vegetables with each meal even if it was only potatoes and peas! I was giving everyone what he or she wanted; it was definitely the easy life.

In 2004 I discovered I had food intolerances that had caused me to suffer from irritable bowel syndrome. At this stage I weighed in at a hefty 14 stone and a size 22. Being only 5ft 2" this was fast developing into a major problem for me, a potential ticking time bomb. I had already been suffering many joint problems and gynaecological medical problems throughout my 42 years and had a partial hysterectomy at the age of 33 due to endometriosis. I had been prescribed strong painkillers and hormone therapies, which also seemed to assist me in piling on the pounds. Once all my medical issues had been dealt with I realised that the food intolerances to wheat and dairy had been exacerbating the endometriosis and irritable bowel symptoms.

The pleasant side affect of excluding these two products from my diet was that I shed 2 stone relatively quickly. The bloated and griping stomach pains diminished and in fact all the irritable bowel symptoms miraculously disappeared within a couple of weeks, although the diarrhoea, gas and heartburn stopped within a week. I also found that my concentration was better. I no longer had that fuzzy head feeling that I had every morning that sometimes lasted well into my day.

I spent the next two years half-heartedly concentrating on my fitness and stamina. I joined a fitness class which I attended once a week to help motivate me and to increase flexibility in my joints. This was great in helping me feel more in control, but my weight at the start was still 12 stone and a size 16. By becoming more conscious of exercise and what I was putting into my mouth I found that I still struggled to lose just half a stone. I became obsessed with my weight; I would get on the scales every day and be surprised and then irritated by the fact that I hadn't lost any weight again. I would then ask myself questions such as, why couldn't I lose weight? I was still a size 16 weighing 11 and a half stone. I just couldn't seem to shift any more weight. I would stand in front of the mirror grabbing handfuls of fleshy fat and telling my reflection how disgusting it was. Every time I tried on a new outfit I would tell myself how fat I was and how gross it is followed by how unattractive I was. You might have guessed that at the time I didn't like myself much, in fact not at all! I hated the fact that I felt I was a failure, that I didn't take enough care of myself. I would ask myself, 'How could you let yourself get this big in the first place?'

Then I discovered the secret to being slim and healthy lay dormant within me! I could hardly believe it. What exactly was this going to mean to me? This was a revelation. I learnt that I was THINKING FAT, yes, thinking fat, instead of thinking, 'thin, slim, trim,' I was asking myself the wrong type of question, Questions that disempowered me, questions that would keep me in my current position of being obese.

I had no idea that I had been previously programming my body to be fat by asking these disempowering questions. I learnt to change my mindset. It wasn't easy at first. Learning to change my mindset meant challenging my existing beliefs about my whole being, my whole world.

Once I achieved my goal I started to wonder why this information is not more widely available. It's so simple and easy to follow, hence the book you are reading, *Ditch the Scales*. I wanted to know why more people didn't know this stuff. There is no excuse. I wanted to find a way to bring it to a wider audience. I became really passionate about how I could help others to lose weight simply by using their own powerful thought processes. So I started to research in depth different weight loss methods and practices. Looking at what it would take for me to be successful in my goal to not only be slim and healthy myself but also to enable and empower others to follow the same path if they choose to.

I was amazed by my discoveries. I soon discovered that it is possible to lose 32 lbs in as many days and keep it off permanently in a healthy way, by eating the right type of foods. I discovered that by asking myself the right type of questions I could change the way I felt inside. I could change everything about me that wasn't yet how I felt it could be. This new information was very enlightening and empowering for me, easily the most powerful information I've ever had the good fortune to stumble across. I knew then that I must find a way to make it more widely available, talked about or promoted. You really can think yourself slim from within, without the need for will power; it is effortless once you understand the principles and it's as easy as you wish to make it. I have used what I've learnt to make massive changes in my life, and you can also find the key to your own success within these pages.

The most important thing I've learned is that taking full responsibility for treating myself with more respect would give me the results I had always craved, a beautiful lean body and the confidence to be me. I now follow an alkalising lifestyle, which has been a revolution to my body and me personally.

Exploding the Myths

Initially we need to look at the myths surrounding mainly women of a certain age and weight loss. As you were growing up you will have heard many so-called facts and figures about weight loss, you may have even taken them for your own truth. There are many myths but I'd like to just mention four here. If you want to check on other popular myths to do with weight loss do an Internet search, there's no shortage. These myths may have been your beliefs and may have been the foundation of your life for many years. The types of beliefs I'm talking about here are the following myths that particularly refer to women over a certain age. These myths are dressed within our culture and are very insidious; the few below affect primarily women but could be applied equally to anyone.

- **Myth 1** - women over a certain age find it harder to lose weight because your metabolism slows down. I'd like to say this is pure bullshit! Excuse my French, but I have proven this one not entirely true. I was over forty when I changed my lifestyle. I did it by eating more of the right food and increasing the amount of exercise taken. Yes, your metabolism does slow down but that doesn't stop you from losing weight, do you really want to buy into this one?

- **Myth 2** – Women on HRT are always overweight because the hormone therapy makes you put on weight. Yeah! I believed this one for many years, it's also pure bullshit! I have lost over three stone and I'm on HRT, and will be untill I decide to stop. My mum subscribed to this belief for more than twenty years untill I showed her the way. She has also reduced her weight by more than three stones.

- **Myth 3** – Having a hysterectomy makes you put on weight. You've guessed it, bullshit! I've had a full hysterectomy due to endometriosis & large ovarian cysts. That means no ovaries and no uterus and I've still lost over three stone! You can too, if you start to ask yourself a different set of questions.

- **Myth 4** – When you've had children it's harder to lose weight. Sorry, ladies, this one is utter bullshit too. Why do we as women feel the need to give up on looking after our selves when we get to a certain age or start a family?

So, it's safe to say that I've discovered for myself by proving that it's a fallacy that women over a certain age or those on HRT cannot lose weight easily. I now have the most amazing body, my skin is fantastic and I look and feel fifteen years younger. Ladies, like me, you don't have to accept these myths or stories as your reality. We can choose to accept a different set of belief and realities. We can look and feel 10 – 15 - 20 years younger if we decide that is what we want and take the necessary actions to achieve it. You can, like me, achieve or even surpass your wildest expectations effortlessly.

Getting ready

You too can achieve outstanding results and live life with the body and confidence you desire. I would like to be your guide, coach and mentor on your journey to achieving your ideal body and self-image. As your guide, mentor and coach, I promise to challenge you and the beliefs that you currently hold about yourself, your past and your potential. Throughout this book I will encourage and support your quest to become healthy and furthermore I will enable you to celebrate your achievement and successes and build on them to support your development. I am totally committed to your success, In return I expect from you **100% commitment** to fully participate in each exercise and to follow your desire to become healthy and develop the most amazing body you can.

I cannot emphasise enough that it really is as easy as asking yourself a different set of questions and using the resulting answers to transform your lifestyle. The exercises and techniques used in this book are designed to stimulate, motivate and challenge you into making massive changes in your current values and beliefs, propelling you to achieving unstoppable self-confidence. I have coached clients to their ideal body image and weight who had for years believed they were meant to be fat. They could never remember being anything else.

To gain maximum impact from *Ditch the Scales* it will be necessary for you to work sequentially through the book as each new exercise builds on the knowledge and insights gained in the last. Also I would recommend that you set aside a certain time each day to complete the exercises, taking a maximum of thirty minutes at a time to allow for a period of reflection after, so that you gain full benefit of the new insights you discover and act on the new strategies you develop. What's really important here is that you give yourself the time to really try on the strategies and new beliefs you develop and test them for yourself.

There will of course be times when you just want to throw the book. There will be times when you will wonder if it's worth it or if you are doing the exercises correctly. I'd like to reassure you that there is no right or wrong way of completing the exercises; all the answers must be meaningful to you and each individual will respond differently to each exercise. I challenge you to keep going, giving up is no longer an option. When the going gets tough or you're thinking to yourself, what's the point and your inner voice is saying, 'You've never been successful before, what's different this time?' Believe me you will get those voices in your head trying to dissuade you from continuing, this is quite normal, acknowledge your inner voice, you will learn to use it to your advantage.

The following **Ralph Waldo Emerson** quote really puts it all in perspective:

"A hero is no braver than an ordinary man, but he is braver five minutes longer."

Before we get started there are a few things I need you to do. The first is to keep an open mind. I would like you to put aside your ordinary thinking and trust in the process, recognise and accept the past for what it is, the past. The second is that you are 100% committed to creating for yourself a healthier body. Thirdly keep a success journal or diary of your developments if you prefer not to write in this book so that you can track the changes, no matter how small. There are spaces in the book to write in or you can use your separate journal/diary. It's so important to recognise your achievements no matter how inconsequential they seem at the time. Also, it's great to be able to record the thought processes that occur and change during the course of following the ditch the scales programme.

Commitment Statement

I am willing to be your guide, coach and mentor through some amazing life changes. Are you ready?

Below is a coaching agreement for you to sign and date with today's date. This is a contract between us, it is also a record of your commitment to yourself.

I .... promise to fully participate in my commitment to live a healthier life; I will do whatever it takes to achieve my goal to create my beautiful, healthy body and lifestyle.

Signed ....

Date ....

I, Donna Still, promise to play full out in my commitment to challenge you to make the changes you desire for yourself and your life.

How it works

We've already established that you have in the past tried dieting, bought gym memberships, read other weight loss books and even attended slimming club meetings and you were still unable or unmotivated to stick with your eating and exercise plan. You may have realised by now that it's not your body that's holding you back. It could possibly be the negative self-talk, your inner voice that surfaces every time you try something new or different.

So…let's start by asking ourselves the following questions and look more closely at how we will approach this journey together.

How would you like to view yourself?

When you look in the mirror what would you like to see? I would take a guess that you've given yourself so much negative self-talk that you don't actually believe that it's possible anymore for you to change.

We will look together at your current self-image and develop ways in which you can change your internal self-talk to a more positive inner voice that will support you so you can overcome anything life throws at you. Ridding yourself of constant cravings, binge eating, over eating, comfort eating and wallowing forever along with the necessity to measure your self-esteem by what the scales tell you.

How do you view your body?

Once you've looked in the mirror, what do you say to yourself? We will look even closer at the negative self-talk and how that has in the past been affecting your results. Looking at what's great and what can be improved, I will assist you in developing strategies that will create results whilst fitting in with your lifestyle. I cannot stress enough the importance of concentrating on the positive aspects of your body – on what you do like, what you feel are your strong features and developing a strong sense of what you are about to create. How will achieving the body image of your dreams make you feel?

How do you view food?

What do you really believe food is? What does food mean to you? You will through taking part in the exercises develop an understanding of the behaviours that have led you to where you are now. You will learn how to develop and create new strategies that you can use daily to support you in healthy ways. These tools and strategies can change your body shape and size in a few short months without the need to resort to surgery or starving yourself. You will devise strategies that will support you for a lifetime, so you never have to worry about calorie counting or weighing yourself ever again.

By the end of this book, if you have worked through all the exercises you will have discovered deep within you a power that is so incredible that it will drive you to achieve and surpass your wildest expectations and dreams. You will have developed a strong sense of identity, of who you really are and fully understand what motivates and moves you into action. You will never again accept anyone else's negative explanation of who you are. Your reality will be one of your making, your results will become your reality, you will be self assured and confident in you abilities to achieve anything you set you mind to. You will have developed so much confidence you will have difficulty believing you bought in to the old ways of behaving. You will be unstoppable. You will be outstanding. **And unleash your hidden power.**

It all starts with creating a healthy self-image. The road map for your success, the healthy body that you will develop all starts with acceptance, acceptance that you are currently in the perfect place to begin... it doesn't matter any more what you've done in the past. It doesn't matter that you've failed before, now is different. It really doesn't matter at all how many times you didn't quite make it to the finish post. What's important NOW is that you concentrate on the positive aspects about yourself, we all have them, but we oftentimes forget to think about or celebrate them. It's all too easy to just beat ourselves up with our inner voice's negative self-talk and carry on doing what we've always done, getting the same results as we always have. This is a familiar story for many people and I'm sure it is for you too. How can we expect anything to change on the outside if we don't change what's going on inside?

How do you view yourself?

Self Image

According to Dr Maxwell Maltz, It's a well-known fact that a person will not rise above their image of himself/herself. (Psycho-cybernetics) How is your self-image? Where is this thing we call self-image located? If I were to ask you, what would your answer be? Do you even like yourself?

Our culture seems to produce very few examples of beauty in any other way than a stick thin body shape, and as young girls we were pressured into seeing one's body shape as the route to being valued. Due to celebrities and role models, our society is set up this way. The result has been that you have felt compelled to spend many years following faddy diet programmes that just served to help you pile on the pounds and make you feel even worse about yourself. If you have always thought of yourself as fat, thick, lazy, stupid, then you will be. If you have told yourself in the past that it's impossible for you to lose weight then it will be. Whatever you create in your mind is what you manifest on the outside; it's a self-fulfilling prophecy.

Our Western culture, Christian teachings and parental conditioning all serve to teach us throughout our childhood that to feel good about ourselves is VAIN or even worse, MORALLY WRONG and SELFISH. We have been encouraged all our lives to develop humility and meekness in order to be 'good people'. Even those whose families are not religious will have still received those same messages through the very teachings of our culture.

We were all born of course with a very large bank account of self-esteem, but on our journey to adulthood our accounts can become severely depleted. This happens because we have the need to feel good about ourselves. In our experiences we are sometimes ridiculed or reprimanded by the very people we love and trust, we then crave approval so naturally we start to look outside ourselves for approval and expect others to give it to us. This is our first insidious mistake as humans. True self-worth/esteem can only be self-generated. It CANNOT be conferred on you by anyone or anything else. It is not determined by peer approval, economic status or cultural successes.

Fiona Harrold explains that: "True self worth is a sense of internal composure that gives you complete freedom; **when you have it your life choices will spring from genuine desires and talents, rather than the need to achieve or impress."** You will know inside, your internal guidance system, (your inner voice) will work perfectly well, you can tap into it at any time!

To achieve the results we have talked about so far in this book we first have to take control of our psychology. What we think and feel minute to minute has a major impact on our daily lives on every level. You may not at the moment even be consciously making any decisions about your self worth. But you can be sure it's affecting many areas of your life. I'd like you to answer the following questions very honestly, working through them quickly, they are not meant to be agonised over. You already know the answers. Remember you started out life with a full account of 100.

Q How do I rate my self worth right now? (Out of 100)

....

Q If my rating is less than 100, the three reasons for this are:

....

....

....

Q Look at the responses above and ask yourself, 'What specifically stops me from liking myself more?'

....

....

....

....

....

....

....

Q Now that you have your first insights into what you feel might be stopping you from liking yourself more. Ask yourself, 'What are three ways that I hold myself back through not having enough belief in myself?'

....

....

....

Q To gain an even deeper understanding of yourself ask, 'What are three things that I do to be liked by others?' The answers to this question will enable you to immediately make the necessary changes and start taking back your personal power.

....

....

....

Q Now that you know what hidden tactics you have been using to be liked by other people it would be useful for you to understand also the things that you tolerate in your life that drive you crazy and sap your energy. Ask yourself, 'What three things do I tolerate or put up with that if I changed today would make a difference in my life NOW?'

....

....

....

Now you know these insights into your past actions, it's time to do something about it. You have the choice. You can make those changes today or tomorrow. Right now decide when you will make those changes. You will no longer tolerate these three things and see how much more interesting your life becomes as a result. How is your life now different?

We all want to feel good about ourselves. Having answered the set of questions above you will have a clearer picture of what has been driving you up until now and where you have been giving away some of your personal power. This is the start of your journey. By making subtle changes in your thought processes the people around you will start to notice! Revel in it.

Feeling good within yourself is a state of being in which you feel profoundly comfortable with who you are, being able to generate immense enthusiasm and optimism for life. Make another decision now about feeling good within yourself. You really are the best ally you can have, so it makes sense to make peace with yourself and get comfortable in your own skin! It's OK to have had failures in the past, it's OK not to have all the answers and it's OK to let go of things that have been hanging on to you and sticking like glue. Unstick them now and leave them in a safe place. Maybe you could create a box or a room in your mind to put them in, somewhere outside of you. Give it a name so that if later on you decide you want to go back to the old way of behaving you can pick them up again. Although I can assure you that you will never want to go back to acting or thinking in the same way ever again.

I'd like you to take another honesty check; if you imagine your life in terms of a plant and imagine right now that you have all the potential to be a strong, beautiful plant and at the moment you are the seed – full of potential. Like all plants for it to reach its fullest potential it requires certain things to happen. First it requires nurturing, watering, more nurturing, feeding, warmth and light, all these things are required in order to reach the expected potential of being a strong beautiful plant.

As humans we require the same nurturing process of life and living. Ask yourself the following question:

@ How much support do I really offer myself in my life (on a scale of 0 – 100)?

You may have found that you have not been very supportive of your own actions up until now. You may have even realised that you have many wounds gained from events during your life. What are the benefits of these wounds? And why do you keep opening them? If you had an open surface wound, you wouldn't rub salt in it, would you? Why do you insist on opening old wounds and doing the equivalent of rubbing salt in them? What benefits do you really gain from them?

Ⓠ You have had the benefit of your inner voice; you may have experienced two conflicting voices almost like having two people one sitting on each shoulder, talking into each ear, a good guy and a bad guy. It may even just be two different tones of voice, one loud and one soft that has prevented you from saying and doing or achieving things in the past. It may have had a negative affect on your life and caused you great turmoil. All your internal negative self-talk has previously prevented you from achieving your goals so ask yourself, **if my score is less than 100, what is the reason it is not yet 100?** What exactly is your inner voice saying to you now? Write the first thing that pops into your head.

....

....

....

....

....

....

Upgrading your self-esteem/confidence enables you to develop responsibility for yourself and your actions, it is neither self indulgent, self-centred nor arrogant, it will have a positive effect on you and everyone around you.

You may have noticed that people who have a high self-esteem are happy people; they are often the ones who are able to generate feelings of affinity and contribution towards others because they have taken care of themselves and the responsibility for generating their own happiness. People with a high self-esteem are often more sociable, flexible and creative and are able to tolerate life's little irritations and frustrations, being able to come up with creative solutions. They are generally full of feelings of well being, more loving and forgiving towards themselves or others.

The first step is to LOVE YOURSELF. Fiona Harrold puts it so eloquently in her book, *Be your Own Life Coach*, **"Generosity of spirit flows from an eternal spring of self-acceptance, self respect and personal comfort. Generosity and 'bigness' of character can only flourish when we have provided for ourselves and have plenty over to share."**

It's never too late to re-educate yourself; you have the power within to make the necessary changes to create unquestionable and unstoppable self-esteem and blooming self-confidence. The following question will help you to understand how fantastic life can become simply by deciding and committing to doing whatever it takes to achieve your outcomes.

⊙ How would my life be different if I really and truly believed in myself?

What would really be happening in your life if you really and truly believed in yourself? So ask yourself the question again. How would my life be different if I truly believed in myself? You know deep down you can have this vision for your life and make it your reality. What stories have you been telling yourself up to this point about why you never achieve your desired outcomes?

So what's your story?

You may or may not already be aware that you have a programme, an unconscious pattern of behaving running in the background of your life that has till now dictated your behaviour. Your brain is like a massive super computer and came with no manual and no instructions. Your programme has been running without your conscious awareness. This means you may have picked up erroneous programmes that have been causing you pain, turmoil and possibly trauma. We are going to uncover your operating system and obliterate the old systems that are no longer of any benefit to you so that you are free to develop new beliefs about yourself and make new choices.

"That's all very well for you to say," I hear, but, "how will just answering a few questions stop me from hitting the fridge and help me lose weight? How will it stop all those ugly past experiences from ruining my future plans, as they have done in the past? It can't be that easy, can it? "

I expect you're saying to yourself, "My experiences have shaped and moulded me into the person I am today; I can't change just like that, can I? I've been carrying these thoughts and feelings around for a long time, in fact an entire lifetime; I can't just stop them, can I? It's just the way I am." If you are saying any of these things to yourself then read on, you may not be surprised to hear. They are just your...

EXCUSES! EXCUSES! Yes EXCUSES!

Stop blaming others, events or circumstances for your current weight problem. Let's get things clear right now; we have to take responsibility for ourselves. We must take responsibility for our actions; you must take complete responsibility for yourself. It is only by taking control of yourself, for yourself that you will be able to achieve the positive outcome just waiting to be yours.

By taking responsibility, I mean, not blaming others, events or circumstances for being FAT. "You are Fat because you OVER EAT, or COMFORT EAT, or BINGE EAT, or make the wrong choices and eat the WRONG type of foods." You may even be fat because you believe that you were just built that way. You may also believe that you don't deserve to be thin! It could be any one of a number of reasons.

You may even be making excuses for yourself right now, saying to yourself that you don't eat much at all. Who are you kidding? That may even be the problem, you don't eat enough and your body is constantly in starvation mode. Maybe you don't drink enough water to keep your body hydrated. It may be that when you were young, someone close to you called you, 'fat,' or even told you that it was difficult to lose weight. You may even feel that you don't deserve to be slim or look fantastic. You may have had a previous partner that humiliated you in some way that somewhere along the line you stopped respecting yourself. This may come as a surprise to you, but you can choose how you represent all those past experiences to yourself with the right strategies and techniques.

You may have also seen adverts in newspapers and magazines showing images of the, 'perfect figure' and feel that you don't match up. I have news for you; there is no such thing as the perfect figure. We are all individuals, completely unique. No two people are the same, or can be the same. They may exhibit similarities but they are not the same; this richness of difference is what makes us, the human race, so fascinating.

Answering the following three questions will open the door to some of the root causes as to why you decided that you no longer had any respect for yourself, again it's not necessary to agonise over them. You really do already know the answers. Just put it down, you will feel so much better once you have admitted and acknowledged this to yourself. There's nowhere else to hide, you can no longer hide from yourself and giving up is no longer an option. No one said this was going to be easy, just write it down.

Q For what three things do I blame or resent myself for? Just write in the first three things that pop into your awareness.

....

....

....

....

....

....

To give you an example, Shelagh discovered many valuable insights as to why she always had previously struggled with losing weight when answering this question which were brought up for discussion during the coaching programme. The one that affected change in her behaviour most was the realisation that for many years she had been punishing herself for an event that had happened when she was just 16, a sexual attack that she was completely powerless to do anything about at the time. Due to the horrific events, her mother turned to drink as a way of blocking out the pain, thus adding to the intensity and compounding the pain felt by Shelagh and destroying family life as they had previously known it.

Shelagh at the tender age of 16 had taken on board the responsibility for the event and felt that it was all her fault. if she hadn't been raped then everything would have been OK!. Resenting and hating herself for years following the traumatic life changing event, Shelagh had taken on a new belief - I don't deserve to be happy. The event was so powerful and consuming that she now found it very difficult to think back to how she was prior to the event. She could only think of how much she hated and resented who she was and had no respect for herself. Consequently the personal and professional relationships she developed were representative of this. Her relationship with her life partner was abusive and she felt the necessity at work to take on everyone else's problems. Once these issues had been worked through during her coaching session Shelagh was able to recover her self-respect and forgive herself for the past event, which then left her free to make new choices.

For the next step towards a healthy life we need to continue with developing a healthy mind and discover what has really been holding you back and limiting your choices. Don't be a prisoner of your memories. We all have stuff hidden away in a closet in the deepest darkest recesses of our unconscious minds. We hang on to these events, letting them dictate who we are and who we become. We become scared that someone will find us out, so scared that we have to keep visiting it, opening the door and checking if it's still there, oh no! It is. Why can't I get rid of this feeling, thought or event that keeps haunting me? What would I do if someone else found out? What if they find out that that I'm human just like everyone else? Would they judge me? Or maybe you did something you now consider unthinkable and have not gone back and made amends. Now is the time to get it out in the open. To bare your soul to yourself, so that you can re-assess the event and get a new or different perspective on it. Our intention is to deal with the past event and let go of it. **Permanently.**

Firmly place these old thoughts and beliefs about yourself in your very own special place, the one you developed earlier outside yourself, the place where they now belong, so you no longer have to check on them regularly and live in fear of being judged because of them.

On first reading this you may now be thinking that there isn't any hidden stuff in your closet, that's great if that is the case. Ask yourself, am I really and truly being completely honest with myself? If you have a completely clean closet then what is holding you back from achieving your dreams and aspirations? Especially your long-held goal of effortless weight loss? Why have you spent years yo-yo dieting? You may need to give yourself time to reflect on this question for a while and trust in your unconscious mind to bring it to your awareness.

The unconscious mind is very clever at protecting us from being hurt, which is its primary role, so it buries the pain deep, very deep. However it's never completely gone as it's there under the surface, gnawing away. Put the book away for a couple of days. Once you have mulled the question over you will find that your unconscious mind will eventually bring into your conscious awareness the one thing that you have been hiding from. It may be one thing or it may be several. When the reason becomes apparent to you, and it will, write it below. Whatever it is, this will be the right answer for you at this time, so give yourself a chance to be honest with yourself for a change; the resulting positive effect will be like a weight lifting from your shoulders, freeing you to move forward and get on with your life.

❑ For what three things can I not forgive myself?

....

....

....

....

....

When Celia asked this question of herself, she came to the understanding that she had not forgiven herself for her messy divorce. The resulting behaviour was affecting her relationships with her children and herself until she was able to forgive her past demons. Indeed until this was done Celia couldn't move on. The resulting effects of hanging on to feeling bad about how she had failed as a wife and mother were the deep rooted causes that led her to overeat and find solace in food.

Q Now that you have uncovered some of your unthinkables, ask yourself in what three ways do I now punish myself for these past events?

Q When you look at the resulting answers what changes can you make today that will impact your life and help you to achieve your outcome of ridding yourself of the necessity of looking in that closet? What changes must you initiate right now so that you can replace these old ways of behaving? What differences will you be noticing in your self-confidence by making these changes? What will you no longer have to tolerate? How much do you want this change?

As an individual it's of the utmost importance that you must learn to respect yourself.

> *"If you don't set a baseline standard for what you'll accept in life, you'll find it easy to slip into behaviours and attitudes or a quality of life that's far below what you deserve"*
> *– Anthony Robbins.*

Now you have so much new knowledge about yourself it's time to take responsibility for your future. As you work through the following exercises you will discover further ways in which you can more effectively use your past experiences to bring you a new set of positive results and really start living and enjoying life to the full. We will look at your current belief system. How it was formed and how you can use it to make powerful changes in your life that will astound you and those around you. Take a short period of time to reflect on the amazing things you have discovered about yourself. Make notes below of five major changes you have made since embarking on this awesome journey. Make sure you date them. You are now in a great position to look at and make changes to your current belief system, the belief system that has been locking you into the fat cycle.

Beliefs about yourself

Beliefs are the rules you live your life by, they are the reasons you do what you do.. The reason you have achieved what you have in your life to date. They are your reality. Beliefs are also the stories that you tell yourself about what you perceive to be true. Beliefs are formed from the moment we start learning, however they are not always of our choosing, we pick them up from our parents, our friends or colleagues, religion and so on.

Beliefs can be changed. Beliefs are only your perceived reality. To understand how you formed your beliefs we will look at several areas but first we'll look at a time when you used to believe something to be true and now you don't. I bet you can think of an example of something that you used to believe but no longer do, such as Father Christmas or the tooth fairy. When you were younger you believed them to be true until you discovered there was another theory. After a period of time when you heard the new information several times you may have begin to wonder whether you existing theory was correct. Once you had looked at the facts as you saw them at the time you formed a new belief, that's what we are going to do here. Looking at what you used to believe, taking into account the new facts and experience and then forming a new belief, trying it out for a while and seeing if it works for you.

The first step to recognising where and when your particular beliefs were formed involves thinking about your spiritual beliefs and practices. A religion that condemns you as an unworthy sinner and requires you to spend the rest of your life atoning for your wrong doings is not exactly a great place to start feeling good about yourself as a human being. Even if your family didn't attend church regularly, the ideas are embedded within our culture and tend to seep in without our even realising it. The reason I've pointed this out is not because I want you to give up your religious beliefs but to develop a sense of questioning the parts that imply that you are intrinsically bad.

What about your beliefs as a person? Who do you think you really are? What would you be saying to me if I asked that question right now? Do you believe you are intrinsically good? Yes or no? Do you believe you are capable of so much more than you ever dreamed possible? Yes or no?

Again ask yourself the following questions you may think that you are repeating yourself here. You may wish to put down the same answer as before, you may also have realised that there are even more important and urgent areas that require attention now that you already have some insight into your old beliefs.

Ask yourself, **what have I been tolerating in my life?** Let it all out, write everything down that really irritates you everything that niggles you, everything which drives you to distraction yet you do absolutely nothing about it because you believed that it was not in your power to change it. You'll be surprised by what has been affecting you on a daily basis. When I asked Celia this question, she became very emotional which is what everyone does when they realise that these things. These niggles, these irritations have been dragging her down, holding her back. What are the things you have been tolerating? What really niggles you? What are the thorns in your side? Who or what is the pain in your neck? What irritates you to boiling point so you feel that you could explode at any minute yet you choose to do nothing about it? Take the whole of the next page and just get it all out. You may find this easy or you may find this the hardest thing you've ever done. Do it now.

❷ Use this space to write in your new answers to the previous question, what have you been tolerating in your life? We have asked this question before. There is a very good reason to ask you again. You will have a very different answer this time. One that has been deeper rooted than the earlier response.

I bet once you got going it wasn't very hard at all to write a long list. It's all very well knowing what irritates and upsets you but what are you going to do with this information. You've probably thought about the answers a thousand times before. I expect you have even previously come up with relevant solutions to your problems and challenges before but never actually followed them through. Instead you've slipped back into the 'you,' that everyone else expects, resisting the temptation to upset others just in case they judge you in some way.

Julie mentioned that at work every time there was an opportunity for internal promotion she would not apply for it even though she was more than qualified for the role. Her reason for this was she felt that she wouldn't be considered because of her size. This self-limiting thought was affecting her ability to proceed up the career ladder in her profession. She was then irritated by those who achieved promotion with lesser qualifications this was really eating away at her self-confidence and her ability to interact with others in a professional manner.

Julie had developed a pattern of behaving that was so automatic she felt it was part of who she was, part of her identity because she couldn't think of a time when she didn't react in this particular way. Julie's number one issue though was saying no to extra work towards the end of the day. The negative effect of the extra work meant that she would be late home so her children were in bed when she got home, leaving her little or no quality time with them through out the week. This irritated her and made her feel very guilty which was leading to her feeling resentful towards her job and her children.

The new standard that Julie decided to set was firstly to make sure that her boss knew how important it was for her to be home in time to be with her children before they went to bed, then planning and organising her work for the day so that there were no surprises lurking for her at the end, and speaking to her work colleagues, impressing upon them that if they required her input they would need to have the reports to her by a certain time each day. Julie found at first that this was alien to her, however everyone at home and work benefited from the new criteria.

The positive effect of this new standard enabled Julie to spend quality time with her children in the evenings, also gaining more respect from her work colleagues. Julie's self-confidence began to blossom and everyone knew where they stood. Obviously there were teething troubles in the beginning but with persistence and perseverance everyone got the message and Julie had her quality time with her children. Julie then no longer felt the need to sit and comfort eat each evening with bags of crisps, cakes and ice cream.

Ⓠ You may have gathered by now, the only way to change **your** future results is to change the actions that got you to be where you didn't want to be in the first place. For example if you wanted to go to Scotland for your holiday you wouldn't look at brochures for Cornwall, would you! Look at the answers you have given above and assign them each a number starting with No. 1 being the one that if you changed it today, if you stopped tolerating this right now, this instant, would make the biggest change to your life today. The next stage in the process is to decide what you are willing to do to stop this situation or events happening. You have the power to STOP old habits and **CHANGE**, make it different. Ask yourself, **what would I need to do to change its effect on me or to eliminate it completely?** The answers to these questions may at first seem a little uncomfortable, but it's like anything new, it takes time to try it on, see if it fits. Some responses will work better for you than others. It is completely up to you. The best way to deal with this now is just to write it all down.

Now you are ready to ask, **what would I be willing to do to set a new standard for self-respect and respect from others?** Once you have created your new standard let everyone know that from now on this is how it will be. How will you do this? You could write it out neatly and stick it to the fridge if it's personal or somewhere prominent so that everyone can see you mean business. I'm sure you can think of many other ways that would be beneficial to you and those around you. I must warn you, there will be fall out at first. Remember your new standard is not only about how others treat you but also about how you will treat them; you will need to be firm and retain your inner calm, knowing that they will come round eventually on your terms or it's no deal. Get tough on them, get tough on yourself and stick to your new standard. Others have a vested interest in keeping things the same as they always were because otherwise it will mean that they themselves will have to work harder and look at their own actions and behaviours, and why would they want to do that! Keep in mind that most people have their own closets they can't bear to look into! So again, what would you be willing to do to set a new standard for self-respect and respect from others?

Sitting comfortably, just imagine in your mind's eye for the next few minutes what impact these changes would have in your life. Actually ask yourself, **what impact would making these changes have on my life right now and in the future?** Write it down in the space below: the full impact making these changes would have both in your personal life and your professional life.

❑ We can often be quite different at work and at home, in fact most of us have quite different personas for each role we participate in. Think about that for a moment, you may have a job that requires you to be tough, yet at home you are Mrs Softy and let your family walk all over you. Ask yourself, **what new boundaries do I need to set at work and at home?** Maybe you find yourself with an increased workload because you have had trouble-saying NO. These new boundaries will become your benchmark standard. By setting clear boundaries you are sending a clear message to those around about how you wish to be treated. If we don't let them know exactly how we wish them to treat us, then how will they know? We can't expect other people to read our minds. This also goes for how we treat ourselves and what we say to ourselves. **What new boundaries do I need to set at work and at home?**

....

....

....

....

....

....

....

....

Reflecting on the information above, **what new boundaries will I implement from today, right away?** Elaine joined the programme to end her see-saw battle with weight loss. She noticed that she had for as long as she could remember been a member of the self-beaters club, in fact it had been such a long membership that she could no longer remember a time when she said anything positive to herself where her weight and body image was concerned. This was having a negative effect on both her personal and professional relationships.

Starting off just keeping a note in her journal of the language she was using daily to represent certain areas of her life and looking at the effects on her self-confidence of the subsequent actions and attitudes caused by her language, Elaine picked out a couple of words and phrases that she was using most often and that were having the most negative effect. She then substituted them for more positive alternatives She continued to keep a note in her journal of how the new words affected her behaviour and attitudes.

The most negative words and phrases that Elaine used were substituted for more positive ones.

Q Make a list of your negative words and phrases and opposite write their positive alternative. Use the positive words and phrases for at least a week and notice the changes. Make sure you note them down in your journal.

OLD Negative word or phrase	NEW Positive word or phrase

Q Now it's your turn, what new boundaries will you implement from today, right now, which will enable you to reach nearer to your goals, dreams and aspirations?

How committed are you to following through on these actions? (On a scale of 1-10)

....

Make sure you follow through and take this action today. It may seem uncomfortable at first; remember to place your old beliefs in your museum and you will soon enjoy the feelings created within, especially when you start to see the results you intended. Your confidence will also get a fantastic boost.

If I were to ask you if you believed you were a good person, what would you say now? Would you have difficulty in answering this question or can you find many examples of great things you have done or achieved in your lifetime? So here's the question, can you list ten indications that show your goodness as a person or shows what a great person you are?

....

....

....

....

....

....

....

....

....

....

....

....

If you have found this exercise challenging perhaps you need to give yourself more opportunities to demonstrate acts of tolerance, respect and kindness. Practice random acts of kindness and senseless acts of beauty for the next seven days and write below or in your journal or diary each day the effects it has on you, what you feel inside, the response from others etc. These will serve you in very deep and meaningful ways. We all gain huge benefits from small acts of kindness, just a few kind words, a friendly look, a helping hand. Contributing to someone else selflessly doesn't have to cost you huge amounts of time or effort but you gain huge benefits.

Q You will also begin to notice the nice things that others say about you and to you. You will also notice that other people want to spend more time with you because you generate warm feelings in them too! Write in the space below some of the great comments you've heard about you. You may also want to write these comments and place them where you can see them on a regular basis, use them as a tonic, as a pick-me-up for those times when negative self-talk seeps in.

Forgiveness

Earlier I asked you what three things can you not forgive yourself for. The next stage in this wonderful process is to **forgive yourself**, to give yourself a clean slate so that you no longer punish yourself or others for yours or their mistakes, to accept that you are human and that you may not have always achieved the results you were hoping for or indeed expecting.

The most common problem for most people is low level guilt and jealousy which eats away at your self-esteem just below the skin. It manages to seep into every part of your life, simmering and festering just below the surface. All the time you see yourself as bad or feel guilty you'll just put the brakes on the positive feelings that tell you you deserve great things. You've probably noticed that you catch yourself saying things like, that's great for her/him, but I could never have that or be so successful or do something as amazing as that, almost sneering as you say it through gritted teeth. These types of negative self-talk emanate from your feelings of worthiness. It's time for a mind detox. Ask yourself these two questions and write down the answers.

Q What are the three major things I do not forgive myself for and why? Are they the same as before or have you uncovered something different?

You may find that you require more time to reflect on this question as often once we've given an answer there is another more deep rooted issue that comes to the fore, and that's great, however it works for you. Now having purged the depths of your unconscious mind, you need to look at the events you've written above and ask yourself, is my interpretation of the events still correct? Maybe it's just that you were having an 'off day' and that clouded your perception, when in actual fact you never did anything wrong to feel guilty about at all. Maybe with hindsight you are able to see the event from a different perspective. If you decide after all that you were in the wrong then please make amends, make that phone call, write that letter and send that bouquet of flowers.

Now is the time to **forgive yourself for anything that happened in your past** that you feel responsible for and anyone who you feel wronged you in any way, shape or form. If it's not possible to make amends in person, write them a long letter. You don't even need to send it; just the sheer act of purging the unconscious mind is enough to clear it up. When you look at the event with the life experience you now have, what can you learn? What changes happen in your perception of the past challenges or events? What new information have you gleaned from looking at the issue in a detached way? What new facts do you have about each situation that will assist your learning and development?

Remember it's **THE PAST** and we learn from the past, it's time now to let go. By developing your ability to take each experience without clouding the event with emotional baggage you will be able to turn it into a positive learning experience. Any situation you encounter from today, you will have the ability to look at it objectively and ask what have I learnt from this situation or event? How can I use it to further my development or enhance my experience?

> **YOU CANNOT CHANGE THE EVENT OR SITUATION. It is gone. You can, however, change how you represent the event or situation to yourself now, and this will have the most profound effect on your entire life, past present and future.**

> **FORGIVE YOURSELF AND ALL THOSE WHO HAVE EVER CAUSED YOU PAIN IN ANY WAY WHATSOEVER.**

It's only by doing the forgiving part that you will release yourself. I expect you have heard the saying, 'what you resist will persist,' you will then become free to create what ever you want to be. Infinite potential becomes yours for the taking.

WRITE DOWN HERE THE NAMES OF ALL THOSE WHO YOU FORGIVE. Look at each event, what learning can you take from it? Get it all out of your system now.

@ **Remember to thank them for providing you with positive learning experiences.** The reason for doing this NOW is to clear all negativity, so that you can move forward with clear positive perceptions and associations with your past experiences. It's not always easy to look for the positive when we are running away, licking our wounds! So keep going, when you hit a block let your conscious mind relax and let the un-conscious take over. You will be amazed at what insights you unearth. It may help for you to play some relaxing or inspirational music while completing this exercise. This exercise can be very liberating; you'll soon realise that you are free to choose how you represent these previously negative experiences, and you can choose to learn from them. **Do it NOW.** And start writing.

Name	what positive benefit have I gained from the experience
e.g. Mum	I forgive you for ********** and thank you for showing me that I have tenacity of spirit

By developing your ability to take positive learning experiences from any situation you will quickly understand that these events are just events. If you stick to the facts and not cloud them with emotions or emotional reactions you are able to look at what the event has taught you.

You decide how you represent and remember any event or experience. Each person has his or her own individual view on any situation. Who's to say whose perspective is the truth? All viewpoints are representative of each person's perception or reality. What new choices do you have now? Reflect for a while on the new insights you have gained about your past experiences. You have the basis for developing your new true identity and really allow yourself to shine. Give yourself the chance now to be who you want to become. You can decide. You have given yourself permission to be all you can be.

Q What new choices do you now have?

@ You no longer have to accept the old way of thinking; you can choose to believe something new about yourself. What would that something new be? Think of as many new ways of being and write them here, write them in such a way that you can use them every day as affirmations to increase your confidence at any time when you become aware of the old thoughts creeping in. Write them positively, use only positive words, write them very neatly, keep them close by you either in your purse or in a more prominent position so you can look at them whenever you have a free moment. As an example you might come up with something like I accept and like myself or I am capable of connecting with others or even, I am at the beginning of great things. I'm sure you have no shortage of affirmations that are suited to you and your development.

What you have just written is the basis of a powerful new set of beliefs about yourself, about your identity, about your very being, about the person you are becoming, the person you are from this very moment on. Remember, you may find it really useful to write your affirmations out neatly on a piece of card and keep them with you at all times or even write them out large and put them in a really prominent place to remind you of who you are at your core.

There's only one way you can make lasting change and that's by understanding that you must feel what you're creating in your body. Really feel it deep within your gut. You might already know these types of feelings as your intuitive sensibilities, your intuitive inner guidance system. It is there within you even if you no longer feel it or recognise it.   When we talk about inner voices we are really talking about our intuitive guidance system which lets us know whether something feels right or not. Our ego, however, is not really concerned with what is right or wrong; it's only interested in satiating our hunger for material objects. This inner conflict can be controlled by using the short sentences you developed as affirmations. These sentences will support you until they form part of your belief system. Their purpose is to build on what you already know to be true on the inside of you. They will assist you in becoming congruent with those strong inner feelings so that they show on the outside in everything that you do.

Review your progress so far

Whenever we are changing old habits and beliefs, It's very important to take time to reflect and review your progress so far and to really appreciate the quality of the new choices and resources you now have available to you, as a result of your actions. what incredible new insights do you have about your self? How can you use these to further your resolve and create better outcomes for your life? what is the single most positive benefit you have received so far?

Write in this space any new insights you've had as a result of the responses you have given so far.

Controlling your inner conflict

You're already aware there is only one sure fire way to make a lasting change and that's by understanding now that you must **feel** what you are creating throughout your entire nervous system. When you feel something deep inside, you have that knowing inside that penetrates to your core and a belief that it can and will become your reality. You really believe and you are CERTAIN.

These are your intuitive feelings; we are going to look at ways of further developing your intuitive feelings so that you can be guided by your very own inner guidance system. Your inner guidance system is known to you as your gut feelings or intuition. You may have stopped trusting in your own intuitive sensibilities, the following set of exercises are designed specifically to rescue and revitalise your intuition.

When we talk about intuition we are really talking about our inner voice, you know the one that lets you know when you are on the right track, the voice that protects you from doing the wrong thing. The other half of the voice is your ego, the part of you that is only interested in material gain and negative interference. Have you ever wondered why at times you have so much inner conflict that you are overcome with inertia and nothing is achieved?

This inner conflict can be controlled using affirmations. These are sentences that convey a thought or a feeling. You already know a very well known one that was used initially as an experiment with the war wounded soldiers it goes, 'Every day in every way I'm getting better and better.' It was found to be very effective in helping the speedy recovery of patients who had been patched up after being seriously wounded during World War II.

I expect you can think of others.

You will gain many positive benefits by using affirmations on a daily basis; in the beginning you may feel an emotional struggle while you are repeating them. If your ego fights you all the way, this is quite normal. Affirmations are a way of talking directly to your unconscious mind. The purpose of this exercise to build on what your intuitive sensibilities you already know to be true on the inside and assist you in becoming fully congruent with this self-image. Therefore the initial discomfort is quite normal; I can assure you that you will get used to feeling great about yourself and find yourself repeating affirmations to yourself at every opportunity or whenever you see a mirror. I urge you to persevere as just the mere action of repeating them every day will change your future, reading these as instructed you cannot not make a change.

For the greatest success you will need to repeat the process every day for the next 30 days. Stand or sit comfortably in front of the mirror look yourself directly in the eye and repeat the following:-

- I am responsible for the achievement of my desires.

- I am responsible for my choices and actions.

- I am responsible for the level of consciousness I bring to my work.

- I am responsible for the level of consciousness I bring to my relationships.

- I am responsible for my behaviour with other people, co-workers, associates, customers, spouse, children, and friends.

- I am responsible for how I prioritise my time.

- I am responsible for the quality of my communications.

- I am responsible for my personal happiness.

- I am responsible for choosing the values by which I live.

You have discovered so much about how in the past you may have been powerless to resist the labels put on you by others however after at least 30 days of repeating the above affirmations combined with the ones you developed in the previous chapter you will no longer be dependent on others for your inner guidance. You will be unstoppable, free to make your own choices and decisions. Free to choose a healthier lifestyle, free to decide what you will accept as your own truth. Free to embody the spirit of the words you have been repeating to be who you really are.

Remember to make time to repeat these sentences every day, first thing in the morning and last thing at night before you go to bed. What you will notice as you become more aware of your resourcefulness and start making new choices with new found inner resources, is that you will begin to focus on being healthier and you will be! Pareto's principle states that 20% of what you focus on creates 80% of your results. You will begin to find it easy to concentrate on the more positive aspects of yourself and your body because positive actions are what will be stimulating your unconscious mind to assist you in creating the dream body of your desire.

Setting powerful & motivating goals

Recapping on what we've covered so far, firstly you have accepted the past for what it is, the past, you have moved on through forgiveness and letting go of those past events or situations that had previously held you back in the previous chapters. The letting go happened when you acknowledged and accepted the past experiences and events so that they now no longer haunt you but are utilised in a way that helps you to grow exponentially personally and professionally. Essentially you have taken all the positive learnings from the past experiences and moved on.

Because you've taken the time and had a really good long, hard look into what has previously stood in the way of you achieving your desired outcome of living a healthy lifestyle, you will want to assess whether your initial goals are still powerful enough and motivating you in the right direction. I'm sure you've heard it a thousand times before but goal setting really is the driving force to achieving outstanding success.

So what is a goal? I'm sure you know already that the goal is the end vision, the dream, your ultimate desire, the outcome you wish to achieve. I'm sure you have set many goals in the past that have fallen by the wayside and never been accomplished. I'm also certain that you have set other goals that you have achieved quite easily. So what was the difference between the two?

Your goal is like the 'rudder' or the 'steering wheel' of your life. Whether you are consciously aware or not your dreams and desires are guiding you. Wouldn't it be fantastic if you could harness this power and really make it work for you?

The book *Psycho-Cybernetics* opens with the following statement:

"If you aren't achieving everything you want in life, it is probably because your goals are ineffectively communicated to, or rejected by your self-image, and your servo-mechanism is under-utilised or uninspired." – *Maxwell Maltz*

A statement full of jargon but in a nutshell what it really means is that your servo-mechanism according to Maltz is your internal guidance system, the one that guides you, the one that informs you if you are right or wrong. The one that lets you know whether you really believe you are worth the effort. The system that you have now taken control of by letting go and learning from past events and are shaping exactly as you want it with your daily meaningful affirmations.

But what exactly does this mean to me, I can hear your thinking. Let us briefly explore the possibilities of this statement. We can make the assumption that the way you were before embarking on the earlier exercises within this book had been unconsciously conditioned and programmed by your past experiences, that is why you have completed the exercises in a particular order. You are then left asking the question, what do I need to do to change my past results? How do I change my past results so that I can achieve my aspirations of leading a healthy life?

To start this powerful driving process you are going to develop a set of goals or outcomes that are so compelling you can't wait to get out of bed every morning to start working on them. To achieve your goals there is a particular process and steps you need to take so we will work through them in order. Just so that you know this process can be used for any area of your life but here we are concentrating on you setting powerfully stimulating goals for a healthy life.

Step one – DREAM

Forget about what's realistic, even dream the things that you think are so ridiculous and far-fetched. What is your dream, your vision? It really doesn't matter whether you actually believe at this stage it's possible or not; all you need to do now is dream BIG, dream. We really do live in a no limit world. Use all your senses, all your imagination. What does your dream look like? What does it sound like? What does it feel like? What does it taste like? And what does it smell like? Ramp it up and double those feelings, bigger, brighter, and louder. When you have finished dreaming write it down here. You may like to keep a board that contains images of what you wish your outcome to be. Keep it in a prominent place, look at it every day.

In the past you may have gone through this initial stage of dreaming and even got as far as writing it down, put it in a drawer, then nothing! You never set it as a goal, as a must for you to achieve. You may have even shared it with someone else and they told you it wasn't possible for you, or it was too hard or maybe you have even thought yourself that it would be great but you didn't have the resources within. Feelings of defeat and powerlessness ensued. You then believed that it wasn't possible for you to achieve your dreams. What's different now? You do already know that you can achieve your dreams, don't you? I expect there is a little voice in your head saying right now that this goal is so far away from where you are now that it's not possible to achieve, and that's right.

Think of this dream, this vision of where you aim to go, as like looking at your destination on a road map. When you want to go anywhere new you need to have a destination in mind otherwise how will you know what roads you need to take on your journey there? If you didn't have a destination you would end up driving around aimlessly, wouldn't you? Maybe that's how your life has been up till now. Do you really want to be going in no particular direction? Your dream, your vision can become your goal and this is your destination, the place you want to end up in, and you only achieve this by being determined and focused on where you want to go.

Step two – Clarity

When your dream actually becomes clearly defined you are more able to work out the best route to take to reach your destination. For example if you wanted to go to Australia you wouldn't get on a plane to Iceland, would you!

❷ To reach your destination you need clarity about why you want to get to this certain destination. Looking at your dream, your vision, what exactly is the reason you want to achieve this outcome? What will you gain from the experience of achieving or accomplishing your particular vision? What will you become? How will it benefit you now and into the future?

In the past you may not have actually achieved your desired outcomes because you felt defeated even before you gave your dream the opportunity to grow. Before you had given yourself the possibility to nurture your dream into a worthwhile goal you may have thought or heard that it was impossible to achieve so you gave up simply because you perceived that it might be to difficult to achieve.

What is really fantastic about right now is you now have all the skills and resources available to you. Your previous defeats are a positive aspect of this as without these earlier failures you would not have the skills and resources right now to achieve and nurture your goal. Setting your dream as a clearly defined goal will lead to accomplishment of your vision. Defeat therefore is a necessary stage of accomplishment. Accomplishment means success; the more failures you have had the more rewarding is your final result.

To achieve your outcome you will need to develop the determination to achieve your goal; without this, your dream will be forever stuck in your imagination. I will explain accomplishment/success in more detail so that you really understand the point I'm making about defeat being a vital component of the success cycle so that you can break out of the 'fat cycle' and develop your very own unique success cycle.

On an earlier camping trip we had taken a bottle of wine to enjoy on a balmy summer evening under the stars. When we came to opening the bottle we realised that we had left the corkscrew at home. We didn't have a corkscrew to open the bottle. At first we felt defeated and briefly looked at the alternatives available to us, but we really wanted a glass of wine so instead of deciding to drink something else we started to look at alternative ways we could remove the cork from the bottle. We became determined to get that glass of wine whatever it was going to take.

So to sum it up our dream was to, 'enjoy a glass of wine.' We felt defeated when we realised that we didn't have the means to open the bottle. After considering briefly what other drinks were available to us we turned our attention back to the wine, as we really did prefer the idea of drinking a glass of wine and that cork was standing in the way of what we wanted. We really wanted and needed the bottle open so I said to myself, I'm not going to let that little cork stand in the way of something that I really really want, a glass of wine. I am so much bigger than that cork! I've accomplished and overcome more challenging and difficult things in the past so I'm not going to let a little diddy cork hold me back. I will have that cork out. This is the determination stage. What had happened here was I began to believe that I could open the bottle with or without a corkscrew. My dream when added to the belief turned into a goal. I now believed that I could open the bottle and my goal was very clear. I no longer felt the emotion of defeat, in fact I felt the feelings of empowerment because I had considered the challenges I had previously overcome and knew with certainty that I wasn't going to be beaten by a little cork.

I looked around at likely alternative implements to the corkscrew. By the door to the tent was a spare tent peg, I thought I could use this to open the bottle but as yet I wasn't sure how. I picked up the tent peg and pushed it into the cork, pushing the cork down into the bottle. This enabled the cork to stay whole and wouldn't taint the wine. I then used the tent peg to hold the cork out of the way and poured the wine into the glass. Finally we sat down and enjoyed our glass of wine.

What I had done was become determined to enjoy a glass of wine. I had used my imagination to use a tool for a job for which it was not created and that I had never even previously considered it for. I was implementing the plan my imagination had supplied. When I drank the wine I experienced accomplishment, a real feeling of satisfaction and success.

This series of events can take place over any time frame using any event or outcome, no matter how small or large. Success in all its forms always follows this same chain of events. So you now know that the process starts with the **dream** which suffers some sort of initial **defeat** which then grows into **belief** which follows on with the setting of a clearly defined **goal**. Because you now have a clearly defined goal and the belief that you can achieve your goal you enable your **imagination** to develop possible solutions that drives you on developing the **determination** to achieve **accomplishment** of your goal.

Step three – Realistic

There are other considerations when turning your dreams into goals and goals into real success. It would be helpful to remember that if your goal is really just too far-fetched and you deep down believe that it is completely impossible for you to achieve in your entire life time, then your chance of success is limited.

To achieve accomplishment of your goal you need to know what your deeper motivation is, that is why I asked you to fill out the question in step two. What you have written down in your response is what is driving your deeper motivation for achieving accomplishment of your dream. It's the magic that will drive you forward, the juice that will power you with the necessary determination and desire to turn your dream into a worthwhile goal and achieve its full and final outcome one of fruition and success.

❓ To bring your dream of being healthy and slim into your reality you must have desire, without desire your dream will always stay a dream. So how much do you really want your outcome of being slim and healthy? What will your success really mean to you? take a few minutes and write your answer below.

So far you have your dream, you know why you want to achieve your desire, you have a clearly defined goal and a target date by which to achieve your outcome.

It's time to take a minute and check that you are clearly focused on your well-formed outcome. Answer the following questions as a check to enable you to achieve real clarity for yourself on why you want to create change. What sometimes happens is we want change but never quite seem to achieve it fully. By answering the following 10 questions it will also serve to root out any conflicting values. (We will look at your values later in this book). The next set of questions has little in the way of explanation as they are quite straightforward. What is important here is for you to note down what is coming into your conscious awareness. Some of the questions may baffle you, initially rendering it necessary for you to read them several times, they are meant to. You may even need to put the book down for a couple of days and come back to it and that's great. I would like to encourage you to just write down the first answer that pops into your head.

So here are the questions.

Q What wouldn't happen if I did achieve this outcome? Write down what comes into your mind's eye.

....

....

....

....

Q What about this is most important?

....

....

....

....

....

Q What would happen if I did achieve this outcome?

Q What about this is most important? This is about checking to see if you really do want this outcome for yourself.

Q What wouldn't happen if I didn't achieve this outcome?

Q What about this is most important?

Q What would happen if I didn't achieve this outcome?

Q What about this is most important?

Q What effect will this new outcome have on the rest of my family?

Q What about this is most important?

Super size your self-confidence

You are now ready to super size your self-confidence. You may have worked out by now that the single most important ingredient is for you to like yourself. People who like themselves are more light hearted and optimistic; they are comfortable with themselves and are easy to be with; they're the ones at parties who are surrounded with a crowd, the ones that everyone is attracted to.

Q So, do you really like you? What would it take for you to like yourself?

....

....

....

....

....

....

Q Ask yourself, 'What are ten top qualities about me that I like?'

....

....

....

....

....

....

◎ Name three things that you now believe really mark you out as unique...

◎ Three things that I've previously failed to notice or appreciate about myself that others tell me...

Q Two things that I wouldn't want to change about myself...

Q The main reason I am now proud to be me is?

Congratulations, what a fantastic success you are. you've covered an incredible amount of ground on the most challenging part of your journey and you're still with me. Thank you for sticking with it and showing yourself that you really are a tenacious spirit. You deserve that huge smile on your face and feelings of a strong inner knowing that you really can achieve your dream of being healthy. To celebrate your fantastic success, think of something positive that you can do today as an extra special reward for your achievements so far.

I expect your mind is now brimming with new ideas and a deep satisfaction as you look at how all the powerful insights and resources you've re discovered and recovered, they really can and will help you accelerate your progress and more importantly all this will assist you in changing both your spiritual and physical body.

No journey to success is complete without the necessary steps to get you there. You have your big goal, your dream, your vision and you have a date by which you wish to achieve it, you now need to break it down into manageable steps so that you at no time feel overwhelmed by your vision. All great marathon runners know that to achieve their big target of being able to run 26.2 miles, they need first to break down the goal into manageable sized goals. Mini-goals if you like. These mini-goals are the steps you need to take. So a short distance runner who wished to undertake a marathon would need to set a series of smaller more achievable targets so they can reach their bigger goal. So for instance they would start with the end date, this is the date they will complete their 26 mile run. Next they would work out a strategy that allows them to develop from their current ability of running, say, 200 metres. This at first seems like an impossible task, but broken down into stages or chunks that can be ticked off makes it easier to keep up momentum. So they might start by adding an extra 100 meters or just add extra time to their daily running schedule until they reached their target distance of 26 miles. Also they would keep a check on their technique and time, making the fine-tuning adjustments that were necessary. Another thing any great athlete always factors in are rest days and celebration points or milestones so that when they are reached, they celebrate in some important way.

To help you on your journey you will need to complete the following questions. These will help you formulate which areas are the most important for you to work on. Being able to prioritise is another important requisite of achieving the success of your goals.

After reading the next paragraph you have two options, the first is to write in the chart below or you can take a blank page and create a map that offers you the most encouragement. The choice is yours.

NOW stand in front of your mirror NAKED, or at least in your underwear. I found this really challenging at first because even though I had been working on my psychology I still didn't like my physical body at all.

⊘ Take a long hard look at your body look at all the curves, the shapes. Ask yourself, what is great about my body? Be honest with yourself! This may take a few goes, as you are changing habits and attitudes of a lifetime. It will help to have your book handy to write down all the **positive** points that you notice. Note down **everything** you notice, from your hair, right down to your toenails. This will have the immediate effect of making you feel better about yourself.

Body part   **What's great about it?**
e.g. hair   great colour

The next step is to make a list of all the aspects of your body that are, 'not yet as you would like them to be'. Look at each area, start with your feet and work up every inch of your unique frame. As you do this exercise write next to it how you would want it to be.

Body part not yet as you would like it to be! e.g. Thick calves

How would you prefer it to be? toned calves

Write down, what it would feel like if you achieved the results you have just listed in the 'not yet as you would like it' question. Take about two or three minutes to visualise and really experience each one in your mind then write it down.

◉ How would I walk? How would I stand? What would I wear? What would my partner say as I achieve my outcome of becoming healthy? What will it do for my relationships? How will my personal and professional relationships change for the better? What would my friends be saying to me as I achieve my outcome?

In a minute I want you to put the book down and do the following exercise, but first read through the next paragraph then shut your eyes and spend just ten minutes imagining and feeling these comments you have just written down being said to you now. How would you respond? How would you feel inside? Really feel those feelings. Then pick up your journal again and write all this down.

Every day read this vision of your future to yourself in the mirror. Congratulate yourself on your achievements so far.

Remember to do this! Because as you acknowledge your achievements you build momentum, and that momentum creates massive shifts within you as your self-esteem and confidence grows and develops. As you start to fully associate with these inner feelings and believe that they are your reality you will see the massive results. The images, feelings and sounds you just experienced whilst visualising all need to be recorded here. Do it NOW.

If you are finding it difficult to actually visualise yourself achieving the successful outcomes you desire then perhaps you need to reinforce the importance of your self-image using this prescription, one which I myself found very useful for my own development in Maxwell Maltz's book *Psycho-Cybernetics*.

The Self-image surgery – 30-day challenge will cement your focus and direct your attention daily until it becomes a part of who you are.

*Start each day with; **"I am beginning the day in a new and better way."** Then consciously decide that throughout the day:*

1. I will be as cheerful as possible.

2. I will act a little more friendly toward other people.

3. I am going to be less critical and a little more tolerant of other people, their faults, failings and mistakes. I will place the best possible interpretation on their actions.

4. In so far as possible, I am going to act as if successes were inevitable and I am already the sort of personality I want to be. I will practice acting like and feeling like this new personality.

5. I will not let my own opinion colour facts in a pessimistic or negative way.

6. I will practice smiling at least three times during the day.

7. Regardless of what happens I will react as calmly and as intelligently as possible.

8. I will ignore completely and close my mind to all those pessimistic and negative 'facts,' which I can do nothing to change.

Devote just ten or fifteen minutes EVERY DAY writing out your goal,
Reading it out aloud as you visualise it in perfect detail.
Feel as you would feel if it were already a reality TODAY
Smell the environment you have created, experience it with all your senses.
As an aide-memoire to help your visualisation, cut out pictures from magazines that show your desired outcome and keep them close by so that your end result is never far from your mind's eye.

Close your eyes to the outer world and open them to the inner world of pictures and continuous development of your goals.

Focus, Habits and Attitudes

Keeping yourself on track

With the passing of days and weeks since you embarked on this amazing journey your beliefs and values will have changed. You may have noticed that you have become more congruent and confident with whom you wish to become. You have worked through all the previous exercises and as you are already aware it takes daily practice and determination to make the kind of changes you've already achieved for yourself. I can't emphasise enough how important it is for you to continue with the great strides you've achieved so far. To help you accelerate the rate at which you move forward you will need to start to really laser your focus. You want to look even closer at your daily habits and concentrate on developing the attitudes that will guarantee you the results you desire. In order for your success to endure, be consistent and long-lasting you must keep a constant eye on where you place your focus and how your habits and attitudes are developing. Consistently directing your attention to all three will guarantee your results.

Stick to the facts at all times, those which can be changed. Never allow yourself to be drawn back into the old ways of behaving. Always look forward. We all know that for all challenges there are solutions. Your new focus and determination to follow through on your commitment to yourself will enable you to develop the new habits and attitudes more in tune with your new way of thinking. This new way of thinking and behaving will not only change the way you view and treat yourself, it will also positively affect the way others treat you. You will really begin to enjoy the encouraging positive praise for your fantastic efforts and results.

I have divided the next vital stage of your incredible journey into three sections, the first being focus, followed by habits and attitudes. My intention is to assist you in developing your positive focus, a healthy balanced attitude and new habits that will support your vision of how you want to develop. As you work through each section you may find yourself repeating responses and that's exactly right. You may even find that you have so many more resources available to you now that you find it effortless to develop your new strategy.

Focus

⊙ Ask yourself, **What focus is necessary for the successful accomplishment of my goal to achieve a healthier me?** Write a list of all the things you think you would be regularly focusing on if you had **already achieved your goal**. You already know the answers to this question, so just get on and write the first thing that comes to mind. When you get to the point when you can't think of anything else write down at least two more responses. Write your answers positively, for example: I am enjoying mealtimes with enthusiasm. I am positively enjoying life even when the unexpected happens.

Q What would be the new inner self-talk be? What's going on in your head? What would you be saying to yourself? What strong new personal messages do you want to send your unconscious mind? When I asked myself this question my response was, I am healthy and whole now. I regularly stand in front of the mirror and repeat this sentence to my reflection. I'm sure you can think of many more alternatives suitable for your own lifestyle.

Q To understand where you currently focus ask, **What is my current focus?** Be honest here! What do you really focus on while you're going about your daily chores? Is it on lack of speed of achievement or abundance of choices? Have you been telling yourself that you are denying yourself pleasure by denying yourself and not eating that last chocolate or finishing off the kid's dinners? Are you telling yourself that it's difficult to lose weight and sustain the results long term? Or are you being really positive and relishing the new resources you've exposed in your personality?

Q If you haven't yet cracked this new way of thinking, **what do you need to change in your life from today to create the necessary focus for the effortless achievement of your goal of being healthier?** What must you do to create the necessary strategies to support you? Think about what would be helpful to you in achieving your goal? What would give you intense pleasure and help move you forward? It's only by creating a positive forward looking environment that you will be able to propel yourself forward into the life you desire.

What would you need to do to sustain the positive changes you've created for your life? What are the little things you will need to do each day to keep yourself on track?

There's an old Chinese proverb:

"A journey of 1,000 miles begins with a single step." *– Lao Tzu*

◎ The answer to transform your life lies in your taking action. Just one tiny step at a time is enough to create an enormous shift in your direction. The tiny actions will gather momentum so you become unstoppable. If you need an example, when I was at this stage I set myself the task of regularly visualising my outcome as if I had already achieved it, something that I've continued. This is what you're aiming for. To have your strategies become part of your daily routines, part of your very being, it's now who you are. List yours here:

It may be helpful for you to achieve the outcomes in the last question if you break down the actions into ever-smaller processes. So you are then able to take the necessary baby steps forward. The process is then, write down the action, then write next to it the one thing you can do towards achieving it today and so on. E.g. join a fitness class. What do I need to do? Action - Phone the health club. Then what do I need to do? Action - Find out time of classes. Then what do I need to do? Arrange my day to make time to attend class. Then what do I need to do? Etc. you get the picture. This way you realise that it's no longer impossible, but quite simply straight forward. Create a list of steps for each of your planned activities.

Action	What I need to do & When am I going to achieve this by?
1	
2	
3	
4	
5	
6	
7	

Q It's all very well having a list of actions that you can easily take but all too often they are not acted on. So **what are you really willing to do?** Again, be really honest with yourself, it's no good coming up with a list of actions if you don't believe you can achieve them or if you already know they don't excite you. You need to be really personal with yourself; it's time for you to really take responsibility for your actions. By actually following through on your actions listed above you will achieve your goal. By checking your commitment on a scale of 1-10, with 1 being the lowest and 10 being absolutely committed, where would you place your current level of commitment to achieving your desired outcome?

Action	What am I willing to do?
1	
2	
3	
4	
5	
6	
7	

Q If your commitment to any of the above actions is less than a 10, what would it take to become a 10?

Action	What would it take for my Commitment to be level 10?
1	
2	
3	
4	
5	
6	
7	

Attitudes

Your attitudes towards yourself and your abilities have been developed over years of conditioning by life events and society. Conditioning is simply the things you have repeatedly learnt, heard, been told or assumed to be true while you have been growing and developing as a person. You've taken onboard a huge amount of information in your formative years and developed attitudes and ideas of your own based on this past conditioning. This could have been from your parents, peers, work colleagues or friends. I'm sure you've said or done something and immediately known who specifically you gained that thought or attitude from. Some of these thoughts, actions and attitudes may be deeply entrenched in your personality, in who you've become. This sometimes leads us to hold erroneous beliefs about ourselves. You may even believe that it is just the way you are. You couldn't be more wrong. You learned these patterns of behaving and now you can unlearn them. All it takes is perseverance which you have proven to yourself many times already that you have in abundance. ⊙ Replacing your old attitudes with new ones that will support your development towards your goal is the next stage in this exciting process. Take time now to review your key learning insights. What new beliefs do you have about yourself and your abilities since embarking on the ditch the scales programme and fully participating in the exercises?

To make the integration of your above key learning points effortless and be able to develop a new attitude as and when you desire, it is important for you to be in the moment. Being in the moment, put quite simply, is to be in the here and now. When you start to be present in the moment you start to notice the things that make you tick. What's really important is for you to notice the things that had acted as a trigger for your past results. To release yourself from this past or old behaviour patterns you must first acknowledge this old conditioning as you become aware of it. By acknowledging the behaviour and the effects on you in the past, you become able to use what you have learned from it to develop a new attitude.

There are six stages to this process:

1. Acknowledge the old behaviour

2. Analyse what has caused it. These are your triggers. However don't spend too long on this area. You only need enough information to start making a change.

3. Understand the effect on your future if you don't change the behaviour NOW

4. Look at what beliefs have led you to this point.

5. Break the old pattern. This is a very liberating process; you could stand in front of the mirror, tell yourself out loud that the old pattern of ******* is bullshit (or another similar phrase), what I really believe is, ******(substitute with new belief). Repeat this out loud to your reflection at least 10 times, do it with passion, say it with great intensity. If you are having difficulty in breaking old behaviour patterns that no longer serve you, develop an action that would put you off the old behaviour so that you can no longer possibly repeat it ever again. Scramble the pattern, visualise yourself operating with this new attitude. I expect if you let your imagination, you could think of many other ways to achieve the same result. For example, what if you caught yourself looking in one of your children's bedrooms for their chocolate stash? Or the urge to jump on the scales every time you see them? What could you do or say to yourself that would act as a pattern/behaviour interrupt that would prevent you from carrying out what was previously the unconscious action?

6. Visualise in minute detail the positive outcome you desire, every vivid,

glorious technicolour detail. How does it feel? How does it sound? Make it large, make it bright, Hold that image in your mind. Step physically into your visualised outcome. Engage fully with it; imagine yourself celebrating your success.

Take **Immediate Massive Action** now. Break down your task into specific, manageable tasks.

⊜ In line with your vision, **what attitude would best support your focus?** In your quest for a healthier body what would be the best attitude to develop to support you? Write it down here.

....

....

....

....

....

....

....

⊜ **What is your current attitude?** C'mon, be honest! It doesn't matter if you think it stinks, we all have to start somewhere and by far the best place to start, is acknowledging the place we're at now. It's only by accepting that in the past, we didn't always have the necessary attitude to achieve our goals, but now we know we can do something about it. So what is your current attitude?

....

....

....

....

....

....

Q Are you willing and able to create the necessary attitude you need?
Write below what your new attitude will now be for each of the areas outlined in your goals list. Your goals list is the list of actions you decided were important for you to do in order to achieve your long-term goal of becoming healthy. Decide that from this point on this is how you will be.

Goal	My new attitude from this day on will be...
1	
2	
3	
4	
5	
6	
7	

Habits

Habits are the routines that you do every day without thinking about them. The results you've achieved in your life up till now are the consequence of your continual habits. We are looking in this section at how those habits affect you.

❶ You have already developed the tools for creating sustainable lasting change, use the tools available to you from the earlier chapters to assist you. **Ask yourself, what habits are vital for me to maintain my focus and to accomplish my goals in my quest for a healthier body?**

....

....

....

....

....

....

....

....

....

❶ If there were one habit that would help me maintain my focus and attitude, what would it be?

....

....

....

....

....

....

Q What else would help me?

_____

_____

_____

_____

_____

_____

_____

_____

Q What habits do I currently have that do not support me, or my goal/vision of a healthier life?

_____

_____

_____

_____

_____

_____

_____

_____

_____

_____

_____

Now the moment of truth. Be honest. Even after all I had learnt I still found that there were certain times and foods that really had me on my knees. What is your biggest downfall? Maybe you had in the past a craving for a particular brand or flavour of crisps or chocolate. You don't need me to tell you, you already know, don't you? Write them down here.

What can you do to change this?

Q When are you at your most tired?

Q What can you do to alleviate this?

Q In the past what were the times/circumstances/events that triggered your comfort eating?

Q How might you change the way you represent this time/circumstance/event to yourself?

Q What strategies have you used previously when you have been following diets & regimes that worked for a little while?

Q How can you use and refine those particular strategies that worked to help move you towards your goal?

Ⓠ What habits do you have already that you believe will really support you in your goal/vision? Think about what you do already that helps to keep you on track. Sometimes it may be a routine that you use in another area of your life that you can transfer into a new context.

Ⓠ What is it specifically about that habit that helps keep you on track?

Q What habits do you need to create? If there were one habit that you could develop that would deliver your vision, what would it be?

Q What else could you do?

Q How will this new habit really support you?

Having looked at the minutiae of your life, you now have an even clearer picture of how you operate on a daily, minute by minute basis. You have an understanding of the times and triggers that could potentially end all your efforts. Use these insights to move you forward so that you never again have to accept anything less than you can be.

The new set of strategies you are about to create are to be the basis of your new rules, a blueprint containing the action steps that will elevate you to your new healthier body goal. For you to be the most effective you need to plan how you will achieve your goal, so list the actions in order of your priority. E.g. step 1 by let's say the end of today, put the date in the target date section. Remember your goals need to be SMART – specific, measurable, action oriented, realistic and timed! See the example below. You can carry on like this but remember you don't need to do everything at once. As always, remember the process, **decide, plan, commit, and TAKE ACTION**

"It is in the moments of your decision that your destiny is shaped."

– Tony Robbins

Step	By target date
1 e.g. cut out caffeine from my diet	The end of today 10/01/07
2	
3	
4	
5	
6	
7	
8	
9	
10	
11	
12	
13	
14	

What to eat and how you view food

You won't find anything on nutrition or what you should be eating in this next section. You will, however, find a set of tools that will help you nail your dream and help you sustain your vision of having a healthy body and lifestyle. What's really important is for you to take a long hard look at what you've previously been eating to achieve your current results and what you know you must be eating to achieve the results you desire.

By completing all the exercises and staying with the programme you have shown already that you have taken full responsibility and ownership for your results. Gaining full control of your mind is the major linchpin to your success. You are guiding and directing your mind towards the results you must achieve and away from the pain it would cause you if you didn't achieve your goal of a healthy life.

Having a clear healthy mind is the most important part of the whole process. Your desire to achieve a particular outcome will be successful only if you know why you want it and have developed a way that works for you, to get it. So far we've looked at how you can change your perception of what's going on in your life now and what has happened in your past, in the same way you can change the perception and associations with certain foods. When you change how you perceive your world everything changes, it cannot not change! Things that once seemed difficult become effortless. When you have changed what is at your core, you really can achieve everything anything you want. You develop an unquestionable belief in yourself and more importantly unstoppable motivation to do anything it takes to achieve your goals.

You've done a lot of work on your mindset and you are ready to implement changes in your eating habits. What you put into your body and how you maintain your physiology will have a profound effect on your end results. By now it will not be a surprise to you to know that if you do what you've always done, you will get the same results as you always got! Looking more closely at your particular eating habits, rituals and beliefs surrounding food itself will enable you to untangle your past conditioning.

It's not my intention to tell you what to eat or how much exercise you should take. It is only my intention to inform you of what I did to achieve my own goal of achieving a healthier fitter, leaner body.

I am not a nutritionist; I only know what worked for me, which was alkalising my blood/body. I am willing to assist and support you in developing an eating plan suitable for you. For only you know what's right for you. I was willing to do what ever it took to achieve my goals, are you? I would recommend having a blood analysis as this helps to discover a whole host of issues that could be affecting your weight. Also a visit to your GP for a well woman check is advisable.

On my own journey I found it useful to start with a complete Detox. This meant excluding everything from my diet that could be potential toxins such as, caffeine, sugar, vinegars, salt, white flour, eggs and anything that had once had a face. Also included was removing the rituals of tea, coffee and alcohol. I had made a commitment to be the healthiest I could be. Coffee and wine had been a part of who I was for so long that it seemed a little daunting at first. The way I got over those initial negative thoughts was to tell myself that it was only for ten days, then I would make a further decision as to how I wanted to continue.

In our house my husband and I had a mealtime ritual of having a glass or two of fine wine with our evening meal, which usually ended with us consuming the whole bottle of wine between us. During the first ten days of the cleanse amazing things began to happen, because I had made the decision in advance there was no question that I was going to let a drop of wine or coffee pass my lips. I found it relatively easy to refuse in my mind, but, the physical reality, or my, 'auto pilot mode,' led me to pour just a small amount of wine into a glass and I sipped it as if it were poison. Needless to say it wasn't long before I didn't feel the need to indulge or feel that I was missing out! I no longer needed to prop up this mealtime ritual.

Once you have made decisions and are committed to making the necessary changes to your diet, it will be important for you to plan ahead. Don't leave it to chance, take it as fact that most people will not understand your requirements so if you're going out to a restaurant, phone ahead to check they can cater for you. Most are very helpful and always try to find something on their menu that can accommodate you. I've become expert at picking apart restaurant menus and creating my own dishes. Of course this only works where food is prepared fresh and not ready meals out of packets.

Planning your menu for the week at home is ultra important too. Initially I wasn't very good at this. I would look in the cupboard each day and make something from what I had rather than plan, shop then create! Plan your lunchtimes, if you are lucky enough to have a canteen at work then you are sure to find healthy options. If you are taking a packed lunch then make sure that you take foods that will sustain you for the afternoon.

The first thing I tried was a 10-day cleanse. I was now eating to maintain health and increase my energy levels. For the first 10 days I cut completely from my diet caffeine, alcohol, meat, chocolate (I had a passion for green & blacks dark chocolate), vinegar, sugars and salt. I had 2 years earlier eliminated wheat and dairy products.

I was making sure that my diet consisted mainly of green leafy vegetables, fruit, nuts and seeds. I began to create nutritionally rich meals that were either protein or carbohydrate oriented this was really beneficial and the positive results were almost immediate.

Each day starts in the morning by drinking a cup of hot water with a slice of organic wax free lemon in it, followed by eating fruit during the morning until midday. Then, I would tuck into the biggest salad you'd ever seen covered with nuts and seeds. In the evenings I would (and still do) make a vegetable based family dinner and add meat to the meal for the rest of the family.

The other major difference in my life now is that I drink in excess of 3 litres of water per day. Contrary to the belief that I must spend all my time in the toilet, I don't. I find that it helps with concentration and the elimination of waste products from the body. Dr Young, in his book *The PH Miracle for Life* recommends that you require 1 litre of water per 30lbs of body weight to maintain normal bodily functions. This is something that I have maintained myself.

I never weigh myself and have no interest in weight, only in how I feel inside. Although I do get asked on a regular basis how much I weigh, I just respond with the answer, "I have no idea and no desire to know because weight is not an indicator of health!"

There are a couple of great books that I would recommend for further reading; both cover nutritional and exercise advice. They are *The PH Miracle for Weight Loss* by Dr Robert Young and *Detox for Life* by Carole Vorderman. Both also have fantastic recipes along with good honest hints and tips on nutrition.

To maintain my healthy body I loosely follow an alkalising lifestyle. which consists mainly of fruit, vegetables, nuts, rice & oats and the occasional fish along with 3 litres per day of 'greens' drink. I do occasionally have potatoes but I find that they sit heavy in my stomach and make me feel very lethargic. I still find food very exciting and have become even more creative when preparing meals for the family and myself. It's become fun to disguise vegetables to get them down the kids! And to make cakes without eggs! Now there's a challenge!

Someone who has become the friend at the end of the phone whenever I need advice about nutritional matters is Errol Denton, a certified Nutritional Microscopist with a background in Traditional Chinese Medicine as well as having been a personal trainer and athlete. Denton states, "Since there is only one root cause of all sickness and disease, live blood analysis can help all situations. The benefits of having a blood analysis is likened to satellite navigation for good health, it gives you the opportunity to see for yourself the true state of your health and the opportunity to be in control of your own health." The positive benefits of alkalising are stated as follows, "increased energy levels, greater concentration, and most crucially a sense of well being along with an increase in the length and quality of life. The philosophy is to remove all acid forming foods from your diet and replace them with alkaline foods. Results can be seen within a few days or weeks for most people."

I found alkalising very easy to follow, and I appreciate that, for you it may seem like massive changes, So let's look at what you are prepared to do in order for you to feel and look fantastic and reach your goal of having a fitter healthier lifestyle.

❂ What foods or food groups do I currently crave? (I craved sweet things; I was definitely addicted to sugar. What about you?)

Q What strategies have I used to deny myself in the past?

Q What benefit do I gain by denying myself this food?

Q What do I feel I benefit from eating this certain type of food?

Q What would be the benefit of not eating this particular food type? Maybe you've experienced side effects such as bloating etc. so by not eating this particular food you will alleviate any previous issues associated with it.

Q How does this behaviour serve me? (By continuing to eat a food that causes you obvious distress)

Q What new strategy can I develop to breakthrough this old pattern?

Q What else could I do?

Q How will I view this situation in future?

Q What will I do instead?

Q How will I view this food in future?

Review your progress

How will your life be different now having almost completed this programme? what positive benefits have you received? spend a few minutes reflecting and creating in your minds eye your positive future containing and utilising all the new skills and strategies you've developed. when you have created this vision for yourself take a few more minutes to write it down, capture every minute detail. what will it look like? what will it sound like? what will it feel like? what will it smell like? what will it taste like? capture it all so that you have a clear focus and direction.

Physical exercise

As you've already discovered, changing old habits can feel a little strange at first; your ego will try to keep pulling you back into what you've always done because it's safe there! However this is not the only consideration here. The people around you, those you love may also have a vested interested in your staying the same as you've always been. It can be a little unnerving for families especially when mum is growing in confidence and reducing in size. You will notice straight away their negativity when it rears it ugly head. You will be ready. You have a full understanding of the what's, the why's and the wherefores about yourself and your old eating habits and what had previously triggered you into those old patterns of behaviour. You will be making massive shifts in your psychology and language so that you can now offer yourself support from within. There remains one final process that pays results far in excess of the energy exerted and that is exercise. Without exercise how can you achieve a beautifully toned svelte body? Sculpt your body to be exactly as you want it and exercise is the only way to achieve your results.

I'm not a fitness instructor but I do know THAT YOUR PHYSIOLOGY IS REALLY IMPORTANT. I know that I got to lose all that weight and created a beautifully shaped body with no saggy skin by combining everything we've talked about so far with taking regular exercise. If you haven't exercised before you will need to get the OK from your GP, just to give you the go ahead.

I joined a local fitness class, going once a week to start with then increasing it to three times per week. I was determined not to end up with saggy, drooping skin. I chose this method originally for the anonymity in a group, no one was looking at me, they were all only interested in worrying about themselves and the classes were the most fun for me. I tried the exercise videos at home but as soon as the phone rang I would make an excuse to myself and stop, not going back and finishing it off.

Think about the type of exercise you might enjoy doing. What would really motivate you to take part on a regular basis especially on a cold dark winter's eve? You could try something new, maybe go swimming, take up jogging, join a local class. The most important thing is that you enjoy it and go especially on the days when you feel you can't be bothered, you will be rewarded tenfold on those days.

Francesca Flin, Advance fitness instructor & Personal Trainer of Flin's Fitness recommends that, "If you are new to exercise then its always better to start with something low impact. This is so you can gauge how your body feels and ease it gently into exercise. Low impact exercise includes walking, swimming, dancing or anything that's easy on the joints to start."

You'll know when it's time to increase the level of intensity. The benefits of adding exercise to your daily routine are many. The immediate one is enhanced mood and feeling more positive. We all know how great we feel after a bout of exercise that has made us huff and puff a little. It makes me grin from ear to ear! Other benefits are increased heart and lung capacity, increased muscle tone and body shape. The return of feminine curves! Of course if you have been eating sensibly too then you will have a flatter stomach and start to feel more comfortable in your clothes within 3-6 weeks. The American College of Sports Medicine recommend five sessions per week of at least 30 minutes strenuous activity, by strenuous they mean huff & puff type to maintain optimum health.

Deepak Chopra in his book *Ageless Body, Timeless Mind* states that exercise or lack of it, is one of the determining factors of aging. Added to the benefits received from taking regular exercise are your body will look younger and more toned, it will actually be physically younger. American Scientific research referred to by Chopra in his book has shown that even sedentary 75 year olds can increase their muscle tone and greatly reduce the effects of aging on their bodies by taking regular exercise. The other aspect of course is that exercise helps the body to eliminate toxins more effectively. Eliminating toxins that are stored in fat will show on your surface, by giving you radiant skin, build lean muscle tissue, and last but not least release happy endorphins into your blood system that increase your pleasure sensations.

To stay youthful your body requires you to take regular exercise, imagine how it would make you feel inside when your acquaintances guess your age and they think it's actually 5 -10 years younger than you really are! Wow! Wouldn't that make it all worthwhile?

How can you plan exercise into your daily habits?

Q What form of exercise would you like to take part in? List them below, any types of sport that you think you might like to try. Maybe it's something that you've never done before or maybe it's something that you did for a while but stopped because life got in the way. What form of exercise would have you gagging for your trainers?

Q Once you've looked at what type of exercise you'd like to participate in, how much time per week are you prepared to spend actually doing it?

Q I am prepared to spend...

@ How am I going to fit this into my daily schedule?

@ What will need to change in order for me to take action and participate in my chosen activity?

@ What will be the benefits to me of this newfound activity?

Q How committed am I to making these changes? (On a scale of 1-10.)

Q If the answer to the previous question were less than a ten, what would make it a 10?

FANTASTIC!

You have travelled far on your journey of self discovery.
You have now created a very clear blueprint for your continued success
and the healthy life style and body you really do deserve.

I truly wish your life to be filled with the joy and comfort
of being happy in your own skin. I have really enjoyed
being your coach and mentor and look forward
to hearing from you soon.

With love & light as always

Donna

XOX

Final Thoughts

So what do you do now?

The only reason people fail at losing weight is because they give up!

Practice, patience and application are three words that spring to mind, sadly in todays society it's all about instant gratification – sometimes people don't get the results they want right away so they give up, they quit, thinking it's not working for them. Ironically this is just before it starts to work and achieve the results they desired. If only they had continued to persevere rather than giving up on themselves.

The idea of giving up seems to be a behaviour we learn as adults. I think most people have a fear of failure or a fear of not being enough. We don't have those fears as children. Did you learn to ride a bike as a child? I'm sure when you were learning to ride you fell of hundreds of times, did that stop you from getting back on and trying again? No, of course not! Did your parents ever say to you, "Ah well it's not meant to be?" No, of course they didn't, they encouraged and supported you to keep at it. You persevered learning from your mistakes and eventually learned to ride without your stabilisers, and finally without even thinking about it.

At first it may seem like you've a mountain to climb and be very daunting, you may even think that the exercises do not apply to you, however, once you know the secret to your own 'operating system' you can use your incredible inner power to support you whilst taking positive action and create the healthy body you deserve.

If you would like more details on individual and group coaching and training programmes offered please contact me through:

www.ditchthescales.com

I look forward to hearing about your future success.

warmest regards,
Donna

Sources

Awaken the giant within
Anthony Robbins. Pocket Books (1991)

Unlimited Power
Anthony Robbins. Pocket Books (1986)

PH Miracle for weight loss
Dr Robert Young & Shelly Redford Young. The winner Press (2006)

Be your own life coach.
Fiona Harrold. Coronet Books (2001)

Ageless body, Timeless mind
Deepak Chopra. Random House, (1993)

The new psycho-cybernetics
Maxwell Maltz MD FICS. Souveneir Press (2002)

www.bbc.co.uk/Science

Printed in the United Kingdom
by Lightning Source UK Ltd.
129042UK00001B/286-525/P

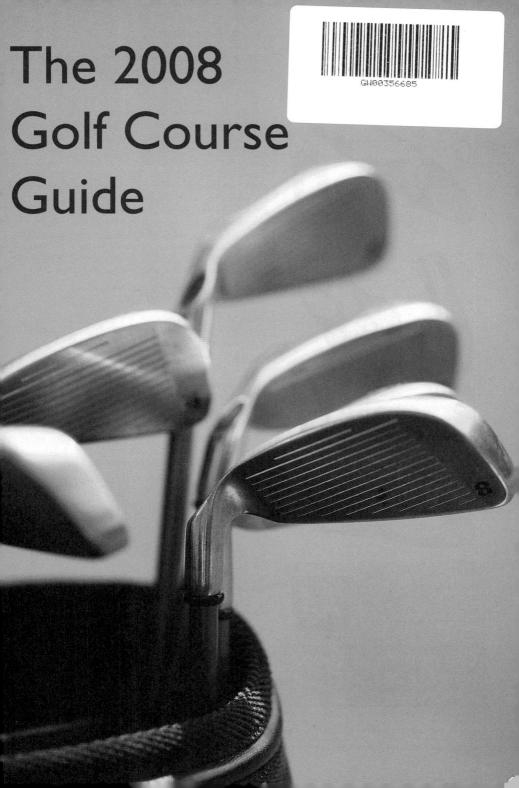

The 2008
Golf Course
Guide

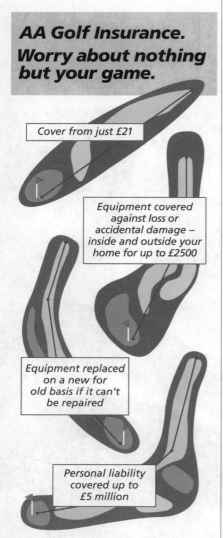

22nd edition published 2007
Published by AA Publishing, which is a trading name of Automobile Association Developments Limited, whose registered office is: Fanum House, Basingstoke, Hampshire RG21 4EA Registered number 1878835

Advertisement Sales: advertisingsales@theAA.com
Editorial: lifestyleguides@theAA.com

The Automobile Association would like to thank the following photographers, companies and picture libraries for their assistance in the preparation of this book.

Abbreviations for the picture credits are as follows: (t) top; (b) bottom; (l) left; (r) right; (AA) AA World Travel Library.

AA: 3br (Jim Carnie), 408; Corbis: front cover, 1, 3tr, 3bl, 4tl, 4b, 6tl, 7tr, 8tl, 9tr, 9b, 12tl, 13tr, 14tl, 14br, 15tr, 16tl, 19, 307, 379, 465, 483tr, 484tl, 485tr, 486tl, 487tr, 488tl, 489tr, 490tl, 491tr, 492tl;
Lhara O' Connor, Old Head Golf Links: 15

Every effort has been made to trace the copyright holders, and we apologise in advance for any accidental errors. We would be happy to apply the corrections in the following edition of this publication.

Typeset/repro by Servis Filmsetting Ltd, Manchester
Printed and bound in Italy by Printer Trento S.r.l

A CIP catalogue record for this book is available from the British Library
ISBN-10: 0-7495-5297-2
ISBN-13: 978-0-7495-5297-8
A03279

Maps prepared by the Mapping Services Department of The Automobile Association. © Automobile Association Developments Limited 2007

This product includes mapping data licensed from Ordnance Survey® with the permission of the Controller of Her Majesty's Stationery Office. © Crown copyright 2007 All rights reserved. Licence number 100021153

This product includes mapping based upon data licensed from Ordnance Survey of Northern Ireland® reproduced by permission of the Chief Executive, acting on behalf of the Controller of Her Majesty's Stationery Office. © Crown copyright 2007 Permit number 60230

Republic of Ireland mapping based on Ordnance Survey Ireland Permit number MP000106 © Ordnance Survey Ireland and Government of Ireland.

Contents

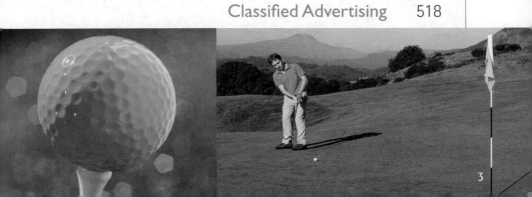

Welcome

Welcome to the AA Golf Course Guide 2008. Besides covering more courses and clubs than ever before, this fully-updated and revised edition has several new features to help you make the most of playing golf in the UK and Ireland.

Golf is one of the most democratic of sports. Unlike football or rugby, amateur players always have the opportunity of following in the actual footsteps of the some of the most famous names in the game.

On pages 12-13 you'll find the Championship Course finder which will give you at-a-glance information about the top courses (feature pages and extensive descriptions can be found within the main gazetteer). Throughout the guide, courses of particular merit or interest are highlighted and on page 14 there's a special feature on a few of the more unique courses. Whether you're an armchair golf enthusiast or enjoy the thrill of seeing the game live, there's also a selection of dates and events to look forward to in the upcoming golfing calendar (see page 16).

This guide also contains more AA-recommended Hotels and Guest Accommodation establishments. After most entries you'll find details of local hotels complete with their ratings. See pages 6-9 for more details on how to use this information.

The expanded index section now means there are several ways to find a course to play. To browse by place name see pages 493-502, or if you know a specific course you could try the brand new Course Name Index on pages 503-517. Alternatively, if you just want to practice your swing, there's the Driving Range index on pages 483-492.

So, if you are interested in reliving the glories of a well-known golfing moment, looking to organise a golfing trip with friends or just feel like playing a few holes down the back nine of your local municipal course, you'll be able to find a place to play and stay in the AA Golf Course Guide 2008.

To recommend a new course for the guide, please write to:
The Editor, AA Golf Course Guide
Fanum House Floor 14
Basingstoke, Hampshire RG21 4EA

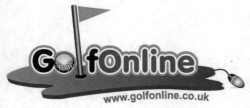
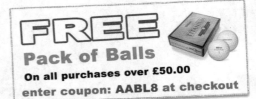
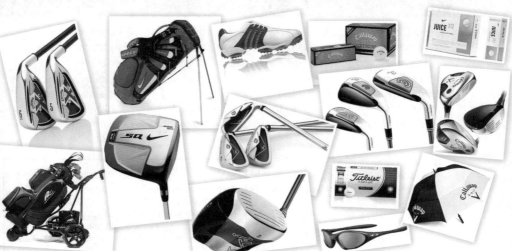
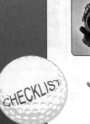
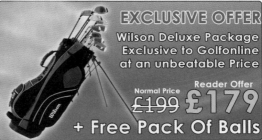
     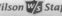

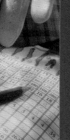

How to Use the Guide

The golf courses in the AA Golf Course Guide are selected by the AA and their entry is free of charge. The guide is updated every year for new courses, changes, closures and new features, and an AA recommended accommodation follows most entries. To avoid disappointment we recommend that you phone before visiting a golf course; please mention the guide when you make an enquiry. The country directories are arranged alphabetically by county, then by town or village name. The town or village locations are shown on the atlas and listed in the index. A sample entry is explained below.

❶ Town name and map reference
The atlas at the end of the guide shows the locations of the courses. The map reference includes the atlas page number and the National Grid reference. The grid references for the Republic of Ireland are unique to this atlas.

❷ Club name and contact details
Where the club name appears in italic we have been unable to verify current course details with the club. You should check any details with the club before your visit.

❸ Description The description highlights the significant features of the course or courses.

❹ Course statistics The number of holes, distance, par, Standard Scratch Score, Course Record, and the number of club members.

❺ Visitor information Playing days, booking requirements or restrictions are noted. A small number of courses in the guide are not open to visitors and we have included their details for information only.

❻ Society information Booking requirements or restrictions for societies.

❼ Green fees The most up-to-date green fees are given, including any variations or restrictions. Where green fees are not confirmed you should contact the club for current rates. An asterisk * denotes 2007 fees.

❽ Professional The name of the club professional(s).

---

❶ HARTLEY WINTNEY   MAP 04 SU75

❷ Hartley Wintney London Rd RG27 8PT
☎ 01252 844211 (Sec/Gen Mgr) 📠 01252 844211
e-mail: office@hartleywintneygolfclub.com
web: www.hartleywintneygolfclub.com
❸ Easy walking parkland and partly wooded course in pleasant countryside. Provides a challenging test for golfers of all abilities with many mature trees and water hazards.

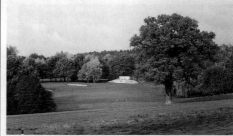

❹ *18 holes, 6240yds, Par 71, SSS 71, Course record 63.*
Club membership 750.
❺ Visitors Mon-Sun & BHs Booking required Sat, Sun & BHs. Handicap certificate. Dress code. **❻ Societies** Booking required **❼ Green Fees** £45 per day, £30 per 18 holes (£50/£35 weekends and Bank holidays). **❽ Prof** Martin Smith **❾ Facilities** ⑪ 🏌 ☐ 🏐 ⅄ 🍴 🎁 ✦ **⑪ Leisure** indoor teaching studio. **❿ Conf** facs Corporate Hospitality Days **⑪ Location** NE of village on A30
⑫ Hotel ★★★ 78% HL The Elvetham, HARTLEY WINTNEY - 01252 844871 41 en suite 29 annexe en suite

---

❾ Facilities See the key to symbols on page 7.

❿ Conference facilities The available conference facilities are noted, and corporate hospitality days.

⑪ Location The location of the club is given in relation to the nearest town or motorway junction.

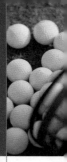

Many golf courses are in rural locations and we do not provide detailed directions in the guide. You should contact the club for further details, or use he AA Route Planner at www.theAA.com.

12 Accommodation An AA recognised hotel is provided for most entries. This does not imply that the hotel offers special terms for the golf club, though in some cases the golf course is in the grounds of the hotel. The Star rating, Quality Assessment (%) score and AA Rosette restaurant award appear as applicable. Contact details and the number of rooms are given. Where there is no nearby AA recognised hotel, an AA guest accommodation is recommended. See pages 8-9 for details of AA ratings. Where golf courses offer club accommodation the bed symbol appears under Facilities. Unless the club accommodation has an AA Star classification, the only AA recognised accommodation is the hotel or guest house that follows the entry.

Golf courses and hotels in the guide can illustrate their entry with a photograph or an advertisement.

Championship courses

Major championship courses have a full-page entry in the guide with an extensive description. A list of championship courses can be found on pages 12-13. A selection of AA recognised hotels is given for these courses in the main directory.

Selected courses

Green boxes in the guide highlight selected courses considered to be of particular merit or interest. These may include historic clubs, particularly testing or enjoyable courses, or those in holiday areas popular with visiting golfers. The selection is not exhaustive nor totally objective, but it is independent - courses cannot pay to have an entry in the guide, nor can they pay to have a highlighted entry. Highlighted courses do not represent any formal category on quality or other grounds.

Key to symbols

☎	Phone number
🖹	Fax number
€	Euro (Republic of Ireland)
🚫	No credit card
🍴	Lunch
🍽	Dinner
🍺	Bar snacks
☕	Tea/coffee
🍺	Bar open midday and evenings
◇	Accommodation at club
👕	Changing rooms
🏠	Well stocked shop
⛳	Clubs for hire
🛺	Motorized cart/trolley for hire
🚙	Buggies for hire
🛒	Trolley for hire
🏌	Driving range
★	AA Star Hotel
U	Hotel not yet rated by the AA
◉	AA Rosettes indicate an award for food

Links to other sections of the book

AA Hotel & Guest Accommodation

The AA inspects and rates establishments under two different accommodation schemes. Guest houses, B&Bs, farmhouses and inns are rated under the Guest Accommodation Scheme and hotels are rated under the Hotel Scheme. Establishments recognised by the AA pay an annual fee according to the rating and the number of bedrooms.

Star Quality

Stars shown in the guide indicate where the accommodation has been rated by the AA under a new common standard rating agreed between the AA, VisitBritain, VisitScotland and Visit Wales. Under the new common standards, guests can be confident that, for example, a guest house anywhere in the UK and Ireland will offer consistent quality and facilities. The new system also uses a brief description to classify the establishment (abbreviations for these designators are described in the box opposite).

The Inspection Process

Establishments applying for AA recognition are visited by a qualified AA accommodation inspectors as a mystery guest. Inspectors stay overnight to make a thorough test of the accommodation, food, and hospitality. After paying the bill the following morning, they identify themselves and ask to be shown around the premises. The inspector completes a full report, resulting in a recommendation for the appropriate star rating. After this first visit, the establishment will receive an annual visit to check that standards are maintained. If it changes hands, the new owners must re-apply for rating, as standards can change.

AA Hotel Classification

★ In a one-Star hotel you should expect relatively informal yet competent service and an adequate range of facilities, including a television in the lounge or bedroom, and a reasonable choice of hot and cold dishes. The majority of bedrooms are en suite with a bath or shower room always available.

★★ Run by professionally presented staff and offers at least one restaurant or dining room for breakfast and dinner.

★★★ Three-Star hotels have direct-dial phones, a wide selection of drinks in the bar, and last orders for dinner no earlier than 8pm.

★★★★ A four-Star hotel is characterised by uniformed, well-trained staff, additional services, a night porter and a serious approach to cuisine.

★★★★★ Finally, and most luxurious of all, five-Star hotels offer many extra facilities, attentive staff, top-quality rooms and a full concierge service. A wide selection of drinks, including cocktails, are available in the bar, and the impressive menu reflects the hotel's own style of cooking.

% The Quality Assessment score appears after the Star rating for hotels in this guide. This is an additional assessment made by AA hotel inspectors, covering everything the hotel has to offer, including hospitality. The Quality Assessment score allows a quick comparison between hotels with the same Star rating: the higher the score the better the hotel.

★ Red stars highlight the very best hotels in Britain and Ireland across all ratings. Such hotels offer outstanding levels of quality, comfort, cleanliness and customer care, and serve food of at least one-Rosette standard. No Quality Assessment score is shown for hotels with red Stars.

AA Guest Accommodation Classification

Guests can expect to find the following minimum standards at all levels:
- Pleasant and helpful welcome and service, and sound standards of housekeeping and maintenance
- Comfortable accommodation equipped to modern standards

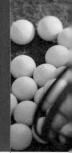

- Bedding and towels changed for each new guest, and at least weekly if the room is taken for a long stay
- Adequate storage, heating, lighting and comfortable seating
- A sufficient hot water supply at reasonable times
- A full cooked breakfast. (If this is not provided, the fact must be advertised and a substantial continental breakfast must be offered.)

There are additional requirements for an establishment to achieve three, four or five Stars:

- Three Stars and above - access to both sides of all beds for double occupancy.
- Three Stars and above – bathrooms/shower rooms cannot be shared by the proprietor.
- Three Stars and above (from January 1 2008) – a washbasin in every guest bedroom (either in the bedroom or the en suite/private facility).

- Four Stars (from January 1 2008) – half of the bedrooms must be en suite or have private facilities.
- Five Stars (from January 1 2008) – all bedrooms must be en suite or have private facilities.

Designators

B&B	Private house managed by owner
GH	Guest house, a larger B&B
GA	Guest Accommodation
INN	Traditional inn with pub atmosphere
FH	B&B on working farm
HL	Hotel
SHL	Small hotel managed by owner
RR	Restaurant with rooms
THH	Town House Hotel
CHH	Country House Hotel
MH	Metro Hotel
BUD	Budget Hotel

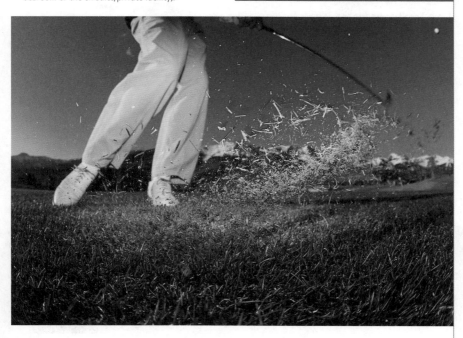

Find it with theAA.com

www.theAA.com

Go to **theAA.com** for maps and the **Route Planner** to help you find AA listed guest houses, hotels, pubs and restaurants – more than 12,000 establishments

Simply enter your postcode and the establishment postcode given in this guide and click **Get route**. Check your details and you are on your way. Or, search on the home page for a Hotel/B&B or a Pub/Restaurant by location or establishment name. Scroll down the list of finds for the interactive map and local routes.

You can also do postcode searches on www.ordnancesurvey.co.uk and www.multimap.com, and the latter provides useful aerial views of your destination.

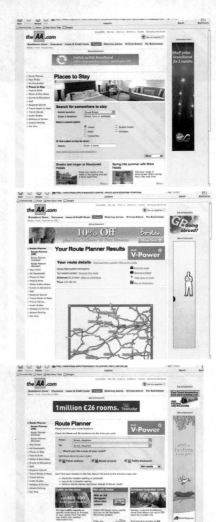

Discover new horizons with Britain's largest travel publisher

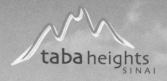

taba heights
SINAI

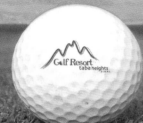

Golf Resort
taba heights
SINAI

In the Heart of
Natural Luxury
golf with a view of three countries

i iconeg.com

Discover Taba Heights, a complete leisure destination located at one of the most beautiful spots on the Sinai peninsula.

- 5 and 4-star Luxury Hotels
- 18-hole USPGA Golf Course
- 5 km of Natural Beachfront
- Innovative Dine-Around Program
- Spas and Leisure Activities
- Adventure and Excursions
- International Sailing Marina
- A short flight from Europe
- 400 km from Cairo, 225 km from Sharm El Sheikh
- Easy access to Jordan, Israel and all of Egypt

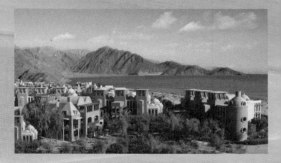

golf@tabaheights.com
www.tabaheights.com

Championship Courses

Name	Location	Course(s)	Map Ref	Page
Sunningdale	Sunningdale, Berkshire	Old Course: 18 holes, 6308yds, Par 70 New Course: 18 holes, 6443yds, Par 71	Map 04 SU96	27
Woburn	Little Brickhill, Buckinghamshire	Duke's Course: 18 holes, 6973yds, Par 72 Duchess Course: 18 holes, 6651yds, Par 72 Marquess Course: 18 holes, 7214yds, Par 72	Map 04 SP93	33
St Mellion	St Mellion, Cornwall	Nicklaus Course: 18 holes, 6592yds, Par 72 The Old Course: 18 holes, 5782yds, Par 68	Map 04 SX36	55
Marriot Hanbury Manor	Ware, Hertfordshire	18 holes, 7052yds, Par 72	Map 05 TL31	137
Royal St George's	Sandwich, Kent	18 holes, 7102, Par 70	Map 05 TR35	147
Royal Lytham & St Annes	Lytham St Annes, Lancashire	18 holes, 6882yds, Par 71	Map 07 SD32	157
The National Golf Centre	Woodhall Spa, Lincolnshire	The Hotchkin: 18 holes, 7080yds, Par 73 The Bracken: 18 holes, 6735yds, Par 73	Map 08 TF16	171
Royal Liverpool	Hoylake, Merseyside	18 holes, 6440yds, Par 72	Map 07 SJ28	181
Royal Birkdale	Southport, Merseyside	18 holes, 6726yds, Par 72	Map 07 SD31	183
Wentworth	Virginia Water, Surrey	West Course: 18 holes, 7301yds, Par 73 East Course: 18 holes, 6201yds, Par 68 Edinburgh Course: 18 holes, 7004yds, Par 72	Map 04 TQ06	237
Walton Heath	Walton-on-the-Hill, Surrey	Old Course: 18 holes, 6836yds, Par 72 New Course: 18 holes, 6613yds, Par 72	Map 04 TQ25	241
East Sussex National	Uckfield, East Sussex	East Course: 18 holes, 7138yds, Par 72 West Course: 18 holes, 7154yds, Par 72	Map 05 TQ42	247
The Belfry	Wishaw, Warwickshire	The Brabazon: 18 holes, 6724yds, Par 72 PGA National: 18 holes, 6639yds, Par 71 The Derby: 18 holes, 6057yds, Par 69	Map 07 SP19	259
Marriott Forest of Arden	Meriden, West Midlands	Arden Course: 18 holes, 6707yds, Par 72 Aylesford Course: 18 holes, 5801, Par 69	Map 04 SP28	263
Carnoustie Golf Links	Carnoustie, Angus	Championship: 18 holes, 6941yds, Par 72 Burnside: 18 holes, 6028, Par 68 Buddon Links: 18 holes, 5420yds, Par 66	Map 12 NO53	315

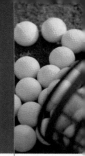

Name	Location	Course(s)	Map Ref	Page
Murfield: The Honourable Company of Edinburgh Golfers	Gullane, East Lothian	Murfield Course: 18 holes, 6673yds, Par 70	Map 12 NT68	327
Marriott Dalmahoy	Edinburgh, Edinburgh	East Course: 18 holes, 7055yds, Par 73 West Course: 18 holes, 5168yds, Par 68	Map 11 NT27	333
St Andrews Links	St Andrews, Fife	Old Course: 18 holes, 6609yds, Par 72 New Course: 18 holes, 6604yds, Par 71 Jubilee Course: 18 holes, 6742yds, Par 72 Eden Course: 18 holes, 6112yds, Par 70 Strathyrum Course: 18 holes, 5094yds, Par 69 Balgove Course: 9 holes, 1530yds, Par 30	Map 12 NO51	341
Gleneagles Hotel	Auchterarder, Perth and Kinross	King's Course: 18 holes, 6471yds, Par 70 Queen's Course: 18 holes, 5965yds, Par 68 PGA Centenary Course: 18 holes, 6787yds, Par 73	Map 11 NN91	359
Royal Troon	Troon, South Ayrshire	Old Course: 178 holes, 6641yds, Par 71 Portland: 18 holes, 6289yds, Par 71 Craigend: 9 holes	Map 10 NS33	367
Westin Turnberry Resort	Turnberry, South Ayrshire	Ailsa Course: 18 holes, 6440yds Kintyre Course: 18 holes, 6376yds, Par 71 Arran Course: 9 holes, 1996, Par 31	Map 10 NS20	369
Aberdovey	Aberdyfi, Gwynedd	18 holes, 6454yds, Par 71	Map 06 SN69	391
Marriott St Pierre Hotel	Chepstow, Monmouthshire	Old Course: 18 holes, 6733yds, Par 71 Mathern Course: 18 holes, 5732, Par 68	Map 03 ST59	395
Celtic Manor Resort	Newport, Celtic Manor Resort	Roman Road: 18 holes, 6030yds, Par 70 Coldra Woods: 18 holes, 3539yds, Par 71 Wentwood Hills: 18 holes, 6211yds, Par 71	Map 03 ST38	399
Royal Portrush	Co Antrim	Dunluce: 18 holes, 6641yds, Par 72 Valley: 18 holes, 6054yds, Par 70	Map 01 C6	409
Royal County Down	Newcastle, Co Down	Championship Course: 18 holes, 7181yds, Par 71 Annesley: 18 holes, 4681yds, Par 66	Map 01 D5	415
The Links	Portmarnock, Co Dublin	Old Course: 18 holes, 6567metres, Par 72 New Course: 9 holes, 3082metres, Par 37	Map 01 D4	435
Ballybunion	Ballybunion, Co Kerry	Old Course: 18 holes, 6083metres Cashen: 18 holes, Par 72	Map 01 A3	441
The K Club	Straffan, Co Kildare	Palmer Course: 18 holes, 6526mtrs, Par 74 Smurfit Course: 18 holes, 6636mtrs, Par 72	Map 01 D4	443
Mount Juliet Hotel	Thomastown, Co Kilkenny	18 holes, 6639metres, Par 72	Map 01 C3	447
Druids Glen Golf Club	Kilcoole, Co Wicklow	18 holes, 5987metres, Par 71	Map 01 D3	463

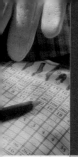

Golf Extremes
Play a round against the elements

The highest, the most remote and the windiest – these courses each have a unique place in the sporting landscape of the UK and Ireland. See their respective gazetteer entries for more details about opening times and course facilities.

Leadhills
South Lanarkshire (page 371)
Set among the Lowther Hills at 400 metres above sea level, this is the highest golf course in Scotland. The testing course runs east from the village of Leadhills uphill towards the moorland slopes of Shiel Gair Rig. Could be nippy in winter.

Whalsay
Shetland Islands (page 378)
The most northerly golf course in Britain is on the same latitude as Bergen in Norway. A large part of the course goes round the rugged north-east tip of the island, offering spectacular holes in an exposed but highly scenic setting. The fairways are defined by marker posts.

Mullion
Cornwall (page 52)
Founded in 1895, the clifftop and links course lies on dramatic National Trust coastline and has sweeping views over Mount's Bay. A steep downhill on 6th and the 10th descends to the beach with a deep ravine alongside the green. This is the second-most southerly course in the British Isles.

West Monmouthshire
Nantyglo, Blaenau Gwent (page 380)
Established in 1906, the West Monmouthshire is the highest British course, with the 14th tee at 461 metres above sea level. The mountain and heathland course has plenty of views, hard walking and natural hazards. Brace yourself for the testing 3rd hole, par 5, and 7th hole, par 4.

Kilkee
County Clare (page 422)
This established course on the west coast of Ireland follows the cliffs of Kilkee Bay. Its mature championship greens offer a great variety of challenges – seaside holes, clifftop holes, and holes with crafty water hazards. The spectacular 3rd hole hugs the cliff top, but the real test is the ever-present Atlantic breeze. Don't forget your waterproofs.

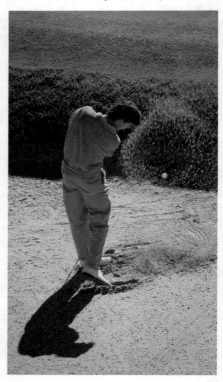

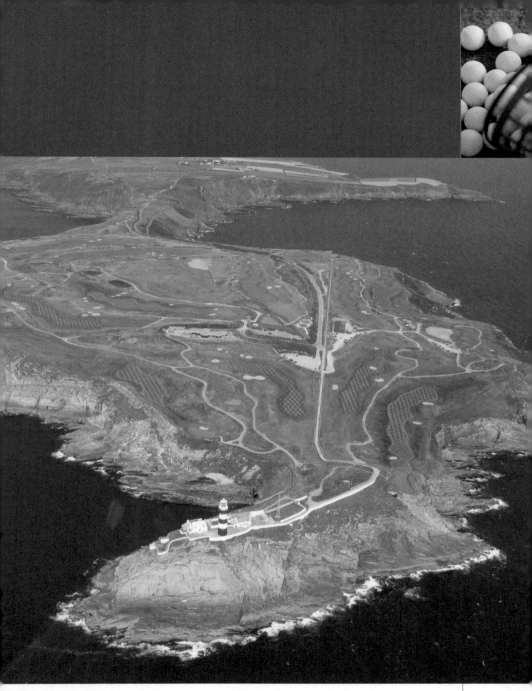

Old Head Kinsale, County Cork (page 426)

The Old Head course has a spectacular location on a lighthouse promontory jutting out into the Atlantic.
As well as the sea and cliffs, you have to contend with strong prevailing winds – a fine test for serious golfers.

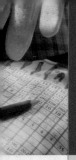

Dates & Events

The tables below provides a list of events to look out for over the next golfing year. The page references link to details about the course in the main gazetteer. All dates were correct at the time of going to press.

Event	Date	Location and course	Page
Walker Cup	8-9 September 2007	Royal County Down	415
Home Internationals Matches	12-14 September 2007	Dunbar Golf Club	326
Quinn Direct British Masters	20-23 September 2007	The Belfry	259
Ladies European Tour: De Vere Ladies Scottish Open	21-23 September 2007	De Vere Cameron House, The Carrick on Loch Lomond	373
European Tour, Alfred Dunhill Links Championship	1-8 October 2007	St Andrew's	341
HSBC World Match Play Championship	11-14 October 2007	Wentworth	237
Curtis Cup	30 May-1 June 2008	St Andrews, Old Course	341
English Seniors Championship	4-6 June 2008	Wildernesse and Knole Park	146
Ladies British Open Amateur Championship	11-15 June 2008	North Berwick	329
British Amateur Championship	16-21 June 2008	Westin Turnberry Resort, Ailsa & Kintyre courses	369
Junior Open Championship	July 2008 (tbc)	Hesketh	184
137th British Open Championship	17-20 July 2008	Royal Birkdale	183
Senior British Open Championship	24-27 July 2008	Royal Troon, Old Course	367
English Amateur Championship	28 July-2 Aug 2008	Woodhall Spa	171
Boys Home Internationals	5-7 August 2008	Royal County Down	415
Seniors Open Amateur Championship	6-8 August 2008	Royal Cinque Ports & Prince's	140
Boys Amateur Championship	11-16 August 2008	Little Aston	265
British Mid-Amateur Championship	13-17 August 2008	Royal St David's	392
Home International Matches	10-12 September 2008	Muirfield	327

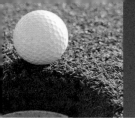
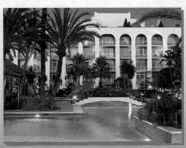
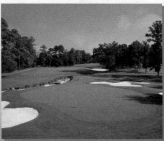
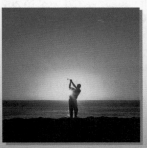

Would you like to slash your handicap by 30% in under 6 weeks?

Sound impossible? Discover the full power of your mental game and achieve astounding results, immediately.

Do you ever find yourself:

- Getting frustrated or even angry over mis-hits?
- Being easily distracted by other golfers?
- Worrying about missing your next shot or putt?
- Getting concerned about the effect missing your next shot will have on your score?
- Following a bad shot with further bad shots?
- Losing concentration after a superb shot and mis-hitting your next shot?
- Worrying about how other golfers will think of you unless you hit your next shot perfectly?
- Trying to control or steer your shots?
- Losing concentration for no apparent reason?

If you answered 'yes' to any of the above, then **Unleash Your Inner Golfer** will help you find significant improvements, quickly and easily.

The top tour professionals have understood the importance of the mental game for years, so much so that most of them now employ sports psychologists.

Try **Unleash Your Inner Golfer** for 6 weeks and if you're not 100% satisfied with the results, just return the CDs for a full, no quibbles, money-back refund.

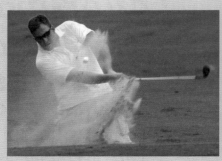

"A strong mental game is a crucial ingredient of success for golfers at every level" - David Leadbetter

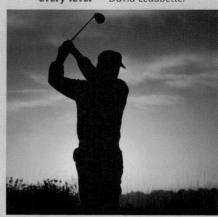

"Golf is 100% mental and 100% physical, and the two factions of golf cannot and should not be separated" - Ben Hogan

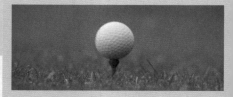

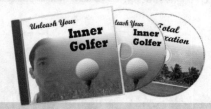

2 CD Set, only £35

Quote AA030 for an extra 15% discount.
For more information, visit:
www.UnleashYourInnerGolfer.com
Tel: 0118 946 3227 Email: info@UnleashYourInnerGolfer.co.uk

"No matter what a player's handicap, the scores will always be lower if the golfer thinks well" - Tom Kite

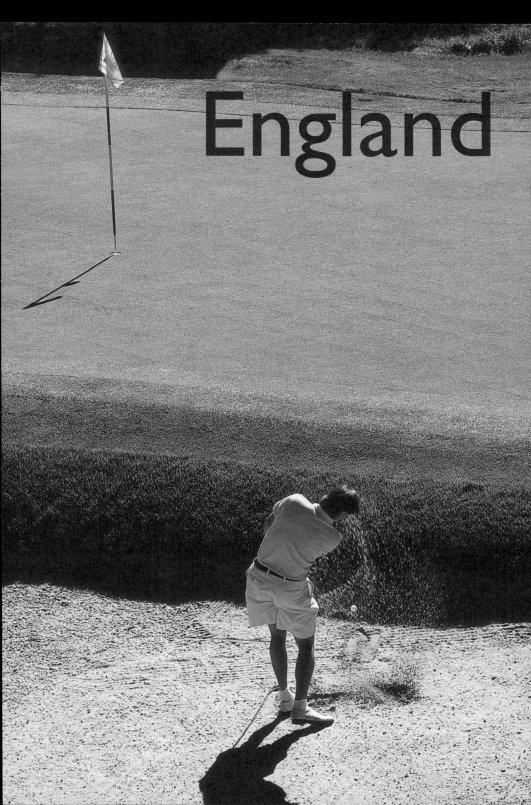

England

England

BEDFORDSHIRE

ASPLEY GUISE
MAP 04 SP93

Aspley Guise & Woburn Sands West Hill MK17 8DX
☎ 01908 583596 📠 01908 583596 (Secretary)
A fine undulating course in expansive heathland interspersed with many attractive clumps of gorse, broom and bracken. Some well-established silver birch is a feature. The really tough 7th, 8th and 9th holes complete the first half.
18 holes, 6079yds, Par 71, SSS 70, Course record 65.
Club membership 590.
Visitors may play Mon-Sun except BHs. Advance booking required Sat & Sun). Handicap certificate required. Dress code. **Societies** advance booking required. **Green Fees** not confirmed. **Prof** Colin Clingan **Course Designer** Sandy Herd **Facilities** ⚑ 🍴 🍺 ⛳🟊 🏋 🛍 🏌 🛒 ✏
Conf Corporate Hospitality Days **Location** M1 junct 13, 2m W
Hotel ★★★ 70% HL Best Western Moore Place Hotel, The Square, ASPLEY GUISE ☎ 01908 282000 35 en suite 27 annexe en suite

BEDFORD
MAP 04 TL04

Bedford Great Denham Golf Village, Carnoustie Dr, Biddenham MK40 4FF
☎ 01234 320022 📠 01234 320023
e-mail: thebedford@btopenworld.com
web: www.kolvengolf.com
American-style course with 89 bunkers, eight large water features and large contoured USPGA specification greens. Built on sand and gravel the course is open all year round.
18 holes, 6471yds, Par 72, SSS 72, Course record 63.
Club membership 500.
Visitors may play Mon-Sun & BHs. Advance booking required Sat, Sun & BHs. Dress code. **Societies** Booking required. **Green Fees** £40 per 18 holes (£60 weekends). **Prof** Zac Thompson **Course Designer** David Pottage **Facilities** ⚑ 🍴 🍺 ⛳🟊 🏋 🛍 🏌 🛒 ✏ **Conf** facs Corporate Hospitality Days **Location** 2.5m W of Bedford off A428
Hotel BUD Innkeeper's Lodge Bedford, 403 Goldington Rd, BEDFORD ☎ 0845 112 6056 47 en suite

Bedford & County Green Ln, Clapham MK41 6ET
☎ 01234 352617 📠 01234 357195
web: www.bedfordandcountygolfclub.co.uk
A mature, undulating parkland course established in 1912 with views over Bedford and surrounding countryside. Beware of the brook that discreetly meanders through the 7th, 10th, 11th and 15th holes. The testing Par 4 15th is one of the most challenging holes in the area.
18 holes, 6420yds, Par 70, SSS 70, Course record 66.
Club membership 600.
Visitors may play Mon-Fri except BHs. Handicap certificate required. Dress code. **Societies** advance booking required. **Green Fees** not confirmed. ✆ **Prof** R Tattersall **Facilities** ⚑ 🍴 🍺 ⛳🟊 🏋 🛍 ✏ **Conf** Corporate Hospitality Days **Location** 2m N off A6 in Clapham
Hotel BUD Premier Travel Inn Bedford, Priory Country Park, Barkers Ln, BEDFORD ☎ 08701 977030 32 en suite

Bedfordshire Spring Ln, Stagsden MK43 8SR
☎ 01234 822555 📠 01234 825052
e-mail: martin.bond@bedfordshiregolf.com
web: www.bedfordshiregolf.com
A challenging 18-hole course on undulating terrain with established trees and woods and water hazards. Magnificent views.

18 holes, 6565yds, Par 70, SSS 71, Course record 65.
Academy Course: 9 holes, 1354yds, Par 28, SSS 28.
Club membership 700.
Visitors Mon-Fri. Booking required. Must contact in advance. **Societies** Booking required. **Green Fees** £40 per day, £30 per 18 holes. 9 hole course £6 (£8 weekends). **Prof** David Armor **Course Designer** Cameron Sinclair **Facilities** ⚑ 🍴 by prior arrangement 🍺 ⛳🟊 🏋 🛍 🏌 🛒 ✏ 🏌 **Conf** facs Corporate Hospitality Days **Location** 3m W of Bedford on A422 at Stagsden
Hotel BUD Travelodge Bedford Marston Morstaine, Beancroft Rd Junction, MARSTON MORETAINE ☎ 08700 850 950 54 en suite

Mowsbury Cleat Hill, Kimbolton Rd, Ravensden MK41 8BJ
☎ 01234 772700 📠 01234 772700
Parkland municipal course in rural surroundings. Long and testing 14-bay driving range and squash facilities.
18 holes, 6182yds, Par 72, SSS 69. Club membership 390.
Visitors Mon-Sun & BHs. Dress code. **Societies** Booking required. **Green Fees** £14.30 per round (£18.70 weekends). **Prof** Malcolm Summers **Course Designer** Hawtree **Facilities** ⚑ 🍴 by prior arrangement 🍺 ⛳🟊 🏋 🛍 🏌 🛒 ✏ **Leisure** squash. **Location** 2m N of town centre on B660
Hotel BUD Innkeeper's Lodge Bedford, 403 Goldington Rd, BEDFORD ☎ 0845 112 6056 47 en suite

CHALGRAVE
MAP 04 TL02

Chalgrave Manor Dunstable Rd LU5 6JN
☎ 01525 876556 & 876554
e-mail: steve@chalgravegolf.co.uk
web: www.chalgravegolf.co.uk
Undulating parkland course set in 150 acres of Bedfordshire countryside. No two consecutive holes play in the same direction. Four holes have water hazards including the signature tenth hole, playing 130yds across water to a sloping green. The Par 5 9th, at 621yds, is one of the longest holes in the country.
18 holes, 6382yds, Par 72, SSS 70, Course record 68.
Club membership 550.
Visitors may play Mon-Sun & BHs. Advance booking required Sat, Sun & BHs. Dress code. **Societies** Booking required. **Green Fees** £20 per round (£30 weekends & bank holidays). **Prof** Martin Heanve **Course Designer** M Palmer **Facilities** ⚑ 🍴 by prior arrangement 🍺 ⛳🟊 🏋 🛍 🏌 ✏ **Conf** facs Corporate Hospitality Days **Location** M1 junct 12, A5120 through Toddington, signed 1m
Hotel ★★★ 72% HL Old Palace Lodge, Church St, DUNSTABLE ☎ 01582 662201 68 en suite

COLMWORTH
MAP 04 TL15

Colmworth & North Bedfordshire New Rd MK44 2NN
☎ 01234 378181 📠 01234 376678
e-mail: colmworth@btopenworld.com
web: www.colmworthgolfclub.co.uk
An easy walking course with well-bunkered greens, opened in 1991. The course is often windy and plays longer than the yardage suggests. Water comes into play on three holes.
18 holes, 6435yds, Par 72, SSS 71, Course record 69.
Club membership 200.
Visitors Mon-Sun & BHs. Booking required Sat, Sun & BHs. Dress code. **Societies** Booking required. **Green Fees** £17 per 18 holes, £14 per 12 holes, £12 per 9 holes (£25/£18/£15 Sat, Sun & BHs). **Prof** Graham Bithrey **Course Designer** John Glasgow **Facilities** ⚑ 🍴 by prior

Continued

arrangement 🖢 🖵 🍴 ⚘ 🍸 ♢ ♣ 🏂 **Leisure** fishing, Par 3 course.
Conf Corporate Hospitality Days **Location** Off A1 between Bedford & St
Neots
Hotel ★★★ 73% HL The Barns Hotel, Cardington Rd, BEDFORD
☎ 0870 609 6108 48 en suite

DUNSTABLE MAP 04 TL02

Dunstable Downs Whipsnade Rd LU6 2NB
☎ 01582 604472 📠 01582 478700
e-mail: dunstabledownsgc@btconnect.com
web: www.dunstable-golf.co.uk
A fine downland course set on two levels with far-reaching views
and frequent sightings of graceful gliders. The 9th hole is one of the
best short holes in the country.
18 holes, 6320yds, Par 70, SSS 70, Course record 64.
Club membership 600.
Visitors Mon-Fri & BHs. Dress code. **Societies** Welcome. **Green Fees**
£30 per round. ● **Prof** Darren Charlton **Course Designer** James Braid
Facilities ⑪ �📥 🖵 🍴 ⚘ 🛆 ♣ **Conf** Corporate Hospitality Days
Location 2m S off B4541
Hotel ★★★ 72% HL Old Palace Lodge, Church St, DUNSTABLE
☎ 01582 662201 68 en suite

Griffin Chaul End Rd, Caddington LU1 4AX
☎ 01582 415573 📠 01582 415314
e-mail: griffin@griffingolfclub.fsbusiness.co.uk
web: www.vauxhallrecreation.co.uk
18 holes, 6240yds, Par 71, SSS 70.
Location M1 junct 11, after 0.5m exit left at Tesco rdbt, towards Dunstable
Telephone for further details
Hotel ★★★ 72% HL Old Palace Lodge, Church St, DUNSTABLE
☎ 01582 662201 68 en suite

LEIGHTON BUZZARD MAP 04 SP92

Leighton Buzzard Plantation Rd LU7 3JF
☎ 01525 244800 (Office) 📠 01525 244801
e-mail: lbgc.secretary1@btopenworld.com
web: www.leightonbuzzardgolf.net
Mature parkland and heathland with easy walking. The 17th
and 18th holes are challenging tree-lined finishing holes with tight
fairways. The Par 3 11th is the signature hole.

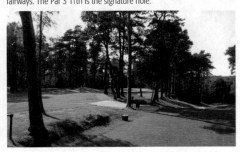

18 holes, 6101yds, Par 71, SSS 70, Course record 63.
Club membership 700.
Visitors may play Mon-Fri. Handicap certificate required. Dress code.
Societies welcome. **Green Fees** Phone. ● **Prof** Maurice Campbell
Facilities ⑪ �🍴 📥 🖵 🍴 ⚘ 🏂 ♣ 🏂 **Conf** facs Corporate Hospitality
Days **Location** 1.5m N of town centre off A4146

Hotel ★★★ 72% HL Old Palace Lodge, Church St, DUNSTABLE
☎ 01582 662201 68 en suite

LOWER STONDON MAP 04 TL13

Mount Pleasant Station Rd SG16 6JL
☎ 01462 850999
e-mail: manager@mountpleasantgolfclub
web: www.mountpleasantgolfclub.co.uk
Undulating meadowland course with three ponds in play and many
tree plantations. A deep ditch, sometimes with water, runs through
the middle of the course and is crossed four times per nine holes. The
main feature of the course is its presentation and superb greens. The
course is seldom closed by bad weather.
9 holes, 6185yds, Par 70, SSS 70, Course record 68.
Club membership 300.
Visitors Mon-Sun & BHs. Booking required. Dress code. **Societies** Booking
required. **Green Fees** £16 per 18 holes, £9 per 9 holes (£20/£11.50
weekends). **Prof** Glen Kemble **Course Designer** Derek Young **Facilities**
⑪ ⚑ by prior arrangement � 📥 🖵 🍴 ⚘ 🍸 ♣ 🏂 **Leisure** undercover
driving nets. **Conf** Corporate Hospitality Days **Location** 0.75m W of A600,
4m N of Hitchin
Hotel ★★★ 74% SHL Redcoats Farmhouse Hotel, Redcoats Green,
HITCHIN ☎ 01438 729500 4 en suite 9 annexe en suite

LUTON MAP 04 TL02

South Beds Warden Hill Rd LU2 7AE
☎ 01582 591500 📠 01582 495381
e-mail: office@southbedsgolfclub.co.uk
web: www.southbedsgolfclub.co.uk
An 18-hole and a nine-hole chalk downland course, slightly undulating.
Galley Hill Course: 18 holes, 6438yds, Par 71, SSS 71,
Course record 64.
Warden Hill Course: 9 holes, 2425yds, Par 32, SSS 32.
Club membership 1000.
Visitors Mon-Sun & BHs. Handicap certificate required for Galley Hill
course. Dress code. **Societies** Booking required. **Green Fees** Phone.
Prof Eddie Cogle **Facilities** ⑪ ⍟ ⍟ 📥 🖵 🍴 ⚘ 🏂 ♣ **Conf** Corporate
Hospitality Days **Location** 3m N of Luton on A6
Hotel BUD Hotel Ibis Luton, Spittlesea Rd, LUTON ☎ 01582 424488
98 en suite

Stockwood Park London Rd LU1 4LX
☎ 01582 413704 (pro shop)
18 holes, 6049yds, Par 69, SSS 69, Course record 67.
Location 1m S
Telephone for further details
Hotel ★★★ 72% HL Hotel St Lawrence, 40A Guildford St, LUTON
☎ 01582 482119 28 en suite

MILLBROOK MAP 04 TL03

Millbrook Millbrook Village MK45 2JB
☎ 01525 840252 📠 01525 406249
e-mail: info@themillbrook.com
web: www.themillbrook.com
Long parkland course on rolling countryside high above the
Bedfordshire plains. Laid out on well-drained sandy soil with many
fairways lined with silver birch, pine and larch. The course provides

Continued

a continuous test of the tee where length and accuracy pay a huge premium.

18 holes, 6966yds, Par 73, SSS 73, Course record 68.
Club membership 560.

Visitors Mon-Fri. Sat, Sun & BHs pm only. Dress code. **Societies** Booking required. **Green Fees** £26 per 18 holes (£35 weekends & BHs pm only). **Prof** Geraint Dixon **Course Designer** William Sutherland **Facilities** ⑪ ⌂ ▽ ¶⟋ ⚲ ☎ ᵠ ♿ ♂ **Conf** facs Corporate Hospitality Days **Location** M1 junct 12/13, A507 Woburn-Ampthill road

Hotel ★★★ 70% HL Best Western Moore Place Hotel, The Square, ASPLEY GUISE ☎ 01908 282000 35 en suite 27 annexe en suite

PAVENHAM   MAP 04 SP95

Pavenham Park MK43 7PE
☎ 01234 822202 📄 01234 826602
e-mail: kolvengolf@ukonline.co.uk
web: www.kolvengolf.com

18 holes, 6400yds, Par 72, SSS 71, Course record 63.
Course Designer Zac Thompson **Location** 1.5m from A6, N of Bedford
Telephone for further details

Hotel BUD Travelodge Bedford Marston Morstaine, Beancroft Rd Junction, MARSTON MORETAINE ☎ 08700 850 950 54 en suite

SANDY   MAP 04 TL14

John O'Gaunt Sutton Park SG19 2LY
☎ 01767 260360 📄 01767 262834
e-mail: admin@johnogauntgolfclub.co.uk
web: www.johnogauntgolfclub.co.uk

Two magnificent parkland courses - John O'Gaunt and Carthagena - covering a gently undulating and tree-lined terrain. The John O'Gaunt course makes the most of numerous natural features, notably a river which crosses the fairways of four holes. The Carthagena course has larger greens, longer tees and from the back tees is a challenging course.

John O'Gaunt Course: 18 holes, 6513yds, Par 71, SSS 71, Course record 64.
Carthagena Course: 18 holes, 5869yds, Par 69, SSS 69.
Club membership 1500.

Visitors may play Mon-Fri. Handicap certificate required. Dress code. **Societies** advance booking required. **Green Fees** not confirmed. ☻ **Prof** Lee Scarbrow **Course Designer** Hawtree **Facilities** ⑪ ⍥ ⌂ ▽ ¶⟋ ⚲ ☎ ♂ ᵠ ♂ **Conf** Corporate Hospitality Days **Location** 3m NE of Biggleswade on B1040

SHEFFORD   MAP 04 TL13

Beadlow Manor Hotel & Golf & Country Club
SG17 5PH
☎ 01525 860800 📄 01525 861345
e-mail: info@beadlowmanor.co.uk
web: www.beadlowmanor.co.uk

A 36-hole golf and leisure complex. The Baroness Manhattan and the Baron Manhattan courses are undulating with water hazards on numerous holes. These are good challenging courses for both the beginner and low handicap player.

Baroness Course: 18 holes, 6072yds, Par 71, SSS 69, Course record 67.
Baron Course: 18 holes, 6619yds, Par 73, SSS 72, Course record 67. Club membership 850.

Visitors contact club for details. **Societies** advance booking required. **Green Fees** not confirmed. **Prof** Gordon Morrison **Facilities** ⑪ ⍥ ⌂ ▽ ¶⟋ ⚲ ☎ ᵠ ♿ ♂ ♂ **Conf** facs Corporate Hospitality Days **Location** On A507

Hotel ★★ HL Firs Hotel, 83 Bedford Rd, HITCHIN ☎ 01462 422322 29 en suite

TILSWORTH   MAP 04 SP92

Tilsworth Dunstable Rd LU7 9PU
☎ 01525 210721/2 📄 01525 210465
e-mail: nick@tilsworthgolf.co.uk
web: www.tilsworthgolf.co.uk

The course is in first-class condition and, although not a long course, is particularly demanding and challenging where the key is straight driving. The course has its own Amen Corner between the 14th and 16th holes, which will challenge all golfers. Panoramic views of three counties from the 6th tee.

18 holes, 5306yds, Par 69, SSS 66, Course record 61.
Club membership 400.

Visitors Mon-Sun & BHs. Advance booking Sat, Sun & BHs. **Societies** Booking required. **Green Fees** £17 for 18 holes (£19.50 weekends/BHs). **Prof** Nick Webb **Facilities** ⑪ ⍥ ⌂ ⌂ ▽ ¶⟋ ⚲ ☎ ᵠ ♿ ♂ ♂ **Conf** facs Corporate Hospitality Days **Location** 0.5m NE off A5, N of Dunstable

Hotel ★★★ 72% HL Old Palace Lodge, Church St, DUNSTABLE ☎ 01582 662201 68 en suite

WYBOSTON   MAP 04 TL15

Wyboston Lakes MK44 3AL
☎ 01480 212625 📄 01480 223000
e-mail: venue@wybostonlakes.co.uk
web: www.wybostonlakes.co.uk

Parkland with narrow fairways and small greens, set around four lakes and a river, which provide the biggest challenge on this very scenic course.

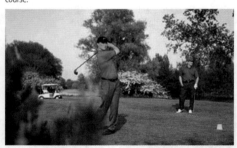

18 holes, 5955yds, Par 70, SSS 69, Course record 65.
Club membership 375.

Visitors may play Mon-Sun & BHs. Advance booking required Sat, Sun & BHs. **Societies** advance booking required. **Green Fees** not confirmed. **Prof** Paul Ashwell **Course Designer** N Oakden **Facilities** ⑪ ⍥ ⌂ ⌂ ▽ ¶⟋ ⚲ ☎ ᵠ ♿ ♂ ♂ **Leisure** heated indoor swimming pool, fishing, sauna, solarium, gymnasium, watersports. **Conf** facs Corporate Hospitality Days **Location** 1m S of St Neots off A1/A428

Hotel ★★★ 73% HL The Barns Hotel, Cardington Rd, BEDFORD ☎ 0870 609 6108 48 en suite

BERKSHIRE

ASCOT
MAP 04 SU96

Berkshire Swinley Rd SL5 8AY
☎ 01344 621495 📠 01344 623328

Two classic heathland courses, with splendid tree-lined fairways, that have remained the same since they were constructed in 1928. The Red Course, on slightly higher ground, is a little longer than the Blue. It has an unusual assortment of holes, six Par 3s, six Par 4s and six Par 5s, the short holes, particularly the 10th and 16th, being the most intimidating. The Blue Course starts with a Par 3 and shares with the 16th the reputation of being the finest holes of the 18.

Red Course: 18 holes, 6379yds, Par 72, SSS 71.
Blue Course: 18 holes, 6260yds, Par 71, SSS 71.
Visitors Mon-Fri except BHs. Booking required. Dress code.
Societies Booking required. **Green Fees** £115 per day, £85 per round.
Prof P Anderson **Course Designer** H Fowler **Facilities** ⑪ 🍴 🏌 ♨ 🏕 🖺 🏊 🍺 🛒 ♨ ☂ **Conf** Corporate Hospitality Days **Location** M3 junct 3, 2.5m NW on A332
Hotel ★★★★ 78% HL Macdonald Berystede Hotel & Spa, Bagshot Rd, Sunninghill, ASCOT ☎ 0870 400 8111 126 en suite

Lavender Park Swinley Rd SL5 8BD
☎ 01344 893344
e-mail: lavenderpark@yahoo.com
web: www.lavenderparkgolf.co.uk

Public parkland course, ideal for the short game featuring challenging narrow fairways. Driving range with nine-hole Par 3 course, floodlit until 10pm.

9 holes, 1102yds, Par 27, SSS 28.
Visitors may play Mon-Sun & BHs. **Societies** welcome. **Green Fees** not confirmed. **Prof** David Johnson **Facilities** ♨ 🍴 🏕 ♨ ☂ **Leisure** snooker. **Location** 1.5m W of Ascot, off the A329 on the B3017
Hotel ★★★★ 78% HL Macdonald Berystede Hotel & Spa, Bagshot Rd, Sunninghill, ASCOT ☎ 0870 400 8111 126 en suite

Mill Ride Mill Ride SL5 8LT
☎ 01344 886777 📠 01344 886820
e-mail: c.sheffield@mill-ride.com
web: www.mill-ride.com

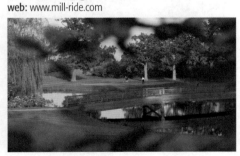

18 holes, 6807yds, Par 72, SSS 72, Course record 64.
Course Designer Donald Steel **Location** 2m W of Ascot
Telephone for further details
Hotel ★★★★ 78% HL Macdonald Berystede Hotel & Spa, Bagshot Rd, Sunninghill, ASCOT ☎ 0870 400 8111 126 en suite

Royal Ascot Winkfield Rd SL5 7LJ
☎ 01344 625175 📠 01344 872330
e-mail: golf@royalascotgc.fsnet.co.uk
web: www.royalascotgolfclub.co.uk
18 holes, 5716yds, Par 68, SSS 68, Course record 65.
Course Designer J H Taylor **Location** 0.5m N on A330
Telephone for further details
Hotel ★★★★ 78% HL Macdonald Berystede Hotel & Spa, Bagshot Rd, Sunninghill, ASCOT ☎ 0870 400 8111 126 en suite

Swinley Forest Coronation Rd SL5 9LE
☎ 01344 874979 (Secretary) 📠 01344 874733
e-mail: swinleyfgc@tiscali.co.uk

An attractive and immaculate course of heather and pine situated in the heart of Swinley Forest. The 17th is as good a short hole as can be found, with a bunkered plateau green, and the 12th is one of the most challenging Par 4s.

18 holes, 6100yds, Par 69, SSS 70, Course record 62.
Club membership 350.
Visitors may play Mon-Fri except BHs. Booking required. Handicap certificate. Dress code. **Societies** Welcome. **Green Fees** £135 per day.
Prof Stuart Hill **Course Designer** Harry Colt **Facilities** ⑪ 🍴 🏌 ♨ 🏕 🖺 🏊 🍺 🛒 ♨ ☂ **Leisure** Video studio. **Conf** Corporate Hospitality Days **Location** 2m S of Ascot, off A30
Hotel ★★★★ 78% HL Macdonald Berystede Hotel & Spa, Bagshot Rd, Sunninghill, ASCOT ☎ 0870 400 8111 126 en suite

BINFIELD
MAP 04 SU87

Blue Mountain Golf Centre Wood Ln RG42 4EX
☎ 01344 300200 📠 01344 360960
e-mail: bluemountain@americangolf.uk.com
web: www.bluemountain-golf.co.uk
18 holes, 6097yds, Par 70, SSS 70, Course record 63.
Location From M4 junct 10, take A329(M) signed Bracknell. 1st exit signed B3408 Binfield. Straight over roundabout and traffic lights to next roundabout. 2nd exit, first left into Wood Lane.
Telephone for further details
Hotel ★★★★ 77% HL Coppid Beech, John Nike Way, BRACKNELL ☎ 01344 303333 205 en suite

CAVERSHAM
MAP 04 SU77

Caversham Heath Chazey Heath RG4 7UT
☎ 0118 947 8600 📠 0118 947 8700
e-mail: info@cavershamgolf.co.uk
web: www.cavershamgolf.co.uk

A course in a beautiful heathland setting which has matured well and rewards golfers of all levels. The course, built to exacting USGA standards, is unusually dry in winter whilst fully irrigated in summer, and therefore offers dependable year-round play.

18 holes, 7151yds, Par 73, SSS 73, Course record 69.
Club membership 600.
Visitors Mon-Fr. Sat, Sun & BHs pm only. Booking required Sat, Sun & BHs. Handicap certificate. Dress code. **Societies** Booking required. **Green Fees** £40 per 18 holes, £26 per 9 holes (£56/£32 Sat & Sun). **Prof** Adam Harrison **Course Designer** David Williams **Facilities** ⑪ 🍴 🏌 ♨ 🏕 🖺 🏊 🍺 🛒 ♨ 🍴 ♨ ☂ **Conf** Corporate Hospitality Days **Location** 2m NE of Caversham on A4074 towards Oxford
Hotel ★★★★ 77% HL Novotel Reading Centre, 25b Friar St, READING ☎ 0118 952 2600 178 en suite

CHADDLEWORTH — MAP 04 SU47

West Berkshire RG20 7DU
☎ 01488 638574 🖹 01488 638781
e-mail: info@thewbgc.co.uk
web: www.thewbgc.co.uk
Challenging and interesting downland course with views of the Berkshire Downs. The course is bordered by ancient woodland and golfers will find manicured fairways with well-constructed greens and strategically placed hazards. The testing 627yd 5th hole is one of the longest Par 5s in southern England. Bunkers are well placed from tees and around the greens to catch any wayward shots.
18 holes, 7022yds, Par 73, SSS 74. Club membership 650.
Visitors Mon-Sun & BHs. Advance booking required Sat, Sun & BHs. Dress code. **Societies** Booking required. **Green Fees** £28 per round (£35 per round weekends & bank holidays). **Prof** Paul Simpson **Facilities** ⓉⓁ⊡ 🏌⛳🛒🏌️ **Conf** Corporate Hospitality Days **Location** 1m S of village off A338
Hotel ★★★ 77% CHH Ramada Hotel & Resort Elcot Park, ELCOT ☎ 01488 658100 56 en suite 17 annexe en suite

COOKHAM — MAP 04 SU88

Winter Hill Grange Ln SL6 9RP
☎ 01628 527613 (Secretary) 🖹 01628 527479
Parkland course set in a curve of the Thames with wonderful views across the river to Cliveden.

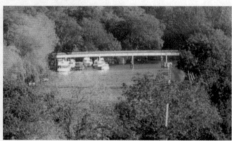

18 holes, 6408yds, Par 72, SSS 71, Course record 63.
Club membership 770.
Visitors Mon-Fri except BHs. Handicap certificate required. Dress code.
Societies Booking required. **Green Fees** £36 per day. **Prof** Roger Frost
Course Designer Charles Lawrie **Facilities** Ⓣ Ⓘ by prior arrangement
Ⓛ⊡🏌⛳🛒🏌️ **Conf** facs Corporate Hospitality Days
Location 1m NW off B4447
Hotel ★★★★ 80% HL Macdonald Compleat Angler, Marlow Bridge, MARLOW ☎ 0870 400 8100 64 en suite

CROWTHORNE — MAP 04 SU86

East Berkshire Ravenswood Ave RG45 6BD
☎ 01344 772041 🖹 01344 777378
e-mail: thesecretary@eastberksgc.fsnet.co.uk
web: www.eastberkshiregolfclub.co.uk
An attractive heathland course with an abundance of heather and pine trees. Walking is easy and the greens are exceptionally good. Some fairways become tight where the heather encroaches on the line of play. The course is testing and demands great accuracy.
18 holes, 6236yds, Par 69, SSS 70, Course record 65.
Club membership 766.

Visitors may play Mon-Fri. Handicap certificate required. Dress code
Societies Booking required. **Green Fees** £60 per day, £40 per round.
 Prof Jason Brant **Course Designer** P Paxton **Facilities** Ⓣ Ⓘ Ⓛ ⊡
🏌⛳🛒🏌️ **Conf** Corporate Hospitality Days **Location** W side of town centre off B3348
Hotel ★★★★★ HL Pennyhill Park Hotel & The Spa, London Rd, BAGSHOT ☎ 01276 471774 26 en suite 97 annexe en suite

DATCHET — MAP 04 SU97

Datchet Buccleuch Rd SL3 9BP
☎ 01753 543887 & 541872 🖹 01753 541872
e-mail: secretary@datchetgolfclub.co.uk
web: www.datchetgolfclub.co.uk
Meadowland course, easy walking.
9 holes, 6087yds, Par 70, SSS 69, Course record 63.
Club membership 430.
Visitors may play Mon-Fri & BHs. Sat & Sun pm only. Dress code.
Societies Booking required. **Green Fees** £25 per 18 holes (£30 weekends & bank holidays). **Prof** Ian Godelman **Course Designer** J H Taylor
Facilities Ⓣ Ⓘ Ⓛ ⊡🏌 🛒🏌️ **Location** NW side of Datchet off B470
Hotel ★★★★ 77% HL Mercure Castle Hotel, 18 High St, WINDSOR ☎ 0870 400 8300 38 en suite 70 annexe en suite

MAIDENHEAD — MAP 04 SU88

Bird Hills Drift Rd, Hawthorn Hill SL6 3ST
☎ 01628 771030 🖹 01628 631023
e-mail: info@birdhills.co.uk
web: www.birdhills.co.uk
A gently undulating course with easy walking and many water hazards. Some challenging holes are the Par 5 6th dog-leg, Par 3 9th surrounded by water and bunkers, and the 16th which is a long uphill Par 4 and a two-tier green.

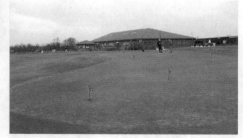

18 holes, 6176yds, Par 72, SSS 69, Course record 65.
Club membership 400.
Visitors Mon-Sun & BHs. Advance booking required. Dress code. **Societies** Booking required. **Green Fees** seasonal charges - ring for details. **Prof** Nick Slimming **Facilities** Ⓣ Ⓘ Ⓛ ⊡🏌⛳🛒🏌️ **Leisure** pool tables.
Conf facs Corporate Hospitality Days **Location** M4 junct 8/9, 4m S on A330
Hotel ★★★ 78% HL Stirrups Country House, Maidens Green, BRACKNELL ☎ 01344 882284 30 en suite

Maidenhead Shoppenhangers Rd SL6 2PZ
☎ 01628 624693 📠 01628 780758
e-mail: manager@maidenheadgolf.co.uk
web: www.maidenheadgolf.co.uk
Pleasant parkland with excellent greens and some challenging holes. The long Par 4 4th and short Par 3 13th are only two of the many outstanding aspects of this course. Fairway irrigation installed 2006.
18 holes, 6364yds, Par 70, SSS 70. Club membership 750.
Visitors Mon-Sun & BHs. Booking required Sat, Sun & BHs. Handicap certificate required. Dress code. **Societies** Booking required.
Green Fees £46 per day, £36 per round (£46 per round weekends).
Prof Steve Geary **Course Designer** Alex Simpson **Facilities** ⊕ ⏺ ⑆ 🏌 ⊡
⤵ ⛳ 🏴‍☠️ 🚗 **Conf** facs Corporate Hospitality Days **Location** S side of town centre off A308
Hotel ★★★★ HL Fredrick's Hotel, Restaurant & Spa, Shoppenhangers Rd, MAIDENHEAD ☎ 01628 581000 34 en suite

Temple Henley Rd, Hurley SL6 5LH
☎ 01628 824795 📠 01628 828119
e-mail: templegolfclub@btconnect.com
web: www.templegolfclub.co.uk
Open parkland with extensive views over the Thames Valley. Firm, relatively fast greens, natural slopes and subtle contours provide a challenging test to golfers of all abilities. Excellent drainage assures play during inclement weather.
18 holes, 6266yds, Par 70, SSS 70. Club membership 480.
Visitors Mon-Sun & BHs. Booking required. Handicap certificate required. Dress code. **Societies** Booking required. **Green Fees** £56 per day; £44 per round (£60/ £50 weekends). **Prof** James Whiteley
Course Designer Willie Park (Jnr) **Facilities** ⊕ ⏺ by prior arrangement ⑆ ⊡ ⤵ ⛳ 🏴‍☠️ 🚗 **Conf** Corporate Hospitality Days **Location** M4 junct 8/9, A404M then A4130, signed Henley
Hotel ★★★★ 80% HL Macdonald Compleat Angler, Marlow Bridge, MARLOW ☎ 0870 400 8100 64 en suite

MORTIMER   MAP 04 SU66

Wokefield Park Wokefield Park RG7 3AE
☎ 0118 933 4072 📠 0118 933 4031
e-mail: wokgolfteam@deverevenues.co.uk
web: www.deverevenues.co.uk
Set in a prime location amid the peaceful and picturesque Berkshire countryside. The course architect has retained the numerous mature trees, and these, together with the winding streams, nine lakes and large bunkers, contribute to the beauty and challenge of this championship course.
18 holes, 6579yds, Par 72, SSS 72, Course record 65. Club membership 350.
Visitors Mon-Fri & BHs. After noon Sat & Sun. Dress code.
Societies Booking required. **Green Fees** £25 (£35 Sat & Sun).
Course Designer Jonathan Gaunt **Facilities** ⊕ ⏺ ⑆ ⊡ ⤵ ⛳ 🚗
🏴‍☠️ ♦ 🚗 🏌 ⛳ **Leisure** heated indoor swimming pool, fishing, sauna, gymnasium, jacuzzi. **Conf** facs Corporate Hospitality Days **Location** M4 junct 11, A33 towards Basingstoke. 1st rdbt, 3rd exit towards Grazeley. After 2.5m right bend, club on right
Hotel ★★★ 70% HL Romans Hotel, Little London Rd, SILCHESTER ☎ 0118 970 0421 11 en suite 14 annexe en suite

NEWBURY   MAP 04 SU46

Donnington Valley Snelsmore House, Snelsmore Common RG14 3BG
☎ 01635 568140 📠 01635 568141
e-mail: golf@donningtonvalley.co.uk
web: www.donningtonvalleygolfclub.co.uk

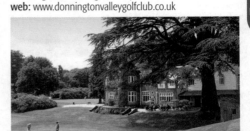

18 holes, 6353yds, Par 71, SSS 71, Course record 71.
Course Designer Mike Smith **Location** 2m N of Newbury
Telephone for further details
Hotel ★★★★ 83% HL Donnington Valley Hotel & Spa, Old Oxford Rd, Donnington, NEWBURY ☎ 01635 551199 111 en suite

Newbury & Crookham Bury's Bank Rd, Greenham RG19 8BZ
☎ 01635 40035 📠 01635 40045
e-mail: steve.myers@newburygolf.co.uk
web: www.newburygolf.co.uk
A traditional English parkland course, whose tree-lined fairways provide a challenge of consistency and accuracy.
18 holes, 5969yds, Par 69, SSS 69, Course record 63. Club membership 750.
Visitors Mon-Fri. Handicap certificate required. Dress code. **Societies** Booking required. **Green Fees** £40 per day; £35 per round. **Prof** David Harris **Course Designer** J H Taylor **Facilities** ⊕ ⏺ ⑆ ⊡ ⤵ ⛳ ⛳
Conf Corporate Hospitality Days **Location** 4m S of M4 off A339
Hotel ★★★ 77% CHH Ramada Hotel & Resort Elcot Park, ELCOT ☎ 01488 658100 56 en suite 17 annexe en suite

READING   MAP 04 SU77

Calcot Park Bath Rd, Calcot RG31 7RN
☎ 0118 942 7124 📠 0118 945 3373
e-mail: info@calcotpark.com
web: www.calcotpark.com
A delightfully picturesque, slightly undulating parkland course just outside the town, which celebrated its 75th anniversary in 2005. The subtle borrows on the greens challenge all categories of golfer. Hazards include streams, a lake and many trees. The 6th is a 503yd Par 5, with the tee shot hit downhill over cross-bunkers to a well-guarded green; the 7th (156yds) is played over the lake to an elevated green and the 13th (also 156yds) requires a carry across a valley to a plateau green.
18 holes, 6216yds, Par 70, SSS 70, Course record 63. Club membership 730.
Visitors may play Mon-Fri. Booking required. Handicap certificate required. Dress code. **Societies** Booking required. **Green Fees** £50 per day/round. Enquire for off peak rates. ⬤ **Prof** Mark Grieve

Continued

Course Designer H S Colt Facilities ⊕ ⫶Ⓞ⫶ ᝰ 🖙 🗗⛳🏊 🖻 ⛯ ✐
Leisure fishing. Conf facs Corporate Hospitality Days Location 1.5m
from M4 junct 12 on A4 towards Reading
Hotel ★★★ 70% HL Best Western Calcot Hotel, 98 Bath Rd, Calcot,
READING ☎ 0118 941 6423 78 en suite

Hennerton Crazies Hill Rd, Wargrave RG10 8LT
☎ 0118 940 1000 🖺 0118 940 1042
web: www.hennertongolfclub.co.uk
Overlooking the Thames Valley, this course has many existing natural
features and a good number of hazards such as bunkers, mature trees
and two small lakes.
18 holes, 4187yds, Par 65, SSS 62, Course record 62.
Club membership 450.
Visitors Mon-Sun & BHs. Dress code. Societies Booking required.
Green Fees £20 per 18 holes, £14 per 9 holes (£30/£18 weekends and bank
holidays). Prof William Farrow Course Designer Col D Beard Facilities ⊕
ᝰ 🖙 🗗🏊 ⛯ ✐ 🖻 ⛯ ✐ Conf Corporate Hospitality Days Location
Signed from A321 Wargrave High St
Hotel ★★ 72% HL Elva Lodge Hotel, Castle Hill, MAIDENHEAD
☎ 01628 622948 26 rms (23 en suite)

Mapledurham Chazey Heath, Mapledurham RG4 7UD
☎ 0118 946 3353 🖺 0118 946 3363
web: www.theclubcompany.com
An 18-hole parkland and woodland course designed by Bob Sandow.
Flanked by hedgerows and mature woods, it is testing for players of
all levels.
18 holes, 5700yds, Par 69, SSS 67, Course record 65.
Club membership 750.
Visitors Mon-Sun & BHs. Advance booking required. Dress code. Societies
Booking required. Green Fees £21.50 per round (£30 Sat & Sun). Prof Tim
Gilpin Course Designer Robert Sandow Facilities ⊕ ⫶Ⓞ⫶ ᝰ 🖙 🗗🏊 🖻
✐ Leisure heated indoor swimming pool, sauna, solarium, gymnasium.
Conf Corporate Hospitality Days Location On A4074 to Oxford
Hotel ★★★ 78% HL The French Horn, SONNING ON THAMES
☎ 0118 969 2204 13 en suite 8 annexe en suite

Reading 17 Kidmore End Rd, Emmer Green RG4 8SG
☎ 0118 947 2909 (Secretary) 🖺 0118 946 4468
e-mail: secretary@readinggolfclub.com
web: www.readinggolfclub.com
Pleasant parkland, part hilly and part flat with interesting views and
several challenging Par 3s. After the opening holes the course moves
across the valley. The Par 4 5th is played from an elevated tee and
although relatively short, the well-placed bunkers and trees come
into play. The 470yd Par 4 12th is a great hole. It has a slight dog-leg
and requires an accurate second shot to hit a well-guarded green.
The finishing hole requires two great shots to have any chance of
reaching par.
18 holes, 6212yds, Par 70, SSS 70, Course record 65.
Club membership 600.
Visitors Mon-Thu. Handicap certificate. Dress code. Societies advance
booking required. Green Fees £50 per day, £35 per round. Prof Scott
Fotheringham Course Designer James Braid Facilities ⊕ ⫶Ⓞ⫶ ᝰ 🖙 🗗
🗗🏊 🖻 🖻 ✐ Leisure indoor nets. Conf Corporate Hospitality Days
Location 2m N off B481
Hotel ★★★ 78% HL The French Horn, SONNING ON THAMES
☎ 0118 969 2204 13 en suite 8 annexe en suite

SINDLESHAM
MAP 04 SU76

Bearwood Mole Rd RG41 5DB
☎ 0118 976 0060
e-mail: barrytustin@btconnect.com
Flat parkland with one water hazard, the 40-acre lake that features on
the challenging 6th and 7th holes.
9 holes, 5610yds, Par 70, SSS 68, Course record 66.
Club membership 500.
Visitors may play Mon-Sun & BHs. Handicap certificate. Dress code. Prof
Bayley Tustin Course Designer Barry Tustin Facilities 🏊 🖻 🖻 ✐ 🌾
Location 1m SW on B3030
Hotel ★★★★ 81% HL Millennium Madejski Hotel Reading, Madejski
Stadium, READING ☎ 0118 925 3500 140 en suite

SONNING
MAP 04 SU77

Sonning Duffield Rd RG4 6GJ
☎ 0118 969 3332 🖺 0118 944 8409
e-mail: secretary@sonning-golf-club.co.uk
web: www.sonning-golf-club.co.uk
A quality parkland course and the scene of many county
championships. Wide fairways, not over-bunkered, and very good
greens. holes of changing character through wooded belts. Four
challenging Par 4s over 450yds.
18 holes, 6366yds, Par 70, SSS 70, Course record 65.
Club membership 750.
Visitors may play Mon-Fri. Handicap certificate required. Dress code.
Societies Booking required. Green Fees £40.50 before 10.30am or
£30.50 after 10.30am. ☜ Prof R McDougall Course Designer J H Taylor
Facilities ⊕ ⫶Ⓞ⫶ ᝰ 🖙 🗗🏊 🖻 ✐ Conf facs Corporate Hospitality
Days Location 1m S off A4
Hotel ★★★ 78% HL The French Horn, SONNING ON THAMES
☎ 0118 969 2204 13 en suite 8 annexe en suite

STREATLEY
MAP 04 SU58

Goring & Streatley RG8 9QA
☎ 01491 873229 🖺 01491 875224
e-mail: secretary@goringgc.org
web: www.goringgc.org
A parkland and moorland course that requires negotiating. Four well-
known holes lead up to the heights of the 5th tee, to which there is
a 300ft climb. Wide fairways, not over-bunkered, with nice rewards
on the way home down the last few holes. A delightful course that
commands magnificent views of the Ridgeway & the River Thames.
18 holes, 6355yds, Par 71, SSS 70, Course record 65.
Club membership 740.
Visitors Mon-Fri. Handicap certificate. Societies Booking required.
Green Fees Phone. Prof Jason Hadland Course Designer Tom Morris
Facilities ⊕ ⫶Ⓞ⫶ ᝰ 🖙 🗗🏊 🖻 ✐ Location N of village off A417
Hotel ★★★★ 73% HL The Swan at Streatley, High St, STREATLEY
☎ 01491 878800 45 en suite

CHAMPIONSHIP COURSE

SUNNINGDALE

Map 04 SU96

Ridgemount Rd SL5 9RR
☎ **01344 621681** 📠 **01344 624154**
web: www.sunningdalegolfclub.co.uk
Old Course: 18 holes, 6308yds, Par 70, SSS 70.
New Course: 18 holes, 6443yds, Par 71,
SSS 72. **Club membership 1000.**
Visitors may play Mon-Thu. Advance booking
required. Handicap certificate required. Dress
code. **Societies** advance booking required.
Green Fees Old Course: £165 per round;
New Course £125 per round. 36 holes £225.
Prof Keith Maxwell **Course Designer** W Park
Facilities Ⓨ 🄻 ▭ 🝑 ⟑ 🛆 🖻 🏌 ⚎ ⚐
Conf Corporate Hospitality Days **Location** 1m
S off A30

Sunningdale Golf Club has two championship
courses, laid out on the most glorious piece of
heathland and both have their own individual
characteristics. The Old Course, founded
in 1900, was designed by Willie Park. It is a
classic course at just 6308yds long, with gorse
and pines, silver birch, heather and
immaculate turf. The New Course was
created by H S Colt in 1922. At 6443yds, it is
a mixture of wood and open heath with long
carries and tight fairways.

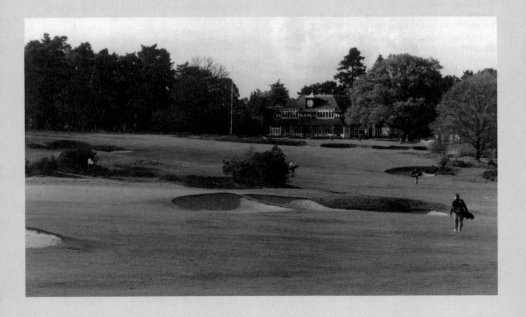

SUNNINGDALE
MAP 04 SU96

Sunningdale see page 27

Hotel ★★★★★ HL Pennyhill Park Hotel & The Spa, London Rd, BAGSHOT ☎ 01276 471774 26 en suite 97 annexe en suite
Hotel ★★★★ 78% HL Macdonald Berystede Hotel & Spa, Bagshot Rd, Sunninghill, ASCOT ☎ 0870 400 8111 Fax 01344 872301 126 en suite
Hotel ★★★★ 77% HL The Royal Berkshire Ramada Plaza, London Rd, Sunninghill, ASCOT ☎ 01344 623322 Fax 01344 627100 63 en suite
Hotel ★★ 67% HL Brockenhurst Hotel, Brockenhurst Rd, SOUTH ASCOT ☎ 01344 621912 Fax 01344 873252 12 en suite 5 annexe en suite

Sunningdale Ladies Cross Rd SL5 9RX
☎ 01344 620507 📄 01344 620507
e-mail: clbsec.slgc@tiscali.co.uk
web: www.sunningdaleladies.co.uk
A short 18-hole course with a typical Surrey heathland layout. A very tight course, making for a challenging game.
18 holes, 3705yds, Par 58, SSS 58, Course record 51.
Club membership 400.
Visitors Mon-Sun & BHs. Booking required. Handicap certificate. Dress code.| **Societies** Welcome. **Green Fees** £27 per round (£32 Sat, Sun & BHs). ⊛ **Facilities** ⓨ ⓫ 🖵 🏲 🏊 ⚌ **Leisure** Practice net. **Location** 1m S off A30
Hotel ★★★★ 78% HL Macdonald Berystede Hotel & Spa, Bagshot Rd, Sunninghill, ASCOT ☎ 0870 400 8111 126 en suite

---

THEALE
MAP 04 SU67

Theale North St RG7 5EX
☎ 0118 930 5331
e-mail: mikelowe1@btinternet.com
web: www.thealegolf.co.uk
Challenging parkland course set in the heart of the Berkshire countrysiide
18 holes, 6395yds, Par 72, SSS 71, Course record 68.
Club membership 300.
Visitors Mon-Sun & BHs. Booking required Sat, Sun & BHs. Dress code.
Societies Booking required. **Green Fees** £30 per day, £18 per 18 holes, £12 per 9 holes. (£40/£25/£16 Sat, Sun & BHs). **Prof** Kevin Hill **Course Designer** Mike Lowe **Facilities** ⓨ ⓫ 🖵 🏲 🏊 ⚐ ⚌ 🎯 **Conf** facs Corporate Hospitality Days **Location** Off M4 junct 12
Hotel ★★★ 70% HL Best Western Calcot Hotel, 98 Bath Rd, Calcot, READING ☎ 0118 941 6423 78 en suite

---

WOKINGHAM
MAP 04 SU86

Downshire Easthampstead Park RG40 3DH
☎ 01344 302030 📄 01344 301020
e-mail: downshiregc@bracknell-forest.gov.uk
web: www.bracknell-forest.gov.uk
Beautiful municipal parkland course with mature trees. Water hazards come into play on the 14th & 18th holes, & especially on the short 7th, a testing downhill 169yds over the lake. Pleasant easy walking. Challenging holes: 7th (Par 4), 15th (Par 4), 16th (Par 3). Rated as one of the finest municipal courses in the country.
18 holes, 6416yds, Par 73, SSS 71. Club membership 1000.
Visitors Mon-Sun & BHs. Dress code. **Societies** Booking required. **Green Fees** £19.45 per 18 holes Mon-Thu, £21.45 Fri, £25.95 Sat, Sun & BHs.
Prof Wayne Owers/Rhys Iolo **Facilities** ⓨ ⓫ 🖵 🏲 🏊 ⚐ 🎯 ⚌ ⚌

Leisure 9 hole pitch & putt, power tees. **Conf** facs Corporate Hospitality Days **Location** 3m SW of Bracknell. M4 junct 10, signs for Crowthorne
Hotel ★★★★ 77% HL Coppid Beech, John Nike Way, BRACKNELL ☎ 01344 303333 205 en suite

Sand Martins Finchampstead Rd RG40 3RQ
☎ 0118 9792711 📄 0118 977 0282
e-mail: info@sandmartins.com
web: www.sandmartins.com

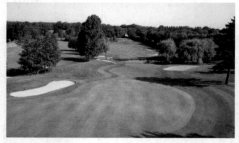

18 holes, 6212yds, Par 70, SSS 70, Course record 65.
Course Designer Edward Fox **Location** 1m S of Wokingham
Telephone for further details
Hotel ★★★ 70% HL The Waterloo Hotel, Duke's Ride, CROWTHORNE ☎ 0870 609 6111 79 en suite

---

BRISTOL

BRISTOL
MAP 03 ST57

Bristol and Clifton Beggar Bush Ln, Failand BS8 3TH
☎ 01275 393474 📄 01275 394611
e-mail: mansec@bristolgolf.co.uk
web: www.bristolgolf.co.uk
Utilising the aesthetics and hazards of a former quarry, a valley, stone walls and spinneys of trees, the course is a stern challenge but one always in tip top condition, due in summer to the irrigation and in winter to the natural draining land upon which it is situated. Par 3s from 120 to 220yds, dog-legs which range from the gentle to the brutal and a collection of natural obstacles and hazards add to the charm of the layout.
18 holes, 6387yds, Par 70, SSS 71, Course record 63.
Club membership 850.
Visitors may play Mon-Sun & BHs. Booking required. Handicap certificate. Dress code. **Societies** Booking required. **Green Fees** £40 per day (£45 weekends). **Prof** Paul Mitchell **Facilities** ⓨ 🍴 ⓫ 🖵 🏲 🏊 🏁 ⚐ ⚌ ⚌ 🎯 **Leisure** chipping green, practice bunkers. **Conf** facs Corporate Hospitality Days **Location** M5 junct 19, A369 for 4m, onto B3129, club 1m on right
Hotel ★★★ 70% HL Redwood Hotel & Country Club, Beggar Bush Ln, Failand, BRISTOL ☎ 0870 609 6144 112 en suite

Filton Golf Course Ln, Filton BS34 7QS
☎ 0117 969 4169 📄 0117 931 4359
e-mail: thesecretary@filtongolfclub.co.uk
web: www.filtongolfclub.co.uk
Interesting and challenging mature parkland course situated on high ground north of the city. Extensive views can be enjoyed from the course to the Concorde and Severn bridges.
18 holes, 6173yds, Par 70, SSS 70, Course record 61.
Club membership 750.
Visitors Mon-Fri & BHs. Booking required. Handicap certificate required. Dress code **Societies** Booking required. **Green Fees** £32 per round.
Prof D Kelley **Facilities** ⊕ ♚◎⌾ ⚑ ⌶ ⚐ ⚑ 🍴 ⚬ 🏌 **Conf** Corporate Hospitality Days **Location** M5 junct 15, off A38
Hotel BUD Premier Travel Inn Bristol (Filton), Shield Retail Park, Gloucester Rd North, Filton, BRISTOL ☎ 0870 9906456 60 en suite

Henbury Henbury Hill, Westbury-on-Trym BS10 7QB
☎ 0117 950 0044 & 950 2121 (Prof) 📄 0117 959 1928
e-mail: thesecretary@henburygolfclub.co.uk
web: www.henburygolfclub.co.uk
A parkland course tree-lined and on two levels. The River Trym comes into play on the 7th drop-hole with its green set just over the stream. The last nine holes have the beautiful Blaise Castle woods for company.
18 holes, 6007yds, Par 69, SSS 70, Course record 65.
Club membership 825.
Visitors Mon-Fri except BHs. Booking required. Handicap certificate. Dress code. **Societies** Booking required. **Green Fees** £30 per day.
Prof Nick Riley **Facilities** ⊕ ◎ by prior arrangement ♚ ⚐ 🍴 ⚐ ⚑
🍴 ⚬ 🏌 **Conf** facs Corporate Hospitality Days **Location** 3m NW of city centre on B4055 off A4018
Hotel ★★★ 66% HL Henbury Lodge Hotel, Station Rd, Henbury, BRISTOL ☎ 0117 950 2615 12 en suite 9 annexe en suite

Knowle West Town Ln, Brislington BS4 5DF
☎ 0117 977 0660 📄 0117 972 0615
e-mail: mike@knowlegolfclub.co.uk
web: www.knowlegolfclub.co.uk
Parkland with nice turf. The first five holes climb up and down hill but the remainder are on a more even plane.

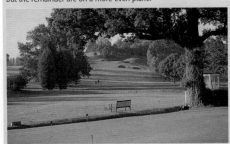

18 holes, 6006yds, Par 69, SSS 69, Course record 61.
Club membership 700.
Visitors may play Mon-Sun & BHs. Advance booking required. Handicap certificate required. Dress code. **Societies** advance booking required. **Green Fees** not confirmed. ⊕ **Prof** Robert Hayward
Course Designer Hawtree/J H Taylor **Facilities** ⊕ ◎ ♚ ⚐ 🍴 ⚐ ⚑ 🍴
🍴 ⚬ 🏌 **Location** 3m SE of city centre off A37
Hotel ★★★ 82% CHH Hunstrete House Hotel, HUNSTRETE
☎ 01761 490490 25 en suite

Shirehampton Park Park Hill, Shirehampton BS11 0UL
☎ 0117 982 2083 📄 0117 982 5280
e-mail: info@shirehamptonparkgolfclub.co.uk
web: www.shirehamptonparkgolfclub.co.uk
Lovely parkland course with views across the Avon Gorge.
18 holes, 5453yds, Par 67, SSS 66, Course record 63.
Club membership 622.
Visitors may play Mon-Fri. Handicap certificate . Dress code. **Societies** Booking required. **Green Fees** £36 per day, £22 per round. **Prof** Brent Ellis
Facilities ⊕ ♚ ⚐ 🍴 ⚐ ⚑ 🍴 ⚬ 🏌 **Location** M5 junct 18, 2m E on B4054
Hotel ★★★ 70% HL Redwood Hotel & Country Club, Beggar Bush Ln, Failand, BRISTOL ☎ 0870 609 6144 112 en suite

Shortwood Lodge Carsons Rd, Mangotsfield BS16 9LW
☎ 0117 956 5501 📄 0117 957 3640
e-mail: info@shortwoodlodge.com
web: www.shortwoodlodge.com
An easy walking parkland course with well-placed bunkers.
18 holes, 5337yds, Par 68, SSS 66, Course record 61.
Club membership 400.
Visitors Mon-Sun & BHs. **Societies** Booking required. **Green Fees** £14
(£16 weekends & BHs). **Prof** Craig Trewin **Course Designer** John Day
Facilities ⊕ ◎ ♚ ⚐ 🍴 ⚐ ⚑ 🍴 ⚬ 🏌 **Conf** Corporate Hospitality Days **Location** 6m NE of city centre off B4465
Hotel BUD Premier Travel Inn Bristol East, 200/202 Westerleigh Rd, Emersons Green, BRISTOL ☎ 08701 977042 40 en suite

Woodlands Trench Ln, Almondsbury BS32 4JZ
☎ 01454 619319 📄 01454 619397
e-mail: info@woodlands-golf.com
web: www.woodlands-golf.com
Situated on the edge of the Severn Valley, bordered by Hortham Brook and Shepherds Wood, this interesting parkland course features five testing Par 3s set around the course's five lakes, notably the 206yd 5th hole which extends over water.
18 holes, 6068yds, Par 70, SSS 69. Club membership 45.
Visitors Mon-Sun & BHs. **Societies** Welcome. **Green Fees** £14 per round
(£16 weekends & bank holidays). **Prof** L Riddiford **Facilities** ⊕ ◎ ♚ ⚐
🍴 ⚐ ⚑ 🍴 ⚬ 🏌 **Leisure** fishing. **Conf** facs Corporate Hospitality Days
Location M5 junct 16, A38 towards Bradley Store
Hotel ★★ 69% HL The Bowl Inn, 16 Church Rd, Lower Almondsbury, BRISTOL ☎ 01454 612757 11 rms (2 en suite) 2 annexe en suite

BUCKINGHAMSHIRE

AYLESBURY   MAP 04 SP81

Aylesbury Golf Centre Hulcott Ln, Bierton HP22 5GA
☎ 01296 393644
Parkland with magnificent views to the Chiltern Hills. A good test of golf with out of bounds coming into play on nine of the holes, plus a number of water hazards and bunkers.
18 holes, 5965yds, Par 71, SSS 69. Club membership 200.
Visitors Mon-Sun & BHs. Booking required Sat, Sun & BHs. Dress code.
Societies Booking required. **Green Fees** Phone. **Prof** Richard Wooster
Course Designer T S Benwell **Facilities** ⊕ ◎ ♚ ⚐ 🍴 ⚐ ⚑ 🍴 ⚬ 🏌
Conf Corporate Hospitality Days **Location** 1m N of Aylesbury on A418
Hotel BUD Premier Travel Inn Aylesbury, Buckingham Rd, AYLESBURY
☎ 08701 977019 64 en suite

Aylesbury Park
Andrews Way, Off Coldharbour Way, Oxford Rd HP17 8QQ
☎ 01296 399196
e-mail: info@aylesburyparkgolf.com
web: www.aylesburyparkgolf.com
Parkland with mature trees, located just south-west of Aylesbury.
18 holes, 6166yds, Par 70, SSS 69, Course record 66.
Club membership 379.
Visitors Mon-Sun & BHs. Dress code. **Societies** Booking required. **Green Fees** £20 per round (£25 Sat & Sun). **Prof** John Scheu **Course Designer** M Hawtree **Facilities** ⊕ ⚑ 🖵 🛍 ⚑ ⚑ 🍴 🍴 🍴 **Leisure** 9 hole Par 3 course. **Location** 0.5m SW of Aylesbury, on the A418
Hotel ★★★★ HL Hartwell House Hotel Restaurant & Spa, Oxford Rd, AYLESBURY ☎ 01296 747444 30 en suite 16 annexe en suite

Chiltern Forest
Aston Hill, Halton HP22 5NQ
☎ 01296 631267 📠 01296 632709
e-mail: secretary@chilternforest.co.uk
web: www.chilternforest.co.uk
The course nestles in the Chiltern Hills above Aylesbury with stunning views of the surrounding countryside and meanders around challenging wooded terrain. Although not a long course the tightly wooded holes and smallish greens present a challenge to all standards of golfer.
18 holes, 5765yds, Par 70, SSS 69, Course record 65.
Club membership 650.
Visitors Mon-Fri. Handicap certificate required. Dress code.
Societies Booking required. **Green Fees** £40 per day, £34 per round.
Facilities ⊕ 🍴 ⚑ 🖵 🛍 ⚑ 🍴 **Conf** Corporate Hospitality Days
Location off A41 between Tring and Aylesbury
Hotel BUD Innkeeper's Lodge Aylesbury East, London Rd, ASTON CLINTON
☎ 0845 112 6094 11 en suite

Ellesborough
Wendover Rd, Butlers Cross HP17 0TZ
☎ 01296 622114 📠 01296 622114
e-mail: admin@ellesboroughgolf.co.uk
web: www.ellesboroughgolf.co.uk
Once part of the property of Chequers, and under the shadow of the famous Coombe monument at the Wendover end of the Chilterns. A downland course, it is rather hilly with most holes enhanced by far-ranging views over the Aylesbury countryside.
18 holes, 6360yds, Par 71, SSS 71, Course record 64.
Club membership 700.
Visitors Mon-Fri except BHs. Booking required. Handicap certificate. Dress code. **Societies** Booking required. **Green Fees** £50 per day; £30 per round. 🖥 **Prof** Mark Squire **Course Designer** James Braid **Facilities** ⊕ ⚑ 🖵 🍴 ⚑ 🛍 🍴 **Conf** Corporate Hospitality Days **Location** 1m W of Wendover on B4010 towards Princes Risborough
Hotel BUD Innkeeper's Lodge Aylesbury South, 40 Main St, Weston Turville, AYLESBURY ☎ 0845 112 6095 16 en suite

BEACONSFIELD
MAP 04 SU99

Beaconsfield
Seer Green HP9 2UR
☎ 01494 676545 📠 01494 681148
e-mail: secretary@beaconsfieldgolfclub.co.uk
web: www.beaconsfieldgolfclub.co.uk
An interesting and, at times, testing tree-lined and parkland course which frequently plays longer than appears on the card. Each hole differs to a considerable degree and here lies the charm. Walking is easy, except perhaps the 6th and 8th. Well bunkered.
18 holes, 6506yds, Par 72, SSS 71, Course record 63.
Club membership 900.
Visitors Mon-Fri except BHs. Handicap certificate. Dress code.
Societies Booking required. **Green Fees** £60 per day; £50 per round. 🖥
Prof Michael Brothers **Course Designer** H S Colt **Facilities** ⊕ 🍴 ⚑ 🖵 🍴 🛍 ⚑ 🍴 🍴 **Conf** Corporate Hospitality Days **Location** M40 junct 2, next to Seer Green railway station
Hotel BUD Innkeeper's Lodge Beaconsfield, Aylesbury End, BEACONSFIELD ☎ 0845 112 6096 32 en suite

BLETCHLEY
MAP 04 SP83

Windmill Hill
Tattenhoe Ln MK3 7RB
☎ 01908 631113 & 366457 (Sec) 📠 01908 630034
Windmill Hill Golf Course: 18 holes, 6720yds, Par 73, SSS 72, Course record 68.
Course Designer Henry Cotton **Location** W side of town centre on A421
Telephone for further details
Hotel BUD Campanile, 40 Penn Rd, Fenny Stratford, Bletchley, MILTON KEYNES ☎ 01908 649819 80 en suite

BUCKINGHAM
MAP 04 SP63

Buckingham
Tingewick Rd MK18 4AE
☎ 01280 815566 📠 01280 821812
e-mail: admin@buckinghamgolfclub.co.uk
web: www.buckinghamgolfclub.co.uk
Undulating parkland with a stream and river affecting eight holes.
18 holes, 6162yds, Par 71, SSS 70, Course record 66.
Club membership 740.
Visitors may play Mon-Fri. Dress code. **Societies** Booking required.
Green Fees £45 per day, £35 per 18 holes. 🖥 **Prof** Greg Hannah
Course Designer Peter Jones **Facilities** ⊕ 🍴 ⚑ 🖵 🍴 🛍 ⚑ 🍴 🍴
Leisure snooker room. **Conf** Corporate Hospitality Days **Location** 1.5m W on A421
Hotel ★★★ 66% HL Best Western Buckingham Hotel, Buckingham Ring Rd, BUCKINGHAM ☎ 01280 822622 70 en suite

BURNHAM
MAP 04 SU98

Burnham Beeches
Green Ln SL1 8EG
☎ 01628 661448 📠 01628 668968
e-mail: enquiries@bbgc.co.uk
web: www.bbgc.co.uk
Wooded parkland on the edge of the historic Burnham Beeches Forest with a good variety of holes.
18 holes, 6449yds, Par 70, SSS 71, Course record 66.
Club membership 670.
Visitors Mon-Fri exepr BHs. Handicap certificate. Dress code. **Societies** Booking required. **Green Fees** not confirmed. 🖥 **Prof** Ronnie Bolton
Course Designer J H Taylor **Facilities** ⊕ 🍴 ⚑ 🖵 🍴 🛍 ⚑ 🍴 🍴 **Conf** Corporate Hospitality Days **Location** 0.5m NE of Burnham
Hotel ★★★ 72% HL Burnham Beeches Hotel, Grove Rd, BURNHAM ☎ 0870 609 6124 82 en suite

Lambourne
Dropmore Rd SL1 8NF
☎ 01628 666755 📠 01628 663301
A championship standard 18-hole parkland course. Undulating terrain with many trees and several lakes, notably on the tricky 7th hole which has a tightly guarded green reached via a shot over a lake. Seven Par 4s over 400yds with six picturesque lakes, excellent drainage and full irrigation.
Continued

18 holes, 6798yds, Par 72, SSS 73, Course record 67.
Club membership 650.
Visitors may play Mon-Fri. Advance booking required. Handicap certificate. Dress code. **Societies** Booking required. **Green Fees** £60 per round. **Prof** David Hart **Course Designer** Donald Steel **Facilities** ⑪ ⑩ ⚐ ▣ ♨ ⚒ △ 🖩 ⛴ ⚸ ⚐ ✦ **Leisure** sauna. **Conf** facs Corporate Hospitality Days **Location** M4 junct 7 or M40 junct 2, towards Burnham
Hotel ★★★ 72% HL Burnham Beeches Hotel, Grove Rd, BURNHAM ☎ 0870 609 6124 82 en suite

---

CHALFONT ST GILES   MAP 04 SU99

Harewood Downs Cokes Ln HP8 4TA
☎ 01494 762184 📄 01494 766869
e-mail: secretary@hdgc.co.uk
web: www.hdgc.co.uk
A testing undulating parkland course with sloping greens and plenty of trees.
18 holes, 6028yds, Par 69, SSS 69, Course record 63.
Club membership 600.
Visitors Mon-Sun & BHs. Handicap certificate. Dress code. **Societies** Booking required. **Green Fees** £40 per round (/£45 Sat, Sun & BHs). ⚇ **Prof** G C Morris **Course Designer** J H Taylor **Facilities** ⑪ ⑩ ⚐ by prior arrangement ▣ ⚐ ▣ △ 🖩 ⛴ ⚸ ✦ **Conf** Corporate Hospitality Days **Location** 2m E of Amersham on A413
Hotel ★★★ 72% HL The Crown, High St, AMERSHAM ☎ 01494 721 541 19 en suite 18 annexe en suite

Oakland Park Threehouseholds HP8 4LW
☎ 01494 871277 & 877333 (pro) 📄 01494 874692
e-mail: info@oaklandparkgolf.co.uk
web: www.oaklandparkgolf.co.uk
Parkland with mature trees, hedgerows and water features, designed to respect the natural features of the land and lakes while providing a good challenge for players at all levels.
18 holes, 5246yds, Par 67, SSS 66, Course record 66.
Club membership 650.
Visitors may play Mon-Fri. Sat, Sun & BHs pm only. Booking required. Dress code. **Societies** Booking required. **Green Fees** £25 per 18 holes (£30 weekends & bank holidays). **Prof** Alistair Thatcher **Course Designer** Johnathan Gaunt **Facilities** ⑪ ⑩ ▣ ⚐ ▣ △ 🖩 ⛴ ⚸ ⚐ ✦ **Conf** facs Corporate Hospitality Days **Location** M40 junct 2, 3m N
Hotel ★★★ 72% HL The Crown, High St, AMERSHAM ☎ 01494 721 541 19 en suite 18 annexe en suite

---

CHARTRIDGE   MAP 04 SP90

Chartridge Park HP5 2TF
☎ 01494 791772 📄 01494 786462
e-mail: ian@cpgc.co.uk
web: www.cpgc.co.uk
A family run, easy walking parkland course set high in the beautiful Chiltern Hills, affording breathtaking views.
18 holes, 5516yds, Par 69, SSS 67, Course record 65.
Club membership 700.
Visitors may play Mon-Sun except BHs. Advance booking required. Handicap certificate required. Dress code. **Societies** advanced booking required. **Green Fees** not confirmed. **Course Designer** John Jacobs **Facilities** ⑪ ▣ ⚐ ▣ ⚐ △ 🖩 ⛴ ⚸ ✦ **Conf** facs Corporate Hospitality Days **Location** 3m NW of Chesham
Hotel ★★★ 72% HL The Crown, High St, AMERSHAM ☎ 01494 721 541 19 en suite 18 annexe en suite

---

CHESHAM   MAP 04 SP90

Chesham & Ley Hill Ley Hill Common HP5 1UZ
☎ 01494 784541 📄 01494 785506
e-mail: secretary@cheshamgolf.co.uk
web: www.cheshamgolf.co.uk
Wooded parkland on hilltop with easy walking.
9 holes, 5296yds, Par 67, SSS 65, Course record 62.
Club membership 350.
Visitors may play Mon-Fri. Dress code. **Societies** advance booking required. **Green Fees** not confirmed. ⚇ **Prof** James Short **Facilities** ⑪ ⑩ ▣ ⚐ △ **Leisure** practice net. **Conf** facs **Location** 2m E of Chesham, off A41 on B4504 to Ley Hill
Hotel ★★★ 72% HL The Crown, High St, AMERSHAM ☎ 01494 721 541 19 en suite 18 annexe en suite

---

DAGNALL   MAP 04 SP91

Whipsnade Park Studham Ln HP4 1RH
☎ 01442 842330 📄 01442 842090
e-mail: whipsnadeparkgolfc@btopenworld.com
web: www.whipsnadeparkgolf.co.uk
Parkland on downs adjoining Whipsnade Zoo. Easy walking, good views and great test of golf.
18 holes, 6800yds, Par 73, SSS 72, Course record 66.
Club membership 500.
Visitors may play Mon-Fri. Sat, Sun & BHs after 1pm. Advance booking required. Dress code. **Societies** Booking required. **Green Fees** £40 per day; £30 per round. **Prof** Mark Day **Facilities** ⑪ ⑩ ⚐ by prior arrangement ▣ ⚐ ▣ △ 🖩 ⛴ ⚸ ✦ **Conf** Corporate Hospitality Days **Location** 1m E off B4506 between Dagnall
Hotel ★★★ 72% HL Old Palace Lodge, Church St, DUNSTABLE ☎ 01582 662201 68 en suite

---

DENHAM   MAP 04 TQ08

Buckinghamshire Denham Court Dr UB9 5PG
☎ 01895 835777 📄 01895 835210
e-mail: enquiries@buckinghamshiregc.co.uk
web: www.buckinghamshiregc.com
The course runs in two loops of nine starting and finishing at the clubhouse. The fairways wander through three distinct areas incorporating woodland, lakes and rivers and undulating links style land, providing a variety of golfing terrain calling for careful thought on every shot. The greens are constructed to USGA specification with excellent drainage and smooth true putting surfaces.
18 holes, 6880yds, Par 72, SSS 73, Course record 62.
Club membership 550.
Visitors may play Mon-Sun & BHs. Advance booking required. Dress code. **Societies** Booking required. **Green Fees** £90 per 18 holes (£100 Fri-Sun & BHs). **Prof** Paul Schunter **Course Designer** John Jacobs **Facilities** ⑪ ⑩ ▣ ⚐ ▣ ⚐ △ 🖩 ⛴ ⚸ ⚐ ✦ **Conf** facs Corporate Hospitality Days **Location** M25 junct 16, signed Uxbridge
Hotel ★★★ 77% HL Barn Hotel, West End Rd, RUISLIP ☎ 01895 636057 59 en suite

Denham Tilehouse Ln UB9 5DE
☎ 01895 832022 📠 01895 835340
e-mail: club.secretary@denhamgolfclub.co.uk
web: www.denhamgolfclub.co.uk
18 holes, 6462yds, Par 70, SSS 71, Course record 66.
Course Designer H S Colt **Location** 0.5m N of North Orbital Road, 2m
from Uxbridge
Telephone for further details
Hotel ★★★ 77% HL Barn Hotel, West End Rd, RUISLIP
☎ 01895 636057 59 en suite

FLACKWELL HEATH MAP 04 SU89

Flackwell Heath Treadaway Rd, High Wycombe
HP10 9PE
☎ 01628 520929 📠 01628 530040
e-mail: secretary@flackwellheathgolfclub.co.uk
web: www.flackwellheathgolfclub.co.uk
Open sloping heath and tree-lined course on hills overlooking the
Chilterns. Some good challenging Par 3s and several testing small
greens.
18 holes, 6211yds, Par 71, SSS 70, Course record 63.
Club membership 700.
Visitors Mon-Sun & BHs. Booking required. Handicap certificate. Dress
code. **Societies** booking required **Green Fees** £36 per round. ◉ **Prof** Paul
Watson **Course Designer** J H Taylor **Facilities** ⊕ ⚑ 🍴 ⌂ ☴ ⚑ ☴ ⚑ ✆ ✆
Conf facs Corporate Hospitality Days **Location** E side of High Wycombe,
NE side of town centre
Hotel BUD Premier Travel Inn High Wycombe, Thanestead Farm, London
Rd, Loudwater, HIGH WYCOMBE ☎ 08701 977135 81 en suite

GERRARDS CROSS MAP 04 TQ08

Gerrards Cross Chalfont Park SL9 0QA
☎ 01753 883263 (Sec) & 885300 (Pro) 📠 01753 883593
e-mail: secretary@gxgolf.co.uk
web: www.gxgolf.co.uk
A wooded parkland course that has been modernised in recent years
and is now a very pleasant circuit with infinite variety and fine views.

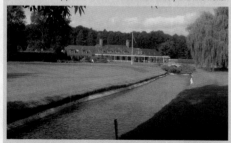

18 holes, 6212yds, Par 69, SSS 70, Course record 64.
Club membership 700.
Visitors Mon-Fri. Handicap certificate. Dress code. **Societies** Booking
required. **Green Fees** £55 per day, £45 per round. **Prof** Matthew
Barr **Course Designer** Bill Pedlar **Facilities** ⊕ ⚑ ⌂ 🍴 ☴ ⚑ ✆ ✆
Location NE side of town centre off A413
Hotel ★★ 71% HL The Ethorpe Hotel, Packhorse Rd, GERRARDS CROSS
☎ 01753 882039 32 en suite

HIGH WYCOMBE MAP 04 SU89

Hazlemere Penn Rd, Hazlemere HP15 7LR
☎ 01494 719300 📠 01494 713914
e-mail: enquiries@hazlemeregolfclub.co.uk
web: www.hazlemeregolfclub.co.uk
Undulating parkland course located in the Chiltern Hills in an area of
outstanding natural beauty. Deceiving in its yardage and a challenge to
golfers of all standards.
18 holes, 5833yds, Par 70, SSS 69, Course record 61.
Club membership 600.
Visitors Mon-Fri except BHs. Booking required. Dress code. **Societies**
Welcome. **Green Fees** Phone. **Prof** G Cousins/C Barsberg **Course
Designer** Terry Murray **Facilities** ⊕ ⚑ ⌂ 🍴 ☴ ⚑ ☴ ⚑ **Conf** facs
Location On B474 , 2m NE of High Wycombe
Hotel ★★★ 72% HL The Crown, High St, AMERSHAM ☎ 01494 721 541
19 en suite 18 annexe en suite

IVER MAP 04 TQ08

Iver Hollow Hill Ln, Langley Park Rd SL0 0JJ
☎ 01753 655615 📠 01753 654225
9 holes, 6288yds, Par 72, SSS 72, Course record 66.
Location M4 junct 5, 1.5m SW off B470
Telephone for further details
Hotel ★★★★ 75% HL Slough/Windsor Marriott Hotel, Ditton Rd, Langley,
SLOUGH ☎ 0870 400 7244 382 en suite

Richings Park Golf & Country Club North Park
SL0 9DL
☎ 01753 655370 & 655352(pro shop) 📠 01753 655409
e-mail: info@richingspark.co.uk
web: www.richingspark.co.uk
Set among mature trees and attractive lakes, this testing Par 70
parkland course provides a suitable challenge to golfers of all abilities.
Well-irrigated greens and abundant wildlife.
18 holes, 6144yds, Par 70, SSS 69, Course record 63.
Club membership 500.
Visitors may play Mon-Sun & BHs. Advance booking required Fri-Sun &
BHs. Handicap certificate required. Dress code. **Societies** advanced booking
required. **Green Fees** not confirmed. **Prof** Ben Tarry **Course Designer**
Alan Higgins **Facilities** ⊕ 🍴 ⚑ ⌂ 🍴 ☴ ⚑ ☴ ⚑ ✆ ✆ ⚑ **Conf** facs
Corporate Hospitality Days **Location** M4 junct 5, A4 towards Colnbrook, left
at lights, Sutton Lane, right at next lights North Park
Hotel ★★★ 79% HL Courtyard by Marriott Slough/Windsor, Church St,
SLOUGH ☎ 0870 400 7215 & 07153 551551 📠 0870 400 7315 150 en suite

Thorney Park Thorney Mill Rd SL0 9AL
☎ 01895 422095 📠 01895 431307
e-mail: sales@thorneypark.com
web: www.thorneypark.com
An 18-hole parkland course which will test both the beginner and
established golfer. Fairway irrigation ensures lush green fairways and
smooth putting surfaces. Many interesting holes including the testing
Par 4 9th which needs a long drive to the water's edge and a well-hit
iron onto the bunker-guarded green. The back nine finishes with two
water holes, the 17th, a near island green and the shot of 150yds
makes this a picturesque hole. The 18th has more water than grass.
18 holes, 5765yds, Par 69, SSS 68, Course record 69.
Club membership 350.

Continued

CHAMPIONSHIP COURSE

BUCKINGHAMSHIRE — LITTLE BRICKHILL

WOBURN

Map 04 SP93

MK17 9LJ
☎ **01908 370756** 📠 **01908 378436**
e-mail: **enquiries@woburngolf.com**
web: **www.discoverwoburn.co.uk**
Duke's Course: 18 holes, 6973yds, Par 72, SSS 74, Course record 62.
Duchess Course: 18 holes, 6651yds, Par 72, SSS 72.
Marquess Course: 18 holes, 7214yards, Par 72, SSS 74.
Visitors Mon-Fri except BHs. Booking required. Handicap certificate required. Dress code.
Societies Booking required. **Green Fees** May-Oct £140-£155 per day including lunch. Nov-Feb £75/ Mar £95/ Apr £115. Aug & Oct £105-£120 per round including lunch. **Prof** Luther Blacklock
Course Designer Charles Lawrie/Peter Alliss & others **Facilities** ⚑ 🍴 🖥 🏌 ⛳ 🛒 🚐 🚗 🏌 🎯
Conf Corporate Hospitality Days **Location** M1 junct 13, 4m W off A5130

Easily accessible from the M1, Woburn is famed not only for its golf courses but also for the magnificent stately home and wildlife park, which are both well worth a visit. Charles Lawrie of Cotton Pennink designed two great courses here among trees and beautiful countryside. From the back tees they are rather long for the weekend amateur golfer. The Duke's Course is a tough challenge for golfers at all levels. The Duchess Course, although relatively easier, still demands a high level of skills to negotiate the fairways guarded by towering pines. A third course, the Marquess, opened in June 2000 and has already staged the British Masters twice. The town of Woburn and the abbey are in Bedfordshire, while the golf club is over the border in Buckinghamshire.

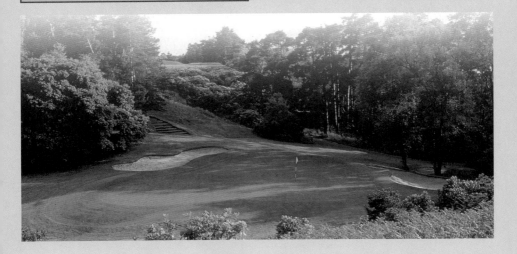

Visitors may play Mon-Sun & BHs. Booking required. Dress code. **Societies** Booking required. **Green Fees** £23 per 18 holes (£28 per round weekends). **Prof** Andrew Killing **Course Designer** David Walker **Facilities** ⊕ ⏐◯⏐ ℠ ☐ ❡ ⏐ ⚐ ⚲ ⛟ ⛳ ✆ **Conf** facs Corporate Hospitality Days **Location** M4 junct 5, left onto A4, left onto Sutton Ln, right for Thorney Mill Rd
Hotel ★★★★ 75% HL Slough/Windsor Marriott Hotel, Ditton Rd, Langley, SLOUGH ☎ 0870 400 7244 382 en suite

---

LITTLE BRICKHILL   MAP 04 SP93

Woburn Golf & Country Club   see page 33

Hotel ★★★ 79% HL The Inn at Woburn, George St, WOBURN ☎ 01525 290441 50 en suite 7 annexe en suite
Hotel ★★★ 70% HL Best Western Moore Place Hotel, The Square, ASPLEY GUISE ☎ 01908 282000 Fax 01908 281888 35 en suite 27 annexe en suite
Hotel ★★ 63% HL The Bell Hotel & Inn, 21 Bedford St, WOBURN ☎ 01525 290280 Fax 01525 290017 24 en suite

---

LITTLE CHALFONT   MAP 04 SU99

Little Chalfont Lodge Ln HP8 4AJ
☎ 01494 764877
Gently undulating parkland surrounded by mature trees.
9 holes, 5752yds, Par 70, SSS 68, Course record 66.
Club membership 300.
Visitors Mon-Sun & BHs. **Societies** Booking required. **Green Fees** £14 per 18 holes (£16 weekends). **Prof** M Dunne **Course Designer** J M Dunne **Facilities** ⊕ ⏐◯⏐ ℠ ☐ ❡ ⏐ ⚲ ⛟ ✆ **Leisure** one motorised cart for hire by arrangement. **Conf** facs Corporate Hospitality Days **Location** M25 junct 18, on A404
Hotel ★★★ 72% HL The Crown, High St, AMERSHAM ☎ 01494 721 541 19 en suite 18 annexe en suite

---

LOUDWATER   MAP 04 SU89

Wycombe Heights Golf Centre Rayners Ave HP10 9SZ
☎ 01494 816686 📄 01494 816728
e-mail: sales@wycombeheightsgc.co.uk
web: www.wycombeheightsgc.co.uk
An impressive tree-lined parkland course with panoramic views of the Chilterns. The final four holes are particularly challenging. A delightful 18 hole Par 3 course and floodlit driving range complement the High Course.

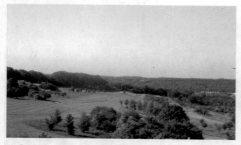

High Course: 18 holes, 6265yds, Par 70, SSS 71, Course record 64. Club membership 600.
Visitors Mon-Sun & BHs. Dress code. **Societies** Booking required. **Green Fees** £18 per round (£25 Sat, Sun & BHs). **Prof** Joe McKie **Course Designer** John Jacobs **Facilities** ⊕ ⏐◯⏐ ℠ ☐ ❡ ⏐ ⚲ ⛟ ✆ ⛳ ✆ ⚐ **Leisure** Par 3 course. **Conf** facs Corporate Hospitality Days

Location M40 junct 3, A40 towards High Wycombe. 0.5m right onto Rayners Ave at lights
Hotel BUD Premier Travel Inn High Wycombe, Thanestead Farm, London Rd, Loudwater, HIGH WYCOMBE ☎ 08701 977135 81 en suite

---

MARLOW   MAP 04 SU88

Harleyford Harleyford Estate, Henley Rd SL7 2SP
☎ 01628 816161 📄 01628 816160
e-mail: info@harleyfordgolf.co.uk
web: www.harleyfordgolf.co.uk
Set in 160 acres, this Donald Steel designed course, founded in 1996, makes the most of the natural rolling contours of the beautiful parkland of the historic Harleyford Estate. A challenging course to golfers of all handicaps. Stunning views of the Thames Valley.

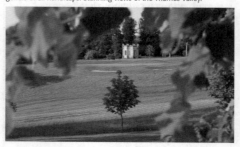

18 holes, 6708yds, Par 72, SSS 72, Course record 68.
Club membership 750.
Visitors Mon-Sun except BHs. Booking required. Handicap certificate. Dress code. **Societies** Booking required. **Green Fees** £45 per round (£65 weekends). **Prof** Mark Burroughes **Course Designer** Donald Steel **Facilities** ⊕ ⏐◯⏐ ℠ ☐ ❡ ⏐ ⚲ ⛟ ✆ ⛳ ✆ ⚐ **Conf** facs Corporate Hospitality Days **Location** S side A4156 Marlow-Henley road
Hotel ★★★★ 85% HL Danesfield House Hotel & Spa, Henley Rd, MARLOW-ON-THAMES ☎ 01628 891010 87 en suite

---

MENTMORE   MAP 04 SP91

Mentmore Golf & Country Club LU7 0UA
☎ 01296 662020 📄 01296 662592
Two 18-hole courses - Rosebery and Rothschild - set within the wooded estate grounds of Mentmore Towers. Gently rolling parkland course with mature trees and lakes and two interesting feature holes; the long Par 5 (606 yds) 9th on the Rosebery course with fine views of the Chilterns and the Par 4 (340yd) 14th on the Rothschild course, in front of the Towers.
Rosebery Course: 18 holes, 6777yds, Par 72, SSS 72, Course record 68.
Rothschild Course: 18 holes, 6700yds, Par 72, SSS 72.
Club membership 1100.
Visitors Mon-Sun except BHs. Dress code. **Societies** Welcome. **Green Fees** £40 per 18 holes (£50 Sat & Sun). **Prof** Alister Halliday **Course Designer** Bob Sandow **Facilities** ⊕ ⏐◯⏐ ℠ ☐ ❡ ⏐ ⚲ ⛟ ✆ ⛳ ✆ ⚐ **Leisure** hard tennis courts, heated indoor swimming pool, fishing, sauna, gymnasium. **Conf** facs Corporate Hospitality Days **Location** 4m S of Leighton Buzzard
Hotel ★★★ 72% HL Old Palace Lodge, Church St, DUNSTABLE ☎ 01582 662201 68 en suite

MILTON KEYNES   MAP 04 SP83

Abbey Hill Monks Way, Two Mile Ash MK8 8AA
☎ 01908 562408
e-mail: steve.tompkins@ukonline.co.uk

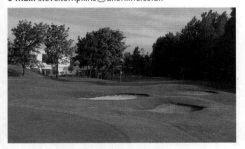

18 holes, 6122yds, Par 71, SSS 69, Course record 71.
Location 2m W of town centre off A5
Telephone for further details
Hotel ★★★ 70% HL Quality Hotel & Suites Milton Keynes, Monks Way,
Two Mile Ash, MILTON KEYNES ☎ 01908 561666 88 en suite

Three Locks Great Brickhill MK17 9BH
☎ 01525 270050 📠 01525 270470
e-mail: info@threelocksgolfclub.co.uk
web: www.threelocksgolfclub.co.uk
Parkland course offering a challenge to beginners and experienced
golfers, with water coming into play on ten holes. Magnificent views.
18 holes, 6036yds, Par 70, SSS 69, Course record 60.
Club membership 300.
Visitors may play Mon-Sun & BHs. Dress code. **Societies** Booking
required. **Green Fees** £30 per day, £19 per round (£37/£25 weekends
& bank holidays). **Prof** G Harding **Course Designer** MRM Sandown
Facilities ⑪ ⅄ ⌷ ♐ ⌵ ⚑ ⇩ ⚐ **Leisure** fishing. **Location** A4146
between Leighton Buzzard & Bletchley
Hotel BUD Campanile, 40 Penn Rd, Fenny Stratford, Bletchley, MILTON
KEYNES ☎ 01908 649819 80 en suite

PRINCES RISBOROUGH   MAP 04 SP80

Whiteleaf Upper Icknield Way, Whiteleaf HP27 0LY
☎ 01844 274058 📠 01844 275551
e-mail: whiteleafgc@tiscali.co.uk
web: www.whiteleafgolfclub.co.uk
A picturesque nine-hole course on the edge of the Chilterns. Good
views over the Vale of Aylesbury. A short challenging course requiring
great accuracy.
9 holes, 5391yds, Par 66, SSS 66, Course record 64.
Club membership 300.
Visitors Mon-Fri except BHs. Advance booking required Tue. Dress code.
Societies Welcome, **Green Fees** £17.50 per 18 holes, £12 per 9 holes.
⊛ **Prof** Ken Ward **Facilities** ⑪ ⅄ ⌷ ♐ ⌵ ⚑ ⚐ **Conf** Corporate
Hospitality Days **Location** 1m NE off A4010
Hotel ★★★ 68% HL Best Western Kings Hotel, Oxford Rd, HIGH
WYCOMBE ☎ 01494 609090 43 en suite

STOKE POGES   MAP 04 SU98

Farnham Park Park Rd SL2 4PJ
☎ 01753 643332 & 647065 📠 01753 647065
e-mail: farnhamparkgolfclub@btinternet.com
web: www.farnhampark.co.uk
Fine, public parkland course in a tree-lined setting.
18 holes, 6172yds, Par 71, SSS 70, Course record 68.
Club membership 300.
Visitors Mon-Sun & BHs. Dress code. **Societies** Booking required.
Green Fees £15 per round (£21 weekends). **Prof** Nigel Whitton
Course Designer Hawtree **Facilities** ⑪ ⅃⑩ ⅄ ⌷ ♐ ⌵ ⚑ ⇩ ⚐
Location W side of village off B416
Hotel ★★★★ 75% HL Slough/Windsor Marriott Hotel, Ditton Rd, Langley,
SLOUGH ☎ 0870 400 7244 382 en suite

Stoke Poges Stoke Park, Park Rd SL2 4PG
☎ 01753 717171 📠 01753 717181
e-mail: info@stokeparkclub.com
web: www.stokeparkclub.com
Course 1: 18 holes, 6721yds, Par 71, SSS 72,
Course record 65.
Course 2: 18 holes, 6551yds, Par 72, SSS 73.
Course 3: 18 holes, 6318yds, Par 71, SSS 70.
Course Designer Harry Shapland Colt **Location** Off A4 at Slough onto
B416 Stoke Poges Ln, club 1.5m on left
Telephone for further details
Hotel ★★★★ 75% HL Slough/Windsor Marriott Hotel, Ditton Rd,
Langley, SLOUGH ☎ 0870 400 7244 382 en suite

STOWE   MAP 04 SP63

Silverstone Silverstone Rd MK18 5LH
☎ 01280 850005 📠 01280 850156
e-mail: proshop@silverstonegolfclub.co.uk
18 holes, 6472yards, Par 72, SSS 71, Course record 65.
Course Designer David Snell **Location** From Silverstone signs to Grand
Prix track. Club 1m past entrance on right
Telephone for further details
Hotel ★★★★ 74% HL Villiers Hotel, 3 Castle St, BUCKINGHAM
☎ 01280 822444 46 en suite

Where to stay, where to eat?
Visit www.theAA.com

35

WAVENDON

MAP 04 SP93

Wavendon Golf Centre Lower End Rd MK17 8DA
☎ 01908 281811 🖹 01908 281257
e-mail: wavendon@jack-barker.co.uk
web: www.jack-barker.co.uk
Pleasant parkland course set within mature oak and lime trees and incorporating several small lakes as water hazards. Easy walking.

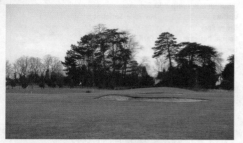

18 holes, 5570yds, Par 69, SSS 68. Club membership 300.
Visitors may play Mon-Sun & BHs. **Societies** Booking required.
Green Fees Phone. **Prof** Greg Iron **Course Designer** J Drake/N Elmer
Facilities ⑪ ⑩ ⅃ ☷ ☷ ⅂ ☷ ☷ ☷ ⅃ ☷ **Leisure** 9 hole Par 3 course.
Conf facs **Location** M1 junct 13, off A421
Hotel ★★★ 70% HL Best Western Moore Place Hotel, The Square, ASPLEY
GUISE ☎ 01908 282000 35 en suite 27 annexe en suite

WESTON TURVILLE

MAP 04 SP81

Weston Turville Golf New Rd HP22 5QT
☎ 01296 424084 🖹 01296 395376
e-mail: westonturvillegc@btconnect.com
web: www.westonturvillegolfclub.co.uk
18 holes, 6008yds, Par 69, SSS 69, Course record 68.
Location 2m SE of Aylesbury, off A41
Telephone for further details
Hotel BUD Innkeeper's Lodge Aylesbury South, 40 Main St, Weston Turville,
AYLESBURY ☎ 0845 112 6095 16 en suite

WEXHAM STREET

MAP 04 SU98

Wexham Park SL3 6ND
☎ 01753 663271 🖹 01753 663318
e-mail: info@wexhamparkgolfcourse.co.uk
web: www.wexhamparkgolfcourse.co.uk
Gently undulating parkland. Three courses, an 18 hole, a challenging nine hole, and another nine hole suitable for beginners.

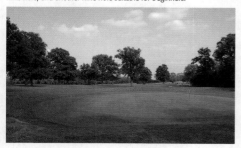

Blue: 18 holes, 5346yds, Par 68, SSS 66.
Red: 9 holes, 2822yds, Par 34.
Green: 9 holes, 2233yds, Par 32. Club membership 950.
Visitors Mon-Sun & BHs. Dress code. **Societies** Booking required. **Green
Fees** £15 for 18 holes, £8.50 for 9 holes (£22/£12 Sat & Sun). **Prof** John
Kennedy **Course Designer** E Lawrence/D Morgan **Facilities** ⑪ ⅃ ☷ ⅃ ☷
☷ ☷ ☷ ☷ **Conf** Corporate Hospitality Days **Location** 0.5m S
Hotel ★★★★ 75% HL Slough/Windsor Marriott Hotel, Ditton Rd, Langley,
SLOUGH ☎ 0870 400 7244 382 en suite

WING

MAP 04 SP82

Aylesbury Vale Stewkley Rd LU7 0UJ
☎ 01525 240196 🖹 01525 240848
e-mail: info@avgc.co.uk
web: avgc.co.uk
This gently undulating course is set amid tranquil countryside.
There are five ponds to pose the golfer problems, notably on the
Par 4 420yd 13th - unlucky for some - where the second shot is all
downhill with an inviting pond spanning the approach to the green. In
addition there is a practice putting green.
18 holes, 6612yds, Par 72, SSS 72, Course record 67.
Club membership 515.
Visitors Mon-Sun & BHs. Booking required. Dress code. **Societies** Booking
required. **Green Fees** £21 (£30 Sat & Sun, £22 after 11am). **Prof** Terry
Bunyan **Course Designer** D Wright **Facilities** ⑪ ⑩ ⅃ ☷ ⅃ ☷ ☷ ☷
☷ ☷ ☷ **Conf** facs Corporate Hospitality Days **Location** 2m NW of
Leighton Buzzard on unclassified Stewkley road, between Wing & Stewkley
Hotel ★★★ 72% HL Old Palace Lodge, Church St, DUNSTABLE
☎ 01582 662201 68 en suite

CAMBRIDGESHIRE

BAR HILL

MAP 05 TL36

Menzies Cambridgeshire Bar Hill CB3 8EU
☎ 01954 780098 & 249971 🖹 01954 780010
e-mail: cambridge@menzies-hotels.co.uk
web: www.bookmenzies.com
Mature undulating parkland course with tree-lined fairways, easy
walking. Challenging opening and closing holes with water on the
right and out of bounds on the left of both.
18 holes, 6575yds, Par 71, SSS 72, Course record 68.
Club membership 600.
Visitors Mon-Sun & BHs. Booking required Sat, Sun & BHs. Dress code.
Societies Booking required. **Green Fees** £30 per round (£40 weekends
& bank holidays). Winter £25/£30. **Prof** Mike Clemons **Facilities** ⑪ ⑩
⅃ ☷ ⅃ ☷ ☷ ☷ ☷ ☷ **Leisure** hard tennis courts, heated indoor
swimming pool, sauna, solarium, gymnasium. **Conf** facs Corporate
Hospitality Days **Location** M11/A14, then B1050 (Bar Hill)
Hotel ★★★★ 80% HL Hotel Felix, Whitehouse Ln, CAMBRIDGE
☎ 01223 277977 52 en suite

BOURN

MAP 05 TL35

Bourn Toft Rd CB3 7TT
☎ 01954 718958 🖹 01954 718908
e-mail: proshop@bourn-golf-club.co.uk
web: www.club-noticeboard.com/bourn
Meadow and parkland with many water features and some very
challenging holes.

Continued

18 holes, 6417yards, Par 72, SSS 71. Club membership 600.
Visitors may play Mon-Sun & BHs. Dress code. **Societies** welcome.
Green Fees not confirmed. ❸ **Prof** Craig Watson **Course Designer** J
Hull **Facilities** ⊕ ⊺◎⊺ ⬚ ⬚ ⊓ ⬚ ⬚ ✆ ♣ ✔ ☂ **Leisure** heated indoor
swimming pool, sauna, solarium, gymnasium. **Conf** facs Corporate
Hospitality Days
Hotel BUD Travelodge Cambridge Lolworth, Huntingdon Rd, LOLWORTH
☎ 08700 850 950 36 en suite

BRAMPTON   MAP 04 TL27

Brampton Park Buckden Rd PE28 4NF
☎ 01480 434700 🖹 01480 411145
e-mail: admin@bramptonparkgc.co.uk
web: www.bramptonparkgc.co.uk
Set in truly attractive countryside, bounded by the River Great Ouse
and bisected by the River Lane. Great variety with mature trees, lakes
and water hazards. One of the most difficult holes is the 4th, a Par 3
island green, 175yds in length.
18 holes, 6300yds, Par 71, SSS 72, Course record 62.
Club membership 650.
Visitors Contact club for details. **Societies** Welcome. **Green Fees** Phone.
Prof Alisdair Currie **Course Designer** Simon Gidman **Facilities** ⊕
⊺◎⊺ ⬚ ⬚ ⊓ ⬚ ⬚ ♢ ✆ ♣ ✔ ☘ **Conf** facs Corporate Hospitality Days
Location Signs from A1 or A14 to RAF Brampton
Hotel ★★★★ 75% HL Huntingdon Marriott Hotel, Kingfisher Way,
Hinchingbrooke Business Park, HUNTINGDON ☎ 01480 446000
150 en suite

CAMBRIDGE   MAP 05 TL45

Gog Magog Shelford Bottom CB2 4AB
☎ 01223 247626 🖹 01223 414990
e-mail: secretary@gogmagog.co.uk
web: www.gogmagog.co.uk
Situated just outside the centre of the university town, Gog
Magog, established in 1901, is known as the nursery of Cambridge
undergraduate golf. The chalk downland courses are on high
ground, and it is said that if you stand on the highest point and
could see far enough to the east the next highest ground would be
the Ural Mountains. The courses are open but there are enough
trees and other hazards to provide plenty of problems. Views from
the high parts are superb. The nature of the ground ensures good
winter golf. The area has been designated a Site of Special Scientific
Interest.
Old Course: 18 holes, 6398yds, Par 70, SSS 70,
Course record 62.
Wandlebury: 18 holes, 6735yds, Par 72, SSS 72,
Course record 67. Club membership 1400.
Visitors Mon-Fri except BHs. Advance booking required. Handicap
certificate required. Dress code. **Societies** Booking required.
Green Fees £60 per day, £45 per round (£65 per round weekends and
bank holidays). ❸ **Prof** Ian Bamborough **Course Designer** Hawtree
Ltd **Facilities** ⊕ ⊺◎⊺ ⬚ ⬚ ⊓ ⬚ ⬚ ✆ ✔ ♣ ✔ ☘ **Conf** Corporate
Hospitality Days **Location** 3m SE on A1307
Hotel ★★★ 78% HL Best Western The Gonville Hotel, Gonville Place,
CAMBRIDGE ☎ 01223 366611 & 221111 🖹 01223 315470 73 en suite

ELY   MAP 05 TL58

Ely City 107 Cambridge Rd CB7 4HX
☎ 01353 662751 (Office) 🖹 01353 668636
e-mail: elygolf@lineone.net
web: www.elygolf.co.uk.
Slightly undulating parkland with water hazards formed by lakes
and natural dykes. Demanding Par 4 5th hole (467yds), often into
a headwind, and a testing Par 3 2nd hole (160yds) played over two
ponds. Magnificent views of the cathedral.
18 holes, 6627yds, Par 72, SSS 72, Course record 65.
Club membership 750.
Visitors Mon-Sun & BHs. Handicap certificate required. Dress code.
Societies Booking required. **Green Fees** £34 per day (£40 weekends).
Prof Andrew George **Course Designer** Sir Henry Cotton **Facilities** ⊕ ⊺◎⊺
⬚ ⬚ ⊓ ⬚ ⬚ ♣ ✔ **Conf** Corporate Hospitality Days **Location** S of
city on A10
Hotel ★★★ 72% HL Lamb Hotel, 2 Lynn Rd, ELY ☎ 01353 663574
31 en suite

GIRTON   MAP 05 TL46

Girton Dodford Ln CB3 0QE
☎ 01223 276169 🖹 01223 277150
e-mail: secretary@girtongolfclub.sagehost.co.uk
web: www.club-noticeboard.co.uk
Flat, open, easy walking parkland with many trees and ditches.
18 holes, 6012yds, Par 69, SSS 69, Course record 66.
Club membership 800.
Visitors Mon-Fri except BHs. Booking required. Dress code.
Societies Booking required. **Green Fees** £25 weekdays. ❸ **Prof** Scott
Thomson **Course Designer** Allan Gow **Facilities** ⊕ ⊺◎⊺ ⬚ ⬚ ⊓ ⬚ ⬚
♣ ✔ **Location** 3m from Cambridge. Just off A14 junct 31
Hotel ★★★★ 80% HL Hotel Felix, Whitehouse Ln, CAMBRIDGE
☎ 01223 277977 52 en suite

HEMINGFORD ABBOTS   MAP 04 TL27

Hemingford Abbots Cambridge Rd PE28 9HQ
☎ 01480 495000 & 493900 🖹 01480 4960000
9 holes, 5468yds, Par 68, SSS 68, Course record 69.
Course Designer Ray Paton **Location** A14 Hemingford Abbots turn,
between St Ives
Telephone for further details
Hotel ★★★ 80% HL The Old Bridge Hotel, 1 High St, HUNTINGDON
☎ 01480 424300 24 en suite

LONGSTANTON　　　　　MAP 05 TL36

Cambridge Station Rd CB4 5DR
☎ 01954 789388
Undulating parkland with bunkers and ponds.
18 holes, 6736yds, Par 72, SSS 73. Club membership 300.
Visitors Mon-Sun & BHs. Booking required. Dress code. **Societies**
Welcome. **Green Fees** £14 per 18 holes (£18 Sat & Sun). **Prof** Geoff
Huggett/A Engelman **Facilities** ⑪ ⑩ ⓛ ➷ ☶ ⚐ ⚘ ⚑ ⛳ ⚑ **Leisure**
fishing, hot air ballons. **Conf** facs Corporate Hospitality Days
Hotel BUD Travelodge Cambridge Swavesey, Cambridge Rd, SWAVESEY
☎ 08700 850 950　36 en suite

MARCH　　　　　MAP 05 TL49

March Frogs Abbey, Grange Rd PE15 0YH
☎ 01354 652364 🖹 01354 658142
e-mail: secretary@marchgolfclub.co.uk
web: www.marchgolfclub.co.uk
A nine-hole parkland course with a particularly challenging Par 3 9th
hole, with out of bounds on the right and high hedges to the left.
9 holes, 6204yds, Par 70, SSS 70, Course record 65.
Club membership 367.
Visitors contact club for details. Dress code. **Societies** advance booking
required. **Green Fees** not confirmed. ⓦ **Prof** Alex Oldham **Facilities** ⚐
⚑⛳ ⚘ & **Location** 0.5m off A141, March bypass
Hotel ★★★ 77% HL Crown Lodge Hotel, Downham Rd, Outwell,
WISBECH ☎ 01945 773391 & 772206 🖹 01945 772668　10 en suite

MELDRETH　　　　　MAP 05 TL34

Malton Malton Rd, Malton SG8 6PE
☎ 01763 262200 🖹 01763 262209
e-mail: desk@maltongolf.co.uk
web: www.maltongolf.co.uk
Set among 230 acres of beautiful undulating countryside. The River
Cam bisects part of the course which is surrounded by woodlands and
wetlands.
18 holes, 6708yards, Par 72, SSS 72, Course record 67.
Visitors may play Mon-Sun & BHs. Advance booking required. Dress code.
Societies Welcome. **Green Fees** £12 per 18 holes (£18 Sat, Sun & BHs)
Twilight after 4pm £8/£12. **Prof** Kevin Evans **Facilities** ⑪ ⑩ ⓛ ⚐⚑ ☶
⚑⛳ ⚘ & **Location** Between Orwell
Hotel ★★★ 81% HL Duxford Lodge Hotel, Ickleton Rd, DUXFORD
☎ 01223 836444　11 en suite　4 annexe en suite

PETERBOROUGH　　　　　MAP 04 TL19

Elton Furze Bullock Rd, Haddon PE7 3TT
☎ 01832 280189 & 280614 (Pro shop) 🖹 01832 280299
e-mail: secretary@eltonfurzegolfclub.co.uk
web: www.eltonfurzegolfclub.co.uk
Elton Furze Golf Club is set in the picturesque surroundings of the
Cambridgeshire countryside. The course has been designed in and
around mature woodland with ponds and slopes, which provides the
golfer with an interesting and enjoyable round of golf.
18 holes, 6279yds, Par 70, SSS 71, Course record 66.
Club membership 620.
Visitors Mon-Fri, weekends only with prior permission **Societies** welcome.
Green Fees not confirmed. **Prof** Glyn Krause **Course Designer** Roger
Fitton **Facilities** ⑪ ⑩ by prior arrangement ⓛ ⚐ ⚑⛳ ☶ ☰ ⚘ ⚑

Conf facs　Corporate Hospitality Days **Location** 4m SW of Peterborough,
off A605/A1
Hotel ★★★★ 72% HL Peterborough Marriott Hotel, Peterborough
Business Park, Lynchwood, PETERBOROUGH ☎ 01733 371111　163 en suite

Orton Meadows Ham Ln, Orton Waterville PE2 5UU
☎ 01733 237478 🖹 01733 332774
e-mail: enquiries@ortonmeadowsgolfcourse.co.uk
web: www.ortonmeadowsgolfcourse.co.uk
Picturesque course with trees, lakes and an abundance of water fowl,
providing some challenges with water featuring on 10 holes.
18 holes, 5269yds, Par 67, SSS 68, Course record 64.
Club membership 650.
Visitors booking required. **Societies** welcome. **Green Fees** £13.80 per
round (£18.50 weekends & bank holidays). **Prof** Stuart Brown
Course Designer D & R Fitton **Facilities** ⑪ ⑩ ⓛ ⚐ ⚑⛳ ☶ ☰ ⚐⚑ ◇ ⚘
Leisure 12 hole pitch & putt. **Location** 3m W of town on A605
Hotel ★★★ 78% HL Best Western Orton Hall Hotel, Orton Longueville,
PETERBOROUGH ☎ 01733 391111　65 en suite

Peterborough Milton Milton Ferry PE6 7AG
☎ 01733 380489 & 380793 (Pro) 🖹 01733 380489
e-mail: miltongolfclub@aol.com
web: www.peterboroughmiltongolfclub.co.uk
Designed by James Braid, this well-bunkered parkland course is set in
the grounds of the Milton Estate, many of the holes being played in
full view of Milton Hall. Challenging holes are the difficult dog-leg 10th
and 15th. Easy walking.
18 holes, 6541yds, Par 71, SSS 72, Course record 69.
Club membership 800.
Visitors Mon-Sun & BHs. Booking required. Handicap certificate. Dress
code. **Societies** Booking required. **Green Fees** £50 per 36 holes, £40
per 18 holes. **Prof** Jasen Barker **Course Designer** James Braid **Facilities** ⑪
⑩ ⓛ ⚐ ⚑⛳ ☶ ☰ ⚘ **Conf** facs　Corporate Hospitality Days
Location 2m W of Peterborough on A47
Hotel BUD Travelodge Peterborough Eye Green, Crowlands Rd,
PETERBOROUGH ☎ 08700 850 950　42 en suite

Thorpe Wood Thorpe Wood, Nene Parkway PE3 6SE
☎ 01733 267701 🖹 01733 332774
e-mail: enquiries@thorpewoodgolfcourse.co.uk
web: www.thorpewoodgolfcourse.co.uk
18 holes, 7086yds, Par 73, SSS 74, Course record 68.
Course Designer Peter Allis/Dave Thomas **Location** 3m W of city centre
on A47
Telephone for further details
Hotel ★★★ 78% HL Best Western Orton Hall Hotel, Orton Longueville,
PETERBOROUGH ☎ 01733 391111　65 en suite

PIDLEY　　　　　MAP 05 TL37

Lakeside Lodge Fen Rd PE28 3DF
☎ 01487 740540 🖹 01487 740852
e-mail: info@lakeside-lodge.co.uk
web: www.lakeside-lodge.co.uk
A well-designed, spacious course incorporating eight lakes, 12,000
trees and a modern clubhouse. The 9th and 18th holes both finish
dramatically alongside a lake in front of the clubhouse. Also nine-hole
Par 3, and 25-bay driving range. The Manor provides an interesting
contrast with its undulating fairways and angular greens.

Continued

Lodge Course: 18 holes, 6885yds, Par 72, SSS 73.
The Manor: 9 holes, 2601yds, Par 34, SSS 33.
The Church: 12 holes, 3290yds, Par 44.
Club membership 1200.
Visitors Mon-Sun & BHs. Advance booking required. Dress code.
Societies Booking required. **Green Fees** £17 per 18 holes (£27 weekends & bank holidays); £10 per 9/12 holes (£13 week ends & bank holidays).
Prof Scott Waterman **Course Designer** A W Headley **Facilities** ⊕ ⌖ ☺ ⅃ ⌂ ⌱ ⌲ ⌳ ⚘ ⚐ ⚑ ⚒ **Leisure** solarium, ten pin bowling. **Conf** facs Corporate Hospitality Days **Location** A141 from Huntingdon, then B1040
Hotel ★★★ 70% HL Slepe Hall Hotel, Ramsey Rd, ST IVES
☎ 01480 463122 16 en suite

RAMSEY   MAP 04 TL28

Old Nene Golf & Country Club Muchwood Ln, Bodsey PE26 2XQ
☎ 01487 815622 🖷 01487 813610
e-mail: info@oldnene.freeserve.co.uk
9 holes, 5605yds, Par 68, SSS 68, Course record 64.
Course Designer R Edrich **Location** 0.75m N of Ramsey towards Ramsey Mereside
Telephone for further details
Hotel ★★★ 80% HL The Old Bridge Hotel, 1 High St, HUNTINGDON
☎ 01480 424300 24 en suite

Ramsey 4 Abbey Ter PE26 1DD
☎ 01487 812600 🖷 01487 815746
e-mail: admin@ramseyclub.co.uk
web: www.ramseyclub.co.uk
Flat parkland with water hazards and well-irrigated greens, mature tees and fairways - a good surface whatever the conditions. The impression of wide-open spaces soon punishes the wayward shot.
18 holes, 6163yds, Par 71, SSS 68, Course record 64.
Club membership 600.
Visitors Mon-Fri except BHs. Booking required Fri. Handicap certificate. Dress code. **Societies** Welcome. **Green Fees** £25 per 18 holes.
Prof Stuart Scott **Course Designer** J Hamilton Stutt **Facilities** ☺ ⌂ ⌱ ⌳ ⌲ ⚘ ⚐ ⚒ **Leisure** snooker tables, bowls rinks. **Location** 12m SE of Peterborough on B1040
Hotel ★★★ 80% HL The Old Bridge Hotel, 1 High St, HUNTINGDON
☎ 01480 424300 24 en suite

ST IVES   MAP 04 TL37

St Ives (Cambs) Westwood Rd PE27 6DH
☎ 01480 468392 🖷 01480 468392
e-mail: stivesgolfclub@zoom.co.uk
Picturesque parkland course.
9 holes, 6180yds, Par 70, SSS 70, Course record 68.
Club membership 500.
Visitors may play Mon-Sun & BHs. Advance booking required. Handicap certificate required. Dress code. **Societies** advance booking required.
Green Fees not confirmed. **Prof** Mark Pond **Facilities** ⊕ ⌖ ☺ ⅃ ⌂ ⌱ ⚘ ⚒ **Conf** facs Corporate Hospitality Days **Location** W side of town centre off A1123
Hotel ★★★ 70% HL Slepe Hall Hotel, Ramsey Rd, ST IVES
☎ 01480 463122 16 en suite

ST NEOTS   MAP 04 TL16

Abbotsley Golf & Squash Club Eynesbury Hardwicke PE19 6XN
☎ 01480 474000 🖷 01480 403280
e-mail: abbotsley@crown-golf.co.uk
Set in 250 acres of idyllic countryside, with two 18-hole courses and a nine-hole Par 3. The Cromwell course is the less challenging of the two, offering a contrast to the renowned Abbotsley course with its holes meandering through woods and streams. One of the most memorable holes is the Abbotsley 2nd hole known as the Mousehole, which requires an accurate tee shot to a green that is protected by a stream and shaded by the many trees that surround it.
Abbotsley Course: 18 holes, 6311yds, Par 73, SSS 72, Course record 69.
Cromwell Course: 18 holes, 6087yds, Par 70, SSS 69, Course record 66. Club membership 550.
Visitors may play Mon-Sun & BHs. Dress code **Societies** advance booking required. **Green Fees** not confirmed. **Prof** Denise Hastings/Steve Connolly **Course Designer** D Young/V Saunders **Facilities** ⊕ ⌖ ☺ ⅃ ⌂ ⌱ ⌲ ⚘ ⚐ ⚑ ⚒ **Leisure** squash, solarium, gymnasium. **Conf** facs Corporate Hospitality Days **Location** Off A1 & A428

St Neots Crosshall Rd PE19 7GE
☎ 01480 472363 🖷 01480 472363
e-mail: office@stneots-golfclub.co.uk
web: www.stneots-golfclub.co.uk
Set in picturesque rolling parkland and divided by the river Kym, the course offers a challenge to all standards of golfer with tree-lined fairways, water hazards and outstanding greens.
18 holes, 6033yds, Par 69, SSS 69, Course record 64.
Club membership 630.
Visitors Mon-Fri. Booking required. Handicap certificate required. Dress code. **Societies** Welcome. **Green Fees** £45 per day; £35 per round.
Prof Paul Toyer **Course Designer** H Vardon **Facilities** ⊕ ⌖ ☺ ⅃ ⌂ ⌱ ⚘ ⚐ ⚒ **Conf** Corporate Hospitality Days **Location** A1 onto B1048 into St Neots

---

THORNEY   MAP 04 TF20

Thorney English Drove, Thorney PE6 0TJ
☎ 01733 270570 🖷 01733 270842
web: www.thorneygolfcentre.com
The 18-hole Fen course is ideal for the beginner, while the Lakes Course has a challenging links-style layout with eight holes around water.
Fen Course: 18 holes, 6104yds, Par 70, SSS 69, Course record 66.
Lakes Course: 18 holes, 6402yds, Par 71, SSS 70, Course record 65. Club membership 500.
Visitors Mon-Sun & BHs. Booking required Sat, Sun & BHs. Dress code. **Societies** Booking required. **Green Fees** Phone. **Prof** Mark Templeman **Course Designer** A Dow **Facilities** ⊕ ⌖ ☺ ⅃ ⌂ ⌱ ⌲ ⚘ ⚐ ⚒ **Leisure** Par 3 course. **Location** Off A47, 7m NE of Peterborough
Hotel BUD Travelodge Peterborough Eye Green, Crowlands Rd, PETERBOROUGH ☎ 08700 850 950 42 en suite

England

TOFT
MAP 05 TL35

Cambridge National Comberton Rd CB23 2RY
☎ 01223 264700 & 264702 📠 01223 264701
e-mail: meridian@golfsocieties.com
web: www.golfsocieties.com
Set in 207 acres to a Peter Allis and Clive Clark design with sweeping fairways, lakes and well-bunkered greens. The 4th hole has bunker complexes, a sharp dog-leg and a river with the green heavily guarded by bunkers. The 9th and 10th holes challenge the golfer with river crossings.
18 holes, 6651yds, Par 73, SSS 72, Course record 72.
Club membership 450.
Visitors Mon-Sun & BHs. Dress code. **Societies** Booking required.
Green Fees £28 per 18 holes (£35 Sat & Sun). **Prof** Craig Watson
Course Designer Peter Alliss/Clive Clark **Facilities** ⑪ ⑩ by prior arrangement 🍴 ⬤ 🏌 ⬤ ⛳ ⬤ **Leisure** indoor golf simulator.
Conf facs Corporate Hospitality Days **Location** 3m W of Cambridge, on B1046

TYDD ST GILES
MAP 09 TH41

Tydd St Giles Golf & Country Club Kirkgate PE13 5NZ
☎ 01945 871007 📠 01945 870566
e-mail: enquiries@tyddgolf.co.uk
web: www.tyddgolf.co.uk
At only ten years old, this is a comparatively new course. All the greens are around 50 yards long so pin positions in the summer months will add approximately 400 yards to the course making the length around 6,700 yards. Even in its early years, it is a challenge for even the most talented of golfers and with a few more years of maturity, this course should become one of the finest in the area.
18 holes, 6264yds, Par 70, SSS 70, Course record 66.
Club membership 600.
Visitors Mon-Sun & BHs.Booking required. Dress code. **Societies** Booking required. **Green Fees** £17 per day (£20 Sat, Sun & BHs). Twilight £10 everyday from 1pm. **Prof** Ashley Howard **Course Designer** Adrian Hurst **Facilities** ⑪ ⑩ 🍴 ⬤ 🏌 ⬤ ⛳ ⬤ **Leisure** fishing. **Conf** facs Corporate Hospitality Days **Location** A1101 N of Wisbech to Long Sutton, turn left into Hannath Rd at Tydd Gate/River
Hotel ★★★ 73% HL Elme Hall Hotel, Elm High Rd, WISBECH
☎ 01945 475566 7 en suite

CHESHIRE

ALDERLEY EDGE
MAP 07 SJ87

Alderley Edge Brook Ln SK9 7RU
☎ 01625 586200
e-mail: honsecretary@aegc.co.uk
web: www.aegc.co.uk
Well-wooded, undulating pastureland course. A stream crosses seven of the nine holes. A challenging course even for the low handicap player.
9 holes, 5823yds, Par 68, SSS 68, Course record 62.
Club membership 400.
Visitors Mon, Wed-Fri, Sun & BHs. Handicap certificate required. Dress code. **Societies** Booking required. **Green Fees** Phone. **Prof** Peter Bowring **Facilities** ⑪ ⑩ 🍴 ⬤ 🏌 ⬤ ⛳ ⬤ **Conf** facs Corporate Hospitality Days **Location** 1m NW on B5085
Hotel ★★★ 83% HL Alderley Edge Hotel, Macclesfield Rd, ALDERLEY EDGE ☎ 01625 583033 50 en suite

ALDERSEY GREEN
MAP 07 SJ45

Aldersey Green CH3 9EH
☎ 01829 782157
e-mail: bradburygolf@aol.com
web: www.alderseygreengolfclub.co.uk
An exciting, tricky, beautiful parkland course set in 200 acres of countryside. With tree-lined fairways and 14 lakes.
18 holes, 6145, Par 70, SSS 69, Course record 72.
Club membership 350.
Visitors Mon-Sun & BHs. Booking required. Dress code. **Societies** Booking required. **Green Fees** £25 per day, £15 per round (£30/£20 weekends).
Prof Stephen Bradbury **Facilities** ⑪ ⑩ 🍴 ⬤ 🏌 ⬤ ⛳ ⬤ **Location** On A41 Whitchurch Rd, 6m S of Chester
Hotel ★★★★ 84% HL De Vere Carden Park, Carden Park, BROXTON ☎ 01829 731000 113 en suite 83 annexe en suite

ALSAGER
MAP 07 SJ75

Alsager Golf & Country Club Audley Rd ST7 2UR
☎ 01270 875700 📠 01270 882207
e-mail: business@alsagergolfclub.com
web: www.alsagergolfclub.com
18 holes, 6225yds, Par 70, SSS 70, Course record 67.
Location M6 junct 16, 2m NE
Telephone for further details
Hotel ★★★ 82% HL Best Western Manor House Hotel, Audley Rd, ALSAGER ☎ 01270 884000 57 en suite

ANTROBUS
MAP 07 SJ68

Antrobus Foggs Ln CW9 6JQ
☎ 01925 730890 📠 01925 730100
web: www.antrobusgolfclub.co.uk
A challenging parkland course where water is the main feature with streams and ponds in play on most holes. Large undulating greens.
18 holes, 6220yards, Par 71, SSS 71, Course record 65.
Club membership 500.
Visitors Mon-Fri, Sun & BHs. Advance booking required. Dress code.
Societies Booking required. **Green Fees** £25 per day (£28 Sun and BHs). **Prof** Paul Farrance **Course Designer** Mike Slater **Facilities** ⑪ ⑩ 🍴 ⬤ 🏌 ⬤ ⛳ ⬤ **Leisure** fishing. **Conf** facs **Location** M56 junct 10, A559 towards Northwich, 2nd left after Birch pub onto Knutsford Rd, 1st left into Foggs Ln
Hotel ★★★ 64% HL The Floatel, Northwich, London Rd, NORTHWICH ☎ 01606 44443 60 en suite

CHESTER
MAP 07 SJ46

Chester Curzon Park CH4 8AR
☎ 01244 677760 📠 01244 676667
e-mail: vfcwood@chestergolfclub.co.uk
web: www.chestergolfclub.co.uk
Meadowland course on two levels contained within a loop of the River Dee. The car park overlooks the racecourse across the river.
18 holes, 6508yds, Par 72, SSS 71, Course record 66.
Club membership 820.
Visitors may play Mon, Tue, Thu & Fri. Advance booking required. Handicap certificate required. Dress code. **Societies** advance booking required.
Green Fees not confirmed. ◉ **Prof** Scott Booth **Facilities** ⑪ ⑩ 🍴 ⬤ 🏌 ⬤ ⛳ ⬤ **Location** 1m W of city centre
Hotel ★★★ 80% HL Grosvenor Pulford Hotel, Wrexham Rd, Pulford, CHESTER ☎ 01244 570560 73 en suite

De Vere Carden Park Hotel CH3 9DQ
☎ 01829 731000 📠 01829 731032
e-mail: golf.carden@devere-hotels.com
web: www.devere.co.uk
A superb golf resort set in 750 acres of beautiful Cheshire countryside.
Facilities include the mature parkland Cheshire Course, the Nicklaus
Course, the nine-hole Par 3 Azalea Course, Golf School and a luxurious
clubhouse.
Cheshire: 18 holes, 6824yds, Par 72, SSS 72,
Course record 63.
Nicklaus: 18 holes, 7045yds, Par 72, SSS 72,
Course record 63. Club membership 250.
Visitors Mon-Sun & BHs. Dress code. **Societies** Booking required. **Green
Fees** Phone. **Prof** Alastair Taylor **Course Designer** Jack Nicklaus (Nicklaus
course) **Facilities** ⑪ 🍴 🍺 🖳 🍴 🏌 🚶 🏠 🎯 🚑 🏆 **Leisure** hard
tennis courts, heated indoor swimming pool, sauna, solarium, gymnasium,
residential golf school, snooker room. **Conf** facs Corporate Hospitality Days
Location S of City on A41, right at Broxton rdbt onto A534 signed Wrexham.
Situated 1.5m on left
Hotel ★★★★ 84% HL De Vere Carden Park, Carden Park, BROXTON
☎ 01829 731000 113 en suite 83 annexe en suite

Eaton Guy Ln, Waverton CH3 7PH
☎ 01244 335885 📠 01244 335782
e-mail: office@eatongolfclub.co.uk
web: www.eatongolfclub.co.uk
Parkland with a liberal covering of mature trees and new planting
enhanced by natural water hazards.

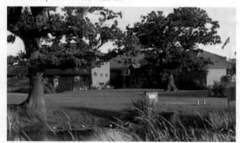

18 holes, 6562yds, Par 72, SSS 71, Course record 68.
Club membership 550.
Visitors Mon, Tue, Thu-Sun & BHs. Advance booking required. Handicap
certificate Dress code. **Societies** Booking required. **Green Fees** £35 per
round (£40 Sat, Sun & BH). Winter rates £30/£35. 🏌 **Prof** William Tye
Course Designer Donald Steel **Facilities** ⑪ 🍴 🍺 🖳 🍴 🏌 🚶 🏠 🎯 🚑
🏆 **Conf** Corporate Hospitality Days **Location** 3m SE of Chester off A41
Hotel ★★★★★ HL The Chester Grosvenor & Spa, Eastgate, CHESTER
☎ 01244 324024 80 en suite

Upton-by-Chester Upton Ln, Upton-by-Chester CH2 1EE
☎ 01244 381183 📠 01244 376955
Pleasant, tree-lined parkland. Not easy for low-handicap players to
score well. Testing holes are 2nd (Par 4), 14th (Par 4) and 15th (Par 3).
18 holes, 5807yds, Par 69, SSS 68, Course record 63.
Club membership 750.
Visitors Mon-Sun except BHs. Booking required Wed-Sun. Dress code.
Societies Booking required. **Green Fees** £35 per day, £25 per round. **Prof**

Stephen Dewhurst **Course Designer** Bill Davies **Facilities** ⑪ 🍴 🍺 🖳 🍴
🚶 🏠 🎯 🚑 🚑 **Conf** Corporate Hospitality Days **Location** N side off A5116
Hotel Hoole Hall Hotel, Warrington Rd, Hoole Village, CHESTER
☎ 01244 408800 0870 6096126 📠 01244320251 94 en suite

Vicars Cross Tarvin Rd, Great Barrow CH3 7HN
☎ 01244 335595 📠 01244 335686
e-mail: secretary@vcgc.fsnet.co.uk
web: www.vicarscrossgc.co.uk
18 holes, 6446yds, Par 72, SSS 71, Course record 64.
Course Designer J Richardson **Location** 4m E on A51
Telephone for further details
Hotel ★★★★ 80% HL Rowton Hall Country House Hotel, Whitchurch Rd,
Rowton, CHESTER ☎ 01244 335262 38 en suite

CONGLETON   MAP 07 SJ86

Astbury Peel Ln, Astbury CW12 4RE
☎ 01260 272772 📠 01260 276420
e-mail: admin@astburygolfclub.com
web: www.astburygolfclub.com
Parkland course in open countryside, bisected by a canal. The
testing 12th hole involves a long carry over a tree-filled ravine. Large
practice area.
18 holes, 6296yds, Par 71, SSS 70, Course record 61.
Club membership 720.
Visitors Mon-Fri except BHs. Handicap certificate. Dress code **Societies**
Welcome. **Green Fees** £30 per round. 🏌 **Prof** Ashley Salt **Facilities** ⑪ 🍺
🖳 🍴 🏌 🏠 🚑 **Location** 1.5m S between A34 A527
Inn ★★★★ INN Egerton Arms, Astbury Village, CONGLETON
☎ 01260 273946 6 en suite

Congleton Biddulph Rd CW12 3LZ
☎ 01260 273540
Superbly-manicured parkland course with views over three counties
from the balcony of the clubhouse.
9 holes, 5103yds, Par 68, SSS 65. Club membership 400.
Visitors Booking required. Handicap certificate. Dress code. **Societies**
Welcome. **Green Fees** Mon-Fri £24 per round (£36 Sat & Sun). 🏌 **Prof**
Andrew Preston **Facilities** ⑪ 🍴 🍺 🖳 by prior arrangement 🍴 🏌 🏠 🚑
Conf Corporate Hospitality Days **Location** 1.5m SE on A527
Inn ★★★★ INN Egerton Arms, Astbury Village, CONGLETON
☎ 01260 273946 6 en suite

CREWE   MAP 07 SJ75

Crewe Fields Rd, Haslington CW1 5TB
☎ 01270 584099 📠 01270 256482
e-mail: secretary@crewsgolfclub.co.uk
web: www.crewegolfclub.co.uk
Undulating parkland.
18 holes, 6424yds, Par 71, SSS 71, Course record 63.
Club membership 674.
Visitors Tue. Booking required. Dress code. **Societies** Booking
required. **Green Fees** £36 per day (£16 winter). 🏌 **Prof** David Wheeler
Course Designer James Braid **Facilities** ⑪ 🍴 🍺 🖳 🍴 🏌 🚶 🏠 🚑
Location 2.25m NE off A534
Hotel ★★★ 78% HL Hunters Lodge Hotel, Sydney Rd, Sydney, CREWE
☎ 01270 539100 57 en suite

Queen's Park Queen's Park Dr CW2 7SB
☎ 01270 666724 📄 01270 569902
e-mail: crewe@americangolf.co.uk
9 holes, 4920yds, Par 68, SSS 64, Course record 67.
Location Located behind Queen's Park. Well signposted
Telephone for further details
Hotel ★★★ 78% HL Hunters Lodge Hotel, Sydney Rd, Sydney, CREWE
☎ 01270 539100 57 en suite

Wychwood Park Wychwood Park, Weston CW2 5GP
☎ 01270 829247 (manager) & 829248 (pro)
📄 01270 829201
e-mail: jcann@deverevenues.co.uk
web: www.deverevenues.co.uk
Parkland style course opened in 2002, built to USGA standards, with
water features on many holes and wildlife protected areas.
18 holes, 6736yds, Par 72, SSS 73. Club membership 570.
Visitors Mon-Sun & BHs. Booking required. Handicap certificate. Dress
code. **Societies** Booking required **Green Fees** £50 per 18 holes (£60 Sat
& Sun). **Prof** Frank Kiddie **Course Designer** Hawtree & Co **Facilities**
⑪ 🍴 🍺 ♨ 🏌 ⚒ ♦ ✎ 🍴 ✎ **Leisure** sauna, gymnasium.
Conf facs Corporate Hospitality Days **Location** M6 junct 16, A500 for
Nantwich, A531 for Keeleo
Hotel ★★★ 74% HL The Crewe Arms Hotel, Nantwich Rd, CREWE
☎ 01270 213204 59 en suite

DELAMERE   MAP 07 SJ56

Delamere Forest Station Rd CW8 2JE
☎ 01606 883264 & 883800 📄 01606 889444
e-mail: info@delameregolf.co.uk
web: www.delameregolf.co.uk
Played mostly on undulating open heath there is great charm in the
way this course drops down into the occasional pine sheltered valley.
Six of the first testing nine holes are from 420 to 455yds in length.

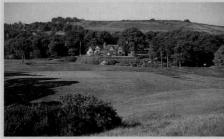

18 holes, 6348yds, Par 72, SSS 71, Course record 65.
Club membership 500.
Visitors may play Tue-Fri. Dress code. **Societies** Booking required.
Green Fees not confirmed. ☻ **Prof** Ellis B Jones **Course Designer** H
Fowler **Facilities** ⑪ 🍴 by prior arrangement 🍺 ♨ 🏌 ⚒ 🍴 ♦ ✎ ✎
Conf Corporate Hospitality Days **Location** 1.5m NE, off B5152
Hotel ★★★ 78% CHH Willington Hall, Willington, TARPORLEY
☎ 01829 752321 10 en suite

DISLEY   MAP 07 SJ98

Disley Stanley Hall Ln SK12 2JX
☎ 01663 764001 📄 01663 762678
e-mail: secretary@disleygolfclub.co.uk
web: www.disleygolfclub.co.uk
Straddling a hilltop site above Lyme Park, this undulating parkland
and moorland course affords good views and requires accuracy
of approach to almost all the greens which lie on either a ledge or
plateau. Testing holes are the 3rd and 4th.

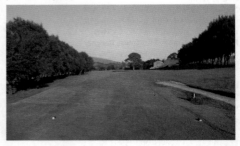

18 holes, 6015yds, Par 70, SSS 69, Course record 63.
Club membership 650.
Visitors may play Mon-Wed, Fri-Sun & BHs. Booking required Fri-Sun
& BHs. Handicap certificate. Dress code. **Societies** Booking required.
Green Fees £28 per day (£40 Sat & Sun). **Prof** Andrew Esplin
Course Designer James Braid **Facilities** ⑪ 🍴 🍺 ♨ 🏌 ⚒ 🍴 ♦
Conf facs Corporate Hospitality Days **Location** NW side of village off A6
Hotel ★★★ 75% HL Best Western Moorside Grange Hotel & Spa,
Mudhurst Ln, Higher Disley, DISLEY ☎ 01663 764151 98 en suite

ELLESMERE PORT   MAP 07 SJ47

Ellesmere Port Chester Rd, Childer Thornton CH66 1QF
☎ 0151 339 7689 📄 0151 339 7502
18 holes, 6432yds, Par 71, SSS 70.
Course Designer Cotton, Pennick & Lawrie **Location** NW side of town
centre. M53 junct 5, A41 for Chester, club 2m on left
Telephone for further details
Hotel ★★★ 75% HL Quality Hotel Chester, Berwick Rd, Little Sutton,
ELLESMERE PORT ☎ 0151 339 5121 75 en suite

FRODSHAM   MAP 07 SJ57

Frodsham Simons Ln WA6 6HE
☎ 01928 732159 📄 01928 734070
e-mail: alastair@frodshamgolf.co.uk
web: www.frodshamgolfclub.co.uk
Undulating parkland with pleasant views from all parts. Emphasis
on accuracy over the whole course, the long and difficult Par 5 18th
necessitating a drive across water to the green. Crossed by two
footpaths so extreme care needed.
18 holes, 6328yds, Par 70, SSS 70, Course record 63.
Club membership 700.
Visitors may play Mon-Fri except BHs. Advance booking required. Dress
code. **Societies** advance booking required. **Green Fees** not confirmed.
Prof Graham Tonge **Course Designer** John Day **Facilities** ⑪ 🍴 🍺 ♨ 🏌
🏌 ⚒ ♦ ✎ **Leisure** snooker. **Location** M56 junct 12, 1.5m SW, signs for
Forest Hills Hotel, Golf Club 1st left on Simons Ln
Hotel ★★★ 77% HL Forest Hills Hotel & Leisure Complex, Overton Hill,
FRODSHAM ☎ 01928 735255 58 en suite

HELSBY   MAP 07 SJ47

Helsby Towers Ln WA6 0JB
☎ 01928 722021 📠 01928 725384
e-mail: secathgc@aol.com
web: www.helsbygolfclub.org
This gentle but challenging parkland course was originally designed by James Braid. With a wide variety of trees and natural water hazards interspersed throughout the course, it is an excellent test of golfing ability. The last six holes are reputed to be perhaps among the most difficult home stretch in Cheshire, with the last being a Par 3 of 205yds to a narrow green guarded by bunkers. A wide variety of wildlife lives around the several ponds which are features to be noted (and hopefully avoided).
18 holes, 6221yds, Par 70, SSS 70, Course record 65.
Club membership 640.
Visitors Mon-Fri except BHs. Dress code. **Societies** Booking required.
Green Fees £27.50 per round. **Prof** Matthew Jones **Course Designer**
James Braid (part) **Facilities** ⊕ ⊗ ⓘ ⌷ ⌷ ⊥ ⌷ 🕳 ⚡ ⌀ **Conf** Corporate
Hospitality Days **Location** M56 junct 14, 1m. 6m from Chester
Hotel ★★★★★ HL The Chester Grosvenor & Spa, Eastgate, CHESTER
☎ 01244 324024 80 en suite

KNUTSFORD   MAP 07 SJ77

Heyrose Budworth Rd, Tabley WA16 0HZ
☎ 01565 733664 📠 01565 734578
e-mail: info@heyrosegolfclub.com
web: www.heyrosegolfclub.com
An 18-hole course in wooded and gently undulating terrain. The Par 3 16th (237yds), bounded by a small river in a wooded valley, is an interesting and testing hole - one of the toughest Par 3s in Cheshire. Several water hazards. Both the course and the comfortable clubhouse have attractive views.
18 holes, 6499yds, Par 73, SSS 71, Course record 66.
Club membership 600.
Visitors may play Mon-Sun & BHs. Advance notice required. Dress code.
Societies must contact in advance. **Green Fees** not confirmed. **Prof** Philip
Bills **Course Designer** C N Bridge **Facilities** ⊕ ⊗ ⓘ ⌷ ⌷ ⌷ ⊥ 🕳 ⚡
⚡ 🛒 ⚡ ⊱ **Leisure** practice bunker, practice nets. **Conf** facs Corporate
Hospitality Days **Location** M6 junct 19, 1m, follow tourist signs
Hotel ★★★★ 78% HL Cottons Hotel & Spa, Manchester Rd, KNUTSFORD
☎ 01565 650333 109 en suite

High Legh Park Warrington Rd, Mere & High Legh
WA16 0WA
☎ 01565 830888 📠 01565 830999

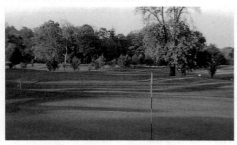

Championship: 18 holes, 6715yds, Par 72.
South: 18 holes, 6281yds, Par 70.
North: 18 holes, 6472yds, Par 70.

Location M6 junct 20, A50 to High Legh
Telephone for further details
Hotel ★★★★ 78% HL Cottons Hotel & Spa, Manchester Rd, KNUTSFORD
☎ 01565 650333 109 en suite

Knutsford Mereheath Ln WA16 6HS
☎ 01565 633355
9 holes, 6288yds, Par 70, SSS 70.
Location N side of town centre off A50
Telephone for further details
Hotel ★★★★ 78% HL Cottons Hotel & Spa, Manchester Rd, KNUTSFORD
☎ 01565 650333 109 en suite

Mere Golf & Country Club Chester Rd, Mere
WA16 6LJ
☎ 01565 830155 📠 01565 830713
e-mail: enquiries@meregolf.co.uk
web: www.meregolf.co.uk
A gracious parkland championship course designed by James Braid in the Cheshire sand belt, with several holes close to a lake. The round has a tight finish with four testing holes.

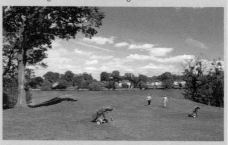

18 holes, 6817yds, Par 71, SSS 73, Course record 64.
Club membership 550.
Visitors Mon, Tue & Thu except BHs. Booking required. Handicap certificate. Dress code. **Societies** Booking required **Green Fees** £70 per day (£50 Oct-Mar). **Prof** Peter Eyre **Course Designer** James Braid/George Duncan **Facilities** ⊕ ⊗ ⓘ ⌷ ⌷ ⌷ ⊥ 🕳 ⚡ ⚡ 🛒 ⊱
Leisure hard tennis courts, heated indoor swimming pool, squash, sauna, solarium, gymnasium. **Conf** facs Corporate Hospitality Days
Location M6 junct 19, 1m E. M56 junct 7, 1m W
Hotel ★★★★ 78% HL Cottons Hotel & Spa, Manchester Rd,
KNUTSFORD ☎ 01565 650333 109 en suite

Peover Plumley Moor Rd, Lower Peover WA16 9SE
☎ 01565 723337 📠 01565 723311
e-mail: mail@peovergolfclub.co.uk
web: www.peovergolfclub.co.uk
Tees and greens have been positioned to maximise the benefits of the natural contours of the land. An excellent mix of holes varying in design and character, with many dog-legs and water hazards, and a river that three of the fairways cross, including the 1st.
18 holes, 6702yds, Par 72, SSS 72, Course record 69.
Club membership 400.
Visitors booking required. Dress code. **Societies** Welcome. **Green Fees** Phone. **Prof** Mark Twiss **Course Designer** P A Naylor **Facilities** ⊕ ⊗ ⓘ ⌷ ⌷ 🕳 ⊥ 🛒 ⚡ ⌀ **Conf** facs Corporate Hospitality Days **Location** M6 junct 19, A556 onto Plumley Moor Rd
Hotel ★★ 80% HL The Longview Hotel & Restaurant, 55 Manchester Rd, KNUTSFORD ☎ 01565 632119 13 en suite 19 annexe en suite *Continued*

England

LYMM
MAP 07 SJ68

Lymm Whitbarrow Rd WA13 9AN
☎ 01925 755020 📄 01925 755020
e-mail: lymmgolfclub@btconnect.com
web: www.lymm-golf-club.co.uk
First ten holes are gently undulating with the Manchester Ship Canal running alongside the 6th hole. The remaining holes are comparatively flat.
18 holes, 6341yds, Par 71, SSS 70. Club membership 800.
Visitors Mon-Wed, Fri-Sun & BHs. Handicap certificate. Dress code.
Societies Booking required. **Green Fees** £32 per round. 🏌 **Prof** Steve McCarthy **Facilities** 🏌🍴🛒🗄🍷🍸🚶🏨🏌 **Location** 0.5m N off A6144
Hotel ★★★ 72% HL The Lymm Hotel, Whitbarrow Rd, LYMM
☎ 0870 1942121   14 en suite   48 annexe en suite

MACCLESFIELD
MAP 07 SJ97

Macclesfield The Hollins SK11 7EA
☎ 01625 423227 📄 01625 260061
e-mail: secretary@maccgolfclub.co.uk
web: maccgolfclub.co.uk
Hillside heathland course situated on the edge of the Pennines with excellent views across the Cheshire Plain. The signature hole is the 410yd 3rd, which drops majestically to a plateau green situated above a babbling brook. The temptation is to over-club, thus bringing the out of bounds behind into play. The 7th hole is aptly named Seven Shires as seven counties can be seen on a clear day, as well as the mountains.
18 holes, 5714yds, Par 70, SSS 68, Course record 63.
Club membership 620.
Visitors Mon-Fri except BHs. Booking required. Handicap certificate. Dress code. **Societies** Booking required **Green Fees** £30 per day (£40 weekends and bank holidays). 🏌 **Prof** Tony Taylor **Course Designer** Hawtree & Son
Facilities 🏌🍴🛒🗄🍷🍸🚶🏨🏌🏌 **Conf** Corporate Hospitality Days
Location SE side of town centre off A523
Hotel ★★★ 75% HL Best Western Hollin Hall, Jackson Ln, Kerridge, Bollington, MACCLESFIELD ☎ 01625 573246   54 en suite

Shrigley Hall Hotel Shrigley Park, Pott Shrigley SK10 5SB
☎ 01625 575626 📄 01625 575437
e-mail: shrigleyhall@paramount-hotels.co.uk
web: www.shrigleyhall.co.uk

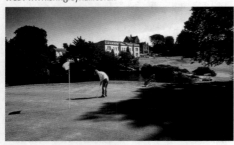

18 holes, 6281yds, Par 71, SSS 71, Course record 68.
Course Designer Donald Steel **Location** Off A523 Macclesfield-Stockport road
Telephone for further details
Hotel ★★★★ 74% HL Shrigley Hall Hotel Golf & Country Club, Shrigley Park, Pott Shrigley, MACCLESFIELD ☎ 01625 575757   150 en suite

Tytherington Dorchester Way, Tytherington SK10 2JP
☎ 01625 506000 📄 01625 506040
e-mail: tytherington.events@clubhaus.com
web: www.clubhaus.com
18 holes, 6765yds, Par 72, SSS 74.
Course Designer Dave Thomas/Patrick Dawson **Location** 1m N of Macclesfield off A523
Telephone for further details
Hotel ★★★★ 74% HL Shrigley Hall Hotel Golf & Country Club, Shrigley Park, Pott Shrigley, MACCLESFIELD ☎ 01625 575757   150 en suite

NANTWICH
MAP 07 SJ65

Reaseheath Reaseheath College CW5 6DF
☎ 01270 625131 📄 01270 625665
e-mail: chrisb@reaseheath.ac.uk
web: www.reaseheath.ac.uk
The course here is attached to Reaseheath College, which is one of the major centres of green-keeper training in the UK. It is a short nine-hole parkland course with challenging narrow fairways, bunkers and a water hazard, all of which make accuracy essential.
9 holes, 1882yds, Par 62, SSS 58, Course record 55.
Club membership 600.
Visitors Mon-Sun & BHs. Booking required. Dress code. **Societies** Booking required. **Green Fees** £10 per day (£8 Oct-Mar). 🏌 **Course Designer** D Mortram **Facilities** 🚶 **Conf** facs **Location** 1.5m NE of Nantwich, off A51
Hotel ★★★★ 84% HL Rookery Hall, Main Rd, Worleston, NANTWICH
☎ 01270 610016   30 en suite   16 annexe en suite

OSCROFT
MAP 07 SJ56

Pryors Hayes Willington Rd CH3 8NL
☎ 01829 741250 & 740140 📄 01829 749077
e-mail: info@pryors-hayes.co.uk
web: www.pryorshayes.com
A picturesque 18-hole parkland course set in the heart of Cheshire. Gently undulating fairways demand accurate drives, and numerous trees and water hazards make the course a challenging test of golf.
18 holes, 6054yds, Par 69, SSS 69, Course record 65.
Club membership 530.
Visitors Mon-Sun & BHs. Booking required. Dress code. **Societies** Booking required. **Green Fees** £30 per round (£40 weekends). **Prof** Martin Redrup
Course Designer John Day **Facilities** 🏌🍴🛒🗄🍷🍸🚶🏨🏌🏌
Location Between A51 & A54, 6m E of Chester
Hotel ★★★ 71% HL Macdonald Blossoms Hotel, St John St, CHESTER
☎ 0870 400 8108   64 en suite

POYNTON
MAP 07 SJ98

Davenport Worth Hall, Middlewood Rd SK12 1TS
☎ 01625 876951 📄 01625 877489
e-mail: elaine@davenportgolf.co.uk
web: www.davenportgolf.co.uk
Gently undulating parkland. Extensive view over the Cheshire plain from elevated 18th tee. Testing 1st hole, Par 4. Several long Par 3s, water hazards and tree-lined fairways make this a challenging test of golf.
18 holes, 6034yds, Par 69, SSS 69, Course record 64.
Club membership 700.

Continued

Visitors Mon-Sun & BHs. Advance booking required. Handicap certificate required. Dress code. **Societies** Booking required. **Green Fees** Phone. ⊕ **Prof** Tony Stevens **Facilities** ⑪ by prior arrangement ⑩ by prior arrangement ⬛ ⬜⬛⬜ ⬛ ⬛ ⬛ **Leisure** snooker. **Conf** facs Corporate Hospitality Days **Location** 1m E off A523
Hotel ★★★ 75% HL Best Western Moorside Grange Hotel & Spa, Mudhurst Ln, Higher Disley, DISLEY ☎ 01663 764151 98 en suite

PRESTBURY — MAP 07 SJ97

Prestbury Macclesfield Rd SK10 4BJ
☎ 01625 828241 ▤ 01625 828241
e-mail: office@prestburygolfclub.com
web: www.prestburygolfclub.com
Undulating parkland with many plateau greens. The 9th hole has a challenging uphill three-tier green and the 17th is over a valley. Host to county and inter-county championships, including hosting an Open qualifying event annually until 2008.

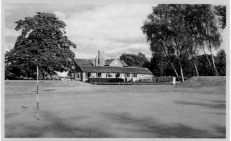

18 holes, 6371yds, Par 71, SSS 71, Course record 64.
Club membership 730.
Visitors Mon-Fri except BHs. Booking required Tue & Thu. Dress code.
Societies Booking required. **Green Fees** £50 per day. **Prof** Nick Summerfield **Course Designer** Harry S Colt **Facilities** ⑪ ⑩ ⬛ ⬜⬛⬜ ⬛ ⬛ ⬛ **Conf** Corporate Hospitality Days **Location** S side of village off A538
Hotel ★★★★ 80% HL De Vere Mottram Hall, Wilmslow Rd, Mottram St Andrew, Prestbury, WILMSLOW ☎ 01625 828135 131 en suite

RUNCORN — MAP 07 SJ58

Runcorn Clifton Rd WA7 4SU
☎ 01928 574214 ▤ 01928 574214
e-mail: secretary@runcorngolfclub.ltd.uk
Easy walking parkland with tree-lined fairways. Fine views over Mersey and Weaver valleys. Testing holes: 7th Par 5; 14th Par 5; 17th Par 4.
18 holes, 6048yds, Par 69, SSS 69, Course record 63.
Club membership 570.
Visitors Mon & Wed-Fri except BHs. Booking required. Handicap certificate required. Dress code. **Societies** Booking required. **Green Fees** Phone. ⊕ **Prof** Kevin Hartley **Facilities** ⑪ ⑩ by prior arrangement ⬛ ⬜⬛⬜ ⬛ ⬛ ⬛ **Location** 1.25m S of Runcorn Station

SANDBACH — MAP 07 SJ76

Malkins Bank Betchton Rd, Malkins Bank CW11 4XN
☎ 01270 765931 ▤ 01270 764730
e-mail: phil.pleasance@congleton.gov.uk
web: www.congleton.gov.uk
This parkland course has a different challenge around every corner. The four Par 3s on the course are all a challenge, especially the signature hole 14th. Trees in all directions make the short Par 3 a really exciting hole. In fact, holes 12, 13 and 14 are the Amen Corner of Malkins Bank. Three very tricky holes, yet for straight hitters low scores are possible.
18 holes, 6005yds, Par 70, SSS 69, Course record 65.
Club membership 500.
Visitors may play Mon-Sun & BHs. Booking required. Dress code. **Societies** Booking required. **Green Fees** £11 per 18 holes (£13per 18 holes, £9.50 per 9 holes Sat & Sun). **Prof** D Hackney **Course Designer** Hawtree **Facilities** ⑪ ⑩ ⬛ ⬜⬛⬜ ⬛ ⬛ ⬛ **Location** 1.5m SE off A533
Hotel ★★★ 70% HL The Chimney House Hotel, Congleton Rd, SANDBACH ☎ 0870 609 6164 48 en suite

SANDIWAY — MAP 07 SJ67

Sandiway Chester Rd CW8 2DJ
☎ 01606 883247 (Secretary) ▤ 01606 888548
e-mail: info@sandiwaygolf.fsnet.co.uk
web: www.sandiwaygolf.co.uk
Delightful undulating wood and heathland course with long hills up to the 8th, 16th and 17th holes. Many dog-leg and tree-lined holes give opportunities for the deliberate fade or draw. True championship test and one of the finest inland courses in north-west England.
18 holes, 6404yds, Par 70, SSS 71, Course record 65.
Club membership 750.
Visitors Mon-Sun & BHs. Handicap certificate. Dress code. **Societies** Booking required. **Green Fees** £55 per day, £45 per round (£60 per round weekends). ⊕ **Prof** William Laird **Course Designer** Ted Ray **Facilities** ⑪ ⑩ ⬛ ⬜⬛⬜ ⬛ ⬛ ⬛ **Conf** Corporate Hospitality Days **Location** 2m W of Northwich on A556
Hotel ★★★★ HL Nunsmere Hall Country House Hotel, Tarporley Rd, SANDIWAY ☎ 01606 889100 36 en suite

SUTTON WEAVER — MAP 07 SJ57

Sutton Hall Aston Ln WA7 3ED
☎ 01928 790747 ▤ 01928 759174
Undulating parkland on south-facing slopes of the Weaver valley. A challenge to all levels of play.
18 holes, 6608yards, Par 72, SSS 72, Course record 69.
Club membership 750.
Visitors Booking required. **Societies** Welcome. **Green Fees** Phone. **Prof** Jamie Hope **Course Designer** Ace Golf Associates **Facilities** ⑪ ⑩ ⬛ ⬜⬛⬜ ⬛ ⬛ ⬛ **Location** M56 junct 12, follow signs for A56 to Warrington, on entering Sutton Weaver take 1st turn right
Hotel ★★★ 77% HL Forest Hills Hotel & Leisure Complex, Overton Hill, FRODSHAM ☎ 01928 735255 58 en suite

England

TARPORLEY MAP 07 SJ56

Portal Golf & Country Club Cobbler's Cross Ln
CW6 0DJ
☎ 01829 733933 📠 01829 733928
e-mail: portalgolf@aol.com

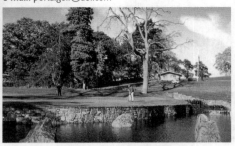

Championship Course: 18 holes, 7037yds, Par 73, SSS 74,
Course record 64.
Premier Course: 18 holes, 6508yds, Par 71, SSS 72,
Course record 64.
Arderne Course: 9 holes, 1724yds, Par 30.
Course Designer Donald Steel **Location** Off A49
Telephone for further details
Hotel ★★★ 72% HL The Wild Boar, Whitchurch Rd, Beeston, TARPORLEY
☎ 01829 260309 37 en suite

WARRINGTON MAP 07 SJ68

Birchwood Kelvin Close, Science Park North, Birchwood
WA3 7PB
☎ 01925 818819 (Club) & 816574 (Pro) 📠 01925 822403
e-mail: birchwoodgolfclub.com@lineone.net
web: www.birchwoodgolfclub.org
Pilgrims: 18 holes, 6727yds, Par 71, SSS 73,
Course record 66.
Progress: 18 holes, 6359yds, Par 71, SSS 72.
Mayflower (ladies course): 18 holes, 5849yds, Par 74,
SSS 74.
Course Designer T J A Macauley **Location** M62 junct 11, signs for Science
Park North, course 2m
Telephone for further details
Hotel ★★★ 75% HL The Rhinewood Country House Hotel, Glazebrook
Ln, Glazebrook, WARRINGTON ☎ 0161 775 5555 32 en suite

Leigh Kenyon Hall, Broseley Ln, Culcheth WA3 4BG
☎ 01925 762943 (Secretary) 📠 01925 765097
e-mail: golf@leighgolf.fsnet.co.uk
web: www.leighgolf.co.uk
This compact parkland course has benefited in recent years from
intensive tree planting and extra drainage. An interesting course to
play with narrow fairways making accuracy from the tees essential.
18 holes, 5853yds, Par 69, SSS 69, Course record 64.
Club membership 850.
Visitors Mon-Sun & BHs. Booking required. Dress code **Societies**
Booking required. **Green Fees** Summer: £30 per day, £28 per 18 holes.
Winter £15 per 18 holes. ☻ **Prof** Andrew Baguley **Course Designer**
Harold Hilton **Facilities** ⑪ ◖◍ ⓑ ◰ 甲 ⓵ ◮ 🖴 ℰ **Conf** Corporate
Hospitality Days **Location** 5m NE off A579
Hotel ★★★ 77% HL Best Western Fir Grove Hotel, Knutsford Old Rd,
WARRINGTON ☎ 01925 267471 52 en suite

Poulton Park Dig Ln, Cinnamon Brow, Padgate WA2 0SH
☎ 01925 822802 & 825220 📠 01925 822802
e-mail: secretary@poultonparkgolfclub.com
web: www.poultonparkgolfclub.co.uk
A short but rather testing course which runs between houses and the
motorway embankment. Easy walking with water coming into play
on four holes, which together with trees and out of bounds require
straight hitting. The 7th/16th hole has a brook in front of the green
which demands respect or you may lose your ball. The 4th, 13th
and 17th can also wreck a scorecard. If you can play well here, you
should be able to play well anywhere.
9 holes, 5587yds, Par 68, SSS 67, Course record 66.
Club membership 350.
Visitors Mon-Sun & BHs. Booking required Tue, Sat, Sun & BHs. Dress code.
Societies Booking required. **Green Fees** £20 per day, £18 winter (£22
Sat, Sun & BHs). ☻ **Prof** Ian Orrell **Facilities** ⑪ ◖◍ ⓑ ◰ 甲 ⓵ ◮ 🖴 ℰ
Conf Corporate Hospitality Days **Location** M6 junct 12, follow Woolston
Grange Av parallel to motorway across 6 rdbts onto Crab Lane. Cross mini-
rdbt and car park on right. M62 junct 11, follow A574 to Warrington. Cross
M6 and turn right into Crab Lane.
Hotel ★★★ 77% HL Best Western Fir Grove Hotel, Knutsford Old Rd,
WARRINGTON ☎ 01925 267471 52 en suite

Walton Hall Warrington Rd, Higher Walton WA4 5LU
☎ 01925 263061 (bookings) 📠 01925 263061
Set in a picturesque parkland setting with fine views from the 13th tee.
It has many mature trees, and a lot of water comes into play on seven
of the holes. Three Par 3s are over 200yds.
18 holes, 6647yds, Par 72, SSS 73, Course record 70.
Club membership 250.
Visitors may play Mon-Sun & BHs. Advance booking required. Dress
code. **Societies** must contact in writing. **Green Fees** not confirmed.
☻ **Prof** John Jackson **Course Designer** Peter Alliss/Dave Thomas
Facilities ⑪ ◰ 甲 ⓵ ◮ 🖴 ◆ **Location** M56 junct 11, 2m
Hotel ★★★★ 77% HL De Vere Daresbury Park, Chester Rd, Daresbury,
WARRINGTON ☎ 01925 267331 183 en suite

Warrington Hill Warren, London Rd, Appleton WA4 5HR
☎ 01925 261775 (Secretary) 📠 01925 265933
e-mail: secretary@warrington-golf-club.co.uk
web: www.warrington-golf-club.co.uk
18 holes, 6305yds, Par 72, SSS 70, Course record 61.
Course Designer James Braid **Location** M56 junct 10, 1.5m N on A49
Telephone for further details
Hotel ★★★★ 77% HL The Park Royal Hotel, Stretton Rd, Stretton,
WARRINGTON ☎ 01925 730706 146 en suite

WIDNES MAP 07 SJ58

Mersey Valley Golf & Country Club Warrington Rd,
Bold Heath WA8 3XL
☎ 0151 4246060 📠 0151 2579097
e-mail: chrismgerrard@yahoo.co.uk
web: www.merseyvalley golfclub.co.uk
Parkland with very easy walking.
18 holes, 6374yards, Par 72, SSS 71, Course record 68.
Club membership 500.
Visitors may play Mon-Sun & BHs. Advance booking required. Dress
code. **Societies** Booking required. **Green Fees** £30 per day, £20 per round
(£40/£25 weekends and bank holidays). **Prof** Andy Stevenson **Course
Designer** R Bush **Facilities** ⑪ ⓑ ◰ 甲 ⓵ ◮ 🖴 ℰ ◆ ℰ **Leisure** fishing.
Continued

Conf facs Corporate Hospitality Days **Location** M62 junct 7, A57 towards Warrington, club 2m on left
Hotel ★★★ 67% HL The Hillcrest Hotel, 75 Cronton Ln, WIDNES
☎ 0870 609 6174   50 en suite

St Michael Jubilee Dundalk Rd WA8 8BS
☎ 0151 424 6230 ▤ 0151 495 2124
e-mail: dchapmam@aol.com
18 holes, 5925yds, Par 69, SSS 67.
Location W side of town centre off A562
Telephone for further details
Hotel BUD Travelodge Widnes, Fiddlers Ferry Rd, WIDNES
☎ 08700 850 950   32 en suite

Widnes Highfield Rd WA8 7DT
☎ 0151 424 2440 & 424 2995 ▤ 0151 495 2849
e-mail: email@widnes-golfclub.co.uk
web: www.widnes-golfclub.co.uk
18 holes, 5719yds, Par 69, SSS 68, Course record 64.
Location M62 junct 7, A57 to Warrington, right at lights onto Wilmere Ln, right at T-junct. 1st left at rdbt onto Birchfield Rd, right after 3rd pelican crossing onto Highfield Rd, right before lights
Telephone for further details
Hotel BUD Travelodge Widnes, Fiddlers Ferry Rd, WIDNES
☎ 08700 850 950   32 en suite

WILMSLOW   MAP 07 SJ88

De Vere Mottram Hall Wilmslow Rd, Mottram St Andrew SK10 4QT
☎ 01625 828135 ▤ 01625 829312
e-mail: dmhgolf@devere-hotels.com
web: www.deveregolf.co.uk
Championship-standard course - flat meadowland on the front nine and undulating woodland on the back nine, with well-guarded greens. The course is unusual as each half opens and closes with Par 5s. Good test for both professional and novice golfers alike.
18 holes, 7006yds, Par 72, SSS 74, Course record 63.
Club membership 250.
Visitors may play Mon-Sun & BHs. Advance booking required. Handicap certificate required. Dress code. **Societies** advance notice required. **Green Fees** not confirmed. **Prof** Matthew Turnock **Course Designer** Dave Thomas **Facilities** ⑪ ⑩ ⓛ ☐ ⑪ ☖ ☎ ☖ ◇ ✦ ▨ ✦ **Leisure** hard tennis courts, heated indoor swimming pool, squash, sauna, solarium, gymnasium, day store & drying room, satellite navigation buggies. **Conf** facs Corporate Hospitality Days **Location** On A538 between Wilmslow and Prestbury
Hotel ★★★★ 80% HL De Vere Mottram Hall, Wilmslow Rd, Mottram St Andrew, Prestbury, WILMSLOW ☎ 01625 828135   131 en suite

Styal Station Rd, Styal SK9 4JN
☎ 01625 531359 ▤ 01625 416373
e-mail: gtraynor@styalgolf.co.uk
web: www.styalgolf.co.uk
Well-designed flat parkland course with USGA specification greens. Challenging and enjoyable test for all standards of golfer. The Par 3 course is widely regarded as one of the finest short courses in the country.
18 holes, 6238yds, Par 70, SSS 70, Course record 63.
Club membership 800.
Visitors Mon-Sun & BHs. Booking required.Sat, Sun & BHs. Dress code.
Societies Booking required. **Green Fees** £23 per round (£28 weekends).

Prof Simon Forrest **Course Designer** Tony Holmes **Facilities** ⑪ ⑩ ⓛ ☐ ⑪ ☖ ☎ ◇ ✦ ▨ ✦ **Leisure** Par 3 9 hole course. **Conf** facs Corporate Hospitality Days **Location** M56 junct 5, 5 mins from Wilmslow/Manchester Airport
Hotel ★★★ 72% HL Best Western Belfry House Hotel, Stanley Rd, HANDFORTH ☎ 0161 437 0511   81 en suite

Wilmslow Great Warford, Mobberley WA16 7AY
☎ 01565 872148 ▤ 01565 872172
e-mail: info@wilmslowgolfclub.co.uk
web: www.wilmslowgolfclub.co.uk
Peaceful parkland in the heart of the Cheshire countryside offering golf for all levels.
18 holes, 6607yds, Par 72, SSS 72, Course record 62.
Club membership 800.
Visitors contact club for details. Handicap certificate required. Dress code. **Societies** advance booking required. **Green Fees** not confirmed.
Prof John Nowicki **Facilities** ⑪ ⑩ ⓛ ☐ ⑪ ☖ ☎ ☖ ◇ ✦ **Conf** Corporate Hospitality Days **Location** 2m SW off B5058
Hotel ★★★ 83% HL Alderley Edge Hotel, Macclesfield Rd, ALDERLEY EDGE ☎ 01625 583033   50 en suite

WINSFORD   MAP 07 SJ66

Knights Grange Grange Ln CW7 2PT
☎ 01606 552780
e-mail: knightsgrangewinsford@valeroyal.gov.uk
web: www.valeroyal.gov.uk/leisure
An 18-hole course set in beautiful Cheshire countryside on the town outskirts. The front nine is mainly flat but players have to negotiate water, ditches and other hazards along the way. The back nine takes the player deep into the countryside, with many of the tees offering panoramic views. A lake known as the Ocean is a feature of many holes - a particular hazard for slicers of the ball. There are also many mature woodland areas to catch the wayward drive.
18 holes, 5921yds, Par 70, SSS 68.
Visitors Mon-Sun & BHs. **Societies** Booking required **Green Fees** £9.80 per 18 holes (£12 weekends). **Course Designer** Steve Dawson **Facilities** ☐ ☖ ⑪ ✦ **Leisure** hard and grass tennis courts. **Location** N side of town off A54
Hotel BUD Travelodge Middlewich, MIDDLEWICH ☎ 08700 850 950   32 en suite

WINWICK   MAP 07 SJ69

Alder Root Alder Root Ln WA2 8R2
☎ 01925 291919 ▤ 01925 291961
e-mail: admin@alderroot.wanadoo.co.uk
web: www.alderroot.com
A woodland course, flat in nature but with many undulations. Several holes have water hazards. One of the most testing nine-hole courses in the north-west.
9 holes, 5837yds, Par 69, SSS 68, Course record 67.
Club membership 400.
Visitors Mon-Sun & BHs. Booking required Sat, Sun & BHs. Dress code.
Societies Welcome. **Green Fees** Phone. **Prof** C McKevitt **Course Designer** Mr Lander/Mr Millington **Facilities** ⑪ ⓛ ☐ ⑪ ☖ ☎ ◇ ✦ **Location** M62 junct 9, A49 N for 800yds, left at lights right into Alder Root Ln
Hotel ★★ 74% HL Paddington House Hotel, 514 Old Manchester Rd, WARRINGTON ☎ 01925 816767   37 en suite

CORNWALL & ISLES OF SCILLY

BODMIN   MAP 02 SX06

Lanhydrock Hotel Lostwithiel Rd PL30 5AQ
☎ 01208 262570 📄 01208 262579
e-mail: info@lanhydrockhotel.com
web: www.lanhydrockhotel.com
An acclaimed parkland and moorland course adjacent to the National
Trust property of Lanhydrock House. Nestling in a picturesque wooded
valley of oak and birch, this undulating course provides an exciting and
enjoyable challenge.

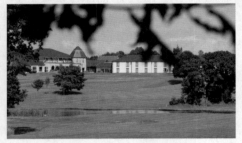

18 holes, 6100yds, Par 70, SSS 70, Course record 66.
Club membership 300.
Visitors Mon-Sun & BHs. Booking required. Dress code. **Societies** Booking
required. **Green Fees** £45 per day, £22-£32 per round. **Prof** Colin Willis
Course Designer Hamilton Stutt **Facilities** ⑪ ⑩ ⬛ ⬜ ⅋ ⬜ ⬛ ♻
⬛ ⅋ ⅀ **Conf** facs Corporate Hospitality Days **Location** 1m S of Bodmin
off B3268
Hotel ★★★ 73% HL Best Western Restormel Lodge Hotel, Castle Hill,
LOSTWITHIEL ☎ 01208 872223 24 en suite 12 annexe en suite

BUDE   MAP 02 SS20

Bude & North Cornwall Burn View EX23 8DA
☎ 01288 352006 📄 01288 356855
e-mail: secretary@budegolf.co.uk
web: www.budegolf.co.uk
A traditional links course established in 1891. Situated in the centre
of Bude with magnificent views to the sea. A challenging course with
super greens and excellent drainage enables course to be playable
throughout the year off regular tees and greens.
18 holes, 6057yds, Par 71, SSS 70. Club membership 800.
Visitors Mon-Sun & BHs. Dress code. **Societies** Booking required.
Green Fees £27 per day (£27 per round weekends & bank holidays).
Prof John Yeo **Course Designer** Tom Dunn **Facilities** ⑪ ⑩ ⬛ ⬜ ⅋ ⬜ ⬛
⬛ ⅋ ⬛ ⅋ **Leisure** snooker room. **Conf** facs Corporate Hospitality Days
Location N side of town

Hotel ★★★ 74% HL Camelot Hotel, Downs View, BUDE ☎ 01288 352361
24 en suite

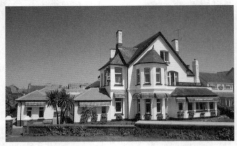

BUDOCK VEAN   MAP 02 SW73

Budock Vean Hotel on the River Mawnan Smith
TR11 5LG
☎ 01326 252102 (shop) 📄 01326 250892
e-mail: relax@budockvean.co.uk
web: www.budockvean.co.uk
Set in 65 acres of mature grounds with a private foreshore to the
Helford River, this 18-tee undulating parkland course has a tough
Par 4 5th hole (456yds) which dog-legs at halfway around an oak tree.
The 16th hole measures 572yds, Par 5.

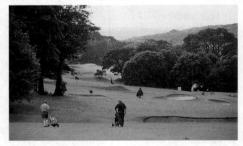

9 holes, 5255yds, Par 68, SSS 66, Course record 58.
Club membership 200.
Visitors Mon-Sun & BHs. Booking required. Handicap certificate. Dress
code. **Societies** Booking required. **Green Fees** £23 per day (£27 Sat,
Sun & BHs). **Prof** Tony Ramsden/David Short **Course Designer** James
Braid **Facilities** ⑪ ⑩ by prior arrangement ⬛ ⬜ ⅋ ⬜ ⬛ ♻ ⅋
⬛ ⅋ **Leisure** hard tennis courts, heated indoor swimming pool, fishing,
sauna, boating facilities, health spa, outdoor hot tub. **Conf** facs Corporate
Hospitality Days **Location** 1.5m SW of Mawnan Smith
Hotel ★★★★ 71% CHH Budock Vean-The Hotel on the River, MAWNAN
SMITH ☎ 01326 252100 & 0800 833927 📄 01326 250892 57 en suite

CAMBORNE   MAP 02 SW64

Tehidy Park TR14 0HH
☎ 01209 842208 📠 01209 842208
e-mail: secretary-manager@tehidyparkgolfclub.co.uk
web: www.tehidyparkgolfclub.co.uk
A well-maintained parkland course providing good holiday golf and a
challenge for golfers of all abilities.

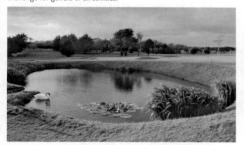

18 holes, 6241yds, Par 71, SSS 71, Course record 62.
Club membership 850.
Visitors Mon-Sun & BHs. Handicap certificate required. Dress code
Societies Booking required. **Green Fees** £25.50 per day (£30.50 weekends
& bank holidays). ☻ **Prof** Jonathan Lamb **Course Designer** C K Cotton
Facilities ⑪ ⑩ 🖢 ☑ 🎱 ⚒ 🖪 ⚒ **Conf** Corporate Hospitality
Days **Location** On Portreath-Pool road, 2m S of Camborne
Hotel ★★★ 77% HL Penventon Park Hotel, REDRUTH ☎ 01209 203000
68 en suite

CAMELFORD   MAP 02 SX18

Bowood Park Hotel Lanteglos PL32 9RF
☎ 01840 213017 📠 01840 212622
e-mail: info@bowoodpark.org
web: www.bowoodpark.org
A rolling parkland course set in 230 acres of ancient deer park once
owned by the Black Prince; 27 lakes and ponds test the golfer and
serve as a haven for wildlife.
18 holes, 6736yds, Par 72, SSS 72, Course record 68.
Club membership 350.
Visitors Mon-Sun & BHs. Booking required. Handicap certificate. Dress
code. **Societies** Booking required. **Green Fees** £40 per day, £30 Apr
& Oct. **Prof** Tony Nash **Course Designer** Sandow **Facilities** ⑪ ⑩ 🖢
☑ 🎱 ⚒ 🖪 ⚒ 🖪 ⚒ **Leisure** fishing. **Conf** facs Corporate
Hospitality Days **Location** Through Camelford, 0.5m turn right Tintagel/
Boscastle B3266, 1st left at garage
Hotel ★★★ 73% HL Bowood Park Hotel & Golf Course, Lanteglos,
CAMELFORD ☎ 01840 213017 31 en suite

CARLYON BAY   MAP 02 SX05

Carlyon Bay Hotel Beach Rd PL25 3RD
☎ 01726 814250 📠 01726 814250
e-mail: golf@carlyonbay.com
web: www.carlyonbay.com
A championship-length, clifftop parkland course, running east
to west and back again - and also uphill and down a fair bit. The
fairways stay in excellent condition all year as they have since the
course was laid down in 1925. Magnificent views from the course

across St Austell Bay; particularly from the 9th green, where an
approach shot remotely to the right will plummet over the cliff edge.

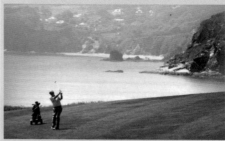

18 holes, 6597yds, Par 72, SSS 71, Course record 63.
Club membership 500.
Visitors may play Mon-Sun & BHs. Booking required. Handicap
certificate. Dress code. **Societies** Booking required. **Green Fees** from
£25-£42 per round depending on season. £10 for extra round. **Prof** Mark
Rowe **Course Designer** Hamilton Stutt **Facilities** ⑪ ⑩ 🖢 ☑ 🎱 ⚒
🖪 ⚒ ⚒ **Leisure** hard tennis courts, outdoor and indoor heated
swimming pools, sauna, solarium, 9 hole Par 3 course. **Conf** Corporate
Hospitality Days **Location** 3m SE of St Austell off A390, signposted
Hotel ★★★★ 80% HL Carlyon Bay Hotel, Sea Rd, Carlyon Bay, ST
AUSTELL ☎ 01726 812304 87 en suite

CONSTANTINE BAY   MAP 02 SW87

Trevose PL28 8JB
☎ 01841 520208 📠 01841 521057
e-mail: info@trevose-gc.co.uk
web: www.trevose-gc.co.uk
Well-known links course with early holes close to the sea on
excellent springy turf. A championship course affording varying
degrees of difficulty appealing to both the professional and higher
handicap player. It is a good test with well-positioned bunkers,
and a meandering stream, and the wind playing a decisive role in
preventing low scoring. Hosts for the English Amateur Stroke Play
championship 2007.

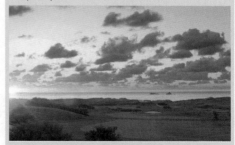

Championship Course: 18 holes, 6863yds, Par 72,
SSS 73, Course record 66. New Course: 9 holes,
3031yds, Par 35. Short Course: 9 holes, 1360yds, Par 29.
Club membership 1650.
Visitors may play Mon-Sun & BHs. Advance booking required. Handicap
certificate required. Dress code. **Societies** advance booking required.
Green Fees not confirmed. **Prof** Gary Lenaghan **Course Designer** H S
Colt **Facilities** ⑪ ⑩ 🖢 ☑ 🎱 ⚒ 🖪 ⚒ ⚒ **Leisure**

Continued

hard tennis courts, heated outdoor swimming pool, self catering accommodation & a la carte restaurant, snooker room. **Conf** facs Corporate Hospitality Days **Location** 4m W of Padstow on B3276, to St Merryn, 500yds past x-rds turn, signed
Hotel ★★★★ 74% HL Treglos Hotel, CONSTANTINE BAY
☎ 01841 520727 42 en suite

FALMOUTH   MAP 02 SW83

Falmouth Swanpool Rd TR11 5BQ
☎ 01326 311262 📠 01326 317783
e-mail: falmouthgc@onetel.com
web: www.falmouthgolfclub.com
Stunning sea and coastal views. The course has been adjusted to make it fairer, while still a good test of golf. Excellent greens and a well-drained course which rarely closes.

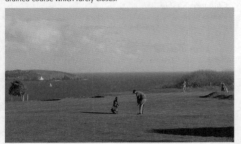

18 holes, 6037yds, Par 71, SSS 70. Club membership 500.
Visitors may play Mon-Sun & BHs. Advance booking required. Dress code. **Societies** advance booking required. **Green Fees** not confirmed. **Prof** Nick Rogers **Facilities** ⑨ ⚑ ▣ ⌨ ⚑ ⚑ ⚑ ⚑ ⚑ ⚑ **Conf** Corporate Hospitality Days **Location** SW of town centre
See advert on opposite page
Hotel ★★★★ 78% HL Royal Duchy Hotel, Cliff Rd, FALMOUTH
☎ 01326 313042 43 en suite

HOLYWELL BAY   MAP 02 SW75

Holywell Bay TR8 5PW
☎ 01637 830095 📠 01637 831000
e-mail: golf@trevornick.co.uk
web: www.holywellbay.co.uk/golf
Situated beside a family fun park with many amenities. The course is an 18-hole Par 3 with excellent sea views. Fresh Atlantic winds make the course hard to play and there are several tricky holes, particularly the 18th over the trout pond. The site also has an excellent 18-hole Pitch and Putt course for the whole family.
18 holes, 2784yds, Par 61, Course record 58. Club membership 100.
Visitors may play Mon-Sun & BHs. **Societies** welcome. **Green Fees** not confirmed. **Course Designer** Hartley **Facilities** ⑨ ⚑ ▣ ⌨ ⚑ ⚑
⚑ **Leisure** heated outdoor swimming pool, fishing, touring & camping facilities. **Location** Off A3075 Newquay-Perranporth road
Hotel ★★★ 72% HL Barrowfield Hotel, Hilgrove Rd, NEWQUAY
☎ 01637 878878 81 en suite

LAUNCESTON   MAP 02 SX38

Launceston St Stephens PL15 8HF
☎ 01566 773442 📠 01566 777506
e-mail: secretarylgc@tiscali.co.uk
web: www.launcestongolfclub.co.uk
Highly rated course with magnificent views over the historic town and moors. Noted for superb greens and lush fairways.
18 holes, 6407yds, Par 70, SSS 71, Course record 65. Club membership 800.
Visitors Mon-Sun & BHs. Handicap certificate required. Dress code. **Societies** Welcome. **Green Fees** £35 per day, £28 per round. **Prof** John Tozer **Course Designer** Hamilton Stutt **Facilities** ⑨ ⚑ ▣ ⌨ ⚑ ⚑ ⚑ ⚑
⚑ ⚑ **Leisure** practice nets. **Conf** facs Corporate Hospitality Days **Location** NW of town centre on B3254
Hotel ★★ 69% SHL Eagle House Hotel, Castle St, LAUNCESTON
☎ 01566 772036 14 en suite

Trethorne Kennards House PL15 8QE
☎ 01566 86903 📠 01566 880925
e-mail: reservations@trethornegolfclub.com
web: www.trethornegolfclub.com
Rolling parkland course with well maintained fairways and computer irrigated greens. Plenty of trees and natural water hazards make this well respected course a good challenge.

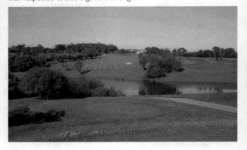

18 holes, 6178yds, Par 71, SSS 71, Course record 69. Club membership 250.
Visitors may play Mon-Sun & BHs. Booking required Sat & Sun. Dress code. **Societies** Booking required. **Green Fees** £22 per round, £32 Sat & Sun. **Prof** Chris Brewer **Course Designer** Frank Frayne **Facilities** ⑨ ⚑
⚑ ▣ ⌨ ⚑ ⚑ ⚑ ⚑ ⚑ ⚑ ⚑ **Leisure** leisure farm and tenpin bowling. **Conf** facs Corporate Hospitality Days **Location** Off junct A30, 3m W of Launceston
Hotel ★★ 69% SHL Eagle House Hotel, Castle St, LAUNCESTON
☎ 01566 772036 14 en suite

LELANT MAP 02 SW53

West Cornwall TR26 3DZ
☎ 01736 753401 📠 01736 758468
e-mail: secretary@westcornwallgolfclub.co.uk
web: www.westcornwallgolfclub.co.uk
A seaside links with sandhills and lovely turf adjacent to the Hayle estuary and St Ives Bay. A real test of the player's skill, especially Calamity Corner starting at the 5th on the lower land by the River Hayle.

18 holes, 5884yds, Par 69, SSS 69, Course record 63.
Club membership 813.
Visitors Mon-Sun & BHs. Handicap certificate required. Dress code.
Societies advance booking required. **Green Fees** £28 per day (£33 weekends & BHs). **Prof** Jason Broadway **Course Designer** Reverend Tyack **Facilities** ⑪ ⑩ ⌁ ☷ ⚑ ⛳ ⚑ ☍ ⚑ **Location** N side of village off A3074

Hotel ★★ 79% HL Pedn-Olva Hotel, West Porthminster Beach, ST IVES ☎ 01736 796222 31 en suite

LOOE MAP 02 SX25

Looe Bindown PL13 1PX
☎ 01503 240239 📠 01503 240864
e-mail: enquiries@looegolfclub.co.uk
web: www.looegolfclub.co.uk
Designed by Harry Vardon in 1935, this downland and parkland course commands panoramic views over south-east Cornwall and the coast. Easy walking.

18 holes, 5940yds, Par 70, SSS 69, Course record 64.
Club membership 420.
Visitors may play Mon-Sun & BHs. Advance booking required. Dress code.
Societies Booking required. **Green Fees** not confirmed. **Prof** Jason Bowen
Course Designer Harry Vardon **Facilities** ⑪ ⌁ ☷ ⚑ ⛳ ⚑ ☍ ⚑ ⛳
Conf Corporate Hospitality Days **Location** 3.5m NE off B3253
Hotel ★★★ 64% HL Hannafore Point Hotel, Marine Dr, West Looe, LOOE ☎ 01503 263273 37 en suite

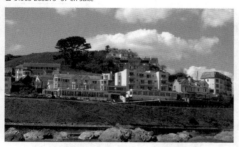

See advert on page 52

LOSTWITHIEL MAP 02 SX15

Lostwithiel Hotel, Golf & Country Club Lower Polscoe
PL22 0HQ
☎ 01208 873550 📠 01208 873479
e-mail: reception@golf-hotel.co.uk
web: www.golf-hotel.co.uk
This 18-hole course is one of the most varied in the county, designed to take full advantage of the natural features of the landscape,
Continued

combining two distinct areas of hillside and valley. The challenging front nine has magnificent views of the surrounding countryside, while the picturesque back nine runs through parkland flanked by the River Fowey.

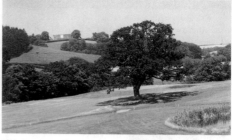

18 holes, 5984yds, Par 72, SSS 71, Course record 67.
Club membership 500.
Visitors Mon-Sun & BHs. Booking required Fr-Sun & BHs. Dress code.
Societies Welcome. **Green Fees** £26 per round (£30 Sat & Sun). Reductions during winter months. **Prof** Andrew Hooper **Course Designer** S Wood **Facilities** ⑪ ⑩ ⌁ ☷ ⚑ ⛳ ⚑ ☍ ⚑ ⛳ **Leisure** hard tennis courts, heated indoor swimming pool, fishing, gymnasium, indoor golf simulator. **Conf** facs Corporate Hospitality Days **Location** 1m from Lostwithiel off A390

Hotel ★★★ 66% HL Lostwithiel Hotel Golf & Country Club, Lower Polscoe, LOSTWITHIEL ☎ 01208 873550 27 en suite

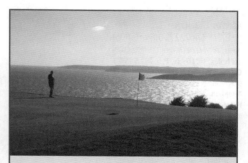

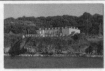
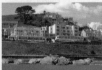
MAWGAN PORTH · MAP 02 SW86

Merlin TR8 4DN
☎ 01841 540222 📠 01841 541031
web: www.merlingolfcourse.co.uk
18 holes, 6210yds, Par 71, SSS 71.
Course Designer Ross Oliver **Location** On Newquay-Padstow coast road.
After Mawgan Porth signs for St Eval, course on right
Telephone for further details
Hotel ★★★★ 75% HL Bedruthan Steps Hotel, MAWGAN PORTH
☎ 01637 860555 & 860860 📠 01637 860714 101 en suite

MULLION · MAP 02 SW61

Mullion Cury TR12 7BP
☎ 01326 240685 (sec) & 241176 (pro) 📠 01326 241527
e-mail: secretary@mulliongolfclub.plus.com
Founded in 1895, a clifftop and links course with panoramic views
over Mounts Bay. A steep downhill slope on 6th and the 10th
descends to the beach with a deep ravine alongside the green.
Second most southerly course in the British Isles.
18 holes, 6083yds, Par 70, SSS 70. Club membership 800.
Visitors Mon-Sun & BHs. Handicap certificate required. Dress code.
Societies Booking required. **Green Fees** £30 per day, £25 per
round (£35/£30 weekends & bank holidays). **Prof** Ian Harris
Course Designer W Sich **Facilities** ⊕ ⃝ ◎ ⑤ ⑤ ⑦ ⑦ ⃝ ⑤ ⑤ ⑤
Leisure indoor computerised teaching academy. **Location** 1.5m NW of
Mullion, off A3083
Hotel ★★★ 77% HL Polurrian Hotel, MULLION ☎ 01326 240441
39 en suite

NEWQUAY · MAP 02 SW86

Newquay Tower Rd TR7 1LT
☎ 01637 874354 📠 01637 874066
e-mail: newquaygolf@btconnect.com
web: www.newquaygolfclub.co.uk
One of Cornwall's finest seaside links with magnificent views over the
Atlantic Ocean. Open to the unpredictable nature of the elements and
possessing some very demanding greenside bunkers, the prerequisite
for good scoring at Newquay is accuracy.
18 holes, 6150yds, Par 69, SSS 69, Course record 63.
Club membership 600.
Visitors contact club for details. Handicap certificate required. Dress code.
Societies Booking required. **Green Fees** £30 per day; £25 per round
(£30 per round weekends and bank holidays). **Prof** Mark Bevan **Course
Designer** H Colt **Facilities** ⊕ ⃝ ◎ ⑤ ⑤ ⑦ ⑤ ⑤ ⑤ ⑤ ⑤ **Leisure** Snooker.
Conf Corporate Hospitality Days **Location** W side of town
Hotel ★★★ 78% HL Best Western Hotel Bristol, Narrowcliff, NEWQUAY
☎ 01637 875181 74 en suite

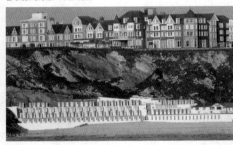

PADSTOW

See **Constantine Bay**

PERRANPORTH · MAP 02 SW75

Perranporth Budnic Hill TR6 0AB
☎ 01872 573701
e-mail: office.pgc@tiscali.co.uk
web: www.perranporthgolfclub.com
There are three testing Par 5 holes on the links course (2nd, 5th, 11th).
This seaside links course has magnificent views of the North Cornwall
coastline, and excellent greens. The drainage of the course, being
sand-based, is also exceptional.

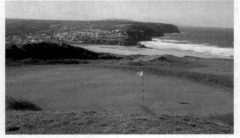

18 holes, 6272yds, Par 72, SSS 72, Course record 62.
Club membership 650.

Continued

Visitors Mon-Sun & BHs. Booking required. Dress code. **Societies** Booking required. **Green Fees** £30 per round (£35 per round weekends and bank holidays). Additional £5 for extra holes. **Prof** D Michell **Course Designer** James Braid **Facilities** ⑪ ⎀ 🍴 📶 ☐ ﹂ 🏌 🚶 ◇ ✔ 🏌 ✔ **Conf** Corporate Hospitality Days **Location** 0.75m NE on B3285
Hotel ★★★ 70% HL Rosemundy House Hotel, Rosemundy Hill, ST AGNES
☎ 01872 552101 46 en suite

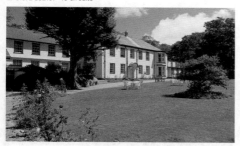

PORTWRINKLE   MAP 02 SX45

Whitsand Bay Hotel Golf & Country Club PL11 3BU
☎ 01503 230276 ▤ 01503 230329
e-mail: whitsandbayhotel@btconnect.com
web: www.whitsandbayhotel.co.uk
Testing seaside course laid out on cliffs overlooking Whitsand Bay. Easy walking after first hole. The Par 3 3rd hole is acknowledged as one of the most attractive holes in Cornwall.
18 holes, 6030yds, Par 69, SSS 68, Course record 62.
Club membership 400.
Visitors may play Mon-Sun & BHs. Dress code. **Societies** Booking required. **Green Fees** £22 per round (£28 weekends). **Prof** Steve Dougan **Course Designer** Fernie **Facilities** ⑪ ⎀ 🍴 📶 ☐ ﹂ 🏌 🚶 🏌 ✔ 🚶 ✔ **Leisure** heated indoor swimming pool, sauna, solarium, gymnasium, spa centre.
Conf Corporate Hospitality Days **Location** from Tamar Bridge, turn left at Treulefoot roundabout for Polbathic. After 2m turn right to Crafthole then Portwrinkle. Golf course on right.
Hotel ★★★ 74% HL Whitsand Bay Hotel & Golf Club, PORTWRINKLE
☎ 01503 230276 32 en suite

PRAA SANDS

Praa Sands Germoe Cross Roads TR20 9TQ
☎ 01736 763445 ▤ 01736 763399
e-mail: praasandsgolf@aol.com
A beautiful parkland course, overlooking Mount's Bay with outstanding sea views from every tee and green.

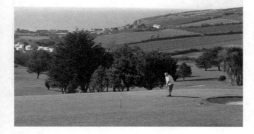

---

9 holes, 4122yds, Par 62, SSS 60, Course record 59.
Club membership 220.
Visitors contact club for details. **Societies** welcome. **Green Fees** not confirmed. ⊕ **Course Designer** R Hamilton **Facilities** ⑪ ⎀ 🍴 ☐ ﹂ 🏌 🚶 🏌 ✔ **Leisure** pool, darts. **Location** A394 between Penzance & Helston
Inn ★★★★ INN Harbour Inn, Commercal Rd, PORTHLEVEN
☎ 01326 573876 10 en suite

ROCK   MAP 02 SW97

St Enodoc PL27 6LD
☎ 01208 863216 ▤ 01208 862976
e-mail: enquiries@st-enodoc.co.uk
web: www.st-enodoc.co.uk
Classic links course with huge sand hills and rolling fairways. James Braid laid out the original 18 holes in 1907 and changes were made in 1922 and 1935. On the Church, the 10th is the toughest Par 4 on the course and on the 6th is a truly enormous sand hill known as the Himalayas. The Holywell is not as exacting as the Church; it is less demanding on stamina but still a real test of skill for golfers of any handicap.
Church Course: 18 holes, 6406yds, Par 69, SSS 70, Course record 64.
Holywell Course: 18 holes, 4142yds, Par 63, SSS 61.
Club membership 1300.
Visitors may play Mon-Fri, Sun & BHS. Handicap certificate required.
Societies advance booking required. **Green Fees** Church Course:£65 per day, £50 per round (£60 per round Sun). Holywell Course: £25 per day, £16 per round. **Prof** Nick Williams **Course Designer** James Braid **Facilities** ⑪ ⎀ 🍴 ☐ ﹂ 🏌 🚶 🏌 ✔ ✔ 🚩 **Location** W side of village
Hotel ★★★ 70% HL Old Custom House Inn, South Quay, PADSTOW
☎ 01841 532359 24 en suite

ST AUSTELL   MAP 02 SX05

Porthpean Porthpean PL26 6AY
☎ 01726 64613 ▤ 01726 71643
e-mail: ktuckerpgc@aol.com
web: www.porthpean-golf.co.uk
18 holes, 5210yds, Par 67, SSS 66.
Location 1.5m from St Austell bypass
Telephone for further details
Hotel ★★ 78% HL The Pier House, Harbour Front, Charlestown, ST AUSTELL ☎ 01726 67955 28 en suite

St Austell Tregongeeves Ln PL26 7DS
☎ 01726 74756 📠 01726 71978
18 holes, 6089yds, Par 69, SSS 69, Course record 64.
Location 1m W of St Austell on A390
Telephone for further details
Hotel ★★★ 77% HL Porth Avallen Hotel, Sea Rd, Carlyon Bay, ST AUSTELL
☎ 01726 812802 28 en suite

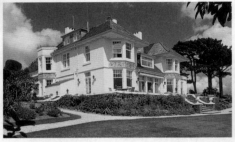

Porth Avallen Hotel

Hotel ★★★★ BB Wisteria Lodge, Boscundle, Tregrehan, ST AUSTELL
☎ 01726 810800 Fax 0871 661 6213 5 en suite

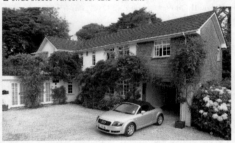

Wisteria Lodge

ST IVES
MAP 02 SW54

Tregenna Castle Hotel, Golf & Country Club
TR26 2DE
☎ 01736 797381 📠 01736 796066
e-mail: hotel@tregenna-castle.co.uk
web: www.tregenna-castle.co.uk
Parkland course surrounding a castellated hotel and overlooking St Ives Bay and harbour.
14 holes, 1846yds, Par 42, SSS 42. Club membership 140.
Visitors Mon-Sun & BHs. **Societies** Welcome. **Green Fees** £15 per round.
Course Designer Abercrombie **Facilities** ⑪ 🎱 ⚑ 🏊 🖥 🍴 🕯 ⚕ ◇ ✐
Leisure hard tennis courts, outdoor and indoor heated swimming pools, squash, sauna, solarium, gymnasium, badminton court, spa. **Conf** facs Corporate Hospitality Days **Location** Off A30 past Hayle onto A3074
Hotel ★★★ 71% HL Tregenna Castle Hotel, ST IVES ☎ 01736 795254
81 en suite

ST JUST (NEAR LAND'S END) MAP 02 SW33

Cape Cornwall Golf & Country Club Cape Cornwall
TR19 7NL
☎ 01736 788611 📠 01736 788611
e-mail: info@capecornwall.com
web: www.capecornwall.com

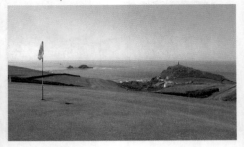

18 holes, 5632yds, Par 69, SSS 68, Course record 64.
Course Designer Bob Hamilton **Location** 1m W of St Just
Telephone for further details
Hotel ★★ 69% HL The Old Success Inn, Sennen Cove, SENNEN
☎ 01736 871232 12 en suite

ST MELLION
MAP 02 SX36

St Mellion Hotel, Golf & Country Club see page 55

Hotel ★★★ 72% HL St Mellion International, ST MELLION
☎ 01579 351351 39 annexe en suite
Hotel ★★ 81% HL The Well House Hotel, St Keyne, LISKEARD
☎ 01579 342001 Fax 01579 343891 9 en suite
Hotel ★★★ 67% HL China Fleet Country Club, SALTASH ☎ 01752 848668
Fax 01752 848456 40 en suite

ST MINVER
MAP 02 SW97

Roserrow Golf & Country Club Roserrow PL27 6QT
☎ 01208 863000 📠 01208 863002
e-mail: info@roserrow.co.uk
web: www.roserrow.co.uk/golf
Challenging Par 72 course in an undulating wooded valley.
Stunning views over the Cornish countryside and out to Hayle Bay.
Accommodation and numerous facilities on site.

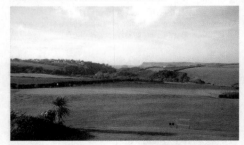

18 holes, 6551yds, Par 72, SSS 72, Course record 68.
Club membership 450.

Continued

CHAMPIONSHIP COURSE

ST MELLION

Map 02 SX36

PL12 6SD
☎ **01579 351351** 📠 **01579 350537**
e-mail: **stmellion@crown-golf.co.uk**
web: **www.st-mellion.co.uk**
Nicklaus Course: 18 holes, 6592yds, Par 72, SSS 74, Course record 63.
The Old Course: 18 holes, 5782yds, Par 68, SSS 68, Course record 60.
Club membership 1000.
Visitors Mon-Sun & BHs. Advance booking required. Dress code. **Societies** Booking required.
Green Fees Nicklaus Course: £85 per day, £59 per round: Old Course:£70 per day, £40 per round. **Prof** David Moon **Course Designer** Old Course H J Stutt/Jack Nicklaus **Facilities** ⓣ ⚭ ♨ 🖥 🍴 🏌 👜 🏕 ⛳ ✦ ♟ ✦ **Leisure** hard tennis courts, heated indoor pool, squash, sauna, solarium, gym. **Conf** facs Corporate Hospitality Days **Location** A38 to Saltash, onto A388 to Callington

Set among 450 acres of glorious Cornish countryside, St Mellion with its two outstanding courses is heralded as the premier golf and country club in the south-west. The Old Course is perfect for golfers of all abilities. Complete with well-sited bunkers, strategically tiered greens and difficult water features, this is definitely not a course to be overlooked. But if you really want to test your game, then head to the renowned Nicklaus Course, designed by the great man himself. On its opening in 1998 Jack declared, 'St Mellion is potentially the finest golf course in Europe'. The spectacularly sculptured fairways and carpet greens of the Nicklaus Course are a challenge and an inspiration to all golfers.

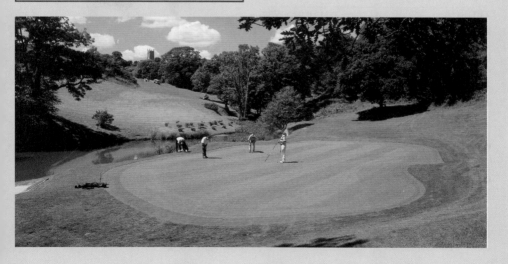

Visitors Tue, Fri, Sat & BHs. Booking required Sat, Sun & BHs. Dress code. **Societies** Booking required. **Green Fees** £27.50 (£20 winter). **Prof** John Witcomb **Facilities** ⊕ ⦿ ⚑ ⬚ ⛳ ⌁ ✆ ♦ ✓ 🛒 ✔ 🏌 **Leisure** hard tennis courts, heated indoor swimming pool, sauna, solarium, gymnasium, outdoor bowling green. **Conf** facs Corporate Hospitality Days **Location** Off B3314 between Wadebridge

Hotel ★★★ 75% HL The Bedford Arms Hotel, CHENIES ☎ 01923 283301 10 en suite 8 annexe en suite

SALTASH MAP 02 SX45

China Fleet Country Club PL12 6LJ
☎ 01752 848668 ▤ 01752 848456
e-mail: golf@china-fleet.co.uk
web: www.china-fleet.co.uk
Parkland with river views. The 14th tee shot has to carry a lake of some 150yds.

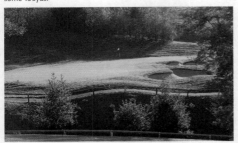

18 holes, 6551yds, Par 72, SSS 72, Course record 69.
Club membership 600.
Visitors Mon-Sun & BHs. Booking required except BHs. Handicap certificate. Dress code. **Societies** Booking required. **Green Fees** Phone. **Prof** Damien McEvoy **Course Designer** Hawtree **Facilities** ⊕ ⦿ ⚑ ⬚ ⛳ ⌁ ✆ ♦ ✓ 🛒 ✔ 🏌 **Leisure** hard tennis courts, heated indoor swimming pool, squash, sauna, solarium, gymnasium, Beauty & hairdresser. **Conf** facs Corporate Hospitality Days **Location** 1m from the Tamar Bridge

Hotel ★★★ 67% HL China Fleet Country Club, SALTASH ☎ 01752 848668 40 en suite

TRURO MAP 02 SW84

Killiow Park Kea TR3 6AG
☎ 01872 270246 ▤ 01872 240915
e-mail: sec@killiow.co.uk
web: www.killiowgolf.co.uk
A picturesque and testing parkland course in the grounds of Killiow Estate, with mature trees, water hazards, small greens and tight fairways making this a challenge for golfers of all abilities. Five holes are played across or around water. Floodlit, all-weather driving range and practice facilities.
18 holes, 6141yds, Par 72, SSS 71. Club membership 500.
Visitors Mon-Sun & BHs. Dress code. **Societies** Welcome. **Green Fees** £25 per 18 holes. Reduced winter rates. **Facilities** ⊕ ⦿ ⚑ ⬚ ⛳ ⌁ ✆ ✓ 🛒 ✔ **Leisure** 3 hole academy course. **Conf** Corporate Hospitality Days **Location** 3m SW of Truro, off A39

Hotel ★★★ 81% HL Alverton Manor, Tregolls Rd, TRURO ☎ 01872 276633 32 en suite

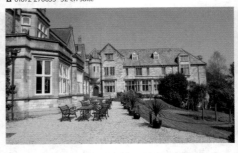

Truro Treliske TR1 3LG
☎ 01872 278684 (manager) ▤ 01872 225972
e-mail: trurogolfclub@tiscali.co.uk
web: www.trurogolfclub.co.uk
A picturesque and gently undulating parkland course with lovely views of the cathedral city of Truro and the surrounding countryside. The 5306yd course offers a great challenge to golfers of all standards and ages. The many trees and shrubs offer open invitations for wayward balls, and with many fairways boasting out of bounds markers, play needs to be safe and sensible. Fairways are tight and the greens small and full of character, making it difficult to play to one's handicap.
18 holes, 5306yds, Par 66, SSS 66, Course record 59.
Club membership 800.
Visitors Mon-Sun & BHs. Handicap certificate required. Dress code. **Societies** Booking required. **Green Fees** £25 per day (£30 weekends & bank holidays). ⊕ **Prof** Nigel Bicknell **Course Designer** Colt, Alison & Morrison **Facilities** ⊕ ⦿ ⚑ ⬚ ⛳ ⌁ ✆ ✓ **Conf** Corporate Hospitality Days **Location** 1.5m W on A390 towards Redruth, adjacent to Treliske Hospital

Hotel ★★★ 81% HL Alverton Manor, Tregolls Rd, TRURO ☎ 01872 276633 32 en suite

Hotel ★★★ GH Gwel-Tek Lodge Guest House, 41 Treyew Rd, TRURO ☎ 01872 276843 Fax 01872 242574 7 en suite

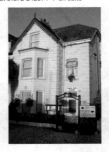

WADEBRIDGE MAP 02 SW97

St Kew St Kew Highway PL30 3EF
☎ 01208 841500 ▤ 01208 841500
e-mail: fjb@stkewgolfclub.fsnet.co.uk
web: www.thisisnorthcornwall.com
9 holes, 4550yds, Par 64, SSS 62, Course record 63.
Course Designer David Derry **Location** 2m N of Wadebridge main A39
Telephone for further details
Hotel ★★★ 70% HL Old Custom House Inn, South Quay, PADSTOW ☎ 01841 532359 24 en suite

CUMBRIA

ALSTON MAP 12 NY74

Alston Moor The Hermitage, Middleton in Teesdale Rd CA9 3DB
☎ 01434 381675 & 381354 (Sec) 📄 01434 381675
Parkland and Fell, in process of upgrading to full 18 holes, stunning views of the North Pennines.
10 holes, 5518yds, Par 68, SSS 66, Course record 67. Club membership 170.
Visitors Mon-Sun & BHs. Dress code. **Societies** Welcome. **Green Fees** Phone. ⊛ **Facilities** ⊑ ⊓ ⚑ **Location** 1 S of Alston on B6277
Hotel ★★ 76% HL Nent Hall Country House Hotel, ALSTON
☎ 01434 381584 18 en suite

APPLEBY-IN-WESTMORLAND MAP 12 NY62

Appleby Brackenber Moor CA16 6LP
☎ 017683 51432 📄 017683 52773
e-mail: enquiries@applebygolfclub.co.uk
web: www.applebygolfclub.co.uk
This remotely situated heather and moorland course offers interesting golf with the rewarding bonus of several long Par 4 holes that will be remembered and challenging Par 3s. There are superb views of the Pennines and the Lakeland hills. Renowned for the excellent greens and very good drainage.
18 holes, 5901yds, Par 68, SSS 68, Course record 61. Club membership 800.
Visitors Mon-Sun & BHs. **Societies** Booking required. **Green Fees** £28 per day, £22 per round (£34/£27 Sat, Sun & BHs). ⊛ **Prof** James Taylor **Course Designer** Willie Fernie **Facilities** ⊕ ⊙ ⊑ ⊓ ⚑ 🏌 ⛾ ✦ **Leisure** buggy for disabled use. **Conf** Corporate Hospitality Days
Location 2m E of Appleby 0.5m off A66
Hotel ★★★ 85% HL Best Western Appleby Manor Country House Hotel, Roman Rd, APPLEBY-IN-WESTMORLAND ☎ 017683 51571
23 en suite 7 annexe en suite

ASKAM-IN-FURNESS MAP 07 SD27

Dunnerholme Duddon Rd LA16 7AW
☎ 01229 462675 & 467421 📄 01229 462675
e-mail: dunnerholmegolfclub@btinternet.com
Unique 10-hole (18-tee) links course with view of the Cumbrian mountains and Morecambe Bay. Two streams run through and around the course, providing water hazards on the 1st, 2nd, 3rd and 9th holes. The Par 3 6th is the feature hole on the course, playing to an elevated green on Dunnerholme Rock, an imposing limestone outcrop jutting out into the estuary.
10 holes, 6138yds, Par 72, SSS 69. Club membership 450.
Visitors may play Mon & Wed-Fri. Handicap certificate required. Dress code. **Societies** apply in writing to the secretary. **Green Fees** not confirmed. ⊛
Facilities ⊑ ⊓ ⚑ **Location** 1m N on A595
Hotel ★★ 64% HL Lisdoonie Hotel, 307/309 Abbey Rd, BARROW-IN-FURNESS ☎ 01229 827312 12 en suite

BARROW-IN-FURNESS MAP 07 SD26

Barrow Rakesmoor Ln, Hawcoat LA14 4QB
☎ 01229 825444
e-mail: barrowgolf@supanet.com
Pleasant course laid out on two levels of meadowland, with extensive views of the nearby Lakeland fells and west to the Irish Sea. Upper level is affected by easterly winds.
18 holes, 6010yds, Par 71, SSS 70, Course record 65. Club membership 520.
Visitors may play Mon-Sun & BHs. Advance booking required. Handicap certificate required. Dress code. **Societies** advance booking required. **Green Fees** not confirmed. ⊛ **Prof** Mike Newton **Course Designer** A M Duncan **Facilities** ⚑ **Location** M6 junct 35, A590 towards Barrow. 2m to K Papermill, left to top of hill
Hotel ★★★ 77% HL Clarence House Country Hotel & Restaurant, Skelgate, DALTON-IN-FURNESS ☎ 01229 462508 7 en suite 12 annexe en suite

Furness Central Dr LA14 3LN
☎ 01229 471232 📄 01229 475100
e-mail: furnessgolfclub@chessbroadband.co.uk
web: www.furnessgolfclub.co.uk
Links golf with a fairly flat first half but a much sterner second nine played across subtle sloping ground. There are good views of the Lakes, North Wales and the Isle of Man.
18 holes, 6363yds, Par 71, SSS 71, Course record 65. Club membership 600.
Visitors may play Mon-Fri & BHs. Restricted Sat & Sun. Booking required. Handicap certificate. Dress code. **Societies** Booking required. **Green Fees** £25 per day. ⊛ **Facilities** ⊕ ⊙ ⊑ ⊓ ⚑ **Location** 1.75 W of town centre off A590 to Walney Island
Hotel ★★ 64% HL Lisdoonie Hotel, 307/309 Abbey Rd, BARROW-IN-FURNESS ☎ 01229 827312 12 en suite

BOWNESS-ON-WINDERMERE MAP 07 SD49

Windermere Cleabarrow LA23 3NB
☎ 015394 43123 📄 015394 43123
e-mail: windermeregc@btconnect.com
web: www.windermeregolfclub.net
Located in the heart of the Lake District, just 2m from Windermere. The course offers some of the finest views in the country. Not a long course but makes up for its lack of distance with heather and tight undulating fairways. The 6th hole has nerve-racking but exhilarating blind shots - 160yds over a rocky face to a humpy fairway with a lake to avoid on the second shot.
18 holes, 5122yds, Par 67, SSS 65, Course record 58. Club membership 890.
Visitors may play Mon-Sun & BHs. Advance booking required. Handicap certificate required. Dress code. **Societies** welcome. **Green Fees** not confirmed. **Prof** W S M Rooke **Course Designer** G Lowe **Facilities** ⊕ ⊙ ⊑ ⊓ ⚑ 🏌 ✦ **Leisure** snooker. **Conf** Corporate Hospitality Days **Location** B5284 1.5m from Bowness
Hotel ★★★ 78% HL Best Western Famous Wild Boar Hotel, Crook, WINDERMERE ☎ 015394 45225 36 en suite

BRAMPTON · MAP 12 NY56

Brampton Tarn Rd CA8 1HN
☎ 016977 2255 📠 01900 822917
e-mail: secretary@bramptongolfclub.com
web: www.bramptongolfclub.com
Undulating heathland course set in rolling fell country. A number of particularly fine holes, the pick of which may arguably be the lengthy 3rd and 11th. The challenging nature of the course is complemented by unspoilt panoramic views of the Lake District, Pennines and southern Scotland.

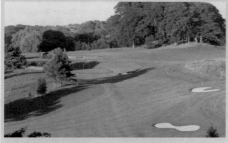

18 holes, 6407yds, Par 72, SSS 71, Course record 64.
Club membership 800.
Visitors Mon-Sun & BHs. Advance booking required Fri-Sun & BHs. Handicap certificate. Dress code. **Societies** Booking required. **Green Fees** £35 per day £28 round (£42/£35 Sat, Sun & BHs). **Prof** Stewart Wilkinson **Course Designer** James Braid **Facilities** ⊕ 🍴 🐐 ♨ ⛳🔥 ⚒ 🏠 🚩 ⚐ 🎣 ⚒ 🏌 **Leisure** games room. **Conf** Corporate Hospitality Days **Location** 1.5m SE of Brampton on B6413
Hotel ★★★ HL Farlam Hall Hotel, BRAMPTON ☎ 016977 46234
11 en suite 1 annexe en suite

CARLISLE · MAP 11 NY35

Carlisle Aglionby CA4 8AG
☎ 01228 513029 (secretary) 📠 01228 513303
e-mail: secretary@carlislegolfclub.org
web: www.carlislegolfclub.org
Majestic, long-established parkland course with great appeal providing a secure habitat for red squirrels and deer. A complete but not too severe test of golf, with fine turf, natural hazards, a stream and many beautiful trees; no two holes are similar.
18 holes, 6263yds, Par 71, SSS 70, Course record 63.
Club membership 700.
Visitors may play Mon, Wed-Sun & BHs. Booking required. Handicap certificate. Dress code. **Societies** Booking required. **Green Fees** £50 per day; £35 per round. **Prof** Graeme Lisle **Course Designer** Mackenzie Ross **Facilities** ⊕ 🍴 🐐 ♨ ⛳🔥 🏠 🚩 ⛴ 🎣 ⚒ **Conf** facs Corporate Hospitality Days **Location** M6 junct 43, 0.5m E on A69
Hotel ★★★ 77% HL Crown Hotel, Wetheral, CARLISLE ☎ 01228 561888
49 en suite 2 annexe en suite

Stony Holme Municipal St Aidans Rd CA1 1LS
☎ 01228 625511 📠 01228 625511
e-mail: stephenli@carlisle-city.gov.uk
web: ww.carlisleleisure.com

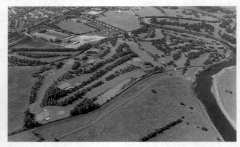

18 holes, 5783yds, Par 69, SSS 68, Course record 64.
Location M6 junct 43, A69, 2m W
Telephone for further details
Hotel ★★★ 66% HL The Crown & Mitre, 4 English St, CARLISLE
☎ 01228 525491 74 en suite 20 annexe en suite

See advert on opposite page

COCKERMOUTH · MAP 11 NY13

Cockermouth Embleton CA13 9SG
☎ 017687 76223 & 76941 📠 017687 76941
e-mail: secretary@cockermouthgolf.co.uk
web: www.cockermouthgolf.co.uk
Fell course, fenced, with exceptional views of Lakeland hills and valleys and the Solway Firth. A hard climb on the 3rd and 11th holes. Testing holes: 10th and 16th (rearranged by James Braid).

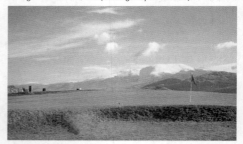

18 holes, 5496yds, Par 69, SSS 66, Course record 62.
Club membership 600.
Visitors may play Mon-Sun & BHs. Booking required Wed, Thu, Sat, Sun & BHs. Dress code. **Societies** Welcome. **Green Fees** £20 per day (£25 weekends and bank holidays). Winter £15/£20. 🐐 **Course Designer** J Braid **Facilities** 🐐 ⚐ 🔥 🏌 🎣 **Conf** Corporate Hospitality Days **Location** 3m E off A66
Hotel ★★★ 81% HL The Trout Hotel, Crown St, COCKERMOUTH
☎ 01900 823591 47 en suite

CROSBY-ON-EDEN MAP 12 NY45

Eden CA6 4RA
☎ 01228 573003 🖹 01228 818435
e-mail: info@edengolf.co.uk
web: www.edengolf.co.uk
Open, championship-length parkland course following the River Eden. Tight tree lined fairways and numerous natural water hazards mark this course out as a great test of golf. The nine hole Hadrian's course is set in natural undulating surroundings and has a contrasting style to the main 18.

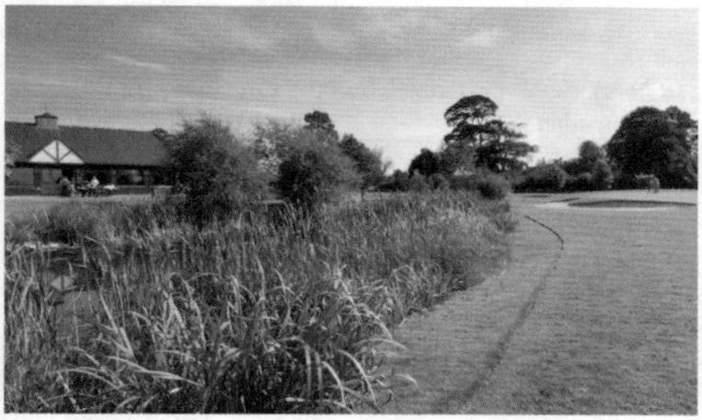

18 holes, 6432yds, Par 72, SSS 71, Course record 64. Club membership 700.
Visitors Mon-Sun & BHs. Booking required. Dress code. **Societies** Booking required. **Green Fees** Eden Course £28 (£32 Sat, Sun & BHs). Hadrian's £12/£15. **Prof** Steve Harrison **Course Designer** A G M Wannop **Facilities** **Leisure** hard tennis courts. **Conf** facs Corporate Hospitality Days **Location** M6 junct 44, 5m on A689 towards Brampton
Hotel BUD Travelodge Carlisle Todhills, A74 Southbound, Todhills, CARLISLE ☎ 08700 850 950 40 en suite

GRANGE-OVER-SANDS MAP 07 SD47

Grange Fell Fell Rd LA11 6HB
☎ 015395 32536
e-mail: grangefellgc@aol.com
A fell course with no excessive climbing and dependant on how straight you hit the ball. Fine views in all directions.
9 holes, 5292yds, Par 70, SSS 66, Course record 65. Club membership 300.
Visitors may play Mon & Wed-Sat except BHs. Dress code. **Green Fees** £15 per day (£20 weekends & bank holidays). **Course Designer** A B Davy **Facilities** **Location** 1m W on Grange-Over-Sands/Cartmel
Hotel ★★★ 80% HL Netherwood Hotel, Lindale Rd, GRANGE-OVER-SANDS ☎ 015395 32552 32 en suite

Grange-over-Sands Meathop Rd LA11 6QX
☎ 015395 33180 or 33754 🖹 015395 33754
e-mail: grangegolfclub@tiscali.co.uk
web: www.grangegolfclub.co.uk
Interesting parkland course with well-sited tree plantations, ditches and water features which has recently been drained and extended. The five Par 3s are considered to be some of the best in the area.
18 holes, 6120yds, Par 70, SSS 69, Course record 64. Club membership 650.
Visitors may play Mon, Wed, Fri, Sun & BHs. Tue & Thu pm only. Advance booking required Tue, Thu, Sun & BHs. Handicap certificate required. Dress code. **Societies** Booking required. **Green Fees** £35 per day; £28 per round.

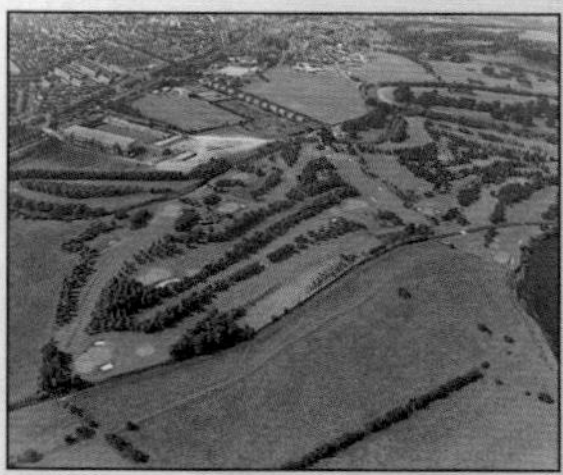

Stony Holme Golf Course, Carlisle

With the magnificent back drop of the Lakeland fells, this mature, flat, easy-walking parkland course is a challenge to any golfer. The Pavilion was fully refurbished in 2006 and offers new changing rooms, a fully stocked shop and the Riverside Restaurant and Bar serves delicious home cooked food. Golf Packages for visiting groups are available and a pay as you play system is in operation.

St. Aidans Road, Carlisle, Cumbria.
Tel: 01228 625511
www.carlisleleisure.com

OUTDOOR RECREATION
CARLISLE CITY COUNCIL
www.carlisle.gov.uk

Prof Nick Lowe **Course Designer** Mackenzie (part) **Facilities** **Conf** Corporate Hospitality Days **Location** NE of town centre off B5277
Hotel ★★★ 67% HL Graythwaite Manor Hotel, Fernhill Rd, GRANGE-OVER-SANDS ☎ 015395 32001 & 33755 🖹 015395 35549 24 en suite

KENDAL MAP 07 SD59

Carus Green Burneside Rd LA9 6EB
☎ 01539 721097 🖹 01539 721097
e-mail: info@carusgreen.co.uk
web: www.carusgreen.co.uk
Flat 18-hole course surrounded by the rivers Kent and Mint with an open view of the Kentmere and Howgill fells. The course is a mixture of relatively easy and difficult holes. These rivers come into play on five holes and there are also a number of ponds and bunkers.
18 holes, 5691yds, Par 70, SSS 68, Course record 65. Club membership 600.
Visitors Mon-Sun & BHs. Booking required. Dress code. **Societies** Booking required. **Green Fees** £18 per round (£20 weekends & bank holidays). **Prof** D Turner/N Barron **Course Designer** W Adamson **Facilities** **Conf** Corporate Hospitality Days **Location** 1m from Kendal centre
Hotel ★★★ 70% HL Riverside Hotel Kendal, Beezon Rd, Stramongate Bridge, KENDAL ☎ 01539 734861 47 en suite

Kendal The Heights LA9 4PQ
☎ 01539 723499 (pro) 🖹 01539 736466
e-mail: secretary@kendalgolfclub.co.uk
web: www.kendalgolfclub.co.uk
Elevated parkland and fell course with breathtaking views of Lakeland fells and the surrounding district.
18 holes, 5737yds, Par 70, SSS 68, Course record 65.
Club membership 552.
Visitors may play Mon-Fri, Sun & BHs. Booking required Sun & BHs. required. Dress code. **Societies** Booking required. **Green Fees** £36 per day, £28 per round (£44/£34 weekends). **Prof** Peter Scott **Facilities** ⑪ 🎿🍴 🕳 ⌦ 🗑 ⚲ ⚑ ✦ 🎒 ✦ **Leisure** Golf clinic with computer analysis. **Location** 1m W of town centre, turn left at town hall and follow signposts
Hotel ★★★ 81% HL Best Western Castle Green Hotel in Kendal, KENDAL ☎ 01539 734000 100 en suite

---

KESWICK   MAP 11 NY22

Keswick Threlkeld Hall, Threlkeld CA12 4SX
☎ 017687 79324 🖹 017687 79861
e-mail: secretary@keswickgolf.com
web: www.keswickgolf.com
18 holes, 6225yds, Par 71, SSS 72, Course record 68.
Course Designer Eric Brown **Location** 4m E of Keswick, off A66
Telephone for further details
Hotel ★★★ 70% HL Keswick Country House Hotel, Station Rd, KESWICK ☎ 0845 458 4333 74 en suite

---

KIRKBY LONSDALE   MAP 07 SD67

Kirkby Lonsdale Scaleber Ln, Barbon LA6 2LJ
☎ 015242 76365 🖹 015242 76503
e-mail: klgolf@dial.pipex.com
web: www.klgolf.dial.pipex.com
Parkland on the east bank of the River Lune and crossed by Barbon Beck. Mainly following the lie of the land, the gently undulating course uses the beck to provide water hazards.
18 holes, 6542yds, Par 72, SSS 71, Course record 67.
Club membership 600.
Visitors Mon-Sun & BHs. Advance booking required. Dress code. **Societies** Booking required. **Green Fees** £30 per day (£35 weekends & bank holidays). ⊛ **Prof** Chris Barrett **Course Designer** Bill Squires **Facilities** ⑪ 🎿🍴 🕳 ⌦ 🗑 🛋 ⚲ ⚑ ✦ **Conf** Corporate Hospitality Days **Location** 3m NE of Kirkby Lonsdale on A683
Hotel ★★ 72% HL The Whoop Hall, Burrow with Burrow, KIRKBY LONSDALE ☎ 015242 71284 24 rms (23 en suite)

MARYPORT   MAP 11 NY03

Maryport Bankend CA15 6PA
☎ 01900 812605 🖹 815626
e-mail: maryportgcltd@one-tel.com
A tight seaside links course exposed to Solway breezes. Fine views across Solway Firth. Course comprises nine links holes and nine parkland holes, and small streams can be hazardous on several holes. The first three holes have the seashore on their left and an errant tee shot can land in the water. Holes 6-14 are parkland in quality, gently undulating and quite open. holes 15-18 revert to links.
18 holes, 5982yds, Par 70, SSS 69, Course record 65.
Club membership 539.
Visitors may play Mon-Sun & BHs. Advance booking required for Thu, Sat, Sun & BHs. Handicap certificate required. Dress code. **Societies** advance

booking required. **Green Fees** not confirmed. ⊛ **Facilities** ⑪ 🍴 🕳 ⌦ 🗑 🛋 ⚲ ⚑ ✦ **Location** 1m N on B5300
Hotel ★★★ 85% HL Washington Central Hotel, Washington St, WORKINGTON ☎ 01900 65772 46 en suite

---

PENRITH   MAP 12 NY53

Penrith Salkeld Rd CA11 8SG
☎ 01768 891919 🖹 01768 891919
e-mail: golf@penrithgolfclub.co.uk
A beautiful and well-balanced course, always changing direction, and demanding good length from the tee. It is set on rolling moorland with occasional pine trees and some fine views.
18 holes, 6047yds, Par 69, SSS 69, Course record 63.
Club membership 850.
Visitors may play Mon-Sun & BHs. Handicap certificate required. Dress code. **Societies** telephone in advance. **Green Fees** not confirmed. ⊛ **Prof** Garry Key **Facilities** 🛋 ⚲ ⚑ ✦ **Conf** facs **Location** M6 junct 41, A6 to Penrith, left after 30mph sign

---

ST BEES   MAP 11 NX91

St Bees Peckmill, Beach Rd CA27 0EJ
☎ 01946 824300
10 holes, 5306yds, Par 66, SSS 66, Course record 64.
Location 0.5m W of village off B5345
Telephone for further details
Hotel ★★★ 75% HL Ennerdale Country House Hotel, CLEATOR ☎ 01946 813907 30 en suite

---

SEASCALE   MAP 06 NY00

Seascale The Banks CA20 1QL
☎ 019467 28202 🖹 019467 28042
e-mail: seascalegolfclub@aol.com
web: www.seascalegolfclub.co.uk
A tough links requiring length and control. The natural terrain is used to give a variety of holes and considerable character. Undulating greens add to the challenge. Fine views of the western fells, the Irish Sea and the Isle of Man.
18 holes, 6416yds, Par 71, SSS 71, Course record 64.
Club membership 700.
Visitors may play Mon, Tue, Thu-Sun & BHs. Booking required. Handicap certificate. Dress code. **Societies** Booking required. **Green Fees** £33 per day; £28 per round (£38/£33 Sat, Sun & BHs). **Course Designer** Willie Campbell **Facilities** ⑪ 🎿🍴 🕳 ⌦ 🗑 🛋 ⚲ ⚑ ✦ **Conf** facs **Location** NW side of village off B5344
Hotel ★★ 74% HL Low Wood Hall Hotel & Restaurant, NETHER WASDALE ☎ 019467 26100 7 en suite 6 annexe en suite

---

SEDBERGH   MAP 07 SD69

Sedbergh Dent Rd LA10 5SS
☎ 015396 21551 (Club) 🖹 015396 21551
e-mail: info@sedberghgolfclub.co.uk
web: www.sedberghgolfclub.co.uk
A tree-lined parkland course with superb scenery in the Yorkshire Dales National Park. Undulating fairways cross or are adjacent to the Dee and Rawthey rivers. Well guarded greens and many water features make the course a test for golfers of all abilities.

Continued

9 holes, 5624yds, Par 70, SSS 68, Course record 66.
Club membership 250.
Visitors contact club for details. Dress code. **Societies** advance booking required. **Green Fees** not confirmed. ◉ **Course Designer** W G Squires
Facilities ⊕ ⌷ ☷ ⚒ 🖧 ⛾ 🏌 **Leisure** fishing. **Conf** facs Corporate Hospitality Days **Location** 1m S off A683
Hotel BUD Premier Travel Inn Kendal (Killington Lake), Killington Lake, Motorway Service Area, Killington, KENDAL ☎ 08701 977145 36 en suite

SILECROFT   MAP 06 SD18

Silecroft Silecroft, Millom LA18 4NX
☎ 01229 774250
e-mail: silecroftgcsoc@aol.com
Seaside links course parallel to the coast of the Irish Sea with spectacular views inland of Lakeland hills. Looks deceptively easy but an ever present sea breeze ensures a sporting challenge.
9 holes, 5896yds, Par 68, SSS 68, Course record 66.
Club membership 240.
Visitors may play Mon-Fri. By-arrangement Sat, Sun & BHs. Handicap certificate. Dress code. **Societies** Booking required. **Green Fees** £15 per day (£20 weekends & bank holidays). ◉ **Facilities** ⚒ **Location** 3m W of Millom

SILLOTH   MAP 11 NY15

Silloth on Solway The Clubhouse CA7 4BL
☎ 016973 31304 📠 016973 31782
e-mail: office@sillothgolfclub.co.uk
web: www.sillothgolfclub.co.uk
Billowing dunes, narrow fairways, heather and gorse and the constant subtle problems of tactics and judgement make these superb links on the Solway an exhilarating and searching test. The 13th is a good long hole. Superb views.
18 holes, 6041yds, Par 72, SSS 69, Course record 59.
Club membership 700.
Visitors Mon-Sun & BHs. Booking required. Handicap certificate. Dress code. **Societies** Booking required. **Green Fees** £37 per day (£50 per round weekends). **Prof** J Graham **Course Designer** David Grant/Willie Park Jnr **Facilities** ⊕ 🍴 ☷ ⌷ 🖧 ⚒ 🏠 ⛾ **Conf** facs **Location** S side of village off B5300
Hotel Golf Hotel, Criffel St, SILLOTH ☎ 016973 31438 22 en suite

ULVERSTON   MAP 07 SD27

Ulverston Bardsea Park LA12 9QJ
☎ 01229 582824 📠 01229 588910
e-mail: enquiries@ulverstongolf.co.uk
web: www.ulverstongolf.co.uk
Undulating parkland course overlooking Morecambe Bay with extensive views to the Lakeland Fells.
18 holes, 6201yds, Par 71, SSS 70, Course record 64.
Club membership 808.
Visitors may play Mon-Fri. Advance booking required. Handicap certificate required. Dress code. **Societies** advance booking required.
Green Fees not confirmed. **Prof** P A Stoller **Course Designer** A Herd/H S Colt **Facilities** ⊕ 🍴 ☷ ⌷ 🖧 ⚒ 🏠 🏌 **Leisure** practice ball dispensing machine. **Conf** Corporate Hospitality Days **Location** 2m S off A5087
Hotel ★★★ 73% HL Whitewater Hotel, The Lakeland Village, NEWBY BRIDGE ☎ 015395 31133 35 en suite

WINDERMERE
See **Bowness-on-Windermere**

WORKINGTON   MAP 11 NY02

Workington Branthwaite Rd CA14 4SS
☎ 01900 67828 📠 01900 607123
e-mail: golf@workingtongolfclub.freeserve.co.uk
18 holes, 6217yds, Par 72, SSS 70, Course record 65.
Course Designer James Braid **Location** 1.75m E off A596
Telephone for further details
Hotel ★★★ 85% HL Washington Central Hotel, Washington St, WORKINGTON ☎ 01900 65772 46 en suite

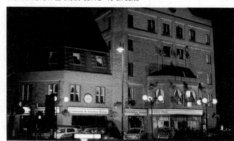

DERBYSHIRE

ALFRETON   MAP 08 SK45

Alfreton Wingfield Rd, Oakerthorpe DE55 7LH
☎ 01773 832070
11 holes, 5393yds, Par 67, SSS 66, Course record 66.
Location 1m W on A615
Telephone for further details
Hotel ★★★★ 77% HL Renaissance Derby/Nottingham Hotel, Carter Ln East, SOUTH NORMANTON ☎ 01773 812000 & 0870 4007262
📠 01773 580032 & 0870 4007362 158 en suite

ASHBOURNE   MAP 07 SK14

Ashbourne Wyaston Rd DE6 1NB
☎ 01335 347960 (pro shop) 📠 01335 347937
e-mail: sec@ashbournegc.fsnet.co.uk
web: www.ashbournegolfclub.co.uk
With fine views over surrounding countryside, the course uses natural contours and water features.
18 holes, 6308yds, Par 71, SSS 71. Club membership 650.
Visitors may play Mon-Sun except BHs. Booking required. Dress code. **Societies** Booking required. **Green Fees** £40 for 36 holes, £28 per 18 holes (£35 per 18 holes Sat & Sun). ◉ **Prof** Andrew Smith
Course Designer D Hemstock **Facilities** ⊕ 🍴 ☷ ⌷ 🖧 ⚒ 🏠 ⛾
Leisure snooker table. **Location** Off Wyaston Rd, club signed
Hotel ★★★ 80% CHH Callow Hall, Mappleton Rd, ASHBOURNE
☎ 01335 300900 16 en suite

BAKEWELL   MAP 08 SK26

Bakewell Station Rd DE45 1GB
☎ 01629 812307
web: www.bakewellgolfclub.org.uk
Hilly parkland course with plenty of natural hazards to test the golfer.
Magnificent views across the Wye Valley.
9 holes, 5240yds, Par 68, SSS 66, Course record 68.
Club membership 340.
Visitors Mon-Sun & BHs. Booking required Tue, Sat & BHs. Handicap
certificate. Dress code. **Societies** Booking required. **Green Fees** Phone. ☺
Facilities ⑪ ⑩⬤ ⅃ ⬤ ⎅ ⅃ ⬤ **Conf** Corporate Hospitality Days
Location E side of town off A6
Hotel ★★★ 70% HL Rutland Arms Hotel, The Square, BAKEWELL
☎ 01629 812812 18 en suite 17 annexe en suite

BAMFORD   MAP 08 SK28

Sickleholme Saltergate Ln S33 0BN
☎ 01433 651306 ▤ 01433 659498
e-mail: sickleholme.gc@btconnect.com.
web: www.sickleholme.co.uk
Undulating downland course in the lovely Peak District, with rivers and
ravines and spectacular scenery.
18 holes, 6064yds, Par 69, SSS 69, Course record 62.
Club membership 700.
Visitors may play Mon-Sun & BHs. Advance booking required. Handicap
certificate required. Dress code. **Societies** advanced booking required.
Green Fees not confirmed. ☺ **Prof** P H Taylor **Facilities** ⑪ ⑩⬤ ⅃ ⬤ ⎅ ⅃
⬤ ⬤ ✓ **Conf** Corporate Hospitality Days **Location** 0.75m S on A6013
Hotel ★★ 72% HL Yorkshire Bridge Inn, Ashopton Rd, Hope Valley,
BAMFORD ☎ 01433 651361 14 en suite

BREADSALL   MAP 08 SK33

Marriot Breadsall Priory Hotel & Country Club Moor
Rd, Morley DE7 6DL
☎ 01332 836016 ▤ 01332 836089
e-mail: ian.knox@marriothotels.com
Set in 200 acres of mature undulating parkland, the Priory Course is
built on the site of a 13th-century priory. Full use has been made of
natural features and fine old trees. A degree of accuracy is required to
play small protected greens along tree lined fairways. Signature hole
is the 16th. In contrast the Moorland Course is a sand based course
allowing all year round play to full greens. Slighter wider fairways allow
for more attacking tee shots but beware of well-placed bunkers, trees
and rough. At the 13th the tee shot is narrow with trees and bushes
lining the fairway.
Priory Course: 18 holes, 6120yds, Par 72, SSS 69,
Course record 63.
Moorland Course: 18 holes, 6028yds, Par 70, SSS 69.
Club membership 900.
Visitors Mon-Sun & BHs. Dress code. **Societies** Booking required.
Green Fees from £45. **Prof** Darren Steels **Course Designer** D Steel
Facilities ⑪ ⑩⬤ ⅃ ⬤ ⎅ ⅃ ⬤ ⎅ ✓ ✿ **Leisure** hard tennis courts,
heated indoor swimming pool, sauna, solarium, gymnasium. **Conf** facs
Corporate Hospitality Days **Location** 0.75m W
Hotel ★★★★ 75% HL Marriott Breadsall Priory Hotel& Country Club,
Moor Rd, MORLEY ☎ 01332 832235 12 en suite 100 annexe en suite

BUXTON   MAP 07 SK07

Buxton & High Peak Waterswallows Rd SK17 7EN
☎ 01298 26263 & 23453 ▤ 26333
e-mail: admin@bhpgc.co.uk
web: www.bhpgc.co.uk
Bracing, well-drained meadowland course, the highest in Derbyshire.
Challenging course where wind direction is a major factor on
some holes; others require blind shots to sloping greens.
18 holes, 5966yds, Par 69, SSS 69. Club membership 650.
Visitors By prior arrangment only. **Societies** Booking required. **Green
Fees** £30 per day, £24 per round (£36/£30 weekends & bank holidays).
Prof John Lines **Course Designer** J Morris **Facilities** ⑪ ⑩⬤ by prior
arrangement ⬤ ⎅ ⅃ ⬤ ⎅ ✓ ⬤ ✓ **Conf** facs Corporate Hospitality
Days **Location** 1m NE off A6
Hotel ★★★★ 73% HL Paramount Palace Hotel, Palace Rd, BUXTON
☎ 01298 22001 122 en suite

Cavendish Gadley Ln SK17 6XD
☎ 01298 79708 ▤ 01298 79708
e-mail: admin@cavendishgolfcourse.com
web: www.@cavendishgolfcourse.com
This parkland and moorland course with its comfortable clubhouse
nestles below the rising hills. Generally open to the prevailing west
wind, it is noted for its excellent surfaced greens which contain many
deceptive subtleties. Designed by Dr Alastair McKenzie, good holes
include the 8th, 9th and 18th.

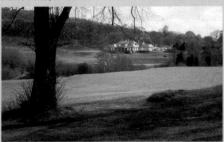

18 holes, 5721yds, Par 68, SSS 68, Course record 61.
Club membership 650.
Visitors Mon-Sun & BHs. Booking required Sat & Sun. Handicap
certificate required. Dress code. **Societies** Booking required. **Green Fees**
Phone. **Prof** Simon Townend **Course Designer** Dr Mackenzie **Facilities**
⑪ by prior arrangement ⑩⬤ by prior arrangement ⬤ ⎅ ⅃ ⬤ ⎅ ⅃ ⬤
✓ ✓ **Conf** Corporate Hospitality Days **Location** 0.75m W of town
centre off A53
Hotel ★★★ 78% HL Best Western Lee Wood Hotel, The Park, BUXTON
☎ 01298 23002 35 en suite 5 annexe en suite

CHAPEL-EN-LE-FRITH   MAP 07 SK08

Chapel-en-le-Frith The Cockyard, Manchester Rd
SK23 9UH
☎ 01298 812118 & 813943 (sec) ▤ 01298 814990
e-mail: info@chapelgolf.co.uk
web: www.chapelgolf.co.uk
Scenic parkland surrounded by spectacular mountain views. A new
longer and challenging front nine, a testing short Par 4 14th and
possibly the best last three-hole finish in Derbyshire.

Continued

18 holes, 6434yds, Par 72, SSS 71, Course record 71.
Club membership 570.
Visitors Mon-Sun & BHs. Dress code. **Societies** Booking required.
Green Fees Phone. **Prof** David J Cullen **Course Designer** David Williams
Facilities ⑪ ⑩ ⓵ ⓵ ⓵ ⓵ ⓵ ⓵ **Conf** Corporate Hospitality Days
Location On B5470
Hotel ★★★ 78% HL Best Western Lee Wood Hotel, The Park, BUXTON
☎ 01298 23002   35 en suite   5 annexe en suite

CHESTERFIELD   MAP 08 SK37

Chesterfield Walton S42 7LA
☎ 01246 279256 ᐧ 01246 276622
e-mail: secretary@chesterfieldgolfclub.co.uk
web: www.chesterfieldgolfclub.co.uk
A varied and interesting, undulating parkland course with trees
picturesquely adding to the holes and the outlook alike. Stream hazard
on the back nine.
18 holes, 6281yds, Par 71, SSS 70, Course record 64.
Club membership 600.
Visitors Mon-Fri except BHs. Booking required. Handicap certificate. Dress
code. **Societies** Welcome. **Green Fees** £40 per day; £32 per round (£40
per round weekends). ⑧ **Prof** Mike McLean **Facilities** ⑪ ⑩ ⓵
⓵ ⓵ **Leisure** snooker/pool. **Conf** Corporate Hospitality Days **Location** 2m
SW off A632
Hotel ★★★ 66% HL Sandpiper Hotel, Sheffield Rd, Sheepbridge,
CHESTERFIELD ☎ 01246 450550   46 en suite

Grassmoor Golf Centre North Wingfield Rd, Grassmoor
S42 5EA
☎ 01246 856044 ᐧ 01246 853486
e-mail: enquiries@grassmoorgolf.co.uk
web: www.grassmoorgolf.co.uk
An 18-hole heathland course with interesting and challenging water
features, testing greens and testing Par 3s.
18 holes, 5723yds, Par 69, SSS 69, Course record 67.
Club membership 450.
Visitors Mon-Sun & BHs. Booking required. Dress code **Societies** Booking
required. **Green Fees** £12 per 18 holes (£15 weekend & BH). **Prof** Gary
Hagues **Course Designer** Hawtree **Facilities** ⑪ ⓵ ⓵ ⓵ ⓵ ⓵ ⓵
⓵ ⓵ ⓵ **Conf** Corporate Hospitality Days **Location** M1 junct 29, 4m off
B6038 between Chesterfield and Grassmor
Hotel ★★★ 66% HL Sandpiper Hotel, Sheffield Rd, Sheepbridge,
CHESTERFIELD ☎ 01246 450550   46 en suite

Stanedge Walton Hay Farm, Stonedge, Ashover S45 0LW
☎ 01246 566156
e-mail: graemecooper@tiscali.co.uk
web: www.stanedgegolfclub.co.uk
Moorland course in hilly situation open to strong winds. Some
tricky short holes with narrow fairways, so accuracy is paramount.
Magnificent views over four counties. Extended course now open.
10 holes, 5786yds, Par 69, SSS 68, Course record 68.
Club membership 310.
Visitors may play Mon-Fri. Dress code. **Societies** Booking required.
Green Fees £15 per round. ⑧ **Facilities** ⓵ ⓵ ⓵ ⓵ **Conf** Corporate
Hospitality Days **Location** 5m SW off B5057 near Famous Red Lion pub
Hotel ★★ 83% HL The Red House Country Hotel, Old Rd, Darley Dale,
MATLOCK ☎ 01629 734854   7 en suite   3 annexe en suite

Tapton Park Tapton Park, Tapton S41 0EQ
☎ 01246 239500 & 273887
Municipal parkland course with some fairly hard walking. The 625yd
(Par 5) 5th is a testing hole.
Tapton Main: 18 holes, 6104yds, Par 72, SSS 69.
Dobbin Clough: 9 holes, 2613yds, Par 34, SSS 34.
Club membership 300.
Visitors Mon-Sun & BHs. Booking required. Dress code. **Societies** Booking
required. **Green Fees** £12 per 18 holes, £7 per 9 holes (£13.50/£8 Fri-Sun
& BHs). **Prof** Andrew Carnall **Facilities** ⑪ ⑩ ⓵ ⓵ ⓵ ⓵ ⓵ ⓵
⓵ **Leisure** 9 hole Par 3 course. **Conf** facs Corporate Hospitality Days
Location 0.5m E of Chesterfield station
Hotel ★★★ 66% HL Sandpiper Hotel, Sheffield Rd, Sheepbridge,
CHESTERFIELD ☎ 01246 450550   46 en suite

CODNOR   MAP 08 SK44

Ormonde Fields Golf & Country Club Nottingham Rd
DE5 9RG
☎ 01773 570043 (Secretary) ᐧ 01773 742987
Parkland course with undulating fairways and natural hazards. There is
a practice area.
18 holes, 6502yds, Par 71, SSS 72, Course record 68.
Club membership 500.
Visitors Mon-Sun & BHs. Booking required. Dress code. **Societies** Booking
required. **Green Fees** £25 per 18 holes (£30 weekend & bank holidays).
⑧ **Prof** Richard White **Course Designer** John Fearn **Facilities** ⑪ ⑩ ⓵
⓵ ⓵ ⓵ ⓵ ⓵ **Conf** facs Corporate Hospitality Days **Location** 1m
SE on A610
Hotel ★★★★ 71% HL Makeney Hall Hotel, Makeney, Milford, BELPER
☎ 01332 842999   28 en suite   18 annexe en suite

DERBY   MAP 08 SK33

Allestree Park Allestree Hall, Duffield Rd, Allestree
DE22 2EU
☎ 01332 550616 ᐧ 01332 541195
Public course, picturesque and undulating, set in 300-acre park with
views across Derbyshire.
18 holes, 5806yds, Par 68, SSS 68, Course record 61.
Club membership 220.
Visitors Mon-Sun & BHs. Booking required. **Societies** welcome. **Green
Fees** not confirmed. **Prof** Leigh Woodward **Facilities** ⑪ ⓵ ⓵ ⓵ ⓵ ⓵ ⓵
⓵ **Leisure** fishing, pool table. **Conf** Corporate Hospitality Days **Location** N
of Derby, A38 onto A6 N, course 1.5m on left
Hotel ★★★★ 75% HL Marriott Breadsall Priory Hotel& Country Club,
Moor Rd, MORLEY ☎ 01332 832235   12 en suite   100 annexe en suite

Mickleover Uttoxeter Rd, Mickleover DE3 9AD
☎ 01332 518662 ᐧ 01332 516011
Undulating parkland course of two loops of nine holes, in a pleasant
setting and affording splendid country views. There is a premium in
hitting tee shots in the right place for approaches to greens, some
of which are on elevated plateaux. Some attractive Par 3s which are
considered to be very exacting.
18 holes, 5702yds, Par 68, SSS 68, Course record 64.
Club membership 800.
Visitors Mon-Fri, Sun.& BHs. Booking required.Sun & BHs. Dress code.
Societies Booking required. **Green Fees** Phone. **Prof** Tim Coxon
Course Designer J Pennink **Facilities** ⑪ ⑩ ⓵ ⓵ ⓵ ⓵ ⓵ ⓵ ⓵ ⓵ ⓵
Conf Corporate Hospitality Days **Location** 3m W of Derby on A516/B5020

Sinfin Wilmore Rd, Sinfin DE24 9HD
☎ 01332 766462 📠 01332 769004
e-mail: phil.dews@derby.gov.uk
web: www.sinfingolfcourse.co.uk
Municipal parkland course with tree-lined fairways; an excellent test of golf and famous for its demanding Par 4s. Generally a flat course, it is suitable for golfers of all ages.
18 holes, 6163yds, Par 70, SSS 70, Course record 65.
Club membership 244.
Visitors contact course for details. **Societies** Welcome. **Green Fees** not confirmed. **Prof** Daniel Delaney **Facilities** ⓦ🍴🍺🖥️🏌️🏖️🛄🚩🏌️✦
Location 2.5m S of city centre
Hotel ★★★ 67% HL International Hotel, 288 Burton Rd, DERBY
☎ 01332 369321 41 en suite 21 annexe en suite

DRONFIELD   MAP 08 SK37

Hallowes Hallowes Ln S18 1UR
☎ 01246 411196 📠 01246 413753
e-mail: john.oates@hallowesgolfclub.org
web: www.hallowesgolfclub.org
Attractive moorland and parkland in the Derbyshire hills. Several testing Par 4s and splendid views.
18 holes, 6319yds, Par 71, SSS 71, Course record 64.
Club membership 630.
Visitors Mon-Fri & Sun except BHs. Booking required. Handicap certificate. Dress code. **Societies** Welcome. **Green Fees** £40 per day; £35 per round.
♿ **Prof** Philip Dunn **Facilities** ⓦ🍴🍺🖥️🏌️🏖️🛄🚩🏌️✦ **Leisure** short game facility, snooker. **Conf** Corporate Hospitality Days **Location** S side of town, off B6057 onto Cemetery Rd and Hallowes Rise/Drive
Hotel ★★★ 66% HL Sandpiper Hotel, Sheffield Rd, Sheepbridge, CHESTERFIELD ☎ 01246 450550 46 en suite

---

DUFFIELD   MAP 08 SK34

Chevin Golf Ln DE56 4EE
☎ 01332 841864 📠 01332 844028
e-mail: secretary@chevingolf.fsnet.co.uk
web: www.chevingolf.co.uk
A mixture of parkland and moorland, this course is rather hilly which makes for some hard walking, but with most rewarding views of the surrounding countryside. The 8th hole, aptly named Tribulation, requires an accurate tee shot, and is one of the most difficult holes in the county.
18 holes, 6057yds, Par 69, SSS 69, Course record 64.
Club membership 750.
Visitors Mon-Fri & Sun except BHs.Booking required Sun. Handicap certificate . Dress code. **Societies** Welcome. **Green Fees** Phone. ♿
Prof Willie Bird **Course Designer** J Braid **Facilities** 🖥️🛄🚩🏌️✦✦
Conf facs Corporate Hospitality Days **Location** N side of town off A6
Hotel ★★★★ 71% HL Makeney Hall Hotel, Makeney, Milford, BELPER
☎ 01332 842999 28 en suite 18 annexe en suite

GLOSSOP   MAP 07 SK09

Glossop and District Hurst Ln, off Sheffield Rd SK13 7PU
☎ 01457 865247(club house)
Moorland course in good position, excellent natural hazards. Difficult closing hole (9th & 18th).
11 holes, 5800yds, Par 68, SSS 68, Course record 64.
Club membership 350.

Visitors may play Mon, Tue, Thu, Fri except BHs. **Societies** advance booking required. **Green Fees** not confirmed. ♿ **Prof** Daniel Marsh **Facilities** ⓦ🍴🍺🖥️🏌️🏖️🛄🚩✦ **Conf** Corporate Hospitality Days
Location 1m E off A57 from town centre
Hotel ★★ 80% HL Wind in the Willows Hotel, Derbyshire Level, GLOSSOP
☎ 01457 868001 12 en suite

HORSLEY   MAP 08 SK34

Horsley Lodge Smalley Mill Rd DE21 5BL
☎ 01332 780838 📠 01332 781118
e-mail: enquiries@horsleylodge.co.uk.
web: www.horsleylodge.co.uk.
Parkland course set in 180 acres of Derbyshire countryside, has some very challenging holes. Also floodlit driving range. Big undulating greens designed by former World Champion Peter McEvoy.

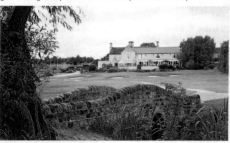

18 holes, 6400yds, Par 71, SSS 71, Course record 65.
Club membership 650.
Visitors Mon-Sun & BHs. Booking required for Sat & Sun. Dress code **Societies** Welcome. **Green Fees** £25 per 18 holes. **Prof** Mark Whithorn
Course Designer Bill White **Facilities** ⓦ🍴🍺🖥️🏌️🏖️🛄🚩✦♿🍺
✦🏌️ **Leisure** fishing. **Conf** facs Corporate Hospitality Days **Location** 4m NE of Derby, off A38 at Belper then follow tourist signs
Hotel ★★★★ 75% HL Marriott Breadsall Priory Hotel& Country Club, Moor Rd, MORLEY ☎ 01332 832235 12 en suite 100 annexe en suite

---

KEDLESTON   MAP 08 SK34

Kedleston Park DE22 5JD
☎ 01332 840035 📠 01332 840035
e-mail: secretary@kedleston-park-golf-club.co.uk
web: www.kedlestonparkgolf.co.uk
The course is laid out in flat mature parkland with fine trees and background views of historic Kedleston Hall (National Trust). Many testing holes are included in each nine and there is an excellent modern clubhouse.
18 holes, 6430yds, Par 72, SSS 71. Club membership 697.
Visitors Mon, Tue, Thu-Sun & BHs. Booking required Sat, Sun & BHs. Handicap certificate. Dress code. **Societies** Booking required. **Green Fees** £55 per day; £45 per round. **Prof** Paul Wesselingh **Course Designer** James Braid **Facilities** ⓦ🍴🍺🖥️🏌️🏖️🛄🚩✦♿🍺✦
Leisure sauna. **Conf** Corporate Hospitality Days **Location** Signposted Kedleston Hall from A38
Hotel ★★★ 67% HL International Hotel, 288 Burton Rd, DERBY
☎ 01332 369321 41 en suite 21 annexe en suite

LONG EATON
MAP 08 SK43

Trent Lock Golf Centre Lock Ln, Sawley NG10 2FY
☎ 0115 946 4398 📄 0115 946 1183
e-mail: trentlockgolf@aol.com
Main course has two Par 5, five Par 3 and eleven Par 4 holes, plus water features and three holes adjacent to the river. A challenging test of golf. A 22-bay floodlit golf range is available.
Main Course: 18 holes, 5848yds, Par 69, SSS 68, Course record 67.
9 hole: 9 holes, 2911yds, Par 36. Club membership 500.
Visitors Mon-Sun & BHs. Booking required Sat & Sun. Dress code. **Societies** Booking required. **Green Fees** 18 hole course: £17.50 per round (£22.50 weekends). 9 hole course: £6 per round (£7.50 per round weekends). **Prof** M Taylor **Course Designer** E McCausland **Facilities** ⊕ ⑩ ⓑ ⌷ ⚑ 🔱 ⚐ 🖉 🐟 🗲 **Leisure** club fitting centre. **Conf** facs Corporate Hospitality Days
Hotel ★★★ 67% HL Novotel Nottingham/Derby, Bostock Ln, LONG EATON ☎ 0115 946 5111 108 en suite

MATLOCK
MAP 08 SK36

Matlock Chesterfield Rd, Matlock Moor DE4 5LZ
☎ 01629 582191 📄 01629 582135
web: www.matlockgolfclub.co.uk
Moorland course with fine views of the beautiful Peak District.
18 holes, 5996yds, Par 70, SSS 69, Course record 63.
Club membership 700.
Visitors Mon-Sun except BHs. Booking required Sat & Sun. Handicap certificate. Dress code. **Societies** Booking required. **Green Fees** £35 per day, £29 per round. **Course Designer** Tom Williamson **Facilities** ⊕ ⑩ ⓑ ⌷ 🔱 ⚐ 🖉 **Location** 1.5m NE of Matlock on A632
Hotel ★★★ 81% CHH Riber Hall, MATLOCK ☎ 01629 582795 3 en suite 11 annexe en suite

MORLEY
MAP 08 SK34

Morley Hayes Main Rd DE7 6DG
☎ 01332 780480 & 782000 (shop) 📄 01332 781094
e-mail: golf@morleyhayes.com
web: www.morleyhayes.com
Peaceful pay and play course set in a splendid valley and incorporating charming water features and woodland. Floodlit driving range. Challenging nine-hole short course (Tower Course).

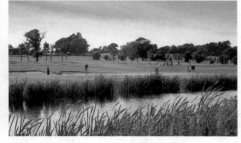

Manor Course: 18 holes, 6726yds, Par 72, SSS 72, Course record 63.
Tower Course: 9 holes, 1614yds, Par 30.

Visitors Mon-Sun & BHs. Booking required. Dress code. **Societies** Booking required. **Green Fees** not confirmed. **Prof** Mark Marriott **Facilities** ⊕ ⑩ ⓑ ⌷ 🔱 ⚐ ◇ 🖉 🗲 **Conf** facs Corporate Hospitality Days
Location On A608 4m N of Derby
Hotel ★★★★ 73% HL The Morley Hayes Hotel, Main Rd, MORLEY ☎ 01332 780480 32 en suite

NEW MILLS
MAP 07 SK08

New Mills Shaw Marsh SK22 4QE
☎ 01663 743485 📄 01663 743485
web: www.newmillsgolfclub.com
Moorland course with panoramic views and first-class greens.
18 holes, 5604yds, Par 69, SSS 67, Course record 62.
Club membership 483.
Visitors contact club for details. **Societies** welcome. **Green Fees** not confirmed. ⊕ **Prof** Carl Cross **Course Designer** Williams **Facilities** ⊕ ⑩ ⓑ ⌷ 🔱 ⚐ 🖉 🗲 **Conf** Corporate Hospitality Days
Location 0.5m N off B6101
Hotel ★★★ 75% HL Best Western Moorside Grange Hotel & Spa, Mudhurst Ln, Higher Disley, DISLEY ☎ 01663 764151 98 en suite

RENISHAW
MAP 08 SK47

Renishaw Park Club House, Mill Ln S21 3UZ
☎ 01246 432044 & 435484 📄 01246 432116
web: www.renishawparkgolf.co.uk
Part parkland and part meadowland with easy walking.
18 holes, 6107yds, Par 71, SSS 70, Course record 64.
Club membership 750.
Visitors Mon-Sun except BHs. Handicap certificate required. Dress code. **Societies** Booking required. **Green Fees** Phone. ⊕ **Prof** Nigel Parkinson **Course Designer** Sir George Sitwell **Facilities** ⊕ ⑩ ⓑ ⌷ 🔱 ⚐ 🖉 **Conf** Corporate Hospitality Days **Location** M1 junct 30, 1.5m W
Hotel ★★★ 70% HL Sitwell Arms Hotel, Station Rd, RENISHAW ☎ 01246 435226 & 437327 📄 01246 433915 30 en suite

RISLEY
MAP 08 SK43

Maywood Rushy Ln DE72 3ST
☎ 0115 939 2306 & 9490043 (pro)
18 holes, 6424yds, Par 72, SSS 71, Course record 70.
Course Designer P Moon **Location** M1 junct 25
Telephone for further details
Hotel BUD Days Inn Donington, Welcome Break Services, A50 Westbound, SHARDLOW ☎ 01332 799666 47 en suite

SHIRLAND
MAP 08 SK45

Shirland Lower Delves DE55 6AU
☎ 01773 834935 📄 01773 832515
e-mail: office@shirlandgolfclub.co.uk
web: www.shirlandgolfclub.co.uk
Rolling parkland and tree-lined course with extensive views of Derbyshire countryside.
18 holes, 6072yds, Par 71, SSS 70, Course record 67.
Club membership 250.
Visitors may play Mon-Fri & BHs. Sat & Sun after 1pm. Dress code. **Societies** Booking required. **Green Fees** Phone. **Prof** Neville Hallam **Facilities** ⊕ ⑩ ⓑ ⌷ 🔱 ⚐ 🖉 🗲 **Conf** facs Corporate Hospitality Days **Location** S side of village off A61

Hotel ★★★★ 77% HL Renaissance Derby/Nottingham Hotel, Carter Ln East, SOUTH NORMANTON ☎ 01773 812000 & 0870 4007262 📠 01773 580032 & 0870 4007362 158 en suite

---

STANTON BY DALE — MAP 08 SK43

Erewash Valley DE7 4QR
☎ 0115 932 2984 📠 0115 944 0061
e-mail: secretary@erewashvalley.co.uk
web: www.erewashvalley.co.uk
Parkland and meadowland course overlooking valley and M1. Unique 4th and 5th in Victorian quarry bottom; 5th testing Par 3.
18 holes, 6557yds, Par 72, SSS 71, Course record 67.
Club membership 750.
Visitors advance booking required. Handicap certificate required. **Societies** contact in advance. **Green Fees** not confirmed. ⊕ **Prof** M J Ronan **Course Designer** Hawtree **Facilities** ⊕ ⑩ ⚑ 🖵 ⛴ ⚒ 🥄 🏆 🏌 🍴 🏆
Location 1m W. M1 junct 25, 2m
Hotel BUD Days Hotel Derby, Derbyshire C C Ground, Pentagon Roundabout, Nottingham Rd, DERBY ☎ 01332 363600 100 en suite

---

UNSTONE — MAP 08 SK37

Birch Hall Sheffield Rd S18 4DB
☎ 01246 291979 📠 01246 412912
Very testing woodland/moorland course demanding respect and a good straight game if one is to walk away with a respectable card. Sloping fairways gather wayward drives into thick gorse and deep ditches. Signature holes are the tough 6th and scenic 13th, the latter begs a big-hitter to go for a shot to the green.
18 holes, 6379yds, Par 73, SSS 71, Course record 72.
Club membership 320.
Visitors may play Mon-Sun & BHs. Advance booking required. Dress code. **Societies** advance booking required. **Green Fees** not confirmed. ⊕ **Prof** Pete Ball **Course Designer** D Tucker **Facilities** ⚒ 🍴 **Location** Off A61 between Sheffield , outskirts of Unstone
Hotel ★★★ 66% HL Sandpiper Hotel, Sheffield Rd, Sheepbridge, CHESTERFIELD ☎ 01246 450550 46 en suite

---

DEVON

AXMOUTH — MAP 03 SY29

Axe Cliff Squires Ln EX12 4AB
☎ 01297 21754 📠 01297 24371
e-mail: davidquinn@axecliff.co.uk
web: www.axecliff.co.uk
One of the oldest courses in Devon, established in 1884. An undulating links course with spectacular coastal views over the Jurassic coastline of Lyme Bay. Good natural drainage gives excellent winter play. A challenge to golfers of all levels.
18 holes, 6000yds, Par 70, SSS 70, Course record 64.
Club membership 327.
Visitors Mon-Sun & BHs. Dress code. **Societies** Welcome. **Green Fees** £17 per day (£22 weekends & bank holidays). Twilight after 4.30pm £10. Reduced winter rates. **Prof** Mark Dack **Course Designer** James Braid **Facilities** ⊕ ⑩ ⚑ 🖵 ⛴ ⚒ 🥄 🏌 🏆 **Conf** Corporate Hospitality Days
Location 0.75m S on B3172
Hotel ★★ 81% HL Swallows Eaves, COLYFORD ☎ 01297 553184
8 en suite

BIGBURY-ON-SEA — MAP 03 SX64

Bigbury TQ7 4BB
☎ 01548 810557 (Secretary) 📠 01548 810207
web: www.bigburygolfclub.com
Clifftop pasture and parkland with easy walking. Exposed to winds, but with fine views over the sea and River Avon. The 7th hole is particularly tricky.
18 holes, 5896yds, Par 70, SSS 69, Course record 65.
Club membership 850.
Visitors may play Mon-Sun & BHs. Handicap certificate required. Dress code. **Societies** Welcome. **Green Fees** £30 per day (£35 weekends). ⊕ **Prof** Simon Lloyd **Course Designer** J H Taylor **Facilities** ⊕ ⑩ by prior arrangement ⚑ 🖵 ⛴ ⚒ 🥄 🏌 🍴 🏆 **Conf** Corporate Hospitality Days
Location 1m S on B3392 between Bigbury and Bigbury-on-Sea
Hotel ★★★★ 79% HL Thurlestone Hotel, THURLESTONE ☎ 01548 560382 64 en suite

---

BLACKAWTON — MAP 03 SX85

Dartmouth Golf & Country Club TQ9 7DE
☎ 01803 712686 📠 01803 712628
e-mail: info@dgcc.co.uk
web: www.dgcc.co.uk
The nine-hole course and the 18-hole Championship Course are both worth a visit and not just for the beautiful views. The Championship is one of the most challenging courses in the West Country with 12 water hazards and a daunting Par 5 4th hole that visitors will always remember. The spectacular final hole, looking downhill and over a water hazard to the green, can be difficult to judge and has been described as one of the most picturesque finishing holes in the country.
Championship Course: 18 holes, 6663yds, Par 72, SSS 72, Course record 64.
Dartmouth Course: 9 holes, 4791yds, Par 66, SSS 64.
Club membership 600.
Visitors may play Mon-Sun & BHs. Advance booking required. Dress code. **Societies** Booking required **Green Fees** Championship: £38 (£48 weekends). Dartmouth: £15 (£16 weekends). **Course Designer** Jeremy Pern **Facilities** ⊕ ⑩ ⚑ 🖵 ⛴ ⚒ 🥄 🏌 🍴 🏆 **Leisure** heated indoor swimming pool, sauna, solarium, gymnasium, Massage & beauty treatments. **Conf** facs Corporate Hospitality Days **Location** A38 from Buckfastleigh. Follow brown leisure signs for Woodlands Leisure Park. 800yds beyond park turn left into club.
Hotel ★★★ 70% HL Stoke Lodge Hotel, Stoke Fleming, DARTMOUTH ☎ 01803 770523 25 en suite

---

BUDLEIGH SALTERTON — MAP 03 SY08

East Devon Links Rd EX9 6DG
☎ 01395 443370 📠 01395 445547
e-mail: secretary@edgc.co.uk
web: www.edgc.co.uk
An interesting course with downland turf, much heather and gorse, and superb views over the bay. Laid out on cliffs 250 to 400 feet above sea level, the early holes climb to the cliff edge. The downhill 17th has a heather section in the fairway, leaving a good second to the green. In addition to rare orchids, the course enjoys an abundance of wildlife including deer and peregrine falcons.
18 holes, 6231yds, Par 70, SSS 70, Course record 61.
Club membership 850.

Continued

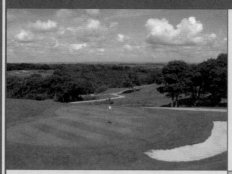
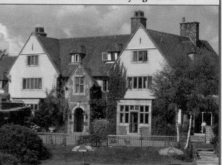

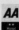

Visitors may play Mon-Sun & BHs. Advance booking required. Handicap certificate required. Dress code. **Societies** Booking required. **Green Fees** £48 per 27/36 holes; £36 per 18 holes. **Prof** Trevor Underwood **Facilities** ⊕ ⊚ ⊾ ⊡ ᛏ ♨ ⚐ ⌇ 🖭 ∦ **Conf** Corporate Hospitality Days **Location** W side of town centre

Hotel ★★★ 75% HL Royal Beacon Hotel, The Beacon, EXMOUTH ☎ 01395 264886 60 en suite

CHITTLEHAMHOLT MAP 03 SS62

Highbullen Hotel EX37 9HD
☎ 01769 540561 📄 01769 540492
e-mail: info@highbullen.co.uk
web: www.highbullen.co.uk

Mature parkland with water hazards and outstanding views to Exmoor and Dartmoor. An easy walking course with some outstanding holes. Excellent greens, which will hold a well-flighted ball, invite you to shoot for the heart of the green past well-maintained bunkers that have been intelligently placed to add to the golfing challenge.

18 holes, 5755yds, Par 68, SSS 67. Club membership 150.
Visitors may play Mon-Sun & BHs. Dress code. **Societies** advance booking required. **Green Fees** not confirmed. **Prof** Paul Weston **Course Designer** M Neil/ J Hamilton **Facilities** ⊕ ⊚ ⊾ ⊡ ᛏ ♨ ⚐ ⌇ ◇ ∦ 🖭 ⌇ **Leisure** hard and grass tennis courts, outdoor and indoor heated swimming pools, fishing, sauna, gymnasium, golf simulator. **Conf** facs Corporate Hospitality Days **Location** 0.5m S of village
Hotel ★★★ CHH Northcote Manor, BURRINGTON ☎ 01769 560501 11 en suite

CHRISTOW MAP 03 SX88

Teign Valley EX6 7PA
☎ 01647 253026 📄 01647 253026
e-mail: julia@teignvalleygolf.co.uk
web: www.teignvalleygolf.co.uk

A scenically spectacular 18-hole course set beside the River Teign in Dartmoor National Park. Offering a good challenge to both low and high handicap golfers, it features two lakeside holes, rolling fairways and fine views.

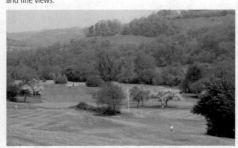

18 holes, 5913yds, Par 70, SSS 69. Club membership 500.
Visitors Mon-Fri & Sun except BHs. Booking required Sun. Dress code.
Societies Welcome. **Green Fees** from £20 per round (£28 Sun). **Prof** Scott Amiet **Course Designer** P Nicholson **Facilities** ⊕ ⊚ ⊾ ⊡ ᛏ ♨ ⚐ ◇ ∦ 🖭 ⌇ **Leisure** gymnasium. **Conf** facs **Location** A38 Teign Valley exit, Exeter/Plymouth Expressway signs on B3193
Hotel ★★★ 75% HL Lord Haldon Hotel, Dunchideock, EXETER ☎ 01392 832483 23 en suite

See advert on opposite page

CHULMLEIGH MAP 03 SS61

Chulmleigh Leigh Rd EX18 7BL
☎ 01769 580519 📄 01769 580519
e-mail: chulmleighgolf@aol.com
web: www.chulmleighgolf.co.uk

Situated in a scenic area with views to distant Dartmoor, this undulating meadowland course offers a good test for the most experienced golfer and is enjoyable for newcomers to the game. Short 18-hole summer course with a tricky 1st hole; in winter the course is changed to nine holes and made longer for players to extend their game.

Summer Course: 18 holes, 1407yds, Par 54, SSS 54,
Course record 48. Club membership 110.
Visitors may play Mon-Sun & BHs. **Societies** Booking required.
Green Fees £8.50 per 18 holes, £7.50 before 10am. **Course Designer** John Goodban **Facilities** ⊾ ⊡ ᛏ ♨ ⚐ ◇ ∦ **Location** SW side of village just off A377
Hotel ★★★ CHH Northcote Manor, BURRINGTON ☎ 01769 560501 11 en suite

CHURSTON FERRERS MAP 03 SX95

Churston Dartmouth Rd TQ5 0LA
☎ 01803 842751 & 842218 📄 01803 845738
e-mail: manager@churstongc.freeserve.co.uk
web: www.churstongolfclublimited.co.uk
18 holes, 6219yds, Par 70, SSS 70, Course record 64.
Location NW side of village on A379
Telephone for further details
Hotel ★★★ 70% HL Berry Head Hotel, Berry Head Rd, BRIXHAM ☎ 01803 853225 32 en suite

See advert on page 51

CREDITON MAP 03 SS80

Downes Crediton Hookway EX17 3PT
☎ 01363 773025 & 774464 📄 01363 775060
e-mail: secretary@downescreditongc.co.uk
web: www.downescreditongc.co.uk

Parkland with water features. Flat front nine. Hilly and wooded back nine.

18 holes, 5954yds, Par 70, SSS 69. Club membership 700.
Visitors may play Mon-Sun & BHs. Booking required. Handicap certificate. Dress code. **Societies** Booking required. **Green Fees** £28 per day (£32 weekends). **Prof** Barry Austin **Facilities** ⊕ ⊚ ⊾ ⊡ ᛏ ♨ ⚐ ∦ **Conf** Corporate Hospitality Days **Location** 1.5m SE off A377
Hotel ★★★ 71% HL Barton Cross Hotel & Restaurant, Huxham, Stoke Canon, EXETER ☎ 01392 841245 9 en suite

CULLOMPTON MAP 03 ST00

Padbrook Park EX15 1RU
☎ 01884 836100 📄 01884 836101
e-mail: padbrookpark@fsmail.net
web: www.padbrookpark.co.uk

A nine-hole, 18-tee parkland course with many water and woodland hazards and spectacular views. The dog-leg 2nd and pulpit 7th are particularly challenging to golfers of all standards. Greens to USPGA specification.

9 holes, 6108yds, Par 70, SSS 69, Course record 65.
Club membership 280.

Continued

Visitors Mon-Sun & BHs. Dress code. **Societies** Booking required. **Green Fees** £18 per 18 holes, £13 per 9 holes (£21/£16 weekends). **Prof** Robert Thorpe/Richard Coffin **Course Designer** Bob Sandow **Facilities** ⓪ ⑩⬤ ▯ ♨ ▯ ⚒ ⬚ ⑰⬥ ✿ ▰ ⚒ ▰ **Leisure** fishing, solarium, gymnasium, indoor bowling centre. **Conf** facs Corporate Hospitality Days **Location** M5 junct 28, 1m on S edge of town

Hotel ★★★ 77% HL Padbrook Park, CULLOMPTON ☎ 01884 836100 40 en suite

DAWLISH WARREN   MAP 03 SX97

Warren EX7 0NF
☎ 01626 862255 & 864002 📄 01626 888005
e-mail: secretary@dwgc.co.uk
web: www.dwgc.co.uk
Typical flat, genuine links course lying on spit between sea and Exe estuary. Picturesque scenery, a few trees but much gorse. Testing in windy conditions. The 7th hole provides the opportunity to go for the green across a bay on the estuary.

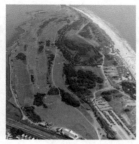

*18 holes, 5954yds, Par 69, SSS 69, Course record 65.
Club membership 600.*
Visitors may play Mon-Sun & BHs. Handicap certificate required. Dress code. **Societies** Booking required. **Green Fees** £30 per day (£35 weekends & bank holidays). Rates exclusive of £1 players' insurance. **Prof** Darren Prowse **Course Designer** James Braid **Facilities** ⓪ ⑩⬤ ▯ ▯ ▯ ♨ ⚒ ⬚ ⑰⬥ ✿ **Conf** facs **Location** E side of village
Hotel ★★★ 77% HL Langstone Cliff Hotel, Dawlish Warren, DAWLISH ☎ 01626 868000 62 en suite 4 annexe en suite

DOWN ST MARY   MAP 03 SS70

Waterbridge EX17 5LG
☎ 01363 85111
web: www.waterbridgegc.co.uk
A testing course of nine holes set in a gently sloping valley. The Par of 32 will not be easily gained, with one Par 5, three Par 4s and five Par 3s, although the Course record holder has Par 29. The 3rd hole which is a raised green is surrounded by water and the 4th (439yds) is demanding for beginners.

9 holes, 3910yds, Par 64, SSS 64. Club membership 120.
Visitors may play Mon-Sun & BHs. **Societies** advance booking required.
Green Fees not confirmed. **Prof** David Ridyard **Course Designer** D Taylor **Facilities** ⓪ ▯ ▯ ⑰ ▯ ⬚ ▯ ⑰⬥ ✿ **Conf** Corporate Hospitality Days **Location** A377 from Exeter towards Barnstaple, 1m past Copplestone
Hotel ★★★ CHH Northcote Manor, BURRINGTON ☎ 01769 560501 11 en suite

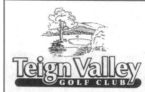
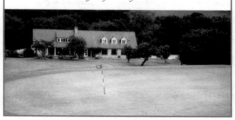
EXETER   MAP 03 SX99

Exeter Golf & Country Club Topsham Rd, Countess Wear EX2 7AE
☎ 01392 874139 📄 01392 874914
e-mail: golf@exetergcc.fsnet.co.uk
web: www.exetergcc.com
Sheltered parkland with some very old trees and known as the flattest course in Devon. Situated in the grounds of a fine mansion, which is now the clubhouse. The 15th and 17th are testing Par 4 holes. Small, well-guarded greens.
*18 holes, 5980yds, Par 69, SSS 69, Course record 62.
Club membership 800.*
Visitors Mon-Sun & BHs. Booking required. Handicap certificate. Dress code.
Societies Booking required. **Green Fees** £44 per day; £36 per round (£48 Sat, Sun & BHs). **Prof** Gary Milne **Course Designer** J Braid **Facilities** ⓪ ⑩⬤ ▯ ▯ ⑰ ▯ ⬚ ⑰⬥ ✿ **Leisure** hard tennis courts, outdoor and indoor heated swimming pools, squash, sauna, solarium, gymnasium, jacuzzi. **Conf** facs Corporate Hospitality Days **Location** SE side of city centre off A379
Hotel ★★★ 73% HL Buckerell Lodge Hotel, Topsham Rd, EXETER ☎ 01392 221111 54 en suite

Woodbury Park Hotel, Golf & Country Club
Woodbury Castle, Woodbury EX5 1JJ
☎ 01395 233500 📄 01395 233384
e-mail: golfbookings@woodburypark.co.uk
web: www.woodburypark.co.uk
Irrigated 18-hole Oaks championship course and excellent nine-hole Acorns course set in 500 acres of wooded parkland with stunning views. *Continued*

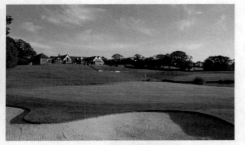

Woodbury Park Hotel, Golf & Country Club

Oaks: 18 holes, 6578yds, Par 72, SSS 72, Course record 66. Acorn: 9 holes, 2297yds, Par 32, SSS 32. Club membership 700.
Visitors may play Mon-Sun & BHs. Advance booking required. Handicap certificate required. Dress code. **Societies** advance booking required. **Green Fees** not confirmed. **Prof** Alan Richards **Course Designer** J Hamilton-Stutt **Facilities** ⚙ ⏐◎⏐ ⏐▙ � ▭ ⏐┒ ▵ ⏐ ◈ ✔ ✚ ◈ ✚ **Leisure** hard tennis courts, heated indoor swimming pool, squash, fishing, sauna, gymnasium, health spa. **Conf** facs Corporate Hospitality Days **Location** M5 junct 30, A3052
Hotel ★★★★ 72% HL Woodbury Park Hotel Golf & Country Club, Woodbury Castle, WOODBURY ☎ 01395 233382 56 en suite

---

HIGH BICKINGTON   MAP 02 SS52

Libbaton EX37 9BS
☎ 01769 560269 & 560167 📄 01769 560342
e-mail: gerald.hemiman@tesco.net
web: www.libbaton.golfclub.com
Parkland on undulating land. Water comes into play on 11 of the 18 holes, as well as a quarry, ditches, trees and eight raised greens. Not a heavily bunkered course, but those present are well positioned and the sharp sand they contain makes them tricky. Five Par 5s could easily get you thinking this course is only for big hitters but as with many good courses, sound course management is the key to success.
18 holes, 6481yds, Par 73, SSS 71, Course record 72. Club membership 500.
Visitors Mon-Sun & BHs. Dress code. **Societies** Booking required. **Green Fees** £20 per 18 holes (£26 weekends). **Prof** Andrew Norman **Course Designer** Col Badham **Facilities** ⚙ ⏐◎⏐ ⏐▙ ▭ ⏐┒ ▵ ⏐ ◈ ✔ ▥ ◈ ✚ **Conf** facs Corporate Hospitality Days **Location** B3217 1m of High Bickington, off A377
Hotel ★★★ CHH Northcote Manor, BURRINGTON ☎ 01769 560501 11 en suite

---

HOLSWORTHY   MAP 02 SS30

Holsworthy Killatree EX22 6LP
☎ 01409 253177 📄 01409 253177
e-mail: hgcsecretary@aol.com
web: www.holsworthygolfclub.co.uk
Pleasant parkland with gentle slopes, numerous trees and a few strategic bunkers. Small greens offer a good test for players of all abilities.
18 holes, 6059yds, Par 70, SSS 69, Course record 64. Club membership 500.
Visitors Mon-Sun & BHs. Booking required. Dress code. **Societies** Booking required. **Green Fees** Phone. **Prof** Alan Johnston **Facilities** ⚙ ⏐◎⏐ ⏐▙ ▭ ⏐┒ ▵ ▭ ⏐┒ ◈ ✔ ▥ ◈ ✚ **Conf** facs Corporate Hospitality Days **Location** 1.5m W on A3072 towards Bude

Hotel ★★★ 77% HL Falcon Hotel, Breakwater Rd, BUDE ☎ 01288 352005 29 en suite

---

HONITON   MAP 03 ST10

Honiton Middlehills EX14 9TR
☎ 01404 44422 & 42943 📄 01404 46383
e-mail: secretary@honitongolfclub.fsnet.co.uk
web: honitongolfclub.fsnet.co.uk
Founded in 1896, this level parkland course is situated on a plateau 850ft above sea level. Easy walking and good views. The 4th hole is a testing Par 3. The 17th and 18th provide a challenging finish. A premium is placed on accuracy especially from the tee.
18 holes, 5897yds, Par 69, SSS 68, Course record 63. Club membership 800.
Visitors Mon-Sun & BHs. Booking advised. Handicap certificate required. Dress code. **Societies** Welcome. **Green Fees** £26 per day (£30 weekends & bank holidays). Twilight and winter rates on application. ✆ **Prof** Adrian Cave **Facilities** ⚙ ⏐◎⏐ ⏐▙ ▭ ⏐┒ ▵ ▭ ⏐┒ ◈ ✔ **Leisure** hardstanding for touring caravans with services. **Conf** Corporate Hospitality Days **Location** 1.25m SE of Honiton, turn towards Farway at Tower Cross on A35
Hotel ★★ 80% SHL Home Farm Hotel & Restaurant, Wilmington, HONITON ☎ 01404 831278 7 en suite 5 annexe en suite

---

ILFRACOMBE   MAP 02 SS54

Ilfracombe Hele Bay EX34 9RT
☎ 01271 862176 & 863328 📄 01271 867731
e-mail: ilfracombegolfclub@btinternet.com
web: www.ilfracombegolfclub.com
A challenging coastal heathland course with views over the Bristol Channel and South Wales from every hole.
18 holes, 5596yds, Par 69, SSS 67, Course record 66. Club membership 520.
Visitors Mon-Sun & BHs. Booking required. **Societies** Booking required. **Green Fees** £25 per round (£30 weekends & bank holidays). **Prof** Mark Davies **Course Designer** T K Weir **Facilities** ⚙ ⏐◎⏐ ⏐▙ ▭ ⏐┒ ▵ ▭ ⏐┒ ◈ ✔ ▥ ◈ ✚ **Location** 1.5m E of Ilfracombe, off A399
Hotel ★★ 74% HL Elmfield Hotel, Torrs Park, ILFRACOMBE ☎ 01271 863377 11 en suite 2 annexe en suite

---

IPPLEPEN   MAP 03 SX86

Dainton Park Totnes Rd, Ipplepen TQ12 5TN
☎ 01803 815000
e-mail: info@daintonparkgolf.co.uk
web: www.daintonparkgolf.co.uk
A challenging parkland course in typical Devon countryside, with gentle contours, tree-lined fairways and raised tees. Water hazards make the two opening holes particularly testing. The 8th, a dramatic 180yd drop hole surrounded by sand, is one of four tough Par 3s on the course.
18 holes, 6400yds, Par 71, SSS 71, Course record 69. Club membership 700.
Visitors may play Mon-Sun & BHs. Booking required. Dress code. **Societies** Booking required. **Green Fees** £22 per round (£25 weekends). **Prof** Jason Fullard **Course Designer** Adrian Stiff **Facilities** ⚙ ⏐◎⏐ ⏐▙ ▭ ⏐┒ ▵ ▭ ⏐┒ ◈ ✔ ▥ **Leisure** gymnasium, fitness gym. **Conf** Corporate Hospitality Days **Location** 2m S of Newton Abbot on A381
Hotel ★★ 72% MET Best Western Queens Hotel, Queen St, NEWTON ABBOT ☎ 01626 363133 26 en suite

IVYBRIDGE MAP 02 SX65

Dinnaton Blachford Rd PL21 9HU
☎ 01752 690020 & 892512 📠 01752 698334
e-mail: info@mccaulays.com
web: www.mccaulays.com
9 holes, 4089yds, Par 64, SSS 60.
Course Designer Cotton & Pink **Location** Off A38 at Ivybridge junct
towards town centre, 1st rdbt brown signs for club 1m
Telephone for further details
Hotel ★★ 76% HL Glazebrook Country House Hotel, SOUTH BRENT
☎ 01364 73322 10 en suite

MORETONHAMPSTEAD MAP 03 SX78

Bovey Castle TQ13 8RE
☎ 01647 445009 📠 01647 440961
e-mail: richard.lewis@boveycastle.com
web: www.boveycastle.com
This enjoyable parkland course has enough hazards to make any
golfer think. Most hazards are natural such as the Rivers Bowden and
Bovey which meander through the first eight holes.
18 holes, 6303yds, Par 70, SSS 70, Course record 63.
Club membership 320.
Visitors may play Mon-Sun & BHs. Advance booking required. Dress
code. **Societies** Booking required **Green Fees** £100 per round.
Prof Richard Lewis **Course Designer** J Abercrombie **Facilities** ⑪ ⑩
🕭 🖵 🖫 ⚒ 🖝 ♢ ✔ 🖢 ✔ 🟊 **Leisure** hard and grass tennis courts,
outdoor and indoor heated swimming pools, fishing, sauna, solarium,
gymnasium. **Conf** facs Corporate Hospitality Days **Location** 2m W of
Moretonhampstead, off B3212
Hotel ★★★★★ 84% HL Bovey Castle, Dartmoor National Park, North
Bovey, MORETONHAMPSTEAD ☎ 01647 445000 58 en suite 7 annexe
en suite

MORTEHOE MAP 02 SS44

Mortehoe & Woolacombe EX34 7EH
☎ 01271 870667 & 870566
e-mail: malcolm_wilkinson@northdevon.gov.uk
Easewell: 9 holes, 4690yds, Par 66, SSS 63,
Course record 66.
Course Designer D Hoare **Location** 0.25m before Mortehoe on station
road
Telephone for further details
Hotel ★★★ 88% HL Watersmeet Hotel, Mortehoe, WOOLACOMBE
☎ 01271 870333 25 en suite

NEWTON ABBOT MAP 03 SX87

Hele Park Golf Centre Ashburton Rd TQ12 6JN
☎ 01626 336060
e-mail: info@heleparkgolf.co.uk
web: www.heleparkgolf.co.uk
Gently undulating parkland course with views stretching to Dartmoor.
A fair test of golf with water in play on 3 holes.
9 holes, 5228yds, Par 68, SSS 65, Course record 63.
Club membership 400.
Visitors Mon-Sun & BHs. Booking required. Dress code. **Societies** Booking
required. **Green Fees** £20 per 18 holes, £11.50 per 9 holes. (£22/£12.50
Sat, Sun & BHs). **Prof** Duncan Arnold **Course Designer** M Craig **Facilities**

⑪ 🕭 🖵 🖫 ⚒ 🖝 ♞ ✔ 🖢 ✔ 🟊 **Conf** Corporate Hospitality Days
Location W of town off A383 Newto Abbot to Ashburton road.
Hotel ★★★ 71% HL Passage House Hotel, Hackney Ln, Kingsteignton,
NEWTON ABBOT ☎ 01626 355515 38 en suite

Newton Abbot (Stover) Bovey Rd TQ12 6QQ
☎ 01626 352460 (Secretary) 📠 01626 330210
e-mail: info@stovergolfclub.co.uk
web: www.stovergolfclub.co.uk
Mature wooded parkland with water coming into play on eight holes.
18 holes, 5764yds, Par 69, SSS 68, Course record 63.
Club membership 800.
Visitors Mon & Wed-Sun except BHs. Booking required Thu. Handicap
certificate. Dress code. **Societies** Booking required. **Green Fees** £32 per
round/day. **Prof** Malcolm Craig **Course Designer** James Braid **Facilities** ⑪
⑩ 🕭 🖵 🖫 ⚒ 🖝 ✔ **Conf** Corporate Hospitality Days **Location** 3m N of
Newton Abbot on A382. Bovey Tracey exit on A38
Hotel ★★ 72% MET Best Western Queens Hotel, Queen St, NEWTON
ABBOT ☎ 01626 363133 26 en suite

OKEHAMPTON MAP 02 SX59

Ashbury Golf Hotel Higher Maddaford EX20 4NL
☎ 01837 55453 📠 01837 55468
web: www.ashburygolfhotel.co.uk
The courses occupy a lightly wooded parkland setting in rolling Devon
countryside on the foothills of Dartmoor National Park. Extra hazards
have been added to the natural ones already present, with over 100
bunkers and 18 lakes. The courses are open throughout the year with
either larger main greens or purpose built alternate ones.

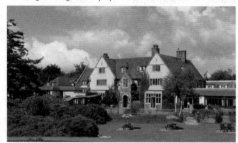

Oakwood: 18 holes, 5400yds, Par 68, SSS 66,
Course record 65.
Pines: 18 holes, 5628yds, Par 69, SSS 67.
Beeches: 18 holes, 5351yds, Par 68, SSS 66.
Club membership 170.
Visitors may play Mon-Thu. Advance booking required. Handicap certificate
required. Dress code. **Societies** advance booking required. **Green Fees** not
confirmed. **Course Designer** David Fensom **Facilities** ⑪ 🕭 🖵 🖫 ⚒ 🖝
🖞 ♢ 🖢 ✔ 🟊 **Leisure** hard tennis courts, heated indoor swimming pool,
fishing, sauna, Par 3 course, indoor bowls, snooker. **Location** Off A3079
Okehampton-Holsworthy
Hotel ★★ 71% HL Ashbury Hotel, Higher Maddaford, Southcott,
OKEHAMPTON ☎ 01837 55453 69 en suite 30 annexe en suite

See advert on page 67

Okehampton Tors Rd EX20 1EF
☎ 01837 52113 📠 01837 52734
e-mail: okehamptongc@btconnect.com
web: www.okehamptongc.co.uk
A good combination of moorland, woodland and river makes this one of the prettiest, yet testing courses in Devon.
18 holes, 5268yds, Par 68, SSS 66, Course record 66.
Club membership 600.
Visitors Contact club for details. **Societies** Welcome. **Green Fees** £30 per day; £25 per round (£30 Sat & Sun). **Prof** Ashley Moon **Course Designer** J F Taylor **Facilities** ⚑ 🍴 ♂ **Location** 1m S off A30, signed from town centre
Hotel ★★ 71% HL White Hart Hotel, Fore St, OKEHAMPTON
☎ 01837 52730 & 54514 📠 01837 53979 19 en suite

PLYMOUTH   MAP 02 SX45

Elfordleigh Colebrook, Plympton PL7 5EB
☎ 01752 336428 (hotel) & 348425 (golf shop)
📠 01752 344581
e-mail: reception@elfordleigh.co.uk
web: www.elfordleigh.co.uk
Undulating, scenic parkland course set deep in the secluded Plym valley and offering a true challenge to all levels of player. The 11th hole, Par 3 is one of the best in the South West area.
18 holes, 5664yds, Par 69, SSS 67, Course record 66.
Club membership 500.
Visitors may play Mon-Sun & BHs. Handicap certificate required. Dress code. **Societies** advance booking required. **Green Fees** not confirmed. **Prof** Nick Cook **Course Designer** J H Taylor **Facilities** ⑪ 🍴 ⚑ 🖥 🍴 ⚒ 🏋 ♦ ♂ ⚑ ♂ **Leisure** hard tennis courts, heated indoor swimming pool, squash, sauna, solarium, gymnasium, golf tuition breaks. **Conf** facs Corporate Hospitality Days **Location** 2m NE off A374, follow signs from Plympton town centre
Hotel ★★★ 73% HL Elfordleigh Hotel Golf Leisure, Colebrook, Plympton, PLYMOUTH ☎ 01752 336428 34 en suite

Staddon Heights Plymstock PL9 9SP
☎ 01752 402475 📠 01752 401998
e-mail: roger.brown@btconnect.com
web: www.staddon-heights.co.uk
Cliff top course affording spectacular views across Plymouth Sound, Dartmoor and Bodmin Moor.
18 holes, 6164yds, Par 70, SSS 70, Course record 66.
Club membership 750.
Visitors Mon-Sun & BHs. Booking required Wed, Thu & Sun. Handicap certificate. Dress code. **Societies** Welcome. **Green Fees** £25 (£30 Sat & Sun). ⊕ **Prof** Ian Marshall **Course Designer** Hamilton Stutt **Facilities** ⑪ 🍴 ⚑ 🖥 🍴 ⚒ 🏋 ♂ **Conf** facs **Location** 5m SW of city centre
Hotel ★★★ 79% CHH Langdon Court Hotel, Down Thomas, PLYMOUTH
☎ 01752 862358 18 en suite

SAUNTON   MAP 02 SS43

Saunton EX33 1LG
☎ 01271 812436 📠 01271 814241
e-mail: info@sauntongolf.co.uk
web: www.sauntongolf.co.uk
Two traditional championship links courses. The opening 4 holes of the East course total over one mile in length. The Par 3 5th and 13th holes are short but testing with undulating features and

the 16th is notable. On the West course club selection is paramount as positioning the ball is the key to success. The loop on the back nine, comprising the 12th, 13th and 14th is as testing as it is pleasing to the eye.

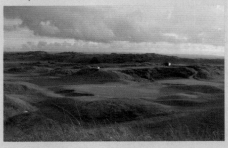

East Course: 18 holes, 6427yds, Par 71, SSS 71, Course record 64.
West Course: 18 holes, 6138yds, Par 71, SSS 70, Course record 63. Club membership 1450.
Visitors Mon-Sun & BHs. Booking required. Handicap certificate. Dress code. **Societies** Booking required. **Green Fees** £85 per day; £60 per round. **Prof** A T MacKenzie **Course Designer** F Pennick/W H Fowler **Facilities** ⑪ 🍴 by prior arrangement ⚑ 🖥 🍴 ⚒ 🏋 ♂ ⚑ ♂ 🏋 **Conf** Corporate Hospitality Days **Location** S side of village off B3231
Hotel ★★★★ 79% HL Saunton Sands Hotel, SAUNTON
☎ 01271 890212 92 en suite

SIDMOUTH   MAP 03 SY18

Sidmouth Cotmaton Rd EX10 8SX
☎ 01395 513451 & 516407 📠 01395 514661
e-mail: secretary@sidmouthgolfclub.co.uk
web: www.sidmouthgolfclub.co.uk
Situated on the side of Peak Hill, offering beautiful coastal views OF Lyme Bay and Sidmouth. Sheltered, undulating fairways and superb greens.
18 holes, 5100yds, Par 66, SSS 65, Course record 59.
Club membership 700.
Visitors Mon-Sun & BHs. Dress code. **Societies** Booking required **Green Fees** £28 per round. **Prof** Chris Haigh **Course Designer** J H Taylor **Facilities** ⑪ 🍴 ⚑ 🖥 🍴 ⚒ 🏋 ♂ ♂ **Conf** Corporate Hospitality Days **Location** W side of town centre
Hotel ★★★★ 83% HL Victoria Hotel, The Esplanade, SIDMOUTH
☎ 01395 512651 61 en suite

SOUTH BRENT   MAP 03 SX66

Wrangaton (S Devon) Golf Links Rd, Wrangaton TQ10 9HJ
☎ 01364 73229 📠 01364 73229
e-mail: wrangatongolf@btconnect.com
web: www.wrangatongolfclub.co.uk
Unique 18-hole course with nine holes on moorland and nine holes on parkland. The course lies within Dartmoor National Park. Spectacular views towards sea and rugged terrain. Natural fairways and hazards include bracken, sheep and ponies.

Continued

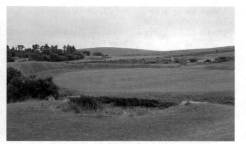

Wrangaton (S Devon)

18 holes, 6065yds, Par 70, SSS 69, Course record 66.
Club membership 680.
Visitors Mon-Sun & BHs. Booking required. Handicap certificate. Dress code. **Societies** Booking required. **Green Fees** Phone. **Prof** Glenn Richards **Course Designer** D M A Steel **Facilities** ⑪ ⑩ by prior arrangement ⓑ ▯ ↑⌾ ⏦ ⛳ ☎ ⛏ ✄ **Location** 2.25m SW off A38, between South Brent and Ivybridge
Hotel ★★ 76% HL Glazebrook Country House Hotel, SOUTH BRENT
☎ 01364 73322   10 en suite

SPARKWELL   MAP 02 SX55

Welbeck Manor & Sparkwell Golf Course Blacklands PL7 5DF
☎ 01752 837219 🖷 01752 837219
9 holes, 2886yds, Par 68, SSS 68, Course record 68.
Course Designer John Gabb **Location** 1m N of A38 Plymouth-Ivybridge road
Telephone for further details

TAVISTOCK   MAP 02 SX47

Hurdwick Tavistock Hamlets PL19 0LL
☎ 01822 612746 🖷 01822 612746
An executive parkland course with many bunkers and fine views. Executive golf originated in America and the concept is that a round should take no longer than 3 hours while offering a solid challenge.
18 holes, 5302yds, Par 68, SSS 67, Course record 67.
Club membership 110.
Visitors may play Mon-Sun & BHs. Dress code. **Societies** advance booking required. **Green Fees** not confirmed. ☺ **Course Designer** Hawtree **Facilities** ⓑ ▯ ↑⌾ ⏦ ☎ ⛏ ✄ **Location** 1m N of Tavistock on the Brentor Road
Hotel ★★★ 70% HL Bedford Hotel, 1 Plymouth Rd, TAVISTOCK
☎ 01822 613221   29 en suite

Tavistock Down Rd PL19 9AQ
☎ 01822 612344 🖷 01822 612344
e-mail: tavygolf@hotmail.org
web: www.tavistockgolfclub.org.uk
Set on Whitchurch Down in south-west Dartmoor with easy walking and magnificent views over rolling countryside into Cornwall. Downland turf with some heather, and interesting holes on undulating ground.
18 holes, 6495yds, Par 71, SSS 71, Course record 60.
Club membership 700.
Visitors may play Mon-Fri. Handicap certificate. Dress code **Societies** Booking required. **Green Fees** £28 per day/round (£36 weekends

and bank holidays). ☺ **Prof** D Rehaag **Course Designer** H Fowler
Facilities ⑪ ⑩ ⓑ ▯ ↑⌾ ⏦ ☎ ⛏ ✄ **Conf** Corporate Hospitality Days
Location 1m SE of town centre, on Whitchurch Down
Hotel ★★★ 70% HL Bedford Hotel, 1 Plymouth Rd, TAVISTOCK
☎ 01822 613221   29 en suite

TEDBURN ST MARY   MAP 03 SX89

Fingle Glen Golf Hotel EX6 6AF
☎ 01647 61817 🖷 01647 61135
e-mail: fingle.glen@btinternet.com
web: www.fingleglen.com
Fingle Glen has been extended in recent years into a fine 18 hole parkland course.
18 holes, 5878yds, Par 70, SSS 68, Course record 63.
Club membership 650.
Visitors may play Mon-Sun & BHs. Dress code. **Societies** welcome **Green Fees** not confirmed. **Prof** Stephen Gould **Course Designer** Bill Pile **Facilities** ⑪ ⑩ ⓑ ▯ ↑⌾ ⏦ ♡ ✄ ⛳ ☎ ⛏ **Conf** facs Corporate Hospitality Days **Location** 5m W of Exeter, off A30
Hotel ★★★ 73% HL St Olaves Hotel, Mary Arches St, EXETER
☎ 01392 217736   15 en suite

TEIGNMOUTH   MAP 03 SX97

Teignmouth Haldon Moor TQ14 9NY
☎ 01626 777070 🖷 01626 777304
e-mail: tgc@btconnect.com
web: www.teignmouthgolfclub.co.uk
This fairly flat heathland course is high up with fine panoramic views of sea, moors and river valley. Good springy turf with some heather and an interesting layout makes for very enjoyable holiday golf. Designed by Dr A MacKenzie, the world famous architect who also designed Augusta GC USA.
18 holes, 6200yds, Par 69, SSS 69, Course record 63.
Club membership 900.
Visitors Mon-Sun & BHs. Handicap certificate required. Dress code. **Societies** Booking required. **Green Fees** £40 per day. **Prof** Rob Selley **Course Designer** Dr Alister Mackenzie **Facilities** ⑪ ⑩ ⓑ ▯ ↑⌾ ⏦ ☎ **Conf** facs Corporate Hospitality Days **Location** 2m NW off B3192
Hotel ★★ 68% HL Cockhaven Manor Hotel, Cockhaven Rd, BISHOPSTEIGNTON ☎ 01626 775252   12 en suite

THURLESTONE   MAP 03 SX64

Thurlestone TQ7 3NZ
☎ 01548 560405 🖷 01548 562149
e-mail: secretary@thurlestonegc.co.uk
web: www.thurlestonegc.co.uk
Situated on the edge of the cliffs with downland turf and good greens. The course, after an interesting opening hole, rises to higher land with fine sea views, and finishes with an excellent 502yd downhill hole to the clubhouse.
18 holes, 6340yds, Par 71, SSS 70, Course record 65.
Club membership 770.
Visitors Mon-Sun & BHs. Booking required. Handicap certificate. Dress code. **Green Fees** £36 per day/round. **Prof** Peter Laugher **Course Designer** Harry S Colt **Facilities** ⑪ ⑩ by prior arrangement ⓑ ▯ ↑⌾ ⏦ ☎ ⛏ ✄ **Leisure** hard and grass tennis courts. **Location** S side of village
Hotel ★★★★ 79% HL Thurlestone Hotel, THURLESTONE
☎ 01548 560382   64 en suite

England

TIVERTON
MAP 03 SS91

Tiverton Post Hill EX16 4NE
☎ 01884 252187 📄 01884 251607
e-mail: tivertongolfclub@lineone.net
web: www.tivertongolfclub.co.uk
Parkland with many different species of tree, and lush pastures that ensure some of the finest fairways in the south-west. The undulating ground provides plenty of variety and there are a number of interesting holes which visitors will find a real challenge.
18 holes, 6236yds, Par 71, SSS 71, Course record 65. Club membership 750.
Visitors Mon-Fri & Sun. Booking required. Handicap certificate. Dress code. **Societies** Booking required. **Green Fees** £32 per 18 holes. 🌐
Prof Michael Hawton **Course Designer** Braid **Facilities** ⑪ ◐ 🖿 ☐ 🕽🎽 🏊 🛋 🏌 **Conf** Corporate Hospitality Days **Location** 3m E of Tiverton. M5 junct 27, through Sampford Peverell & Halberton
Hotel ★★★ 72% HL Best Western The Tiverton Hotel, Blundells Rd, TIVERTON ☎ 01884 256120 69 en suite

TORQUAY
MAP 03 SX96

Torquay 30 Petitor Rd, St Marychurch TQ1 4QF
☎ 01803 314591 📄 01803 316116
e-mail: info@torquaygolfclub.org.uk
web: www.torquaygolfclub.org.uk
Unusual combination of cliff and parkland golf, with wonderful views over the sea and Dartmoor.
18 holes, 6164yds, Par 69, SSS 69, Course record 63. Club membership 725.
Visitors Mon-Sun except BHs. Booking required Sat, Sun & BHs. Handicap certificate. Dress code. **Societies** Booking required. **Green Fees** £33 per day (£35Sat & Sun). **Prof** Martin Ruth **Facilities** ⑪ ◐ 🖿 ☐ 🕽🎽 🏊 🛋 🏌 🏌 🛋 🏌 **Location** 1.25m N
Hotel ★★ 63% HL Norcliffe Hotel, 7 Babbacombe Downs Rd, Babbacombe, TORQUAY ☎ 01803 328456 26 en suite

TORRINGTON (GREAT)
MAP 02 SS41

Torrington Weare Trees, Great Torrington EX38 7EZ
☎ 01805 622229 & 623878 📄 01805 623878
e-mail: theoffice@torringtongolf.fsnet.co.uk
web: twww.torringtongolfclub.co.uk
Attractive and challenging nine-hole course. Free draining to allow play all year round. Excellent greens and outstanding views.
9 holes, 4423yds, Par 64, SSS 62, Course record 58. Club membership 420.
Visitors Mon, Thu, Fri & BHs. Other days pm only. Booking required. Dress code. **Societies** Booking required. **Green Fees** £20 per day, £15 per round. 🌐 **Facilities** ⑪ 🖿 ☐ 🕽🎽 🏊 🎽 🏌 **Location** 1m W of Torringdon
Hotel ★★★ 75% HL Royal Hotel, Barnstaple St, BIDEFORD ☎ 01237 472005 32 en suite

WESTWARD HO!
MAP 02 SS42

Royal North Devon Golf Links Rd EX39 1HD
☎ 01237 473817 📄 01237 423456
e-mail: info@royalnorthdevongolfclub.co.uk
web: www.royalnorthdevongolfclub.co.uk
Oldest links course in England with traditional links features and a museum in the clubhouse.

18 holes, 6665yds, Par 72, SSS 72, Course record 65. Club membership 1150.
Visitors Mon-Sun & BHs. Booking required. Handicap certificate. Dress code. **Societies** Booking required. **Green Fees** £44 per day; £38 per round (£50/£44 weekends & bank holidays). **Prof** Iain Parker
Course Designer Old Tom Morris **Facilities** ⑪ ◐ 🖿 ☐ 🕽🎽 🏊 🛋 🏌 🏌 **Leisure** Museum of Golf Memorabilia, snooker. **Conf** facs Corporate Hospitality Days **Location** N side of village off B3236
Guesthouse ★★★ GH Culloden House, Fosketh Hill, WESTWARD HO! ☎ 01237 479421 5 en suite

WOOLFARDISWORTHY
MAP 02 SS32

Hartland Forest EX39 5RA
☎ 01237 431442 📄 01237 431734
e-mail: hfgolf@googlemail.com
web: www.hartlandforestgolf.co.uk
Exceptionally varied course with water hazards on 12 holes and gentle slopes.
18 holes, 6004yds, Par 71, SSS 69. Club membership 100.
Visitors Mon-Sun & BHs. **Societies** Booking required. **Green Fees** £25 for 18 holes, £15 for 9 holes. **Course Designer** A Cartwright **Facilities** ⑪ 🖿 ☐ 🕽🎽 🏊 🛋 🏌 ◇ 🛋 🏌 **Leisure** hard tennis courts, heated indoor swimming pool, fishing, sauna, gymnasium. **Conf** Corporate Hospitality Days **Location** 4m S of Clovelly Cross, 1.7m E of A39
Hotel ★★★ 74% CHH Penhaven Country House, Rectory Ln, PARKHAM ☎ 01237 451388 & 451711 📄 01237 451878 12 en suite

YELVERTON
MAP 02 SX56

Yelverton Golf Links Rd PL20 6BN
☎ 01822 852824 📄 01822 854869
e-mail: secretary@yelvertongc.co.uk
web: www.yelvertongc.co.uk
An excellent course on Dartmoor with plenty of gorse and heather. Tight lies in the fairways, fast greens and challenging hazards. Three of the best holes in Devon (12th, 13th and 16th) and outstanding views.
18 holes, 6353yds, Par 71, SSS 71, Course record 64. Club membership 650.
Visitors Mon-Fri, Sun & BHs. Handicap certificate. Dress code. **Societies** Booking required. **Green Fees** £34 per day. **Prof** Tim McSherry **Course Designer** Herbert Fowler **Facilities** ⑪ ◐ 🖿 ☐ 🕽🎽 🏊 🛋 🏌 🏌 **Leisure** indoor golf academy. **Conf** facs Corporate Hospitality Days **Location** 1m S of Yelverton, off A386
Hotel ★★★ 74% HL Moorland Links Hotel, YELVERTON ☎ 01822 852245 44 en suite

DORSET

ASHLEY HEATH
MAP 04 SU10

Moors Valley Horton Rd BH24 2ET
☎ 01425 479776
e-mail: golf@eastdorset.gov.uk
web: www.moors-valley.co.uk/golf
Skilfully designed by Hawtree, this mature heathland and woodland course is scenically set within a wildlife conservation area, exuding peace and tranquillity. Each hole has its own character, the back seven being in particular very special. The course is renowned for its greens.
18 holes, 6337yds, Par 72, SSS 70, Course record 67.

Continued

Visitors Mon-Sun & BHs. Booking required. Dress code. **Societies** Booking required. **Green Fees** £22 per round. **Course Designer** Hawtree & Son **Facilities** ⓘ 🍴 by prior arrangement 🏌 ⌨ ⛳ 🏊 ⛵ 🍴 **Leisure** fishing, 4 hole game improvement course, bike hire, aerial assault course. **Conf** facs Corporate Hospitality Days **Location** 1.5m from A331/A338 rdbt, signed
Hotel BUD Travelodge Ringwood, St Leonards, RINGWOOD
☎ 08700 850 950

BEAMINSTER   MAP 03 ST40

Chedington Court South Perrott DT8 3HU
☎ 01935 891413 🖨 01935 891217
e-mail: admincgc@btconnect.com
web: www.chedingtongolfclub.co.uk
This beautiful 18-hole parkland course is set on the Dorset-Somerset borders with mature trees and interesting water hazards. A challenge from the first hole, Par 5, blind drive to the elevated tee on the 15th, and the closing holes can be tricky.

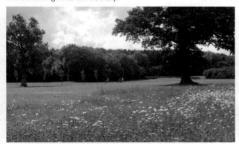

18 holes, 5924yds, Par 70, SSS 70, Course record 68.
Club membership 403.
Visitors Mon-Sun & BHs. Dress code. **Societies** Booking required. **Green Fees** Phone. **Prof** Steve Ritchie **Course Designer** David Hemstock/Donald Steel **Facilities** ⓘ 🍴 🏌 ⌨ ⛳ 🏊 ⛵ 🍴 **Conf** Corporate Hospitality Days **Location** 5m NE of Beaminster on A356 Dorchester-Crewkerne
Hotel ★★★ 77% HL Bridge House Hotel, 3 Prout Bridge, BEAMINSTER
☎ 01308 862200   9 en suite   5 annexe en suite

BERE REGIS   MAP 03 SY89

Dorset Golf & Country Club BH20 7NT
☎ 01929 472244 🖨 01929 471294
e-mail: admin@dorsetgolfresort.com
web: www.dorsetgolfresort.com
Lakeland/Parkland is the longest course in Dorset. Designed by Martin Hawtree with numerous interconnected water features, carefully planned bunkers and sculptured greens. A player who completes a round within handicap has every reason to celebrate. The Woodland course, although shorter, is equally outstanding with rhododendron and tree-lined fairways.
Lakeland/Parkland Course: 18 holes, 6580yds, Par 72, SSS 73, Course record 69.
Woodland Course: 9 holes, 5032yards, Par 66, SSS 64.
Club membership 600.
Visitors may play Mon-Sun & BHs. Advance booking required. Dress code. **Societies** advance booking required. **Green Fees** not confirmed. **Prof** Scott Porter **Course Designer** Martin Hawtree **Facilities** ⓘ 🍴 🏌

⌨ 🍴 🏌 ⌨ ⛳ ⛵ 🍴 **Leisure** fishing. **Conf** facs Corporate Hospitality Days **Location** 5m from Bere Regis on Wool Road
Hotel ★★ 72% CHH Kemps Hotel, East Stoke, WAREHAM
☎ 01929 462563   4 en suite   10 annexe en suite

BLANDFORD FORUM   MAP 03 ST80

Ashley Wood Wimborne Rd DT11 9HN
☎ 01258 452253 🖨 01258 450590
e-mail: generalmanager@ashleywoodgolfclub.com
web: www.ashleywoodgolfclub.com
The course is one of the oldest in the country. The first record of play on Keyneston Down was in 1896, and part of the ancient course is played over Buzbury Rings, a prehistoric hill fort with magnificent views over the Stour and Tarrant valleys. Constructed on downland, the fairways are undulating and, apart from the 3rd hole with a short sharp hill, all holes are easy walking. Four holes are played within the ancient woodland of Ashley Woods. The natural chalk provides excellent drainage.

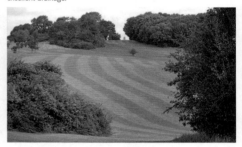

18 holes, 6284yds, Par 70, SSS 70, Course record 66.
Club membership 670.
Visitors Mon-Sun & BHs. Handicap certificate. Dress code. **Societies** Booking required. **Green Fees** £42 per day, £26.50 per 18 holes after 10am (£31.50 per 18 holes weekends). 🏌 **Prof** Jon Shimmons **Course Designer** P Tallack **Facilities** ⓘ 🍴 by prior arrangement 🏌 ⌨ 🍴 🏊 ⛵ 🍴 **Conf** Corporate Hospitality Days **Location** 2m E on B3082
Hotel ★★★ 72% HL Best Western Crown Hotel, West St, BLANDFORD FORUM ☎ 01258 456626   32 en suite

BOURNEMOUTH   MAP 04 SZ09

The Club at Meyrick Park Central Dr, Meyrick Park BH2 6LH
☎ 01202 786000 🖨 01202 786020
e-mail: meyrickpark.lodge@theclubcompany.com
web: www.theclubcompany.com
Picturesque municipal parkland course founded in 1890.
18 holes, 5600yds, Par 69, SSS 69.
Visitors may play Mon-Sun & BHs. Advance booking required. Dress code. **Societies** advance booking required. **Green Fees** not confirmed. **Prof** Andy Britton **Facilities** ⓘ 🍴 🏌 ⌨ 🍴 🏊 ⛵ 🍴 **Leisure** heated indoor swimming pool, sauna, solarium, gymnasium, spa and steam room. **Conf** facs
Hotel ★★★ 67% HL Burley Court Hotel, Bath Rd, BOURNEMOUTH
☎ 01202 552824 & 556704 🖨 01202 298514   38 en suite

England

Iford Golf Centre Riverside Av, off Castle Ln East BH7 7ES
☎ 01202 436436 📠 01202 436400
e-mail: info@ifordgolfcentre.co.uk
web: www.ifordgolfcentre.co.uk
A well drained meadowland course beside the river Stour with many mature trees and lakes on five holes. Enjoyable for intermediates and beginners off yellow or white tees and a test for any golfer off the back blue tees. Greens are superb and need careful reading.
Bridge Course: 18 holes, 6277yards, Par 72, SSS 69.
Club membership 300.
Visitors Mon-Fri & BHs. Booking required. Dress code. **Societies** Booking required. **Green Fees** £16.80 per 18 holes (£20 per 18 holes weekends). Par 3 course from £3. **Prof** Lawrence Moxon **Course Designer** John Jacobs Golf Associates **Facilities** ⑪ ⑩ 🍴 🖥 ☂ 🐴 ⬤ 🎯 🏌 ⛳ **Leisure** 9 hole Par 3 course. **Conf** facs Corporate Hospitality Days **Location** Off A338 onto A3060 for Christchurch, past Tesco, left onto Riverside Av
Hotel BUD Innkeeper's Lodge Bournemouth, Cooper Dean Roundabout, Castle Ln East, BOURNEMOUTH ☎ 0845 112 6085 28 en suite

Knighton Heath Francis Av, West Howe BH11 8NX
☎ 01202 572633 📠 01202 590774
e-mail: khgc@btinternet.com
Undulating heathland course on high ground inland from Poole.
18 holes, 6084yds, Par 70, SSS 69. Club membership 700.
Visitors may play Mon-Thu. Advance booking required. Handicap certificate required. Dress code. **Societies** advance booking required. **Green Fees** not confirmed. ⬤ **Prof** Paul Brown **Facilities** ⑪ ⑩ 🍴 🖥 ☂ 🐴 ⬤ 🎯
Location N side of Poole, junct A348 signed at rdbt
Guesthouse ★★★★ GA Ashton Lodge, 10 Oakley Hill, WIMBORNE ☎ 01202 883423 5 rms (2 en suite)

Queen's Park Queens Park Dr West BH8 9BY
☎ 01202 437807 📠 01202 396817
e-mail: queenspark@bournemouth.gov.uk
web: www.littledowncentre.co.uk/qpgolf
Mature parkland with undulating tree-lined fairways. A demanding test of golf, with each hole having a unique character.
18 holes, 6132yds, Par 71, SSS 69, Course record 69.
Club membership 370.
Visitors Mon-Sun & BHs. Booking required. Dress code. **Societies** Booking required. **Green Fees** £15 per round (£21 Sat, Sun & BHs). Reduced winter rates. **Facilities** ⑪ ⑩ 🍴 🖥 ☂ 🐴 ⬤ 🎯 🏌 ⛳ **Conf** facs Corporate Hospitality Days **Location** 2m NE of Bournemouth town centre off A338
Hotel ★★★ 75% HL Queens Hotel, Meyrick Rd, East Cliff, BOURNEMOUTH ☎ 01202 554415 109 en suite

Solent Meads Rolls Dr, Hengistbury Head BH6 4NA
☎ 01202 420795
e-mail: solentmeads@yahoo.co.uk
web: www.solentmeads.com
An 18-hole Par 3 links course overlooking Hengistbury Head with fine views of Christchurch Harbour and the Isle of Wight. Expect a sea breeze. One of the driest courses in the county.
18 holes, 2182yards, Par 54.
Visitors Mon-Sun & BHs. **Societies** welcome. **Green Fees** £7.70 per 18 holes. ⬤ **Prof** Warren Butcher **Facilities** ⑪ 🍴 🖥 ☂ 🐴 🎯 🏌
Leisure 9 hole pitch & putt. **Conf** Corporate Hospitality Days
Location from A35 take B3509 (signposted Tuckton/Southbourne). At 2nd

roundabout go straight ahead and take 1st left (Broadway). After 0.75m turn left into Rolls Drive.
Hotel BUD Premier Travel Inn Christchurch West, Barrack Rd, CHRISTCHURCH ☎ 08701 977063 42 en suite

---

BRIDPORT   MAP 03 SY49

Bridport & West Dorset The Clubhouse, Burton Rd DT6 4PS
☎ 01308 421491 & 421095 📠 01308 421095
e-mail: secretary@bridportgolfclub.org.uk
web: www.bridportgolfclub.org.uk
Seaside links course on the top of the east cliff, with fine views over Lyme Bay and surrounding countryside. The signature 6th hole, known as Port Coombe, is only 133yds but dropping from the top of the cliff to a green almost at sea level far below. Fine sea views along the Chesil Bank to Portland Bill and across Lyme Bay.
18 holes, 5875yds, Par 70, SSS 68. Club membership 600.
Visitors Mon-Sun & BHs. Dress code. **Societies** Booking required. **Green Fees** £28 per day; £22 after 2pm, £14 after 5pm. **Prof** David Parsons
Course Designer Hawtree **Facilities** ⑪ 🍴 🖥 ☂ 🐴 ⬤ 🎯 🏌 ⛳
Leisure pitch & putt (holiday season). **Conf** Corporate Hospitality Days
Location 1m E of Bridport on B3157
Hotel ★★★ 68% HL Haddon House Hotel, West Bay, BRIDPORT ☎ 01308 423626 & 425323 📠 01308 427348 12 en suite

---

BROADSTONE   MAP 03 SZ09

Broadstone (Dorset) Wentworth Dr BH18 8DQ
☎ 01202 692595 📠 01202 642520
e-mail: admin@broadstonegolfclub.com
web: www.broadstonegolfclub.com
Undulating and demanding heathland course with the 2nd, 7th, 13th and 16th being particularly challenging holes.

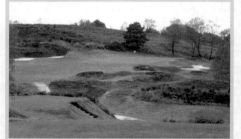

18 holes, 6349yds, Par 70, SSS 70, Course record 63.
Club membership 620.
Visitors Mon-Sun except BHs. Booking required. Handicap certificate. Dress code. **Societies** Booking required. **Green Fees** £72 per 27/36 holes, £48 per round (£62 per round weekends). **Prof** Matthew Wilson **Course Designer** Colt/Dunn **Facilities** ⑪ ⑩ 🍴 🖥 ☂ 🐴 ⬤ 🎯 🏌 ⛳ **Conf** Corporate Hospitality Days **Location** N side of village off B3074
Guesthouse ★★★★ GA Ashton Lodge, 10 Oakley Hill, WIMBORNE ☎ 01202 883423 5 rms (2 en suite)

CHRISTCHURCH
MAP 04 SZ19

Dudmoor Farm Dudmoor Farm Rd, Off Fairmile Rd BH23 6AQ
☎ 01202 473826 ☐ 01202 480207
A testing Par 3 and 4 woodland course in an Area of Outstanding Natural Beauty.
9 holes, 1562 yds, Par 31.
Visitors Mon-Sun & BHs. **Societies** Booking required. **Green Fees** £8.50 per 9/18 holes (£9.50 weekends & bank holidays). ⊛ **Facilities** ⊡ ⊥ ⊶
✦ **Leisure** squash, adjoining riding stables. **Location** Private road off B3073 Christchurch-Hurn road
Hotel ★★★ 80% HL Best Western Waterford Lodge Hotel, 87 Bure Ln, Friars Cliff, CHRISTCHURCH ☎ 01425 272948 & 278801 ☐ 01425 279130 18 en suite

DORCHESTER
MAP 03 SY69

Came Down Higher Came DT2 8NR
☎ 01305 813494 (manager) ☐ 01305 815122
e-mail: manager@camedowngolfclub.co.uk
web: www.camedowngolfclub.co.uk
Scene of the West of England championships on several occasions, this fine course lies on a high plateau commanding glorious views over Portland. Three Par 5 holes add interest to a round. The turf is of the springy, downland type.
18 holes, 6255yds, Par 70, SSS 70. Club membership 750.
Visitors Mon-Sun & BHs. Handicap certificate required. Dress code.
Societies Booking required. **Green Fees** £32 per day weekdays (£38 Sat & Sun). **Prof** Nick Rodgers **Course Designer** J H Taylor/H S Colt
Facilities ⊕ ⊺⊙⊦ ⊫ ⊡ ⊶⊓ ⊥ ⊜ ✦ ✦ **Location** 2m S off A354
Guesthouse ★★★★★ GH Yalbury Cottage Hotel & Restaurant, Lower Bockhampton, DORCHESTER ☎ 01305 262382 8 en suite

FERNDOWN
MAP 04 SU00

Dudsbury 64 Christchurch Rd BH22 8ST
☎ 01202 593499 ☐ 01202 594555
e-mail: golf@dudsburygolfclub.co.uk
web: www.dudsburygolfclub.co.uk
Set in 160 acres of beautiful Dorset countryside rolling down to the River Stour. Wide variety of interesting and challenging hazards, notably water which comes into play on 14 holes. The well-drained greens are protected by large bunkers and water hazards. A feature hole is the 16th where the green is over two lakes; the more aggressive the drive, the greater the reward.
Championship Course: 18 holes, 6904yds, Par 71, SSS 73, Course record 64. Club membership 600.
Visitors Mon-Sun & BHs. Handicap certificate required. Dress code.
Societies Booking required. **Green Fees** £45 per 36 holes; £35 per 18 holes (£50/£40 weekend and bank holidays). **Prof** Steve Pockneall
Course Designer Donald Steel **Facilities** ⊕ ⊺⊙⊦ ⊫ ⊡ ⊶⊓ ⊥ ⊜ ✦ ✦
✦ **Leisure** fishing, 6 Hole Par 3 short game Academy Course. **Conf** facs Corporate Hospitality Days **Location** 3m N of Bournemouth on B3073
Hotel BUD Premier Travel Inn Bournemouth/ Ferndown, Ringwood Rd, Tricketts Cross, FERNDOWN ☎ 08701 977102 32 en suite

Ferndown 119 Golf Links Rd BH22 8BU
☎ 01202 874602 ☐ 01202 873926
e-mail: ferndowngc@lineone.net
web: www.ferndown-golf-club.co.uk
Fairways are gently undulating among heather, gorse and pine trees, giving the course a most attractive appearance. There are a number of dog-leg holes.
Championship Course: 18 holes, 6505yds, Par 71, SSS 71, Course record 63.
Presidents Course: 9 holes, 5604yds, Par 70, SSS 68. Club membership 600.
Visitors Booking required. Handicap certificate. Dress code. **Societies** Booking required. **Green Fees** Championship: £80 per day, £60 per round. **Prof** Neil Plke **Course Designer** Harold Hilton **Facilities** ⊕ ⊺⊙⊦ ⊫ ⊡ ⊶⊓ ⊥ ⊜ ⊜ ✦ **Conf** Corporate Hospitality Days **Location** S side of town centre off A347
Hotel BUD Premier Travel Inn Bournemouth/ Ferndown, Ringwood Rd, Tricketts Cross, FERNDOWN ☎ 08701 977102 32 en suite

Ferndown Forest Forest Links Rd BH22 9PH
☎ 01202 876096 ☐ 01202 894095
e-mail: golf@ferndownforestgolf.co.uk
web: www.ferndownforestgolf.co.uk
Flat parkland dotted with mature oaks, several interesting water features, and some tight fairways.
18 holes, 5068yds, Par 68, SSS 67, Course record 69. Club membership 400.
Visitors Mon-Sun & BHs. Booking required. Dress code. **Societies** Booking required. **Green Fees** £16 per round (£18 Sat, Sun & BHs). **Prof** Graham Howell **Course Designer** Guy Hunt/Richard Graham **Facilities** ⊕ ⊺⊙⊦ ⊫ ⊡ ⊶⊓ ⊥ ⊜ ⊜ ✦ ✦ ⊜ ✦ **Conf** facs Corporate Hospitality Days **Location** Off A31 N of Ferndown, follow signs to Dorset Police Headquarters
Hotel BUD Premier Travel Inn Bournemouth/ Ferndown, Ringwood Rd, Tricketts Cross, FERNDOWN ☎ 08701 977102 32 en suite

HALSTOCK
MAP 03 ST50

Halstock Common Ln BA22 9SF
☎ 01935 891689 & 891968 (pro shop) ☐ 01935 891839
e-mail: halstock.golf@feeuk.com
18 holes, 4481yds, Par 66, SSS 63, Course record 63.
Location 6m S of Yeovil
Telephone for further details
Hotel ★★★★ CHH Summer Lodge, EVERSHOT ☎ 01935 482000 10 en suite 14 annexe en suite

HIGHCLIFFE
MAP 04 SZ29

Highcliffe Castle 107 Lymington Rd BH23 4LA
☎ 01425 272210 ☐ 01425 272953
Picturesque parkland with easy walking.
18 holes, 4776yds, Par 64, SSS 63, Course record 58. Club membership 450.
Visitors Mon-Sun & BHs. Handicap certificate. Dress code.
Societies Booking required. **Green Fees** £26 per round (£36 weekends). ⊛ **Facilities** ⊕ ⊺⊙⊦ by prior arrangement ⊫ ⊡ ⊶⊓ ⊥ **Conf** Corporate Hospitality Days **Location** SW side of town on A337
Hotel ★★★ 80% HL Best Western Waterford Lodge Hotel, 87 Bure Ln, Friars Cliff, CHRISTCHURCH ☎ 01425 272948 & 278801 ☐ 01425 279130 18 en suite

HURN — MAP 04 SZ19

Parley Parley Green Ln BH23 6BB
☎ 01202 591600 🖹 01202 579043
e-mail: info@parleygolf.co.uk
web: www.parleygolf.co.uk
Flat testing parkland course with few hazards including Par 5s.
Renowned 5th hole, bordering the River Stour.

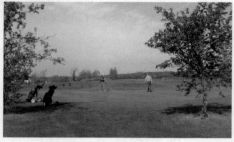

9 holes, 4938yds, Par 68, SSS 64, Course record 69.
Club membership 200.
Visitors may play Mon-Sun & BHs. Dress code **Societies** Welcome.
Green Fees £12 for 18 holes, £9 for 9 holes (£13/£10.50 Sat, Sun & BHs).
Prof Richard Hill **Course Designer** P Goodfellow **Facilities** ⑪ ⑩ by prior
arrangement ⓑ ⬚ ⑪ ⚐ ⛹ ☕ 🏌 **Conf** Corporate Hospitality Days
Location On B3073 opp Bournemouth airport
Hotel BUD Premier Travel Inn Bournemouth/ Ferndown, Ringwood Rd,
Tricketts Cross, FERNDOWN ☎ 08701 977102 32 en suite

LYME REGIS — MAP 03 SY39

Lyme Regis Timber Hill DT7 3HQ
☎ 01297 442963 🖹 01297 444368
e-mail: secretary@lymeregisgolfclub.co.uk
web: www.lymeregisgolfclub.co.uk
Undulating cliff-top course with magnificent views of Golden Cap and
Lyme Bay.

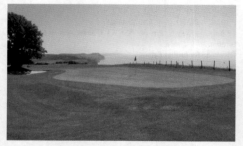

18 holes, 6283yds, Par 71, SSS 70, Course record 65.
Club membership 575.
Visitors Mon-Wed, Fri-Sun & BHs. Handicap certificate. Dress code.
Societies Booking required. **Green Fees** £34 per day. **Prof** Duncan Driver
Course Designer Donald Steel **Facilities** ⑪ ⑩ ⓑ ⬚ ⑪ ⛹ ☕ 🏌 ☕
🏌 **Location** W end of Charmouth bypass (A5), take A3052 to Lyme Regis.
1.5m from A3052/A35 rdbt
Hotel ★★★ 75% HL Hotel Alexandra, Pound St, LYME REGIS
☎ 01297 442010 25 en suite 1 annexe en suite

LYTCHETT MATRAVERS — MAP 03 SY99

Bulbury Woods Bulbury Ln BH16 6HR
☎ 01929 459574 🖹 01929 459000
e-mail: general@bulbury-woods.co.uk
Parkland with a mixture of American and traditional style greens
and extensive views over the Purbecks and Poole harbour. A
comprehensive programme of tree planting coupled with ancient
woodland ensures a round that is picturesque as well as providing
interest and challenge.
18 holes, 6002yds, Par 71, SSS 69. Club membership 450.
Visitors may play Mon-Sun & BHs. Advance booking required. Dress
code. **Societies** advance booking required. **Green Fees** not confirmed.
Facilities ⑪ ⑩ ⓑ ⬚ ⑪ ⛹ ☕ 🏌 ☕ 🏌 **Conf** Corporate Hospitality Days
Location A35 Poole-Dorchester, 3m from Poole centre
Hotel ★★★ 72% HL Springfield Country Hotel & Leisure Club, Grange Rd,
WAREHAM ☎ 01929 552177 48 en suite

POOLE — MAP 04 SZ09

Parkstone Links Rd, Parkstone BH14 9QS
☎ 01202 707138 🖹 01202 706027
e-mail: admin@parkstonegolfclub.co.uk
web: www.parkstonegolfclub.co.uk
Very scenic heathland course with views of Poole Bay. Designed
in 1909 by Willie Park Jnr and enlarged in 1932 by James Braid. The
result of this highly imaginative reconstruction was an intriguing and
varied test of golf set among pines and heather fringed fairways
where every hole presents a different challenge.
18 holes, 6241yds, Par 72, SSS 70, Course record 63.
Club membership 700.
Visitors Mon-Sun & BHs. Booking required. Handicap certificate. Dress
code. **Societies** Booking required. **Green Fees** £80 per day; £55 per
round (£90/£65 Sat, Sun & BHs). **Prof** Martyn Thompson **Course
Designer** Willie Park Jnr **Facilities** ⑪ ⓑ ⬚ ⑪ ⛹ ☕ 🏌 ☕ 🏌 **Conf**
Corporate Hospitality Days **Location** E side of town centre off A35
Hotel ★★★ 68% HL Arndale Court Hotel, 62/66 Wimborne Rd, POOLE
☎ 01202 683746 39 en suite

SHERBORNE — MAP 03 ST61

Sherborne Higher Clatcombe DT9 4RN
☎ 01935 814431 🖹 01935 814218
web: www.sherbornegolfclub.co.uk
Beautiful mature parkland to the north of Sherborne on the
Dorset-Somerset border, with extensive views. Recently extended
to 6414yds.
18 holes, 6414yds, Par 72, SSS 71, Course record 62.
Club membership 600.
Visitors Booking required. **Societies** Wwelcome. **Green Fees** £30 per
day, £25 per round (£36 per round weekends). **Prof** Alistair Tresidder
Course Designer James Braid (part) **Facilities** ⑪ ⑩ ⓑ ⬚ ⑪ ⛹ ☕ 🏌
Location 2m N off B3145
Hotel ★★★ 73% HL Eastbury Hotel, Long St, SHERBORNE
☎ 01935 813131 21 en suite

STURMINSTER MARSHALL   MAP 03 ST90

Sturminster Marshall Moor Ln BH21 4AH
☎ 01258 858444 📠 01258 858262
e-mail: mike@sturminstermarshallgolfclub.co.uk
web: www.sturminstermarshallgolfclub.co.uk
Privately owned club with pay & play facilities set in beautiful Dorset countryside. Played off 18 different tees the course is ideal for golfers of all standards.
9 holes, 3850yds, Par 64, SSS 59, Course record 65.
Club membership 200.
Visitors Mon-Sun & BHs. Dress code. **Societies** Booking required. **Green Fees** £15 per 18 holes; £10 per 9 holes. **Prof** M Dodd/Tracy Loveys **Course Designer** John Sharkey/David Holdsworth **Facilities** ⊕ ⏃⌒ ⍩ ⟊ ⟋ ⌕ ⊒
⚞ 🏌 ✦ **Leisure** children's golf school, ladies academy. **Conf** Corporate Hospitality Days **Location** On A350, signed from village
Hotel ★★★ 72% HL Best Western Crown Hotel, West St, BLANDFORD FORUM ☎ 01258 456626   32 en suite

SWANAGE   MAP 04 SZ07

Isle of Purbeck BH19 3AB
☎ 01929 450361 & 450354 📠 01929 450501
e-mail: iop@purbeckgolf.co.uk
web: www.purbeckgolf.co.uk
A heathland course sited on the Purbeck Hills with grand views across Swanage and Poole Harbour. holes of note include the 5th, 8th, 14th, 15th, and 16th where trees, gorse and heather assert themselves. The very attractive clubhouse is built of local stone.

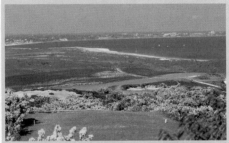

Purbeck Course: 18 holes, 6295yds, Par 70, SSS 70, Course record 66.
Dene Course: 9 holes, 4014yds, Par 60.
Club membership 500.
Visitors Booking required. **Societies** Booking required. **Green Fees** Phone. **Prof** Ian Brake **Course Designer** H Colt **Facilities** ⊕ ⏃⌒ by prior arrangement 🏌 ⍩ ⟊ ⟋ ⌕ ⚞ ✦ **Location** 2.5m N on B3351
Hotel ★★★ 71% HL The Pines Hotel, Burlington Rd, SWANAGE ☎ 01929 425211   49 en suite

VERWOOD   MAP 04 SU00

Crane Valley The Club House BH31 7LE
☎ 01202 814088 📠 01202 813407
e-mail: general@crane-valley.co.uk
web: www.crane-valley.co.uk
Two secluded parkland courses set amid rolling Dorset countryside and mature woodland. The 6th nestles in the bend of the River Crane and there are four long Par 5s ranging from 499 to 545yds.

Valley: 18 holes, 6445yds, Par 72, SSS 71, Course record 65.
Woodland: 9 holes, 2060yds, Par 33, SSS 30.
Club membership 700.
Visitors Booking required ifor Valley course. Woodland course is pay and play. **Societies** Booking required. **Green Fees** Valley: £25 per round (£35 weekends and bank holidays) Woodland: £10 for 18 holes, £5.50 for 9 holes (£12/£6.50 weekends). **Prof** Darrel Ranson **Course Designer** Donald Steel **Facilities** ⊕ ⏃⌒ 🏌 ⍩ ⟊ ⟋ ⌕ ⚞ ✦ ⚞ ✦ **Conf** facs Corporate Hospitality Days **Location** 6m W of Ringwood on B3081
Guesthouse ★★★ GA The Fenland Guest House, 79 Hill Ln, SOUTHAMPTON ☎ 023 8022 0360 8 rms (5 en suite)

WAREHAM   MAP 03 SY98

Wareham Sandford Rd BH20 4DH
☎ 01929 554147 📠 01929 557993
e-mail: warehamgolf@tiscali.co.uk
web: www.warehamgolfclub.com
At the entrance to the Purbeck Hills with splendid views over Poole Harbour and Wareham Forest. A mixture of undulating parkland and heathland fairways. A challenge for all abilities.
18 holes, 5766yds, Par 69, SSS 68, Course record 66.
Club membership 400.
Visitors Mon-Sun & BHs. Handicap certificate. Dress code. **Societies** Booking required. **Green Fees** £36 per day, £25 per round. **Facilities** ⊕ 🏌 ⍩ ⟊ ⟋ ⚞ ✦ **Location** 0.5m N of Wareham on A351
Hotel ★★★ 72% HL Springfield Country Hotel & Leisure Club, Grange Rd, WAREHAM ☎ 01929 552177   48 en suite

WEYMOUTH   MAP 03 SY67

Weymouth Links Rd DT4 0PF
☎ 01305 773981 (Manager) & 773997 (Pro)
📠 01305 788029
e-mail: weymouthgolfclub@aol.com
web: www.weymouthgolfclub.co.uk
A seaside parkland course, almost 100 years old, situated in the heart of the town. The 5th is played off an elevated tee over copse.
18 holes, 5996yds, Par 70, SSS 69, Course record 60.
Club membership 750.
Visitors may play Mon-Sun except BHs. Advance booking required. Handicap certificate required. Dress code. **Societies** advanced booking required. **Green Fees** not confirmed. ⊛ **Prof** Des Lochrie **Course Designer** James Braid **Facilities** ⊕ ⏃⌒ 🏌 ⍩ ⟊ ⟋ ⌕ ⚞ ✦ ⚞ ✦ ✦ **Conf** Corporate Hospitality Days **Location** N side of town centre off B3157
Hotel ★★★ 67% HL Hotel Rex, 29 The Esplanade, WEYMOUTH ☎ 01305 760400   31 en suite

WIMBORNE   MAP 03 SZ09

Canford Magna Knighton Ln BH21 3AS
☎ 01202 592552 📠 01202 592550
e-mail: admin@canfordmagnagc.co.uk
web: www.canfordmagnagc.co.uk
Lying in 350 acres of Dorset countryside, the Canford Magna Golf Club provides 45 holes of challenging golf for the discerning player. The 18-hole Parkland and Riverside courses are quite different and the new nine-hole Knighton course demands the same level of playing skill. For those wishing to improve their handicap, the Golf Academy offers a

Continued

covered driving range, pitching greens, a chipping green and bunkers, together with a 6-hole Par 3 academy course.
Parkland: 18 holes, 6519yds, Par 71, SSS 71, Course record 65.
Riverside: 18 holes, 6214yds, Par 70, SSS 70, Course record 63.
Knighton: 9 holes, 1377yds, Par 27, Course record 26.
Club membership 1000.
Visitors Mon-Sun & BHs. Booking required. Dress code. **Societies** Booking required **Green Fees** Parkland £23 per round (£26.50 Sat & Sun). Riverside £18/£21 Knighton £7/£8. **Prof** Martin Cummins **Course Designer** Howard Swan **Facilities** ⑪ 🍴 ⬛ ⬜ ↻ 🛒 🏌 ⚐ 🏌 🏴 **Conf** facs Corporate Hospitality Days **Location** On A341
Guesthouse ★★★★ GA Ashton Lodge, 10 Oakley Hill, WIMBORNE ☎ 01202 883423 5 rms (2 en suite)

CO DURHAM

BARNARD CASTLE

MAP 12 NZ01

Barnard Castle Harmire Rd DL12 8QN
☎ 01833 638355 📠 01833 695551
e-mail: sec@barnardcastlegolfclub.org.uk
web: www.barnardcastlegolfclub.org.uk
Flat parkland in open countryside. Plantations and natural water add colour and interest to this classic course.

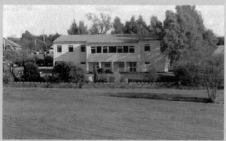

18 holes, 6406yds, Par 73, SSS 71, Course record 63.
Club membership 650.
Visitors Mon-Sun & BHs. Booking required Sat, Sun & BHs. Dress code. **Societies** Welcome. **Green Fees** £22 per round (£35 Sat, Sun & BHs). ☺ **Prof** Darren Pearce **Course Designer** A Watson **Facilities** ⑪ 🍴 ⬛ ⬜ ↻ ⬛ 🛒 ⚐ 🏌 **Conf** Corporate Hospitality Days **Location** 1m N of town centre on B6278
Hotel ★★ HL Rose & Crown Hotel, ROMALDKIRK ☎ 01833 650213 7 en suite 5 annexe en suite

BEAMISH

MAP 12 NZ25

Beamish Park DH9 0RH
☎ 0191 370 1382 📠 0191 370 2937
e-mail: bpgc@beamishparkgc.fsbusiness.co.uk
web: www.beamishgolfclub.co.uk
Parkland course designed by Henry Cotton and W Woodend.
18 holes, 6183yds, Par 71, SSS 70, Course record 64.
Club membership 630.
Visitors may play Mon-Fri except BHs. Advance booking required. Handicap certificate required **Societies** advance booking required. **Green Fees** not

confirmed. **Prof** Chris Cole **Course Designer** H Cotton **Facilities** ⚐ 🛒 ⚐ 🍴 ⚐ **Conf** Corporate Hospitality Days **Location** 1m NW off A693
Hotel ★★★ 74% HL Beamish Park Hotel, Beamish Burn Rd, BEAMISH ☎ 01207 230666 47 en suite

BILLINGHAM

MAP 08 NZ42

Billingham Sandy Ln TS22 5NA
☎ 01642 533816 & 557060 (Pro) 📠 01642 533816
e-mail: billinghamgc@onetel.com
web: www.billinghamgolfclub.com
Undulating parkland with water hazards.
18 holes, 6346yds, Par 71, SSS 70, Course record 62.
Club membership 1050.
Visitors Mon-Sun & BHs. Booking required Sat, Sun & BHs. Dress code. **Societies** Booking required. **Green Fees** £26 per day. ☺ **Prof** Michael Ure **Course Designer** F Pennick **Facilities** ⑪ 🍴 ⬛ ⬜ ↻ 🛒 ⚐ 🏌 🏴 ⚐
Location 1m W of town centre
Hotel Best Western Parkmore Hotel & Leisure Park, 636 Yarm Rd, Eaglescliffe, STOCKTON-ON-TEES ☎ 01642 786815 55 en suite

Wynyard Wellington Dr, Wynyard Park TS22 5QJ
☎ 01740 644399 📠 01740 644599
e-mail: chris@wynyardgolfclub.co.uk
Built against the delightful backdrop of the Wynyard estate, the Wellington Course combines a fine blend of rolling parkland and mature woodland. It represents the ultimate in challenge and excitement for both the novice and the highly experienced player.
Wellington: 18 holes, 7063yds, Par 72, SSS 73, Course record 63. Club membership 350.
Visitors Mon-Sun & BHs. Booking required Wed, Fri-Sun & BHs. Handicap certificate. Dress code. **Societies** Booking required. **Green Fees** £60 per 18 holes. **Prof** Chris Mounter **Course Designer** Hawtree **Facilities** ⑪ 🍴 ⬛ ⬜ ↻ 🛒 ⚐ 🏌 ⚐ 🏌 🏴 **Leisure** David Leadbetter Golf Academy. **Conf** facs Corporate Hospitality Days **Location** off A689 between A19 & A1
Hotel ★★★★ 72% HL Thistle Middlesbrough, Fry St, MIDDLESBROUGH ☎ 0870 333 9141 132 en suite

BISHOP AUCKLAND

MAP 08 NZ22

Bishop Auckland High Plains, Durham Rd DL14 8DL
☎ 01388 661618 📠 01388 607005
e-mail: enquiries@bagc.co.uk
web: www.bagc.co.uk
A parkland course with many well-established trees offering a challenging round. A small ravine adds interest to several holes including the short 7th, from a raised tee to a green surrounded by a stream, gorse and bushes. Pleasant views over the Wear Valley and over the residence of the Bishop of Durham. Has the distinction of having five Par 5 holes and five Par 3s.
18 holes, 6379yds, Par 72, SSS 70, Course record 63.
Club membership 950.
Visitors Mon-Sun except BHs. Booking required Tue, Sat & Sun. Handicap certificate. Dress code. **Societies** Booking required. **Green Fees** £30 per day, £25 per round. **Prof** David Skiffington **Course Designer** James Kay **Facilities** ⑪ 🍴 ⬛ ⬜ ↻ 🛒 ⚐ 🏌 ⚐ **Leisure** snooker. **Conf** facs Corporate Hospitality Days **Location** 1m NE on A689
Hotel ★★★ 77% CHH BW Whitworth Hall Hotel, Whitworth Hall Country Park, SPENNYMOOR ☎ 01388 811772 29 en suite

BURNOPFIELD
MAP 12 NZ15

Hobson Hobson NE16 6BZ
☎ 01207 270941 📄 01207 271069
Meadowland course with very easy walking.
18 holes, 6403yds, Par 69, SSS 68, Course record 65.
Club membership 700.
Visitors contact club for details. Dress code. **Societies** advance booking
required. **Green Fees** not confirmed. **Prof** Jack Ord **Facilities** ⊕ ⫟ ⬛ ⌷
🏐 ⚘ 🛏 ⚘ ⚘ ✓ **Location** 0.75m S on A692
Hotel ★★★ 74% HL Beamish Park Hotel, Beamish Burn Rd, BEAMISH
☎ 01207 230666 47 en suite

CHESTER-LE-STREET
MAP 12 NZ25

Chester-le-Street Lumley Park DH3 4NS
☎ 0191 388 3218 (Secretary)
e-mail: clsgc@ukonline.co.uk
web: www.clsgc.co.uk
Parkland course in castle grounds, good views, easy walking.
18 holes, 6437yds, Par 71, SSS 70, Course record 67.
Club membership 650.
Visitors Mon-Fri. Booking required. Handicap certificate. Dress code.
Societies Welcome. **Green Fees** £30 per day, £25 per round (£35/£30
weekends). ⊕ **Prof** David Fletcher **Course Designer** J H Taylor **Facilities**
⊕ ⫟ ⬛ ⌷ 🏐 ⚘ ⚘ ✓ **Conf** Corporate Hospitality Days
Location 0.5m E off B1284
Hotel ★★★ 79% HL Ramside Hall Hotel, Carrville, DURHAM
☎ 0191 386 5282 80 en suite

Roseberry Grange Grange Villa DH2 3NF
☎ 0191 3700670 📄 0191 3700224
e-mail: grahamstephenson@chester-le-street.gov.uk
web: www.chester-le-street.gov.uk
Parkland course providing a good test of golf for all abilities. Fine
panoramic views of County Durham.
18 holes, 6152yds, Par 71, SSS 69. Club membership 620.
Visitors Mon-Sun & BHs. Booking required. Dress code. **Societies** Booking
required. **Green Fees** £15 per round (£20 Sat & Sun). **Prof** Chris Jones
Course Designer Durham County Council **Facilities** ⊕ ⫟ ⬛ ⌷ 🏐
🏐 ✓ ⚘ **Location** 5m W of Chester-le-Street. Off A694 into West Pelton,
signed
Hotel ★★★ 74% HL George Washington Golf & Country Club, Stone
Cellar Rd, High Usworth, WASHINGTON ☎ 0191 402 9988 103 en suite

CONSETT
MAP 12 NZ15

Consett & District Elmfield Rd DH8 5NN
☎ 01207 505060 (secretary) 📄 01207 505060
e-mail: consettgolfclub@btconnect.com
web: www.consettgolfclub.com
Undulating parkland and moorland course with views across the
Derwent Valley to the Cheviot Hills.
18 holes, 6080yds, Par 71, SSS 69, Course record 63.
Club membership 650.
Visitors Mon-Sun & BHs. Booking required. Handicap certificate. Dress
code. **Societies** Booking required. **Green Fees** £25 per day (£30 weekends
and bank holidays). ⊕ **Prof** Shaun Cowell **Course Designer** Harry Vardon
Facilities ⊕ ⫟ ⬛ ⌷ 🏐 ⚘ 🛏 **Leisure** snooker room.
Conf Corporate Hospitality Days **Location** N side of town on A691

CROOK
MAP 12 NZ13

Crook Low Jobs Hill DL15 9AA
☎ 01388 762429 📄 01388 762137
e-mail: secretary@crookgolfclub.co.uk
web: www.crookgolfclub.co.uk
Meadowland and parkland on an elevated position with natural
hazards and varied holes. Panoramic views over Durham and the
Cleveland Hills.
18 holes, 6102yds, Par 70, SSS 69, Course record 64.
Club membership 550.
Visitors Mon-Sat & BHs. Sat after 2.30pm. Booking required Sat &
Sun. Dress code. **Societies** Booking required. **Green Fees** Phone.
⊛ **Prof** Gordon Cattrell **Facilities** ⊕ ⫟ ⬛ ⌷ 🏐 ⚘ 🛏 ⚘ ✓ ⚘
Conf facs Corporate Hospitality Days **Location** 0.5m E off A690
Hotel ★★ 71% HL Helme Park Hall Hotel, FIR TREE ☎ 01388 730970
13 en suite

DARLINGTON
MAP 08 NZ21

Blackwell Grange Briar Close, Blackwell DL3 8QX
☎ 01325 464458 📄 01325 464458
e-mail: secretary@blackwellgrangegolf.com
web: www.blackwellgrangegolf.com
One of the most attractive courses in north-east England. Clever use
of the trees on this easy walking course gives a feeling of having the
course to oneself. Three ponds add to the variety of holes on offer.
18 holes, 5621yds, Par 68, SSS 67, Course record 63.
Club membership 1000.
Visitors Mon-Sun & BHs. Booking required Wed, Sat, Sun & BHs. Handicap
certificate. Dress code. **Societies** Welcome. **Green Fees** £35 per day; £25
per round (£35 per round Sat, Sun & BHs). ⊛ **Prof** Joanne Furby
Course Designer F Pennink **Facilities** ⊕ ⫟ ⬛ ⌷ 🏐 ⚘ 🛏 ⚘ ✓
Conf Corporate Hospitality Days **Location** 1.5m SW off A66 into Blackwell,
signed
Hotel ★★★ 68% HL The Blackwell Grange Hotel, Blackwell Grange,
DARLINGTON ☎ 0870 609 6121 & 01325 509955 📄 01325 380899 99 en s
uite 11 annexe en suite

Darlington Haughton Grange DL1 3JD
☎ 01325 355324 📄 01325 488126
e-mail: darlington.golfclub@virgin.net
18 holes, 6181yds, Par 70, SSS 69, Course record 65.
Course Designer Dr Alistair McKenzie **Location** N side of town centre
off A1150
Telephone for further details
Hotel ★★★ 79% HL Headlam Hall, Headlam, Gainford, DARLINGTON
☎ 01325 730238 18 en suite 22 annexe en suite

Hall Garth Golf & Country Club Hotel Coatham
Mundeville DL1 3LU
☎ 01325 379710 📠 01325 310083
web: www.foliohotels.com/hallgarth
A 6621 yard course with mature trees and Victorian deer folly. The
challenging 165 yard Par 3 3rd requires teeing over water, whilst
the 500 yard Par 5 6th hole features the picturesque River Swale
running alongside the fairway and the green.

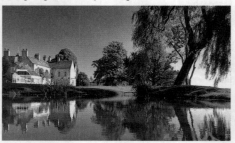

9 holes, 6621yds, Par 72, SSS 72.
Visitors Mon-Sun & BHs. Dress code. **Societies** Booking required. **Green
Fees** £10 per 18 holes (£12 Sat & Sun). Reduced fees for hotel residents.
Course Designer Brian Moore **Facilities** ⓦ ⑩ ⓛ ⓓ ⓟ ⓘ ⓐ ⓢ ⓟ
♦ ⓕ **Leisure** heated indoor swimming pool, fishing, sauna, solarium,
gymnasium. **Conf** facs Corporate Hospitality Days **Location** 0.5m from
A1(M), junct 59 off A167
Hotel ★★★ 73% HL, Hall Garth Hotel, Coatham Mundeville,
DARLINGTON ☎ 0870 6096131 40 en suite 11 annexe en suite

Headlam Hall Headlam, Gainford DL2 3HA
☎ 01325 730238 📠 01325 730790
e-mail: admin@headlamhall.co.uk
web: www.headlamhall.co.uk
Course set over the mature rolling pastureland of Headlam Hall.
Abundance of natural features including rig and fur, woodland, streams
and ponds, making the course both challenging to the player and
pleasing to the eye. Each hole has its own character but the 7th Pond
Hole is particularly special with a stepped green protruding into a
picturesque pond with woodland lining the back.
9 holes, 2075yards, Par 31, SSS 56. Club membership 200.
Visitors may play Mon-Sun & BHs. Booking required Sat & Sun. Dress Code.
Societies Booking required. **Green Fees** £18 per 18 holes, £12 per 9 holes.
Winter: £15/£10. **Prof** Steven Carpenter **Course Designer** Ralph Givens
Facilities ⓦ ⑩ ⓛ ⓓ ⓟ ⓘ ⓐ ⓢ ⓟ ♦ ⓕ ⓕ **Leisure** hard tennis courts,
heated indoor swimming pool, fishing, sauna, gymnasium. **Conf** facs
Corporate Hospitality Days **Location** 8m W of Darlington, off A67
Hotel ★★★ 79% HL Headlam Hall, Headlam, Gainford, DARLINGTON
☎ 01325 730238 18 en suite 22 annexe en suite

Stressholme Snipe Ln DL2 2SA
☎ 01325 461002 📠 01325 461002
web: www.darlington.gov.uk
Picturesque municipal parkland course, long but wide, with 98 bunkers
and a Par 3 hole played over a river.
18 holes, 6431yds, Par 71, SSS 70, Course record 69.
Club membership 450.
Visitors Mon-Sun & BHs. Booking required. Dress code. **Societies**
Welcome. **Green Fees** £22 per day, £14 per round (£27.25/£16 weekends).
Prof Ralph Givens **Facilities** ⓦ ⑩ ⓛ ⓓ ⓟ ⓘ ⓐ ⓢ ⓟ ⓕ ⓕ **Conf** facs
Corporate Hospitality Days **Location** SW of town centre on A67

Hotel ★★★ 68% HL The Blackwell Grange Hotel, Blackwell Grange,
DARLINGTON ☎ 0870 609 6121 & 01325 509955 📠 01325 380899 99 en s
uite 11 annexe en suite

DURHAM   MAP 12 NZ24

Brancepeth Castle Brancepeth Village DH7 8EA
☎ 0191 378 0075 📠 0191 378 3835
e-mail: enquiries@brancepeth-castle-golf.co.uk
web: www.brancepeth-castle-golf.co.uk
Parkland course overlooked at the 9th hole by beautiful Brancepeth
Castle.

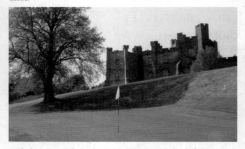

18 holes, 6400yds, Par 70, SSS 70, Course record 64.
Club membership 780.
Visitors Mon-Sun & BHs. Booking required. Dress code. **Societies** Booking
required. **Green Fees** £40 per day, £35 per round (£50 per round Sat, Sun
& BHs). **Prof** David Howdon **Course Designer** H S Colt **Facilities** ⓦ ⑩
ⓛ ⓓ ⓘ ⓐ ⓢ ⓟ ⓕ **Conf** facs Corporate Hospitality Days **Location** 4m
from Durham A690 towards Crook, left at x-rds in Brancepath, left at Castle
Gates, 400yds
Hotel ★★★★ 75% HL Durham Marriott Hotel, Royal County, Old Elvet,
DURHAM ☎ 0191 386 6821 142 en suite 8 annexe en suite

Durham City Littleburn, Langley Moor DH7 8HL
☎ 0191 378 0069 📠 0191 378 4265
e-mail: durhamcitygolf@lineone.net
web: www.durhamcitygolf.co.uk
Undulating parkland course bordered on several holes by the River
Browney.
18 holes, 6326yds, Par 71, SSS 70, Course record 66.
Club membership 750.
Visitors Mon-Sun & BHs. Booking required Sat, Sun & BHs. Handicap
certificate. Dress code. **Societies** Welcome. **Green Fees** £30 (£40 Sat, Sun
& BHs). **Prof** Steve Corbally **Course Designer** C Stanton **Facilities** ⓦ ⑩
ⓛ ⓓ ⓘ ⓐ ⓢ ⓢ ⓕ **Conf** Corporate Hospitality Days **Location** 2m W of
Durham City, turn left off A690 into Littleburn Ind Est
Hotel ★★★★ 75% HL Durham Marriott Hotel, Royal County, Old Elvet,
DURHAM ☎ 0191 386 6821 142 en suite 8 annexe en suite

Mount Oswald South Rd DH1 3TQ
☎ 0191 386 7527 📠 0191 386 0975
e-mail: information@mountoswald.co.uk
web: www.mountoswald.co.uk
Picturesque parkland that gently undulates through the Durham
countryside. The easy walking course attracts golfers of all levels and
abilities.
18 holes, 5991yds, Par 71, SSS 69. Club membership 200.

Continued

Visitors Mon-Sun & BHs. Booking required Sat, Sun & BHs. Dress code. **Societies** Welcome. **Green Fees** £15.25 per round (£17.50 weekends & bank holidays). Reduced winter rates. **Prof** Chris Calder **Facilities** ⑪ ⑩ 🍴 ⌁ 🏌 🏋 🛠 ✎ 🛍 ✎ ⚑ **Conf** facs Corporate Hospitality Days **Location** On A177, 1m SW of city centre **Hotel** ★★★ 79% HL Ramside Hall Hotel, Carrville, DURHAM ☎ 0191 386 5282 80 en suite

Ramside Hall Carrville DH1 1TD
☎ 0191 386 9514 📠 0191 386 9519
e-mail: golf@ramsidegolfclub.fsnet.co.uk
web: www.ramsidehallhotel.co.uk

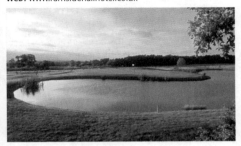

Princes: 9 holes, 3235yds, Par 36, SSS 36.
Bishops: 9 holes, 3285yds, Par 36.
Cathedral: 9 holes, 2874yds, Par 34.
Course Designer Jonathan Gaunt **Location** 500yds from junct A1
Telephone for further details
Hotel ★★★ 79% HL Ramside Hall Hotel, Carrville, DURHAM ☎ 0191 386 5282 80 en suite

---

EAGLESCLIFFE   MAP 08 NZ41

Eaglescliffe and District Yarm Rd TS16 0DQ
☎ 01642 780238 (office) 📠 01642 780238
e-mail: eaglescliffegcsec@tiscali.co.uk
web: www.eaglescliffegolfclub.co.uk
Undulating wooded parkland with views over the River Tees to the Cleveland Hills. A tee on the riverbank makes for a daunting tee shot at the 14th signature hole.
18 holes, 6275yds, Par 72, SSS 70, Course record 64.
Club membership 970.
Visitors Mon-Sun & BHs. Booking required Tue, Sat, Sun & BHs. Handicap certificate. Dress code. **Societies** Welcome. **Green Fees** £40 per day; £32 per round (£55/£40 Sun). ⊕ **Prof** Graeme Bell **Course Designer** J Braid/H Cotton **Facilities** ⑪ ⑩ 🍴 ⌁ 🏌 🏋 🛠 ✎ ⚑ **Conf** Corporate Hospitality Days **Location** On E side of A135 between Yarm -on-Tees
Hotel ★★★★ 79% HL Best Western Parkmore Hotel & Leisure Park, 636 Yarm Rd, Eaglescliffe, STOCKTON-ON-TEES ☎ 01642 786815 55 en suite

---

HARTLEPOOL   MAP 08 NZ53

Castle Eden Castle Eden TS27 4SS
☎ 01429 836510 📠 01429 836510
e-mail: derek.livingston@btinternet.com
Beautiful parkland course alongside a nature reserve. Hard walking but trees provide wind shelter.

---

18 holes, 6262yds, Par 70, SSS 70, Course record 64.
Club membership 750.
Visitors Mon-Fri except BHs. Booking required Sat, Sun & BHs. Handicap certificate. Dress code. **Societies** Booking required. **Green Fees** £28 (£36 Sat, Sun & BHs). ⊕ **Prof** Peter Jackson **Course Designer** Henry Cotton **Facilities** ⑪ ⑩ 🍴 ⌁ 🏌 🏋 🛠 ✎ 🛍 ✎ **Leisure** snooker. **Location** 2m S of Peterlee on B1281 off A19
Hotel BUD Premier Travel Inn Hartlepool, Maritme Av, Hartlepool Marina, HARTLEPOOL ☎ 08701 977127 40 en suite

Hartlepool Hart Warren TS24 9QF
☎ 01429 274398 📠 01429 274129
e-mail: hartlepoolgolf@btconnect.com
web: www.hartlepoolgolfclub.co.uk
A seaside course, half links, overlooking the North Sea. A good test and equally enjoyable to all handicap players. The 10th, Par 4, demands a precise second shot over a ridge and between sand dunes to a green down near the edge of the beach, alongside which several holes are played.
18 holes, 6200yds, Par 70, SSS 70, Course record 62.
Club membership 700.
Visitors Mon-Sat except BHs. Booking required. Dress code. **Societies** Booking required. **Green Fees** £34 per day (£44 weekends). **Prof** Graham Laidlaw **Course Designer** Partly Braid **Facilities** ⑪ ⑩ 🍴 ⌁ 🏌 ⌁ 🛠 ✎ **Location** N of Hartlepool, off A1086
Hotel BUD Premier Travel Inn Hartlepool, Maritme Av, Hartlepool Marina, HARTLEPOOL ☎ 08701 977127 40 en suite

---

MIDDLETON ST GEORGE   MAP 08 NZ31

Dinsdale Spa Neasham Rd DL2 1DW
☎ 01325 332297 📠 01325 332297
Mainly parkland on high land above the River Tees with views of the Cleveland Hills. Water hazards in front of the 15th tee and green; the prevailing west wind affects the later holes. There is a practice area by the clubhouse.
18 holes, 6107yds, Par 71, SSS 69, Course record 65.
Club membership 870.
Visitors Mon & Wed-Fri except BHs. Booking required. Handicap certificate. Dress code. **Societies** Booking required. **Green Fees** £25 per day. ⊕ **Prof** Martyn Stubbings **Facilities** ⑪ ⑩ 🍴 ⌁ 🏌 🛠 ✎ **Conf** Corporate Hospitality Days **Location** 1.5m SW
Hotel ★★★ 74% HL Best Western Croft, Croft-on-Tees, DARLINGTON ☎ 01325 720319 20 en suite

---

NEWTON AYCLIFFE   MAP 08 NZ22

Oakleaf Golf Complex School Aycliffe Ln DL5 6QZ
☎ 01325 310820 📠 01325 318918
A parkland course in a country setting with established trees, streams and lakes, the signature hole being the 15th. Excellent views.
18 holes, 5568yds, Par 70, SSS 67, Course record 67.
Club membership 450.
Visitors Mon-Sun & BHs. Booking required. Dress code. **Societies** Booking required. **Green Fees** Phone. **Prof** Ernie Wilson **Facilities** ⑪ ⑩ 🍴 ⌁ 🏌 🛠 ✎ ⚑ **Leisure** squash, fishing. **Location** 6m N of Darlington, off A6072
Hotel ★★★★ 75% HL Paramount Redworth Hall Hotel, REDWORTH ☎ 01388 770600 100 en suite

Woodham Golf & Country Club Burnhill Way DL5 4PN
☎ 01325 320574 (Office) 315257 (Pro Shop)
📄 01325 315254
18 holes, 6688yds, Par 73, SSS 72, Course record 66.
Course Designer James Hamilton Stutt **Location** A1 onto A689 towards
Bishop Auckland, 0.5m from Rushford
Telephone for further details
Hotel BUD Premier Travel Inn Durham (Newton Aycliffe), Great North Rd,
NEWTON AYCLIFFE ☎ 08701 977085 44 en suite

SEAHAM   MAP 12 NZ44

Seaham Dawdon SR7 7RD
☎ 0191 513 0837 & 581 2354
e-mail: seahamgc@onetel.com
web: www.seahamgolfclub.co.uk
Heathland links course with several holes affected by strong winds.
18 holes, 6017yds, Par 70, SSS 69, Course record 64.
Club membership 600.
Visitors Mon-Fri except BHs. Dress code. **Societies** Booking required.
Green Fees £25 per day. 🅮 **Prof** Andrew Blunt **Facilities** ⑪ 🚾 ☑ 🏐 ⚒
🍴 🏌 🏌 **Location** 3m E of A19, exit for Seaham
Hotel ★★★★ 75% HL Sunderland Marriott Hotel, Queen's Pde, Seaburn,
SUNDERLAND ☎ 0191 529 2041 82 en suite

SEATON CAREW   MAP 08 NZ52

Seaton Carew Tees Rd TS25 1DE
☎ 01429 266249 📄 01429 267952
e-mail: seatoncarewgolf@btconnect.com
web: www.seatoncarewgolfclub.co.uk
A championship links course taking full advantage of its dunes,
bents, whins and gorse. Renowned for its Par 4 17th; just enough
fairway for an accurate drive followed by another precise shot to a
pear-shape sloping green that is severely trapped.
The Old Course: 18 holes, 6622yds, Par 72, SSS 72.
Brabazon Course: 18 holes, 6857yds, Par 73, SSS 73.
Club membership 700.
Visitors Mon-Fri. Limited play Sat, Sun & BHs. Booking required.
Handicap certificate. Dress code. **Societies** Booking required. **Green
Fees** Phone. 🅮 **Prof** Mark Rogers **Course Designer** McKenzie
Facilities ⑪ 🍴 🚾 ☑ 🏐 ⚒ 🏌 🍴 🏌 🏌 **Conf** Corporate Hospitality
Days **Location** SE side of village off A178
Hotel BUD Premier Travel Inn Hartlepool, Maritme Av, Hartlepool Marina,
HARTLEPOOL ☎ 08701 977127 40 en suite

SEDGEFIELD   MAP 08 NZ32

Knotty Hill Golf Centre TS21 2BB
☎ 01740 620320 📄 01740 622227
e-mail: khgc21@btopenworld.com
web: www.knottyhillgolfcentre.co.uk
The 18-hole Princes Course is set in rolling parkland with many holes
routed through shallow valleys. Several holes are set wholly or partially
within woodland and water hazards abound. Bishops Course is a
developing 18-hole course with varied water features on attractive
terrain. Several holes are routed through mature woodland.
Princes Course: 18 holes, 6433yds, Par 72, SSS 71.
Bishops Course: 18 holes, 5976yds, Par 70.
Visitors may play Mon-Sun & BHs. **Societies** advance booking required.
Green Fees not confirmed. 🅮 **Course Designer** C Stanton **Facilities** ⑪

🍴 🚾 ☑ ⚒ 🏐 🏌 🏌 **Leisure** gymnasium, tuition range. **Conf** facs
Corporate Hospitality Days **Location** A1(M) junct 60, 1m N of Sedgefield
on A177
Hotel ★★★ 80% HL Best Western Hardwick Hall Hotel, SEDGEFIELD
☎ 01740 620253 51 en suite

STANLEY   MAP 12 NZ15

South Moor The Middles, Craghead DH9 6AG
☎ 01207 232848 📄 01207 284616
e-mail: bryandavison@southmoorgc.freeserve.co.uk
web: www.southmoorgolfclub.com
Moorland course with natural hazards, designed by Dr A MacKenzie
in 1926 and still one of the most challenging of its type in north east
England. Out of bounds features on 11 holes from the tee, and the
testing Par 5 12th hole is uphill and usually against a strong headwind.
18 holes, 6271yds, Par 72, SSS 70, Course record 66.
Club membership 500.
Visitors Mon-Sun & BHs. Handicap certificate. Dress code. **Societies**
Booking required. **Green Fees** £20 per day (£27 Sat, Sun & BHs). 🅮
Prof Shaun Cowell **Course Designer** Dr Alistair Mackenzie **Facilities** ⑪
🍴 🚾 ☑ 🏐 ⚒ 🏌 🏌 🏌 **Leisure** snooker table. **Conf** Corporate
Hospitality Days **Location** 1.5m SE on B6313
Hotel ★★★ 74% HL Beamish Park Hotel, Beamish Burn Rd, BEAMISH
☎ 01207 230666 47 en suite

STOCKTON-ON-TEES   MAP 08 NZ41

Norton Norton TS20 1SU
☎ 01642 676385 📄 01642 608467
An interesting parkland course with long drives from the 7th and 17th
tees. Several water hazards.
18 holes, 5855yds, Par 70.
Visitors Mon-Sun & BHs. Dress code. **Societies** Welcome.
Green Fees £11.50 per 18 holes (£13.50 weekends and bank holidays).
🅮 **Course Designer** T Harper **Facilities** ☑ 🏌 **Leisure** bowling green.
Conf Corporate Hospitality Days **Location** In Norton 2m N off A19
Hotel Best Western Parkmore Hotel & Leisure Park, 636 Yarm Rd,
Eaglescliffe, STOCKTON-ON-TEES ☎ 01642 786815 55 en suite

Teesside Acklam Rd, Thornaby TS17 7JS
☎ 01642 616516 & 673822 (pro) 📄 01642 676252
e-mail: teessidegolfclub@btconnect.com
web: www.teessidegolfclub.com
Flat, easy walking parkland.
18 holes, 6535yds, Par 72, SSS 71, Course record 64.
Club membership 700.
Visitors Mon-Sun & BHs. Booking required. Handicap certificate. Dress
code. **Societies** Booking required. **Green Fees** Phone. 🅮 **Prof** Ken Hall
Facilities ⑪ 🍴 🚾 ☑ 🏐 ⚒ 🏐 🏌 **Conf** facs Corporate Hospitality Days
Location 1.5m SE on A1130, off A19 at Mandale interchange
Hotel Best Western Parkmore Hotel & Leisure Park, 636 Yarm Rd,
Eaglescliffe, STOCKTON-ON-TEES ☎ 01642 786815 55 en suite

ESSEX

ABRIDGE
MAP 05 TQ49

Abridge Golf and Country Club Epping Ln,
Stapleford Tawney RM4 1ST
☎ 01708 688396 📄 01708 688550
e-mail: info@abridgegolf.com
web: www.abridgegolf.com
Easy walking parkland. The quick drying course is a challenge for all
levels. This has been the venue of several professional tournaments.
Abridge is a golf and country club and has all the attendant facilities.
18 holes, 6704yds, Par 72, SSS 72, Course record 67.
Club membership 600.
Visitors may play Mon & Wed-Fri except BHs, Tue, Sat & Sun pm only.
Advance booking required. Handicap certificate required. Dress code.
Societies advance booking required. **Green Fees** not confirmed.
Prof Stuart Layton **Course Designer** Henry Cotton **Facilities** ⑪ ⓑ ☐
🖈 ⚐ 🏌 ⚑ Ⓛ **Leisure** swimming pool, 3 snooker tables.
Conf facs Corporate Hospitality Days **Location** 1.75m NE
Hotel BUD Premier Travel Inn Romford West, Whalebone Ln North,
Chadwell Heath, ROMFORD ☎ 0870 9906450 40 en suite

BASILDON
MAP 05 TQ78

Basildon Clay Hill Ln, Kingswood SS16 5JP
☎ 01268 533297 📄 01268 284163
e-mail: basildongc@onetel.net.uk
web: www.basildongolfclub.org.uk
18 holes, 6236yds, Par 72, SSS 70.
Course Designer A Cotton **Location** 1m S off A176
Telephone for further details
Hotel BUD Innkeeper's Lodge Basildon/Wickford, Runwell Rd, WICKFORD
☎ 0845 112 6055 24 en suite

BENFLEET
MAP 05 TQ78

Boyce Hill Vicarage Hill, South Benfleet SS7 1PD
☎ 01268 793625 & 752565 📄 01268 750497
e-mail: secretary@boycehillgolfclub.co.uk
web: www.boycehillgolfclub.co.uk
Hilly parkland with good views.
18 holes, 6003yds, Par 68, SSS 69, Course record 61.
Club membership 700.
Visitors Mon-Fri except BHs. Handicap certificate. Dress code. **Societies**
Booking required. **Green Fees** £45 per 27/36 holes, £35 per 18 holes. ⊛
Prof Graham Burroughs **Course Designer** James Braid **Facilities** ⑪ ⓞⓁ ⓑ
☐ 🖈 ⚐ 🏌 ⚑ **Location** 0.75m NE of Benfleet Station
Hotel ★★★ HL Balmoral Hotel, 34 Valkyrie Rd, Westcliff-on-Sea,
SOUTHEND-ON-SEA ☎ 01702 342947 34 rms (14 en suite)

BILLERICAY
MAP 05 TQ69

The Burstead Tye Common Rd, Little Burstead CM12 9SS
☎ 01277 631171 📄 01277 632766
18 holes, 6275yds, Par 71, SSS 70, Course record 69.
Course Designer Patrick Tallack **Location** M25 onto A127, off A176
Telephone for further details
Hotel ★★★ 72% HL Chichester Hotel, Old London Rd, Wickford,
BASILDON ☎ 01268 560555 2 en suite 32 annexe en suite

Stock Brook Golf & Country Club Queens Park Av,
Stock CM12 0SP
☎ 01277 653616 & 650400 📄 01277 633063
e-mail: events@stockbrook.com
web: www.stockbrook.com
Set in 250 acres of picturesque countryside the 27 holes comprise
three undulating 9s, offering the challenge of water on a large number
of holes. Any combination can be played, but the Stock and Brook
courses make the 18-hole, 6750 yard championship course. There are
extensive clubhouse facilities.
Stock & Brook Courses: 18 holes, 6728yds, Par 72, SSS 72,
Course record 66.
Manor Course: 9 holes, 2997yds, Par 35.
Visitors may play Mon-Fri. Sat, Sun & BHs pm only. Dress code. **Societies**
Booking required. **Green Fees** Phone. **Prof** Craig Laurence **Course**
Designer Martin Gillet **Facilities** ⑪ ⓞⓁ ⓑ ☐ 🖈 Ⓛ ⚐ 🏌 ⚑ 🏌 ⚑
Leisure hard tennis courts, heated indoor swimming pool, sauna, solarium,
gymnasium, bowls. **Conf** facs Corporate Hospitality Days
Hotel ★★★★ 80% HL Marygreen Manor Hotel, London Rd,
BRENTWOOD ☎ 01277 225252 4 en suite 52 annexe en suite

BRAINTREE
MAP 05 TL72

Braintree Kings Ln, Stisted CM77 8DD
☎ 01376 346079 📄 01376 348677
e-mail: manager@braintreegolfclub.co.uk
web: www.braintreegolfclub.co.uk
Parkland with many rare mature trees. Good Par 3s with the 14th
- Devils Lair - regarded as one of the best in the county.
18 holes, 6228yds, Par 70, SSS 70, Course record 64.
Club membership 750.
Visitors may play Mon, Wed-Sat except BHs, Tue & Sun pm only. Booking
required. Handicap certificate. Dress code. **Societies** Booking required.
Green Fees £45 per day, £35 per round (£65/£50 Sat, Sun & BHs). ⊛
Prof Tony Parcell **Course Designer** Hawtree **Facilities** ⑪ ⓞⓁ ⓑ ☐ 🖈 Ⓛ
ⓑ 🏌 ⚑ 🏌 **Conf** Corporate Hospitality Days **Location** 1m E, off A120
Hotel ★★★ 72% HL White Hart Hotel, Bocking End, BRAINTREE
☎ 01376 321401 31 en suite

Unex Towerlands Panfield Rd CM7 5BJ
☎ 01376 326802 📄 01376 552487
e-mail: info@towerlands.com
web: www.unextowerlands.com
Undulating, grassland course, nine holes with 18 tees.
9 holes, 5559yds, Par 68. Club membership 250.
Visitors Mon-Sat & BHs, Sun pm only. Booking required. Dress code.
Societies Booking required. **Green Fees** Phone. **Prof** Warren Sargent
Course Designer G Shiels **Facilities** ⓑ ☐ 🖈 Ⓛ ⚑ **Location** On B1053
Hotel ★★★ 72% HL White Hart Hotel, Bocking End, BRAINTREE
☎ 01376 321401 31 en suite

BRENTWOOD
MAP 05 TQ59

Bentley Ongar Rd CM15 9SS
☎ 01277 373179 📄 01277 375097
e-mail: info@bentleygolfclub.com
web: www.bentleygolfclub.com
Mature parkland course with water hazards.
18 holes, 6703yds, Par 72, SSS 72. Club membership 580.

Continued

Visitors Mon-Sun & BHs. Booking required. Handicap certificate. Dress code. **Societies** Welcome. **Green Fees** £27.50 per 18 holes (£40 weekends). **Prof** Nick Garrett **Course Designer** Howard Swann **Facilities** ⑪ ⑩ ⚐ ▯ 🏌 ⛳ 🏌 & ✆ **Conf** Corporate Hospitality Days **Location** 3m NW on A128

Hotel ★★★ 77% HL BW Weald Park Hotel, Golf & Country Club, Coxtie Green Rd, South Weald, BRENTWOOD ☎ 01277 375101 32 annexe en suite

Hartswood King George's Playing Fields, Ingrave Rd CM14 5AE
☎ 01277 218850 📠 01277 218850
Municipal parkland course, easy walking.
18 holes, 6192yds, Par 70, SSS 69, Course record 68.
Club membership 250.
Visitors contact club for details. Dress code. **Societies** advance booking required. **Green Fees** not confirmed. **Prof** Stephen Cole **Course Designer** H Cotton **Facilities** ▵ 🏌 ✆ **Location** 0.75m SE of Brentwood town centre on A128 from A127

Hotel ★★★ 77% HL BW Weald Park Hotel, Golf & Country Club, Coxtie Green Rd, South Weald, BRENTWOOD ☎ 01277 375101 32 annexe en suite

Warley Park Magpie Ln, Little Warley CM13 3DX
☎ 01277 224891 📠 01277 200679
e-mail: enquiries@warleyparkgc.co.uk
web: www.warleyparkgc.co.uk
Parkland with numerous water hazards, reasonable walking. There is also a golf practice ground.
1st & 2nd: 18 holes, 5985yds, Par 69, SSS 67,
Course record 66.
1st & 3rd: 18 holes, 5925yds, Par 71, SSS 69,
Course record 65.
2nd & 3rd: 18 holes, 5917yds, Par 70, SSS 69,
Course record 65. Club membership 800.
Visitors may play Mon-Wed except BHs. Advance booking required. Handicap certificate required. Dress code. **Societies** advance booking required. **Green Fees** not confirmed. **Prof** Kevin Smith **Course Designer** Reg Plumbridge **Facilities** ⑪ ⑩ by prior arrangement ⚐ ▯ 🏌 ▵ ⛳ 🏌 ✆ 🏌 **Conf** facs Corporate Hospitality Days **Location** M25 junct 29, A127 E onto B186, 0.5m N

Hotel ★★★ 77% HL BW Weald Park Hotel, Golf & Country Club, Coxtie Green Rd, South Weald, BRENTWOOD ☎ 01277 375101 32 annexe en suite

Weald Park Hotel, Golf & Country Club Coxtie Green Rd, South Weald CM14 5RJ
☎ 01277 375101 📠 01277 374888
e-mail: info@wealdpark.net
web: www.bw-wealdparkhotel.co.uk
Tranquil parkland course with many mature oak trees, lakes, ponds and plentiful wildlife. The undulating terrain and the numerous hedges and ponds make this Par 71 course a fair test of golf for all abilities.
18 holes, 6285yds, Par 71, SSS 70, Course record 65.
Club membership 400.
Visitors Mon-Sun & BHs. Dress code. **Societies** Booking required. **Green Fees** £25 per 18 holes (£35 Sat & Sun). **Prof** Mike Leitch **Course Designer** Reg Plumbridge **Facilities** ⑪ ⑩ ⚐ ▯ 🏌 ▵ ⛳ ◇ 🏌 **Conf** facs **Location** 3m from M25

Hotel ★★★ 77% HL BW Weald Park Hotel, Golf & Country Club, Coxtie Green Rd, South Weald, BRENTWOOD ☎ 01277 375101 32 annexe en suite

---

BULPHAN   MAP 05 TQ68

Langdon Hills Lower Dunton Rd RM14 3TY
☎ 01268 548444 📠 01268 490084
e-mail: info@golflangdon.co.uk
web: www.golflangdon.co.uk
Well situated with the Langdon Hills on one side and dramatic views across London on the other, the centre offers an interchangeable 27-hole course and a modern refurbished clubhouse.
Langdon & Bulphan Course: 18 holes, 6760yds, Par 72,
SSS 72, Course record 67.
Bulphan & Horndon Course: 18 holes, 6537yds, Par 73,
SSS 72.
Horndon & Langdon Course: 18 holes, 6279yds, Par 71,
SSS 71. Club membership 800.
Visitors Mon-Fri except BHs. Sat & Sun pm only. Booking required. Dress code. **Societies** Booking required. **Green Fees** £20 per 18 holes, £12.50 per 9 holes (£30/£17.50 weekends). **Prof** Terry Moncur **Course Designer** Howard Swan **Facilities** ⑪ ⑩ ⚐ ▯ 🏌 ▵ ◇ 🏌 ⛳ 🏌 **Conf** facs Corporate Hospitality Days **Location** Off A13 onto B1007

Hotel ★★★★ 80% HL Marygreen Manor Hotel, London Rd, BRENTWOOD ☎ 01277 225252 4 en suite 52 annexe en suite

---

BURNHAM-ON-CROUCH   MAP 05 TQ99

Burnham-on-Crouch Ferry Rd, Creeksea CM0 8PQ
☎ 01621 782282 📠 01621 784489
e-mail: burnhamgolf@hotmail.com
Undulating meadowland riverside course, easy walking and stunning views. Challenging for all standards of player.
18 holes, 6056yds, Par 70, SSS 69, Course record 66.
Club membership 580.
Visitors may play Mon-Wed, Fri except BHs, Thu, Sat & Sun pm only. Advance booking required. Handicap certificate required. Dress code. **Societies** advance booking required. **Green Fees** not confirmed.
🌐 **Course Designer** Swan **Facilities** ⑪ ⚐ ▯ 🏌 ▵ 🏌 ⛳ 🏌
Location 1.25m W off B1010
Hotel ★★ 69% HL The Oakland Hotel, 2-6 Reeves Way, SOUTH WOODHAM FERRERS ☎ 01245 322811 34 en suite

---

CANEWDON   MAP 05 TQ99

Ballards Gore Gore Rd SS4 2DA
☎ 01702 258917 📠 01702 258571
e-mail: secretary@ballardsgore.com
web: www.ballardsgore.com
Parkland with lakes. Will test every club in the bag and club management.
18 holes, 6874yds, Par 73, SSS 73, Course record 69.
Club membership 500.
Visitors Mon-Fri. Sat, Sun & BHs after noon. Handicap certificate. Dress code. **Societies** Booking required. **Green Fees** £35 per day/round. **Prof** Gary McCarthy **Course Designer** Arthur Elvin **Facilities** ⑪ ⚐ ▯ 🏌 ▵ ⛳ 🏌 **Leisure** snooker room. **Location** 2m NE of Rochford
Guesthouse ★★★★ GA Ilfracombe House, 9-13 Wilson Rd, SOUTHEND-ON-SEA ☎ 01702 351000 20 en suite

CANVEY ISLAND   MAP 05 TQ78

Castle Point Somnes Av SS8 9FG
☎ 01268 510830 & 511149 📄 01268 511758
18 holes, 6176yds, Par 71, SSS 69, Course record 66.
Location SE of Basildon, A130 to Canvey Island
Telephone for further details
Hotel ★★★ 72% HL Chichester Hotel, Old London Rd, Wickford,
BASILDON ☎ 01268 560555 2 en suite 32 annexe en suite

CHELMSFORD   MAP 05 TL70

Channels Belstead Farm Ln, Little Waltham CM3 3PT
☎ 01245 440005 📄 01245 442032
e-mail: info@channelsgolf.co.uk
web: www.channelsgolf.co.uk
The Channels course is built on land from reclaimed gravel pits, 18
very exciting holes with plenty of lakes providing an excellent test of
golf. Belsteads, a nine-hole course, is mainly flat but has three holes
where water has to be negotiated.

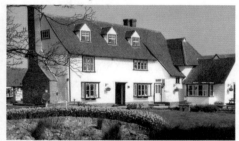

Channels Course: 18 holes, 6413yds, Par 71, SSS 71,
Course record 65.
Belsteads: 9 holes, 2467yds, Par 34, SSS 32.
Club membership 800.
Visitors Channels Course: Mon-Fri except BHs. Belsteads; Mon-Sun & BHs.
Dress code. **Societies** Booking required. **Green Fees** Phone. **Prof** Ian
Sinclair **Course Designer** Cotton & Swan **Facilities** ⑪ ⑩ ⓵ 占 ♡ 🕈 ⌐ ᾩ
🖢 ◇ 🖋 🖐 🖋 🏌 **Leisure** fishing, 9 hole pitch & putt course. **Conf** facs
Corporate Hospitality Days **Location** 2m NE on A130
Hotel ★★★ 75% HL The County Hotel, Bar & Restaurant, Rainsford Rd,
CHELMSFORD ☎ 01245 455700 54 en suite

Chelmsford Widford Rd CM2 9AP
☎ 01245 256483 📄 01245 256483
e-mail: office@chelmsfordgc.co.uk
web: www.chelmsfordgc.co.uk
An undulating parkland course, hilly in parts, with three holes in
woods and four difficult Par 4s. From the reconstructed clubhouse
there are fine views over the course and the wooded hills beyond.
18 holes, 5981yds, Par 68, SSS 69, Course record 61.
Club membership 650.
Visitors Mon-Fri except BHs. Handicap certificate required. Dress code.
Societies Booking required. **Green Fees** £40 per round. ◉ **Prof** Mark
Welch **Course Designer** Tom Dunn **Facilities** ⑪ 占 ♡ 🕈 ⌐ 🖢 🖋 🖐
🖋 🏌 **Location** 1.5m S of town centre off A12
Hotel ★★★ 75% HL Pontlands Park Country Hotel, West Hanningfield
Rd, Great Baddow, CHELMSFORD ☎ 01245 476444 36 en suite

Regiment Way Back Ln, Little Waltham CM3 3PR
☎ 01245 362210 & 361100 📄 01245 442032
e-mail: info@channelsgolf.co.uk
web: www.regimentway.co.uk
A nine-hole course with alternate tee positions, offering a Par 64 18-
hole course. Fully automatic tee and green irrigation plus excellent
drainage ensure play at most times of the year. The course is
challenging but at the same time can be forgiving.

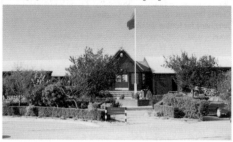

9 holes, 4887yds, Par 65, SSS 64. Club membership 265.
Visitors Mon-Sun & BHs. Booking required Sat & Sun. **Societies** Booking
required. **Green Fees** £15 per 18 holes, £11 per 9 holes. **Prof** David
March/Mark Sharman **Course Designer** R Stubbings/R Clark **Facilities** ⑪
⑩ 占 ♡ 🕈 ⌐ 🖢 ᾩ ♛ ꟼ 🖢 🖋 🏌 **Conf** facs Corporate Hospitality Days
Location off A130 N of Chelmsford
Hotel BUD Premier Travel Inn Chelmsford (Borehamwood), Main Rd,
Boreham, CHELMSFORD ☎ 0870 9906394 78 en suite

CHIGWELL   MAP 05 TQ49

Chigwell High Rd IG7 5BH
☎ 020 8500 2059 📄 020 8501 3410
e-mail: info@chigwellgolfclub.co.uk
web: www.chigwellgolfclub.co.uk
A course of high quality, mixing meadowland with parkland. For
those who believe 'all Essex is flat' the undulating nature of Chigwell
will be a refreshing surprise. The greens are excellent and the
fairways tight with mature trees.
18 holes, 6296yds, Par 71, SSS 70, Course record 66.
Club membership 800.
Visitors may play Mon, Wed, Thu & Tue pm only. Advance booking
required. Handicap certificate required. Dress code. **Societies** advance
booking required. **Green Fees** not confirmed. ◉ **Prof** James Fuller
Course Designer Hawtree/Taylor **Facilities** ⑪ ⑩ 占 ♡ 🕈 ⌐ 🖢 ᾩ ♛ ꟼ 🖋
Conf facs Corporate Hospitality Days **Location** 0.5m S on A113
Hotel BUD Premier Travel Inn Romford Central, Mercury Gardens,
ROMFORD ☎ 08701 977220 64 en suite

Woolston Manor Abridge Rd IG7 6BX
☎ 0208 500 2549 📄 0208 501 5452
e-mail: golf@woolstonmanor.co.uk
web: www.woolstonmanor.co.uk
Manor Course: 18 holes, 6510yards, Par 72, SSS 72,
Course record 67.
Course Designer Neil Coles **Location** M11 junct 5, 1m
Telephone for further details
Hotel BUD Premier Travel Inn Romford West, Whalebone Ln North,
Chadwell Heath, ROMFORD ☎ 0870 9906450 40 en suite

CHIGWELL ROW
MAP 05 TQ49

Essex Golf Centre Romford Rd, Chigwell Row IG7 4QW
☎ 020 8500 2131 📠 020 8501 5196
e-mail: info@essexgolfcentres.com
web: www.essexgolfcentres.com
No 1 Course: 18 holes, 5687yds, Par 70, SSS 67,
Course record 65.
No 2 Course: 18 holes, 6238yds, Par 71, SSS 71.
Course Designer Taylor & Hawtree **Location** 0.5m S on A1112
Telephone for further details
Hotel ★★ 62% SHL Ridgeway Hotel, 115/117 The Ridgeway, North
Chingford, LONDON ☎ 020 8529 1964 20 en suite

CLACTON-ON-SEA
MAP 05 TM11

Clacton West Rd CO15 1AJ
☎ 01255 421919 📠 01255 424602
e-mail: secretary@clactongolfclub.com
web: www.clactongolfclub.com
The course covers 110 acres and runs alongside the sea wall and then
inland. Easy walking layout, part open and part woodland. The course
is well bunkered and a unique feature is the fleets, ditches and streams
that cross and border many of the fairways, demanding accuracy and
good striking.
18 holes, 6448yds, Par 71, SSS 71, Course record 67.
Club membership 650.
Visitors may play Mon-Fri except BHs. Booking required. Handicap
certificate. Dress code. **Societies** Booking required. **Green Fees** £35
per day, £25 per round (£45/£30 weekends and bank holidays). **Prof** S J
Levermore **Course Designer** Jack White **Facilities** ⓣ ⓘ ⓔ 🔹 🛢 🔧 🎿 🛢
🍴 ⚒ **Leisure** practice nets available. **Location** 1.25m SW of town centre
Hotel ★★ 69% HL Esplanade Hotel, 27-29 Marine Pde East, CLACTON-
ON-SEA ☎ 01255 220450 29 en suite

COLCHESTER
MAP 05 TL92

Birch Grove Layer Rd, Kingsford CO2 0HS
☎ 01206 734276
e-mail: maureen@birchgrove.fsbusiness.co.uk
web: www.birchgrovegolfclub.co.uk
A pretty, undulating course surrounded by woodland - small but
challenging with excellent greens. Challenging 6th hole cut through
woodland with water hazards and out of bounds.
9 holes, 4532yds, Par 66, SSS 63, Course record 66.
Club membership 250.
Visitors may play Mon, Wed-Sat & BHs. Tue & Sun pm only. Dress code.
Societies Booking required. **Green Fees** £15 for 18 holes; £10 for 9 holes.
🌐 **Course Designer** L A Marston **Facilities** ⓣ ⓘ ⓔ 🔹 🛢 🔧 🎿 🛢 ⚒
Conf facs Corporate Hospitality Days **Location** 2.5m S on B1026
Hotel ★★★ 79% HL Best Western The Rose & Crown Hotel, East St,
COLCHESTER ☎ 01206 866677 38 en suite

Colchester Braiswick CO4 5AU
☎ 01206 853396 📠 01206 852698
e-mail: secretary@colchestergolfclub.com
web: www.colchestergolfclub.co.uk
Fairly flat yet scenic parkland, with tree-lined fairways and small copses.
Mainly level walking.
18 holes, 6347yds, Par 70, SSS 70, Course record 63.
Club membership 700.

Visitors Mon-Sun except BHs. Booking required Tue, Sat & Sun. Handicap
certificate. Dress code. **Societies** Booking required. **Green Fees** Phone.
🌐 **Prof** Mark Angel **Course Designer** James Braid **Facilities** ⓣ ⓘ ⓔ 🔹
🛢 🔧 🎿 🛢 ⚒ 🎿 **Location** 1.5m NW of town centre on B1508 (West
Bergholt Rd)
Hotel ★★★ 79% HL Best Western The Rose & Crown Hotel, East St,
COLCHESTER ☎ 01206 866677 38 en suite

Lexden Wood Bakers Ln CO3 4AU
☎ 01206 843333 📠 01206 854775
e-mail: info@lexdenwood.com
web: www.lexdenwood.com
Challenging 18-hole, parkland course with many water features. A mix
of undulating and flat land with testing greens. Also a nine-hole pitch
and putt course, and a floodlit driving range. The course has recently
undergone a major redevelopment.
18 holes, 6000yds, Par 67, SSS 70, Course record 63.
Club membership 500.
Visitors Mon-Sun & BHs. Booking required Sat, Sun & BHs. Dress code.
Societies Booking required. **Green Fees** £22 (£30 weekends and bank
holidays, £25 after 11am). **Prof** Phil Grice **Course Designer** J Johnson
Facilities ⓣ ⓘ ⓔ 🔹 🛢 🔧 🎿 🛢 ⚒ 🎿 🎿 **Leisure** 9 hole Par 3. **Conf**
facs Corporate Hospitality Days **Location** A12 towards Colchester Central,
follow tourist signs
Hotel ★★★ 79% HL Best Western The Rose & Crown Hotel, East St,
COLCHESTER ☎ 01206 866677 38 en suite

Stoke-by-Nayland Keepers Ln, Leavenheath CO6 4PZ
☎ 01206 262836 📠 01206 263356
e-mail: mary.saward@stokebynayland.com
web: www.stokebynaylandclub.co.uk
Two 18-hole Championship courses, 'The Gainsborough' and 'The
Constable'. Created in the 1970s, both courses are well established and
feature mature woodland, undulating fairways and picturesque water
features which include 4 large natural lakes. The 18th hole on both
courses presents a challenging and spectacular finish with tee-offs over
the largest of the lakes to a green resting in front of the clubhouse. The
courses are best between March and October but are open all year
round and offer winter buggy paths on the Gainsborough course.

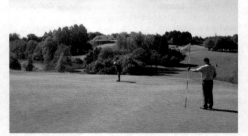

Gainsborough Course: 18 holes, 6498yds, Par 72, SSS 71,
Course record 66.
Constable Course: 18 holes, 6544yds, Par 72, SSS 71,
Course record 67. Club membership 1200.
Visitors Mon-Sun & BHs. Booking required. Dress code. **Societies**
Welcome. **Green Fees** £35 per round (£45 Sat, Sun & BHs). **Prof** Kevin
Lovelock **Course Designer** Howard Swan **Facilities** ⓣ ⓘ ⓔ 🔹 🛢 🔧
🎿 🛢 ⚒ 🎿 🎿 🎿 ⚒ 🎿 **Leisure** heated indoor swimming pool, squash,

Continued

fishing, sauna, solarium, gymnasium. **Conf** facs Corporate Hospitality Days **Location** 1.5m NW of Stoke-by-Nayland on B1068
Hotel ★★★ CHH Maison Talbooth, Stratford Rd, DEDHAM
☎ 01206 322367 10 en suite

EARLS COLNE MAP 05 TL82

Colne Valley Station Rd CO6 2LT
☎ 01787 224343 & 220770 📠 01787 224126
e-mail: info@colnevalleygolfclub.co.uk
web: www.colnevalleygolfclub.co.uk
Opened in 1991, this surprisingly mature parkland course belies its tender years. Natural water hazards, and well-defined bunkers, along with USGA standard greens offer year round playability, and a stimulating test for all abilities.
18 holes, 6301yds, Par 70, SSS 71, Course record 68.
Club membership 500.
Visitors Mon-Sun & BHs. Dress code. **Societies** Booking required.
Green Fees £25 per 18 holes (£30 weekends). **Prof** Peter Garlick **Course Designer** Howard Swan **Facilities** ⑪ ⦿ ⓘⓘ ⓛ ⌦ ⌗⫴ ⚴ ⌂ ☞ 🏌 ⚲ **Leisure** fishing. **Conf** facs Corporate Hospitality Days **Location** Off A1124
Hotel ★★★ 75% HL White Hart Hotel, Market End, COGGESHALL
☎ 01376 561654 18 en suite

Essex Golf & Country Club CO6 2NS
☎ 01787 224466 📠 01787 224410
e-mail: essexgolfops@theclubcompany.com
web: www.the clubcompany.com
Created on the site of a World War II airfield, this challenging course contains 10 lakes and strategically placed bunkering. Also a nine-hole course and a variety of leisure facilities.
County Course: 18 holes, 7019yds, Par 73, SSS 73, Course record 67.
Garden Course: 9 holes, 2190yds, Par 34, SSS 34.
Club membership 700.
Visitors may play Mon-Sun & BHs. Advance booking required. Dress code. **Societies** advance booking required. **Green Fees** not confirmed. **Prof** Lee Cocker/Paul Grotier **Course Designer** Reg Plumbridge **Facilities** ⑪ ⦿ ⓛ ⌦ ⌗⫴ ⚴ ⌂ ☞ ◇ ⚴ 🏌 ⚲ **Leisure** hard tennis courts, heated indoor swimming pool, fishing, sauna, solarium, gymnasium, video golf tuition studio. **Conf** facs Corporate Hospitality Days **Location** Signed off A120 onto B1024
Hotel ★★★ 75% HL White Hart Hotel, Market End, COGGESHALL
☎ 01376 561654 18 en suite

EPPING MAP 05 TL40

Epping Fluxs Ln CM16 7PE
☎ 01992 572282 📠 01992 575512
e-mail: neilsjoberg@hotmail.com
web: www.eppinggolfcourse.org.uk
Undulating parkland with extensive views over Essex countryside and excellent fairways. Incorporates many water features designed to use every club in the bag. Some driveable Par 4s, and the spectacular 18th Happy Valley is rarely birdied. Open all year.
18 holes, 5405yds, Par 68, SSS 65, Course record 67.
Club membership 350.
Visitors Mon-Sun & BHs. Booking required Sat, Sun & BHs. Dress code. **Societies** Booking required. **Green Fees** £20 per day; £14 per round (£23/£17 weekends & bank holidays). 🆓 **Course Designer** Sjoberg **Facilities** ⑪ ⓛ ⌦ ⌗⫴ ⚴ ⌂ ☞ ⚴ 🏌 **Conf** facs Corporate Hospitality

Days **Location** M11 junct 7, 2.5m on B1393, left in Epping High Rd towards station
Hotel BUD Travelodge Harlow North Weald, A414 Eastbound, Tylers Green, North Weald, HARLOW ☎ 08700 850 950 60 en suite

Nazeing Middle St, Nazeing EN9 2LW
☎ 01992 893798 📠 01992 893882
e-mail: secretary@nazeinggolfclub.co.uk
web: www.nazeinggolfclub.co.uk
Parkland course built with American sand-based greens and tees and five strategically placed lakes. One of the most notable holes is the difficult Par 3 13th with out of bounds and a large lake coming into play.
18 holes, 6617yds, Par 72, SSS 72, Course record 68.
Club membership 400.
Visitors Mon-Sun & BHs. Booking required. Dress code. **Societies** Booking required. **Green Fees** Mon £18 per round; Tue-Thu £22, Fri £25 (£30 weekends & BHs). **Prof** Robert Green **Course Designer** M Gillete **Facilities** ⑪ ⦿ ⓛ ⌦ ⌗⫴ ⚴ ⌂ ☞ ⚴ 🏌 **Conf** facs Corporate Hospitality Days **Location** M25 junct 26, near Waltham Abbey
Hotel ★★★★ 78% HL Waltham Abbey Marriott Hotel, Old Shire Ln, WALTHAM ABBEY ☎ 01992 717170 162 en suite

FRINTON-ON-SEA MAP 05 TM22

Frinton 1 The Esplanade CO13 9EP
☎ 01255 674618 📠 01255 682450
e-mail: frintongolf@lineone.net
web: www.frintongolfclub.com
Deceptive, flat seaside links course providing fast, firm and undulating greens that will test the best putters, and tidal ditches that cross many of the fairways, requiring careful placement of shots. Its open character means that every shot has to be evaluated with both wind strength and direction in mind. Easy walking.
Long Course: 18 holes, 6265yds, Par 71, SSS 70, Course record 63. Short Course: 9 holes, 3062yds, Par 60, SSS 60. Club membership 850.
Visitors contact club for details. Handicap certificate required. Dress code. **Societies** advance booking required. **Green Fees** not confirmed. **Prof** Peter Taggart **Course Designer** Willy Park Jnr/Harry Colt **Facilities** ⑪ by prior arrangement ⓛ by prior arrangement ⌦ ⌗⫴ ⚴ ⌂ ☞ ⚴ 🏌 **Leisure** indoor practice nets. **Conf** facs Corporate Hospitality Days **Location** SW of town centre
Hotel BUD Premier Travel Inn Clacton-On-Sea, Crown Green Roundabout, Colchester Rd, Weeley, CLACTON-ON-SEA ☎ 08701 977064 40 en suite
Hotel ★★ 71% HL Hotel Continental, 28/29 Marine Pde, Dovercourt, HARWICH ☎ 01255 551298 Fax 01255 551698 14 en suite

GOSFIELD MAP 05 TL72

Gosfield Lake The Manor House, Hall Dr CO9 1RZ
☎ 01787 474747 📠 01787 476044
e-mail: gosfieldlakegc@btconnect.com
web: www.gosfield-lake-golf-club.co.uk
Parkland with bunkers, lakes and water hazards. Designed by Sir Henry Cotton, Howard Swan. Also a nine-hole course; ideal for beginners and improvers.
Lakes Course: 18 holes, 6615yds, Par 72, SSS 72, Course record 68.

Continued

Meadows Course: 9 holes, 4180yds, Par 64, SSS 61.
Club membership 650.
Visitors Mon-Fri & BHs, Sat/Sun pm only. Booking required. Dress code.
Societies Welcome. **Green Fees** Lakes £35 per round, Meadows £17 per round. ● **Prof** Richard Wheeler **Course Designer** Henry Cotton/Howard Swan **Facilities** ⑪ ⑥ ⚑ ⌨ ⅋ ⚑ ⅄ ⌷ ⚐ ♥ ⚑ **Leisure** sauna.
Conf Corporate Hospitality Days **Location** 1m W of Gosfield off B1017
Hotel ★★★ 72% HL White Hart Hotel, Bocking End, BRAINTREE
☎ 01376 321401 31 en suite

HARLOW
MAP 05 TL41

Canons Brook Elizabeth Way CM19 5BE
☎ 01279 421482 ◱ 01279 626393
web: www.canonsbrook.com
Challenging parkland course designed by Henry Cotton. Accuracy is the key requiring straight driving from the tees, especially on the Par 5 11th to fly a gap with out of bounds left and right before setting up the shot to the green.
18 holes, 6800yds, Par 73, SSS 72, Course record 65.
Club membership 650.
Visitors Mon-Fri. Dress code. **Societies** Booking required.
Green Fees Phone. **Prof** Alan McGinn **Course Designer** Henry Cotton
Facilities ⑪ ⑥ ⚑ ⌨ ⌷ ⅋ ⅄ ⌷ ⚐ ♥ ⚑ **Conf** facs Corporate Hospitality Days **Location** M11 junct 7, 3m NW
Hotel ★★★ 64% HL The Green Man, Mulberry Green, Old Harlow, HARLOW ☎ 01279 442521 55 annexe en suite

North Weald Rayley Ln, North Weald CM16 6AR
☎ 01992 522118 ◱ 01992 522881
e-mail: info@northwealdgolfclub.co.uk
web: www.northwealdgolfclub.co.uk
Although only opened in November 1995, the blend of lakes and meadowland give this testing course an air of maturity.
18 holes, 6377yds, Par 71, SSS 71, Course record 64.
Club membership 500.
Visitors Mon-Fri. Sat/Sun & BHs pm only. Dress code. **Societies** advance booking required. **Green Fees** not confirmed. **Prof** David Rawlings
Course Designer David Williams **Facilities** ⑪ ⑥ ⚑ ⚑ ⌷ ⅄ ⚑ ♥ ⚑
♥ ♟ **Leisure** fishing, gymnasium. **Conf** facs Corporate Hospitality Days
Location M11 exit 7, A414 2m towards Chipping Ongar
Hotel BUD Travelodge Harlow North Weald, A414 Eastbound, Tylers Green, North Weald, HARLOW ☎ 08700 850 950 60 en suite

HARWICH
MAP 05 TM23

Harwich & Dovercourt Station Rd, Parkeston CO12 4NZ
☎ 01255 503616 ◱ 01255 503323
Flat parkland with easy walking. The 234yd Par 3 9th hole to an invisible green is a real experience.
9 holes, 5900yds, Par 70, SSS 69, Course record 59.
Club membership 420.
Visitors Mon-Fri & BHs. Sat & Sun after 11am. Handicap certificate required.
Dress code. **Societies** Booking required. **Green Fees** £22 per 18 holes; £14 per 9 holes. ● **Facilities** ⑪ ⑥ by prior arrangement ⚑ ⌷ ⅄ ⌷ ⚐ ♥
Conf Corporate Hospitality Days **Location** Off A120 near Ferry Terminal
Hotel ★★★ 83% HL The Pier at Harwich, The Quay, HARWICH
☎ 01255 241212 7 en suite 7 annexe en suite

INGRAVE
MAP 05 TQ69

Thorndon Park CM13 3RH
☎ 01277 810345 ◱ 01277 810645
e-mail: office@thorndonpark.com
web: www.thorndonparkgolfclub.com
Course is playable even at the wettest time of the year. holes stand on their own surrounded by mature oaks, some of which are more than 700 years old. The lake in the centre of the course provides both a challenge and a sense of peace and tranquillity. The Palladian Thorndon Hall, site of the old clubhouse, is the magnificent backdrop to the closing hole.
18 holes, 6512yds, Par 71, SSS 71, Course record 68.
Club membership 600.
Visitors Mon-Fri except BHs. Booking required. Handicap certificate.
Dress code. **Societies** Booking required. **Green Fees** Phone. **Prof** Brian White **Course Designer** Colt/Alison **Facilities** ⑪ ⚑ ⌷ ⅄ ⌷ ⚐ ♥ ♥
Conf Corporate Hospitality Days **Location** W side of village off A128
Hotel ★★★ 77% HL BW Weald Park Hotel, Golf & Country Club, Coxtie Green Rd, South Weald, BRENTWOOD ☎ 01277 375101 32 annexe en suite

LOUGHTON
MAP 05 TQ49

High Beech Wellington Hill IG10 4AH
☎ 020 8508 7323
9 holes, 1477, Par 27, Course record 25.
Location M25 junct 26
Telephone for further details
Hotel ★★★★ 78% HL Waltham Abbey Marriott Hotel, Old Shire Ln, WALTHAM ABBEY ☎ 01992 717170 162 en suite

Loughton Clays Ln, Debden Green IG10 2RZ
☎ 020 8502 2923
Nine-hole parkland course on the edge of Epping Forest. A good test of golf.
9 holes, 4652yds, Par 66, SSS 63, Course record 69.
Club membership 150.
Visitors Mon-Sun & BHs. **Societies** Booking required. **Green Fees** £14 per 18 holes; £8.50 per 9 holes (£16/£9.50 Sat, Sun & BHs). **Facilities** ⚑ ⌷
⌷ ⅄ ⚐ ♥ **Location** 1.5m SE of Theydon Bois
Hotel ★★★★ 78% HL Waltham Abbey Marriott Hotel, Old Shire Ln, WALTHAM ABBEY ☎ 01992 717170 162 en suite

MALDON
MAP 05 TL80

Forrester Park Beckingham Rd, Great Totham CM9 8EA
☎ 01621 891406 ◱ 01621 891406
Set in undulating parkland in the Essex countryside and commanding some beautiful views across the River Blackwater. Accuracy is more important than distance and judgement more important than strength on this traditional club course. There is a separate 10-acre practice ground.
18 holes, 6073yds, Par 71, SSS 69, Course record 69.
Club membership 1000.
Visitors Mon, Thu, Fri & BHs. Other days pm only. Booking required.
Dress code. **Societies** Booking required. **Green Fees** £12-£22 depending on time/day. **Prof** Gary Pike **Course Designer** T R Forrester-Muir
Facilities ⑪ ⚑ ⌷ ⅄ ⌷ ♥ ⚐ ♥ ♟ **Leisure** hard tennis courts, heated indoor swimming pool. **Conf** facs Corporate Hospitality Days **Location** 3m NE of Maldon off B1022
Hotel ★★ 76% HL Benbridge Hotel, Holloway Rd, The Square, Heybridge, MALDON ☎ 01621 857666 & 853667 ◱ 01621 841966 13 en suite

Maldon Beeleigh, Langford CM9 6LL
☎ 01621 853212 📄 01621 855232
e-mail: maldon.golf@virgin.net
Flat parkland in a triangle of land bounded by the River Chelmer and the Blackwater Canal. Small greens provide a test for iron shots and the short game. Testing Par 3 14th (166yds) demanding particular accuracy to narrow green guarded by bunkers and large trees.
9 holes, 6253yds, Par 71, SSS 70, Course record 66.
Club membership 380.
Visitors may play Mon, Wed-Fri. Advance booking required. Handicap certificate required. Dress code. **Societies** welcome. **Green Fees** not confirmed. 🏌 **Prof** John Edgington **Course Designer** Thompson of Felixstowe **Facilities** ⑪ ⓘ 🍺 ♨ 🎱 ⚐ 🏌 **Location** 1m NW off B1019
Hotel ★★★ 75% HL Pontlands Park Country Hotel, West Hanningfield Rd, Great Baddow, CHELMSFORD ☎ 01245 476444 36 en suite

---

ORSETT   MAP 05 TQ68

Orsett Brentwood Rd RM16 3DS
☎ 01375 891352 📄 01375 892471
e-mail: enquiries@orsettgolfclub.co.uk
web: www.club-noticeboard.co.uk/orsett
18 holes, 6614yds, Par 72, SSS 72, Course record 65.
Course Designer James Braid **Location** Junct A13 , S towards Chadwell St Mary
Telephone for further details

PURLEIGH   MAP 05 TL80

Three Rivers Stow Rd, Cold Norton CM3 6RR
☎ 01621 828631 📄 01621 828060
web: www.threeriversclub.com
Set in landscaped wooded parkland, Kings Course is fully matured with 18-holes, affording good valley views over the Crouch, Blackwater and Roach rivers that give the club its name. With ponds and dog-legs among the challenges it is ideal for seasoned golfers. The Jubilee Course offers an alternative in both style and challenge with all weather tees and greens built to USGA specification.
Kings Course: 18 holes, 6403yds, Par 72, SSS 71, Course record 66.
Jubilee Course: 18 holes, 4501yds, Par 64, SSS 62.
Club membership 900.
Visitors may play Mon-Sun except BHs. Booking required. Handicap certificate. Dress code. **Societies** Welcome. **Green Fees** Kings £22 per 18 holes (£28 weekends & BHs). Jubilee £11.50/£13.50. **Prof** K Clark/C Lawrence **Course Designer** Hawtree **Facilities** ⑪ ⓘ 🍺 ⚐ 🎱 ♨ 🎱 🏌 🍺 🏌 **Leisure** sauna, solarium, gymnasium. **Conf** facs Corporate Hospitality Days **Location** 2.5m from South Woodham Ferrers
Hotel ★★★ 75% HL Pontlands Park Country Hotel, West Hanningfield Rd, Great Baddow, CHELMSFORD ☎ 01245 476444 36 en suite

---

ROCHFORD   MAP 05 TQ89

Rochford Hundred Hall Rd SS4 1NW
☎ 01702 544302 📄 01702 541343
e-mail: admin@rochfordhundredgolfclub.co.uk
web: www.rochfordhundredgolfclub.co.uk
Parkland with ponds and ditches as natural hazards.
18 holes, 6292yds, Par 72, SSS 71, Course record 64.
Club membership 800.

Visitors Mon-Fri except BHs. Handicap certificate required. Dress code.
Societies Booking required. **Green Fees** £40 per day/round. 🏌 **Prof** Graham Hill **Course Designer** James Braid **Facilities** ⑪ ⓘ 🍺 ⚐ 🏌 🎱 ♨ **Location** W on B1013
Guesthouse ★★★★ GA Ilfracombe House Hotel, 9-13 Wilson Rd, SOUTHEND-ON-SEA ☎ 01702 351000 20 en suite

---

SAFFRON WALDEN   MAP 05 TL53

Saffron Walden Windmill Hill CB10 1BX
☎ 01799 522786 📄 01799 520313
e-mail: office@swgc.com
web: www.swgc.com
Undulating parkland in the former deer park of Audley End House. Fine views over rolling countryside. Two Par 3 signature holes, the 5th and 18th.
18 holes, 6632yds, Par 72, SSS 72, Course record 63.
Club membership 950.
Visitors Mon, Wed-Fri except BHs. Tue pm only. Booking required. Handicap certificate Dress code. **Societies** Booking required. **Green Fees** £50 per day, £40 per 18 holes. **Prof** Philip Davis **Facilities** ⑪ ⓘ 🍺 ⚐ 🎱 ♨ 🎱 🏌 🏌 **Conf** Corporate Hospitality Days **Location** N side of town centre off B184
Hotel ★★★ 74% HL The Crown House, GREAT CHESTERFORD ☎ 01799 530515 8 en suite 14 annexe en suite

---

SOUTHEND-ON-SEA   MAP 05 TQ88

Belfairs Eastwood Rd North, Leigh on Sea SS9 4LR
☎ 01702 525345 & 520202
web: www.southend.gov.uk
Municipal parkland course. Tight second half through thick woods, easy walking.
18 holes, 5840yds, Par 70, SSS 68, Course record 68.
Club membership 350.
Visitors may play Mon-Sun & BHs. Advance booking required. Dress code. **Societies** advance booking required. **Green Fees** not confirmed. 🏌 **Prof** Steve Spittles **Course Designer** H S Colt **Facilities** ⑪ by prior arrangement ⓘ by prior arrangement ⚐ 🎱 ♨ 🏌 **Leisure** hard tennis courts. **Location** Off A127/A13
Hotel ★★★ HL Balmoral Hotel, 34 Valkyrie Rd, Westcliff-on-Sea, SOUTHEND-ON-SEA ☎ 01702 342947 34 rms (14 en suite)

Thorpe Hall Thorpe Hall Av, Thorpe Bay SS1 3AT
☎ 01702 582205 📄 01702 584498
e-mail: sec@thorpehallgc.co.uk
web: www.thorpehallgc.co.uk
Tree-lined parkland with narrow fairways, where placement rather than length is essential.
18 holes, 6290yds, Par 71, SSS 70, Course record 62.
Club membership 995.
Visitors may play Mon-Fri except BHs. Advance booking required. Handicap certificate required. Dress code. **Societies** advance booking required. **Green Fees** not confirmed. 🏌 **Prof** Bill McColl **Course Designer** Various **Facilities** ⑪ ⓘ by prior arrangement 🍺 ⚐ 🎱 ♨ 🎱 🏌 🏌 **Leisure** squash, sauna, snooker room. **Conf** facs **Location** 2m E off A13
Hotel ★★★ HL Balmoral Hotel, 34 Valkyrie Rd, Westcliff-on-Sea, SOUTHEND-ON-SEA ☎ 01702 342947 34 rms (14 en suite)

SOUTH OCKENDON   MAP 05 TQ58

Belhus Park Belhus Park RM15 4QR
☎ 01708 854260 📄 01708 854260
18 holes, 5589yds, Par 69, SSS 68, Course record 67.
Course Designer Capability Brown **Location** Off B1335, brown tourist signs to course
Telephone for further details
Hotel BUD Hotel Ibis Thurrock, Weston Av, WEST THURROCK
☎ 01708 686000 102 en suite

Top Meadow Fen Ln, North Ockendon RM14 3PR
☎ 01708 852239
e-mail: info@topmeadow.co.uk
web: www.topmeadow.co.uk
18 holes, 6348yds, Par 72, SSS 71, Course record 68.
Course Designer Burns/Stock **Location** M25 junct 29, A127 towards Southend, B186 towards Ockendon
Telephone for further details
Hotel BUD Travelodge Brentwood East Horndon, EAST HORNDON
☎ 08700 850 950 45 en suite

STANFORD LE HOPE   MAP 05 TQ68

St Clere's Hall London Rd SS17 0LX
☎ 01375 361565 📄 01375 361565
18 holes, 6474yds, Par 72, SSS 71, Course record 71.
Course Designer A Stiff **Location** 5m from M25 on A13, Stanford turn towards Linford, St Clere on left
Telephone for further details

STAPLEFORD ABBOTTS   MAP 05 TQ59

Stapleford Abbotts Horsemanside, Tysea Hill RM4 1JU
☎ 01708 381108 📄 01708 386345
e-mail: staplefordabbotts@americangolf.uk.com
web: www.staplefordabbotts@americangolf.co.uk
Abbotts Course: 18 holes, 6501yds, Par 72, SSS 71.
Priors Course: 18 holes, 5735yds, Par 70, SSS 69.
Course Designer Henry Cotton/Howard Swan **Location** 1m E of Stapleford Abbotts, off B175
Telephone for further details
Hotel ★★★★ 80% HL Marygreen Manor Hotel, London Rd, BRENTWOOD ☎ 01277 225252 4 en suite 52 annexe en suite

STOCK   MAP 05 TQ69

Crondon Park Stock Rd CM4 9DP
☎ 01277 843027 📄 01277 841356
e-mail: paul@crondon.com
web: www.crondon.com
Undulating parkland with many water hazards, set in the Crondon valley.
18 holes, 6627yards, Par 72, SSS 72, Course record 67.
Club membership 700.
Visitors Mon-Fri. Booking required. Dress code. **Societies** Welcome. **Green Fees** Phone. **Prof** Chris Wood/Freddie Sunderland **Course Designer** Mr M Gillet **Facilities** ⊕ ⑩ ⚑ ⚑ ♨ ⚑ ⚑ ⚑ ⚑ ✔ ⚑
Conf facs Corporate Hospitality Days **Location** On B1007, between Stock and Ingatestone
Hotel ★★★★ 71% CHH Greenwoods Hotel Spa & Retreat, Stock Rd, STOCK ☎ 01277 829990 39 en suite

THEYDON BOIS   MAP 05 TQ49

Theydon Bois Theydon Rd CM16 4EH
☎ 01992 812460 (pro) & 813054 (office)
📄 01992 815602
e-mail: theydonboisgolf@btconnect.com
web: www.theydongolf.co.uk
The course was originally nine holes built into Epping Forest. It was later extended to 18 holes which were well-planned and well-bunkered but in keeping with the Forest tradition. The old nine in the Forest are short and have two bunkers between them, but even so a wayward shot can be among the trees. The autumn colours here are truly magnificent.

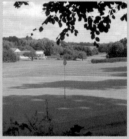

18 holes, 5490yds, Par 68, SSS 67, Course record 64.
Club membership 600.
Visitors Mon, Tue & Fri except BHs. Dress code. **Societies** Booking required. **Green Fees** £30 per round. **Prof** R Hall **Course Designer** James Braid **Facilities** ⊕ ⑩ ⚑ ⚑ ♨ ⚑ ⚑ ⚑ ✔ **Location** M25 junct 26, 2m
Hotel BUD Travelodge Harlow North Weald, A414 Eastbound, Tylers Green, North Weald, HARLOW ☎ 08700 850 950 60 en suite

TOLLESHUNT KNIGHTS   MAP 05 TL91

Five Lakes Hotel, Golf, Country Club & Spa
Colchester Rd CM9 8HX
☎ 01621 868888 & 862426 📄 869696
e-mail: golfoffice@fivelakes.co.uk
web: www.fivelakes.co.uk
Set in 320 acres, the two 18-hole courses both offer their own particular challenges. The Lakes, a PGA championship course, offers generous fairways with water features. The Links has narrow fairways and strategically placed bunkers.

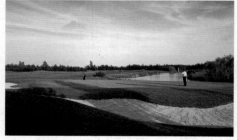

Links Course: 18 holes, 6181yds, Par 71, SSS 70, Course record 67.

Continued

*Lakes Course: 18 holes, 6751yds, Par 72, SSS 72,
Course record 63. Club membership 430.*
Visitors may play Mon-Sun & BHs. Advance booking required. Dress code.
Societies advance booking required. **Green Fees** not confirmed. **Prof** Gary
Carter **Course Designer** Neil Coles **Facilities** ⑪ ℡ ⚑ 🏌 ⬚ 🍴 ⬥ ♨
⬥ 🏌 ⬥ 🏌 **Leisure** hard tennis courts, heated indoor swimming pool,
squash, sauna, solarium, gymnasium, snooker, badminton, fitness studio.
Conf facs Corporate Hospitality Days **Location** 1.75m NE on B1026, 15
mins from A12 Kelvedon exit. Brown tourist signs
Hotel ★★★★ 77% HL Five Lakes Hotel, Golf, Country Club & Spa,
Colchester Rd, TOLLESHUNT KNIGHTS ☎ 01621 868888 114 en suite
80 annexe en suite

TOOT HILL   MAP 05 TL50

Toot Hill School Rd CM5 9PU
☎ 01277 365523 🖷 01277 364509
Pleasant course with several water hazards and sand greens.
*18 holes, 6053yds, Par 70, SSS 69, Course record 65.
Club membership 400.*
Visitors Contact club for details. Dress code. **Societies** Welcome. **Green
Fees** £25 per round(£30 weekends). **Prof** Mark Bishop **Course Designer**
Martin Gillett **Facilities** ⑪ ℡ ⚑ 🏌 ⬚ 🍴 ⬥ ♨ 🏌 ⬥ 🏌 **Conf** facs
Location 7m SE of Harlow off A414
Hotel ★★★ 64% HL The Green Man, Mulberry Green, Old Harlow,
HARLOW ☎ 01279 442521 55 annexe en suite

WITHAM   MAP 05 TL81

Benton Hall Golf & Country Club Wickham Hill
CM8 3LH
☎ 01376 502454 🖷 01376 521050
e-mail: benton.retail@theclubcompany.com
web: www.theclubcompany.com
Set in rolling countryside surrounded by dense woodland, this
challenging course provides a severe test even to the best golfers. The
River Blackwater dominates the front nine and natural lakes come into
play on five other holes. A multi-million pound refurbishment of the
existing clubhouse completed in June 2006 to incorporate health and
fitness facilities.

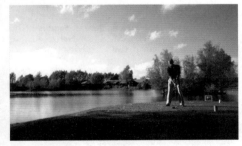

*18 holes, 6574yds, Par 72, SSS 72, Course record 64.
Club membership 600.*
Visitors Mon-Sun & BHs. Booking required. Dress code. **Societies** Booking
required. **Green Fees** Phone. **Prof** Colin Fairweather **Course Designer**
Alan Walker/Charles Cox **Facilities** ⑪ ℡ ⚑ 🏌 ⬚ 🍴 ⬥ ♨ 🏌
Leisure heated indoor swimming pool, sauna, gymnasium, 9 hole Par 3
course. **Conf** facs Corporate Hospitality Days **Location** Off A12 at Witham,
signed
Hotel ★★★ 72% HL White Hart Hotel, Bocking End, BRAINTREE
☎ 01376 321401 31 en suite

WOODHAM WALTER   MAP 05 TL80

Bunsay Downs Little Baddow Rd CM9 6RU
☎ 01245 222648 🖷 01245 223989
Attractive 9-hole public course, challenging for all abilities. Also
undulating and lengthy Par 3 course.
*9 holes, 2932yds, Par 70, SSS 68.
Badgers: 9 holes, 1319yds, Par 54. Club membership 400.*
Visitors may play Mon-Sun & BHs. Dress code. **Societies** advance booking
required. **Green Fees** not confirmed. **Prof** Henry Roblin **Course Designer**
John Durham **Facilities** ⑪ ⚑ 🏌 ⬚ 🍴 ⬥ ♨ 🏌 **Location** 2m from
Danbury on A414, signed
Hotel ★★★ 75% HL The County Hotel, Bar & Restaurant, Rainsford Rd,
CHELMSFORD ☎ 01245 455700 54 en suite

Warren CM9 6RW
☎ 01245 223258 🖷 01245 223989
e-mail: enquiries@warrengolfclub.co.uk
web: www.warrengolfclub.co.uk
Attractive parkland with natural hazards and good views.
*18 holes, 6263yds, Par 70, SSS 70, Course record 62.
Club membership 765.*
Visitors Mon-Sun exept BHs. Booking required Wed, Sat & Sun. Handicap
certificate. Dress code. **Societies** Booking required. **Green Fees** Phone.
Prof David Brooks **Facilities** ⑪ ⚑ 🍴 ⬚ ♨ 🏌 ⬥ ♨ 🏌
Location 0.5m SW
Hotel ★★★ 75% HL The County Hotel, Bar & Restaurant, Rainsford Rd,
CHELMSFORD ☎ 01245 455700 54 en suite

GLOUCESTERSHIRE

ALMONDSBURY   MAP 03 ST68

Bristol St Swithins Park, Blackhorse Hill BS10 7TP
☎ 01454 620000 🖷 01454 202700
e-mail: info@bristolgolfclub.co.uk
web: www.bristolgolfclub.co.uk
An undulating course set in 200 acres of parkland with magnificent
views of the Severn estuary and surrounding countryside.
*18 holes, 6111yds, Par 70, SSS 69, Course record 63.
Club membership 800.*
Visitors Mon-Sun & BHs. Booking required. Dress code **Societies** Booking
required. **Green Fees** £30 per 18 holes (£40 Sat, Sun & BHs). **Prof** Jon
Palmer **Course Designer** Pierson **Facilities** ⑪ ℡ ⚑ 🏌 ⬚ 🍴 ⬥ ♨ ⬥
⬥ 🏌 **Leisure** Par 3 academy course. **Conf** facs Corporate Hospitality Days
Location M5 junct 17, 100yds
Hotel ★★★ 66% HL Henbury Lodge Hotel, Station Rd, Henbury, BRISTOL
☎ 0117 950 2615 12 en suite 9 annexe en suite

CHELTENHAM   MAP 03 SO92

Cotswold Hills Ullenwood GL53 9QT
☎ 01242 515264 🖷 01242 515317
e-mail: contactus@cotswoldhills-golfclub.com
web: www.cotswoldhills-golfclub.com
A gently undulating course with open aspects and views of the
Cotswolds.
*18 holes, 6557yds, Par 72, SSS 71, Course record 67.
Club membership 750.*
Visitors contact club for details. Handicap certificate required. Dress code.
Societies advance notice required. **Green Fees** not confirmed. **Prof** James

Continued

Latham **Course Designer** M D Little **Facilities** 🍴 🍽 🍸 ☕ 🍷 👔 🏪 🏌 🚗 🏌 **Conf** Corporate Hospitality Days **Location** 3m SE on A435
Hotel ★★★★ 73% HL Paramount Cheltenham Park Hotel, Cirencester Rd, Charlton Kings, CHELTENHAM ☎ 01242 222021 33 en suite 110 annexe en suite

Lilley Brook Cirencester Rd, Charlton Kings GL53 8EG
☎ 01242 526785 📠 01242 256880
e-mail: secretary@lilleybrook.co.uk
web: www.lilleybrook.co.uk
Undulating parkland with magnificent views of Cheltenham and the surrounding countryside.
18 holes, 6212yds, Par 69, SSS 70, Course record 61. Club membership 900.
Visitors may play Mon-Fri. Sat/Sun & BHs subject to availability. Advance booking required. Handicap certificate required. Dress code. **Societies** Booking required. **Green Fees** Phone. **Prof** Karl Hayler **Course Designer** Mackenzie **Facilities** 🍴 🍽 🍸 ☕ 🍷 👔 🏪 🛒 🏌 🚗 🏌 **Conf** facs Corporate Hospitality Days **Location** 2m S of Cheltenham on A435
Hotel ★★★ 77% SHL Charlton Kings Hotel, London Rd, Charlton Kings, CHELTENHAM ☎ 01242 231061 13 en suite

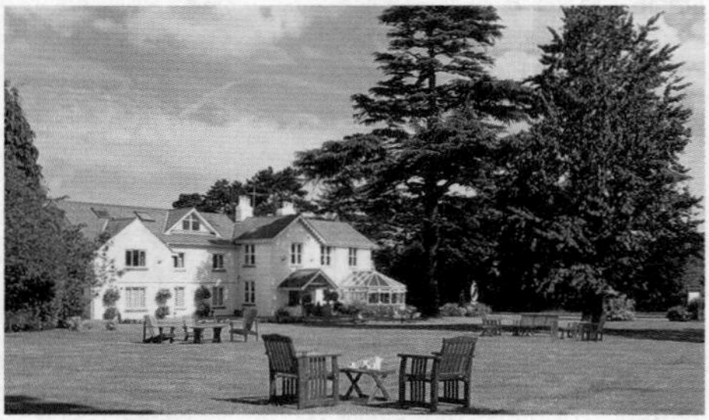

Shipton Shipton Oliffe, Andoverford GL54 4HT
☎ 01242 890237 📠 01242 820336
9 holes, 2516yds, Par 35, SSS 63, Course record 33.
Location On A436, S of A40 junct
Telephone for further details
Hotel ★★★★ 73% HL Paramount Cheltenham Park Hotel, Cirencester Rd, Charlton Kings, CHELTENHAM ☎ 01242 222021 33 en suite 110 annexe en suite

CHIPPING SODBURY MAP 03 ST78

Chipping Sodbury Trinity Ln BS37 6PU
☎ 01454 319042 📠 01454 320052
e-mail: info@chippingsodburygolfclub.co.uk
web: www.chippingsodburygolfclub.co.uk
Founded in 1905, a parkland course of championship proportions on the edge of the Cotswolds. The easy walking terrain, delicately interrupted by a medley of waterways and lakes, is complimented by a stylish clubhouse.
Beaufort Course: 18 holes, 6912yds, Par 73, SSS 73, Course record 65. Club membership 800.
Visitors may play Mon-Fri except BHs. Dress code. **Societies** Welcome. **Green Fees** £32 per round. **Prof** Mike Watts **Course Designer** Hawtree **Facilities** 🍴 🍽 🍸 ☕ 🍷 👔 🏪 🛒 🏌 🚗 🏌 **Leisure** 6 hole academy course. **Conf** facs Corporate Hospitality Days **Location** 0.5m N
Hotel ★★ 78% HL Best Western Compass Inn, TORMARTON ☎ 01454 218242 & 218577 📠 01454 218741 26 en suite

CIRENCESTER MAP 04 SP00

Cirencester Cheltenham Rd, Bagendon GL7 7BH
☎ 01285 652465 📠 01285 650665
e-mail: info@cirencestergolfclub.co.uk
web: www.cirencestergolfclub.co.uk
Undulating open Cotswold course with excellent views.

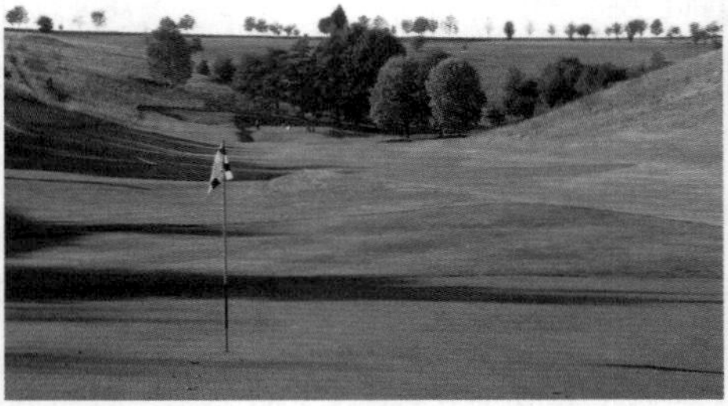

18 holes, 6055yds, Par 70, SSS 69, Course record 65. Club membership 800.
Visitors may play Mon-Sun & BHs. Handicap certificate required. Dress code. **Societies** advance booking required. **Green Fees** not confirmed. **Prof** Ed Goodwin **Course Designer** J Braid **Facilities** 🍴 🍽 🍸 ☕ 🍷 👔 🏪 🏌 🚗 🏌 ⛳ **Leisure** 6 hole Par 3 Academy course. **Conf** facs Corporate Hospitality Days **Location** 2m N of Cirencester on A435
Hotel ★★★ 79% HL Best Western Stratton House Hotel, Gloucester Rd, CIRENCESTER ☎ 01285 651761 39 en suite

CLEEVE HILL MAP 03 SO92

Cleeve Hill GL52 3PW
☎ 01242 672025 📠 01242 67444
e-mail: hugh.fitzsimons@btconnect.com
web: www.cleevehillgolfcourse.com
Undulating and open heathland course affected by crosswinds. Situated on the highest point of the Cotswolds with fine views over Cheltenham racecourse, the Malvern Hills and the Bristol Channel. An ideal setting to enjoy a challenging round of golf.
18 holes, 6448yds, Par 72, SSS 71, Course record 66. Club membership 600.
Visitors Mon-Sun & BHs. Booking required. Dress code. **Societies** Booking required. **Green Fees** £15 per round (£20 Sat & Sun). **Prof** Dave Finch **Facilities** 🍴 🍽 🍸 ☕ 👔 🏪 🛒 🏌 **Conf** facs Corporate Hospitality Days **Location** 1m NE on B4632
Hotel ★★★ 70% HL The Prestbury House Hotel, The Burgage, Prestbury, CHELTENHAM ☎ 01242 529533 7 en suite 8 annexe en suite

COALPIT HEATH MAP 03 ST68

The Kendleshire Henfield Rd BS36 2TG
☎ 0117 956 7007 📠 0117 957 3433
e-mail: info@kendleshire.com
web: www.kendleshire.com
Opened in 1997, the course has 27 holes with water coming into play on 18 holes. Notable holes are the 11th, the 16th and the 27th. The 11th is a short hole with an island green set in a 3-acre lake and the 16th has a second shot played over water. The course is never short of interest and the greens have been built to USGA specification.

Continued

18 holes, 6567, Par 71, SSS 72, Course record 63.
18 holes, 6249, Par 71, SSS 70, Course record 68.
18 holes, 6353, Par 70, SSS 70, Course record 68.
Club membership 900.
Visitors Mon-Sun & BHs. Booking required. Dress code.
Societies Booking required. **Green Fees** £35 per round (£40 weekends).
Prof Tony Mealing **Course Designer** A Stiff/P McEvoy **Facilities** ⊕ ℐᴑ⌁
🝆 ⌷🝆 🛆 🏢 🝚 🝎 🝋 **Conf** facs Corporate Hospitality Days
Location M32 junct 1, on Avon Ring Road
Hotel ★★★★ 72% HL Jurys Bristol Hotel, Prince St, BRISTOL
☎ 0117 923 0333 192 en suite

CODRINGTON MAP 03 ST78

Players Club BS37 6RZ
☎ 01454 313029 📄 01454 323446
e-mail: enquiries@theplayersgolfclub.com
web: www.theplayersgolfclub.com
This Adrian Stiff designed layout can measure up to 7607yds. Often
described as an inland links, the rolling sand based fairways encounter
an unusual mix of gorse and water.
Championship: 18 holes, 6847yards, Par 72, SSS 72,
Course record 63. Club membership 2000.
Visitors may play Mon-Sun & BHs. Booking required. Dress code.
Societies Booking required. **Green Fees** £90 anytime. **Prof** Mark Brookes
Course Designer Adrian Stiff **Facilities** ⊕ ℐᴑ⌁ 🝆 ⌷🝆 🛆 🏢 🝚 🝎 🝋
Leisure fishing, 9 hole Par 3 course. **Conf** facs Corporate Hospitality Days
Location M4 junct 18, 1m on B4465
Hotel ★★ 78% HL Best Western Compass Inn, TORMARTON
☎ 01454 218242 & 218577 📄 01454 218741 26 en suite

COLEFORD MAP 03 SO51

Forest Hills Mile End Rd GL16 7QD
☎ 01594 810620 📄 01594 810823
e-mail: foresthills@btopenworld.com
web: foresthillsgolfclub.co.uk
18 holes, 6740yds, Par 72, SSS 68, Course record 64.
Course Designer A Stiff
Telephone for further details
Hotel Best Western The Speech House, COLEFORD ☎ 01594 822607
15 en suite 22 annexe en suite

Forest of Dean Golf Club & Bells Hotel Lords Hill
GL16 8BE
☎ 01594 832583 📄 01594 832584
e-mail: enquiries@bells-hotel.co.uk
web: www.bells-hotel.co.uk
Established in 1973 and now matured into an extremely pleasant
parkland course. Well bunkered with light rough, a few blind tee shots
and water in play on several holes.
18 holes, 6033yds, Par 70, SSS 69, Course record 63.
Club membership 375.
Visitors may play Mon-Sun & BHs. Dress code. **Societies** advance booking
required. **Green Fees** not confirmed. **Prof** Paul Davies **Course Designer**
John Day **Facilities** ⊕ ℐᴑ⌁ 🝆 ⌷🝆 🛆 🏢 🝚 🝎 🝋 **Leisure** hard
tennis courts, gymnasium, bowling green. **Conf** facs **Location** 0.25m from
Coleford town centre on B4431 Coleford-Parkend road
Hotel Best Western The Speech House, COLEFORD ☎ 01594 822607
15 en suite 22 annexe en suite

DURSLEY MAP 03 ST79

Stinchcombe Hill Stinchcombe Hill GL11 6AQ
☎ 01453 542015 📄 01453 549545
e-mail: secretary@stinchcombehill.plus.com
web: www.stinchcombehillgolfclub.com
High on the hill with splendid views of the Cotswolds, the River
Severn and the Welsh hills. A downland course with good turf, some
trees and an interesting variety of greens. Protected greens make this
a challenging course in windy conditions.
18 holes, 5734yds, Par 68, SSS 68, Course record 63.
Club membership 550.
Visitors Mon-Sun & BHs. Booking required. Handicap certificate
required. Dress code. **Societies** Booking required. **Green Fees** £34 per
day, £28 per 18 holes (£42/£36 weekends and bank holidays). 🝚
Prof Paul Bushell **Course Designer** Arthur Hoare **Facilities** ⊕ ℐᴑ⌁ by
prior arrangement 🝆 ⌷🝆 🛆 🏢 🝋 **Conf** Corporate Hospitality Days
Location 1m W off A4135
Hotel ★★★ 68% HL Prince of Wales Hotel, BERKELEY ROAD
☎ 01453 810474 43 en suite

DYMOCK MAP 03 SO73

Dymock Grange The Old Grange, Leominster Rd
GL18 2AN
☎ 01531 890840 📄 01531 890860
Old Course: 9 holes, 5786yards, Par 72, SSS 70,
Course record 71. New Course: 9 holes, 3390yards, Par 60,
SSS 60.
Course Designer Cufingham **Location** On B4215 Leominster road
Telephone for further details

GLOUCESTER MAP 03 SO81

Brickhampton Court Golf Complex Cheltenham Rd,
Churchdown GL2 9QF
☎ 01452 859444 📄 01452 859333
e-mail: info@brickhampton.co.uk
web: www.brickhampton.co.uk
Rolling parkland featuring lakes, streams, strategic white-sand bunkers,
plantations - but no steep hills.

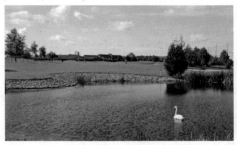

Spa: 18 holes, 6449yds, Par 71, SSS 71, Course record 65.
Glevum: 9 holes, 1859yds, Par 31. Club membership 860.
Visitors may play Mon-Sun & BHs. Dress code. **Societies** advance
booking required. **Green Fees** not confirmed. **Prof** Bruce Wilson
Course Designer Simon Gidman **Facilities** ⊕ ℐᴑ⌁ 🝆 ⌷🝆 🛆 🏢 🝚 🝎
🏢 🝎 🝋 **Conf** facs Corporate Hospitality Days **Location** M5 junct 11, A40
towards Gloucester, at Elmbridge Court rdbt B4063 signed Churchdown, 2m
Hotel ★★★ 70% HL Macdonald Hatherley Manor, Down Hatherley Ln,
GLOUCESTER ☎ 0870 1942126 52 en suite

Ramada Gloucester Matson Ln, Robinswood Hill
GL4 6EA
☎ 01452 525653 📠 01452 307212
web: www.gloucestergolf.com
Undulating, wooded course, built around a hill with superb views
over Gloucester and the Cotswolds. The 12th is a drive straight up a
hill, nicknamed 'Coronary Hill'.
18 holes, 6170yds, Par 70, SSS 69, Course record 65.
Club membership 600.
Visitors Mon-Sun & BHs. Dress code. **Societies** Welcome. **Green Fees**
Phone. **Prof** Keith Wood **Facilities** ⑪ ⑩ ⓛ ⬜ ⬜ 🏋 ⬜ 🍴 ◇ ◊ 🍴
◊ 🍴 **Leisure** hard tennis courts, heated indoor swimming pool, squash,
sauna, solarium, gymnasium, 9 hole Par 3 course. **Location** 2.5m SE of
Gloucester, off B4073
Hotel ★★★ 68% HL Ramada Hotel & Resort Gloucester, Matson Ln,
Robinswood Hill, GLOUCESTER ☎ 01452 525653 97 en suite

Rodway Hill Newent Rd, Highnam GL2 8DN
☎ 01452 384222 📠 01452 313814
e-mail: info@rodway-hill-golf-course.co.uk
web: www.rodway-hill-golf-course.co.uk
A challenging 18-hole course with superb panoramic views. Testing
front five holes and the Par 3 13th and Par 5 16th affected by strong
crosswinds off the River Severn.
18 holes, 6040yds, Par 70, SSS 69, Course record 66.
Club membership 400.
Visitors Mon-Sun & BHs. Boking required. Dress code. **Societies** Booking
required. **Green Fees** £15 per 18 holes, £9 per 9 holes (£17-£18/£9-£10
Sat & Sun). **Prof** Chris Murphy **Course Designer** John Gabb **Facilities**
⑪ ⑩ ⓛ ⬜ ⬜ 🏋 ⬜ ⬜ ◊ 🍴 **Conf** Corporate Hospitality Days
Location 2m outside Gloucester on B4215
Hotel ★★★ 70% HL Macdonald Hatherley Manor, Down Hatherley Ln,
GLOUCESTER ☎ 0870 1942126 52 en suite

LYDNEY MAP 03 SO60

Lydney Lakeside Av GL15 5QA
☎ 01594 841186
e-mail: jongerrymills@pitch60.freeserve.co.uk
web: www.members.tripod.co.uk/kenfar.lgc
Flat parkland and meadowland course with prevailing wind along
fairways.
9 holes, 5298yds, Par 66, SSS 66, Course record 63.
Club membership 240.
Visitors Mon-Sat except BHs. Dress code. **Societies** Booking required.
Green Fees £11 per day/round. ◉ **Facilities** 🍴 ⬜ **Location** SE side of
town centre
Hotel ★★★ 72% HL Best Western The Speech House, COLEFORD
☎ 01594 822607 15 en suite 22 annexe en suite

MINCHINHAMPTON MAP 03 SO80

Minchinhampton (New Course) New Course GL6 9BE
☎ 01453 833866 📠 01453 837360
e-mail: alan@mgcnew.co.uk
web: www.mgcnew.co.uk
Set high on the Cotswolds, both courses offer scenic countryside and
outstanding tests of golf.The Cherington is a testing inland links course
and an Open Qualifying venue from 2002-2007. The Avening is a
parkland course offering a different but no less challenging experience.
Avening: 18 holes, 6263yds, Par 70, SSS 70,
Course record 61. *Continued*

Cherington: 18 holes, 6430yds, Par 71, SSS 71,
Course record 61. Club membership 1200.
Visitors may play Mon-Sun & BHs. Advance booking required. Handicap
certificate required. Dress code. **Societies** Booking required. **Green Fees**
£50 per day £40 per round (£60/£50 weekends & bank holidays) **Prof**
Chris Steele **Course Designer** Hawtree & Son **Facilities** ⑪ ⑩ ⓛ ⬜ ⬜
🍴 ⬜ ⬜ 🍴 🚗 ◊ 🍴 **Conf** Corporate Hospitality Days **Location** B4014
from Nailsworth into Avening, left at Cross pub towards Minchinhampton,
club 0.25m on right
Hotel ★★★ 75% HL Best Western Hare & Hounds Hotel, Westonbirt,
TETBURY ☎ 01666 880233 & 881000 📠 01666 880241 24 en suite
7 annexe en suite

Minchinhampton (Old Course) Old Course GL6 9AQ
☎ 01453 832642 & 836382 📠 01453 832642
e-mail: alan@mgcold.co.uk
web: www.mgcold.co.uk
An open grassland course 600 feet above sea level. The numerous
humps and hollows around the greens test the golfer's ability to play
a variety of shots - often in difficult windy conditions. Panoramic
Cotswold views. Two of the Par 3s, the 8th and the 16th, often require
an accurate long iron or wood depending on the strength and
direction of the wind.
18 holes, 6088yds, Par 71, SSS 69. Club membership 550.
Visitors contact course for details. **Societies** Welcome. **Green Fees** £15
per 18 holes (£18 weekends and bank holidays). **Prof** Peter Dangerfield
Facilities ⑪ ⓛ ⬜ 🍴 ⬜ ⬜ 🍴 ◊ **Location** 1m NW
Hotel ★★ 72% HL Egypt Mill Hotel, NAILSWORTH ☎ 01453 833449
10 en suite 18 annexe en suite

NAUNTON MAP 04 SP12

Naunton Downs GL54 3AE
☎ 01451 850090 📠 01451 850091
e-mail: admin@nauntondowns.co.uk
web: www.nauntondowns.co.uk
Naunton Downs course plays over beautiful Cotswold countryside. A
valley running through the course is one of the main features, creating
one Par 3 hole that crosses over it. The prevailing wind adds extra
challenge to the Par 5s (which play into the wind), combined with
small undulating greens.
18 holes, 6161yds, Par 71, SSS 69, Course record 67.
Club membership 750.
Visitors Mon-Fri. Sat, Sun & BHs after 11am. Booking required. Dress
code. **Societies** Booking required. **Green Fees** Mon £19, Tue-Fri £22 (£28
weekends and bank holidays). **Prof** Nick Ellis **Course Designer** J Pott
Facilities ⑪ ⑩ ⓛ ⬜ 🍴 ⬜ ⬜ 🍴 ◊ 🚗 🍴 **Leisure** hard tennis courts.
Conf facs Corporate Hospitality Days **Location** B4068 Stow-Cheltenham
Hotel ★★★ CHH Lords of the Manor, UPPER SLAUGHTER
☎ 01451 820243 27 en suite

PAINSWICK MAP 03 SO80

Painswick GL6 6TL
☎ 01452 812180
e-mail: hello@painswickgolf.com
web: www.painswickgolf.com
Downland course set on the Cotswolds at Painswick Beacon, with fine
views. Short course more than compensated by natural hazards and
tight fairways.
18 holes, 4895yds, Par 67, SSS 63, Course record 61.
Club membership 250.

Visitors Mon-Sat except BHs. Booking required Sat. Dress code **Societies** Booking required. **Green Fees** £12-£17.50 per 18 holes (£20 Saturday). **Facilities** ⊕ ⚑ ⬛ ➘ ⬛ ⚑ ⬛ ⚑ ⟋ **Conf** Corporate Hospitality Days **Location** 1m N of Painswick, off A46 to Cheltenham **Hotel** ★★★ 77% HL Hatton Court, Upton Hill, Upton St Leonards, GLOUCESTER ☎ 01452 617412 17 en suite 28 annexe en suite

TEWKESBURY   MAP 03 SO83

Hilton Puckrup Hall Puckrup GL20 6EL
☎ 01684 271550 ▤ 01684 271550
web: www.hilton.co.uk/tewkesbury
Set in 140 acres of undulating parkland with lakes, existing trees and marvellous views of the Malvern hills. There are water hazards at the 5th, and a cluster of bunkers on the long 14th, before the challenging tee shot across the water to the Par 3 18th.

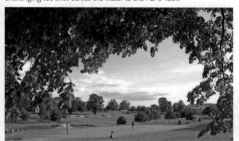

18 holes, 6219yds, Par 70, SSS 68, Course record 63.
Club membership 380.
Visitors Mon-Fri. Sat, Sun & BHs pm only. Booking required. Dress code. **Societies** Booking required. **Green Fees** £30 per round (£35 weekends). **Prof** Mark Fenning **Course Designer** Simon Gidman **Facilities** ⊕ ⚑ ⬛ ⬛ ➘ ⬛ ⚑ ⬛ ⚑ ⟋ ⬛ ⟋ **Leisure** heated indoor swimming pool, sauna, solarium, gymnasium. **Conf** facs Corporate Hospitality Days **Location** 4m N of Tewkesbury on A38
Hotel ★★ 60% HL The Bell Hotel, 52 Church St, TEWKESBURY ☎ 01684 293293 24 en suite

See advert on page 98

Tewkesbury Park Hotel Golf & Country Club
Lincoln Green Ln GL20 7DN
☎ 01684 295405 ▤ 01684 292386
e-mail: tewkesburypark@foliohotels.com
web: www.foliohotels.com/tewkesburypark

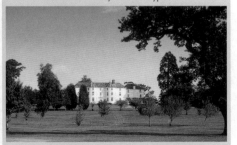

The course offers many interesting and testing holes, with wooded areas and water hazards early in the round, opening up onto spacious fairways on the back nine of the undulating course.

18 holes, 6533yds, Par 73, SSS 72, Course record 66.
Club membership 550.
Visitors Mon-Sun & BHs. Booking required. Dress code.
Societies Booking required. **Green Fees** Phone. **Prof** Marc Cottrell
Course Designer Frank Pennick **Facilities** ⊕ ⚑ ⬛ ⬛ ➘ ⬛ ⚑ ⬛ ⚑ ⟋ ⟋ ⬛ ⟋ ⬛ **Leisure** hard tennis courts, heated indoor swimming pool, squash, sauna, solarium, gymnasium. **Conf** facs Corporate Hospitality Days **Location** 1m SW off A38
Hotel ★★★ 72% HL Tewkesbury Park Hotel Golf & Country Club, Lincoln Green Ln, TEWKESBURY ☎ 0870 609 6101 80 en suite

See advert on page 98

THORNBURY   MAP 03 ST69

Thornbury Golf Centre Bristol Rd BS35 3XL
☎ 01454 281144 ▤ 01454 281177
e-mail: info@thornburygc.co.uk
web: www.thornburygc.co.uk
Two 18-hole pay and play courses designed by Hawtree and set in undulating terrain with views towards the Severn estuary. The Low 18 is a Par 3 with holes ranging from 80 to 207yds and is ideal for beginners. The High course puts to test the more experienced golfer. Excellent 25 bay floodlit driving range.

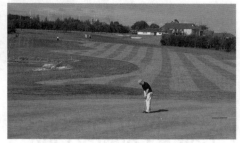

High Course: 18 holes, 6308yds, Par 71, SSS 69.
Low Course: 18 holes, 2195yds, Par 54.
Club membership 510.
Visitors Mon-Sun & BHs. Booking required. Dress code. **Societies** Booking required. **Green Fees** Phone. **Prof** Mike Smedley **Course Designer** Hawtree **Facilities** ⊕ ⚑ ⬛ ⬛ ➘ ⬛ ⚑ ⬛ ⚑ ⬛ ⟋ ⟋ **Conf** facs Corporate Hospitality Days **Location** M5 junct 16, off A38 towards Gloucester
Hotel ★★ 67% HL Thornbury Golf Lodge, Bristol Rd, THORNBURY ☎ 01454 281144 11 en suite

WESTONBIRT   MAP 03 ST88

Westonbirt Westonbirt School GL8 8QG
☎ 01666 880242 & 881338 ▤ 01666 880385
e-mail: doyle@westonbirt.gloucs.sch.uk
web: www.westonbirt.gloucs.sch.uk
Parkland with good views.
9 holes, 4504yds, Par 64, SSS 64. Club membership 287.
Visitors may play Mon-Sun & BHs. Dress code. **Societies** advance booking required. **Green Fees** not confirmed. ⬛ **Facilities** ⊕ ⬛ ⬛ ⟋ **Conf** facs **Location** E side of village off A433
Hotel ★★★ 75% HL Best Western Hare & Hounds Hotel, Westonbirt, TETBURY ☎ 01666 880233 & 881000 ▤ 01666 880241 24 en suite 7 annexe en suite

Hilton Puckrup Hall

Hilton Puckrup Hall is located in the heart of the Gloucestershire countryside and is overlooked by the Malvern Hills. The parkland course measures 6200yd and par 70, strategic bunkering and water hazards provide a challenge to golfers of all abilities.

The Hotel guest rooms allow for every modern convenience, while the hotel's restaurant offers daily and a-la-carte menus. The leisure facilities offer swimming pool, gym, sauna, steam room and beauty treatments

Graham Wallace
Golf Operations Manager
Hilton Puckrup Hall
Tel. 01684 271550   Fax. 01684 271550
email: Graham.Wallace@hilton.com

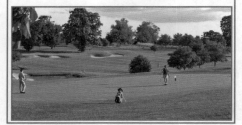

Tewkesbury Park Hotel Golf & Country Club

Lincoln Green Lane, Tewkesbury Gloucestershire, GL20 7DN

Tel: 01684 295405 Fax: 01684 292386
Email: tewkesburypark@foliohotels.com
www.foliohotels.com/tewkesburypark

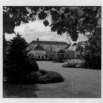
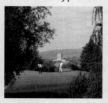

A traditional 176 acre parkland course with wooded areas and water early in your round with welcome relief on later holes with spacious fairways.

80 bedroom hotel and full leisure facilities on site.

folio Hotels

WICK   MAP 03 ST77

Park Resort Tracy Park Estate, Bath Rd BS30 5RN
☎ 0117 937 1800 📠 0117 937 1813
e-mail: info@tpresort.com
web: www.theparkresort.com
Two 18-hole championship courses on the south-western escarpment of the Cotswolds, affording fine views. Both courses present a challenge to all levels of player, with water playing a part on a number of occasions. The elegant clubhouse dates from 1600, set in the 240-acre estate of this golf and country club.
Crown Course: 18 holes, 6201yds, Par 69, SSS 70.
Cromwell Course: 18 holes, 6157yds, Par 71, SSS 70.
Club membership 1000.
Visitors Mon-Sun & BHs. Booking required. Dress code. **Societies** Booking required. **Green Fees** £18-£38 per 18 holes. **Prof** Richard Berry **Facilities** 🏌️ 🍴 🛍️ 🏸 🍽️ 🏊 💆 🎯 ⛳ 🛒 🏌️ **Conf** facs Corporate Hospitality Days **Location** M4 junct 18, then follow A46 towards Bath followed by A420. Course off A420 E of village of Wick
Hotel ★★★ HL The Queensberry Hotel, Russel St, BATH
☎ 01225 447928 820830 📠 01225 446065 29 en suite

WOTTON-UNDER-EDGE   MAP 03 ST79

Cotswold Edge Upper Rushmire GL12 7PT
☎ 01453 844167 📠 01453 845120
e-mail: nnewman@cotswoldedgegolfclub.org.uk
web: www.cotswoldedgegolfclub.org.uk
Meadowland course situated in a quiet Cotswold valley with magnificent views. First half flat and open, second half more varied.
18 holes, 6170yds, Par 71, SSS 71. Club membership 800.
Visitors Contact club for details. **Societies** Booking required. **Green Fees** Phone. 🅿️ **Prof** Rod Hibbitt **Facilities** 🏌️ 🍴 🛍️ 🏸 🍽️ 🏊 💆 🎯 ⛳ **Location** N of town on B4058 Wotton-Tetbury road
Hotel ★★ 72% HL Egypt Mill Hotel, NAILSWORTH ☎ 01453 833449 10 en suite 18 annexe en suite

GREATER LONDON

Those courses which fall within the confines of the London Postal District area (ie have London postcodes - W1, SW1 etc) are listed under the county heading of **London** in the gazetteer (see page 173).

ADDINGTON   MAP 05 TQ36

The Addington 205 Shirley Church Rd CR0 5AB
☎ 020 8777 1055 📠 020 8777 6661
e-mail: info@addingtongolf.com
web: www.addingtongolf.com
This heather and woodland course is considered to be one of the best laid out courses in Southern England with the world famous 13th, Par 3 at 230yds. A good test of golfing ability with no two holes the same.

Continued

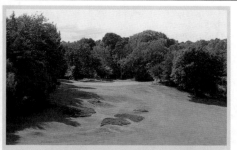

The Addington

18 holes, 6338yds, Par 69, SSS 71, Course record 66.
Visitors Mon-Fri. Restricted play Sat, Sun & BHs. Booking required.
required. Dress code **Societies** Booking required. **Green Fees** Phone.
Prof M Churchill **Course Designer** J F Abercromby **Facilities** ⑪ �⎜ ⅙
⎕ 🍴 ⚘ ⚘ ⚘ 🐾 ⚘ **Conf** Corporate Hospitality Days **Location** M25
junct 7, 3m from Croydon
Hotel ★★★★ 73% HL Selsdon Park Hotel & Golf Club, Addington Rd,
Sanderstead, CROYDON ☎ 020 8657 8811 204 en suite

Addington Court Featherbed Ln CR0 9AA
☎ 020 8657 0281 (booking) & 8651 5270 (admin)
📄 020 8651 0282
e-mail: addington@americangolf.uk.com
Championship Course: 18 holes, 5577yds, Par 68, SSS 67,
Course record 60.
Falconwood: 18 holes, 5472yds, Par 68, SSS 67.
9 Hole: 9 holes, 1804yds, Par 31.
Course Designer Hawtree Snr **Location** 1m S off A2022
Telephone for further details
Hotel ★★★★ 73% HL Selsdon Park Hotel & Golf Club, Addington Rd,
Sanderstead, CROYDON ☎ 020 8657 8811 204 en suite

Addington Palace Addington Park, Gravel Hill CR0 5BB
☎ 020 8654 3061 📄 020 8655 3632
e-mail: johnb@addingtonpalacegolf.co.uk
web: www.addingtonpalacegolf.co.uk
Set in the grounds of Addington Palace, which was the home of the
Archbishops of Canterbury for a number of years. There are a number
of tree-lined fairways and the 17th hole follows one of the original
roads into the Palace and has a fine array of horse chestnut trees. The
course winds its way through tree-lined fairways for the first nine holes.
The second nine holes opens out and needs full concentration to
achieve a good score. The 12th hole is one to remember, over a
fountain and onto a green bunkered on all sides.
18 holes, 6339yds, Par 71, SSS 70, Course record 63.
Club membership 700.
Visitors may play Mon-Fri except BHs. Advance booking required. Dress
code. **Societies** advance booking required. **Green Fees** not confirmed.
Prof Roger Williams **Course Designer** J H Taylor **Facilities** ⑪ ⎜⎜ by prior
arrangement ⅙ ⎕ 🍴 ⚘ ⚘ ⚘ ⚘ **Leisure** snooker. **Conf** Corporate
Hospitality Days **Location** 2m SE of Croydon station on A212
Hotel ★★★★ 73% HL Selsdon Park Hotel & Golf Club, Addington Rd,
Sanderstead, CROYDON ☎ 020 8657 8811 204 en suite

BARNEHURST   MAP 05 TQ57
Barnehurst Mayplace Rd East DA7 6JU
☎ 01322 523746 📄 01322 523860
e-mail: barnehurstgolfcourse@bexley.gov.uk
Public parkland course with well matured greens. Easy walking.
9 holes, 4796yds, Par 70, SSS 67. Club membership 180.
Visitors Mon-Sun & BHs. Dress code. **Societies** Welcome. **Green Fees**
£11.70 for 18 holes, £8.25 for 9 holes (£15.60/£11.50 weekends and bank
holidays). **Course Designer** James Braid **Facilities** ⑪ ⎜⎜ ⅙ ⎕ 🍴 ⚘
⎙ 🍴 ⚘ **Conf** facs Corporate Hospitality Days **Location** 0.75m NW of
Crayford off A2000
Hotel ★★★★ 77% HL Bexleyheath Marriott Hotel, 1 Broadway,
BEXLEYHEATH ☎ 020 8298 1000 142 en suite

BARNET   MAP 04 TQ29
Arkley Rowley Green Rd EN5 3HL
☎ 020 8449 0394 📄 020 8440 5214
e-mail: secretary@arkleygolfclub.co.uk
web: arkleygolfclub.co.uk
Wooded parkland on highest spot in Hertfordshire with fine views.
9 holes, 6046yds, Par 69, SSS 69. Club membership 400.
Visitors Mon, Wed-Fri except BHs. Tue pm only. Dress code.
Societies Booking required. **Green Fees** £32 per day, £25 per round. ⊜
Prof Andrew Hurley **Course Designer** Braid **Facilities** ⑪ ⎜⎜ ⅙ ⎕ 🍴
⅙ ⎙ ⚘ **Conf** Corporate Hospitality Days **Location** Off A1 at Arkley sign
Hotel ★★★ 73% HL Corus hotel Elstree, Barnet Ln, ELSTREE
☎ 0870 609 6151 47 en suite

Old Fold Manor Old Fold Ln, Hadley Green EN5 4QN
☎ 020 8440 9185 📄 020 8441 4863
e-mail: manager@oldfoldmanor.co.uk
web: www.oldfoldmanor.co.uk
Superb heathland course with some fine greens, breathtaking views
and a challenge for all levels of golfer. Slightly undulating in parts, the
course lets you in but gets progressively tougher as it develops.
18 holes, 6447yds, Par 71, SSS 71, Course record 66.
Club membership 560.
Visitors Mon-Fri. Sat, Sun & BHs after 2.30pm. Booking required. Dress
code. **Societies** Booking required. **Green Fees** £45 per 36 holes, £42
per 27 holes, £35 per 18 holes. **Prof** Peter McEvoy **Facilities** ⑪ ⎜⎜ ⅙ ⎕
🍴 ⅙ ⎙ ⚘ ⚘ **Conf** Corporate Hospitality Days **Location** Off A1000
between Barnet & Potters Bar
Hotel ★★★★ 77% HL West Lodge Park Hotel, Cockfosters Rd, HADLEY
WOOD ☎ 020 8216 3900 46 en suite 13 annexe en suite

The Shire London St Albans Rd EN5 4RE
☎ 020 8441 7649 📄 020 8440 2757
e-mail: golf@theshirelondon.com
web: www.theshirelondon.com
A 27-hole golf complex, opened in May 2007 and designed by Seve
Ballesteros, his first full golf course in the UK. The 18-hole Seve
Masters course is a championship style layout with six Par threes, six
Par fours and six Par fives. The 9-hole Seve Challenge course is a mix
of Par fours and threes on a smaller scale, ideal for juniors, beginners
and as a warm-up nine. The complex is also home to the Seve School
Of Natural Golf, a large driving range and practice area, where Seve's
golfing philosophy is unveiled in a world-first teaching package.

Continued

Seve Masters: 18 holes, 7100yds, Par 72, SSS 73.
Seve Challenge: 9 holes, Par 30, SSS 30.
Club membership 400.
Visitors Mon-Sun & BHs. Booking required. Dress code. **Societies** Booking
required. **Green Fees** £40 per 18 holes (£60 Sat, Sun & peak times). **Prof**
Lee Cox **Course Designer** Severiano Ballesteros **Facilities** ⑪ ⅋ ⅃ ⅃ ⅃
⅃ 丄 占 ⅌ ⅋ ⅋ **Leisure** sauna, gymnasium, caddies available,
Severiano Ballesteros School of Natural Golf. **Conf** facs Corporate
Hospitality Days **Location** M25 junct 23 (A1/M25 interchange), take A1081
towards Barnet, Course on right
Hotel ★★★ 73% HL Corus hotel Elstree, Barnet Ln, ELSTREE
☎ 0870 609 6151 47 en suite

BECKENHAM   MAP 05 TQ36

Beckenham Place Park The Mansion, Beckenham Place
Park BR3 2BP
☎ 020 8650 2292 📇 020 8663 1201
18 holes, 5722yds, Par 68, SSS 69.
Location Off A2015
Telephone for further details
Hotel ★★★ 77% HL Best Western Bromley Court Hotel, Bromley Hill,
BROMLEY ☎ 020 8461 8600 114 en suite

Langley Park Barnfield Wood Rd BR3 6SZ
☎ 020 8658 6849 📇 020 8658 6310
e-mail: manager@langleyparkgolf.co.uk
web: www.langleyparkgolf.co.uk
A pleasant but difficult, well-wooded parkland course. Natural
hazards include a lake at the Par 3 18th hole. Although most fairways
are bordered by woodland, they are wide with forgiving rough and
friendly bunkers.
18 holes, 6453yds, Par 69, SSS 71, Course record 65.
Club membership 700.
Visitors Mon-Fri except BHs. Handicap certificate. Dress code.
Societies Booking required. **Green Fees** £60 per day, £40 per round.
Prof Colin Staff **Course Designer** J H Taylor **Facilities** ⑪ ⅋ ⅃ ⅃ ⅃
⅃ 丄 占 ⅌ ⅋ **Conf** Corporate Hospitality Days **Location** 0.5 N of
Beckenham on B2015
Hotel ★★★ 77% HL Best Western Bromley Court Hotel, Bromley Hill,
BROMLEY ☎ 020 8461 8600 114 en suite

BEXLEYHEATH   MAP 05 TQ47

Bexleyheath Mount Rd DA6 8JS
☎ 020 8303 6951
Undulating course.
9 holes, 5162yds, Par 66, SSS 66, Course record 65.
Club membership 330.
Visitors contact club for details. **Societies** welcome. **Green Fees** not
confirmed. ◉ **Facilities** ⅃ **Location** 1m SW
Hotel ★★★★ 77% HL Bexleyheath Marriott Hotel, 1 Broadway,
BEXLEYHEATH ☎ 020 8298 1000 142 en suite

BIGGIN HILL   MAP 05 TQ45

Cherry Lodge Jail Ln TN16 3AX
☎ 01959 572250 📇 01959 540672
e-mail: info@cherrylodgegc.co.uk
web: www.cherrylodgegc.co.uk
Undulating parkland 600ft above sea level with panoramic views of
the surrounding countryside. An enjoyable test of golf for all standards.

The 14th is 434yds across a valley and uphill, requiring two good shots
to reach the green.
18 holes, 6593yds, Par 72, SSS 73, Course record 66.
Club membership 700.
Visitors Mon-Fri except BHs. Handicap certificate. Dress code. **Societies**
Booking required. **Green Fees** £40 per 18 holes. **Prof** Craig Sutherland
Course Designer John Day **Facilities** ⑪ ⅋ ⅃ ⅃ ⅃ 丄 占 ⅌ ⅋ ⅋
Location 1m E of Biggin Hill Airport
Hotel ★★★ 75% HL Best Western Donnington Manor, London Rd,
Dunton Green, SEVENOAKS ☎ 01732 462681 60 en suite

BROMLEY   MAP 05 TQ46

Bromley Magpie Hall Ln BR2 8JF
☎ 020 8462 7014 📇 020 8462 6916
9 holes, 2745yds, Par 70, SSS 67.
Location 2m SE off A21
Telephone for further details
Hotel ★★★ 77% HL Best Western Bromley Court Hotel, Bromley Hill,
BROMLEY ☎ 020 8461 8600 114 en suite

Sundridge Park Garden Rd BR1 3NE
☎ 020 8460 0278 📇 020 8289 3050
e-mail: gm@spgc.co.uk
web: www.spgc.co.uk
The East Course is longer than the West but many think the shorter
of the two courses is the more difficult. The East is surrounded
by trees while the West is more hilly, with good views. Both are
certainly a good test of golf. An Open qualifying course with year
round irrigation of fairways.
East Course: 18 holes, 6516yds, Par 71, SSS 71,
Course record 63.
West Course: 18 holes, 6019yds, Par 69, SSS 69,
Course record 65. Club membership 1200.
Visitors Mon-Fri. Handicap certificate. Dress code. **Societies** Booking
required. **Green Fees** £85 per day, £65 per round **Prof** Stuart Dowsett
Course Designer Willie Park **Facilities** ⑪ ⅋ ⅃ ⅃ ⅃ 丄 占 ⅌ ⅋ ⅋
Conf facs Corporate Hospitality Days **Location** N side of town centre
off A2212
Hotel ★★★ 77% HL Best Western Bromley Court Hotel, Bromley Hill,
BROMLEY ☎ 020 8461 8600 114 en suite

CARSHALTON   MAP 04 TQ26

Oaks Sports Centre Woodmansterne Rd SM5 4AN
☎ 020 8643 8363
web: www.oakssportscentre.co.uk
Public parkland course with floodlit, covered driving range.

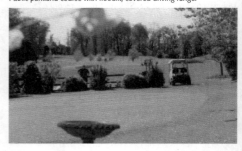

Continued

18 holes: 18 holes, 6054yds, Par 70, SSS 69,
Course record 65.
9 holes: 9 holes, 1497yds, Par 28, SSS 28.
Club membership 432.
Visitors Mon-Fri & BHs. Sat & Sun after noon. Booking required Sat, Sun
& BHs. Dress code. **Societies** Welcome. **Green Fees** £17.40 for 18 holes,
£8.70 for 9 holes (£21/£10.50 weekends). ● **Prof** Horley/Pilkington/
Mulcahy **Facilities** ⑪ ⑩ 🍴 ⚑ ⌨ 🍴 ⚲ 🍴 **Conf** facs
Location 0.5m S on B278
Hotel ★★★ 75% HL Aerodrome Hotel, Purley Way, CROYDON
☎ 020 8710 9000 & 8680 1999 📄 020 8681 6438 105 en suite

CHESSINGTON   MAP 04 TQ16

Chessington Garrison Ln KT9 2LW
☎ 020 8391 0948 📄 020 8397 2068
e-mail: info@chessingtongolf.co.uk
web: www.chessingtongolf.co.uk
Tree-lined parkland course designed by Patrick Tallack, with panoramic
views over the Surrey countryside.
9 holes, 1679yds, Par 30, SSS 28. Club membership 90.
Visitors Mon-Sun & BHs. **Societies** Welcome. **Green Fees** £9 per round
(£11 weekends and bank holidays). **Prof** Mark Janes **Course Designer**
Patrick Tallack **Facilities** ⚑ ⚑ ⌨ 🍴 ⚑ 🍴 ⚲ 🍴 **Leisure** automated
ball teeing facility on driving range. **Conf** facs Corporate Hospitality Days
Location M25 junct 9, 3m N on A243
Hotel BUD Premier Travel Inn Chessington, Leatherhead Rd,
CHESSINGTON ☎ 08701 977057 42 en suite

CHISLEHURST   MAP 05 TQ47

Chislehurst Camden Park Rd BR7 5HJ
☎ 020 8467 6798 📄 020 8295 0874
e-mail: thesecretary@chislehurstgolfclub.co.uk
web: www.chislehurstgolfclub.co.uk
The course was established in 1894 and is dominated by an
imposing 17th century building of great historical interest. The
challenging parkland course has an overall area of less than 70 acres
and accuracy is always more important than distance off the tee. There
are trees, hills and dales and the excellent greens are neither too large
or too flat. Only the 7th hole remains from the original nine-hole
course.
18 holes, 5080yds, Par 66, SSS 65, Course record 61.
Club membership 760.
Visitors Mon-Fri except BHs. Booking required Wed. Handicap certificate
required. Dress code. **Societies** Welcome **Green Fees** £30 per round.
Prof Jonathan Bird **Course Designer** Park **Facilities** ⑪ ⑩ by prior
arrangement ⚑ ⌨ 🍴 ⚑ 🍴 **Leisure** snooker room. **Conf** facs
Hotel ★★★ 77% HL Best Western Bromley Court Hotel, Bromley Hill,
BROMLEY ☎ 020 8461 8600 114 en suite

COULSDON   MAP 04 TQ25

Coulsdon Manor Hotel Coulsdon Court Rd CR5 2LL
☎ 020 8668 0414 📄 020 8668 3118
e-mail: reservations.coulsdon@swallowhotels.com
web: www.swallowhotels.com
Designed by Harry S Colt and set in its own 140 acres of landscaped
parkland.
18 holes, 6037yds, Par 70, SSS 68. Club membership 150.
Visitors may play Mon-Sun & BHs. Advance booking required. Dress code.
Societies advance booking required. **Green Fees** not confirmed. **Prof** Matt

Asbury **Course Designer** Harry Colt **Facilities** ⑪ ⑩ ⚑ ⌨ 🍴 ⚑ 🍴
◇ 🍴 ⚲ **Leisure** hard tennis courts, squash, sauna, solarium, gymnasium.
Conf facs Corporate Hospitality Days **Location** 0.75m E off A23 on B2030
Hotel ★★★★ 73% HL Coulsdon Manor Hotel, Coulsdon Court Rd,
Coulsdon, CROYDON ☎ 020 8668 0414 35 en suite

Woodcote Park Meadow Hill, Bridle Way CR5 2QQ
☎ 020 8668 2788 📄 020 8660 0918
e-mail: info@woodcotepgc.com
web: www.woodcotepgc.com
Slightly undulating parkland.
18 holes, 6720yds, Par 71, SSS 72, Course record 66.
Club membership 700.
Visitors may play Mon-Fri. Booking required. Dress code. **Societies**
Booking required. **Green Fees** £50 per day/round. **Prof** Wraith Grant
Course Designer H S Colt **Facilities** ⑪ ⑩ ⚑ ⌨ 🍴 ⚑ 🍴 ⚲ 🍴
Conf facs Corporate Hospitality Days **Location** 1m N of town centre off
A237
Hotel ★★★ 75% HL Aerodrome Hotel, Purley Way, CROYDON
☎ 020 8710 9000 & 8680 1999 📄 020 8681 6438 105 en suite

CROYDON   MAP 04 TQ36

Croham Hurst Croham Rd CR2 7HJ
☎ 020 8657 5581 📄 020 8657 3229
e-mail: secretary@chgc.co.uk
web: www.chgc.co.uk
Easy walking parkland with tree-lined fairways and bounded by
wooded hills.
18 holes, 6290yds, Par 70, SSS 70. Club membership 800.
Visitors may play Mon Fri except BHs. Advance booking required. Handicap
certificate required. Dress code. **Societies** advance booking required.
Green Fees not confirmed. **Prof** Matthew Paget **Course Designer**
Hawtree/Braid **Facilities** ⑪ ⑩ ⚑ ⌨ 🍴 ⚑ 🍴 ⚲ 🍴 **Conf** facs
Corporate Hospitality Days **Location** 1.5m SE of Croydon on B269
Hotel ★★★★ 73% HL Selsdon Park Hotel & Golf Club, Addington Rd,
Sanderstead, CROYDON ☎ 020 8657 8811 204 en suite

Selsdon Park Hotel Addington Rd, Sanderstead CR2 8YA
☎ 020 8768 3116 📄 020 8651 6171
e-mail: caroline.aldred@principal-hotels.com
web: www.principal-hotels.com
Parkland course in 250 acres of rolling woodland only 12 miles from
the centre of London.
18 holes, 6473yds, Par 73, SSS 71, Course record 63.
Visitors Mon-Sun & BHs. Booking required. Handicap certificate. Dress
code. **Societies** Booking required. **Green Fees** £45 per 18 holes anytime.
Prof Chris Baron **Course Designer** J H Taylor **Facilities** ⑪ ⑩ ⚑ ⌨ 🍴
⚑ 🍴 ⚲ ◇ 🍴 🍴 **Leisure** hard and grass tennis courts, outdoor and
indoor heated swimming pools, squash, sauna, solarium, gymnasium. **Conf**
facs Corporate Hospitality Days **Location** 3m S on A2022
Hotel ★★★★ 73% HL Selsdon Park Hotel & Golf Club, Addington Rd,
Sanderstead, CROYDON ☎ 020 8657 8811 204 en suite

Shirley Park 194 Addiscombe Rd CR0 7LB
☎ 020 8654 1143 ▤ 020 8654 6733
e-mail: secretary@shirleyparkgolfclub.co.uk
web: www.shirleyparkgolfclub.co.uk
The parkland course lies amid fine woodland with good views of
Shirley Hills. The more testing holes come in the middle section of
the course. The remarkable 7th hole calls for a 187yd iron or wood
shot diagonally across a narrow valley to a shelved green set right-
handed into a ridge. The 13th hole, 160yds, is considered to be one
of the finest short holes in the county.
18 holes, 6210yds, Par 71, SSS 69, Course record 64.
Club membership 600.
Visitors may play Mon-Fri except BHs & Sun. Dress code. **Societies**
Booking required. **Green Fees** £40 weekday (£48 Sun). **Prof** Michael
Taylor **Course Designer** Tom Simpson/Herbert Fowler **Facilities** ⑪ ⑩
🝜 ☕ 📠 ♈ 🚻 ♣ 🍴 ♂ **Leisure** snooker. **Conf** Corporate Hospitality
Days **Location** E of town centre on A232
Hotel ★★★★ 73% HL Selsdon Park Hotel & Golf Club, Addington Rd,
Sanderstead, CROYDON ☎ 020 8657 8811 204 en suite

DOWNE   MAP 05 TQ46

High Elms High Elms Rd BR6 7JL
☎ 01689 853232 & 858175 (bookings) ▤ 01689 856326
18 holes, 6210yds, Par 71, SSS 70, Course record 68.
Course Designer Hawthorn **Location** 2m E of A21
Telephone for further details
Hotel ★★★ 77% HL Best Western Bromley Court Hotel, Bromley Hill,
BROMLEY ☎ 020 8461 8600 114 en suite

West Kent Milking Ln BR6 7LD
☎ 01689 851323 ▤ 01689 858693
e-mail: golf@wkgc.co.uk
web: www.wkgc.co.uk
Undulating woodland course close to south London but providing a
quiet rural setting in three valleys.
18 holes, 6426yds, Par 71, SSS 71, Course record 68.
Club membership 700.
Visitors may play Mon-Fri except BHs. Advance booking required. Handicap
certificate required. Dress code. **Societies** Welcome. **Green Fees** £50 per
day; £40 per round. **Prof** Chris Forsyth **Course Designer** H S Colt **Facilities**
⑪ ⑩ 🝜 ☕ 📠 ♈ 🚻 ♣ ♂ **Location** M25 junct 4, A21 towards Bromley,
left signed Downe, through village on Luxted road 0.5m, West Hill on right
Hotel ★★★ 77% HL Best Western Bromley Court Hotel, Bromley Hill,
BROMLEY ☎ 020 8461 8600 114 en suite

ENFIELD   MAP 04 TQ39

Crews Hill Cattlegate Rd, Crews Hill EN2 8AZ
☎ 020 8363 6674 ▤ 020 8363 2343
e-mail: info@crewshillgolfclub.co.uk
web: www.crewshillgolfclub.co.uk
Parkland course in countryside within the M25.
18 holes, 6281yds, Par 70, SSS 70, Course record 65.
Club membership 600.
Visitors may play Mon, Wed-Sun & BHs. Tue after 11.30am. Booking
required Sat, Sun & BHs. Dress code. **Societies** Booking required. **Green
Fees** Phone. **Prof** Neil Wichelow **Course Designer** Harry Colt **Facilities**
⑪ ⑩ by prior arrangement 🝜 ☕ 📠 ♈ 🚻 ♣ 🍴 ♂ **Conf** facs Corporate
Hospitality Days **Location** M25 junct 24, A1005 for Enfield, signed
Hotel ★★★ 83% HL Royal Chace Hotel, The Ridgeway, ENFIELD
☎ 020 8884 8181 92 en suite

Enfield Old Park Rd South EN2 7DA
☎ 020 8363 3970 ▤ 020 8342 0381
e-mail: secretary@enfieldgolfclub.co.uk
web: www.enfieldgolfclub.co.uk
Parkland with tree-lined fairways and a meandering brook that comes
into play on nine holes. There are no hidden or unfair hazards and,
although not easy, the course is highly playable and always attractive.
18 holes, 6154yds, Par 72, SSS 70, Course record 61.
Club membership 600.
Visitors Mon-Sun & BHs. Booking required. Handicap certificate. Dress
code. **Societies** Booking required. **Green Fees** £28 (£36 Sat, Sun & BHs).
Prof Martin Porter **Course Designer** James Braid **Facilities** ⑪ 🝜 ☕ 📠
♈ 🚻 ♣ ♂ **Conf** facs Corporate Hospitality Days **Location** M25 jnct 24,
A1005 to Enfield to rdbt with church on left, right down Slades Hill, 1st left
to end
Hotel ★★★ 83% HL Royal Chace Hotel, The Ridgeway, ENFIELD
☎ 020 8884 8181 92 en suite

Whitewebbs Park Whitewebbs Ln EN2 9HH
☎ 020 8363 4454 ▤ 020 8366 2257
e-mail: gary.sherriff1@btinternet.com
web: www.enfield.gov.uk
This challenging parkland course was first opened for play in 1932 and
is set in over 140 acres of attractive rolling countryside with mature
woodland and the meandering Cuffley brook that comes into play on
four holes.
18 holes, 5782yds, Par 68, SSS 68, Course record 64.
Club membership 350.
Visitors Mon-Sun & BHs. Dress code. **Societies** Booking required.
Green Fees £24 per day, £14.50 per round (£29/£18.50 Sat & Sun).
Prof Gary Sherriff **Facilities** ⑪ ⑩ 🝜 ☕ 📠 ♈ 🚻 ♣ 🍴 ♂ **Location** N of
town centre
Hotel ★★★ 83% HL Royal Chace Hotel, The Ridgeway, ENFIELD
☎ 020 8884 8181 92 en suite

GREENFORD   MAP 04 TQ18

C & L Golf & Country Club Westend Rd, Northolt
UB5 6RD
☎ 020 8845 5662 ▤ 020 8841 5515
18 holes, 4458yds, Par 67, SSS 62, Course record 58.
Course Designer Patrick Tallack **Location** Junct Westend Rd
Telephone for further details

Ealing Perivale Ln UB6 8SS
☎ 020 8997 0937 ▤ 020 8998 0756
e-mail: ealinggolfoffice@aol.com
web: www.ealinggolfclub.com
A classic parkland layout with the river Brent providing a natural hazard
and some of the finest greens around.
18 holes, 6216yds, Par 70, SSS 70, Course record 62.
Club membership 650.
Visitors may play Mon-Sun except BHs. Advance booking required Sat &
Sun. Handicap certificate required. Dress code. **Societies** Booking required.
Green Fees £40 per 18 holes (£50 Sat & Sun). **Prof** Ricky Willison **Course
Designer** H S Colt **Facilities** ⑪ ⑩ by prior arrangement 🝜 ☕ 📠 ♈ 🚻 ♣
♂ 🍴 ♂ **Conf** facs Corporate Hospitality Days **Location** Exit at the Perivale
turn-off on the A40

Horsenden Hill Whitton Av, Woodland Rise UB6 0RD
☎ 020 8902 4555 📱 020 8902 4555
A distinctive picturesque course designed over hilly landscape. Very challenging comprising eight Par 3s (3 over 200yds) and a Par 4 of 292yds. Overlooks the London skyline to Canary Wharf and the London Eye.
9 holes, 1632yds, Par 28, SSS 28. Club membership 135.
Visitors Mon-Sun & BHs. **Societies** Welcome. **Green Fees** £8 per 18 holes, £4.50 per 9 holes (£12.50/£7.50 Sat, Sun & BHs). **Prof** Jeff Quarshie
Facilities ⊕ ⊗ ⟆ ⟆ ⟆ ⟆ ⟆ ⟆ ⟆ **Conf** Corporate Hospitality Days
Location 3m NE on A4090

Lime Trees Park Ruislip Rd, Northolt UB5 6QZ
☎ 020 8842 0442 📱 0208 8420542
9 holes, 5836yds, Par 71, SSS 69.
Location 300yds off A40 at Polish War Memorial, A4180 towards Hayes
Telephone for further details

Perivale Park Stockdove Way UB6 8TJ
☎ 020 8575 7116
Parkland beside the River Brent.
9 holes, 2667yds, Par 68, SSS 67. Club membership 250.
Visitors Mon-Sun & BHs. Booking required Sat & Sun before noon. lWelcome. **Green Fees** £8 per 9 holes (£9 weekends & bank holidays).
Prof Peter Bryant **Facilities** ⟆ ⟆ ⟆ ⟆ ⟆ ⟆ **Location** E side of town centre, off A40
Hotel ★★★ 72% HL Best Western Cumberland Hotel, 1 St Johns Rd, HARROW ☎ 020 8863 4111 31 en suite 53 annexe en suite

---

Hadley Wood Beech Hill EN4 0JJ
☎ 020 8449 4328 & 4486 📱 020 8364 8633
e-mail: gm@hadleywoodgc.com
web: www.hadleywoodgc.com
Parkland on the north-west edge of London. The gently undulating fairways have a friendly width inviting the player to open his shoulders, though the thick rough can be very punishing to the unwary. The course is pleasantly wooded and there are some admirable views.

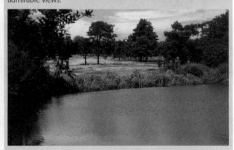

Club membership 650.
Visitors may play Mon-Fri & Sun except BHs. Advance booking required. Handicap certificate required. Dress code. **Societies** advance booking required. **Green Fees** not confirmed. **Prof** Peter Jones
Course Designer Alister Mackenzie **Facilities** ⊕ ⟆ ⟆ ⟆ ⟆ ⟆ ⟆ ⟆ ⟆ ⟆ **Conf** facs Corporate Hospitality Days **Location** M25 junct 24, take A111 to Cockfosters, 2m to 3rd turning right
Hotel ★★★★ 77% HL West Lodge Park Hotel, Cockfosters Rd, HADLEY WOOD ☎ 020 8216 3900 46 en suite 13 annexe en suite

---

Fulwell Wellington Rd, Hampton Hill TW12 1JY
☎ 020 8977 3844 📱 020 8977 7732
e-mail: secretary@fulwellgolfclub.co.uk
web: www.fulwellgolfclub.co.uk
Championship-length parkland course with easy walking. The 575-yd 17th and the water feature 9th are notable.

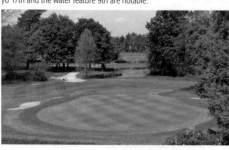

18 holes, 6544yds, Par 71, SSS 71. Club membership 750.
Visitors Mon-Sun & BHs. Booking required Sat, Sun & BHs. Dress code.
Societies Booking required. **Green Fees** £50 per day £40 per round (£55 per round Sat & Sun). **Prof** Nigel Turner **Course Designer** John Morrison
Facilities ⊕ ⟆ ⟆ ⟆ ⟆ ⟆ ⟆ ⟆ ⟆ **Location** 1.5m N on A311
Hotel ★★★★ 71% HL Richmond Hill Hotel, Richmond Hill, RICHMOND UPON THAMES ☎ 020 8940 2247 138 en suite

---

Hampton Court Palace Home Park KT1 4AD
☎ 020 8977 2423 📱 020 8614 4747
e-mail: hamptoncourtpalace@crown-golf.co.uk
web: www.crown-golf.co.uk
Flat course with easy walking situated in the grounds of Hampton Court Palace. Unique blend of parkland and inland links built on a base of sand and gravel, making it one of the finest winter courses in the country.
18 holes, 6513yds, Par 71, SSS 71, Course record 64.
Club membership 750.
Visitors may play Mon-Fri & BHs. Booking required. Dress code. **Societies** Booking required. **Green Fees** £40 Mon-Thu, £45 Fri. **Prof** Edward Litchfield **Course Designer** Willie Park **Facilities** ⊕ ⊗ ⟆ ⟆ ⟆ ⟆ ⟆ ⟆ ⟆ **Conf** facs Corporate Hospitality Days **Location** Off A308 on W side of Kingston Bridge
Hotel ★★★★ 71% HL Richmond Hill Hotel, Richmond Hill, RICHMOND UPON THAMES ☎ 020 8940 2247 138 en suite

---

Playgolf Northwick Park Watford Rd HA1 3TZ
☎ 020 8864 2020 📱 020 8864 4040
e-mail: info@northwickpark.com
web: www.northwickpark.com
The 'Majors' course is an 8-hole golf course (two double greens) where every hole is a full-scale tribute to some of the world's most famous golf holes - including Augusta National, the 8th 'Postage Stamp' hole from Royal Troon, and the 9th from The Belfry. Every hole echoes either a Major championship venue, or a course that has hosted The Ryder Cup or Walker Cup.

Continued

Majors Course: 6 holes, 1409yds, Par 20, Course record 18.
Club membership 200.
Visitors Mon-Sun & BHs. Booking required. **Societies** Booking required.
Green Fees £25 per two rounds, £15 per round. Fees include facilities
on driving range and short game practice area. **Course Designer** Peter
McEvoy **Facilities** ⓞ ⍣ ⌦ ⛳ 🛒 ⚐ 🅟 🏌 **Leisure** gymnasium, short
game practice area, children's golf course. **Conf** facs   Corporate Hospitality
Days **Location** SE of Harrow on A404 Watford road. Follow directions to
Northwick Park Hospital, course adjacent
Hotel ★★★ 72% HL Best Western Cumberland Hotel, 1 St Johns Rd,
HARROW ☎ 020 8863 4111   31 en suite   53 annexe en suite

HILLINGDON   MAP 04 TQ08

Hillingdon 18 Dorset Way UB10 0JR
☎ 01895 233956 & 239810 📠 01895 233956
9 holes, 5490yds, Par 68, SSS 67.
Location W of town off A4020
Telephone for further details
Hotel ★★★ 73% HL Novotel London Heathrow, Cherry Ln, WEST
DRAYTON ☎ 01895 431431   178 en suite

HOUNSLOW   MAP 04 TQ17

Airlinks Southall Ln TW5 9PE
☎ 020 8561 1418 📠 88136284
18 holes, 6000yds, Par 71, SSS 69, Course record 63.
Course Designer P Alliss/D Thomas **Location** M4 junct 3, W of Hounslow
Telephone for further details
Hotel ★★ 67% HL Best Western Master Robert Hotel, 366 Great West Rd,
HOUNSLOW ☎ 020 8570 6261   96 annexe en suite

Hounslow Heath Municipal Staines Rd TW4 5DS
☎ 020 8570 5271 📠 020 8570 5205
18 holes, 5901yds, Par 69, SSS 68, Course record 62.
Course Designer Fraser M Middleton **Location** On A315 towards Bedfont
Telephone for further details
Hotel ★★ 67% HL Best Western Master Robert Hotel, 366 Great West Rd,
HOUNSLOW ☎ 020 8570 6261   96 annexe en suite

ILFORD   MAP 05 TQ48

Ilford Wanstead Park Rd IG1 3TR
☎ 020 8554 2930 📠 020 8554 0822
e-mail: ilfordgolfclub@btconnect.com
web: www.ilfordgolfclub.com
18 holes, 5299yds, Par 67, SSS 66, Course record 61.
Course Designer Whitehead **Location** NW of town centre off A12
Telephone for further details
Hotel BUD Travelodge London Ilford, Clements Rd, ILFORD
☎ 08700 850 950   91 en suite

ISLEWORTH   MAP 04 TQ17

Wyke Green Syon Ln TW7 5PT
☎ 020 8847 0685 (Prof) & 8560 8777 (Sec)
📠 020 8569 8392
e-mail: office@wykegreengolfclub.co.uk
web: www.wykegreengolfclub.co.uk
Fairly flat parkland. Seven Par 4 holes over 420yds.
18 holes, 6182yds, Par 69, SSS 70, Course record 64.
Club membership 650.

Visitors Mon-Fri except BHs. Dress code. **Societies** Booking required.
Green Fees £30 per round; (£35 weekends). **Prof** Neil Smith **Course**
Designer Hawtree **Facilities** ⓞ ⍣ ⌦ ⛳ 🛒 ⚐ 🅟 🏌 🏌 **Conf**   Corporate
Hospitality Days **Location** 0.5m N on B454, off A4 at Gillette Corner
Hotel ★★ 67% HL Best Western Master Robert Hotel, 366 Great West Rd,
HOUNSLOW ☎ 020 8570 6261   96 annexe en suite

KINGSTON UPON THAMES   MAP 04 TQ16

Coombe Hill Golf Club Dr, Coombe Ln West KT2 7DF
☎ 020 8336 7600 📠 020 8336 7601
e-mail: thesecretary@chgc.net
web: www.coombehillgolfclub.com
Charming heathland course featuring a fine display of
rhododendrons during May and June. The course presents a
challenge to golfers of all standards offering superb greens, quality
short holes and a number of testing long holes requiring approach
shots to elevated greens.
18 holes, 6293yds, Par 71, SSS 71, Course record 67.
Club membership 550.
Visitors may play Mon, Tue, Thu-Sun & BHs. Wed pm only. Booking
required. Handicap certificate. Dress code. **Societies** Welcome.
Green Fees £100 per 36 holes, £80 per 18 holes. **Prof** Andy Dunn
Course Designer J F Abercromby **Facilities** ⓞ ⍣ ⌦ ⛳ 🛒 ⚐ 🅟 🏌
🏌 **Leisure** sauna.   **Conf**   Corporate Hospitality Days **Location** 1.75m
E on A238
Hotel BUD Travelodge London Kingston Upon Thames, 21-23 London
Rd, KINGSTON-UPON-THAMES ☎ 08700 850 950   72 en suite

Coombe Wood George Rd, Kingston Hill KT2 7NS
☎ 020 8942 0388 📠 020 8942 5665
e-mail: geoff.seed@coombewoodgolf.com
web: www.coombewoodgolf.com
Mature parkland with seven varied and challenging Par 3s.

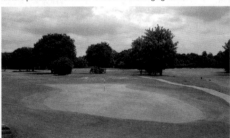

18 holes, 5299yds, Par 66, SSS 66, Course record 59.
Club membership 700.
Visitors Mon, Wed-Sun except BHs. Booking required. Handicap certificate.
Dress code. **Societies** Welcome. **Green Fees** £30 per round (£35 per
round weekends). ⊗ **Prof** Phil Wright **Course Designer** Tom Williamson
Facilities ⓞ ⍣ ⌦ ⛳ 🛒 ⚐ 🅟 🏌 **Conf** facs   Corporate Hospitality
Days **Location** 1.25m NE on A308
Hotel BUD Travelodge London Kingston Upon Thames, 21-23 London Rd,
KINGSTON-UPON-THAMES ☎ 08700 850 950   72 en suite

MITCHAM
MAP 04 TQ26

Mitcham Carshalton Rd, Mitcham Junction CR4 4HN
☎ 020 8648 4280 📠 020 8647 4197
web: www.mitchamgolfclub.co.uk
A wooded heathland course on a gravel base, playing as an inland links course.
18 holes, 5935yds, Par 69, SSS 68, Course record 65.
Club membership 500.
Visitors may play Mon-Fri & BHs. Limited play Sat & Sun. Dress code.
Societies Booking required. **Green Fees** £17 (£22 Sat & Sun, £27 BHs).
Prof Paul Burton **Course Designer** T Scott/T Morris **Facilities** ⑪ 🍽 ⅊
⬜🏐 ⚲ 🏌 🚩 ✆ **Conf** Corporate Hospitality Days **Location** adjacent
Mitcham Junction railway station
Hotel ★★★ 75% HL Aerodrome Hotel, Purley Way, CROYDON
☎ 020 8710 9000 & 8680 1999 📠 020 8681 6438 105 en suite

NEW MALDEN
MAP 04 TQ26

Malden Traps Ln KT3 4RS
☎ 020 8942 0654 📠 020 8336 2219
e-mail: manager@maldengolfclub.com
web: www.maldengolfclub.com
Parkland course with the hazard of the Beverley Brook which affects 4 holes (3rd, 7th, 8th and 12th).
18 holes, 6252yds, Par 71, SSS 70. Club membership 800.
Visitors may play Mon-Fri except BHs. Advance booking required. Dress code. **Societies** advance booking required. **Green Fees** not confirmed.
🏌 **Prof** Robert Hunter **Facilities** ⑪ 🍽 ⅊ ⬜🏐 ⚲ 🏌 ✆ 🚩✆
Conf Corporate Hospitality Days **Location** N of town centre off B283
Hotel BUD Travelodge London Kingston Upon Thames, 21-23 London Rd, KINGSTON-UPON-THAMES ☎ 08700 850 950 72 en suite

NORTHWOOD
MAP 04 TQ09

Haste Hill The Drive HA6 1HN
☎ 01923 825224
18 holes, 5787yds, Par 68, SSS 68, Course record 63.
Location 0.5m S off A404
Telephone for further details
Hotel ★★★ 74% HL Quality Harrow Hotel, 12-22 Pinner Rd, HARROW
☎ 020 8427 3435 79 en suite

Northwood Rickmansworth Rd HA6 2QW
☎ 01923 821384 📠 01923 840150
e-mail: secretary@northwoodgolf.co.uk
web: www.northwoodgolf.co.uk
A high quality parkland course. The course provides a good test of golf to the experienced golfer and can hold many surprises for the unsuspecting. The Par 4 10th hole, Death or Glory, has wrecked many good cards in the past, while the long Par 4 5th hole requires two very good shots to make par.
18 holes, 6535yds, Par 71, SSS 71, Course record 67.
Club membership 650.
Visitors may play Mon, Thu, Fri. Advance booking required. Dress code.
Societies advance booking required. **Green Fees** not confirmed. **Prof** C
J Holdsworth **Course Designer** James Braid **Facilities** ⑪ 🍽 ⅊ ⬜🏐
⚲ 🏌 🚩✆ **Conf** Corporate Hospitality Days **Location** On A404
Hotel ★★★ 74% HL Quality Harrow Hotel, 12-22 Pinner Rd, HARROW
☎ 020 8427 3435 79 en suite

Sandy Lodge Sandy Lodge Ln HA6 2JD
☎ 01923 825429 📠 01923 824319
e-mail: info@sandylodge.co.uk
web: www.sandylodge.co.uk
A links-type, very sandy, heathland course.
18 holes, 6347yds, Par 71, SSS 71, Course record 64.
Club membership 780.
Visitors Mon-Fri. Handicap certificate required. Dress code. **Societies**
Booking required. **Green Fees** £45 per round. **Prof** Jeff Pinsent **Course**
Designer H Vardon **Facilities** ⑪ 🍽 ⅊ ⬜🏐 ⚲ 🏌 🚩 ✆ **Conf**
Corporate Hospitality Days **Location** N of town centre off A4125
Hotel ★★★ 71% HL Best Western The White House, Upton Rd, WATFORD ☎ 01923 237316 57 en suite

ORPINGTON
MAP 05 TQ46

Chelsfield Lakes Golf Centre Court Rd BR6 9BX
☎ 01689 896266 📠 01689 824577
web: www.hannam.mcmail.com
18 holes, 6077yds, Par 71, SSS 69, Course record 64.
Warren: 9 holes, 1188yds, Par 27.
Course Designer M Sandow **Location** M25 junct 4, on A224
Telephone for further details
Hotel ★★★ 77% HL Best Western Bromley Court Hotel, Bromley Hill, BROMLEY ☎ 020 8461 8600 114 en suite

Cray Valley Sandy Ln, St Paul's Cray BR5 3HY
☎ 01689 837909 & 871490 📠 01689 891428
18 hole: 18 holes, 5669yds, Par 70, SSS 67.
9 holes: 9 holes, 2140yds, Par 32.
Location 1m off A20, Critley's Corner junction
Telephone for further details
Hotel ★★★ 77% HL Best Western Bromley Court Hotel, Bromley Hill, BROMLEY ☎ 020 8461 8600 114 en suite

Ruxley Park Golf Centre Sandy Ln, St Paul's Cray
BR5 3HY
☎ 01689 871490 📠 01689 891428
18 holes, 5703yds, Par 70, SSS 68, Course record 63.
Location 2m NE on A223
Telephone for further details
Hotel ★★★ 77% HL Best Western Bromley Court Hotel, Bromley Hill, BROMLEY ☎ 020 8461 8600 114 en suite

PINNER   MAP 04 TQ18

Grims Dyke Oxhey Ln, Hatch End HA5 4AL
☎ 020 8428 4539 🗐 020 8421 5494
e-mail: grimsdykegolfclub@hotmail.com
web: www.club-noticeboard.co.uk/grimsdyke

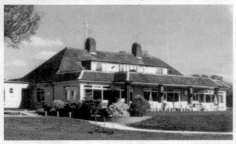

18 holes, 5596yds, Par 69, SSS 67, Course record 61.
Course Designer James Baird **Location** 3m N of Harrow on A4008
Telephone for further details
Hotel ★★★ 72% HL Best Western Cumberland Hotel, 1 St Johns Rd,
HARROW ☎ 020 8863 4111 31 en suite 53 annexe en suite

Pinner Hill Southview Rd, Pinner Hill HA5 3YA
☎ 020 8866 0963 🗐 020 8868 4817
e-mail: phgc@pinnerhillgc.com
web: www.pinnerhillgc.com
On the top of Pinner Hill surrounded by rolling parkland and mature
woods, this peaceful atmosphere will make you feel a million miles
from North West London's suburbia. Two nine-hole loops of mature
fairways and undulating greens will lift and challenge your game.
18 holes, 6392yds, Par 71, SSS 71, Course record 69.
Club membership 710.
Visitors Mon-Sun & BHs. Booking required. Handicap certificate. Dress
code. **Societies** Booking required. **Green Fees** Phone. **Prof** Chris Duck
Course Designer J H Taylor **Facilities** ⊕ �◉ ▣ 🖫 ☐ ⊗ 🖫 ⚐ ⚑ 🍴 ⛳ 🏌 🚗 ⚑
Conf facs Corporate Hospitality Days **Location** 2m NW off A404
Hotel ★★★ 74% HL Quality Harrow Hotel, 12-22 Pinner Rd, HARROW
☎ 020 8427 3435 79 en suite

PURLEY   MAP 05 TQ36

Purley Downs 106 Purley Downs Rd CR2 0RB
☎ 020 8657 8347 🗐 020 8651 5044
e-mail: info@purleydowns.co.uk
web: www.purleydownsgolfclub.co.uk
Hilly downland course which is a good test for golfers.
18 holes, 6262yds, Par 70, SSS 70, Course record 64.
Club membership 750.
Visitors contact club for details. **Societies** welcome. **Green Fees** not
confirmed. **Prof** Graham Wilson **Course Designer** J Taylor/H S Colt
Facilities ⊕ ◉ ▣ 🖫 ☐ ⊗ 🖫 ⚐ ⚑ 🏌 ⛳ **Location** E of town centre off A235
Hotel ★★★ 75% HL Aerodrome Hotel, Purley Way, CROYDON
☎ 020 8710 9000 & 8680 1999 🗐 020 8681 6438 105 en suite

RICHMOND (UPON THAMES) MAP 04 TQ17

Richmond Sudbrook Park, Petersham TW10 7AS
☎ 020 8940 4351 (office) & 8940 7792 (shop)
🗐 8940 8332/7914
e-mail: admin@richmondgolfclub.com
web: www.the richmondgolfclub.com
Beautiful and historic parkland on the edge of Richmond Park
dating from 1891 and extensively modernised in recent years.
The clubhouse is one of the most-distinguished small Georgian
mansions in England.
18 holes, 6100yds, Par 70, SSS 70, Course record 65.
Club membership 650.
Visitors may play Mon-Fri except BHs. Advance booking required Wed.
Handicap certificate required. Dress code. **Societies** advance booking
required. **Green Fees** not confirmed. **Prof** Steve Burridge **Course
Designer** Tom Dunn **Facilities** ⊕ ◉ by prior arrangement 🖫 ☐ 🖫 ⚐ ⚑
🚗 🏌 ⛳ ⚑ ⛳ 🏌 **Conf** facs Corporate Hospitality Days **Location** 1.5m S
off A307 between Kingston & Richmond
Hotel ★★★★ 71% HL Richmond Hill Hotel, Richmond Hill, RICHMOND
UPON THAMES ☎ 020 8940 2247 138 en suite

Royal Mid-Surrey Old Deer Park, Twickenham Rd
TW9 2SB
☎ 020 8940 1894 🗐 020 8939 0150
e-mail: secretary@rmsgc.co.uk
web: www.rmsgc.co.uk
A long playing historic parkland course. The flat fairways are cleverly
bunkered. The 1st hole at 245yds from the medal tees is a tough
Par 3 opening hole. The 18th provides an exceptionally good Par 4
finish with a huge bunker before the green to catch the not quite
perfect long second. The Inner Course, while shorter than the Outer,
offers a fair challenge to all golfers. Again the 18th offers a strong
Par 4 finish with bunkers threatening from the tee. A long second to
a sloping, well-bunkered green will reward the accurate player.
*Outer Course: 18 holes, 6343yds, Par 69, SSS 71,
Course record 62.*
Inner Course: 18 holes, 5544yds, Par 68, SSS 67.
Club membership 1400.
Visitors Mon-Fri except BHs. Booking required. Handicap certificate.
Dress code. **Societies** Booking required. **Green Fees** Phone. **Prof**
Matthew Paget **Course Designer** J H Taylor **Facilities** ⊕ ◉ 🖫 ☐ 🖫 ⚐ ⚑
🚗 🏌 ⚑ ⛳ **Leisure** snooker. **Conf** facs Corporate Hospitality Days
Location 0.5m N of Richmond off A316
Hotel ★★★★ 71% HL Richmond Hill Hotel, Richmond Hill, RICHMOND
UPON THAMES ☎ 020 8940 2247 138 en suite

ROMFORD   MAP 05 TQ58

Maylands Colchester Rd, Harold Park RM3 0AZ
☎ 01708 341777 🗐 01708 343777
e-mail: maylands@maylandsgolf.com
web: www.maylandsgolf.com
Picturesque undulating parkland course.
18 holes, 6361yds, Par 71, SSS 70, Course record 62.
Club membership 550.
Visitors Mon-Fri & BHs. Booking required. Dress code. **Societies** Booking
required. **Green Fees** £40 per round. **Prof** Darren Parker **Course
Designer** H S Colt **Facilities** ⊕ ◉ 🖫 ☐ 🖫 ⚐ ⚑ 🚗 🏌 ⛳ 🏌 **Conf**
Corporate Hospitality Days **Location** M25 junct 28, A12 0.5m towards
London, club on right
Hotel BUD Premier Travel Inn Romford Central, Mercury Gardens,
ROMFORD ☎ 08701 977220 64 en suite

Risebridge Golf Centre Risebridge Chase, Lower
Bedfords Rd RM1 4DG
☎ 01708 741429 🖷 01708 741429
e-mail: pa.jennings@btconnect.com
web: www.jackbarker.com
A well matured parkland golf course, with many challenging holes
especially the long 12th, the Par 4 13th and Par 5 14th with water and
a two tiered green.
18 holes, 6000yds, Par 71, SSS 70, Course record 66.
Club membership 300.
Visitors Mon-Sun & BHs. Dress code. **Societies** Welcome. **Green Fees**
£14 (£19 Sat & Sun). ◉ **Prof** Paul Jennings **Course Designer** Hawtree
Facilities ⓘ ⦿ ⮞ ⛾ ⟊ ⟁ ⌂ ⌖ ✔ ☇ **Location** Between Collier Row
and Harold Hill
Hotel BUD Premier Travel Inn Romford Central, Mercury Gardens,
ROMFORD ☎ 08701 977220   64 en suite

Romford Heath Dr, Gidea Park RM2 5QB
☎ 01708 740986 🖷 01708 752157
18 holes, 6410yds, Par 72, SSS 70, Course record 64.
Course Designer H Colt **Location** 1m NE on A118
Telephone for further details
Hotel BUD Premier Travel Inn Romford Central, Mercury Gardens,
ROMFORD ☎ 08701 977220   64 en suite

RUISLIP   MAP 04 TQ08

Ruislip Ickenham Rd HA4 7DQ
☎ 01895 638081 & 638835 🖷 01895 635780
e-mail: ruislipgolf@btconnect.com
web: www.middlesexgolf.com
Municipal parkland course. Many trees.
18 holes, 5700yds, Par 69, SSS 68, Course record 65.
Club membership 300.
Visitors Mon-Sun & BHs. Booking required. Dress code. **Societies** Booking
required. **Green Fees** £14.50 per 18 holes (£21 Sat, Sun & BHs). **Prof** Paul
Glozier **Course Designer** Sand Herd **Facilities** ⓘ ⦿ ⮞ ⛾ ⟊ ⟁ ⌂ ⌖
☇ ⌯ ☇ ✔ **Location** 0.5m SW on B466 opposite Ruislip underground
station
Hotel ★★★ 74% HL Quality Harrow Hotel, 12-22 Pinner Rd, HARROW
☎ 020 8427 3435   79 en suite

SIDCUP   MAP 05 TQ47

Sidcup 7 Hurst Rd DA15 9AE
☎ 020 8300 2150 🖷 020 8300 2150
e-mail: sidcupgolfclub@tiscali.co.uk
Easy walking parkland with two lakes and the River Shuttle running
through.
9 holes, 5722yds, Par 68, SSS 68. Club membership 370.
Visitors may play Mon-Thu except BHs. Advance booking required.
Handicap certificate required. Dress code. **Societies** advance booking
required. **Green Fees** not confirmed. ◉ **Course Designer** James Braid
Facilities ⓘ ⮞ ⛾ ⟊ ⟁ ⌂ **Location** N of town centre off A222
Hotel ★★★★ 77% HL Bexleyheath Marriott Hotel, 1 Broadway,
BEXLEYHEATH ☎ 020 8298 1000   142 en suite

SOUTHALL   MAP 04 TQ17

West Middlesex Greenford Rd UB1 3EE
☎ 020 8574 3450 🖷 020 8574 2383
e-mail: westmid.gc@virgin.net
web: www.westmiddxgolfclub.co.uk
Gently undulating parkland course founded in 1891, the oldest private
course in Middlesex designed by James Braid.
18 holes, 6119yds, Par 69, SSS 69, Course record 64.
Club membership 600.
Visitors may play Mon-Fri & BHs. Sat & Sun pm only. Booking required Tue,
Thu-Sun & BHs. Dress code. **Societies** Booking required. **Green Fees** Mon:
£16 per round; Tue-Fri: £18, Sat-Sun £25. **Prof** T Talbot **Course Designer**
James Braid **Facilities** ⓘ ⦿ ⮞ ⛾ ⟊ ⟁ ⌂ ⌖ ☇ **Leisure** fishing. **Conf** facs
Corporate Hospitality Days **Location** W of town centre on A4127
Hotel ★★ 67% HL Best Western Master Robert Hotel, 366 Great West Rd,
HOUNSLOW ☎ 020 8570 6261   96 annexe en suite

STANMORE   MAP 04 TQ19

Stanmore 29 Gordon Av HA7 2RL
☎ 020 8954 2599 🖷 020 8954 2599
e-mail: secretary@stanmoregolfclub.co.uk
web: www.stanmoregolfclub.co.uk
A quiet and peaceful parkland course in the suburbs of north-
west London, with incredible views over the Thames basin from
the 3th and 5th tees. The course is short but very challenging as all
the fairways are lined with trees. Accuracy plays a major role and
notable holes are the 2nd, 8th, 11th and 13th. The signature hole is the
Par 4 7th, played over a fir tree from an elevated tee onto the fairway.
18 holes, 5885yds, Par 68, SSS 68, Course record 61.
Club membership 500.
Visitors Mon-Sun & BHs. Booking required Mon, Fri-Sun & BHs. Dress code.
Societies Booking required. **Green Fees** Mon & Fri: £17, Tue-Thu: £25, £35
Sat & Sun. **Prof** J Reynolds **Course Designer** Dr A Mackenzie **Facilities** ⓘ
⦿ ⮞ ⛾ ☇ ⟁ ⌂ ⌖ ☇ **Conf** facs   Corporate Hospitality Days **Location** S
of town centre between Stanmore & Belmont
Hotel ★★★ 74% HL Quality Harrow Hotel, 12-22 Pinner Rd, HARROW
☎ 020 8427 3435   79 en suite

SURBITON   MAP 04 TQ16

Surbiton Woodstock Ln KT9 1UG
☎ 020 8398 3101 (Sec) 🖷 020 8339 0992
e-mail: gill.whitelock@surbitongolfclub.com
web: www.surbitongolfclub.com
Parkland with easy walking.
18 holes, 6055yds, Par 70, SSS 69, Course record 63.
Club membership 700.
Visitors Mon-Fri except BHs. Booking required. Handicap certificate. Dress
code. **Societies** Booking required. **Green Fees** £45 summer, £40 winter. ◉
Prof Paul Milton **Course Designer** Tom Dunn **Facilities** ⓘ ⦿ ⮞ ⛾ ☇
⟁ ⌂ ⌖ ☇ **Location** A3 Hook junct, A309 S 2m, left onto Woodstock Ln
Hotel BUD Premier Travel Inn Chessington, Leatherhead Rd,
CHESSINGTON ☎ 08701 977057   42 en suite

TWICKENHAM   MAP 04 TQ17

Amida Staines Rd TW2 5JD
☎ 0208 783 1698 🖹 0208 783 9475
e-mail: jamie.skinner@amidaclubs.com
web: www.amidaclubs.com
A nine-hole pay and play course situated within 70 acres of
mature parkland with a water feature coming into play on the 2nd
and 3rd holes. The course is mature but has undergone extensive
recent improvement work, including new tees and greens and the
installation of an automated irrigation system.
9 holes, 2788yds, Par 35, SSS 69. Club membership 100.
Visitors Mon-Sun & BHs. Booking required Sat, Sun & BHs. Dress code.
Societies Booking required. **Green Fees** £10 per 9 holes ((£12 Sat,
Sun & BHs). **Prof** Jamie Skinner **Facilities** ⊕ ⏃ ⣷ ⤵ 🖤 ⚐ 🖐 🏌 🏊
Leisure hard tennis courts, heated indoor swimming pool, squash, sauna,
solarium, gymnasium, indoor virtual golf. **Conf** facs Corporate Hospitality
Days **Location** 2m W on A305
Hotel ★★★★ 71% HL Richmond Hill Hotel, Richmond Hill, RICHMOND
UPON THAMES ☎ 020 8940 2247 138 en suite

Strawberry Hill Wellesley Rd, Strawberry Hill TW2 5SD
☎ 020 8894 0165 & 8898 2082
e-mail: secretary@shgc.net
web: www.shgc.net
Parkland with easy walking.
9 holes, 4762yds, Par 64, SSS 63, Course record 59.
Club membership 300.
Visitors Mon-Fri except BHs. Dress code. **Societies** Booking required
Green Fees £25/£18 per day, £18/£11 per 18 holes, £14/£8 per 9 holes.
Prof Peter Buchan **Course Designer** J H Taylor **Facilities** ⊕ ⏃ by prior
arrangement ⣷ ⚐ 🖤 🏌 ⤵ 🏊 **Location** S of town centre off A316, next
to Strawberry Hill railway station
Hotel ★★★★ 71% HL Richmond Hill Hotel, Richmond Hill, RICHMOND
UPON THAMES ☎ 020 8940 2247 138 en suite

UPMINSTER   MAP 05 TQ58

Upminster 114 Hall Ln RM14 1AU
☎ 01708 222788 (Secretary) 🖹 01708 222484
e-mail: secretary@upminstergolfclub.co.uk
web: www.upminstergolfclub.co.uk
The meandering River Ingrebourne features on several holes of this
partly undulating parkland course, situated on one side of the river
valley. It provides a challenge to golfers of all abilities. The clubhouse
is a beautiful Grade II listed building.
18 holes, 6076yds, Par 69, SSS 69, Course record 62.
Club membership 1000.
Visitors Mon, Wed-Fri except BHs. Booking required. Handicap certificate.
Dress code. **Societies** Booking required. **Green Fees** Phone. ⊕ **Prof** Steve
Cipa **Course Designer** W G Key **Facilities** ⊕ ⏃ ⣷ ⚐ 🖤 🏌 ⤵ 🏊 🖐 🏌
Leisure bowling, snooker. **Location** Junct M25 , 2m W
Hotel BUD Premier Travel Inn Romford Central, Mercury Gardens,
ROMFORD ☎ 08701 977220 64 en suite

UXBRIDGE   MAP 04 TQ08

Stockley Park Stockley Park UB11 1AQ
☎ 020 8813 5700 🖹 020 8813 5655
e-mail: s.birch@stockleyparkgolf.com
web: www.stockleyparkgolf.com
Hilly and challenging course set in 240 acres of parkland and designed
by Robert Trent Jones senior. Accessible to a complete range of golfer.
18 holes, 6754yds, Par 72, SSS 71.
Visitors Mon-Sun & BHs. Booking required. Dress code. **Societies** Booking
required. **Green Fees** £25 per round (£37 weekends & bank holidays).
Reduced fees after 2pm (noon winter). **Prof** Stuart Birch **Course Designer**
Robert Trent Jones Snr **Facilities** ⊕ ⏃ ⣷ ⚐ 🖤 🏌 ⤵ 🏊 🖐 **Conf** facs
Corporate Hospitality Days **Location** M4 junct 4, 1m N off A408
Hotel ★★★ 73% HL Novotel London Heathrow, Cherry Ln, WEST
DRAYTON ☎ 01895 431431 178 en suite

Uxbridge The Drive, Harefield Place UB10 8AQ
☎ 01895 237287 🖹 01895 813539
e-mail: higolf@btinternet.com
18 holes, 5750yds, Par 68, SSS 68, Course record 66.
Location 2m N off B467
Telephone for further details
Hotel ★★★ 77% HL Barn Hotel, West End Rd, RUISLIP ☎ 01895 636057
59 en suite

WEMBLEY   MAP 04 TQ18

Sudbury Bridgewater Rd HA0 1AL
☎ 020 8902 3713 🖹 020 8902 3713
e-mail: enquiries@sudburygolfclubltd.co.uk
web: www.sudburygolfclubltd.co.uk
Undulating parkland near the centre of London.

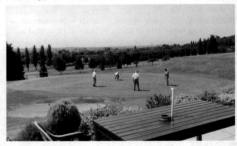

18 holes, 6282yds, Par 69, SSS 70, Course record 63.
Club membership 650.
Visitors Mon-Fri except BHs. Handicap certificate. Dress code. **Societies**
Welcome. **Green Fees** £30 per 18 holes. **Prof** Neil Jordan **Course
Designer** Harry Colt **Facilities** ⊕ ⏃ ⣷ ⚐ 🖤 🏌 ⤵ 🏊 🖐 **Conf** facs
Location SW of town centre on A4090

WEST DRAYTON   MAP 04 TQ07

Heathpark Stockley Rd UB7 9NA
☎ 01895 444232 🖹 01895 444232
9 holes, 2032yds, Par 64, SSS 60, Course record 64.
Course Designer Neal Coles **Location** M4 junct 4, off A408
Telephone for further details
Hotel ★★★★ 74% HL The Pinewood Hotel, Uxbridge Rd, George Green,
SLOUGH ☎ 01753 824848 33 en suite 16 annexe en suite

WOODFORD GREEN MAP 05 TQ49

Woodford Sunset Av IG8 0ST
☎ 020 8504 3330 & 8504 0553 📠 020 8559 0504
e-mail: office@woodfordgolfclub.fsnet.co.uk
web: www.woodfordgolf.co.uk
Forest land course on the edge of Epping Forest. Views over the Lea valley to the London skyline. When played as 18 holes from dual tees, the course is comprised of four Par 3s, two Par 5s and twelve Par 4s. Although fairly short, the tree-lined fairways and subtle undulations provide and excellent test of golfing skill.
9 holes, 5852yds, Par 70, SSS 68, Course record 66.
Club membership 350.
Visitors Mon-Sun & BHs. Booking required Tue, Wed, Sat, Sun & BHs. Dress code. **Societies** Booking required. **Green Fees** £15 per 18 holes; £10 per 9 holes. ◉ **Prof** Jon Robson **Course Designer** Tom Dunn **Facilities** ⊕ ⎆ by prior arrangement ⊑ ⊓ ⏁ ⏄ **Conf** Corporate Hospitality Days **Location** NW of town centre off A104
Hotel ★★ 62% SHL Ridgeway Hotel, 115/117 The Ridgeway, North Chingford, LONDON ☎ 020 8529 1964 20 en suite

GREATER MANCHESTER

ALTRINCHAM MAP 07 SJ78

Altrincham Stockport Rd WA15 7LP
☎ 0161 928 0761 📠 0161 928 8542
e-mail: scott.partington@tclt.co.uk
web: www.altringhamgolfclub.org.uk
Municipal parkland course with easy walking, water on many holes, rolling contours and many trees. Driving range in grounds.
18 holes, 6385yds, Par 71, SSS 69. Club membership 350.
Visitors may play Mon-Sun & BHs. Advance booking required. Dress code. **Societies** advanced booking required. **Green Fees** not confirmed. **Prof** Scott Partington **Facilities** ⊕ ⎋ ⊓ ⏁ ⏄ ⏄ ⏂ **Conf** Corporate Hospitality Days **Location** 0.75m E of town ventre on A560
Hotel ★★★ 77% HL Best Western Cresta Court Hotel, Church St, ALTRINCHAM ☎ 0161 927 7272 137 en suite

Dunham Forest Oldfield Ln WA14 4TY
☎ 0161 928 2605 📠 0161 929 8975
e-mail: email@dunhamforestgolfclub.com
18 holes, 6636yds, Par 72, SSS 72.
Course Designer Dave Thomas **Location** 1.5m W off A56
Telephone for further details
Hotel ★★★ 72% HL Quality Hotel Altrincham, Langham Rd, Bowdon, ALTRINCHAM ☎ 0161 928 7121 91 en suite

Ringway Hale Mount, Hale Barns WA15 8SW
☎ 0161 980 2630 📠 0161 980 4414
e-mail: andrew@ringwaygolfclub.co.uk
web: www.ringwaygolfclub.co.uk
Parkland with interesting natural hazards. Easy walking and good views of the Pennines and the Peak District.
18 holes, 6482yds, Par 71, SSS 71, Course record 65.
Club membership 800.
Visitors Mon, Wed, Thu, Sun & BHs. Booking required. Handicap certificate. Dress code. **Societies** Booking required. **Green Fees** £40 (£50 Sun & BHs). **Prof** Nick Ryan **Course Designer** Colt **Facilities** ⏁ ⏄ ⏂ ⏄ **Conf** Corporate Hospitality Days **Location** M56 junct 6, A538 for 1m signed Hale, right onto Shay Ln
Hotel ★★★ 77% HL Best Western Cresta Court Hotel, Church St, ALTRINCHAM ☎ 0161 927 7272 137 en suite

ASHTON-IN-MAKERFIELD MAP 07 SJ59

Ashton-in-Makerfield Garswood Park, Liverpool Rd WN4 0YT
☎ 01942 719330 📠 01942 719330
18 holes, 6250yds, Par 70, SSS 70, Course record 63.
Location M6 junct 24, 5m W on A580
Telephone for further details
Hotel BUD Premier Travel Inn Wigan South, 53 Warrington Rd, Ashton-in-Makerfield, WIGAN ☎ 0870 9906582 28 en suite

ASHTON-UNDER-LYNE MAP 07 SJ99

Ashton-under-Lyne Gorsey Way, Higher Hurst OL6 9HT
☎ 0161 330 1537 📠 0161 330 6673
e-mail: info@ashtongolfclub.co.uk
A testing, varied moorland course, with large greens. Easy walking.
18 holes, 5754yds, Par 69, SSS 68. Club membership 760.
Visitors Mon-Fri & BHs. Dress code. **Societies** Booking required **Green Fees** £27.50 per day. ◉ **Prof** Colin Boyle **Facilities** ⊕ ⎆ ⎋ ⊑ ⊓ ⏁ ⏂ ⏄ **Conf** facs Corporate Hospitality Days **Location** N off B6194

Dukinfield Lyne Edge, Yew Tree Ln SK16 5DB
☎ 0161 338 2340 📠 0161 303 0205
e-mail: dgclub@tiscali.co.uk
web: www.dukinfieldgolfclub.co.uk
Recently extended, tricky hillside course with several challenging Par 3s and a very long Par 5.
18 holes, 5338yds, Par 67, SSS 66. Club membership 500.
Visitors Contact club for details. **Societies** Welcome. **Green Fees** £20 per day. ◉ **Prof** David Green **Facilities** ⊕ ⎆ ⎋ ⊑ ⊓ ⏁ ⏄ ⏂ ⏄ **Conf** Corporate Hospitality Days **Location** S off B6175
Hotel BUD Premier Travel Inn Manchester (Mottram), Stockport Rd, Mottram, HYDE ☎ 0870 9906334 83 en suite

BOLTON MAP 07 SD70

Bolton Lostock Park, Chorley New Rd BL6 4AJ
☎ 01204 843067 & 843278 📠 01204 843067
e-mail: secretary@boltongolfclub.co.uk
This well-maintained heathland course is always a pleasure to visit. The 12th hole should be treated with respect and so too should the final four holes which have ruined many a card.
18 holes, 6237yds, Par 70, SSS 70, Course record 64.
Club membership 612.
Visitors may play Mon, Wed-Fri except BHs. Booking required. Dress code. **Societies** Booking required. **Green Fees** £35 per day, £30 per round. ◉ **Prof** R Longworth **Facilities** ⊕ ⎆ ⎋ ⊑ ⊓ ⏁ ⏄ ⏂ **Conf** Corporate Hospitality Days **Location** 3m W of Bolton on A673
Hotel BUD Premier Travel Inn Bolton, 991 Chorley New Rd, Horwich, BOLTON ☎ 08701 977282 40 en suite

Breightmet Red Bridge, Ainsworth BL2 5PA
☎ 01204 527381 & 399275 📠 01204 399275
Long parkland course.
18 holes, 6405yds, Par 72, SSS 71, Course record 67.
Club membership 400.
Visitors may play Mon, Tue, Thu, Fri except BHs. Dress code. **Societies** Booking required. **Green Fees** £20 per 18 holes. ◉ **Course Designer** D Griffiths **Facilities** ⊕ ⎆ ⊑ ⊓ ⏁ **Conf** Corporate Hospitality Days **Location** E of town centre off A58
Hotel ★★★★ 76% HL Mercure Last Drop Village Hotel & Spa, Bromley Cross, BOLTON ☎ 0870 1942117 118 en suite 10 annexe en suite

England

Deane Broadford Rd, Deane BL3 4NS
☎ 01204 61944 (professional) & 651808(secretary)
🖹 01204 652047
e-mail: secretary@deanegolfclub.com
Undulating parkland with small ravines on the approach to some holes.
18 holes, 5652yds, Par 68, SSS 67, Course record 64.
Club membership 470.
Visitors Mon-Fri, Sun & BHs. Booking required. Dress code. **Societies**
Booking required. **Green Fees** £25 per round (£30 weekends and bank
holidays). ● **Prof** David Martindale **Facilities** ⊕ ⊗ ⊗ ⊗ ⊗ ⊗ ⊗ ⊗
Conf facs **Location** M61 junct 5, 1m towards Bolton
Hotel BUD Premier Travel Inn Bolton, 991 Chorley New Rd, Horwich,
BOLTON ☎ 08701 977282 40 en suite

Dunscar Longworth Ln, Bromley Cross BL7 9QY
☎ 01204 303321 🖹 01204 303321
e-mail: secretary@dunscargolfclub.fsnet.co.uk
18 holes, 5982yds, Par 71, SSS 69, Course record 63.
Location 2m N off A666
Telephone for further details
Hotel BUD Travelodge Bolton West (M61 Southbound), Bolton West Service
Area, Horwich, BOLTON ☎ 08700 850 950 32 en suite

Great Lever & Farnworth Plodder Ln, Farnworth
BL4 0LQ
☎ 01204 656137 🖹 01204 656137
18 holes, 6044yds, Par 70, SSS 69, Course record 67.
Location M61 junct 4, 1m
Telephone for further details
Hotel ★★★★ 76% HL Mercure Last Drop Village Hotel & Spa, Bromley
Cross, BOLTON ☎ 0870 1942117 118 en suite 10 annexe en suite

Harwood Roading Brook Rd, Harwood BL2 4JD
☎ 01204 522878 & 524233 🖹 01204 524233
e-mail: secretary@harwoodgolfclub.co.uk
web: www.harwoodgolfclub.co.uk
Mainly flat parkland with several water hazards.
18 holes, 5915yds, Par 70, SSS 69, Course record 65.
Club membership 700.
Visitors may play Mon, Tue, Thu, Fri except BHs. Dress code. **Societies**
Booking required. **Green Fees** £25 per round. ● **Prof** C Maroney
Course Designer G Shuttleworth **Facilities** ⊕ ⊗ ⊗ ⊗ ⊗ ⊗ ⊗ ⊗
Location 2.5m NE off B6196
Hotel BUD Premier Travel Inn Bolton, 991 Chorley New Rd, Horwich,
BOLTON ☎ 08701 977282 40 en suite

Old Links Chorley Old Rd, Montserrat BL1 5SU
☎ 01204 842307 🖹 01204 842307 ext 25
e-mail: mail@boltonoldlinksgolfclub.co.uk
web: www.boltonoldlinksgolfclub.co.uk
Championship moorland course.
18 holes, 6469yds, Par 71, SSS 72. Club membership 600.
Visitors Mon, Wed-Fri, Sun & BHs. Handicap certificate. Dress code.
Societies Booking required. **Green Fees** £35 per day (£45 Sat, Sun &
BHs)). ● **Prof** Paul Horridge **Course Designer** Dr Alistair MacKenzie
Facilities ⊕ ⊗ ⊗ ⊗ ⊗ ⊗ ⊗ **Conf** facs **Location** NW of town
centre on B6226
Hotel BUD Travelodge Bolton West (M61 Southbound), Bolton West Service
Area, Horwich, BOLTON ☎ 08700 850 950 32 en suite

Regent Park Links Rd, Chorley New Rd BL6 4AF
☎ 01204 495421 🖹 01204 844620
Parkland course with exceptional moorland views.
18 holes, 6130yds, Par 71, SSS 70, Course record 63.
Club membership 200.
Visitors Mon-Sun & BHs. Booking required. Dress code. **Societies** Booking
required. **Green Fees** £11 per round (£14 Sat & Sun). **Prof** Neil Brazell
Course Designer James Braid **Facilities** ⊕ ⊗ ⊗ ⊗ ⊗ ⊗ ⊗ ⊗ ⊗
Conf facs Corporate Hospitality Days **Location** M61 junct 6, 1m E off A673
Hotel BUD Travelodge Bolton West (M61 Southbound), Bolton West Service
Area, Horwich, BOLTON ☎ 08700 850 950 32 en suite

Turton Wood End Farm, Hospital Rd, Bromley Cross
BL7 9QD
☎ 01204 852235 🖹 01204 856921
e-mail: info@turtongolfclub.com
web: www.turtongolfclub.com
Moorland course with panoramic views. A wide variety of holes which
challenge any golfer's technique.
18 holes, 6124yds, Par 70, SSS 69, Course record 68.
Club membership 550.
Visitors may play Mon, Tue, Thu, Fri, Sun & BHs. Booking required Sun
& BHs. Dress code. **Societies** Booking required. **Green Fees** £26 per
round (£33 Sun & BHs). **Prof** Mark Saunders **Course Designer** Alex Herd
Facilities ⊗ ⊗ ⊗ ⊗ ⊗ **Location** 3m N off A666, follow signs for
'Last Drop Village'
Hotel ★★★★ 76% HL Mercure Last Drop Village Hotel & Spa, Bromley
Cross, BOLTON ☎ 0870 1942117 118 en suite 10 annexe en suite

BRAMHALL   MAP 07 SJ88

Bramall Park 20 Manor Rd SK7 3LY
☎ 0161 485 7101 🖹 0161 485 7101
e-mail: secretary@bramallparkgolfclub.co.uk
web: www.bramallparkgolfclub.co.uk
Attractive parkland with some testing, lengthy Par 4s, especially after
the recent rebunkering of the whole course.
18 holes, 6247yds, Par 70, SSS 70, Course record 63.
Club membership 829.
Visitors Mon-Sun & BHs. Handicap certificate required. Dress code.
Societies Booking required. **Green Fees** £38 per day, £34 per round
(£45/40 weekends & bank holidays). **Prof** M Proffitt **Course Designer**
James Braid **Facilities** ⊕ ⊗ ⊗ ⊗ ⊗ ⊗ ⊗ **Conf** facs Corporate
Hospitality Days **Location** NW of town centre off B5149
Hotel ★★★ 72% HL Best Western Belfry House Hotel, Stanley Rd,
HANDFORTH ☎ 0161 437 0511 81 en suite

Bramhall Ladythorn Rd SK7 2EY
☎ 0161 439 6092 🖹 0161 439 0264
e-mail: office@bramhallgolfclub.com
web: www.bramhallgolfclub.com
Undulating parkland with easy walking.
18 holes, 6347yds, Par 70, SSS 70. Club membership 700.
Visitors Mon-Wed & Fri except BHs. Booking required. Handicap certificate
required. Dress code. **Societies** Booking required. **Green Fees** Phone. ●
Prof Richard Green **Facilities** ⊕ ⊗ ⊗ ⊗ ⊗ ⊗ ⊗ ⊗
Conf Corporate Hospitality Days **Location** E of town centre off A5102
Hotel ★★★ 72% HL Best Western Belfry House Hotel, Stanley Rd,
HANDFORTH ☎ 0161 437 0511 81 en suite

BURY

Bury Unsworth Hall, Blackford Bridge, Manchester Rd BL9 9TJ
☎ 0161 766 4897 📠 0161 796 3480
e-mail: secretary@burygolfclub.com
web: www.burygolfclub.com
Moorland course, difficult in part. Tight and good test of golf.
18 holes, 5961yds, Par 69, SSS 69, Course record 61.
Club membership 650.
Visitors Mon, Wed-Sun & BHs. Booking required Sat, Sun & BHs. Dress code. **Societies** Booking required. **Green Fees** £30 (£35 weekends). **Prof** G Coope **Course Designer** Mackenzie **Facilities** ⑪ ⑩l ⅃ ☐ ⑪ 🐴 ⚑ **Conf** facs Corporate Hospitality Days **Location** 2m N of M60 junct 17 on A56
Hotel ★★★ 72% HL Best Western Bolholt Country Park Hotel, Walshaw Rd, BURY ☎ 0161 762 4000 65 en suite

Lowes Park Hilltop, Lowes Rd BL9 6SU
☎ 0161 764 1231 📠 0161 763 9503
e-mail: lowesparkgc@btconnect.com
web: www.lowesparkgc.co.uk
Moorland with easy walking. Exposed outlook with good views.
9 holes, 6006yds, Par 70, SSS 69, Course record 65.
Club membership 350.
Visitors Tue, Thu, Fri, Sun except BHs. Booking required. Handicap certificate. Dress code. **Societies** Booking required. **Green Fees** £15 (£10 winter). ⑨ **Facilities** ⑪ ⑩l ⅃ ☐ ⑪ 🐴 **Conf** facs Corporate Hospitality Days **Location** N side of town centre off A56
Hotel ★★★ 72% HL Best Western Bolholt Country Park Hotel, Walshaw Rd, BURY ☎ 0161 762 4000 65 en suite

Walmersley Garretts Close, Walmersley BL9 6TE
☎ 0161 764 1429 & 0161 764 7770 📠 0161 764 7770
Moorland hillside course, with wide fairways, large greens and extensive views. Testing holes: 2nd (484 yds) Par 5; 5th Par 4 with severe dog leg and various hazards.
18 holes, 5341yds, Par 69, SSS 67, Course record 65.
Club membership 475.
Visitors may play Mon, Wed-Fri. Sun after 11am. Booking required. Dress code. **Societies** Booking required. **Green Fees** £30 per day. ⑨ **Prof** P Thorpe **Course Designer** S Marnoch **Facilities** ⑪ by prior arrangement ⑩l by prior arrangement ⅃ ☐ 🐴 ⚑ **Conf** Corporate Hospitality Days **Location** 2m N off A56
Hotel ★★★ 72% HL Best Western Bolholt Country Park Hotel, Walshaw Rd, BURY ☎ 0161 762 4000 65 en suite

CHEADLE
MAP 07 SJ88

Cheadle Cheadle Rd SK8 1HW
☎ 0161 491 4452
e-mail: cheadlegolfclub@msn.com
web: www.cheadlegolfclub.com
Parkland with hazards on every hole, from sand bunkers and copses to a stream across six of the fairways.
9 holes, 5006yds, Par 64, SSS 65. Club membership 425.
Visitors may play Mon, Wed-Fri, Sun & BHs. Booking required Sun. Handicap certificate . Dress code. **Societies** Booking required. **Green Fees** £25 (£28 Sun). ⑨ **Prof** D Cain **Course Designer** T Renouf **Facilities** ⑪ ⑩l ⅃ ☐ ⑪ 🐴 ⚑ **Location** S of village off A5149
Hotel ★★★ 72% HL The Wycliffe Hotel, 74 Edgeley Rd, Edgeley, STOCKPORT ☎ 0161 477 5395 14 en suite

DENTON
MAP 07 SJ99

Denton Manchester Rd M34 2GG
☎ 0161 336 3218 📠 0161 336 4751
e-mail: dentongolfclub@btinternet.com
web: www.dentongolfclub.com
Easy walking parkland course with brook running through. One notable hole is called Death and Glory.
18 holes, 6443yds, Par 71, SSS 71, Course record 66.
Club membership 740.
Visitors may play Mon, Wed-Fri & BHs. Dress code. **Societies** Booking required. **Green Fees** Phone. ⑨ **Prof** M Hollingworth **Course Designer** R McCauley **Facilities** ⑪ ⑩l by prior arrangement ⅃ ☐ ⑪ 🐴 ⚑ **Location** M60 junct 24, 1.5m W on A57
Hotel ★★★ 73% HL Old Rectory Hotel, Meadow Ln, Haughton Green, Denton, MANCHESTER ☎ 0161 336 7516 30 en suite 6 annexe en suite

FAILSWORTH
MAP 07 SD80

Brookdale Medlock Rd M35 9WQ
☎ 0161 681 4534 📠 0161 688 6872
e-mail: info@brookdalegolfclub.co.uk
web: www.brookdalegolfclub.co.uk
Challenging parkland course in the Medlock valley with great Pennine views, although only 5m from the centre of Manchester. The river Medlock meanders through the course and features on six of the holes.
18 holes, 5864yds, Par 68, SSS 68, Course record 64.
Club membership 700.
Visitors may play Mon-Fri. Advance booking required. Dress code. **Societies** advance booking required. **Green Fees** not confirmed. ⑨ **Prof** Tony Cuppello **Facilities** ⑪ ⑩l ⅃ ☐ ⑪ 🐴 ⚑ 🛒 ⚑ 🐴 ⚑ **Location** M60/A62 Oldham exit, towards Manchester, left at Nat West bank, left at road end right. Right at minirdbt, 0.5m on left

FLIXTON
MAP 07 SJ79

William Wroe Municipal Pennybridge Ln, Flixton Rd M41 5DX
☎ 0161 748 8680
18 holes, 4395yds, Par 64, SSS 65.
Location E of village off B5158, 3m from Manchester centre
Telephone for further details
Hotel BUD Premier Travel Inn Manchester (Sale), Carrington Ln, Ashton-Upon-Mersey, SALE ☎ 08701 977179 40 en suite

GATLEY
MAP 07 SJ88

Gatley Waterfall Farm, Styal Rd, Heald Green SK8 3TW
☎ 0161 437 2091
e-mail: enquiries@gatleygolfclub.com
web: www.gatleygolfclub.com
Moderately testing parkland course with a tough finish.
9 holes, 5934yds, Par 68, SSS 68, Course record 67.
Club membership 400.
Visitors may play Mon, Wed-Fri, Sun & BHs. Handicap certificate required. Dress code. **Societies** welcome. **Green Fees** not confirmed. **Prof** James Matterson **Facilities** ⑪ ⅃ ☐ ⑪ 🐴 ⚑ **Conf** Corporate Hospitality Days **Location** S of village off B5166
Hotel ★★★ 72% HL Best Western Belfry House Hotel, Stanley Rd, HANDFORTH ☎ 0161 437 0511 81 en suite

England

HAZEL GROVE
MAP 07 SJ98

Hazel Grove Buxton Rd SK7 6LU
☎ 0161 483 3978
Testing parkland course with tricky greens and water hazards coming into play on several holes. Year round play on the greens.
18 holes, 6310yds, Par 71, SSS 70, Course record 62.
Club membership 630.
Visitors may play Mon-Fri. Sat, Sun & BHs by arrangement. Handicap certificate. Dress code. **Societies** Booking required. **Green Fees** Phone.
🏌 **Prof** J Hopley **Course Designer** McKenzie **Facilities** ⓘ ⓘ ⓘ ☞ ⚐ ⛳
⛳ 🏌 ⚐ 🏌 **Leisure** golf electronic teaching system (GASP). **Conf** facs
Corporate Hospitality Days **Location** 1m E off A6
Hotel ★★★ 75% HL Alma Lodge Hotel, 149 Buxton Rd, STOCKPORT
☎ 0161 483 4431 20 en suite 32 annexe en suite

HINDLEY
MAP 07 SD60

Hindley Hall Hall Ln WN2 2SQ
☎ 01942 255131 📠 01942 253871
18 holes, 5913yds, Par 69, SSS 68, Course record 64.
Location M61 junct 6, 3m, 1m N off A58
Telephone for further details
Hotel ★★★ 71% HL Quality Hotel Wigan, Riverway, WIGAN
☎ 01942 826888 88 en suite

HYDE
MAP 07 SJ99

Werneth Low Werneth Low Rd, Gee Cross SK14 3AF
☎ 0161 368 2503 & 336 9496(secretary) 📠 0161 320 0053
e-mail: andrew.dfloyd@btinternet.com
Hard walking but good views of six counties from this undulating moorland course, which is played in a 7-4-7 loop. Exposed to wind with small greens. A good test of golfing skill.
11 holes, 6113yds, Par 70, SSS 70, Course record 64.
Club membership 375.
Visitors Mon, Wed, Fri & Sat. Thu am only. Booking required BHs. Handicap certificate. Dress code. **Societies** Welcome. **Green Fees** Phone. **Prof** Tony Bacchus **Facilities** ⓘ ⓘ ⓘ ⓘ ☞ ⚐ ⛳ **Conf** Corporate Hospitality Days **Location** 2m S of town centre
Hotel ★★ 80% HL Wind in the Willows Hotel, Derbyshire Level, GLOSSOP
☎ 01457 868001 12 en suite

KEARSLEY
MAP 07 SD70

Manor Moss Ln BL4 8SF
☎ 01204 701027 📠 01204 796914
18 holes, 5010yds, Par 66, SSS 64, Course record 65.
Course Designer Jeff Yates **Location** Off A666 Manchester Rd
Telephone for further details
Hotel ★★★ 68% HL Novotel Manchester West, Worsley Brow, WORSLEY 119 en suite

LITTLEBOROUGH
MAP 07 SD91

Whittaker Whittaker Ln OL15 0LH
☎ 01706 378310
Moorland course with outstanding views of Hollingworth Lake Countryside Park and the Pennine Hills.
9 holes, 5632yds, Par 68, SSS 67, Course record 61.
Club membership 240.

Visitors Mon-Sat except BHs. Booking required. Dress code. **Societies** Booking required. **Green Fees** £14 per 18 holes (£18 Sat). Reduced winter rates. ⓐ **Facilities** ⚐ ⛳ **Location** 1.5m from Littleborough off A58
Hotel ★★★★ 77% HL Mercure Norton Grange Hotel & Spa, Manchester Rd, Castleton, ROCHDALE ☎ 0870 1942119 81 en suite

MANCHESTER
MAP 07 SJ89

Blackley Victoria Ave East, Blackley M9 7HW
☎ 0161 643 2980 & 654 7770 📠 0161 653 8300
e-mail: office@blackleygolfclub.com
web: www.blackleygolfclub.com
Parkland course crossed by a footpath. The course has recently been redesigned giving greater challenge and interest including water features.
18 holes, 6168yds, Par 70, SSS 71. Club membership 800.
Visitors may play Mon-Sun & BHs. Advance booking required Thu, Sat, Sun & BHs. Handicap certificate required. Dress code. **Societies** advanced booking required. **Green Fees** not confirmed. ⓐ **Prof** Craig Gould **Course Designer** Gaunt & Marnoch **Facilities** ⓘ ⓘ by prior arrangement ⓘ ⚐ ⛳ ⛳ ⚐ **Conf** Corporate Hospitality Days **Location** 4m N of city centre
Hotel ★★★ 85% HL Malmaison, Piccadilly, MANCHESTER
☎ 0161 278 1000 167 en suite

Chorlton-cum-Hardy Barlow Hall, Barlow Hall Rd, Chorlton-cum-Hardy M21 7JJ
☎ 0161 881 5830 📠 0161 881 4532
e-mail: chorltongolf@hotmail.com
web: www.chorltoncumhardygolfclub.co.uk
Set in the grounds of Barlow Hall, this challenging parkland course winds its way around the way around the banks of the Mersey. The testing opening holes lead up to the stroke 1 7th, an impressive 474yd Par 4, with its elevated green. The course then meanders through parkland culminating at the Par 4 18th.
18 holes, 5994yds, Par 70, SSS 69, Course record 61.
Club membership 700.
Visitors Mon-Sun & BHs. Dress code. **Societies** Booking required.
Green Fees £27 (£32 Sat, Sun & BHs). **Prof** David Valentine **Facilities** ⓘ ⓘ ⓘ ⚐ ⛳ ⛳ ⚐ **Leisure** snooker. **Conf** facs Corporate Hospitality Days **Location** 4m S of Manchester, A5103/A5145
Hotel ★★★ 77% HL Best Western Willow Bank Hotel, 340-342 Wilmslow Rd, Fallowfield, MANCHESTER ☎ 0161 224 0461 117 en suite

Davyhulme Park Gleneagles Rd, Davyhulme M41 8SA
☎ 0161 748 2260 📠 0161 747 4067
e-mail: davyhulmeparkgolfclub@email.com
18 holes, 6237yds, Par 72, SSS 70, Course record 64.
Location Next to Trafford General Hospital
Telephone for further details
Hotel BUD Premier Travel Inn Manchester (Sale), Carrington Ln, Ashton-Upon-Mersey, SALE ☎ 08701 977179 40 en suite

Didsbury Ford Ln, Northenden M22 4NQ
☎ 0161 998 9278 📠 0161 902 3060
e-mail: golf@didsburygolfclub.com
web: www.didsburygolfclub.com
Parkland course.
18 holes, 6273yds, Par 70, SSS 70, Course record 60.
Club membership 750.

Continued

Visitors may play Mon, Tue, Thu, Fri & Sun except BHs. Advance booking required. Dress code. **Societies** advance booking required. **Green Fees** not confirmed. **Prof** Peter Barber **Facilities** ⑪ ⑩ ⓛ ⓑ ⓓ ⓣ ⓛ ⓒ ⓞ ✔ 🚗 **Conf** facs Corporate Hospitality Days **Location** 6m S of city centre off A5145 **Hotel** BUD Travelodge Manchester Didsbury, Kingsway, DIDSBURY ☎ 08700 850 950 62 en suite

Fairfield 'Boothdale', Booth Rd, Audenshaw M34 5QA
☎ 0161 301 4528 📄 0161 301 4254
e-mail: secretary@fairfieldgolf.co.uk
web: fairfield.golf@btconnect.com
Parkland course set around a reservoir. Course demands particularly accurate placing of shots.
18 holes, 5276yds, Par 68, SSS 66, Course record 63.
Club membership 450.
Visitors Mon, Tue, Fri & BHs. Booking required Tue & Fri. **Societies** Booking required. **Green Fees** Phone. ⊛ **Prof** Stephen Pownell **Facilities** ⑪ ⑩ ⓛ ⓓ ⓣ ⓛ ⓒ ⓞ ✔ **Location** 5m E of Manchester off A635 **Hotel** ★★★ 73% HL Old Rectory Hotel, Meadow Ln, Haughton Green, Denton, MANCHESTER ☎ 0161 336 7516 30 en suite 6 annexe en suite

Marriott Worsley Park Hotel & Country Club
Worsley Park, Worsley M28 2QT
☎ 0161 975 2043 📄 0161 975 2058
web: www.marriott.co.uk/golf
Set in 200 acres of parkland with a range of tee positions, eight lakes and 70 strategically placed bunkers and providing an exciting challenge to golfers of all abilities, very often requiring brains rather than brawn to make a successful score.
18 holes, 6611yds, Par 71, SSS 72, Course record 61.
Club membership 400.
Visitors may play Mon-Sun & BHs. Advance booking required. Dress code. **Societies** advance booking required. **Green Fees** not confirmed. **Prof** David Screeton **Course Designer** Ross McMurray **Facilities** ⑪ ⑩ ⓛ ⓓ ⓣ ⓛ ⓒ ⓞ ✔ 🚗 ✔ 🏌 **Leisure** heated indoor swimming pool, sauna, solarium, gymnasium, Short game area. **Conf** facs **Location** M60 junct 13, A585, course 0.5m on left
Hotel ★★★★ 76% HL Marriott Worsley Park Hotel & Country Club, Worsley Park, Worsley, MANCHESTER ☎ 0161 975 2000 158 en suite

Northenden Palatine Rd, Northenden M22 4FR
☎ 0161 998 4738 📄 0161 945 5592
e-mail: manager@northendengolfclub.com
web: www.northendengolfclub.com
Parkland course surrounded by the River Mersey with 18 newly rebuilt USGA specification greens.

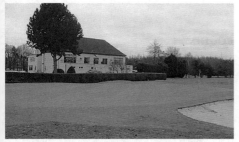

18 holes, 6432yds, Par 72, SSS 71, Course record 64.
Club membership 800.

Visitors Mon-Fri, Sun & BHs. Booking required. Handicap certificate. Dress code. **Societies** Booking required. **Green Fees** £32 per day (£35 weekends & bank holidays). **Prof** J Curtis **Course Designer** Renouf/S Gidman **Facilities** ⑪ ⑩ ⓛ ⓓ ⓣ ⓛ ⓒ ⓞ ✔ **Leisure** indoor teaching facility. **Conf** Corporate Hospitality Days **Location** 6.5m S of city centre on B1567 **Hotel** BUD Travelodge Manchester Didsbury, Kingsway, DIDSBURY ☎ 08700 850 950 62 en suite

Withington 243 Palatine Rd, West Didsbury M20 2UE
☎ 0161 445 9544 📄 0161 445 5210
e-mail: secretary@withingtongolfclub.co.uk
web: www.withingtongolfclub.co.uk
Flat parkland course bordering the River Mersey. Easy walking with an extremely tough finish.
18 holes, 6410yds, Par 71, SSS 71. Club membership 600.
Visitors Booking required Mon-Wed, Fri & Sun. Handicap certificate. Dress code. **Societies** Welcome. **Green Fees** Phone. ⊛ **Prof** S Marr **Facilities** ⑪ ⑩ ⓛ ⓓ ⓣ ⓛ ⓒ ⓞ ✔ **Location** 4m SW of city centre off B5167 **Hotel** BUD Travelodge Manchester Didsbury, Kingsway, DIDSBURY ☎ 08700 850 950 62 en suite

Worsley Stableford Av, Worsley M30 8AP
☎ 0161 789 4202 📄 0161 789 3200
Well-wooded parkland course.
18 holes, 6252yds, Par 71, SSS 70, Course record 65.
Club membership 600.
Visitors contact club for details. **Societies** welcome. **Green Fees** not confirmed. ⊛ **Prof** Ceri Cousins **Course Designer** James Braid **Facilities** ⓛ ⓒ ⓞ 🏌 **Location** 6.5m NW of city centre off A572 **Hotel** ★★★ 68% HL Novotel Manchester West, Worsley Brow, WORSLEY119 en suite

---

MELLOR   MAP 07 SJ98

Mellor & Townscliffe Gibb Ln, Tarden SK6 5NA
☎ 0161 427 2208 (secretary)
web: www.mellorgolf.co.uk
Scenic parkland and moorland course, undulating with some hard walking. Good views. Testing 200yd 9th hole, Par 3.
18 holes, 5925yds, Par 70, SSS 69. Club membership 650.
Visitors may play Mon-Fri, Sun & BHs. Advance booking required. Handicap certificate required. Dress code. **Societies** advance booking required. **Green Fees** not confirmed. ⊛ **Prof** Gary R Broadley **Facilities** ⑪ ⑩ ⓛ ⓓ ⓣ ⓛ ⓒ ⓞ ✔ **Location** 7m SE of Stockport off A626 **Hotel** ★★★ 77% HL Bredbury Hall Hotel & Country Club, Goyt Valley, BREDBURY ☎ 0161 430 7421 150 en suite

---

MIDDLETON   MAP 07 SD80

Manchester Hopwood Cottage, Rochdale Rd M24 6QP
☎ 0161 643 3202 📄 0161 643 9174
e-mail: secretary@mangc.co.uk
web: www.mangc.co.uk
Moorland golf of unique character over a spaciously laid out course with generous fairways sweeping along to large greens. A wide variety of holes will challenge the golfer's technique, particularly the testing last four holes.
18 holes, 6491yds, Par 72, SSS 72, Course record 63.
Club membership 650.

Continued

Visitors Mon-Fri, Sun & BHs. Advance booking required. Handicap certificate. Dress code. **Societies** Booking required. **Green Fees** £45 per day, £35 per round (£50 per round Sun & BHs). **Prof** Brian Connor **Course Designer** Shapland Colt **Facilities** ⑪ ⑩ ⓛ ⌁ ☷ ⌓ ☎
⚘ ⌁ ⚘ ⌁ **Leisure** snooker. **Conf** facs Corporate Hospitality Days **Location** 1m S of M62 junct 20 on A664
Hotel ★★★★ 77% HL Mercure Norton Grange Hotel & Spa, Manchester Rd, Castleton, ROCHDALE ☎ 0870 1942119 81 en suite

New North Manchester Rhodes House, Manchester Old Rd M24 4PE
☎ 0161 643 9033 📠 0161 643 7775
e-mail: tee@nmgc.co.uk
web: www.northmanchestergolfclub.co.uk
Delightful moorland and parkland with several water features. Challenging but fair for the accomplished golfer.
18 holes, 6436yds, Par 71, SSS 71, Course record 69.
Club membership 610.
Visitors Mon-Fri & BHs. Booking required. Handicap certificate. Dress code. **Societies** Booking required. **Green Fees** £32. ☷ **Prof** Jason Peel **Course Designer** J Braid **Facilities** ⑪ ⑩ ⓛ ⌁ ☷ ⌓ ☷ ⚘
Leisure 2 full size snooker tables. **Location** W of town centre off A576

MILNROW   MAP 07 SD91

Tunshill Kiln Ln OL16 3TS
☎ 01706 342095
Testing moorland course with two demanding Par 5s and out of bounds features on eight of the nine holes.
9 holes, 5743yds, Par 70, SSS 68, Course record 64.
Club membership 300.
Visitors Mon-Fri. Booking required. **Societies** apply in writing.
Green Fees not confirmed. ☷ **Facilities** ⑪ by prior arrangement ⑩ by prior arrangement ⓛ by prior arrangement ⌁ by prior arrangement ⌓ ⌁
Location 1m NE M62 exit junct 21 off B6225
Hotel ★★★★ 77% HL Mercure Norton Grange Hotel & Spa, Manchester Rd, Castleton, ROCHDALE ☎ 0870 1942119 81 en suite

---

OLDHAM   MAP 07 SD90

Crompton & Royton Highbarn, Royton OL2 6RW
☎ 0161 624 0986 📠 0161 652 4711
e-mail: secretary@cromptonandroytongolfclub.co.uk
web: www.cromptonandroytongolfclub.co.uk
18 holes, 6214yds, Par 70, SSS 70, Course record 62.
Location 0.5m NE of Royton
Telephone for further details

Oldham Lees New Rd OL4 5PN
☎ 0161 624 4986
18 holes, 5122yds, Par 66, SSS 65, Course record 62.
Location 2.5m E off A669
Telephone for further details

Werneth Green Ln, Garden Suburb OL8 3AZ
☎ 0161 624 1190
e-mail: secretary@wernethgolfclub.co.uk
web: www.wernethgolfclub.co.uk
Semi-moorland course, with a deep gully and stream crossing eight fairways. Testing hole: 3rd (Par 3).

18 holes, 5363yds, Par 68, SSS 66, Course record 61.
Club membership 500.
Visitors may play Mon, Wed, Fri-Sun & BHs. Booking required Sat, Sun & BHs.Dress code. **Societies** Welcome. **Green Fees** £18 per day. ☷
Prof James Matterlon **Course Designer** Sandy Herd **Facilities** ⑪ ⑩ ⓛ
⌓ ⌁ ⌁ ☷ ⌓ ⚘ **Conf** Corporate Hospitality Days **Location** S of town centre off A627

PRESTWICH   MAP 07 SD80

Heaton Park Golf Centre Heaton Park, Middleton Rd M25 2SW
☎ 0161 654 9899 📠 0161 653 2003
An award winning municipal parkland-style course in historic Heaton Park, with rolling hills and lakes, designed by five times Open Champion, JH Taylor. It has some spectacular holes and is a good test of skill for golfers of all abilities.

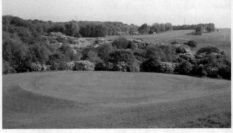

Championship: 18 holes, 5755yds, Par 70, SSS 68.
Visitors may play Mon-Sun & BHs. Advance booking required Sat, Sun & BHs. Dress code. **Societies** Booking required. **Green Fees** £11 (£14.50 Sat & Sun). **Prof** Gary Dermott **Course Designer** J H Taylor **Facilities** ⑪ ⑩ ⓛ ⌓ ⌁ ⌁ ☷ ⌓ ♢ ⚘ **Leisure** fishing, 18 hole Par 3 course.
Conf facs Corporate Hospitality Days **Location** N of Manchester near M60 junct 19
Hotel BUD Premier Travel Inn Manchester West, East Lancs Rd, SWINTON ☎ 0870 9906480 27 en suite

See advert on opposite page

Prestwich Hilton Ln M25 9XB
☎ 0161 773 1404 📠 0161 772 0700
18 holes, 4846yds, Par 65, SSS 65, Course record 60.
Location N of town centre on A6044
Telephone for further details
Hotel ★★★ 68% HL Novotel Manchester West, Worsley Brow, WORSLEY119 en suite

---

ROCHDALE   MAP 07 SD81

Castle Hawk Chadwick Ln, Castleton OL11 3BY
☎ 01706 640841 📠 01706 860587
e-mail: teeoff@castlehawk.co.uk
web: www.castlehawk.co.uk
New Course: 9 holes, 2699yds, Par 34, SSS 34,
Course record 30.
Old Course: 18 holes, 3189yds, Par 55, SSS 55.
Course Designer T Wilson **Location** M62 junct 20, S of Rochdale
Telephone for further details
Hotel ★★★★ 77% HL Mercure Norton Grange Hotel & Spa, Manchester Rd, Castleton, ROCHDALE ☎ 0870 1942119 81 en suite

Marland Park Springfield Park, Bolton Rd OL11 4RE
☎ 01706 656401 (weekends)
18 holes, 5237yds, Par 67, SSS 66, Course record 64.
Location 1.5m SW off A58
Telephone for further details
Hotel ★★★★ 77% HL Mercure Norton Grange Hotel & Spa, Manchester
Rd, Castleton, ROCHDALE ☎ 0870 1942119 81 en suite

Rochdale Edenfield Rd OL11 5YR
☎ 01706 643818 📄 01706 861113
e-mail: rochdale.golfclub@zen.co.uk
Easy walking parkland for enjoyable golf.
18 holes, 6050yds, Par 71, SSS 69, Course record 65.
Club membership 750.
Visitors Mon, Wed, Fri-Sun & BHs. Booking required. Dress code. **Societies**
Booking required. **Green Fees** £22 per day/round (£29 Sat, Sun & BHs). ☺
Prof Andrew Laverty **Course Designer** George Lowe **Facilities** ⑪ ⑩ ﹗
♿ ⚑ ⛳ ﹗ ✔ **Conf** facs Corporate Hospitality Days **Location** 1.75m
W on A680
Hotel ★★★★ 77% HL Mercure Norton Grange Hotel & Spa, Manchester
Rd, Castleton, ROCHDALE ☎ 0870 1942119 81 en suite

ROMILEY   MAP 07 SJ99

Romiley Goose House Green SK6 4LJ
☎ 0161 430 2392 📄 0161 430 7258
e-mail: office@romileygolfclub.org
web: www.romileygolfclub.org
Semi-parkland course on the edge of the Derbyshire Hills, providing a
good test of golf with a number of outstanding holes, notably the 6th,
9th, 14th and 16th. The latter enjoys magnificent views from the tee.

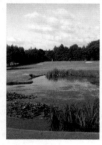

18 holes, 6454yds, Par 70, SSS 71, Course record 66.
Club membership 700.
Visitors Mon-Wed, Fri, Sun & BHs. Booking required. Handicap certificate.
Dress code. **Societies** Booking required. **Green Fees** Phone. ☺ **Prof**
Matthew Ellis **Facilities** ﹗ ⚑ ✔ **Location** E of town centre off B6104
Hotel ★★★ 72% HL The Wycliffe Hotel, 74 Edgeley Rd, Edgeley,
STOCKPORT ☎ 0161 477 5395 14 en suite

SALE   MAP 07 SJ79

Ashton on Mersey Church Ln M33 5QQ
☎ 0161 976 4390 & 962 3727 📄 0161 976 4390
e-mail: golf@aomgc.fsnet.co.uk
web: www.aomgc.co.uk
Parkland with easy walking alongside the River Mersey.
9 holes, 6146yds, Par 71, SSS 69, Course record 66.
Club membership 485.

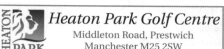

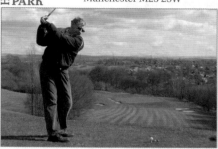

Heaton Park Golf Centre
Middleton Road, Prestwich
Manchester M25 2SW

"Manchester's Best Value, premier pay and play course"
Voted **"Best Municipal course"** in
Golfpunk (Jan/Feb 06), *Esquire* (Aug 06) Magazines.

• 18-Hole Championship Course
• 18-Hole Par-3 Pitch & Putt course
• Fully stocked Pro golf shop
  (Hire equipment available)
• Excellent catering and bar service
• Exceptional society packages available
Find us off junction 19 – M60
To make a booking, please call 0161-654-9899

Visitors may play Mon, Wed-Fri & BHs. Handicap certificate required. Dress
ode. **Societies** advance booking required. **Green Fees** not confirmed.
Prof Mike Williams **Facilities** ⑪ ⑩ by prior arrangement ﹗ ♿ ﹗ ⚑ ⛳
✔ **Leisure** sauna. **Conf** facs **Location** M60 junct 7, 1m W off Glebelands
Rd
Hotel ★★★ 77% HL Best Western Cresta Court Hotel, Church St,
ALTRINCHAM ☎ 0161 927 7272 137 en suite

Sale Golf Rd M33 2XU
☎ 0161 973 1638 (Office) & 973 1730 (Pro)
📄 0161 962 4217
e-mail: mail@salegolfclub.com
web: www.salegolfclub.com
Tree-lined parkland course. Feature holes are the 13th - Watery Gap
- and the Par 3 3rd hole of 210yds over water.
18 holes, 6301yds, Par 70, SSS 69, Course record 63.
Club membership 700.
Visitors Mon-Fri except BHs. Dress code. **Societies** Welcome.
Green Fees £32 per round. **Prof** Mike Stewart **Facilities** ⑪ ﹗ ♿ ﹗ ⚑
⛳ ✔ ✔ **Conf** Corporate Hospitality Days **Location** M60 junct 6, 0.5m NW
of town centre off A6144
Hotel ★★★ 77% HL Best Western Cresta Court Hotel, Church St,
ALTRINCHAM ☎ 0161 927 7272 137 en suite

SHEVINGTON   MAP 07 SD50

Gathurst 62 Miles Ln WN6 8EW
☎ 01257 255235 (Secretary) 📄 01257 255953
A testing parkland course. Slightly hilly.
18 holes, 6016yds, Par 70, SSS 69, Course record 64.
Club membership 630.
Visitors may play Mon, Tue, Thu & Fri except BHs. Booking required.
Handicap certificate. Dress code. **Societies** Booking required. **Green
Fees** £30 per round. 🌐 **Prof** David Clarke **Course Designer** N Pearson
Facilities ⑪ ⑩ ⅃ ☞ ⏚ ⏦ ⏚ ✦ **Location** M6 junct 27, 1m SW of
village on B5375
Hotel ★★★★ 69% HL Macdonald Kilhey Court, Chorley Rd, Standish,
WIGAN ☎ 0870 1942122   62 en suite

STALYBRIDGE   MAP 07 SJ99

Stamford Oakfield House, Huddersfield Rd SK15 3PY
☎ 01457 832126
e-mail: stamford.golfclub@totalise.co.uk
Undulating moorland course.
18 holes, 5701yds, Par 70, SSS 68, Course record 62.
Club membership 600.
Visitors Mon-Fri except BHs. Dress code. **Societies** Booking required.
Green Fees £20 per day. 🌐 **Prof** Brian Badger **Facilities** ⑪ ⑩ ⅃ ☞ ☞ ⏦
⏚ ⏦ ✦ **Conf** facs   Corporate Hospitality Days **Location** 2m NE off A635

STANDISH   MAP 07 SD51

Standish Court Rectory Ln WN6 0XD
☎ 01257 425777 📄 01257 425777
e-mail: golfprostu@hotmail.com
web: www.standishgolf.co.uk
Undulating 18-hole parkland course, not overly long but provides a
good test for all levels of players. The front nine is more open with
room for errors, back nine very scenic through woodland, a number of
tight driving holes. Greens in excellent condition.

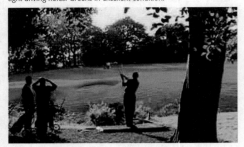

18 holes, 4860yds, Par 68, SSS 64, Course record 63.
Club membership 375.
Visitors Mon-Sun & BHs. Booking required. Dress code. **Societies** Booking
required **Green Fees** Mon/Tue £12.50, Wed-Fri £15 (£20 Sat, Sun & BHs).
Prof Stuart McGrath **Course Designer** P Dawson **Facilities** ⑪ ⅃ ☞ ⏦
⏚ ⏦ ✦ **Conf** facs   Corporate Hospitality Days **Location** E of town centre
on B5239
Hotel ★★★★ 69% HL Macdonald Kilhey Court, Chorley Rd, Standish,
WIGAN ☎ 0870 1942122   62 en suite

STOCKPORT   MAP 07 SJ89

Heaton Moor Mauldeth Rd, Heaton Mersey SK4 3NX
☎ 0161 432 2134 📄 0161 432 2134
e-mail: heatonmoorgolfclub@yahoo.co.uk
web: www.heatonmoorgolfclub.co.uk
Gently undulating parkland with two separate nine holes starting from
the clubhouse. The narrow fairways are challenging.
18 holes, 5970yds, Par 70, SSS 69, Course record 66.
Club membership 700.
Visitors Mon-Fri, Sun & BHs. Booking required. Dress code. **Societies**
Booking required. **Green Fees** Phone. **Prof** Simon Marsh **Facilities** ⑪ ⑩
⅃ ☞ ⏦ ⏚ ⏦ ✦ **Location** N of town centre off B5169
Hotel ★★★ 77% HL Bredbury Hall Hotel & Country Club, Goyt Valley,
BREDBURY ☎ 0161 430 7421   150 en suite

Houldsworth Houldsworth Park, Reddish SK5 6BN
☎ 0161 442 1712 📄 0161 947 9678
e-mail: houldsworthsecretary@hotmail.co.uk
web: www.houldsworthgolfclub.co.uk
Flat, tree-lined parkland course with water hazards. Testing holes 11th
(Par 4) and 13th (Par 5).
18 holes, 6209yds, Par 71, SSS 70, Course record 65.
Club membership 680.
Visitors Mon-Fri except BHs. Handicap certificate. Dress code.
Societies Booking required. **Green Fees** Phone. 🌐 **Prof** Daniel Marsh
Course Designer Dave Thomas **Facilities** ⑪ ⑩ ⅃ ☞ ⏦ ⏚ ⏦ ⏦ ✦
Conf facs **Location** 4m SE of city centre off A6
Hotel ★★★ 77% HL Best Western Willow Bank Hotel, 340-342 Wilmslow
Rd, Fallowfield, MANCHESTER ☎ 0161 224 0461   117 en suite

Marple Barnsfold Rd, Hawk Green, Marple SK6 7EL
☎ 0161 427 2311 & 427 1195(pro) 📄 0161 427 2311
e-mail: marple.golf.club@ukgateway-net
web: www.marplegolfclub.4t.com
18 holes, 5552yds, Par 68, SSS 67, Course record 66.
Location S of town centre
Telephone for further details
Hotel ★★★ 77% HL Bredbury Hall Hotel & Country Club, Goyt Valley,
BREDBURY ☎ 0161 430 7421   150 en suite

Reddish Vale Southcliffe Rd, Reddish SK5 7EE
☎ 0161 480 2359 📄 0161 480 2359
e-mail: admin@rvgc.co.uk
web: www.rvgc.co.uk
Undulating heathland course designed by Dr A MacKenzie and situated
in the Tame valley.
18 holes, 6086yds, Par 69, SSS 69, Course record 64.
Club membership 550.
Visitors Mon-Fri except BHs. Handicap certificate. Dress code. **Societies**
Booking required. **Green Fees** £38 per day, £28 per round. **Prof** Bob
Freeman **Course Designer** Dr A Mackenzie **Facilities** ⑪ ⑩ ⅃ ☞ ⏦
⏚ ⏦ ⏦ ✦ **Conf** facs   Corporate Hospitality Days **Location** Off Reddish
Road, M6 junct 1/27
Hotel ★★★ 72% HL The Wycliffe Hotel, 74 Edgeley Rd, Edgeley,
STOCKPORT ☎ 0161 477 5395   14 en suite

Stockport Offerton Rd, Offerton SK2 5HL
☎ 0161 427 8369 📠 0161 427 8369
e-mail: info@stockportgolf.co.uk
web: www.stockportgolf.co.uk
A beautifully situated course in wide open countryside with views of the Cheshire and Derbyshire hills. It is not too long but requires the player plays all the shots, to excellent greens. Demanding holes include the dog-leg 3rd, 12th and 18th and the 460yd opening hole is among the toughest in Cheshire. Regional qualifying course for Open Championship.
18 holes, 6326yds, Par 71, SSS 71, Course record 64.
Club membership 500.
Visitors may play Mon, Wed-Sun & BHs. Advance booking Wed-Sun & BHs. Handicap certificate required. Dress code. **Societies** advance booking required. **Green Fees** not confirmed. ⊛ **Prof** Mike Peel
Course Designer P Barrie/A Herd **Facilities** ⊕ ⑪ ⓛ ⛄ 🏌 ⛳ 🚕 **Conf** Corporate Hospitality Days **Location** 4m SE on A627
Hotel ★★★ 77% HL Bredbury Hall Hotel & Country Club, Goyt Valley, BREDBURY ☎ 0161 430 7421 150 en suite

---

SWINTON   MAP 07 SD70

Swinton Park East Lancashire Rd M27 5LX
☎ 0161 794 0861 📠 0161 281 0698
e-mail: info@spgolf.co.uk
web: www.spgolf.co.uk
One of Lancashire's longest inland courses. Designed and laid out in 1926 by James Braid.

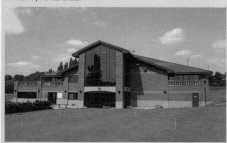

18 holes, 6472yds, Par 73, SSS 71, Club membership 600.
Visitors Mon-Wed & Fri except BHs. Booking required. Handicap certificate. Dress code. **Societies** Booking required. **Green Fees** £30 per day/round. **Prof** James Wilson **Course Designer** James Braid **Facilities** ⊕ ⑪ ⓛ ⛄ 🏌 ⓛ ⛳ 🚕 **Conf** facs Corporate Hospitality Days **Location** Entrance off A580
Hotel ★★★ 68% HL Novotel Manchester West, Worsley Brow, WORSLEY119 en suite

---

UPPERMILL   MAP 07 SD90

Saddleworth Mountain Ash OL3 6LT
☎ 01457 873653 📠 01457 820647
e-mail: secretary@saddleworthgolfclub.org.uk
web: www.saddleworthgolfclub.org.uk
Moorland course, with superb views of Pennines.
18 holes, 6118yds, Par 71, SSS 69, Course record 61.
Club membership 800.
Visitors may play Mon-Fri except BHs. Advance booking Wed & Fri. Handicap certificate required. Dress code. **Societies** advance booking required. **Green Fees** not confirmed. ⊛ **Prof** Robert Johnson

---

Course Designer George Lowe/Dr McKenzie **Facilities** ⊕ ⑪ ⓛ ⛄ 🚕 **Location** E of town centre off A670
Hotel ★★★ 78% HL Best Western Hotel Smokies Park, Ashton Rd, Bardsley, OLDHAM ☎ 0161 785 5000 73 en suite

---

URMSTON   MAP 07 SJ79

Flixton Church Rd, Flixton M41 6EP
☎ 0161 748 2116 📠 0161 748 2116
e-mail: flixtongolfclub@mail.com
web: www.flixtongolfclub.co.uk
Meadowland course bounded by the River Mersey.
9 holes, 6410yds, Par 71, SSS 71. Club membership 430.
Visitors Mon-Fri except BHs. Booking required. Dress code. **Societies** Booking required. **Green Fees** £18. **Prof** Gary Coope **Facilities** ⊕ ⑪ ⓛ ⛄ 🏌 ⓛ ⛳ 🚕 **Conf** facs **Location** S of town centre on B5213
Hotel ★★★★ 76% HL Copthorne Hotel Manchester, Clippers Quay, Salford Quays, MANCHESTER ☎ 0161 873 7321 166 en suite

---

WALKDEN   MAP 07 SD70

Brackley Municipal M38 9TR
☎ 0161 790 6076
A mostly flat testing parkland course. The fairways are forgiving but the greens quite testing.
9 holes, 3003yds, Par 35, SSS 69, Course record 68.
Club membership 65.
Visitors may play Mon-Sun & BHs. **Societies** welcome. **Green Fees** not confirmed. ⊛ **Facilities** ⛳ ⛄ **Location** 2m NW on A6
Hotel ★★★ 68% HL Novotel Manchester West, Worsley Brow, WORSLEY119 en suite

---

WESTHOUGHTON   MAP 07 SD60

Hart Common Wigan Rd BL5 2BX
☎ 01942 813195
A parkland course on green belt land with many water features, including the signature hole, the 7th, which has water all down the left hand side.
18 holes, 5719yards, Par 71, SSS 68. Club membership 400.
Visitors Mon-Sun & BHs. Booking required. Dress code. **Societies** Booking required. **Green Fees** £12 per 18 holes (£16 Sat, Sun & BHs). **Prof** Simon Reeves **Course Designer** Mike Shattock **Facilities** ⊕ ⑪ ⓛ ⛄ 🏌 ⛳ 🚕 ⛳ 🏌 **Leisure** Par 3 Academy course. **Conf** Corporate Hospitality Days **Location** On A58 between Bolton
Hotel ★★★ 71% HL Quality Hotel Wigan, Riverway, WIGAN ☎ 01942 826888 88 en suite

---

Westhoughton Long Island, School St BL5 2BR
☎ 01942 811085 & 608958 📠 01942 811085
e-mail: honsec@westhoughtongc.fsnet.co.uk
18 holes, 5918yds, Par 70, SSS 69, Course record 64.
Course Designer Jeff Shuttleworth **Location** 0.5m NW off A58
Telephone for further details
Hotel ★★★ 71% HL Quality Hotel Wigan, Riverway, WIGAN ☎ 01942 826888 88 en suite

WHITEFIELD   MAP 07 SD80

Stand The Dales, Ashbourne Grove M45 7NL
☎ 0161 766 3197 🖷 0161 796 3234
e-mail: secretary@standgolfclub.co.uk
A semi-parkland course with five moorland holes. Undulating fairways
with views of five counties. A fine test of golf with a very demanding
finish.
18 holes, 6411yds, Par 72, SSS 71, Course record 66.
Club membership 500.
Visitors Mon, Wed, Fri & BHs. **Societies** Welcome. **Green Fees** £35.
Prof Mark Dance **Course Designer** G Lowe/A Herd **Facilities** ⑪ 🍴 ⚑ 🛢
🗗 ⚑ ⛳ 🏌 ✆ **Conf** Corporate Hospitality Days **Location** 1m W off A667
Hotel ★★★ 72% HL Best Western Bolholt Country Park Hotel, Walshaw
Rd, BURY ☎ 0161 762 4000 65 en suite

Whitefield Higher Ln M45 7EZ
☎ 0161 351 2700 🖷 0161 351 2712
e-mail: enquiries@whitefieldgolfclub.com
web: www.whitefieldgolfclub.co.uk
Picturesque parkland course with stunning views and well-watered
greens. Considered to have some of the best Par 3 holes in the North
West. New clubhouse completed 2007.
18 holes, 6063yds, Par 69, SSS 69, Course record 64.
Club membership 540.
Visitors may play Mon-Sat & BHs. Booking required. Dress code. **Societies**
Booking required. **Green Fees** Phone. **Prof** Roy Penney **Facilities** ⑪ 🍴
⚑ 🗗 🏌 ⛳ 🛢 ⚑ 🚩 ✆ 🏌 **Leisure** tennis courts, indoor swing analysis
centre, snooker room. **Conf** Corporate Hospitality Days **Location** M60
junct 17, N of town centre on A665
Hotel ★★★ 85% HL Malmaison, Piccadilly, MANCHESTER
☎ 0161 278 1000 167 en suite

WIGAN   MAP 07 SD50

Haigh Hall Golf Complex Copperas Ln, Haigh WN2 1PE
☎ 01942 831107 🖷 01942 831417
e-mail: hhgen@wiganmgc.gov.uk
web: www.haighhall.net
This golf complex provides all the golfer requires for playing or
practice/tuition facilities. The scenic setting provides an excellent
location for the two courses, an 18 hole and a 9 hole.
Balcarres Course: 18 holes, 6300yards, Par 70, SSS 71.
Crawford Course: 9 holes, 1446yards, Par 28.
Club membership 150.
Visitors contact course for details. Dress code. **Societies** welcome.
Green Fees not confirmed. **Prof** Ian Lee **Course Designer** Steve
Marnoch **Facilities** ⑪ ⚑ 🗗 🏌 ⛳ 🛢 ⚑ ✆ 🏌 **Leisure** golf academy.
Conf Corporate Hospitality Days **Location** M6 junct 27/M61 junct 5 or 6,
signed Haigh Hall
Hotel ★★ 65% HL Bel-Air Hotel, 236 Wigan Ln, WIGAN ☎ 01942 241410
11 en suite

Wigan Arley Hall, Haigh WN1 2UH
☎ 01257 421360 🖷 01257 426500
e-mail: info@wigangolfclub.co.uk
web: www.wigangolfclub.co.uk
Fairly level parkland with outstanding views and magnificent trees. The
fine old clubhouse is the original Arley Hall, and is surrounded by a
medieval moat.
18 holes, 6009yds, Par 70, SSS 69. Club membership 300.

Visitors Wed, Thu, Fri, Sun & BHs. Booking required. Dress code. **Societies**
Booking required. **Green Fees** £30 per round. ◉ **Course Designer** Gaunt
& Marnoch **Facilities** ⑪ 🍴 ⚑ 🗗 🏌 ⛳ **Conf** facs Corporate Hospitality
Days **Location** M6 junct 27, 3m NE off B5238
Hotel ★★★ 71% HL Quality Hotel Wigan, Riverway, WIGAN
☎ 01942 826888 88 en suite

WORSLEY   MAP 07 SD70

Ellesmere Old Clough Ln M28 7HZ
☎ 0161 799 0554 (office) 🖷 0161 790 7322
e-mail: honsec@ellesmeregolf.fsnet.co.uk
web: www.ellesmeregolfclub.co.uk
Parkland with natural hazards and hard walking. Trees and two streams
running through the course make shot strategy an important aspect of
the round. Testing holes: 3rd (Par 5), 9th (Par 3), 15th (Par 5).
18 holes, 6248yds, Par 70, SSS 70, Course record 67.
Club membership 700.
Visitors may play Mon-Fri & Sun except BHs. Advance booking required.
Handicap certificate required. Dress code. **Societies** advance booking
required. **Green Fees** not confirmed. ◉ **Prof** Simon Wakefield **Facilities**
⑪ 🍴 ⚑ 🗗 🏌 ⛳ 🛢 ⚑ ✆ **Conf** Corporate Hospitality Days **Location** N of
village off A580
Hotel ★★★ 68% HL Novotel Manchester West, Worsley Brow,
WORSLEY119 en suite

HAMPSHIRE

ALDERSHOT   MAP 04 SU85

Army Laffans Rd GU11 2HF
☎ 01252 337272 🖷 01252 337562
e-mail: secretary@armygolfclub.com
web: www.armygolfclub.co.uk
The second-oldest course in Hampshire. Picturesque heathland course
with three Par 3s over 200yds.
18 holes, 6550yds, Par 71, SSS 71, Course record 66.
Club membership 750.
Visitors may play Mon-Fri. Handicap certificate required. Dress code.
Societies advance booking required. **Green Fees** not confirmed. **Prof**
Graham Cowley **Facilities** ⑪ 🍴 ⚑ 🗗 🏌 ⛳ 🛢 ⚑ ✆ 🛢 ✆ **Conf** facs
Corporate Hospitality Days **Location** 1.5m N of town centre off A323/A325
Hotel ★★★ 70% HL Potters International Hotel, 1 Fleet Rd, ALDERSHOT
☎ 01252 344000 100 en suite

ALTON   MAP 04 SU73

Alton Old Odiham Rd GU34 4BU
☎ 01420 82042
web: www.altongolfclub.org.uk
9 holes, 5744yds, Par 68, SSS 68, Course record 62.
Course Designer James Braid **Location** 2m N of Alton off B3349 at
Golden Pot
Telephone for further details
Hotel ★★★ 72% HL Alton House Hotel, Normandy St, ALTON
☎ 01420 80033 43 en suite

Worldham Park Cakers Ln, East Worldham GU34 3BF
☎ 01420 543151 📠 01420 544606
e-mail: worldhampark@virgin.net
The course is in a picturesque parkland setting with an abundance of
challenging holes (dog-legs, water and sand). Suitable for all golfing
standards.
18 holes, 6257yds, Par 71, SSS 70. Club membership 400.
Visitors may play Mon-Sun & BHs. Advance booking required. Dress code.
Societies advance booking required. **Green Fees** not confirmed. **Prof**
Anthony Cook **Course Designer** F J Whidborne **Facilities** ⑪ ⦶⌕ by prior
arrangement ⛾ ⬚ ⛳⍻ ⚲ 🏠⛴ 🐾 🐟 ⚷ **Conf** Corporate Hospitality Days
Location B3004, 2 mins from Alton
Hotel ★★★ 74% HL Alton Grange Hotel, London Rd, ALTON
☎ 01420 86565 26 en suite 4 annexe en suite

AMPFIELD   MAP 04 SU42

Ampfield Par Three Winchester Rd SO51 9BQ
☎ 01794 368480
web: www.ampfieldgolf.com
18 holes, 2478yds, Par 54, SSS 53, Course record 49.
Course Designer Henry Cotton **Location** 4m NE of Romsey on A31
Telephone for further details
Hotel ★★★ 72% HL Potters Heron Hotel, Winchester Rd, Ampfield,
ROMSEY ☎ 0870 609 6155 54 en suite

ANDOVER   MAP 04 SU34

Andover 51 Winchester Rd SP10 2EF
☎ 01264 358040 📠 01264 358040
e-mail: secretary@andovergolfclub.co.uk
web: www.andovergolfclub.co.uk
Undulating downland course combining a good test of golf for all abilities
with breathtaking views across Hampshire countryside. Well-guarded
greens and a notable Par 3 9th (225yds) with the tee perched on top of a
hill, 100ft above the green. Excellent drainage on the chalk base.
9 holes, 6096yds, Par 70, SSS 69, Course record 64.
Club membership 450.
Visitors Mon-Sun & BHs. Dress code. **Societies** Booking required. **Green
Fees** £21 per 18 holes (£26 Sat & Sun). **Course Designer** J H Taylor
Facilities ⑪ ⦶⌕ ⛾ ⬚ ⛳⍻ ⚲ 🏠 ⚷ **Conf** facs Corporate Hospitality
Days **Location** 0.5m S on A3057
Hotel ★★★ 63% HL Quality Hotel Andover, Micheldever Rd, ANDOVER
☎ 01264 369111 13 en suite 36 annexe en suite

Hampshire Winchester Rd SP11 7TB
☎ 01264 357555 (pro shop) & 356462 (office)
📠 01264 356606
e-mail: enquiry@thehampshiregolfclub.co.uk
web: www.thehampshiregolfclub.co.uk
Pleasant undulating parkland with fine views and a backdrop of 35,000
young trees and shrubs. The challenging Manor course has two
lakes to catch the unwary. Based on chalk which provides very good
drainage, with a superb finishing hole.
Manor: 18 holes, 6145yds, Par 71, SSS 69,
Course record 67. Club membership 500.
Visitors Mon-Sun & BHs. Booking required. Dress code. **Societies** Booking
required. **Green Fees** £20 per 18 holes (£27 Sat, Sun & BHs). **Prof** Rob
Spurrier **Facilities** ⑪ ⦶⌕ ⛾ ⬚ ⛳⍻ ⚲ 🏠⛴ 🐾 🐟 ⚷ 🐾 **Leisure** 9 hole Par 3
course. **Conf** facs Corporate Hospitality Days **Location** 1.5m S of Andover
on A3057
Hotel ★★★ 63% HL Quality Hotel Andover, Micheldever Rd, ANDOVER
☎ 01264 369111 13 en suite 36 annexe en suite

BARTON-ON-SEA   MAP 04 SZ29

Barton-on-Sea Milford Rd BH25 5PP
☎ 01425 615308 📠 01425 621457
e-mail: admin@barton-on-sea-golf.co.uk
web: www.barton-on-sea-golf.co.uk
A cliff top course with 3 loops of nine giving a great variety and
challenge to golfers of all handicaps. Fine views over the Solent and
Isle of Wight.
9 holes, 3182yds, Par 36.
Needles: 9 holes, 3339yds, Par 36.
Stroller: 9 holes, 3114yds, Par 36. Club membership 750.
Visitors Mon-Sun & BHs. Booking required. Handicap certificate. Dress
code. Must contact in advance. **Societies** Booking required.
Green Fees £44 per day (£55 Sat, Sun & BHs). **Prof** Peter Rodgers
Course Designer Vardon/Colt/Stutt **Facilities** ⑪ ⦶⌕ by prior
arrangement ⛾ ⬚ ⛳⍻ ⚲ 🏠⛴ 🐾 ⚷ **Leisure** snooker tables.
Conf Corporate Hospitality Days **Location** B3058 SE of town
Hotel ★★★★★ HL Chewton Glen Hotel, Christchurch Rd, NEW
MILTON ☎ 01425 275341 58 en suite

BASINGSTOKE   MAP 04 SU65

Basingstoke Kempshott Park RG23 7LL
☎ 01256 465990 📠 01256 331793
e-mail: enquiries@basingstokegolfclub.co.uk
web: www.basingstokegolfclub.co.uk
A well-maintained parkland course. Excellent bunkering requires
good course management from the tee and all clubs will be required
with many long testing Par 4's. A true test of golf, yet fair and
playable for the less experienced golfer.
18 holes, 6350yds, Par 70, SSS 70, Course record 63.
Club membership 700.
Visitors Mon-Fri except BHs. Handicap certificate. Dress code.
Societies Booking required. **Green Fees** £50 per day, £40 per round.
Reduced winter fees. **Prof** Richard Woolley **Course Designer** James
Braid **Facilities** ⑪ ⦶⌕ ⛾ ⬚ ⛳⍻ ⚲ 🏠⛴ 🐾 🐟 ⚷ **Conf** facs Corporate
Hospitality Days **Location** M3 junct 7, 1m SW on A30
Hotel ★★★★ 76% HL Apollo Hotel, Aldermaston Roundabout,
BASINGSTOKE ☎ 01256 796700 125 en suite

Dummer Dummer RG25 2AD
☎ 01256 397888 (office) & 397950 (pro) 📠 01256 397889
e-mail: enquiries@dummergolfclub.com
web: www.dummergolfclub.com
Designed by Peter Alliss, this course is set in 165 acres of fine
Hampshire countryside with panoramic views. The course meanders
around lakes, mature trees and hedgerows. The course combines
large, level teeing areas, undulating fairways, fast true greens and
cleverly positioned bunkers to provide a challenging golf experience.
18 holes, 6500yds, Par 72, SSS 71, Course record 62.
Club membership 650.
Visitors Mon-Sun & BHs. Dress code. **Societies** Welcome. **Green Fees** £30
per round. **Prof** Andrew Fannon **Course Designer** Pete Alliss **Facilities**
⑪ ⦶⌕ ⛾ ⬚ ⛳⍻ ⚲ 🏠⛴ 🐾 🐟 ⚷ 🐾 **Leisure** sauna. **Conf** facs Corporate
Hospitality Days **Location** M3 junct 7, towards Dummer, club 0.25m on left
Hotel BUD Premier Travel Inn Basingstoke South, NORTH WALTHAM
☎ 0870 9906476 28 en suite

Weybrook Park Rooksdown Ln RG24 9NT
☎ 01256 320347 📄 01256 812973
e-mail: weybrookpark@aol.com
web: www.weybrookpark.co.uk
An all year course designed to be enjoyable for all standards of player. Easy walking with fabulous views.
18 holes, 6468yds, Par 71, SSS 71. Club membership 600.
Visitors Mon-Sun except BHs. Booking required Sat & Sun. Dress code. **Societies** Welcome. **Green Fees** Phone. **Prof** Anthony Dillon **Facilities** ⑪ ⑩ 🏌 🖵 🍴 🏌 🏌 🏌 🏌 **Conf** facs Corporate Hospitality Days **Location** 2m W of town centre via A339
Hotel ★★★★ 76% HL Apollo Hotel, Aldermaston Roundabout, BASINGSTOKE ☎ 01256 796700 125 en suite

---

BORDON   MAP 04 SU73

Blackmoor Firgrove Rd, Whitehill GU35 9EH
☎ 01420 472775 📄 01420 487666
e-mail: admin@blackmoorgolf.co.uk
web: www.blackmoorgolf.co.uk
A first-class moorland course with a great variety of holes. Fine greens and wide pine tree-lined fairways are a distinguishing feature. The ground is mainly flat and walking easy.
18 holes, 6164yds, Par 69, SSS 70, Course record 63. Club membership 750.
Visitors Mon-Fri except BHs. Booking required. Handicap certificate. Dress code. **Societies** Booking required. **Green Fees** £49 per 36 holes; £39 per 18 holes. ◉ **Prof** Stephen Clay **Course Designer** H S Colt **Facilities** ⑪ ⑩ by prior arrangement 🏌 🖵 🍴 🏌 🏌 🏌
Conf Corporate Hospitality Days **Location** 6m S from Farnham on A325, through Whitehill, right at rdbt
Hotel ★★★ 72% HL Alton House Hotel, Normandy St, ALTON
☎ 01420 80033 43 en suite

BOTLEY   MAP 04 SU51

Macdonald Botley Park, Golf & Country Club
Winchester Rd, Boorley Green SO32 2UA
☎ 01489 780888 📄 01489 789242
e-mail: info@botleypark.macdonald.hotels.co.uk
18 holes, 6341yds, Par 70, SSS 70, Course record 67.
Course Designer Ewan Murray **Location** 1m NW of Botley on B3354
Telephone for further details
Hotel ★★★★ 77% HL Macdonald Botley Park, Golf & Country Club, Winchester Rd, Boorley Green, BOTLEY ☎ 0870 1942132 100 en suite

---

BROCKENHURST   MAP 04 SU20

Brokenhurst Manor Sway Rd SO42 7SG
☎ 01590 623332 (Secretary) 📄 01590 624691
e-mail: secretary@brokenhurst-manor.org.uk
web: www.brokenhurst-manor.org.uk
An attractive forest course set in the New Forest, with the unusual feature of three loops of six holes each to complete the round. Fascinating holes include the short 5th and 12th, and the 4th and 17th, both dog-legs. A stream also features on seven of the holes.
18 holes, 6222yds, Par 70, SSS 70, Course record 63. Club membership 700.

Visitors Mon-Sun & BHs. Booking required Thu. Handicap certificate. Dress code. **Societies** Booking required. **Green Fees** £67 per day; £49 per round (£78/£60 Sat, Sun & BHs). **Prof** Bruce Parker
Course Designer H S Colt **Facilities** ⑪ ⑩ 🏌 🖵 🍴 🏌 🏌 🏌
Conf Corporate Hospitality Days **Location** 1m S on B3055
Hotel ★★ 65% SHL Watersplash Hotel, The Rise, BROCKENHURST
☎ 01590 622344 23 en suite

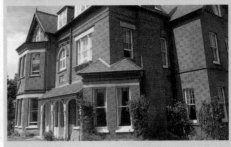

See advert on opposite page

BURLEY   MAP 04 SU20

Burley Cott Ln BH24 4BB
☎ 01425 402431 & 403737 📄 01425 404168
e-mail: secretary@burleygolfclub.co.uk
web: www.burleygolfclub.co.uk
Undulating heather and gorseland. The 7th requires an accurately placed tee shot to obtain Par 4. Played off different tees on second nine.
9 holes, 6151yds, Par 71, SSS 69, Course record 68. Club membership 520.
Visitors Mon-Fri & Sun except BHs. Handicap certificate. Dress code. **Green Fees** Phone. ◉ **Facilities** ⑪ ⑩ 🏌 🖵 🍴 🏌 🏌 **Location** E of village
Hotel ★★★ 72% HL Moorhill House, BURLEY ☎ 01425 403285 31 en suite

---

CORHAMPTON   MAP 04 SU62

Corhampton Shepherds Farm Ln SO32 3GZ
☎ 01489 877279 📄 01489 877680
e-mail: secretary@corhamptongc.co.uk
web: www.corhamptongc.co.uk
Free draining downland course situated in the heart of the picturesque Meon Valley.
18 holes, 6444yds, Par 71, SSS 71. Club membership 800.
Visitors Mon-Fri except BHs. Booking required Mon & Thu. Dress code. **Societies** Booking required. **Green Fees** £50 per 36 holes, £35 per 18 holes. ◉ **Prof** Ian Roper **Facilities** ⑪ ⑩ 🏌 🖵 🍴 🏌 🏌 🏌
Location 1m W of Corhampton off B3035
Hotel ★★ 75% HL Old House Hotel & Restaurant, The Square, WICKHAM
☎ 01329 833049 8 en suite 4 annexe en suite

CRONDALL
MAP 04 SU74

Oak Park Heath Ln GU10 5PB
☎ 01252 850850 📄 01252 850851
e-mail: oakpark@crown-golf.co.uk
Oak Park is a gently undulating parkland course overlooking a pretty village. Woodland is undulating on holes 10 to 13. Panoramic views, mature trees, very challenging; 16-bay floodlit driving range, practice green and practice bunker.
Woodland: 18 holes, 6352yds, Par 70, SSS 70.
Village: 9 holes, 3279yds, Par 36. Club membership 730.
Visitors Booking required. Handicap certificate. Dress code.
Societies Booking required. **Green Fees** Phone. **Prof** Gary Murton
Course Designer Patrick Dawson **Facilities** ⑪ 🍴 🍸 ☕ ⛳ ♨ 🛒 ⚖ 🏌 **Conf** facs Corporate Hospitality Days **Location** 0.5m E of village off A287 Farnham-Odiham

DENMEAD
MAP 04 SU61

Furzeley Furzeley Rd PO7 6TX
☎ 023 9223 1180 📄 023 9223 0921
A well-laid parkland course with many features including several strategically placed lakes which provide a good test set in beautiful scenery. Straight hitting and club selection on the short holes is the key to manufacturing a low score.
18 holes, 4488yds, Par 62, SSS 61, Course record 56.
Club membership 250.
Visitors contact course for details. Dress code. **Societies** advance booking required. **Green Fees** not confirmed. ☕ **Prof** Derek Brown **Course Designer** Mark Sale/Robert Brown **Facilities** ⑪ 🍸 ☕ ⛳ ♨ 🛒 ⚖ **Location** From Waterlooville NW onto Hambledon road, signed
Hotel ★★★ 72% HL Portsmouth Marriott Hotel, Southampton Rd, PORTSMOUTH ☎ 0870 400 7285 174 en suite

DIBDEN
MAP 04 SU40

Dibden Main Rd SO45 5TB
☎ 023 8020 7508 & 8084 5596
web: www.nfdc.gov.uk/golf
Course 1: 18 holes, 5931yds, Par 70, SSS 69,
Course record 64.
Course 2: 9 holes, 1520yds, Par 29.
Course Designer Hamilton Stutt **Location** 2m NW of Dibden Purlieu, off A326 to Hythe
Telephone for further details
Hotel ★★★ 70% HL Best Western Forest Lodge Hotel, Pikes Hill, Romsey Rd, LYNDHURST ☎ 023 8028 3677 28 en suite

EASTLEIGH
MAP 04 SU41

East Horton Golf Centre Mortimers Ln, Fair Oak SO50 7EA
☎ 023 8060 2111 📄 023 8069 6280
e-mail: info@easthortongolf.co.uk
web: www.easthortongolf.co.uk
Greenwood: 18 holes, 5960yds, Par 70, SSS 69.
Course Designer Trevor Pearce **Location** off B3037
Telephone for further details
Hotel BUD Premier Travel Inn Eastleigh, Leigh Rd, EASTLEIGH ☎ 08701 977090 60 en suite

Fleming Park Passfield Av SO50 9NL
☎ 023 8061 2797 📄 023 8065 1686
e-mail: andybunday@dcleisure.co.uk
Parkland and woodland course with stream, Monks Brook, running through. Good greens.
18 holes, 4524yds, Par 65, SSS 62, Course record 62.
Club membership 250.
Visitors Mon-Sun & BHs. **Societies** Booking required. **Green Fees** Phone. **Course Designer** David Miller **Facilities** ⑪ 🍴 🍸 ☕ ⛳ ♨ 🛒 ⚖ **Leisure** hard and grass tennis courts, heated indoor plus outdoor swimming pool, squash, sauna, solarium, gymnasium. **Location** E of town centre
Hotel BUD Travelodge Southampton Eastleigh, Twyford Rd, EASTLEIGH ☎ 08700 850 950 32 en suite

FAREHAM
MAP 04 SU50

Cams Hall Cams Hall Estate PO16 8UP
☎ 01329 827222 📄 01329 827111
e-mail: camshall@americangolf.uk.com
web: americangolf.com
Creek Course: 18 holes, 6244yds, Par 71, SSS 70,
Course record 69.
Park Course: 9 holes, 3247yds, Par 36, SSS 36.
Course Designer Peter Alliss **Location** M27 junct 11, A27
Telephone for further details
Hotel ★★★ 70% HL Lysses House Hotel, 51 High St, FAREHAM ☎ 01329 822622 21 en suite

FARNBOROUGH　　　　MAP 04 SU85

Southwood Ively Rd, Cove GU14 0LJ
☎ 01252 548700 📄 01252 549091
Municipal parkland golf course.
18 holes, 5738yds, Par 69, SSS 68, Course record 61.
Club membership 650.
Visitors may play Mon-Sun & BHs. Advance booking required. **Societies**
advance booking required. **Green Fees** not confirmed. **Prof** Chris Hudson
Course Designer Hawtree & Son **Facilities** ⊕ ⦿ ⓘ ⓛ ⬛ ⬛ ⅋ ⬛ ⬛ ⅋ ⬛
⅋ **Conf** facs Corporate Hospitality Days **Location** 0.5m W
Hotel ★★★ 67% HL Falcon Hotel, 68 Farnborough Rd, FARNBOROUGH
☎ 01252 545378 30 en suite

FLEET　　　　MAP 04 SU85

North Hants Minley Rd GU51 1RF
☎ 01252 616443 📄 01252 811627
e-mail: secretary@north-hants-fleetgc.co.uk
web: www.northhantsgolf.co.uk
Picturesque tree-lined course with much heather and gorse close
to the fairways. The club is currently completing a woodland
management scheme which will give new views and incorporate a
review of fairway and greenside bunkering. A testing first hole to the
course is a 214 yd followed by many other testing holes around the
course. The ground is rather undulating and, though not tiring, does
offer some excellent blind shots, and more than a few surprises in
judging distance.

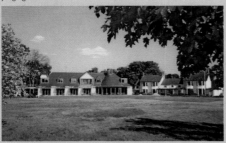

18 holes, 6472yds, Par 70, SSS 72, Course record 65.
Club membership 600.
Visitors Mon-Sun & BHs. Booking required. Handicap certificate. Dress
code. **Societies** Booking required. **Green Fees** Phone. **Prof** Steve
Porter **Course Designer** James Braid **Facilities** ⊕ ⦿ ⓘ ⓛ ⬛ ⬛ ⅋ ⬛ ⬛
⅋ **Conf** Corporate Hospitality Days **Location** 0.25m N of Fleet station
on B3013
Hotel ★★★ 67% HL Falcon Hotel, 68 Farnborough Rd, FARNBOROUGH
☎ 01252 545378 30 en suite

GOSPORT　　　　MAP 04 SZ69

Gosport & Stokes Bay Off Fort Rd, Haslar PO12 2AT
☎ 023 9252 7941
e-mail: secretary@gosportandstokesbaygolfclub.co.uk
web: www.gosportandstokesbaygolfclub.co.uk
A testing links course overlooking the Solent, with plenty of gorse and
short rough. Changing winds.
9 holes, 5995yds, Par 70, SSS 69, Course record 65.
Club membership 400.

Visitors may play Mon-Wed, Fri & BHs. Thu & Sun pm only. Sat restricted.
Dress code. **Societies** Booking required. **Green Fees** £17 Mon-Fri (£22 Sat).
Twilight £8.50. ⊕ **Facilities** ⊕ ⓛ ⬛ ⬛ ⅋ ⬛ ⅋ **Location** A32 S from
Fareham, E onto Fort Rd to Haslar
Hotel ★★★ 70% HL Lysses House Hotel, 51 High St, FAREHAM
☎ 01329 822622 21 en suite

HARTLEY WINTNEY　　　　MAP 04 SU75

Hartley Wintney London Rd RG27 8PT
☎ 01252 844211 (Sec/Gen Mgr) 📄 01252 844211
e-mail: office@hartleywintneygolfclub.com
web: www.hartleywintneygolfclub.com
Easy walking parkland and partly wooded course in pleasant
countryside. Provides a challenging test for golfers of all abilities with
many mature trees and water hazards.

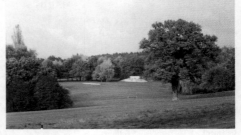

18 holes, 6240yds, Par 71, SSS 71, Course record 63.
Club membership 750.
Visitors Mon-Sun & BHs. Booking required Sat, Sun & BHs. Handicap
certificate. Dress code. **Societies** Booking required. **Green Fees** £45 per
day, £30 per 18 holes (£50/£35 weekends and bank holidays). **Prof** Martin
Smith **Facilities** ⊕ ⓛ ⬛ ⬛ ⅋ ⬛ ⬛ ⅋ **Leisure** indoor teaching studio.
Conf facs Corporate Hospitality Days **Location** NE of village on A30
Hotel ★★★ 78% HL The Elvetham, HARTLEY WINTNEY ☎ 01252 844871
41 en suite 29 annexe en suite

HAYLING ISLAND　　　　MAP 04 SU70

Hayling Links Ln PO11 0BX
☎ 023 9246 4446 📄 023 9246 1119
e-mail: generaloffice@haylinggolf.co.uk
web: www.haylinggolf.co.uk
A delightful links course among the dunes offering fine seascapes
and views of the Isle of Wight. Varying sea breezes and sometimes
strong winds ensure that the course seldom plays the same two
days running. Testing holes at the 12th and 13th, both Par 4. Club
selection is important.
18 holes, 6531yds, Par 71, SSS 71, Course record 65.
Club membership 1000.
Visitors Mon-Fri except BHs. Handicap certificate. Dress code.
Societies Welcome. **Green Fees** £62 per day; £49 per round.
Prof Raymond Gadd **Course Designer** Taylor 1905, Simpson 1933
Facilities ⊕ ⓛ ⬛ ⅋ ⬛ ⬛ ⬛ ⅋ **Conf** facs Corporate Hospitality Days
Location SW side of island at West Town
Hotel ★★★ 75% HL Brookfield Hotel, Havant Rd, EMSWORTH
☎ 01243 373363 40 en suite

KINGSCLERE
MAP 04 SU55

Sandford Springs RG26 5RT
☎ 01635 296800 & 296808 (Pro Shop) 📄 01635 296801
e-mail: alicew@sandfordspringsgolf.co.uk
web: www.sandfordsprings.co.uk
The course has unique variety in beautiful surroundings and offers three distinctive loops of nine holes. There are water hazards, woodlands and gradients to negotiate, providing a challenge for all playing categories.

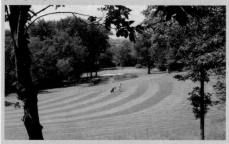

The Park: 9 holes, 2963yds, Par 34.
The Lakes: 9 holes, 3042yds, Par 35.
The Wood: 9 holes, 3180yds, Par 36.
Club membership 700.
Visitors Mon-Fri except BHs. Booking required. Dress code. **Societies** Booking required. **Green Fees** not confirmed. **Prof** Neal Granville **Course Designer** Hawtree & Son **Facilities** ⑪ ⑩ ⅃ ⴹ 🍴 ⅃ ⽿ 🏌 **Conf** facs Corporate Hospitality Days **Location** On A339 between Basingstoke & Newbury
Hotel ★★★★ 76% HL Apollo Hotel, Aldermaston Roundabout, BASINGSTOKE ☎ 01256 796700 125 en suite

KINGSLEY
MAP 04 SU73

Dean Farm GU35 9NG
☎ 01420 489478
Undulating parkland course.
9 holes, 1600yds, Par 31.
Visitors Mon-Sun & BHs. **Societies** Welcome. **Green Fees** Weekdays: £12 per day, £5.50 per 9 holes. **Prof** Matthew Howard **Facilities** ⑪ ⅃ ⴹ 🍴 🍸 ⽿ **Location** W of village off B3004
Hotel ★★★ 74% HL Alton Grange Hotel, London Rd, ALTON ☎ 01420 86565 26 en suite 4 annexe en suite

LECKFORD
MAP 04 SU33

Leckford SO20 6JF
☎ 01264 810320 📄 01264 811122
e-mail: golf@leckfordestate.co.uk
Old Course: 9 holes, 6394yds, Par 72, SSS 71. New Course: 9 holes, 4562yds, Par 66, SSS 62.
Location 1m SW off A3057
Telephone for further details
Hotel ★★★ 63% HL Quality Hotel Andover, Micheldever Rd, ANDOVER ☎ 01264 369111 13 en suite 36 annexe en suite

LEE-ON-THE-SOLENT
MAP 04 SU50

Lee-on-the-Solent Brune Ln PO13 9PB
☎ 023 9255 1170 📄 023 9255 4233
e-mail: enquiries@leeonthesolentgolfclub.co.uk
web: www.leegolf.co.uk
Predominantly heath and oak woodland. While not long in length, still a good test of golf requiring accuracy off the tee to score well. Excellent greens and five very challenging Par 3's.
18 holes, 5962yds, Par 69, SSS 69, Course record 63.
Club membership 725.
Visitors Mon-Sun except BHs. Booking required Sat & Sun. Handicap certificate. Dress code. **Societies** Welcome. **Green Fees** £36 per day/round (£40 Sat & Sun). **Prof** Rob Edwards **Facilities** ⑪ ⑩ ⅃ ⴹ 🍴 ⅃ 🍸 ⽿ **Conf** facs Corporate Hospitality Days **Location** 3m S of Fareham
Hotel ★★★ 70% HL Lysses House Hotel, 51 High St, FAREHAM ☎ 01329 822622 21 en suite

LIPHOOK
MAP 04 SU83

Liphook Wheatsheaf Enclosure GU30 7EH
☎ 01428 723271 & 723785 📄 01428 724853
e-mail: secretary@liphookgolfclub.com
web: www.liphookgolfclub.com
Heathland course with easy walking and fine views.
18 holes, 6167yds, Par 70, SSS 69, Course record 67.
Club membership 800.
Visitors Booking required. Handicap certificate. Dress code. **Societies** Booking required. **Green Fees** £63 per day, £50 per round (£70/£60 Sat, £70 Sun & bank holidays pm only). **Prof** Ian Mowbray **Course Designer** A C Croome **Facilities** ⅃ ⴹ 🍴 ⅃ 🍸 ⽿ ⽿ **Conf** Corporate Hospitality Days **Location** 1m S on B2070
Hotel ★★★★ 77% HL Lythe Hill Hotel & Spa, Petworth Rd, HASLEMERE ☎ 01428 651251 41 en suite

Old Thorns Golf & Country Estate Griggs Green GU30 7PE
☎ 01428 724555 📄 01428 725036
e-mail: sales@oldthorns.com
web: www.oldthorns.com
A challenging 18-hole championship course with rolling hills, undulating greens, demanding water features and magnificent views. A challenge to any level of golfer.
18 holes, 6461yds, Par 72, SSS 72. Club membership 200.
Visitors may play Mon-Sun & BHs. Advance booking required. **Societies** advance booking required. **Green Fees** not confirmed. **Prof** Steven Hall **Course Designer** Peter Alliss **Facilities** ⑪ ⑩ ⅃ ⴹ 🍴 ⅃ 🍸 ⽿ ⽿ **Leisure** hard tennis courts, heated indoor swimming pool, fishing, sauna, solarium, gymnasium. **Conf** Corporate Hospitality Days **Location** Off A3 at Griggs Green, S of Liphook, signed Old Thorns
Hotel ★★★ 79% Old Thorns Hotel Golf & Country Estate, Griggs Green, LIPHOOK ☎ 01428 724555 29 en suite 4 annexe rms (3 en suite)

LYNDHURST   MAP 04 SU20

Bramshaw Brook SO43 7HE
☎ 023 8081 3433 📠 023 8081 3460
e-mail: golf@bramshaw.co.uk
web: www.bramshaw.co.uk
Manor Course: 18 holes, 6527yds, Par 71, SSS 71,
Course record 65.
Forest Course: 18 holes, 5774yds, Par 69, SSS 68,
Course record 65.
Location M27 junct 1, 1m W on B3079
Telephone for further details
Hotel ★★★ 70% HL Bell Inn, BROOK ☎ 023 8081 2214 25 en suite

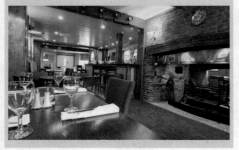

New Forest Southampton Rd SO43 7BU
☎ 023 8028 2752 📠 023 8028 4030
e-mail: tonyatnfgc@aol.com
web: www.newforestgolfclub.co.uk
This picturesque heathland course is laid out in a typical stretch
of the New Forest on high ground a little above the village of
Lyndhurst. The first two holes are somewhat teasing, as is the 485yd
(Par 5) 9th. Walking is easy.
18 holes, 5526yds, Par 69, SSS 67. Club membership 500.
Visitors may play Mon, Wed & Fri. Limited play Tue, Thu, Sat, Sun & BHs.
Booking required. Dress code. **Societies** Welcome.
Green Fees £17 per 18 holes (£23 weekends and bank holidays.
Prof Colin Murray **Facilities** ⊕ 🏠 ⬚ ⊤ ⏇ ⭐ **Conf** Corporate
Hospitality Days **Location** 0.5m NE off A35)
Hotel ★★★ 75% HL Best Western Crown Hotel, High St, LYNDHURST
☎ 023 8028 2922 39 en suite

NEW ALRESFORD   MAP 04 SU53

Alresford Cheriton Rd, Tichborne Down SO24 0PN
☎ 01962 733746 & 733998 (pro shop) 📠 01962 736040
e-mail: secretary@alresfordgolf.demon.co.uk
web: www.alresfordgolf.co.uk
A rolling downland course on well-drained chalk. The five difficult
Par 3s, tree-lined fairways and well-guarded fast greens ensure that the
course offers a true test of skill, even for the most experienced golfer.

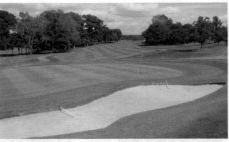

Alresford

18 holes, 5905yds, Par 69, SSS 69, Course record 63.
Club membership 600.
Visitors Mon-Sun except BHs. Dress code. **Societies** Booking required.
Green Fees summer: £30 per 18 holes (£40 Sat & Sun). Winter: £24/£30.
🖲 **Prof** Malcolm Scott **Course Designer** Scott Webb Young **Facilities** ⊕
🍴 by prior arrangement 🏠 ⬚ ⊤ ⏇ 🏠 ⭐ **Conf** Corporate Hospitality
Days **Location** situated 1m S of Alresford on the B3046 with easy access
from the A31 and M3
Hotel ★★ 67% HL Swan Hotel, 11 West St, ALRESFORD ☎ 01962 732302
& 734427 📠 01962 735274 11 rms (10 en suite) 12 annexe en suite

NEW MILTON   MAP 04 SZ29

Chewton Glen Hotel Christchurch Rd BH25 5QS
☎ 01425 275341 📠 01425 272310
e-mail: reservations@chewtonglen.com
web: www.chewtonglen.com
A nine-hole, Par 3 course within the hotel grounds plus a practice area.
Please note - only open to residents of the hotel or as a guest of a
member of the club.
9 holes, 854yds, Par 27. Club membership 150.
Visitors Mon-Sun & BHs. Booking required. **Societies** Welcome. **Green**
Fees Phone. **Facilities** ⊕ 🍴 🏠 ⬚ ⊤ ◇ **Leisure** hard tennis courts,
outdoor and indoor heated swimming pools, sauna, gymnasium, Spa &
health club. **Conf** facs Corporate Hospitality Days **Location** Off A337 W of
town centre
Hotel ★★★★★ HL Chewton Glen Hotel, Christchurch Rd, NEW MILTON
☎ 01425 275341 58 en suite

OVERTON   MAP 04 SU54

Test Valley Micheldever Rd RG25 3DS
☎ 01256 771737 📠 01256 771285
e-mail: info@testvalleygolf.com
web: www.testvalleygolf.com
A downland course with excellent drainage, fine year-round greens
and prominent water and bunker features. On undulating terrain with
lovely views over the Hampshire countryside.
18 holes, 6663yds, Par 72, SSS 69. Club membership 500.
Visitors Mon-Sun & BHs. Booking required. Dress code. **Societies** Booking
required. **Green Fees** £24 per round (£30 weekend). **Prof** Alastair Briggs
Course Designer Don Wright **Facilities** ⊕ 🍴 🏠 ⬚ ⊤ ⏇ 🏠 ⭐ 🛒 ⭐
🏌 **Conf** facs Corporate Hospitality Days **Location** M3 junct 8 southbound,
from A303 take junct signed Overton and follow brown signs. M3 junct 9
northbound, take A34 to A303 signed Basingstoke, leave at junct signed
Overton and follow brown signs .
Hotel ★★★★ 78% HL The Hampshire Court, Centre Dr, Chineham,
BASINGSTOKE ☎ 01256 319700 90 en suite

OWER
MAP 04 SU31

Paultons Golf Centre Old Salisbury Rd SO51 6AN
☎ 023 8081 3992 📠 023 8081 3993
e-mail: paultons@americangolf.uk.com
18 holes, 6238yds, Par 71, SSS 70, Course record 67.
Course Designer J R Smith **Location** M27 junct 2, A36 towards Salisbury,
1st rdbt 1st exit, 1st right at Vine pub
Telephone for further details
Hotel ★★★ 75% HL Bartley Lodge, Lyndhurst Rd, CADNAM
☎ 023 8081 2248 31 en suite

PETERSFIELD
MAP 04 SU72

Petersfield Tankerdale Ln, Liss GU33 7QY
☎ 01730 895165 (office) 📠 01730 894713
e-mail: richard@petersfieldgolfclub.co.uk
web: www.petersfieldgolfclub.co.uk
Gently undulating course of downland and parkland with mature trees
and hedgerows. Very free drainage in an area of outstanding natural
beauty.
18 holes, 6450yds, Par 72, SSS 71, Course record 68.
Club membership 725.
Visitors contact club for details. Handicap certificate. Dress code. **Societies**
Booking required. **Green Fees** £40 per day, £28 per round (£35 per
round Sat, Sun & BHs). ⊕ **Prof** Greg Hughes **Course Designer** M
Hawtree **Facilities** ⚒ 🍴 ✎ 🍴 ✎ **Location** Off the A3(M), between the
Liss/Petersfield exits southbound
Hotel ★★★ 66% HL Southdowns Country Hotel, Dumpford Ln, Trotton,
MIDHURST ☎ 01730 821521 22 en suite

PORTSMOUTH
MAP 04 SU60

Great Salterns Public Course Burrfields Rd PO3 5HH
☎ 023 9266 4549 📠 023 9265 0525
e-mail: portsmouthgolf@aol.com
web: www.portsmouthgolfcentre.co.uk
Easy walking, seaside course with open fairways and testing shots onto
well-guarded, small greens. Testing 13th hole, Par 4, requiring 130yd
shot across a lake.
18 holes, 5575yds, Par 69, SSS 67, Course record 64.
Club membership 700.
Visitors Booking required Sat, Sun & BHs. **Societies** Booking required.
Green Fees Phone. **Prof** Terry Healy **Facilities** ⊕ 🍴 ⚒ 🍴 🍴 ⊕ ✎
Location NE of town centre on A2030
Hotel ★★★★ 72% HL Portsmouth Marriott Hotel, Southampton Rd,
PORTSMOUTH ☎ 0870 400 7285 174 en suite

ROMSEY
MAP 04 SU32

Dunwood Manor Danes Rd, Awbridge SO51 0GF
☎ 01794 340549 📠 01794 341215
e-mail: admin@dunwood-golf.co.uk
web: www.dunwood-golf.co.uk
18 holes, 5767yds, Par 69, SSS 68, Course record 65.
Location 4m NW of Romsey off A27
Telephone for further details
Hotel ★★★ 70% HL Bell Inn, BROOK ☎ 023 8081 2214 25 en suite

Romsey Romsey Rd, Nursling SO16 0XW
☎ 023 8073 4637 📠 023 8074 1036
e-mail: mike@romseygolf.co.uk
web: www.romseygolfclub.com
Parkland and woodland course with narrow tree-lined fairways.
Six holes are undulating, the rest are sloping. There are superb views
over the Test valley. Excellent test of golf for all standards.
18 holes, 5718yds, Par 69, SSS 68, Course record 64.
Club membership 800.
Visitors Mon-Fri except BHs. Dress code. **Societies** Booking required.
Green Fees £38 per day, £32 per round. **Prof** James Pitcher **Facilities** ⊕
🍴 ⚒ 🍴 ⚒ ✎ **Conf** facs Corporate Hospitality Days **Location** 1m
N M27 junct 3 on A3057
Hotel ★★★ 75% HL Chilworth Manor, CHILWORTH ☎ 023 8076 7333
95 en suite

Wellow Ryedown Ln, East Wellow SO51 6BD
☎ 01794 323833 & 322872 📠 01794 323832
web: www.wellowgolfclub.co.uk
Three nine-hole courses set in 217 acres of parkland surrounding
Embley Park, former home of Florence Nightingale.
*Ryedown & Embley: 18 holes, 5939yds, Par 70, SSS 69,
Course record 65.*
Embley & Blackwater: 18 holes, 6295yds, Par 72, SSS 70.
Blackwater & Ryedown: 18 holes, 5819yds, Par 70, SSS 68.
Club membership 600.
Visitors Mon-Sun & BHs. Booking required Sat, Sun & BHs. Dress code.
Societies Booking required. **Green Fees** £20 per 18 holes (£25 Sat, Sun &
BHs). **Prof** Neil Bratley **Course Designer** W Wiltshire **Facilities** ⊕ 🍴 ⚒
🍴 ⚒ 🍴 ✎ **Leisure** gymnasium. **Conf** facs Corporate Hospitality
Days **Location** M27 junct 2, A36 towards Salisbury, 1m right
Hotel ★★★ 75% HL Chilworth Manor, CHILWORTH ☎ 023 8076 7333
95 en suite

ROTHERWICK
MAP 04 SU75

Tylney Park RG27 9AY
☎ 01256 762079 📠 01256 763079
e-mail: martinkimberley@tylneypark.co.uk
web: www.tylneypark.co.uk
Set in historic parkland with many varied mature trees. Fully U.S.G.A.
specified tees, greens and approaches allow year round quality golf.
18 holes, 7017yds, Par 72, SSS 74. Club membership 730.
Visitors Mon-Sun & BHs. Dress code. **Societies** Booking required. **Green
Fees** £43 per day (£60 Sat & Sun). **Prof** Chris de Bruin **Course Designer**
D Steel/T Mackenzie **Facilities** ⊕ 🍴 by prior arrangement ⚒ 🍴 🍴 ⚒
🍴 ⚒ ✎ **Conf** Corporate Hospitality Days **Location** M3 junct 5, 2m
NW of Hook
Hotel ★★★★ HL Tylney Hall Hotel, ROTHERWICK ☎ 01256 764881
35 en suite 77 annexe en suite

ROWLAND'S CASTLE
MAP 04 SU71

Rowland's Castle 31 Links Ln PO9 6AE
☎ 023 9241 2784 📠 023 9241 3649
e-mail: manager@rowlandscastlegolfclub.co.uk
web: www.rowlandscastlegolfclub.co.uk
Reasonably dry in winter, the flat parkland course is a testing one
with a number of tricky dog-legs and bunkers much in evidence. The
Par 4 13th is a signature hole necessitating a drive to a narrow

Continued

fairway and a second shot to a two-tiered green. The 7th, at 522yds, is the longest hole on the course and leads to a well-guarded armchair green.
18 holes, 6630yds, Par 72, SSS 72, Course record 68. Club membership 800.
Visitors may play Sun-Fri & BHs. Advance booking required. Handicap certificate required. Dress code. **Societies** advance booking required. **Green Fees** not confirmed. **Prof** Peter Klepacz **Course Designer** Colt **Facilities** ⓟ ⊙l ⓛ ▭ ⚒ ⚑ ⚐ ✆ **Conf** Corporate Hospitality Days **Location** W of village off B2149
Hotel ★★★ 75% HL Brookfield Hotel, Havant Rd, EMSWORTH ☎ 01243 373363 40 en suite

---

SHEDFIELD   MAP 04 SU51

Marriott Meon Valley Hotel & Country Club Sandy Ln SO32 2HQ
☎ 01329 833455 🖹 01329 834411
It has been said that a golf-course architect is as good as the ground on which he has to work. Here Hamilton Stutt had magnificent terrain at his disposal and a very good and lovely parkland course is the result. There are three holes over water. The hotel provides many sports facilities.
Meon Course: 18 holes, 6520yds, Par 71, SSS 71, Course record 66.
Valley Course: 9 holes, 2721yds, Par 35, SSS 33. Club membership 700.
Visitors Mon-Sun & BHs. Booking required. Dress code.
Societies Welcome. **Green Fees** £44 per 18 holes (£54 Sat, Sun & BHs). **Prof** Neal Grist **Course Designer** Hamilton Stutt **Facilities** ⓟ ⊙l ⓛ ▭ ⚒ ⚑ ✆ ⚐ ✆ ⚑ **Leisure** hard tennis courts, heated indoor swimming pool, sauna, solarium, gymnasium. **Conf** facs Corporate Hospitality Days **Location** M27 junct 7, off A334 between Botley & Wickham
Hotel ★★★★ 74% HL Marriott Meon Valley Hotel & Country Club, Sandy Ln, SHEDFIELD ☎ 01329 833455 113 en suite

---

SOUTHAMPTON   MAP 04 SU41

Chilworth Main Rd, Chilworth SO16 7JP
☎ 023 8074 0544 🖹 023 8073 3166
A course with two loops of nine holes, with a booking system to allow undisturbed play. The front nine is fairly long and undulating and include water hazards. The back nine is tighter and quite a challenge.
Manor Golf Course: 18 holes, 5915yds, Par 69, SSS 69, Course record 68. Club membership 600.
Visitors Mon-Sun & BHs. **Societies** Welcome. **Green Fees** £12 per 18 holes, £6 per 9 holes (£15/£10 Sat, Sun & BHs). **Prof** Darren Newing **Course Designer** J Garner **Facilities** ⓟ ⊙l ⓛ ▭ ⚒ ⚑ ✆ ⚐ **Location** A27 between Chilworth & Romsey
Hotel ★★★ 75% HL Chilworth Manor, CHILWORTH ☎ 023 8076 7333 95 en suite

Southampton Golf Course Rd, Bassett SO16 7LE
☎ 023 8076 0478 & 8076 0546 (booking)
🖹 023 8076 0472
e-mail: golf.course@southampton.gov.uk
18 holes, 6103yds, Par 69, SSS 70.
9 holes, 2395yds, Par 33.
Course Designer Halmree/A P Taylor **Location** 4m N of city centre off A33
Telephone for further details
Hotel ★★ 75% HL The Elizabeth House Hotel, 42-44 The Avenue, SOUTHAMPTON ☎ 023 8022 4327 20 en suite 7 annexe en suite

---

Stoneham Monks Wood Close, Bassett SO16 3TT
☎ 023 8076 9272 🖹 023 8076 6320
e-mail: richard.penley-martin@stonehamgolfclub.org.uk
web: www.stonehamgolfclub.org.uk
Undulating through an attractive parkland and heathland setting with views over the Itchen valley towards Winchester, this course rewards brains over brawn. It is unusual in having 5 Par 5's and 5 Par 3's and no two holes alike. The quality of the course means that temporary greens are never used and the course is rarely closed.

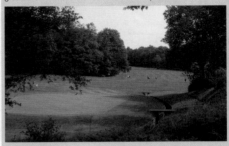

18 holes, 6392yds, Par 72, SSS 70, Course record 63. Club membership 800.
Visitors Mon-Sun & BHs. Booking required. Handicap certificate. Dress code. **Societies** Booking required. **Green Fees** £50 per day, £45 per round (£60/£50 Sat, Sun & BHs). **Prof** Ian Young **Course Designer** Willie Park Jnr **Facilities** ⓟ ⊙l ⓛ ▭ ⚒ ⚑ ✆ ⚐ ✆ **Conf** facs Corporate Hospitality Days **Location** 4m N of city centre off A27
Hotel ★★★ 75% HL Chilworth Manor, CHILWORTH ☎ 023 8076 7333 95 en suite

---

SOUTHWICK   MAP 04 SU60

Southwick Park Naval Recreation Centre Pinsley Dr PO17 6EL
☎ 023 923 80131 🖹 023 9221 0289
e-mail: southwickpark@btconnect.com
web: www.southwickparkgolfclub.co.uk
Set in 100 acres of parkland played around Southwick Park lake. Tight course with good greens and tough finish.
18 holes, 5884yds, Par 69, SSS 69, Course record 64. Club membership 750.
Visitors Mon-Sun except BHs. Booking required Sat & Sun. Dress code. **Societies** Booking required. **Green Fees** £32 per 36 holes, £23 per 18 holes (£28 per 18 holes Sat & Sun). ⊕ **Prof** Eddy Rawlings **Course Designer** C Lawrie **Facilities** ⓟ ⊙l ⓛ ▭ ⚒ ⚑ ✆ ⚐ **Conf** Corporate Hospitality Days **Location** 0.5m SE off B2177
Hotel ★★ 75% HL Old House Hotel & Restaurant, The Square, WICKHAM ☎ 01329 833049 8 en suite 4 annexe en suite

---

TADLEY   MAP 04 SU66

Bishopswood Bishopswood Ln RG26 4AT
☎ 0118 981 2200 🖹 0118 940 8606
e-mail: ddlgoss@aol.com
Wooded parkland with numerous water hazards. Considered to be one of the best nine-hole courses in the UK and venue of the National 9's regional finals.
9 holes, 6474yds, Par 72, SSS 71, Course record 66. Club membership 450.

Continued

Visitors may play Mon-Fri except BHs. Advance booking required. Dress code. **Societies** Booking required. **Green Fees** £19 per 18 holes, £13 per 9 holes. **Prof** Steve Ward **Course Designer** M W Phillips/G Blake **Facilities** ⑪ ⑩ ⚑ ⚑ ♨ ♨ ⚑ ⚑ 🏌 ⚑ ꙮ **Conf** Corporate Hospitality Days **Location** 6m N of Basingstoke off A340

Hotel ★★★ 70% HL Romans Hotel, Little London Rd, SILCHESTER ☎ 0118 970 0421 11 en suite 14 annexe en suite

WATERLOOVILLE — MAP 04 SU60

Portsmouth Crookhorn Ln, Purbrook PO7 5QL
☎ 023 9237 2210 📠 023 9220 0766
e-mail: info@portsmouthgc.com
web: www.portsmouthgc.com
18 holes, 6139yds, Par 69, SSS 70, Course record 64.
Course Designer Hawtree **Location** 2m S off A3
Telephone for further details
Hotel ★★★★ 72% HL Portsmouth Marriott Hotel, Southampton Rd, PORTSMOUTH ☎ 0870 400 7285 174 en suite

Waterlooville Cherry Tree Av, Cowplain PO8 8AP
☎ 023 9226 3388 📠 023 9224 2980
e-mail: secretary@waterloovillegolfclub.co.uk
web: waterloovillegolfclub.co.uk
Easy walking but challenging parkland course, with five Par 5s over 500yds and featuring four ponds and a stream running through. The 13th hole, at 556yds, has a carry over a pond for a drive and a stream crossing the fairway and ending in a very small green.
18 holes, 6602yds, Par 72, SSS 72, Course record 64.
Club membership 800.
Visitors Mon-Fri except BHs. Sat & Sun after 2pm. Booking required Sat & Sun. Handicap certificate. Dress code. **Societies** Booking required. **Green Fees** £44 per day, £34 per round. **Prof** John Hay **Course Designer** Henry Cotton **Facilities** ⑪ ⚑ ⚑ ♨ ♨ ⚑ ⚑ 🏌 ⚑ **Conf** Corporate Hospitality Days **Location** NE of town centre off A3
Hotel ★★★ 75% HL Brookfield Hotel, Havant Rd, EMSWORTH ☎ 01243 373363 40 en suite

WICKHAM — MAP 04 SU51

Wickham Park Titchfield Ln PO17 5PJ
☎ 01329 833342 📠 01329 834798
e-mail: wickham@crown-golf.co.uk
web: www.crown-golf.co.uk
An attractive 18-hole parkland course set in the Meon Valley. Ideal for beginners and established golfers alike. The course is not overly demanding but is challenging enough to provide an enjoyable round of golf.
18 holes, 5898yards, Par 69, SSS 68, Course record 69.
Club membership 600.
Visitors may play Mon-Sun & BHs. Advance booking required. Dress code. **Societies** advance booking required. **Green Fees** not confirmed. **Prof** Scott Edwards **Facilities** ⑪ ⚑ ⚑ ♨ ♨ ⚑ ⚑ 🍴 ⚑ 🏌 **Leisure** chipping area. **Conf** facs Corporate Hospitality Days **Location** M27 junct 9/10
Hotel ★★ 75% HL Old House Hotel & Restaurant, The Square, WICKHAM ☎ 01329 833049 8 en suite 4 annexe en suite

WINCHESTER — MAP 04 SU42

Hockley Twyford SO21 1PL
☎ 01962 713165 📠 01962 713612
e-mail: secretary@hockleygolfclub.com
web: www.hockleygolfclub.com
Downland course with good views.
18 holes, 6500yds, Par 71, SSS 70, Course record 64.
Club membership 750.
Visitors may play Mon-Sun & BHs. Dress code. **Societies** advance booking required. **Green Fees** not confirmed. ⊕ **Prof** Gary Stubbington **Course Designer** James Braid **Facilities** ⑪ ⑩ ⚑ ⚑ ♨ ♨ ⚑ ⚑ 🏌 ⚑ **Conf** Corporate Hospitality Days **Location** M3 junct 11, signed to Twyford
Hotel ★★★★ 71% HL Mercure Wessex Hotel, Paternoster Row, WINCHESTER ☎ 0870 400 8126 94 en suite

Royal Winchester Sarum Rd SO22 5QE
☎ 01962 852462 📠 01962 865048
e-mail: manager@royalwinchestergolfclub.com
web: royalwinchestergolfclub.com
The Royal Winchester course is a sporting downland course centred on a rolling valley, so the course is hilly in places with fine views over the surrounding countryside. Built on chalk downs, the course drains extremely well and offers an excellent playing surface.
18 holes, 6216yds, Par 71, SSS 70, Course record 65.
Club membership 800.
Visitors Mon-Fri except BHs. Booking required. Handicap certificate. Dress code. **Societies** Booking required. **Green Fees** £60 per day, £40 per round. **Prof** Steven Hunter **Course Designer** J H Taylor **Facilities** ⑪ ⑩ by prior arrangement ⚑ ⚑ ♨ ♨ ⚑ ⚑ 🏌 **Conf** Corporate Hospitality Days **Location** 1.5m W off A3090
Hotel ★★★★ HL Lainston House Hotel, Sparsholt, WINCHESTER ☎ 01962 863588 50 en suite

South Winchester Romsey Rd SO22 5QX
☎ 01962 877800 📠 01962 877900
e-mail: swgc@crown-golf.co.uk
web: www.crown-golf.co.uk/southwinchester
18 holes, 7086yds, Par 72, SSS 74, Course record 68.
Course Designer Dave Thomas **Location** M3 junct 11, on A3090 Romsey road
Telephone for further details
Hotel ★★★ 79% HL The Winchester Royal, Saint Peter St, WINCHESTER ☎ 01962 840840 19 en suite 56 annexe en suite

HEREFORDSHIRE

BODENHAM — MAP 03 SO55

Brockington Hall Golf Club & Country House
HR1 3HX
☎ 01568 797877 📠 01568 797877
e-mail: info@brockingtonhall.co.uk
web: www.brockingtonhall.co.uk
A well-maintained course set in attractive countryside with fine greens and defined fairways separated by mixed plantations. A meandering brook runs through the course making it a testing but enjoyable game of golf.
9 holes, 2344yds, Par 66, SSS 63, Course record 32.
Club membership 178.

Continued

Visitors Mon-Sun & BHs. Dress code. **Societies** Booking required. **Green Fees** £11 per 18 holes, £7 per 9 holes (£12/£8 weekends). **Prof** Kevin Davis **Course Designer** Derek Powell **Facilities** ⊕ ⊺◎⊺ 🏌 ⊑ 🍴 🏐 ⚐⚑ ♙ ♠ ♣ **Conf** facs Corporate Hospitality Days **Location** on A417 on outskirts of Bodenham village between Leominster and Hereford.
Hotel ★★★ 72% HL Best Western Talbot Hotel, West St, LEOMINSTER
☎ 01568 616347   20 en suite

CLIFFORD   MAP 03 SO24

Summerhill HR3 5EW
☎ 01497 820451 📄 01497 820451
e-mail: dcbowen@summerhillgolfcourse.co.uk
web: www.summerhillgolfcourse.co.uk
Undulating parkland deep in the Wye Valley on the Welsh border.
9 holes, 2872yds, Par 70, SSS 67, Course record 71.
Club membership 240.
Visitors Mon, Wed, Fri & BHs. Tue pm only, Thu am only, Sat & Sun after noon. Booking required Tue, Thu, Sat, Sun & BHs. Dress code. **Societies** Welcome. **Green Fees** £14 per 18 holes, £10 per 9 holes (£18/12 Sat, Sun & BHs). ♦ **Prof** Andy Gealy **Course Designer** Bob Sandow **Facilities** ⊕ ⊺◎⊺ by prior arrangement 🏌 ⊑ 🍴 ⚐ 🏐 🍴 ♙ ♠ ♣ **Leisure** 3 hole Par 3 course. **Conf** facs Corporate Hospitality Days **Location** 0.5m N from Hay on B4350, on right
Inn ★★★★★ RR The Talkhouse, Pontdolgoch, CAERSWS
☎ 01686 688919   3 en suite

HEREFORD   MAP 03 SO53

Belmont Lodge Belmont HR2 9SA
☎ 01432 352666 📄 01432 358090
e-mail: info@belmont-hereford.co.uk
web: www.belmont-hereford.co.uk
Parkland course designed in two loops of nine. The first nine take the higher ground, offering magnificent views over Herefordshire. The second nine run alongside the River Wye with five holes in play against the river.The course is situated in typically beautiful Herefordshire countryside. The walking is easy on gently rolling fairways with a background of hills and woods and in the distance, the Welsh mountains. Some holes are played through mature cider orchards and there are two lakes to negotiate. A fair but interesting test for players of all abilities.

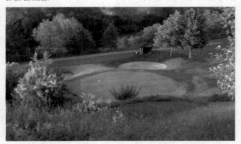

18 holes, 6511yds, Par 72, SSS 71, Course record 66.
Club membership 500.
Visitors may play Mon-Sun & BHs. Booking required Fri-Sun. 14 days booking required BHs. **Societies** Booking required. **Green Fees** £25 per 18 holes (£30 Sat, Sun & BHs). Reduced winter rates. **Prof** Mike Welsh **Course Designer** Bob Sandow **Facilities** ⊕ ⊺◎⊺ 🏌 ⊑ 🍴 ⚐ 🏐 🍴 ♠ ♣

♣ 🏐 ♠ ♣ **Leisure** hard tennis courts, fishing. **Conf** facs Corporate Hospitality Days **Location** 2m S off A465
Hotel ★★★ 72% HL Belmont Lodge & Golf, Belmont, HEREFORD
☎ 01432 352666   30 en suite

Burghill Valley Tillington Rd, Burghill HR4 7RW
☎ 01432 760456 📄 01432 761654
e-mail: info@bvgc.co.uk
web: www.bvgc.co.uk
18 holes, 6239yds, Par 71, SSS 70, Course record 66.
Course Designer M Barnett **Location** 4m NW of Hereford
Telephone for further details
Hotel BUD Premier Travel Inn Hereford, Holmer Rd, Holmer, HEREFORD
☎ 08701 977134   60 en suite

Hereford Municipal Hereford Leisure Centre, Holmer Rd HR4 9UD
☎ 01432 344376 📄 01432 266281
This municipal parkland course is more challenging than first appearance. The well-drained greens are open all year round with good drainage for excellent winter golf.
9 holes, 3060yds, Par 35, SSS 68. Club membership 195.
Visitors may play Mon-Sun & BHs. Advance booking required. **Societies** advance booking required. **Green Fees** not confirmed. **Prof** Gary Morgan **Course Designer** J Leek **Facilities** ⊕ ⊺◎⊺ 🏌 ⊑ 🍴 ⚐ 🏐 🍴 ♠ ♣ **Leisure** squash, gymnasium, Leisure centre. **Location** Within racecourse on A49 Hereford-Leominster
Hotel BUD Premier Travel Inn Hereford, Holmer Rd, Holmer, HEREFORD
☎ 08701 977134   60 en suite

KINGTON   MAP 03 SO25

Kington Bradnor Hill HR5 3RE
☎ 01544 230340 (club) & 231320 (pro shop)
📄 01544 230340 /231320 (pro)
e-mail: kingtongolf@ukonline.co.uk
The highest 18-hole course in England, with magnificent views over seven counties. A natural heathland course with easy walking on mountain turf cropped by sheep. There is bracken to catch any really bad shots but no sand traps. The greens play true and fast and are generally acknowledged as some of the best in the west Midlands.
18 holes, 5980yds, Par 70, SSS 69, Course record 63.
Club membership 510.
Visitors Mon-Sun & BHs. Booking required. Handicap certificate. Dress code. **Societies** Welcome. **Green Fees** £26 per day, £20 per round (£32/£26 Sat, Sun & BHs). ♦ **Prof** Andy Gealy **Course Designer** Major C K Hutchison **Facilities** ⊕ ⊺◎⊺ 🏌 ⊑ 🍴 ⚐ 🏐 🍴 ♙ ♠ ♣ **Location** 0.5m N of Kington off B4355
Hotel ★★★ 72% HL Best Western Talbot Hotel, West St, LEOMINSTER
☎ 01568 616347   20 en suite

LEOMINSTER   MAP 03 SO45

Leominster Ford Bridge HR6 0LE
☎ 01568 610055 📄 01568 610055
e-mail: contact@leominstergolfclub.co.uk
web: www.leominstergolfclub.co.uk
On undulating parkland with the lower holes running alongside the River Lugg and others on the higher part of the course affording fine panoramic views over the surrounding countryside.

Continued

18 holes, 6026yds, Par 70, SSS 69. Club membership 500.
Visitors Mon-Sun & BHs. Booking required. Dress code. **Societies** Booking
required. **Green Fees** £20 per day Mon-Fri, £10 per 18 holes Mon & Fri, £16
Tue-Thu (£30 per day, £25 per round Sat, Sun & BHs). **Prof** Nigel Clarke
Course Designer Bob Sandow **Facilities** ⑪ ⑩ ℔ ☑ ℸ℧ ☒ ☎ ☛ ⚡
Leisure fishing. **Conf** facs Corporate Hospitality Days **Location** 3m S
of Leominster on A49, signed
Hotel ★★★ 72% HL Best Western Talbot Hotel, West St, LEOMINSTER
☎ 01568 616347 20 en suite

ROSS-ON-WYE MAP 03 SO62

Ross-on-Wye Two Park, Gorsley HR9 7UT
☎ 01989 720267 📄 01989 720212
e-mail: admin@therossonwyegolfclub.co.uk
web: www.therossonwyegolfclub.co.uk
This undulating, parkland course has been cut out of a silver birch
forest. The fairways are well-screened from each other and tight, the
greens good and the bunkers have been restructured.
18 holes, 6451yds, Par 72, SSS 71, Course record 68.
Club membership 730.
Visitors Wed-Sun & BHs. Booking required. Handicap certificate. Dress
code. **Societies** Booking required. **Green Fees** £50 per 36 holes; £46
per 27 holes; £40 per round. **Prof** Paul Middleton **Course Designer**
Mr C K Cotton **Facilities** ⑪ ⑩ ℔ ☑ ℸ℧ ☒ ☎ ♐ ⚡ ☛ ♟ **Leisure**
snooker. **Conf** Corporate Hospitality Days **Location** M50 junct 3, on
B4221 N
Hotel ★★★ 80% HL Best Western Pengethley Manor, Pengethley Park,
ROSS-ON-WYE ☎ 01989 730211 11 en suite 14 annexe en suite

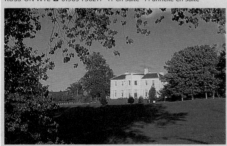

South Herefordshire Twin Lakes HR9 7UA
☎ 01989 780535 📄 01989 780535
e-mail: info@herefordshiregolf.co.uk
web: www.herefordshiregolf.co.uk
Impressive 6672yd parkland course fast maturing into one of
Herefordshire's finest. Magnificent panoramic views of the Welsh
mountains and countryside. Drains well and is playable in any weather.
The landscape has enabled the architect to design 18 individual and
varied holes.
Twin Lakes: 18 holes, 6672yds, Par 71, SSS 72,
Course record 71. Club membership 400.
Visitors Mon-Sun & BHs. Dress code. **Societies** Welcome. **Green Fees**
£20 per 18 holes (£25 Sat & Sun). **Prof** Leo Tarrant **Course Designer** John
Day **Facilities** ⑪ ⑩ ℔ ☑ ℸ℧ ☒ ☎ ♐ ⚡ ☛ ♟ **Conf** Corporate
Hospitality Days **Location** M50 junct 4, to Upton Bishop, right onto B4224,
1m left
Hotel ★★★ 70% CHH Pencraig Court Country House Hotel, Pencraig,
ROSS-ON-WYE ☎ 01989 770306 11 en suite

UPPER SAPEY MAP 03 SO66

Sapey WR6 6XT
☎ 01886 853288 & 853567 📄 01886 853485
e-mail: anybody@sapeygolf.co.uk
web: www.sapeygolf.co.uk
Easy walking parkland with views of the Malvern Hills. The mixture
of long or short holes, including trees, lakes and water hazards, is a
demanding challenge for all golfers.
The Rowan: 18 holes, 5935yds, Par 69, SSS 68,
Course record 63.
The Oaks: 9 holes, 1203, Par 27, SSS 27.
Club membership 400.
Visitors may play Mon-Sat & BHs. Booking required. Dress code.
Societies Booking required. **Green Fees** Rowan: £22 per round (£27 Sat
& Sun). Oaks: £6 (£8 Sat & Sun). **Prof** Chris Knowles **Course Designer**
R McMurray **Facilities** ⑪ ⑩ by prior arrangement ℔ ☑ ℸ℧ ☒ ☎ ♐ ♦
⚡ ☛ ⚡ **Conf** Corporate Hospitality Days **Location** B4203 Bromyard-
Stourport road
Hotel ★★★ 72% HL Best Western Talbot Hotel, West St, LEOMINSTER
☎ 01568 616347 20 en suite

WORMSLEY MAP 03 SO44

Herefordshire Ravens Causeway HR4 8LY
☎ 01432 830219 & 830465 (pro) 📄 01432 830095
e-mail: herefordshire.golf@breath.com
web: www.herefordshiregolfclub.co.uk
Undulating parkland with expansive views of the Clee Hills to the east
and the Black Mountains to the west. Peaceful and relaxing situation.
18 holes, 6078yds, Par 70, SSS 69, Course record 61.
Club membership 750.
Visitors may play Mon-Sun except BHs. Booking required. Handicap
certificate. Dress code **Societies** Booking required. **Green Fees** £30
per day £25 per 18 holes. (£40/£30 Sat & Sun). **Prof** Richard Hemming
Course Designer James Braid **Facilities** ⑪ ⑩ ℔ ☑ ℸ℧ ☒ ☎ ♐ ⚡ ☛
Conf Corporate Hospitality Days **Location** 7m NW of Hereford on B road
to Weobley
Hotel BUD Premier Travel Inn Hereford, Holmer Rd, Holmer, HEREFORD
☎ 08701 977134 60 en suite

HERTFORDSHIRE

ALDBURY MAP 04 SP91

Stocks Hotel & Golf Club Stocks Rd HP23 5RX
☎ 01442 851341 & 851491 (pro) 📄 01442 861253
e-mail: info@stockshotel.co.uk
web: www.stockshotel.co.uk
18 holes, 6804yds, Par 72, SSS 73, Course record 66.
Course Designer Mike Billcliffe **Location** 2m from A41 at Tring, towards
Tring station
Telephone for further details
Hotel ★★★★ 76% HL Pendley Manor Hotel, Cow Ln, TRING
☎ 01442 891891 73 en suite

England

ALDENHAM
MAP 04 TQ19

Aldenham Golf and Country Club Church Ln
WD25 8NN
☎ 01923 853929 📄 01923 858472
e-mail: info@aldenhamgolfclub.co.uk
web: www.aldenhamgolfclub.co.uk
Undulating parkland with woods, water hazards and ditches. Many specimen trees and beautiful views across the countryside.

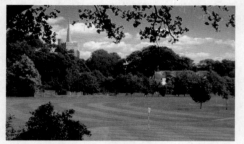

Old Course: 18 holes, 6456yds, Par 70, SSS 71.
White Course: 9 holes, 2350yds, Par 33, SSS 32.
Club membership 500.
Visitors Mon-Sun & BHs. Booking required. Dress code. **Societies** Booking required. **Green Fees** Old Course: £30 per round (£40 Sat, Sun & BHs). White Course £12 (£15 Sat, Sun & BHs). **Prof** Tim Dunstan **Facilities** ⊕ �🍽 ⬚ ⬚ ⬚ ⬚ ⬚ ⬚ ⬚ **Conf** facs Corporate Hospitality Days **Location** M1 junct 5, 0.5m to W of village
Hotel ★★★ 71% HL Best Western The White House, Upton Rd, WATFORD ☎ 01923 237316 57 en suite

BERKHAMSTED
MAP 04 SP90

Berkhamsted The Common HP4 2QB
☎ 01442 865832 📄 01442 863730
e-mail: barryh@berkhamstedgc.co.uk
web: www.berkhamstedgolfclub.co.uk
There are no sand bunkers on this Championship heathland course but this does not make it any easier to play. The natural hazards will test the skill of the most able players, with a particularly testing hole at the 11th, 568yds, Par 5. Fine greens, long carries and heather and gorse.
18 holes, 6605yds, Par 71, SSS 72, Course record 65.
Club membership 700.
Visitors Mon-Sun & BHs. Handicap certificate. Dress code. **Societies** Booking required. **Green Fees** £55 per day, £40 per 18 holes (£50 per 18 holes Sat, Sun & BHs). **Prof** John Clarke **Course Designer** Colt/Braid **Facilities** ⊕ ⬚ ⬚ ⬚ ⬚ ⬚ **Location** 1.5m E
Hotel ★★★★ 76% HL Pendley Manor Hotel, Cow Ln, TRING ☎ 01442 891891 73 en suite

BISHOP'S STORTFORD
MAP 05 TL42

Bishop's Stortford Dunmow Rd CM23 5HP
☎ 01279 654715 📄 01279 655215
e-mail: office@bsgc.co.uk
web: www.bsgc.co.uk
Well-established parkland course, fairly flat, but undulating, with easy walking.

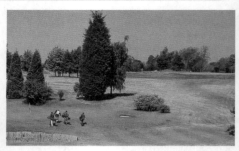

Bishop's Stortford

18 holes, 6404yds, Par 71, SSS 71, Course record 64.
Club membership 900.
Visitors Mon-Fri except BHs. Handicap certificate. Dress code. **Societies** Booking required. **Green Fees** £50 per day, £40 per 18 holes. **Prof** Simon Sheppard **Course Designer** James Braid **Facilities** ⊕ ⬚ ⬚ ⬚ ⬚ ⬚ ⬚ ⬚ ⬚ ⬚ ⬚ **Leisure** snooker tables. **Conf** facs **Location** M11 junct 8, 0.5m W on A1250
Hotel ★★★ 75% HL Best Western Stansted Manor Hotel, Birchanger Ln, BIRCHANGER ☎ 01279 859800 70 en suite

Great Hadham Golf & Country Club Great Hadham Rd, Much Hadham SG10 6JE
☎ 01279 843558 📄 01279 842122
e-mail: info@ghgcc.co.uk
An undulating meadowland and links course offering excellent country views and a challenge with its ever present breeze.
18 holes, 6854yds, Par 72, SSS 73, Course record 67.
Club membership 800.
Visitors may play Mon-Fri, Sat/Sun & BHs pm only. Advance booking required. Dress code. **Societies** advance booking required. **Green Fees** not confirmed. **Prof** Kevin Lunt **Course Designer** Iain Roberts **Facilities** ⬚ ⬚ ⬚ **Leisure** sauna, solarium, gymnasium. **Conf** facs Corporate Hospitality Days **Location** On the B1004, 3m SW of Bishop's Stortford
Hotel ★★★★ 78% HL Down Hall Country House Hotel, Hatfield Heath, BISHOPS STORTFORD ☎ 01279 731441 99 en suite

BRICKENDON
MAP 05 TL30

Brickendon Grange Pembridge Ln SG13 8PD
☎ 01992 511258 📄 01992 511411
e-mail: play@brickendongrangegc.co.uk
web: www.brickendongrangegc.co.uk
Undulating parkland with some fine Par 4s. The 17th hole reputed to be best in the county.
18 holes, 6458yds, Par 71, SSS 71, Course record 67.
Club membership 680.
Visitors Mon-Fri except BHs. Handicap certificate. Dress code. **Societies** Booking required. **Green Fees** £45 per day; £38 per round. 🏌 **Prof** Graham Tippett **Course Designer** C K Cotton **Facilities** ⊕ 🍽 ⬚ ⬚ ⬚ ⬚ ⬚ ⬚ **Conf** facs Corporate Hospitality Days **Location** W of village
Hotel ★★★★ 73% HL Ponsbourne Park Hotel, Newgate St Village, POTTERS BAR ☎ 01707 876191 & 879277 📄 01707 875190 23 en suite 28 annexe en suite

BROOKMANS PARK   MAP 04 TL20

Brookmans Park Golf Club Rd AL9 7AT
☎ 01707 652487 📄 01707 661851
e-mail: info@bpgc.co.uk
web: www.bpgc.co.uk
Undulating parkland with several cleverly constructed holes. But it is a fair course, although it can play long. The 11th, Par 3, is a testing hole which plays across a lake.
18 holes, 6249yds, Par 71, SSS 71, Course record 65. Club membership 750.
Visitors Mon, Wed-Fri except BHs. Booking required. Handicap certificate. Dress code. **Societies** Booking required. **Green Fees** £45 per day; £32 per round. ● **Prof** Ian Jelley **Course Designer** Hawtree/Taylor
Facilities ⚲ ⛳ 🛍 🖥 🍴 🏌 🏐 🍺 🧺 ✓ **Location** N of village off A1000
Hotel ★★★ 75% HL Bush Hall, Mill Green, HATFIELD ☎ 01707 271251 25 en suite

BROXBOURNE   MAP 05 TL30

Hertfordshire Broxbournebury Mansion, White Stubbs Ln EN10 7PY
☎ 01992 466666 & 441268 (pro shop) 📄 01992 470326
e-mail: hertfordshire@crowngolf.co.uk
web: www.crowngolf.co.uk
An 18 hole course of a 'Nicklaus' design set around a Grade II listed clubhouse to full USGA specifications. Considered to be one of the best private courses to appear in recent years.
18 holes, 6388yds, Par 70, SSS 70, Course record 62. Club membership 600.
Visitors Mon-Sun & BHs. Dress code. **Societies** Booking required. **Green Fees** £35 (£40 Sat & Sun). **Prof** Mark Payne **Course Designer** Jack Nicklaus II **Facilities** ⚲ ⛳ 🛍 🖥 🍴 🏌 🏐 🍺 🧺 ✓ 🏐 **Leisure** hard tennis courts, heated indoor swimming pool, fishing, sauna, solarium, gymnasium, jacuzzis. **Conf** facs Corporate Hospitality Days
Location Off A10 for Broxbourne, signs for Paradise Wildlife Park, left at Bell Ln over A10, on right
Hotel ★★★★ 76% HL Cheshunt Marriott Hotel, Halfhide Ln, Turnford, BROXBOURNE ☎ 01992 451245 143 en suite

BUNTINGFORD   MAP 05 TL32

East Herts Hamels Park SG9 9NA
☎ 01920 821978 (office) & 821922 (pro) 📄 01920 823700
e-mail: brian@ehgc.co.uk
web: www.ehgc.co.uk
Mature, attractive, undulating parkland course with magnificent specimen trees.
18 holes, 6456yds, Par 71, SSS 71, Course record 62. Club membership 640.
Visitors may play Mon,Tue, Thu, Fri except BHs. Wed pm only. Handicap certificate. Dress code. **Societies** Booking required. **Green Fees** £43 per day, £32 per round. **Prof** D Field **Facilities** ⚲ ⛳ 🛍 🖥 🍴 🏌 🏐 🍺 ✓ 🏐 **Conf** Corporate Hospitality Days **Location** 1m N of Puckeridge off A10, opposite Pearce's Farm Shop
Hotel ★★★ 71% HL Novotel Stevenage, Knebworth Park, STEVENAGE ☎ 01438 346100 101 en suite

BUSHEY   MAP 04 TQ19

Bushey Golf & Country Club High St WD23 1TT
☎ 020 8950 2215(pro shop) & 8950 2283 (club)
📄 020 8386 1181
e-mail: info@busheycountryclub.com
web: www.busheycountryclub.com
Undulating parkland with challenging 2nd and 9th holes. The latter has a sweeping dog-leg left, playing to a green in front of the clubhouse. For the rather too enthusiastic golfer, Bushey offers its own physiotherapist.

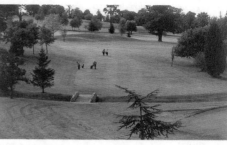

9 holes, 6120yds, Par 70, SSS 69, Course record 67. Club membership 475.
Visitors may play Mon, Tue, Fri except BHs. Wed, Thu, Sat & Sun only. Booking required. Dress code. **Societies** Welcome. **Green Fees** £22 per 18 holes, £14 per 9 holes (£27/£16 Sat & Sun). **Prof** Martin Siggins **Course Designer** Donald Steele **Facilities** ⚲ ⛳ 🛍 🖥 🍴 🍺 🧺 ✓ 🏐 **Leisure** sauna, solarium, gymnasium, health & fitness club.
Conf Corporate Hospitality Days
Hotel ★★★ 73% HL Corus hotel Elstree, Barnet Ln, ELSTREE ☎ 0870 609 6151 47 en suite

Bushey Hall Bushey Hall Dr WD23 2EP
☎ 01923 222253 📄 01923 229759
e-mail: info@golfclubuk.co.uk
web: www.busheyhallgolfclub.co.uk
A tree-lined parkland course, the oldest established club in Hertfordshire.
18 holes, 6099yds, Par 69, SSS 69, Course record 62. Club membership 500.
Visitors Mon-Sun & BHs. Booking required. Handicap certificate. Dress code. **Societies** Booking required. **Green Fees** £26 per 18 holes (£35 Sat, Sun & BHs). **Prof** Ken Wickham **Course Designer** J Braid **Facilities** ⚲ ⛳ by prior arrangement 🛍 🖥 🍴 🏌 🏐 🍺 ✓ 🧺 ✓ 🏐 **Leisure** practice nets.
Conf facs Corporate Hospitality Days **Location** M1 junct 5, A41 Harrow to Bushey, 4th exit at rdbt, club 150yds on left
Hotel ★★★ 73% HL Corus hotel Elstree, Barnet Ln, ELSTREE ☎ 0870 609 6151 47 en suite

CHESHUNT   MAP 05 TL30

Cheshunt Park Cheshunt Park, Park Ln EN7 6QD
☎ 01992 624009 📄 01992 636403
e-mail: golf.leisure@broxbourne.gov.uk
web: www.broxbourne.gov.uk
Municipal parkland course, well bunkered with ponds, easy walking.
18 holes, 6692yds, Par 72, SSS 71. Club membership 350.

Continued

Visitors Mon-Sun & BHs. Booking required. Dress code. Must contact in advance. **Societies** Booking required. **Green Fees** Phone. **Prof** David Banks **Course Designer** P Wawtry **Facilities** ⚙ ⭐ 🍴 🛍 🖤 🎱 🏌 ➢ 🏖 ✂ **Leisure** Club repair service. **Conf** facs Corporate Hospitality Days **Location** 1.5m NW off B156. M25 junct 25, 3m N
Hotel ★★★★ 76% HL Cheshunt Marriott Hotel, Halfhide Ln, Turnford, BROXBOURNE ☎ 01992 451245 143 en suite

CHORLEYWOOD   MAP 04 TQ09

Chorleywood Common Rd WD3 5LN
☎ 01923 282009 📠 01923 286739
e-mail: secretary@chorleywoodgolfclub.co.uk
Very attractive mix of woodland and heathland with natural hazards and good views.
9 holes, 5686yds, Par 68, SSS 67. Club membership 300.
Visitors Mon-Sat except BHs. Booking required. Handicap certificate. Dress code. **Societies** Booking required. **Green Fees** £20 per round; £15 for 9 holes (£25/15 Sat & Sun). ⊕ **Facilities** ⚙ 🛍 🖤 🎱 ✂
Location M25 junct 18, E of village off A404
Hotel ★★★ 75% HL The Bedford Arms Hotel, CHENIES ☎ 01923 283301 10 en suite 8 annexe en suite

ELSTREE   MAP 04 TQ19

Elstree Watling St WD6 3AA
☎ 020 8953 6115 or 8238 6941 📠 020 8207 6390
e-mail: admin@elstree-golf.co.uk
web: www.elstree-golfclub.co.uk
Parkland course incorporating ponds and streams and challenging doglegs.
18 holes, 6556yds, Par 73, SSS 72. Club membership 400.
Visitors Mon-Sun & BHs. Booking required Sat, Sun & BHs. Dress code. **Societies** Booking required. **Green Fees** £40 weekdays (£48 Sat, Sun & BHs). **Prof** Marc Warwick **Course Designer** Donald Steel **Facilities** ⚙ ⭐ 🛍 🖤 🎱 🏌 ➢ 🏖 ✂ 🏖 ✂ **Leisure** snooker, golf academy. **Conf** Corporate Hospitality Days **Location** A5183 between Radlett and Elstree, next to Wagon pub
Hotel ★★★ 73% HL Corus hotel Elstree, Barnet Ln, ELSTREE ☎ 0870 609 6151 47 en suite

ESSENDON   MAP 04 TL20

Hatfield London Country Club Bedwell Park AL9 6HN
☎ 01707 260360 📠 01707 278475
e-mail: info@hatfieldlondon.co.uk
web: www.hatfieldlondon.co.uk
Parkland course with many varied hazards, including ponds, a stream and a ditch. A 19th-century clubhouse.
Old Course: 18 holes, 6808yds, Par 72, SSS 72.
New Course: 18 holes, 6938yds, Par 72, SSS 73.
Club membership 350.
Visitors Mon-Sun & BHs. Booking required. Dress code. **Societies** Booking required. **Green Fees** Old Course £25 (£35 Sat, Sun & BHs). New Course £33 (£50 Sat, Sun & BHs). **Prof** Andrew Clapp **Course Designer** Fred Hawtree **Facilities** ⚙ ⭐ 🛍 🖤 🎱 🏌 ➢ 🏖 ✂ 🏖 ✂ **Leisure** sauna, 9 hole pitch and putt, Japanese bath. **Conf** facs Corporate Hospitality Days **Location** 1m S on B158
Hotel ★★★ 72% HL Quality Hotel Hatfield, Roehyde Way, HATFIELD ☎ 01707 275701 76 en suite

GRAVELEY   MAP 04 TL22

Chesfield Downs Jack's Hill SG4 7EQ
☎ 01462 482929 📠 01462 482930
e-mail: chesfielddowns-manager@crown-golf.co.uk
web: www.crown-golf.co.uk
An undulating, open downland course with an inland links feel.
18 holes, 6648yds, Par 71, SSS 72. Club membership 500.
Visitors Mon-Sun & BHs. Booking required. Dress code. **Societies** must telephone in advance. **Green Fees** not confirmed. **Prof** Jane Fernley **Course Designer** J Gaunt **Facilities** ⚙ ⭐ by prior arrangement 🛍 🖤 🎱 🏌 ➢ 🏖 ✂ 🏖 ✂ **Leisure** par3 9 hole course. **Conf** facs Corporate Hospitality Days **Location** A1 junct 8, B197 to Graveley
Hotel BUD Hotel Ibis Stevenage, Danestrete, STEVENAGE ☎ 01438 779955 98 en suite

HARPENDEN   MAP 04 TL11

Aldwickbury Park Piggottshill Ln AL5 1AB
☎ 01582 760112 📠 01582 760113
e-mail: enquiries@aldwickburyparkgolfclub.com
web: www.aldwickburyparkgolfclub.com
Wooded parkland with lakes and spectacular views across the Lea valley.
18 holes, 6352yds, Par 71, SSS 70, Course record 66.
Club membership 700.
Visitors Mon-Sun & BHs. Booking required. Dress code. **Societies** booking required. **Green Fees** not confirmed. **Prof** Robin Turley **Course Designer** Ken Brown/Martin Gillett **Facilities** ⚙ ⭐ 🛍 🖤 🎱 🏌 ➢ 🏖 ✂ 🏖 ✂ **Leisure** gymnasium, 9 hole Par 3 course, sports injury clinic. **Conf** facs Corporate Hospitality Days **Location** M1 junct 9, off Wheathampstead Rd between Harpenden
Hotel ★★★ 72% HL Harpenden House Hotel, 18 Southdown Rd, HARPENDEN ☎ 01582 449955 17 en suite 59 annexe en suite

Harpenden Hammonds End, Redbourn Ln AL5 2AX
☎ 01582 712580 📠 01582 712725
e-mail: office@harpendengolfclub.co.uk
web: www.harpendengolfclub.co.uk
Gently undulating parkland, easy walking.
18 holes, 6377yds, Par 70, SSS 70, Course record 65.
Club membership 800.
Visitors Tue, Wed & Fri except BHs. Mon pm only. Dress code. **Societies** Booking required. **Green Fees** £45 per day, £35 per round. **Prof** Peter Lane **Course Designer** Hawtree & Taylor **Facilities** ⚙ ⭐ by prior arrangement 🛍 🖤 🎱 🏌 ➢ 🏖 ✂ 🏖 **Conf** Corporate Hospitality Days **Location** 1m S on B487
Hotel ★★★ 72% HL Harpenden House Hotel, 18 Southdown Rd, HARPENDEN ☎ 01582 449955 17 en suite 59 annexe en suite

Harpenden Common Cravells Rd, East Common AL5 1BL
☎ 01582 711328 (pro shop) 📠 01582 711321
e-mail: manager@hcgc.co.uk
web: www.hcgc.co.uk
Flat, easy walking, parkland with good greens. Golf has been played on the common for well over 100 years.
18 holes, 6214yds, Par 70, SSS 70, Course record 64.
Club membership 710.
Visitors may play Mon-Sun. Handicap certificate required. Dress code. **Societies** advance booking required. **Green Fees** not confirmed.

Continued

Prof Danny Fitzsimmons **Course Designer** K Brown **Facilities** ⑱ ⱺ◖ ▐▄
⫿ ⱺ◨ ⩜ ⌂ ⸲ᵐ ✗ **Location** On A1081 0.5m S of Harpenden
Hotel ★★★ 72% HL Harpenden House Hotel, 18 Southdown Rd,
HARPENDEN ☎ 01582 449955 17 en suite 59 annexe en suite

HEMEL HEMPSTEAD   MAP 04 TL00

Boxmoor 18 Box Ln, Boxmoor HP3 0DJ
☎ 01442 242434
web: www.boxmoorgolfclub.co.uk
The second-oldest course in Hertfordshire. Challenging, hilly,
moorland course with sloping fairways divided by trees. Fine views.
Testing holes: 3rd (Par 3), the 4th (Par 4). The 3rd has not been holed in
one since the course was founded in 1890 and the Par for the course
(64) has only been broken once.
9 holes, 4812yds, Par 64, SSS 63, Course record 62.
Club membership 280.
Visitors Mon-Sat & BHs. Sun after 11.30am only. Dress code. **Societies**
Booking required. **Green Fees** £10 per round. ⊛ **Facilities** ▐▄ ⫿ ⱺ◨ ⩜
Location 2m SW on B4505
Hotel ★★ 72% HL The Two Brewers, The Common, CHIPPERFIELD
☎ 01923 265266 20 en suite

Little Hay Box Ln, Bovingdon HP3 0DQ
☎ 01442 833798 📄 01442 831399
e-mail: chris.gordon@dacorum.gov.uk
Semi-parkland, inland links.
18 holes, 6300yds, Par 72, SSS 72.
Visitors Mon-Sun & BHs. Booking required. **Societies** booking required.
Green Fees not confirmed. **Prof** N Allen/M Perry **Course Designer**
Hawtree **Facilities** ⩜ ⌂ᵐ ➹ ✗ ❦ **Location** 1.5m SW off A41 onto
B4505
Hotel ★★★ 78% HL The Bobsleigh Hotel, Hempstead Rd, Bovingdon,
HEMEL HEMPSTEAD ☎ 0870 194 2130 30 en suite 15 annexe en suite

Shendish Manor London Rd, Apsley HP3 0AA
☎ 01442 251806 📄 01442 230683
e-mail: tconcannon@shendish.fsnet.co.uk
web: www.shendish-manor.com
18 holes, 5660yds, Par 70, SSS 67.
Course Designer D Steel **Location** Off A4251
Telephone for further details
Hotel ★★★★ 76% HL Pendley Manor Hotel, Cow Ln, TRING
☎ 01442 891891 73 en suite

KNEBWORTH   MAP 04 TL22

Knebworth Deards End Ln SG3 6NL
☎ 01438 812752 📄 01438 815216
e-mail: knebworth1@btconnect.com
web: www.knebworthgolfclub.com
Easy walking parkland.
18 holes, 6492yds, Par 71, SSS 71, Course record 66.
Club membership 900.
Visitors Mon-Fri except BHs. Handicap certificate. Dress code.
Societies Welcome. **Green Fees** £35 per day/round. **Prof** Garry Parker
Course Designer W Park (Jun) **Facilities** ⑱ ⱺ◖ ▐▄ ⫿ ⱺ◨ ⩜ ⌂ ➸ ✗
Conf Corporate Hospitality Days **Location** N of village off B197
Hotel ★★★ 68% HL Best Western The Roebuck Inn, London Rd,
Broadwater, STEVENAGE ☎ 01438 365445 54 en suite

LETCHWORTH   MAP 04 TL23

Letchworth Letchworth Ln SG6 3NQ
☎ 01462 683203 📄 01462 484567
e-mail: secretary@letchworthgolfclub.com
web: www.letchworthgolfclub.com
Planned more than 100 years ago by Harry Vardon, this is an
adventurous parkland course. To its variety of natural and artificial
hazards is added an unpredictable wind.
18 holes, 6459yds, Par 71, SSS 71, Course record 66.
Club membership 950.
Visitors Mon-Fri. Dress code. **Societies** Booking required.
Green Fees Phone. ⊛ **Prof** Karl Teschner **Course Designer** Harry
Vardon **Facilities** ⑱ ⱺ◖ ▐▄ ⫿ ⱺ◨ ⩜ ⌂ᵐ ✗ ➸ ✗ ❦ **Leisure** 9 hole
Par 3 course. **Conf** Corporate Hospitality Days **Location** S side of town
centre off A505
Hotel ★★★★ 70% HL Cromwell Hotel, High St, Old Town, STEVENAGE
☎ 01438 779954 & 775859 📄 01438 742169 76 en suite

LITTLE GADDESDEN   MAP 04 SP91

Ashridge HP4 1LY
☎ 01442 842244 📄 01442 843770
e-mail: info@ashridgegolfclub.ltd.uk
web: www.ashridgegolfclub.ltd.uk
Classic wooded parkland in area of outstanding natural beauty.
18 holes, 6625yds, Par 72, SSS 71, Course record 63.
Club membership 720.
Visitors Mon-Fri except BHs. Booking required. Dress code.
Societies Booking required. **Green Fees** Phone. **Prof** Peter Cherry
Course Designer Sir G Campbell/C Hutchinson/N V Hotchkin
Facilities ⑱ ⱺ◖ ▐▄ ⫿ ⱺ◨ ⩜ ⌂ ✗ ❦ **Conf** Corporate Hospitality
Days **Location** 5m N of Berkhamsted on B4506
Hotel ★★★ 72% HL Harpenden House Hotel, 18 Southdown Rd,
HARPENDEN ☎ 01582 449955 17 en suite 59 annexe en suite

MUCH HADHAM   MAP 05 TL41

Ash Valley Little Hadham Rd SG10 6HD
☎ 01279 843253 📄 01279 842389
Naturally undulating course with good views extending to Canary
Wharf in London on a clear day. Tough enough for lower handicapped
players but forgiving for the beginner and higher handicapped player.
18 holes, 6586yds, Par 72, SSS 71, Course record 64.
Club membership 150.
Visitors Mon-Sun & BHs. Societies Sat/Sun & BHs. **Societies** welcome.
Green Fees not confirmed. ⊛ **Prof** John Hamilton **Course Designer**
Martin Gillett **Facilities** ⑱ ▐▄ ⫿ ⱺ◨ ⩜ ⌂ ➸ ✗ **Leisure** Par 3 pitch and
putt. **Location** 1.5m S of A120 Little Hadham lights
Hotel ★★★ 70% HL Roebuck Hotel, Baldock St, WARE ☎ 01920 409955
50 en suite

POTTERS BAR   MAP 04 TL20

Potters Bar Darkes Ln EN6 1DE
☎ 01707 652020 📄 01707 655051
e-mail: info@pottersbargolfclub.com
web: www.pottersbargolfclub.com
Undulating parkland.
18 holes, 6279yds, Par 71, SSS 70. Club membership 560.

Continued

Visitors Mon, Tue, Thu & Fri except BHs. Handicap certificate. Dress code **Societies** booking required. **Green Fees** not confirmed. ● **Prof** Gary A'Ris/Julian Harding **Course Designer** James Braid **Facilities** ⑪ ⓛ ☐ ⌂
☒ ➔ ☜ ✦ ⌘ ✓ **Location** M25 junct 24, 1m N
Hotel BUD Days Inn South Mimms, Bignells Corner, POTTERS BAR
☎ 01707 665440 74 en suite

RADLETT   MAP 04 TL10

Porters Park Shenley Hill WD7 7AZ
☎ 01923 854127 📠 01923 855475
e-mail: info@porterspark.fsnet.co.uk
web: www.porterspark.com
18 holes, 6313yds, Par 70, SSS 70, Course record 64.
Course Designer Braid **Location** NE of village off A5183
Telephone for further details
Hotel BUD Innkeeper's Lodge London Borehamwood, Studio Way,
BOREHAM WOOD ☎ 0845 112 6120 55 en suite

REDBOURN   MAP 04 TL11

Redbourn Kinsbourne Green Ln AL3 7QA
☎ 01582 793493 📠 01582 794362
e-mail: enquiries@redbourngolfclub.com
web: www.redbourngolfclub.com
A mature parkland course offering a fair test of golf to all standards. Water comes into play on a number of holes.
Ver Course: 18 holes, 6506yds, Par 70, SSS 71, Course record 67.
Kingsbourne Course: 9 holes, 1361yds, Par 27. Club membership 800.
Visitors Mon-Sun & BHs. Advance booking. Dress code. **Societies** booking required. **Green Fees** not confirmed. **Prof** Stephen Hunter **Facilities** ⑪ ⓛ ☐ ⌂ ☒ ➔ ✦ ⌘ ✓ ☞ **Conf** Corporate Hospitality Days **Location** M1 junct 9, 1m N off A5183
Hotel ★★★ 72% HL Harpenden House Hotel, 18 Southdown Rd, HARPENDEN ☎ 01582 449955 . 17 en suite 59 annexe en suite

RICKMANSWORTH   MAP 04 TQ09

The Grove Chandler's Cross WD3 4TG
☎ 01923 294266 📠 01923 294268
e-mail: golf@thegrove.co.uk
web: www.thegrove.co.uk
A course built to USGA specifications but following the slopes, ridges and mounds that occur naturally within the landscape. The fairway grass encourages crisp ball striking and the greens are superb. Continuous hidden cart path around all holes.
18 holes, 7152yds, Par 72, SSS 74.
Visitors Mon-Sun & BHs. Booking required. **Societies** Booking required. **Green Fees** Phone. **Prof** Spencer Schaub **Course Designer** Kyle Phillips **Facilities** ⑪ ⓛ ☐ ⌂ ☒ ➔ ◇ ✦ ⌘ ✓ ☞ **Leisure** hard tennis courts, outdoor and indoor heated swimming pools, sauna, gymnasium. **Conf** facs Corporate Hospitality Days **Location** M25 junct 19/20, follow signs to Watford, At first large rdbt take exit for A411. Proceed for 0.5m and entrance on right.
Hotel ★★★★★ 89% HL The Grove, Chandler's Cross, RICKMANSWORTH ☎ 01923 807807 227 en suite

Moor Park WD3 1QN
☎ 01923 773146 📠 01923 777109
e-mail: enquiries@moorparkgc.co.uk
web: www.moorparkgc.co.uk
Two parkland courses with rolling fairways - High Course is challenging and will test the best golfer and West Course demands a high degree of accuracy. The clubhouse is a grade 1 listed mansion.

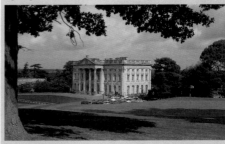

High Golf Course: 18 holes, 6713yds, Par 72, SSS 72, Course record 63.
West Golf Course: 18 holes, 5815yds, Par 69, SSS 68, Course record 60. Club membership 1700.
Visitors Mon-Sun & BHs. Booking required Sat, Sun & BHs. Handicap certificate. Dress code. **Societies** Booking required. **Green Fees** High: £80 per round. West: £50 per round (£120/£80 Sat, Sun & BHs). **Prof** Lawrence Farmer **Course Designer** H S Colt **Facilities** ⑪ ⓘ ⓛ ☐ ⌂ ☒ ➔ ✦ ⌘ ✓ ☞ **Leisure** hard and grass tennis courts, chipping green snooker room. **Conf** facs Corporate Hospitality Days **Location** M25 junct 17/18, off A404 to Northwood
Hotel ★★★ 75% HL The Bedford Arms Hotel, CHENIES ☎ 01923 283301 10 en suite 8 annexe en suite

Rickmansworth Public Course Moor Ln WD3 1QL
☎ 01923 775278
18 holes, 4656yds, Par 65, SSS 63.
Course Designer Colt **Location** 2m S of town off A4145
Telephone for further details
Hotel ★★★ 75% HL The Bedford Arms Hotel, CHENIES ☎ 01923 283301 10 en suite 8 annexe en suite

ROYSTON   MAP 05 TL34

Barkway Park Nuthampstead Rd, Barkway SG8 8EN
☎ 01763 849070
18 holes, 6997yds, Par 74, SSS 74.
Course Designer Vivien Saunders **Location** A10 onto B1368
Telephone for further details
Hotel ★★★ 81% HL Duxford Lodge Hotel, Ickleton Rd, DUXFORD ☎ 01223 836444 11 en suite 4 annexe en suite

Heydon Grange Golf & Country Club Heydon SG8 7NS
☎ 01763 208988 📠 01763 208926
e-mail: enquiries@heydon-grange.co.uk
web: www.heydongrange.co.uk
Three nine-hole parkland courses - the Essex, Cambridgeshire and Hertfordshire - situated in gently rolling countryside. Courses are playable all year round.

Continued

Essex: 9 holes, 2891yds, Par 36, SSS 35, Course record 64.
Cambridgeshire: 9 holes, 3057yds, Par 36, SSS 36.
Hertfordshire: 9 holes, 2937yds, Par 36, SSS 36.
Club membership 250.
Visitors Mon-Sun & BHs. Booking required Sat, Sun & BHs. Dress code.
Societies Booking required. **Green Fees** £20 per 18 holes, £14.50
per 9 holes (£25/£16.50 Sat, Sun & BHs). **Prof** Mike Snow **Course Designer**
Cameron Sinclair **Facilities** ⑪ ⅃ ⌨ ☏ ⊼ 🍴 ⚐ ✆ ⚑ ⚐ **Conf**
Corporate Hospitality Days **Location** M11 junct 10, A505 between Royston
Hotel ★★★ 81% HL Duxford Lodge Hotel, Ickleton Rd, DUXFORD
☎ 01223 836444   11 en suite   4 annexe en suite

Kingsway Cambridge Rd, Melbourn SG8 6EY
☎ 01763 262727 🖹 01763 263298
The Melbourn course is short and deceptively tricky. This nine-hole
course provides a good test for both beginners and experienced
golfers. Out of bounds and strategically placed bunkers come into
play on several holes, in particular the tough Par 3 7th. The Orchard
course is a cleverly designed Par 3 course set among trees. Ideal for
sharpening the short game or as a family introduction to golf.
Melbourn Course: 9 holes, 2455yds, Par 33, SSS 32.
Orchard Course: 9 holes, 727yds, Par 27, SSS 27.
Club membership 150.
Visitors Mon-Sun & BHs. **Societies** Welcome. **Green Fees** Phone.
Prof S Brown/D Hastings/M Sturgess **Facilities** ⑪ ⅃ ⌨ ☏ ⊼ 🍴 ⚐ ✆
⚑ **Location** Off A10
Hotel ★★★ 81% HL Duxford Lodge Hotel, Ickleton Rd, DUXFORD
☎ 01223 836444   11 en suite   4 annexe en suite

Royston Baldock Rd SG8 5BG
☎ 01763 242696 🖹 01763 246910
e-mail: roystongolf@btconnect.com
web: www.roystongolfclub.co.uk
Heathland course on undulating terrain and fine fairways. The 8th, 10th
and 15th are the most notable holes on this all weather course.
18 holes, 6052yds, Par 70, SSS 70, Course record 63.
Club membership 750.
Visitors Mon-Sun & BHs. Dress code. **Societies** Booking required. **Green
Fees** Phone. **Prof** Sean Clark **Course Designer** Harry Vardon **Facilities**
⑪ 🍴 ⅃ ⌨ ☏ ⊼ 🍴 ⚐ ✆ **Conf** facs Corporate Hospitality Days
Location 0.5m W of town centre
Hotel ★★★ 81% HL Duxford Lodge Hotel, Ickleton Rd, DUXFORD
☎ 01223 836444   11 en suite   4 annexe en suite

ST ALBANS   MAP 04 TL10

Abbey View Westminster Lodge Leisure Ctr, Holywell
Hill AL1 2DL
☎ 01727 868227 🖹 01727 848468
e-mail: abbey.view@leisureconnection.co.uk
web: www.leisureconnection.co.uk
Abbey View is a picturesque public course in the centre of the city,
suitable for beginners and those wishing to test their short game. Fine
views of the cathedral.
9 holes, 1411yds, Par 29, Course record 27.
Club membership 140.
Visitors Mon-Sun & BHs. **Societies** Booking required. **Green Fees**
£6.30 (£7.35 Sat, Sun & BHs). **Prof** Mark Flitton **Facilities** ⊼ 🍴 ⚐ ✆
Leisure hard and grass tennis courts, heated indoor swimming pool,
sauna, solarium, gymnasium, crazy golf. **Conf** Corporate Hospitality Days
Location City centre, off Holywell Hill in Verulamium Park
Hotel ★★★★ 74% HL St Michael's Manor, Fishpool St, ST ALBANS
☎ 01727 864444 30 rms (29 en suite)

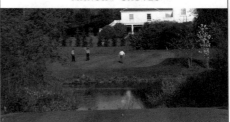

Manor of Groves Hotel, Golf & Country Club is proud to
offer an 18 hole par 71 Championship Golf Course with
US-style sandbedded greens. The course winds its way
around the Hotel and provides a true test of golfing ability.

Our resident PGA Professional is on hand to offer advice
and assistance. In addition to a well-stocked professional
shop, a wide variety of services including tuition, equipment
hire and club repairs are provided for your enjoyment.

Tel: 0870 410 8833   Fax: 0870 417 8833
email: golf@manorofgroves.co.uk
www.manorofgroves.com

Experience the difference

Batchwood Hall Batchwood Dr AL3 5XA
☎ 01727 844250 🖹 01727 858506
e-mail: batchwood@leisureconnection.co.uk
web: www.stalbans.gov.uk
18 holes, 6487yds, Par 71, SSS 71.
Course Designer J H Taylor **Location** 1m NW off A5183
Telephone for further details
Hotel ★★★★ 74% HL St Michael's Manor, Fishpool St, ST ALBANS
☎ 01727 864444 30 rms (29 en suite)

Verulam London Rd AL1 1JG
☎ 01727 853327 🖹 01727 812201
e-mail: gm@verulamgolf.co.uk
web: www.verulamgolf.co.uk
Easy walking parkland with fourteen holes having out of bounds. Water
affects the 12th, 13th and 14th holes. Samuel Ryder was captain here
in 1927 when he began the now celebrated Ryder Cup competition.
18 holes, 6448yds, Par 72, SSS 71, Course record 67.
Club membership 720.
Visitors Mon, Tue, Thu & Fri. Booking required. Handicap certificate. Dress
code. **Societies** Booking required. **Green Fees** Mon: £25 per round, Tue-
Fri: £35. **Prof** Nick Burch **Course Designer** Braid **Facilities** ⑪ 🍴 by prior
arrangement ⅃ ⌨ ☏ ⊼ 🍴 ✆ ⚑ ✆ **Conf** facs Corporate Hospitality
Days **Location** 0.5m from St Albans centre on A1081 London Rd, signed by
railway bridge
Hotel ★★★★ 76% HL Sopwell House, Cottonmill Ln, Sopwell, ST ALBANS
☎ 01727 864477 113 en suite   16 annexe en suite

SAWBRIDGEWORTH · MAP 05 TL41

Manor of Groves Golf & Country Club High Wych CM21 0JU

☎ 01279 603539 📠 01279 726972

e-mail: golf@manorofgroves.co.uk

web: www.manorofgroves.com

The course is set out over 150 acres of established parkland and rolling countryside and is a true test of golf for the club golfer.

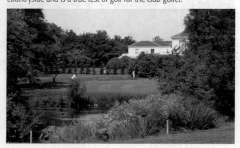

18 holes, 6228yds, Par 71, SSS 70, Course record 63.
Club membership 550.

Visitors Mon-Fri & BHs, Sat/Sun pm only. Dress code. **Societies** booking required. **Green Fees** not confirmed. **Prof** Christian Charlier **Course Designer** S Sharer **Facilities** ⏰ ⏐◎⏐ ⬛ ⬜ ⏛⏐ ⬛ ⬛ ☎ ◈ ∮
⬛ ∮ **Leisure** heated indoor swimming pool, sauna, solarium, gymnasium.
Conf Corporate Hospitality Days **Location** 1.5m west of town centre
Hotel ★★★ 78% HL Manor of Groves Hotel, High Wych,
SAWBRIDGEWORTH ☎ 01279 600777 0870 4108833 📠 01279 600374
80 en suite

See advert on page 135

STANSTEAD ABBOTTS · MAP 05 TL31

Briggens House Hotel Briggens Park, Stanstead Rd SG12 8LD

☎ 01279 793742 📠 01279 793685

web: www.corushotels.com/briggenshouse

9 holes, 2793yds, Par 36, SSS 69, Course record 31.

Location Off A414 Stanstead road

Telephone for further details

STEVENAGE · MAP 04 TL22

Stevenage Golf Centre 6 Aston Ln, Aston SG2 7EL

☎ 01438 880223 & 880424 (pro shop) 📠 01438 880040

Municipal course designed by John Jacobs, with natural water hazards and some wooded areas.

Bragbury Course: 18 holes, 6451yds, Par 72, SSS 71, Course record 63.
Aston Course: 9 holes, 880yds, Par 27, SSS 27.
Club membership 600.

Visitors Mon-Sun & BHs. Booking required. Dress code. **Societies** booking required. **Green Fees** not confirmed. **Prof** Pat Winston **Course Designer** John Jacobs **Facilities** ⏰ ⬛ ⬜ ⏛⏐ ⬛ ◈ ∮ ⏛ **Leisure** Par 3 course. **Conf** Corporate Hospitality Days **Location** 4m SE off B5169
Hotel ★★★ 68% HL Best Western The Roebuck Inn, London Rd,
Broadwater, STEVENAGE ☎ 01438 365445 54 en suite

WARE · MAP 05 TL31

Chadwell Springs Hertford Rd SG12 9LE

☎ 01920 461447 📠 01920 466596

9 holes, 6418yds, Par 72, SSS 71, Course record 68.

Location 0.75m W on A119

Telephone for further details

Hotel ★★★ 70% HL Roebuck Hotel, Baldock St, WARE ☎ 01920 409955
50 en suite

Marriott Hanbury Manor Golf & Country Club see page 137

Hotel ★★★★★ 82% HL Marriott Hanbury Manor Hotel & Country Club,
WARE ☎ 01920 487722 & 0870 400 7222 📠 01920 487692 134 en suite
27 annexe en suite
Hotel ★★★ 70% HL Roebuck Hotel, Baldock St, WARE ☎ 01920 409955
Fax 01920 468016 50 en suite

Whitehill Dane End SG12 0JS

☎ 01920 438495 📠 01920 438891

e-mail: whitehillgolf@btconnect.com

web: www.whitehillgolf.co.uk

Undulating course providing a good test for both the average golfer and the low handicapper. Several lakes in challenging positions.

18 holes, 6618yds, Par 72, SSS 72. Club membership 600.

Visitors Mon-Sun & BHs. Booking required. Dress code. **Societies** Booking required. **Green Fees** £23 Mon-Thu (£30 Fri-Sun & BHs). **Prof** Matt Belsham **Facilities** ⏰ ⏐◎⏐ ⬛ ⬜ ⏛⏐ ⬛ ☎ ∮ ◈ ∮ ⏛ **Leisure** snooker room. **Conf** Corporate Hospitality Days **Location** M25 junct 25 towards Cambridge (A10). Take turn for Ware A1170 and turn right at rdbt. After 2m turn left, proceed for 2m, course on left
Hotel ★★★ 70% HL Roebuck Hotel, Baldock St, WARE ☎ 01920 409955
50 en suite

WATFORD · MAP 04 TQ19

West Herts Cassiobury Park WD3 3GG

☎ 01923 236484 📠 01923 222300

Set in parkland, the course is close to Watford but its tree-lined setting is beautiful and tranquil. Set out on a plateau the course is exceedingly dry. It also has a very severe finish with the 17th, a hole of 378yds, the toughest on the course. The last hole measures over 480yds.

18 holes, 6620yds, Par 72, SSS 72, Course record 65.
Club membership 700.

Visitors Mon-Sun & BHs. Booking required. Dress code. **Societies** Booking required. **Green Fees** £40 per 18 holes (£50 weekends). **Prof** Charles Gough **Course Designer** Tom Morris **Facilities** ⏰ ⏐◎⏐ ⬛
⬜ ⏛⏐ ⬛ ☎ ◈ ∮ ⏛ ⬛ ∮ **Leisure** indoor teaching facility. **Conf** Corporate Hospitality Days **Location** W of town centre off A412
Hotel ★★★ 71% HL Best Western The White House, Upton Rd,
WATFORD ☎ 01923 237316 57 en suite

WELWYN GARDEN CITY · MAP 04 TL21

Mill Green Gypsy Ln AL7 4TY

☎ 01707 276900 & 270542 (Pro shop) 📠 01707 276898

e-mail: millgreen@crown-golf.co.uk

The course plays over the second 9 holes around the lakes and sweeps back through the woods. The first 9 holes are subject to the prevailing winds. The Par 3 9-hole gives a good test for improving the short game. *Continued*

CHAMPIONSHIP COURSE

HERTFORDSHIRE — WARE

MARRIOTT HANBURY MANOR

Map 05 TL31

SG12 0SD
☎ **01920 487722** 🖶 **01920 487692**
e-mail: **golf.hanburymanor@
marriotthotels.co.uk**
web: **www.hanbury-manor.com**
18 holes, 7052yds, Par 72, SSS 74,
Course record 61.
Club membership 850.
Visitors Mon-Sun & BHs. Booking required.
Handicap certificate. Must be hotel resident.
Societies welcome. **Green Fees** Phone.
Course Designer Jack Nicklaus II
Facilities ⑨ ⑩ 🝙 ⬚ 🙾 🏊 🛗 ⛳ ♢ 🛒 ✎ 🏌
Leisure hard tennis courts, heated indoor
swimming pool, sauna, solarium, gymnasium,
Health spa. **Conf** facs Corporate Hospitality
Days **Location** M25 junct 25, 12m N on A10

There can be few golf venues that combine the old and the new so successfully. The old is the site itself, dominated since the 19th century by Hanbury Manor, a Jacobean-style mansion; the wonderful grounds included a nine-hole parkland course designed by the legendary Harry Vardon. The new is the conversion of the estate into the golf and country club; the manor now offers a five-star country house hotel, while Jack Nicklaus II redesigned the grounds for an 18-hole course. The American-style design took the best of Vardon's original and added meadowland to produce a course that looks beautiful and plays superbly. Hanbury Manor has hosted a number of professional events, including the Women's European Open in 1996 and the Men's European Tour's English Open from 1997 to 1999, won respectively by Per Ulrik Johannson, Lee Westwood and Darren Clarke.

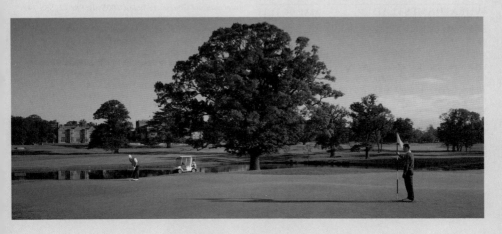

18 holes, 6615yds, Par 72, SSS 72, Course record 64.
Club membership 850.
Visitors may play Mon-Fri. Sat, Sun & BHs after noon only. Booking
required. Dress code. **Societies** Booking required. **Green Fees** Phone.
Prof Ian Parker **Course Designer** Alliss & Clark **Facilities** ⑪ ⑩ ⌵ ⌵ ⌵ ⌵
⌵ ⌵ ⌵ ⌵ ⌵ ⌵ **Leisure** 9 hole Par 3 course. **Conf** facs Corporate
Hospitality Days **Location** Exit 4 of A1(M), A414 to Mill Green
Hotel ★★★ 66% HL Quality Hotel Welwyn, The Link, WELWYN
☎ 01438 716911 96 en suite

Panshanger Golf & Squash Complex Old Herns Ln
AL7 2ED
☎ 01707 333350 📄 01707 390010
e-mail: michaelcorlass@finesseleisure.com
web: www.finesseleisure.com
Picturesque and challenging mature course overlooking Mimram
Valley. Excellent condition all year round.
18 holes, 6347yds, Par 72, SSS 70, Course record 65.
Club membership 400.
Visitors Mon-Sun & BHs. Booking required. Dress code. **Societies** booking
required. **Green Fees** not confirmed. **Prof** Bryan Lewis/Mick Corlass
Course Designer Peter Kirkham **Facilities** ⑪ ⑩ ⌵ ⌵ ⌵ ⌵ ⌵ ⌵ ⌵
⌵ **Leisure** squash, 9 hole pitch and putt. **Conf** facs Corporate Hospitality
Days **Location** 1m N of town centre signed off B1000
Hotel ★★★ 66% HL Quality Hotel Welwyn, The Link, WELWYN
☎ 01438 716911 96 en suite

Welwyn Garden City Mannicotts, High Oaks Rd
AL8 7BP
☎ 01707 325243 📄 01707 393213
e-mail: secretary@welwyngardencitygolfclub.co.uk
web: www.welwyngardencitygolfclub.co.uk
Undulating parkland with a ravine. A former Course record holder is
Nick Faldo.
18 holes, 6114yds, Par 70, SSS 69, Course record 63.
Club membership 930.
Visitors Mon-Fri except BHs. Dress code. **Societies** booking required.
Green Fees not confirmed. **Prof** Richard May **Course Designer** Hawtree
Facilities ⑪ ⑩ by prior arrangement ⌵ ⌵ ⌵ ⌵ ⌵ ⌵ ⌵ **Conf**
Corporate Hospitality Days **Location** A1 junct 6, W of city
Hotel ★★★ 66% HL Quality Hotel Welwyn, The Link, WELWYN
☎ 01438 716911 96 en suite

WHEATHAMPSTEAD   MAP 04 TL11

Mid Herts Lamer Ln, Gustard Wood AL4 8RS
☎ 01582 832242 📄 01582 834834
e-mail: secretary@mid-hertsgolfclub.co.uk
web: www.mid-hertsgolfclub.co.uk
Commonland, wooded with heather and gorse-lined fairways.
18 holes, 6060yds, Par 69, SSS 69, Course record 61.
Club membership 760.
Visitors Mon-Fri. Handicap certificate. Dress code. **Societies** Booking
required. **Green Fees** Phone. **Prof** Barney Puttick **Course Designer** James
Braid **Facilities** ⑪ ⌵ ⌵ ⌵ ⌵ ⌵ ⌵ ⌵ **Conf** facs **Location** 1m N on
B651
Hotel ★★★ 72% HL Harpenden House Hotel, 18 Southdown Rd,
HARPENDEN ☎ 01582 449955 17 en suite 59 annexe en suite

KENT

ADDINGTON   MAP 05 TQ65

West Malling London Rd ME19 5AR
☎ 01732 844785 📄 01732 844795
e-mail: mike@westmallinggolf.com
web: www.westmallinggolf.com
*Spitfire Course: 18 holes, 6142yds, Par 70, SSS 70,
Course record 67.*
*Hurricane Course: 18 holes, 6281yds, Par 70, SSS 70,
Course record 68.*
Course Designer Max Falkner **Location** 1m S off A20
Telephone for further details
Hotel ★★★ 77% HL Grange Moor Hotel, St Michael's Rd, MAIDSTONE
☎ 01622 677623 38 en suite 12 annexe en suite

ASH   MAP 05 TQ66

The London South Ash Manor Estate TN15 7EN
☎ 01474 879899 📄 01474 879912
e-mail: golf@londongolf.co.uk
web: www.londongolf.co.uk
The two courses were designed by Jack Nicklaus: both include a
number of lakes, generous fairways framed with native grasses and
many challenging holes. A state-of-the-art drainage system ensures
continuous play. Visitors may play the International course, the
Heritage is for members and their guests.

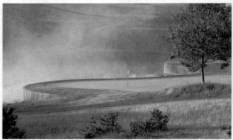

*Heritage Course: 18 holes, 7208yds, Par 72, SSS 75,
Course record 67.*
International Course: 18 holes, 7005yds, Par 72, SSS 74.
Club membership 500.
Visitors International course only. Mon-Sun & BHs. Booking required.
Handicap certificate. Dress code. **Societies** Booking required.
Green Fees International Course : £85 per round (£95 Sat, Sun & BHs).
Prof Paul Stuart **Course Designer** Jack Nicklaus **Facilities** ⑪ ⑩ ⌵ ⌵
⌵ ⌵ ⌵ ⌵ ⌵ ⌵ ⌵ **Leisure** sauna, spa bath. **Conf** facs Corporate
Hospitality Days **Location** A20, 2m from Brands Hatch
Hotel ★★★★ 80% HL Brandshatch Place Hotel & Spa, Brands Hatch
Rd, Fawkham, BRANDS HATCH ☎ 01474 875000 26 en suite 12 annexe
en suite

ASHFORD
MAP 05 TR04

Ashford (Kent) Sandyhurst Ln TN25 4NT
☎ 01233 622655
e-mail: secretary@ashfordgolfclub.co.uk
web: www.ashfordgolfclub.co.uk
Parkland with good views and easy walking. Narrow fairways and
tightly bunkered greens ensure a challenging game for all levels of
golfer.
18 holes, 6263yds, Par 71, SSS 70, Course record 65.
Club membership 672.
Visitors Mon-Sun & BHs. Booking required. Handicap certificate. Dress
code. **Societies** booking required. **Green Fees** not confirmed. ◉
Prof Hugh Sherman **Course Designer** Cotton **Facilities** ⑪ ⤮ ☐ ⋔ ⚑ ⚏
⛁ ✔ ⚏ ✔ **Conf** facs Corporate Hospitality Days **Location** 1m NW M20
junct 9
Hotel ★★★★ 76% HL Ashford International, Simone Weil Av, ASHFORD
☎ 01233 219988 179 en suite

Homelands Golf Centre Ashford Rd, Kingsnorth
TN26 1NJ
☎ 01233 661620
e-mail: info@ashfordgolf.co.uk
web: www.ashfordgolf.co.uk
Challenging nine-hole course designed by Donald Steel to provide
a stern test for experienced golfers and for others to develop their
game. With four Par 3s and five Par 4s it demands accuracy rather than
length. Floodlit driving range.
9 holes, 2205yds, Par 32, SSS 31, Course record 32.
Club membership 400.
Visitors Mon-Sun & BHs. Booking required. Dress code.
Societies Booking required. **Green Fees** Phone. **Prof** Howard Bonaccorsi
Course Designer Donald Steel **Facilities** ⑪ ⑩ ⤮ ☐ ⋔ ⚑ ⛁ ⚏
✔ ⚐ **Location** M20 junct 10, A2070, signed from 2nd rdbt to Kingsnorth
Hotel BUD Premier Travel Inn Ashford Central, Hall Av, Orbital Park,
Sevington, ASHFORD ☎ 08701 977305 60 en suite

BARHAM
MAP 05 TR25

Broome Park The Broome Park Estate CT4 6QX
☎ 01227 830728 🗎 01227 832591
e-mail: golf@broomepark.co.uk
web: www.broomepark.co.uk
Championship-standard parkland course in a valley, with a 350-year-
old mansion clubhouse.
18 holes, 6580yds, Par 72, SSS 71, Course record 66.
Club membership 700.
Visitors may play Mon-Sun & BHs. Booking required. Dress code. **Societies**
Booking required **Green Fees** £40 per round (£50 weekends). **Prof** Tienne
Britz **Course Designer** Donald Steel **Facilities** ⑪ ⑩ ⤮ ☐ ⋔ ⚑ ⛁ ⚏ ✔
⚏ ✔ ⚐ **Leisure** hard tennis courts. **Conf** facs Corporate Hospitality Days
Location 1.5m SE on A260
Hotel ★★★ 88% HL Best Western Abbots Barton Hotel, New Dover Rd,
CANTERBURY ☎ 01227 760341 50 en suite

BEARSTED
MAP 05 TQ85

Bearsted Ware St ME14 4PQ
☎ 01622 738198 🗎 01622 735608
Parkland with fine views of the North Downs.
18 holes, 6437yds, Par 72, SSS 71. Club membership 780.

Visitors Mon-Sun except BHs. Booking required. Handicap certificate. Dress
code. **Societies** booking required. **Green Fees** not confirmed. ◉ **Prof** Tim
Simpson **Facilities** ⑪ ⑩ ⤮ ☐ ⋔ ⚑ ⛁ ⚏ ✔ **Location** M20 junct 7, right
at rdbt, left at minirdbt, left at 2nd minirdbt. Pass Bell pub on right, under
bridge, on left
Hotel ★★★★ 77% HL Marriott Tudor Park Hotel & Country Club, Ashford
Rd, Bearsted, MAIDSTONE ☎ 01622 734334 120 en suite

BIDDENDEN
MAP 05 TQ83

Chart Hills Weeks Ln TN27 8JX
☎ 01580 292222 🗎 01580 292233
e-mail: info@charthills.co.uk
web: www.charthills.co.uk
Created by Nick Faldo, he has truly left his mark on this course.
Signature features include the 200-yard long snake-like Anaconda
Bunker (one of 138) on the 5th and the island green at the short 17th.
18 holes, 7119yds, Par 72, SSS 74, Course record 61.
Club membership 500.
Visitors Mon-Sun & BHs. Booking required. Handicap certificate. Dress
code. **Societies** Booking required.| **Green Fees** Phone. **Prof** James Cornish
Course Designer Nick Faldo **Facilities** ⑪ ⑩ ⤮ ☐ ⋔ ⚑ ⛁ ⚏ ✔ ⚏ ✔
⚐ **Leisure** fishing. **Conf** facs Corporate Hospitality Days **Location** 1m N of
Biddenden off A274
Hotel ★★★ 78% HL Best Western London Beach Hotel & Golf Club,
Ashford Rd, TENTERDEN ☎ 01580 766279 26 en suite

BOROUGH GREEN
MAP 05 TQ65

Wrotham Heath Seven Mile Ln TN15 8QZ
☎ 01732 884800 🗎 01732 887370
18 holes, 5954yds, Par 70, SSS 69, Course record 66.
Course Designer Donald Steel (part) **Location** 2.25m E on B2016
Telephone for further details
Hotel BUD Premier Travel Inn Sevenoaks/Maidstone, London Rd, Wrotham
Heath, WROTHAM ☎ 08701 977227 40 en suite

BRENCHLEY
MAP 05 TQ64

Kent National Golf & Country Club Watermans Ln
TN12 6ND
☎ 01892 724400 🗎 01892 723300
e-mail: info@kentnational.com
web: www.kentnational.com
A rolling parkland course with dramatic views over the Weald of Kent.
The challenging holes are the Par 4 8th with its tough dog-leg, the 10th
where there is a wooded copse with a Victorian bath-house to be
avoided, and the 14th where the approach to the green is guarded by
oak trees.
18 holes, 6693yds, Par 72, SSS 72, Course record 63.
Club membership 620.
Visitors Mon-Sun & BHs. Booking required. Dress code. **Societies** booking
required. **Green Fees** not confirmed. **Prof** Gary Stewart **Course Designer**
T Saito **Facilities** ⑪ ⑩ ⤮ ☐ ⋔ ⚑ ⛁ ⚏ ✔ ⚏ ✔ ⚐ **Leisure** hard tennis
courts. **Conf** facs Corporate Hospitality Days **Location** 3m N of Brenchley
off B2160
Hotel ★★ 64% MET Russell Hotel, 80 London Rd, TUNBRIDGE WELLS
☎ 01892 544833 21 en suite 5 annexe en suite

BROADSTAIRS
MAP 05 TR36

North Foreland Convent Rd, Kingsgate CT10 3PU
☎ 01843 862140 🖺 01843 862663
e-mail: office@northforeland.co.uk
web: www.northforeland.co.uk
A picturesque cliff top course situated where the Thames Estuary widens towards the sea. One of the few courses where the sea can be seen from every hole. Walking is easy and the wind is deceptive. The 8th and 17th, both Par 4, are testing holes. There is also an 18-hole approach and putting course.
18 holes, 6430yds, Par 71, SSS 71, Course record 63.
Club membership 1100.
Visitors Mon-Fri except BHs. Sat & Sun pm only. Handicap certificate. Dress code. **Societies** Booking required. **Green Fees** £51 per day; £34 per round (£76/51 Sat & Sun). Par 3 course £8 (£9.50 Sat & Sun). **Prof** Darren Parris **Course Designer** Fowler & Simpson **Facilities** ⑪ 🍴 ⓑ 🖵 🍴 🏖 🗕 ⛿ 🏌 🏌 **Leisure** hard tennis courts, 18 hole Par 3 course. **Conf** Corporate Hospitality Days **Location** 1.5m N off B2052

CANTERBURY
MAP 05 TR15

Canterbury Scotland Hills, Littlebourne Rd CT1 1TW
☎ 01227 462865 🖺 01227 784277
e-mail: secretary@canterburygolfclub.co.uk
Undulating parkland, densely wooded in places, with elevated tees and challenging drives on several holes.

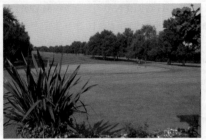

18 holes, 6272yds, Par 71, SSS 70, Course record 64.
Club membership 700.
Visitors Mon-Sun except BHs. Booking required. Handicap certificate. Dress code. **Societies** Booking required. **Green Fees** £48 per day, £38 per round (£58/£48 weekends). **Prof** Paul Everard **Course Designer** Harry Colt **Facilities** ⑪ 🍴 ⓑ 🖵 🍴 🏖 🗕 ⛿ 🏌 🏌 **Conf** facs Corporate Hospitality Days **Location** 1.5m E on A257
Hotel ★★★ 88% HL Best Western Abbots Barton Hotel, New Dover Rd, CANTERBURY ☎ 01227 760341 50 en suite

CHART SUTTON
MAP 05 TQ84

The Ridge Chartway St, East Sutton ME17 3DL
☎ 01622 844382
18 holes, 6254yds, Par 71, SSS 70, Course record 68.
Course Designer Tyton Design **Location** 5m S of Bearsted off A274
Telephone for further details
Hotel ★★★★ 77% HL Marriott Tudor Park Hotel & Country Club, Ashford Rd, Bearsted, MAIDSTONE ☎ 01622 734334 120 en suite

CRANBROOK
MAP 05 TQ73

Hemsted Forest Golford Rd TN17 4AL
☎ 01580 712833 🖺 01580 714274
e-mail: golf@hemstedforest.co.uk
web: www.hemstedforest.co.uk
Scenic parkland with easy terrain, backed by Hemstead Forest. The course lies in a beautiful natural setting and offers a tranquil haven. The clubhouse, a converted oast, is the only one of its kind.
18 holes, 6305yds, Par 70, SSS 71, Course record 64.
Club membership 1500.
Visitors Tue-Sun & BHs. Booking required. Dress code. **Societies** Booking required. **Green Fees** £28 per round (£40 weekends). **Prof** Chris Weston **Course Designer** Commander J Harris **Facilities** ⑪ 🍴 ⓑ 🖵 🍴 🏖 🗕 ⛿ 🏌 **Conf** facs Corporate Hospitality Days **Location** 2m E
Hotel ★★★ 78% HL Best Western London Beach Hotel & Golf Club, Ashford Rd, TENTERDEN ☎ 01580 766279 26 en suite

DARTFORD
MAP 05 TQ57

Birchwood Park Birchwood Rd, Wilmington DA2 7HJ
☎ 01322 662038 & 660554 🖺 01322 667283
e-mail: info@birchwoodparkgc.co.uk
web: www.birchwoodparkgc.co.uk
The main course offers highly challenging play and will test golfers of all abilities. Beginners and those requiring a quick game or golfers wishing to improve their short game will appreciate the Orchard course where holes range from 96 to 258yds.
Parkland: 18 holes, 6364yds, Par 71, SSS 70,
Course record 64.
Orchard: 9 holes, 1349yds, Par 29. Club membership 600.
Visitors Mon-Sun & BHs. Week advance booking. Dress code. **Societies** welcome. **Green Fees** not confirmed. **Course Designer** Howard Swann **Facilities** ⑪ 🍴 ⓑ 🖵 🍴 🏖 🗕 ⛿ 🏌 🏌 **Leisure** sauna, solarium, gymnasium. **Conf** facs Corporate Hospitality Days **Location** B258 between Dartford & Swanley
Hotel ★★★★ 77% HL Bexleyheath Marriott Hotel, 1 Broadway, BEXLEYHEATH ☎ 020 8298 1000 142 en suite

Dartford Heath Ln (Upper), Dartford Heath DA1 2TN
☎ 01322 226455 🖺 01322 226455
e-mail: dartfordgolf@hotmail.com
Challenging parkland course with tight fairways and easy walking.
18 holes, 5909yds, Par 69, SSS 69, Course record 61.
Club membership 700.
Visitors Mon-Fri. Handicap certificate. Dress code. **Societies** Booking required. **Green Fees** £25 per 18 holes. ⊕ **Prof** John Gregory **Course Designer** James Braid **Facilities** ⑪ 🍴 ⓑ 🖵 🍴 🏖 🗕 **Conf** Corporate Hospitality Days **Location** 2m from town centre off A2
Hotel BUD Campanile, 1 Clipper Boulevard West, Crossways Business Park, DARTFORD ☎ 01322 278925 125 en suite

DEAL
MAP 05 TR35

Royal Cinque Ports Golf Rd CT14 6RF
☎ 01304 374007 🖺 01304 379530
e-mail: rcpgcsec@aol.com
web: www.royalcinqueports.com
18 holes, 6899yds, Par 72, SSS 73.
Course Designer James Braid **Location** On seafront at N end of Deal
Telephone for further details

Continued

Hotel ★★★ 82% HL Wallett's Court Country House Hotel & Spa, West Cliffe, St Margarets-at-Cliffe, DOVER ☎ 01304 852424 & 0800 0351628 📠 01304 853430 3 en suite 13 annexe en suite

EDENBRIDGE   MAP 05 TQ44

Sweetwoods Park Cowden TN8 7JN
☎ 01342 850729 (Pro shop) 📠 01342 850866
e-mail: danhowe@sweetwoodspark.com
web: www.sweetwoodspark.com
An undulating and mature parkland course with very high quality greens, testing water hazards and fine views across the Weald from four holes. A good challenge off the back tees. Signature holes include the 2nd, 4th and 14th.

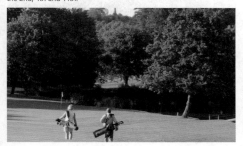

18 holes, 6617yds, Par 72, SSS 72, Course record 63.
Club membership 700.
Visitors Mon-Sun & BHs. Dress code. **Societies** Booking required. **Green Fees** £30 per round (£36 weekends and bank holidays). **Prof** Paul Lyons
Course Designer P Strand **Facilities** ⑪ ⑩ ⴱ ⯅ ⯑ ⱱ 🍴 ⯅ ⯑ ♦ ✔ 🍴
✔ ✈ **Leisure** Sussex College of Golf. **Conf** facs Corporate Hospitality Days
Location 4m E of East Grinstead on A264
Hotel ★★★ HL Gravetye Manor Hotel, EAST GRINSTEAD ☎ 01342 810567 18 en suite

EYNSFORD   MAP 05 TQ56

Austin Lodge Upper Austin Lodge Rd DA4 0HU
☎ 01322 863000 📠 01322 862406
e-mail: linda@pentlandgolf.co.uk
web: www.pentlandgolf.co.uk
A well-drained course designed to lie naturally in three secluded valleys in rolling countryside. Over 7000yds from the medal tees. Practice ground, nets and a putting green add to the features.
18 holes, 7026yds, Par 73, SSS 71, Course record 68.
Club membership 400.
Visitors Mon-Fri & BHs, Sat/Sun pm only. Booking required. Dress code.
Societies booking required. **Green Fees** not confirmed. **Prof** Martin Windsor **Course Designer** P Bevan **Facilities** ⑪ ⑩ ⴱ ⯅ ⯑ 🍴 ⯅ ⯑ ✔
🍴 ✔ ✈ **Location** 6m S of Dartford
Hotel ★★★★ 80% HL Brandshatch Place Hotel & Spa, Brands Hatch Rd, Fawkham, BRANDS HATCH ☎ 01474 875000 26 en suite 12 annexe en suite

FAVERSHAM   MAP 05 TR06

Boughton Brickfield Ln, Boughton ME13 9AJ
☎ 01227 752277 📠 01227 752361
e-mail: greg@pentlandgolf.co.uk
web: www.pentlandgolf.co.uk
Rolling parkland and downland course set in 160 acres of Kent countryside, providing a good test of golf, even for the more accomplished players.
18 holes, 6469yds, Par 72, SSS 71, Course record 68.
Club membership 500.
Visitors Mon-Sun & BHs. Booking required. Dress code. **Societies** booking required. **Green Fees** not confirmed. **Prof** Greg Haenen/Trevor Dungate
Course Designer P Sparks **Facilities** ⑪ ⑩ ⴱ ⯅ ⯑ 🍴 ⯅ ⯑ ✔ 🍴 ✔ 🍴
Location M2 junct 7, Brenley Corner
Hotel ★★★★ HL Eastwell Manor, Eastwell Park, Boughton Lees, ASHFORD ☎ 01233 213000 23 en suite 39 annexe en suite

Faversham Belmont Park ME13 0HB
☎ 01795 890561 📠 01795 890760
e-mail: themanager@favershamgolf.co.uk
web: www.favershamgolf.co.uk
A beautiful inland course laid out over part of a large estate with pheasants walking the fairways quite tamely. Play follows two heavily wooded valleys but the trees affect only the loose shots going out of bounds. Fine views.

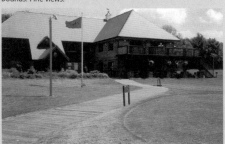

18 holes, 5978yds, Par 70, SSS 69, Course record 62.
Club membership 800.
Visitors Mon-Fri & BHs. Booking required. Dress code. **Societies** Welcome. **Green Fees** £35 per round. ⊛ **Prof** Stuart Rokes **Course Designer** J H Taylor/D Steel **Facilities** ⑪ ⑩ ⴱ ⯅ ⯑ 🍴 ⯅ ⯑ ✔ 🍴 ✔
Conf Corporate Hospitality Days **Location** 3.5m S on Belmont road
Hotel ★★★★ HL Eastwell Manor, Eastwell Park, Boughton Lees, ASHFORD ☎ 01233 213000 23 en suite 39 annexe en suite

FOLKESTONE   MAP 05 TR23

Etchinghill Canterbury Rd, Etchinghill CT18 8FA
☎ 01303 863863 📠 01303 863210
e-mail: deb@pentlandgolf.co.uk
web: www.pentlandgolf.co.uk
A varied course incorporating parkland and an interesting downland landscape with many challenging holes on the back nine.
27 holes, 6101yds, Par 70, SSS 69, Course record 67.
Club membership 600.
Visitors Mon-Sun & BHs. Handicap certificate. Dress code. **Societies** Booking required. **Green Fees** Phone. **Prof** Roger Dowle/Steve Watkins
Course Designer John Sturdy **Facilities** ⑪ ⑩ ⴱ ⯅ ⯑ 🍴 ⯅ ⯑ ✔ 🍴 ✔
✈ **Leisure** 9 hole par3. **Conf** facs **Location** M20 junct 11/12
Hotel ★★★ 75% HL Best Western Clifton Hotel, The Leas, FOLKESTONE ☎ 01303 851231 80 en suite

GILLINGHAM
MAP 05 TQ76

Gillingham Woodlands Rd ME7 2AP
☎ 01634 853017 (office) 🖹 01634 574749
e-mail: golf@gillinghamgolf.idps.co.uk
web: www.gillinghamgolfclub.co.uk
Mature parkland course with views of the estuary.
18 holes, 5495yds, Par 69, SSS 66, Course record 64.
Club membership 900.
Visitors Mon, Wed & Fri. Handicap certificate. Dress code.
Societies Booking required. **Green Fees** £28 per day, £20 per round. 🌐
Prof Andrew Brooks **Course Designer** James Braid/Steel **Facilities** ⑪ ⑩ ⬛ ▱ 🍴 🔄 △ 🛇 ⛳ ✔ **Conf** facs Corporate Hospitality Days **Location** 1.5m SE on A2
Hotel BUD Premier Travel Inn Gillingham, Kent, Will Adams Way, GILLINGHAM ☎ 08701 977105 45 en suite

GRAVESEND
MAP 05 TQ67

Mid Kent Singlewell Rd DA11 7RB
☎ 01474 568035 🖹 01474 564218
e-mail: secretary@mkgc.co.uk
web: www.mkgc.co.uk
A well-maintained downland course with some easy walking and some excellent greens. The first hole is short, but nonetheless a real challenge. The slightest hook and the ball is out of bounds or lost.
18 holes, 6106yds, Par 70, SSS 69, Course record 60.
Club membership 900.
Visitors Mon-Fri except BHs. Handicap certificate. Dress code. **Societies** Welcome. **Green Fees** £50 per day; £35 per round. 🌐 **Prof** Mark Foreman **Course Designer** Frank Pennick **Facilities** ⑪ ⑩ by prior arrangement ⬛ ▱ 🍴 △ 🛇 ✔ ⛳ **Leisure** snooker. **Location** S of town centre off A227
Hotel BUD Premier Travel Inn Gravesend, Wrotham Rd, GRAVESEND ☎ 08701 977118 36 en suite

Southern Valley Thong Ln, Shorne DA12 4LF
☎ 01474 568568 🖹 01474 360366
e-mail: info@southernvalley.co.uk
web: www.southernvalley.co.uk
All year playing conditions on a course landscaped with gorse, bracken and thorn and designed to enhance the views across the Thames Estuary. The course features undulating greens, large trees and rolling fairways with the 9th and 18th holes located close to the clubhouse.
18 holes, 6200yds, Par 69, SSS 69, Course record 62.
Club membership 450.
Visitors Mon-Sun & BHs. Booking required. Dress code. **Societies** booking required. **Green Fees** not confirmed. **Prof** Larry Batchelor **Course Designer** Weller/Richardson **Facilities** ⑪ ⑩ ⬛ ▱ 🍴 △ 🛇 ✔ ⛳ **Conf** facs Corporate Hospitality Days **Location** A2 junct 4, off slip-road left onto Thong Ln, continue 1m
Hotel ★★★ 77% HL Best Western Manor Hotel, Hever Court Rd, GRAVESEND ☎ 01474 353100 59 en suite

HALSTEAD
MAP 05 TQ46

Broke Hill Sevenoaks Rd TN14 7HR
☎ 01959 533225 🖹 01959 532680
e-mail: bhgc@crown-golf.co.uk
web: www.crown-golf.co.uk/brokehill
A challenging game awaits all golfers. The fairways have strategically placed bunkers, some of which come into play off the tee. Five holes

have water hazards including the 18th where a lake has to be carried to get onto the green. Recent design changes have made it one of the most challenging finishing holes in Kent.

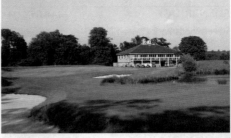

Broke Hill

18 holes, 6469yds, Par 72, SSS 71, Course record 65.
Club membership 480.
Visitors Mon-Sun & BHs. Booking required Fri-Sun & BHs. Dress code.
Societies Booking required. **Green Fees** Mon-Thu £35, Fri £40, Sat & Sun £50, BHs £40. **Prof** Iain Naylor **Course Designer** David Williams **Facilities** ⑪ ⑩ ⬛ ▱ 🍴 △ 🛇 ⚑ ✔ 🛒 🏌 **Leisure** sauna. **Conf** facs Corporate Hospitality Days **Location** M25 junct 4, opp Knockholt station
Hotel ★★★ 75% HL Best Western Donnington Manor, London Rd, Dunton Green, SEVENOAKS ☎ 01732 462681 60 en suite

HAWKHURST
MAP 05 TQ73

Hawkhurst High St TN18 4JS
☎ 01580 754074 & 752396 🖹 01580 754074
e-mail: hawkhurstgolfclub@tiscali.co.uk
web: hawkhurstgolfclub.org.uk
Undulating parkland.
9 holes, 5751yds, Par 70, SSS 68, Course record 69.
Club membership 450.
Visitors Mon, Wed, Fri except BHs. Booking required. Dress code **Societies** booking required. **Green Fees** not confirmed. **Prof** Mike Barton **Course Designer** W A Baldock **Facilities** ⑪ ⑩ ⬛ ▱ 🍴 △ 🛇 ✔ **Leisure** squash, squash. **Conf** facs **Location** W of village off A268
Hotel ★★★ 78% HL Best Western London Beach Hotel & Golf Club, Ashford Rd, TENTERDEN ☎ 01580 766279 26 en suite

HEADCORN
MAP 05 TQ84

Weald of Kent Maidstone Rd TN27 9PT
☎ 01622 890866 🖹 01622 890070
e-mail: info@weald-of-kent.co.uk
Enjoying delightful views over the Weald, this pay and play course features a range of natural hazards, including lakes, trees, ditches and undulating fairways. A good test to golfers of every standard.
18 holes, 6240yds, Par 70, SSS 70, Course record 67.
Club membership 350.
Visitors Mon-Sun & BHs. Dress code. **Societies** Welcome **Green Fees** Phone. **Prof** Paul Fosten **Course Designer** John Millen **Facilities** ⑪ ⑩ ⬛ ▱ 🍴 △ 🛇 ⚑ ◇ ✔ ⛳ **Leisure** training academy. **Conf** facs Corporate Hospitality Days **Location** M20 junct 8, through Leeds village, A274 towards Headcorn, course on left
Hotel ★★★★ 77% HL Marriott Tudor Park Hotel & Country Club, Ashford Rd, Bearsted, MAIDSTONE ☎ 01622 734334 120 en suite

HERNE BAY MAP 05 TR16

Herne Bay Eddington CT6 7PG
☎ 01227 374727
18 holes, 5567yds, Par 68, SSS 68.
Course Designer James Braid **Location** On junct A291
Telephone for further details
Hotel ★★★ 88% HL Best Western Abbots Barton Hotel, New Dover Rd,
CANTERBURY ☎ 01227 760341 50 en suite

HEVER MAP 05 TQ44

Hever Castle Hever Rd, Edenbridge TN8 7NP
☎ 01732 700771 📄 01732 700775
e-mail: mail@hevercastlegolfclub.co.uk
web: www.hevercastlegolfclub.co.uk
Originally part of the Hever Castle estate, set in 250 acres of Kentish
countryside, the Kings and Queens championship course has
matured well and, with the addition of the Princes' nine holes, offers
stunning holes to challenge all golfers. Water plays a prominent
part in the design of the course, particularly around Amen Corner,
holes 11 through 13. The golfer is then met with the lengthy stretch
home, especially up the 17th, a daunting 644yd Par 5, one of Europe's
longest.
Kings & Queens Course: 18 holes, 6761yds, Par 72, SSS 73,
Course record 69.
Princes Course: 9 holes, 2784yds, Par 35.
Club membership 450.
Visitors Mon-Sun & BHs. Booking required. Dress code. **Societies** Booking
required. **Green Fees** KIngs & Queens Course £38.50 summer, £27 winter.
Princes Course £10.50. **Prof** Peter Parks **Course Designer** Dr Nicholas
Facilities ⊕ ⚑ ⮯ ☕ ♨ ☆ ♿ 🏌 **Conf** facs Corporate
Hospitality Days **Location** Off B269 between Oxted and Tonbridge, 0.5m
from Hever Castle
Hotel ★★★★ 74% HL The Spa Hotel, Mount Ephraim, TUNBRIDGE
WELLS ☎ 01892 520331 69 en suite

HILDENBOROUGH MAP 05 TQ54

Nizels Nizels Ln TN11 9LU
☎ 01732 838926 (Bookings) 📄 01732 833764
e-mail: nizels.retail@clubhaus.com
18 holes, 6408yds, Par 72, SSS 71, Course record 65.
Course Designer Donaldson/Edwards Partnership **Location** Off B245
Telephone for further details
Hotel ★★★ 70% HL Best Western Rose & Crown Hotel, 125 High St,
TONBRIDGE ☎ 01732 357966 54 en suite

HOO MAP 05 TQ77

Deangate Ridge Dux Court Rd ME3 8RZ
☎ 01634 251180 📄 01634 250537
Parkland, municipal course designed by Fred Hawtree. 18-hole pitch
and putt.
18 holes, 6300yds, Par 71, SSS 70, Course record 65.
Club membership 500.
Visitors Mon-Sun & BHs. Booking required. Dress code. **Societies**
Welcome. **Green Fees** Phone. **Prof** Richard Fox **Course Designer** Hawtree
Facilities ⊕ ⚑ ⮯ ☕ ♨ ☆ ⛳ ☆ ♿ 🏌 **Leisure** hard tennis courts,
gymnasium. **Location** 4m NE of Rochester off A228
Hotel ★★★★ 74% HL Bridgewood Manor, Bridgewood Roundabout,
Walderslade Woods, CHATHAM ☎ 01634 201333 100 en suite

HYTHE MAP 05 TR13

Hythe Imperial Princes Pde CT21 6AE
☎ 01303 267441 📄 01303 264610
e-mail: hytheimperial@qhotels.co.uk
web: www.qhotels.co.uk
A nine-hole 18-tee links course bounded by the Royal Military Canal
and the English Channel. Although the course is relatively flat, its aspect
offers an interesting and challenging round to a wide range of golfers.
9 holes, 5560yds, Par 68, SSS 66, Course record 62.
Club membership 300.
Visitors Contact hotel for details. Handicap certificate. Dress code.
Societies Welcome. **Green Fees** Phone. **Facilities** ⊕ ⚑ ⮯ ☕ ♨ ☆ ♿ 🍽
⛳ ◇ ♿ **Leisure** hard and grass tennis courts, heated indoor swimming
pool, squash, sauna, solarium, gymnasium, snooker. **Conf** facs Corporate
Hospitality Days **Location** Exit M20 junct 11. Follow into Hythe towards the
town centre. Turn right into Twiss Road. Golf course is in grounds of the
Hythe Imperial
Hotel ★★★★ 75% HL The Hythe Imperial, Princes Pde, HYTHE
☎ 01303 267441 100 en suite

Sene Valley Sene CT18 8BL
☎ 01303 268513 (Manager) 📄 01303 237513
e-mail: senevalleygolf@bt.connect.com
web: www.senevalleygolfclub.co.uk
A two-level downland course, standing 350 feet above the town and
providing interesting golf over an undulating landscape with sea
views. A typical hole that challenges most players, is the Par 3, 11th
which combines a stunning sea view with a testing tee shot to a green
surrounded by bunkers and gorse.
18 holes, 6271yds, Par 71, SSS 70, Course record 65.
Club membership 700.
Visitors Mon-Fri except BHs. Booking required. Dress code. **Societies**
Welcome. **Green Fees** £30 weekdays. Winter rates available. **Prof** Nick
Watson **Course Designer** Henry Cotton **Facilities** ⊕ ⚑ ⮯ ☕ ♨ ☆
⛳ ☆ ♿ **Conf** Corporate Hospitality Days **Location** M20 junct 12, A20
towards Ashford for 3m, left at rdbt, Hythe Rd for 1m
Hotel ★★★ 71% HL Best Western Stade Court, West Pde, HYTHE
☎ 01303 268263 42 en suite

KINGSDOWN MAP 05 TR34

Walmer & Kingsdown The Leas CT14 8EP
☎ 01304 373256 📄 01304 382336
e-mail: info@kingsdowngolf.co.uk
web: www.kingsdowngolf.co.uk
This beautiful downland site is situated near Deal and, being situated
on top of the famous White Cliffs, offers breathtaking views of the
Channel from every hole.

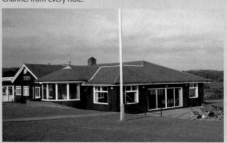

Continued

18 holes, 6471yds, Par 72, SSS 71, Course record 66.
Club membership 640.
Visitors Mon-Fri. Sat, Sun & BHs pm only. Booking required. Handicap
certificate. Dress code. **Societies** Welcome. **Green Fees** £40 per
day; £32 per round (£40 per round Sat, Sun & BHs). **Prof** Jude Read
Course Designer James Braid **Facilities** ⚙🎱🍺🍴🏌🍽🚪🅿🏐🏸
Conf Corporate Hospitality Days **Location** 1.5m E of Ringwould off A258
Dover-Deal road
Hotel ★★★ 74% HL Dunkerleys Hotel & Restaurant, 19 Beach St, DEAL
☎ 01304 375016 16 en suite

LAMBERHURST　　　　MAP 05 TQ63

Lamberhurst Church Rd TN3 8DT
☎ 01892 890591 📄 01892 891140
e-mail: secretary@lamberhurstgolfclub.com
web: www.lamberhurstgolfclub.com
Parkland course crossing the river twice. Fine views.
18 holes, 6423yds, Par 72, SSS 71, Course record 65.
Club membership 650.
Visitors Mon-Fri except BHs. Sat & Sun pm only. Handicap certificate.
Dress code. **Societies** Booking required. **Green Fees** £43 per day, £33
per round. **Prof** Brian Impett **Facilities** ⚙🎱🍺🍴🏌🍽🚪🅿🏐🏸
Conf Corporate Hospitality Days **Location** N of village on B2162
Hotel ★★★★ 74% HL The Spa Hotel, Mount Ephraim, TUNBRIDGE
WELLS ☎ 01892 520331 69 en suite

LITTLESTONE　　　　MAP 05 TR02

Littlestone St Andrew's Rd TN28 8RB
☎ 01797 363355 📄 01797 362740
e-mail: secretary@littlestonegolfclub.org.uk
web: www.littlestonegolfclub.org.uk
Located in the Romney Marshes, this fairly flat seaside links course
calls for every variety of shot. The 8th, 15th, 16th and 17th are
regarded as classics by international golfers. Fast running fairways
and faster greens.
18 holes, 6486yds, Par 71, SSS 72, Course record 66.
Club membership 550.
Visitors Mon-Fri. Booking required. Handicap certificate. Dress code.
Societies booking required. **Green Fees** not confirmed. **Prof** Andrew
Jones **Course Designer** Laidlaw Purves **Facilities** ⚙🍺🍴🏌🍽🚪
🏐🏸🏸 **Leisure** hard tennis courts. **Conf** Corporate Hospitality Days
Location 1m from New Romney off Littlestone road B2070
Hotel ★★★★ 75% HL The Hythe Imperial, Princes Pde, HYTHE
☎ 01303 267441 100 en suite

Romney Warren St Andrews Rd TN28 8RB
☎ 01797 362231 📄 01797 363511
e-mail: info@romneywarrengolfclub.org.uk
web: www.littlestonegolfclub.org.uk
A links-style course, normally very dry. Flat providing easy walking
and play challenged by sea breezes. Although not overly long, narrow
fairways and small greens place a premium on shot selection and
placement.
18 holes, 5126yds, Par 67, SSS 65, Course record 63.
Club membership 300.
Visitors Mon-Sun & BHs. Booking required. Dress code. **Societies** booking
required. **Green Fees** not confirmed. **Prof** Andrew Jones **Course Designer**
Evans/Lewis **Facilities** ⚙🎱🍺🍴🏌🍽🚪🏐🏸 **Location** N of
Littlestone centre
Hotel ★★★★ 75% HL The Hythe Imperial, Princes Pde, HYTHE
☎ 01303 267441 100 en suite

LYDD　　　　MAP 05 TR02

Lydd Romney Rd TN29 9LS
☎ 01797 320808 📄 01797 321482
e-mail: info@lyddgolfclub.co.uk
web: www.lyddgolfclub.co.uk
A links-type course on marshland, offering some interesting challenges,
including a number of eye-catching water hazards, wide fairways and
plenty of semi-rough. A constant breeze makes club selection difficult.
A good test for experienced golfers and an appealing course to the
complete novice.

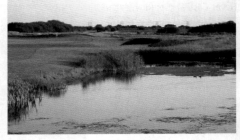

18 holes, 6529yds, Par 71, SSS 71, Course record 65.
Club membership 400.
Visitors Mon-Sun & BHs. Booking required. Dress code. **Societies** Booking
required. **Green Fees** £21 per round (£30 Sat & Sun). **Prof** Richard J
Perkins **Course Designer** Mike Smith **Facilities** ⚙🍺🍴🏌🍽🚪🏐🏸
🏸🏸 **Leisure** 6 hole Academy course. **Conf** facs Corporate Hospitality
Days **Location** A259 onto B2075 by Lydd Airport
Hotel ★★★★ 80% HL The George in Rye, 98 High St, RYE
☎ 01797 222114 24 en suite

MAIDSTONE　　　　MAP 05 TQ75

Cobtree Manor Park Chatham Rd, Sandling ME14 3AZ
☎ 01622 753276 📄 01622 620387
e-mail: sales@medwaygolf.co.uk
web: www.medwaygolf.co.uk
Undulating parkland with some water hazards.
18 holes, 5611yds, Par 69, SSS 69, Course record 66.
Club membership 400.
Visitors Mon-Sun & BHs. Booking required. Dress code. **Societies** Booking
required. **Green Fees** Phone. **Prof** Paul Foston **Course Designer** Lawtree
Facilities ⚙🎱🍺🍴🏌🍽🚪🏐🏸 **Conf** facs Corporate Hospitality
Days **Location** M20 junct 6, 0.25m N on A229
Hotel ★★★ 79% HL Best Western Russell Hotel, 136 Boxley Rd,
MAIDSTONE ☎ 01622 692221 42 en suite

Leeds Castle Ashford Rd ME17 1PL
☎ 01622 767828 & 880467 📄 01622 735616
e-mail: stevepurves@leeds-castle.co.uk
web: www.leeds-castle.co.uk
Situated around Leeds Castle, this is one of the most picturesque
courses in Britain. Redesigned in the 1980s by Neil Coles, it is a
challenging nine-hole course with the added hazard of the castle moat.

Continued

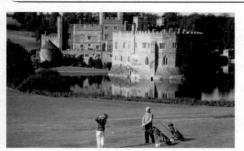

Leeds Castle

9 holes, 2681yds, Par 33, SSS 33, Course record 29.
Visitors Mon-Sun & BHs. Booking required. Dress code. **Societies** booking required. **Green Fees** not confirmed. **Prof** Steve Purves **Course Designer** Neil Coles **Facilities** ⚲ ⚐ 🏠 ⚐ ⚐ **Leisure** Green fees include admission to Leeds Castle's Gardens & Attractions. **Conf** Corporate Hospitality Days **Location** M20 junct 8, 4m E of Maidstone on A20 towards Lenham **Hotel** ★★★★ 77% HL Marriott Tudor Park Hotel & Country Club, Ashford Rd, Bearsted, MAIDSTONE ☎ 01622 734334 120 en suite

Marriott Tudor Park Hotel & Country Club Ashford Rd, Bearsted ME14 4NQ

☎ 01622 734334 📠 01622 735360
e-mail: golf.tudorpark@marriotthotels.co.uk
web: www.marriotthotels.com/tdmgs
The course is set in a 220-acre former deer park with the pleasant undulating Kent countryside as a backdrop. The natural features of the land have been incorporated into this picturesque course to form a challenge for those of both high and intermediate standard. The Par 5 14th is particularly interesting. It can alter your score dramatically should you gamble with a drive to a narrow fairway. This hole has to be carefully thought out from tee to green depending on the wind direction.

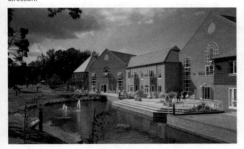

Milgate Course: 18 holes, 6085yds, Par 70, SSS 69, Course record 64. Club membership 750.
Visitors Mon-Sun & BHs. Booking required. Dress code. **Societies** please telephone Golf Events **Green Fees** not confirmed. **Prof** Nick McNally **Course Designer** Donald Steel **Facilities** ⚐ 🏠 ⚐ ⚐ ⚐ ⚐ 🏠 ⚐ ⚐ ⚐ ⚐ ⚐ **Leisure** hard tennis courts, heated indoor swimming pool, sauna, solarium, gymnasium, steam room & spa bath, golf academy. **Conf** facs Corporate Hospitality Days **Location** M20 junct 8, 1.25m W on A20 **Hotel** ★★★★ 77% HL Marriott Tudor Park Hotel & Country Club, Ashford Rd, Bearsted, MAIDSTONE ☎ 01622 734334 120 en suite

NEW ASH GREEN   MAP 05 TQ66

Redlibbets Manor Ln, West Yoke TN15 7HT

☎ 01474 879190 📠 01474 879290
e-mail: redlibbets@golfandsport.co.uk
web: www.redlibbetsmembers.co.uk
Delightful rolling Kentish course cut through an attractive wooded valley.
18 holes, 6639yds, Par 72, SSS 72, Course record 67.
Club membership 500.
Visitors Mon-Fri except BHs. Dress code. **Societies** Booking required.
Green Fees £40. **Prof** Ross Taylor **Course Designer** Jonathan Gaunt **Facilities** ⚐ 🏠 ⚐ ⚐ ⚐ ⚐ **Conf** Corporate Hospitality Days **Location** off A20, close to Brand's Hatch
Hotel ★★★★ 80% HL Brandshatch Place Hotel & Spa, Brands Hatch Rd, Fawkham, BRANDS HATCH ☎ 01474 875000 26 en suite 12 annexe en suite

RAMSGATE   MAP 05 TR36

St Augustine's Cottington Rd, Cliffsend CT12 5JN

☎ 01843 590333 📠 01843 590444
e-mail: sagc@ic24.net
web: www.staugustines.co.uk
A comfortably flat course in this famous bracing championship area of Kent. Neither as long nor as difficult as its lordly neighbours, St Augustine's will nonetheless extend most golfers. Dykes run across the course.
18 holes, 5254yds, Par 69, SSS 66, Course record 61.
Club membership 670.
Visitors Mon-Sun & BHs. Booking required Sat & Sun. Dress code.
Societies Booking required. **Green Fees** Phone. **Prof** Derek Scott **Course Designer** Tom Vardon **Facilities** ⚐ 🏠 ⚐ ⚐ ⚐ ⚐ ⚐ ⚐ ⚐ ⚐ **Location** Off A256 Ramsgate-Sandwich

ROCHESTER   MAP 05 TQ76

Rochester & Cobham Park Park Pale ME2 3UL

☎ 01474 823411 📠 01474 824446
e-mail: rcpgc@talk21.com
web: www.rochesterandcobhamgc.co.uk
A first-rate course of challenging dimensions in undulating parkland. All holes differ and each requires accurate drive placing to derive the best advantage. Open Championship regional qualifying course.
18 holes, 6597yds, Par 71, SSS 72, Course record 64.
Club membership 730.
Visitors Mon-Fri except BHs. Handicap certificate. Dress code.
Societies booking required. **Green Fees** not confirmed. **Prof** Iain Higgins **Course Designer** Donald Steel **Facilities** ⚐ 🏠 ⚐ ⚐ ⚐ ⚐ ⚐ ⚐ ⚐ **Conf** Corporate Hospitality Days **Location** 2.5m W on A2 **Hotel** ★★★★ 74% HL Bridgewood Manor, Bridgewood Roundabout, Walderslade Woods, CHATHAM ☎ 01634 201333 100 en suite

SANDWICH   MAP 05 TR35

Prince's Prince's Dr, Sandwich Bay CT13 9QB
☎ 01304 611118 📄 01304 612000
e-mail: office@princesgolfclub.co.uk
web: www.princesgolfclub.co.uk
With 27 championship holes, Prince's Golf Club has a world-wide
reputation as a traditional links of the finest quality and is a venue
that provides all that is best in modern links golf. One of only 14
courses to be selected to host the Open Championship.

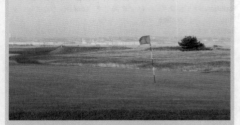

Dunes: 9 holes, 3425yds, Par 36, SSS 36.
Himalayas: 9 holes, 3163yds, Par 35, SSS 35.
Shore: 9 holes, 3347yds, Par 36, SSS 36.
Club membership 310.
Visitors Mon-Sun & BHs. Booking required. Dress code. **Societies**
booking required. **Green Fees** not confirmed. **Prof** Derek Barbour
Course Designer Sir Guy Campbell & J S F Morrison **Facilities** ⑪ 🍴 by
prior arrangement 🏊 ♨ 🎿 🛎 ⚙ ✆ 🛍 ✏ **Leisure** private beach
area. **Conf** facs Corporate Hospitality Days **Location** 2m E via toll road,
signs from Sandwich
Hotel ★★★ 74% HL Dunkerleys Hotel & Restaurant, 19 Beach St, DEAL
☎ 01304 375016 16 en suite

Royal St George's see page 147

Hotel ★★★ 74% HL Dunkerleys Hotel & Restaurant, 19 Beach St, DEAL
☎ 01304 375016 16 en suite

SEAL   MAP 05 TR36

Wildernesse Park Ln TN15 0JE
☎ 01732 761199 📄 01732 763809
e-mail: golf@wildernesse.co.uk
web: www.wildernesse.co.uk
A tight inland course, heavily wooded with tree-lined fairways. Straight
driving and attention to the well-placed bunkers is essential. With few
slopes and easy walking, it is difficult to beat par.
18 holes, 6501yds, Par 72, SSS 71. Club membership 720.
Visitors Mon, Thu & Fri except BHs. Booking required Handicap certificate.
Dress code. **Societies** Booking required. **Green Fees** £48 per round
weekdays. **Prof** Craig Walker **Course Designer** Braid (part) **Facilities** ⑪
🏊 ♨ 🎿 🛎 ⚙ ✆ 🛍 ✏ **Leisure** hard tennis courts. **Conf** Corporate
Hospitality Days **Location** take A25 from Sevenoaks to Seal, turn right into
Park Lane, club entrance on left.
Hotel ★★★ 75% HL Best Western Donnington Manor, London Rd,
Dunton Green, SEVENOAKS ☎ 01732 462681 60 en suite

SEVENOAKS   MAP 05 TQ55

Knole Park Seal Hollow Rd TN15 0HJ
☎ 01732 452150 📄 01732 463159
e-mail: secretary@knoleparkgolfclub.co.uk
web: www.knoleparkgolfclub.co.uk
The course is laid out within the grounds of the Knole Estate and
can rightfully be described as a natural layout. The course designer
has used the contours of the land to produce a challenging course
in all weather conditions and throughout all seasons. While, for most
of the year, it may appear benign, in summer, when the bracken
is high, Knole Park represents a considerable challenge but always
remains a fair test of golf.

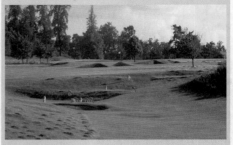

18 holes, 6246yds, Par 70, SSS 70, Course record 62.
Club membership 750.
Visitors Mon-Fri except BHs. Booking required. Handicap certificate.
Dress code. **Societies** Welcome. **Green Fees** £50 per day, £39 per
round. **Prof** Phil Sykes **Course Designer** J A Abercromby **Facilities** ⑪
🍴 🏊 ♨ 🎿 🛎 ⚙ ✆ **Leisure** squash. **Conf** Corporate Hospitality Days
Location NE of town centre off B2019
Hotel ★★★ 75% HL Best Western Donnington Manor, London Rd,
Dunton Green, SEVENOAKS ☎ 01732 462681 60 en suite

SHEERNESS   MAP 05 TQ97

Sheerness Power Station Rd ME12 3AE
☎ 01795 662585 📄 01795 668100
e-mail: thesecretary@sheernessgc.freeserve.co.uk
Semi-links, marshland course, few bunkers, but many ditches and
water hazards.
18 holes, 6390yds, Par 71, SSS 71, Course record 66.
Club membership 650.
Visitors Mon-Sat except BHs. Dress code. **Societies** Booking required.
Green Fees £31 per day, £22 per 18 holes. ⊕ **Prof** L Stanford
Facilities ⑪ 🏊 ♨ 🎿 🛎 ⚙ ✆ 🛍 ✏ **Location** 1.5m E off A249
Hotel ★★★★ 74% HL Bridgewood Manor, Bridgewood Roundabout,
Walderslade Woods, CHATHAM ☎ 01634 201333 100 en suite

CHAMPIONSHIP COURSE

KENT — SANDWICH

ROYAL ST GEORGE'S

Map 05 TR35

CT13 9PB
☎ 01304 613090 📠 01304 611245
e-mail: secretary@royalstgeorges.com
web: www.royalstgeorges.com
18 holes, 7102yds, Par 70, SSS 74,
Course record 67.
Club membership 750.
Visitors Mon, Tue, Thu except BHs.
Booking required. Handicap certificate. Dress
code. **Societies** booking required.
Green Fees £150 per 36 holes, £120
per 18 holes. Reduced winter rates.
Prof A Brooks **Course Designer** Dr Laidlaw
Purves **Facilities** ⑨ by prior arrangement
🖫🕎🏊🍴🏌🛆🗲🏌 **Conf** Corporate
Hospitality Days **Location** 1.5m E of Sandwich.
Enter town for golf courses

Consistently ranked among the leading
golf courses in the world, Royal St George's
occupies a unique place in the history
of golf, playing host in 1894 to the first
Open Championship outside Scotland.
Set among the dunes of Sandwich Bay, the
links provide a severe test for the greatest
of golfers. Only three Open winners (Bill
Rogers in 1981, Greg Norman in 1993 and
Ben Curtis in 2003) have managed to under
Par after 72 holes. The undulating fairways,
the borrows on the greens, the strategically
placed bunkers, and the prevailing winds
that blow on all but the rarest of occasions;
these all soon reveal any weakness in
the player. There are few over the years
who have mastered all the vagaries in
one round. It hosted its thirteenth Open
Championship in 2003, won dramatically
by outsider Ben Curtis.

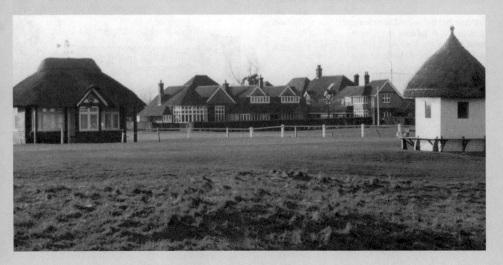

SHOREHAM — MAP 05 TQ56

Darenth Valley Station Rd TN14 7SA
☎ 01959 522922 📠 01959 525089
e-mail: enquiries@dvgc.co.uk
web: www.dvgc.co.uk
Gently undulating parkland in a beautiful Kent valley, with excellent well-drained greens. The course has matured and developed to become a challenge to both high and low handicap golfers.

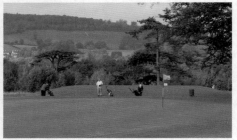

18 holes, 6193yds, Par 72, SSS 71, Course record 64.
Visitors Mon-Sun & BHs. Dress code. **Societies** Booking required. **Green Fees** £32 per 36 holes, £20 per 18 holes (£27 per 18 holes Sat, Sun & BHs). **Prof** Pete Stopford **Course Designer** Michael Cross **Facilities** ⑪ ⑩ ⒧ ▱ ☍ ⑪ ♨ 🍴 🆓 ✔ **Conf** facs Corporate Hospitality Days **Location** 3m N of Sevenoaks off A225 between Otford & Eynsford
Hotel ★★★ 75% HL Best Western Donnington Manor, London Rd, Dunton Green, SEVENOAKS ☎ 01732 462681 60 en suite

SITTINGBOURNE — MAP 05 TQ96

The Oast Golf Centre Church Rd, Tonge ME9 9AR
☎ 01795 473527
e-mail: rmail@oastgolf.co.uk
web: www.oastgolf.co.uk
A Par 3 approach course of nine holes with 18 tees augmented by a 17-bay floodlit driving range and a putting green.
9 holes, 1664yds, Par 54, SSS 54.
Visitors contact centre for details. **Societies** Welcome. **Green Fees** £7.50 for 18 holes, £5.50 for 9 holes. Weekdays £5.50 per am, £7.50 per pm unlimited. **Prof** D Chambers **Course Designer** D Chambers **Facilities** ⒧ ▱ 🍴🝞 ♨ ✔ ✔ **Location** 2m NE, A2 between Bapchild
Hotel ★★★★ 74% HL Bridgewood Manor, Bridgewood Roundabout, Walderslade Woods, CHATHAM ☎ 01634 201333 100 en suite

Sittingbourne & Milton Regis Wormdale, Newington ME9 7PX
☎ 01795 842261
e-mail: sittingbournegc@btconnect.com
web: www.sittingbournegolfclub.com
A downland course with pleasant vistas and renowned for its greens. There are a few uphill climbs, but the course is far from difficult. The back nine holes are challenging.
18 holes, 6291yds, Par 71, SSS 70, Course record 63.
Club membership 715.
Visitors Mon, Tue, Thu & Fri. Wed pm only. Booking required Wed. Dress code. **Societies** Booking required. **Green Fees** £32 per 18 holes. **Prof** John Hearn **Course Designer** Donald Steel **Facilities** ⑪ ⑩ by prior arrangement ⒧ ▱ 🍴 ♨ 🍴 🆓 ✔ **Conf** Corporate Hospitality Days **Location** 0.5m from M2 junct 5, off Chestnut St at Danaway

Hotel ★★★★ 74% HL Bridgewood Manor, Bridgewood Roundabout, Walderslade Woods, CHATHAM ☎ 01634 201333 100 en suite

Upchurch River Valley Golf Centre Oak Ln, Upchurch ME9 7AY
☎ 01634 379592 📠 01634 387784
18 holes, 6237yds, Par 70, SSS 70.
Course Designer David Smart **Location** A2 between Rainham & Newington
Telephone for further details
Hotel ★★★ 79% HL Best Western Russell Hotel, 136 Boxley Rd, MAIDSTONE ☎ 01622 692221 42 en suite

SNODLAND — MAP 05 TQ76

Oastpark Malling Rd ME6 5LG
☎ 01634 242661 📠 01634 240744
A challenging parkland course for golfers of all abilities. The course has water hazards and orchards. Construction of a further nine holes is planned for 2006.
9 holes, 3150yds, Par 35, SSS 35, Course record 71.
Club membership 60.
Visitors Mon-Sun & BHs. **Societies** Booking required. **Green Fees** £7 per day (weekends: £14 per 18 holes, £8 per 9 holes). **Prof** David Porthouse **Course Designer** J D Banks **Facilities** ⒧ ▱ 🍴 ♨ 🍴 🆓 ✔ **Location** M20 junct 4
Hotel ★★★★ 74% HL Bridgewood Manor, Bridgewood Roundabout, Walderslade Woods, CHATHAM ☎ 01634 201333 100 en suite

TENTERDEN — MAP 05 TQ83

London Beach Hotel & Golf Club Ashford Rd TN30 6HX
☎ 01580 766279 📠 01580 763884
e-mail: enquiries@londonbeach.com
web: www.londonbeach.com
Located in a mature parkland setting in the Weald. A test of golf for all abilities of golfer with its rolling fairways and undulating greens.

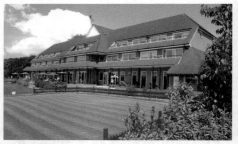

9 holes, 5860yds, Par 70, SSS 69, Course record 66.
Club membership 250.
Visitors Booking required. **Societies** booking required. **Green Fees** not confirmed. **Prof** Mark Chilcott **Course Designer** Golf Landscapes **Facilities** ⑪ ⑩ ⒧ ▱ 🍴 ♨ 🝞 🆓 ✔ 🆓 ✔ **Leisure** fishing, pitch & putt clay pigeon shooting. **Conf** facs Corporate Hospitality Days **Location** M20 Junct 9, A28 towards Tenterden, hotel on right 1m before Tenterden
Hotel ★★★ 78% HL Best Western London Beach Hotel & Golf Club, Ashford Rd, TENTERDEN ☎ 01580 766279 26 en suite

Tenterden Woodchurch Rd TN30 7DR
☎ 01580 763987 (sec) 📄 01580 763430
e-mail: enquiries@tenterdengolfclub.co.uk
web: tenterdengolfclub.co.uk
Set in tranquil undulating parkland with beautiful views, the course is challenging with several difficult holes.
18 holes, 6071yds, Par 70, SSS 69, Course record 61.
Club membership 600.
Visitors Mon-Sun except BHs. Handicap certificate. Dress code.
Societies Booking required. **Green Fees** £34 per day all week, £22 per round (£20 Sat & Sun). Winter £22/£16/£15. **Prof** Kyle Kelsall **Facilities** ⑪ ⑩ ⓑ ⏚ ♀ 🍴 ⚱ 🍴 ♂ **Location** 0.75m E on B2067
Hotel ★★★ 78% HL Best Western London Beach Hotel & Golf Club, Ashford Rd, TENTERDEN ☎ 01580 766279 26 en suite

---

TONBRIDGE   MAP 05 TQ54

Poultwood Higham Ln TN11 9QR
☎ 01732 364039 & 366180 📄 01732 353781
web: www.poultwoodgolf.co.uk
There are two public pay and play parkland courses in an idyllic woodland setting. The courses are ecologically designed, over predominantly flat land offering challenging hazards and interesting playing conditions for all standards of golfer.
18 holes, 5524yds, Par 68, SSS 66.
9 holes, 2562yds, Par 28.
Visitors Mon-Sun & BHs. Booking required. Dress code. **Societies** Booking required. **Green Fees** 18 hole course: £15 (£21Sat, Sun & BHs). 9 hole course:£5.70/£7.40. **Prof** Bill Hodkin **Course Designer** Hawtree **Facilities** ⑪ ⑩ ⓑ ⏚ 🍴 ⚱ ⛳ ♂ **Leisure** squash. **Conf** facs Corporate Hospitality Days **Location** Off A227 3m N of Tonbridge
Hotel ★★★ 70% HL Best Western Rose & Crown Hotel, 125 High St, TONBRIDGE ☎ 01732 357966 54 en suite

---

TUNBRIDGE WELLS (ROYAL) MAP 05 TQ53

Nevill Benhall Mill Rd TN2 5JW
☎ 01892 525818 📄 01892 517861
e-mail: manager@nevillgolfclub.co.uk
web: www.nevillgolfclub.co.uk
The Kent-Sussex border forms the northern perimeter of the course. Open undulating ground, well-wooded with some heather and gorse for the first half. The second nine holes slope away from the clubhouse to a valley where a narrow stream hazards two holes.
18 holes, 6349yds, Par 71, SSS 70, Course record 64.
Club membership 800.
Visitors Mon-Fri except BHs. Booking required. Handicap certificate. Dress code. **Societies** booking required. **Green Fees** not confirmed. ☺ **Prof** Paul Huggett **Course Designer** Henry Cotton **Facilities** ⑪ ⓑ ⏚ 🍴 ⚱ 🍴 ♂ **Location** S of Tunbridge Wells
Hotel ★★★★ 74% HL The Spa Hotel, Mount Ephraim, TUNBRIDGE WELLS ☎ 01892 520331 69 en suite

Tunbridge Wells Langton Rd TN4 8XH
☎ 01892 523034 📄 01892 536918
e-mail: info@tunbridgewellsgolfclub.co.uk
web: www.tunbridgewellsgolfclub.co.uk
Somewhat hilly, well-bunkered parkland course with lake; trees form natural hazards.
9 holes, 4725yds, Par 65, SSS 62, Course record 59.
Club membership 470.

Visitors Mon-Sun & BHs. Booking required. Dress code. **Societies** booking required. **Green Fees** not confirmed. **Facilities** ⑪ ⑩ ⓑ ⏚ 🍴 ⚱ 🍴 ♂ ⚱ 🍴
Location 1m W on A264
Hotel ★★★★ 74% HL The Spa Hotel, Mount Ephraim, TUNBRIDGE WELLS ☎ 01892 520331 69 en suite

---

WESTERHAM   MAP 05 TQ45

Park Wood Chestnut Av, Tatsfield TN16 2EG
☎ 01959 577744 & 577177 (pro-shop) 📄 01959 572702
e-mail: mail@parkwoodgolf.co.uk
web: www.parkwoodgolf.co.uk
Situated in an Area of Outstanding Natural Beauty, flanked by an ancient woodland with superb views across Kent and Surrey countryside. An undulating course, tree lined and with some interesting water features. Playable in all weather conditions.

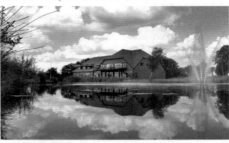

18 holes, 6835yds, Par 72, SSS 72, Course record 66.
Club membership 500.
Visitors Mon-Fri. Sat, Sun & BHs after 11am. Dress code **Societies** Booking required. **Green Fees** Phone. **Prof** Nick Terry **Facilities** ⑪ ⓑ ⏚ 🍴 ⚱ 🍴 ♂ ⚱ 🍴 **Conf** facs Corporate Hospitality Days **Location** A25 onto B2024 Croydon Rd Ln, at Church Hill junct onto Chestnut Av
Hotel ★★★ 75% HL Best Western Donnington Manor, London Rd, Dunton Green, SEVENOAKS ☎ 01732 462681 60 en suite

Westerham Valence Park, Brasted Rd TN16 1LJ
☎ 01959 567100 📄 01959 567101
e-mail: tom.terry@westerhamgc.co.uk
web: www.westerhamgc.co.uk
Originally forestry land with thousands of mature pines. The storms of 1987 created natural fairways and the mature landscape makes the course both demanding and spectacular. A clubhouse with first-class facilities and magnificent views.

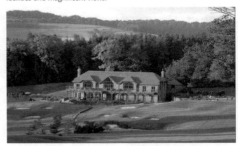

18 holes, 6329yds, Par 72, SSS 72. Club membership 600.

Continued

Visitors Mon-Sun & BHs. Dress code. **Societies** Booking required.
Green Fees £33 per round Mon-Thu, £36 Fri, £40 weekends and bank
holidays. **Prof** J Marshal **Course Designer** D Williams **Facilities** ⑪ ⓑ ⏄
🕈⌷ ⌓ ♨ 🏌 🏌 **Leisure** short game practice area. **Conf** facs Corporate
Hospitality Days **Location** A25 between Westerham & Brasted
Hotel ★★★ 75% HL Best Western Donnington Manor, London Rd,
Dunton Green, SEVENOAKS ☎ 01732 462681 60 en suite

WESTGATE ON SEA   MAP 05 TR37

Westgate and Birchington 176 Canterbury Rd CT8 8LT
☎ 01843 831115
e-mail: wandbgc@tiscali.co.uk
A fine blend of inland and seaside holes which provide a good test of
the golfer despite the apparently simple appearance of the course.
18 holes, 4926yds, Par 64, SSS 64, Course record 60.
Club membership 350.
Visitors Mon-Sun & BHs. Dress code. **Societies** Welcome. **Green Fees**
£17 per day (£20 Sat, Sun & BHs). ⊛ **Prof** Roger Game **Facilities** ⑪ ⓣⓞⓣ
ⓑ ⌷🕈⌷ ⌓ ♨ ⌀ **Conf** Corporate Hospitality Days **Location** E of town
centre off A28

WEST KINGSDOWN   MAP 05 TQ56

Woodlands Manor Tinkerpot Ln, Otford TN15 6AB
☎ 01959 523806 🖹 01959 524398
e-mail: info@woodlandsmanorgolf.co.uk
web: www.woodlandsmanorgolf.co.uk
Two nine-hole layouts with views over an area of outstanding
natural beauty. The course is challenging but fair with varied and
memorable holes of which the 7th, 10th and 18th stand out. Good
playing conditions all year round.

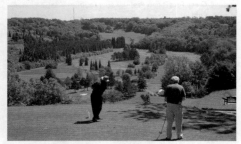

18 holes, 6015yds, Par 69, SSS 69, Course record 64.
Club membership 600.
Visitors Mon-Sun & BHs. Booking required. Dress code. **Societies** booking
required. **Green Fees** not confirmed. **Prof** Philip Womack **Course
Designer** Lyons/Coles **Facilities** ⑪ ⓑ ⌷🕈⌷ ⌓ ♨ ⌀ 🏌 **Conf** facs
Corporate Hospitality Days **Location** A20 through West Kingsdown, right
opp Portbello Inn onto School Ln Ln, clubhouse left
Hotel BUD Premier Travel Inn Sevenoaks/Maidstone, London Rd, Wrotham
Heath, WROTHAM ☎ 08701 977227 40 en suite

WEST MALLING   MAP 05 TQ65

Kings Hill Fortune Way, Discovery Dr, Kings Hill
ME19 4AG
☎ 01732 875040 🖹 01732 875019
e-mail: khatkhgolf@aol.com
web: www.kingshill-golfclub.com
Set in over 200 acres of undulating terrain and features large areas
of protected heath and mature woodland. USGA standard greens
and tees.
18 holes, 6622yards, Par 72, SSS 72. Club membership 530.
Visitors Mon-Sun & BHs. Booking required. Dress code. **Societies**
Welcome. **Green Fees** £30 (£45 Sat, Sun & BHs). **Prof** David Hudspith
Course Designer David Williams Partnership **Facilities** ⑪ ⓣⓞⓣ by prior
arrangement ⓑ ⌷🕈⌷ ⌓ ♨ ⌀ ⌀ 🏌 **Location** M20 junct 4, A228
towards Tonbridge
Hotel BUD Premier Travel Inn Maidstone (Leybourne), Castle Way,
LEYBOURNE ☎ 08701 977170 40 en suite

WHITSTABLE   MAP 05 TR16

Chestfield (Whitstable) 103 Chestfield Rd, Chestfield
CT5 3LU
☎ 01227 794411 & 792243 🖹 01227 794454
e-mail: secretary@chestfield-golfclub.co.uk
web: www.chestfield-golfclub.co.uk
Recent changes have been made to this parkland course with
undulating fairways and fine views of the sea and countryside. These
consist of six new greens and five new tees. The ancient clubhouse,
dating back to the 15th century, is reputed to the oldest building in the
world used for this purpose.
18 holes, 6200yds, Par 70, SSS 70, Course record 66.
Club membership 725.
Visitors Mon-Sun & BHs. Dress code. **Societies** Booking required.
Green Fees £44 per day, £36 per round. **Prof** John Brotherton
Course Designer D Steel/James Braid **Facilities** ⑪ ⓣⓞⓣ ⓑ ⌷🕈⌷ ⌓
♨ ⌀ ⌀ 🏌 **Leisure** half-way house providing snacks/refreshments.
Location 0.5m S by Chestfield Railway Station, off A2990
Hotel BUD Premier Travel Inn Whitstable, Thanet Way, WHITSTABLE
☎ 08701 977269 40 en suite

Whitstable & Seasalter Collingwood Rd CT5 1EB
☎ 01227 272020 🖹 01227 280822
Links course.
9 holes, 5357yds, Par 66, SSS 65, Course record 62.
Club membership 350.
Visitors Mon-Sat except BHs. Booking required. Dress code.
Green Fees not confirmed. ⊛ **Facilities** ⑪ by prior arrangement ⓑ ⌷🕈⌷
⌓ **Location** W of town centre off B2205
Hotel BUD Premier Travel Inn Whitstable, Thanet Way, WHITSTABLE
☎ 08701 977269 40 en suite

LANCASHIRE

ACCRINGTON MAP 07 SD72

Accrington & District Devon Av, Oswaldtwistle BB5 4LS
☎ 01254 231091 📠 01254 350119
e-mail: info@accrington-golf-club.co.uk
web: www.accrington-golf-club.co.uk
Moorland course with pleasant views of the Pennines and surrounding areas. The course is a real test for even the best amateur golfers and has hosted many county matches and championships over its 100 plus years of history.
18 holes, 6060yds, Par 70, SSS 69, Course record 63.
Club membership 600.
Visitors Mon-Fri except BHs. Booking required. Dress code. **Societies** Mon & Fri, booking required. **Green Fees** not confirmed. 🏌 **Prof** Mark Harling **Course Designer** J Braid **Facilities** 🍴 by prior arrangement 🍽 by prior arrangement 🛏 ☕ 🍷 ⛳ 🏪 🚗 🏌 **Conf** Corporate Hospitality Days **Location** Between Accrington & Blackburn
Hotel ★★★★ 74% HL Mercure Dunkenhalgh Hotel & Spa, Blackburn Rd, Clayton-le-Moors, ACCRINGTON ☎ 0870 1942116 78 en suite 97 annexe en suite

Baxenden & District Top o' th' Meadow, Baxenden BB5 2EA
☎ 01254 234555
e-mail: baxgolf@hotmail.com
web: www.baxendengolf.co.uk
Moorland course with panoramic views and a long Par 3 to start.
9 holes, 5740yds, Par 70, SSS 68, Course record 65.
Club membership 340.
Visitors Mon-Sun & BHs. Booking required. Dress code.
Societies Welcome. **Green Fees** £15 per 18 holes (£25 Sat, Sun & BHs). 🏌
Facilities 🍴 🍽 🛏 ☕ 🍷 ⛳ **Conf** facs Corporate Hospitality Days
Location 1.5m SE off A680
Hotel ★★★★ 74% HL Mercure Dunkenhalgh Hotel & Spa, Blackburn Rd, Clayton-le-Moors, ACCRINGTON ☎ 0870 1942116 78 en suite 97 annexe en suite

Green Haworth Green Haworth BB5 3SL
☎ 01254 237580 & 382510 📠 01254 396176
e-mail: golf@greenhaworth.co.uk
web: www.greenhaworthgolfclub.co.uk
Moorland course dominated by quarries and difficult in windy conditions.
9 holes, 5522yds, Par 68, SSS 67, Course record 66.
Club membership 250.
Visitors Mon, Tue, Thu & Fri. Booking required. Handicap certificate. Dress code. **Societies** advance booking. **Green Fees** not confirmed. 🏌
Facilities 🍴 🍽 🛏 ☕ 🍷 ⛳ **Conf** Corporate Hospitality Days
Location 2m S off A680
Hotel ★★★★ 74% HL Mercure Dunkenhalgh Hotel & Spa, Blackburn Rd, Clayton-le-Moors, ACCRINGTON ☎ 0870 1942116 78 en suite 97 annexe en suite

BACUP MAP 07 SD82

Bacup Maden Rd OL13 8HY
☎ 01706 873170 📠 01706 877726
e-mail: secretary@bacupgolfltd.co.uk
Tree-lined moorland course, predominantly flat except climbs to 1st and 10th holes.
9 holes, 6018yds, Par 70, SSS 69, Course record 60.
Club membership 350.
Visitors Wed-Fri & BHs. Sun by arrangement. Booking required. Handicap certificate. Dress code. **Societies** Booking required **Green Fees** £25 per day, £15 per round (£30/£20 Sun & BHs). 🏌 **Facilities** 🍴 by prior arrangement 🍽 by prior arrangement 🛏 ☕ 🍷 ⛳ **Conf** Corporate Hospitality Days **Location** W of town off A671
Hotel ★★★ 78% HL Rosehill House Hotel, Rosehill Av, BURNLEY
☎ 01282 453931 34 en suite

BARNOLDSWICK MAP 07 SD84

Ghyll Skipton Rd BB18 6JH
☎ 01282 842466
e-mail: secretary@ghyllgc.freeserve.com
web: www.ghyllgc.co.uk
Excellent parkland course with outstanding views, especially from the 8th tee where you can see the Three Peaks. Testing 8th hole is an uphill Par 3. Eleven holes in total, nine in Yorkshire and two in Lancashire.
11 holes, 5790yds, Par 68, SSS 66, Course record 62.
Club membership 345.
Visitors Mon, Wed-Sat & BHs. Tue after 3pm. Dress code.
Societies Booking required. **Green Fees** £15 per day (£20 Sat). 🏌
Facilities 🍽 ☕ 🍷 ⛳ **Conf** Corporate Hospitality Days **Location** NE of town on B6252
Hotel ★★★ 74% HL Herriots Hotel, Broughton Rd, SKIPTON
☎ 01756 792781 23 rms (13 en suite)

BICKERSTAFFE MAP 07 SD40

Mossock Hall Liverpool Rd L39 0EE
☎ 01695 421717 📠 01695 424961
Relatively flat parkland with scenic views. USGA greens and water features on four holes.
18 holes, 6272yards, Par 71, SSS 70, Course record 68.
Club membership 580.
Visitors Mon-Sun & BHs. Booking required. Dress code. **Societies** Booking required **Green Fees** £22 per 18 holes (£30 Sat, Sun & BHs). **Prof** Brad Millar **Course Designer** Steve Marnoch **Facilities** 🍴 🍽 🛏 ☕ 🍷 ⛳ 🏪 🏌 **Conf** Corporate Hospitality Days **Location** M58 junct 3

BLACKBURN MAP 07 SD62

Blackburn Beardwood Brow BB2 7AX
☎ 01254 51122 📠 01254 665578
e-mail: sec@blackburngolfclub.com
web: www.blackburngolfclub.com
Parkland on a high plateau with stream and hills. Superb views of Lancashire coast and the Pennines.
18 holes, 6144yds, Par 71, SSS 70, Course record 62.
Club membership 550.
Visitors Mon-Sun & BHs. Booking required Tue, Sat, Sun & BHs. Handicap certificate. Dress code. **Societies** Welcome. **Green Fees** £26 per day (£30 weekends). 🏌 **Prof** Alan Rodwell **Facilities** 🍴 🍽 🛏 ☕ 🍷 ⛳ 🏪 🏌 🚗 🏌 **Conf** facs **Location** 1.25m NW of town centre off A677
Hotel ★★ 85% HL The Millstone at Mellor, Church Ln, Mellor, BLACKBURN ☎ 01254 813333 17 en suite 6 annexe en suite

BLACKPOOL MAP 07 SD33

Blackpool North Shore Devonshire Rd FY2 0RD
☎ 01253 352054 ▤ 01253 591240
e-mail: office@bnsgc.com
web: www.bnsgc.com
Links type course with rolling fairways and good sized greens. Excellent views of the Lake District and Pennine Hills.

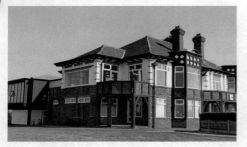

18 holes, 6432yds, Par 71, SSS 71, Course record 62.
Club membership 900.
Visitors Mon-Wed, Fri & Sun & BHs. Booking required Fri & Sun. Handicap certificate. Dress code. **Societies** Booking required. **Green Fees** £37 per day, £29 per round (£44/£35 Sun & BHs). **Prof** Andrew Richardson
Course Designer H S Colt **Facilities** ⑪ ⑩↾ ⓑ ⚐ ↿ ⏌ ⌖ ☎ ⌖ ✦
Leisure Y. **Conf** Corporate Hospitality Days **Location** on A587 N of town centre
Hotel ★★ 69% HL Hotel Sheraton, 54-62 Queens Promenade, BLACKPOOL ☎ 01253 352723 104 en suite

Blackpool Park North Park Dr FY3 8LS
☎ 01253 397916 & 478176 (tee times) ▤ 01253 397916
e-mail: secretary@bpgc.org.uk
web: www.bpgc.org.uk
The course, situated in Stanley Park, is municipal. The golf club (Blackpool Park) is private but golfers may use the clubhouse facilities if playing the course. An abundance of grassy pits, ponds and open dykes.
18 holes, 6087yds, Par 70, SSS 70, Course record 64.
Club membership 650.
Visitors Mon-Fri, Sun & BHs. Dress code. **Societies** Welcome. **Green Fees** £16.50 per round (£19 Sun & BHs). **Prof** Brian Purdie **Course Designer** A.McKenzie **Facilities** ⑪ ⑩↾ ⓑ ⚐ ↿ ⏌ ⌖ ☎ ↾ ✦ **Conf** Corporate Hospitality Days **Location** 1m E of Blackpool Tower
Hotel ★★★ 75% HL Carousel Hotel, 663-671 New South Prom, BLACKPOOL ☎ 01253 402642 92 en suite

De Vere Herons Reach East Park Blackpool FY3 8LL
☎ 01253 766156 & 838866 ▤ 01253 798800
e-mail: dot.kilbride@devere-hotels.com
web: www.deveregolf.co.uk
18 holes, 6628yds, Par 72, SSS 71, Course record 64.
Course Designer Peter Alliss/Clive Clark **Location** Off A587 next to Stanley Park Zoo
Telephone for further details
Hotel ★★★★ 79% HL De Vere Herons' Reach, East Park Dr, BLACKPOOL ☎ 01253 838866 172 en suite

BURNLEY MAP 07 SD83

Burnley Glen View BB11 3RW
☎ 01282 421045 & 451281 ▤ 01282 451281
e-mail: burnleygolfclub@onthegreen.co.uk
web: www.burnleygolfclub.org.uk
Challenging moorland course with exceptional views.
18 holes, 5939yds, Par 69, SSS 69, Course record 62.
Club membership 700.
Visitors Mon-Sun & BHs. Booking required Wed-Sun & BHs. Handicap certificate. Dress code. **Societies** Welcome. **Green Fees** £25 per day (£30 weekends & bank holidays). **Prof** Matthew Baker **Facilities** ⑪ ⑩↾ ⓑ ⚐ ↿ ⏌ ⌖ ☎ ⌖ **Leisure** snooker table. **Conf** facs Corporate Hospitality Days
Location S of town off A646
Hotel ★★★ 78% HL Rosehill House Hotel, Rosehill Av, BURNLEY ☎ 01282 453931 34 en suite

Towneley Towneley Park, Todmorden Rd BB11 3ED
☎ 01282 438473
18 holes, 5811yds, Par 70, SSS 68, Course record 67.
Location 1m SE of town centre on A671
Telephone for further details

CHORLEY MAP 07 SD51

Charnock Richard Preston Rd, Charnock Richard PR7 5LE
☎ 01257 470707 ▤ 01257 791196
e-mail: mail@crgc.co.uk
web: www.charnockrichardgolfclub.co.uk
Flat parkland course with plenty of American-style water hazards. Signature hole the 6th Par 5 with an island green.
18 holes, 6239yds, Par 71, SSS 70, Course record 68.
Club membership 550.
Visitors Mon-Sun & BHs. Booking required. Dress code. **Societies** booking required. **Green Fees** not confirmed. **Prof** Lee Taylor/Alan Lunt
Course Designer Martin Turner **Facilities** ⑪ ⑩↾ ⓑ ⚐ ↿ ⏌ ⌖ ☎ ↾ ✦ ✦ **Leisure** 9 hole pitch & putt. **Conf** facs Corporate Hospitality Days
Location On A49, 0.25m from Camelot Theme Park
Hotel ★★★ 74% HL Best Western Park Hall Hotel, Park Hall Rd, Charnock Richard, CHORLEY ☎ 01257 455000 56 en suite 84 annexe en suite

Chorley Hall o' th' Hill, Heath Charnock PR6 9HX
☎ 01257 480263 ▤ 01257 480722
e-mail: secretary@chorleygolfclub.freeserve.co.uk
web: www.chorleygolfclub.co.uk
18 holes, 6269yds, Par 71, SSS 70, Course record 62.
Course Designer J A Steer **Location** 2.5m SE on A673
Telephone for further details
Hotel ★★★ 78% HL Pines Hotel, 570 Preston Rd, Clayton-Le-Woods, CHORLEY ☎ 01772 338551 37 en suite

Duxbury Jubilee Park Duxbury Hall Rd PR7 4AT
☎ 01257 265380 ▤ 01257 274500
18 holes, 6390yds, Par 71, SSS 70.
Course Designer Hawtree & Sons **Location** 2.5m S off A6
Telephone for further details
Hotel BUD Welcome Lodge Charnock Richard, Welcome Break Service Area, CHORLEY ☎ 01257 791746 100 en suite

England

Shaw Hill Hotel Golf & Country Club Preston Rd, Whittle-Le-Woods PR6 7PP
☎ 01257 269221 🖹 01257 261223
e-mail: info@shaw-hill.co.uk
web: www.shaw-hill.co.uk
A fine heavily wooded parkland course designed by one of Europe's most prominent golf architects and offering a considerable challenge as well as tranquillity and scenic charm. Six holes are protected by water and signature holes are the 8th and the closing 18th played slightly up hill to the imposing club house.
18 holes, 6283yds, Par 72, SSS 71, Course record 65.
Club membership 500.
Visitors Mon-Sat & BHs. Booking required. Handicap certificate. Dress code. **Societies** Booking required. **Green Fees** Mon- Thu £35 per 18 holes, Fri, Sat & BHs £45. **Prof** David Clark **Course Designer** Harry Vardon **Facilities** ⑪ ⑩ 🖥 🖪 🖫 🏊 🖾 🖎 ◇ 🏌 🏌
Leisure heated indoor swimming pool, sauna, solarium, gymnasium, snooker. **Conf** facs Corporate Hospitality Days **Location** 1.5m N on A6
Hotel ★★★ 74% HL Best Western Park Hall Hotel, Park Hall Rd, Charnock Richard, CHORLEY ☎ 01257 455000 56 en suite 84 annexe en suite

---

CLITHEROE   MAP 07 SD74

Clitheroe Whalley Rd, Pendleton BB7 1PP
☎ 01200 422292 🖹 01200 422292
e-mail: secretary@clitheroegolfclub.com
web: www.clitheroegolfclub.com
One of the best inland courses in the country. Clitheroe is a parkland-type course with water hazards and good scenic views, particularly towards Longridge and Pendle Hill.
18 holes, 6326yds, Par 71, SSS 71, Course record 63.
Club membership 700.
Visitors Mon-Wed & Fri except BHs. Booking required. Handicap certificate. Dress code. **Societies** Booking required. **Green Fees** Mon-Thu £45 per day, £35 per 18 holes, Fri £45/£38. ● **Prof** Paul McEvoy **Course Designer** James Braid **Facilities** ⑪ ⑩ 🖥 🖪 🖫 🏊 🖾 🖎 ◇ 🏌 🏌
Conf Corporate Hospitality Days **Location** 2m S of Clitheroe
Hotel ★★★ 71% HL Shireburn Arms Hotel, Whalley Rd, Hurst Green, CLITHEROE ☎ 01254 826518 22 en suite

---

COLNE   MAP 07 SD84

Colne Law Farm, Skipton Old Rd BB8 7EB
☎ 01282 863391 🖹 01282 870547
Moorland course with scenic surroundings.
9 holes, 6053yds, Par 70, SSS 69, Course record 63.
Club membership 440.
Visitors Mon-Wed, Fri & BHs. Dress code. **Societies** Booking required. **Green Fees** £20 per day (£25 weekends and bank holidays). ● **Facilities** ⑪ ⑩ 🖥 🖪 🖫 🏊 **Leisure** snooker. **Conf** Corporate Hospitality Days **Location** 1m E off A56
Hotel ★★★ 67% HL Sparrow Hawk Hotel, Church St, BURNLEY ☎ 01282 421551 35 en suite

---

DARWEN   MAP 07 SD62

Darwen Winter Hill BB3 0LB
☎ 01254 701287 (club) & 704367 (office) 🖹 01254 773833
e-mail: admin@darwengolfclub.com
First 9 holes on parkland, the second 9 on moorland.
18 holes, 6046yds, Par 71, SSS 71. Club membership 600.

Visitors Mon, Wed-Fri, Sun except BHs. Booking required. Dress code.
Societies booking required. **Green Fees** not confirmed. ● **Prof** Wayne Lennon **Facilities** ⑪ ⑩ 🖥 🖪 🖫 🏊 🖾 🖎 **Conf** facs Corporate Hospitality Days **Location** 1m NW
Hotel BUD Travelodge Blackburn (M65), Darwen Motorway services, DARWEN ☎ 08700 850 950

FLEETWOOD   MAP 07 SD34

Fleetwood Princes Way FY7 8AF
☎ 01253 873661 & 773573 🖹 01253 773573
e-mail: fleetwoodgc@aol.com
web: www.fleetwoodgolfclub.org.uk
Championship length, flat seaside links where the player must always be alert to changes of direction or strength of the wind.

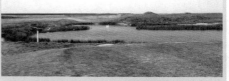

18 holes, 6723yds, Par 72, SSS 72. Club membership 600.
Visitors Mon-Sun & BHs. Booking required. Handicap certificate. Dress code. **Societies** Booking required. **Green Fees** Phone. ● **Prof** S McLaughlin **Course Designer** J A Steer **Facilities** ⑪ ⑩ 🖥 🖪 🖫 🏊 🖾 🖎 **Conf** facs Corporate Hospitality Days **Location** W of town centre
Hotel BUD Premier Travel Inn Blackpool (Bispham), Devonshire Rd, Bispham, BLACKPOOL ☎ 08701 977033 39 en suite

---

GARSTANG   MAP 07 SD44

Garstang Country Hotel & Golf Club Garstang Rd, Bowgreave PR3 1YE
☎ 01995 600100 🖹 01995 600950
e-mail: reception@ghgc.co.uk
web: www.garstanghotelandgolf.com
Fairly flat parkland course following the contours of the Rivers Wyre and Calder and providing a steady test of ability, especially over the longer back nine. Exceptional drainage makes the course playable all year round.

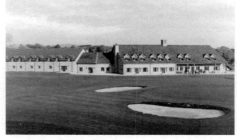

18 holes, 6050yds, Par 68, SSS 68.

Continued

Visitors Mon-Sun & BHs. Booking required. **Societies** Booking required.
Green Fees £15 per round (£17 weekends). **Prof** Robert Head **Course Designer** Richard Bradbeer **Facilities** ⏰ 🍴 ⬛ ⬜ 🏐 ⚑ 🏌 ♂ 🏐 ♂ **Conf** facs Corporate Hospitality Days **Location** 1m S of Garstang on B6430 **Hotel** ★★★ 75% HL Garstang Country Hotel & Golf Club, Garstang Rd, Bowgreave, GARSTANG ☎ 01995 600100 32 en suite

See advert on opposite page

GREAT HARWOOD   MAP 07 SD73

Great Harwood Harwood Bar, Whalley Rd BB6 7TE
☎ 01254 884391
Flat parkland with fine views of the Pendle region.
9 holes, 6404yds, Par 73, SSS 71, Course record 68.
Club membership 400.
Visitors Mon-Sat except BHs. Booking required. Handicap certificate. Dress code. **Societies** welcome mid-week only, apply in writing. **Green Fees** not confirmed. 🌐 **Facilities** ⬛ ⬜ 🏐 ⬜ **Location** E of town centre on A680 **Hotel** ★★★★ 74% HL Mercure Dunkenhalgh Hotel & Spa, Blackburn Rd, Clayton-le-Moors, ACCRINGTON ☎ 0870 1942116 78 en suite 97 annexe en suite

HASLINGDEN   MAP 07 SD72

Rossendale Ewood Ln Head BB4 6LH
☎ 01706 831339 (Secretary) & 213616 (Pro)
📠 01706 228669
e-mail: rgc@golfers.net
web: www.rossendalegolfclub.co.uk
A surprisingly flat parkland course, situated on a plateau with panoramic views and renowned for excellent greens.
18 holes, 6293yds, Par 72, Course record 64.
Club membership 700.
Visitors Mon-Fri, Sun & BHs. Booking required. Handicap certificate. Dress code. **Societies** Booking required. **Green Fees** £40 per day, £30 per round (£45/£35 Sun). 🌐 **Prof** Stephen Nicholls **Facilities** 🏐 🏌 ♂ **Conf** Corporate Hospitality Days **Location** 0.5m S off A56 **Hotel** ★★ 85% HL The Millstone at Mellor, Church Ln, Mellor, BLACKBURN ☎ 01254 813333 17 en suite 6 annexe en suite

HEYSHAM   MAP 07 SD46

Heysham Trumacar Park, Middleton Rd LA3 3JH
☎ 01524 851011 (Sec) & 852000 (Pro) 📠 01524 853030
e-mail: secretary@heyshamgolfclub.co.uk
web: www.heyshamgolfclub.co.uk
A seaside parkland course, partly wooded. The 15th is a 459yd Par 4 nearly always played into the prevailing south west wind.
18 holes, 5999yds, Par 68, SSS 69. Club membership 850.
Visitors Mon-Sun & BHs. Booking required. Handicap certificate. Dress code. **Societies** Booking required. **Green Fees** £35 per day; £30 per round (£40 Sat, Sun & BHs). **Prof** Ryan Done **Course Designer** Alex Herd **Facilities** ⏰ 🍴 ⬛ ⬜ 🏐 🏌 ♂ 🏐 ♂ **Leisure** snooker. **Conf** Corporate Hospitality Days **Location** 0.75m S off A589 **Hotel** ★★★ 68% HL Clarendon Hotel, 76 Marine Rd West, West End Promenade, MORECAMBE ☎ 01524 410180 29 en suite

KNOTT END-ON-SEA   MAP 07 SD34

Knott End Wyreside FY6 0AA
☎ 01253 810576 📠 01253 813446
e-mail: louise@knottendgolfclub.com
web: www.knottendgolfclub.com
Scenic links and parkland course next to the Wyre estuary. The opening five holes run along the river and have spectacular views of the Fylde Coast. Although the course is quite short, the prevailing winds can add to one's score. Over-clubbing can be disastrous with trouble behind most of the smallish and well-guarded greens.
18 holes, 5849yds, Par 69, SSS 68, Course record 63.
Club membership 650.
Visitors Mon-Wed, Fri & BHs. Restricted Tue, Thu, Sun. Booking required. Dress code. **Societies** Booking required. **Green Fees** £33 per day, £31 per round (£43/£39 weekends). **Prof** Paul Walker **Course Designer** James Braid **Facilities** ⏰ 🍴 ⬛ ⬜ 🏐 🏌 ♂ 🏐 ♂ **Leisure** practice net. **Location** W of village off B5377 **Hotel** BUD Travelodge Lancaster (M6), White Carr Ln, Bay Horse, FORTON ☎ 08700 850 950 53 en suite

LANCASTER   MAP 07 SD46

Lancaster Golf Club Ashton Hall, Ashton-with-Stodday LA2 0AJ
☎ 01524 751247 📠 01524 752742
e-mail: office@lancastergc.co.uk
web: www.lancastergc.co.uk
This parkland course is unusual as it is exposed to winds from the Irish Sea. It is situated on the Lune estuary and has some natural hazards and easy walking. There are several fine holes among woods near the old clubhouse. Fine views towards the Lake District.
18 holes, 6282yds, Par 71, SSS 71, Course record 66.
Club membership 925.
Visitors Mon-Fri except BHs. Booking required. Handicap certificate. Dress code. **Societies** Welcome. **Green Fees** £50 per day, £40 per round. **Prof** David Sutcliffe **Course Designer** James Braid **Facilities** ⏰ 🍴 ⬛ ⬜ 🏐 🏌 ♂ 🏐 ♂ **Conf** Corporate Hospitality Days **Location** 3m S on A588 **Hotel** ★★★★ 73% HL Best Western Lancaster House Hotel, Green Ln, Ellel, LANCASTER ☎ 01524 844822 99 en suite

Lansil Caton Rd LA1 3PE
☎ 01524 61233
e-mail: lansilsportsgolfclub@onetel.net
9 holes, 5540yds, Par 70, SSS 67, Course record 68.
Location N of town centre on A683
Telephone for further details
Hotel ★★★★ 73% HL Best Western Lancaster House Hotel, Green Ln, Ellel, LANCASTER ☎ 01524 844822 99 en suite

LANGHO   MAP 07 SD73

Mytton Fold Hotel & Golf Complex Whalley Rd BB6 8AB
☎ 01254 245392 📠 01254 248119
web: www.myttonfold.co.uk
The course has panoramic views across the Ribble Valley and Pendle Hill. Tight fairways and water hazards are designed to make this a challenging course for any golfer.
18 holes, 6155yds, Par 72, SSS 70, Course record 69.
Club membership 450.   *Continued*

Visitors Mon-Fri & BHs. Sat & Sun after 2pm. Booking required. Dress code. **Societies** Booking required. **Green Fees** Mon-Thu £21, Fri-Sun & BHs £23. **Prof** Michael Bardi **Course Designer** Frank Hargreaves **Facilities** ⑪ ⑩ 🍴 ⬛ 🖥 ♦ 🏌 🛄 ✔ 🏌 ✔ **Conf** facs Corporate Hospitality Days **Location** On A59 between Langho
Hotel ★★ 79% HL The Avenue, Brockhall Village, LANGHO
☎ 01254 244811 21 en suite

LEYLAND   MAP 07 SD52

Leyland Wigan Rd PR25 5UD
☎ 01772 436457 📄 01772 435605
e-mail: manager@leylandgolfclub.co.uk
web: www.leylandgolfclub.co.uk
Parkland, fairly flat and usually breezy.
18 holes, 6298yds, Par 70, SSS 70, Course record 67.
Club membership 750.
Visitors Mon-Fri except BHs. Booking required. Handicap certificate. Dress code. **Societies** Booking required. **Green Fees** £25 per day. **Prof** Colin Burgess **Facilities** ⑪ ⑩ 🍴 ⬛ 🖥 ♦ 🏌 ✔ 🏌 ✔ **Conf** facs Corporate Hospitality Days **Location** M6 junct 28, 0.75m
Hotel ★★★ 78% HL Pines Hotel, 570 Preston Rd, Clayton-Le-Woods, CHORLEY ☎ 01772 338551 37 en suite

---

LONGRIDGE   MAP 07 SD63

Longridge Fell Barn, Jeffrey Hill PR3 2TU
☎ 01772 783291 📄 01772 783022
e-mail: secretary@longridgegolfclub.com
web: www.longridgegolfclub.com
One of the oldest clubs in England, which celebrated its 125th anniversary in 2002. A moorland course with panoramic views of the Trough of Bowland, the Fylde coast and Welsh mountains. Small, sloping greens, difficult to read.
18 holes, 5975yds, Par 70, SSS 69, Course record 63.
Club membership 600.
Visitors Mon-Sun & BHs. Booking required. Dress code. **Societies** Booking required. **Green Fees** £35 per day (£40 Sat & Sun). **Prof** Stephen Taylor **Facilities** ⑪ ⑩ 🍴 ⬛ 🖥 ♦ 🏌 ✔ 🏌 ✔ **Leisure** 9 hole Par 3 course. **Conf** facs Corporate Hospitality Days **Location** 8m NE of Preston off B6243
Hotel ★★★ 71% HL Shireburn Arms Hotel, Whalley Rd, Hurst Green, CLITHEROE ☎ 01254 826518 22 en suite

---

LYTHAM ST ANNES   MAP 07 SD32

Fairhaven Oakwood Av FY8 4JU
☎ 01253 736741 (Secretary) 📄 01253 731461
e-mail: secretary@fairhavengolfclub.co.uk
web: www.fairhavengolfclub.co.uk
A flat, but interesting parkland links course of good standard. There are natural hazards as well as numerous bunkers, and players need to produce particularly accurate second shots. Excellent natural drainage ensures year round play. An excellent test of golf for all abilities.
18 holes, 6883yds, Par 74, SSS 73, Course record 64.
Club membership 750.
Visitors Mon-Fri. Restricted Sat, Sun & BHs. Booking required. Handicap certificate. Dress code. **Societies** booking required. **Green Fees** £70 per day, £50 per round (£80/£60 Sat, Sun & BHs). **Prof** Brian Plucknett **Course Designer** J A Steer **Facilities** ⑪ ⑩ 🍴 ⬛ 🖥 ♦ 🏌 ✔ **Leisure** snooker. **Location** E of town centre off B5261

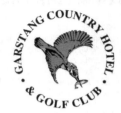

Between Royal Birkdale and Royal Lytham

... is the oasis of the Garstang Country Hotel & Golf Club. Our superb golf course offers a rewarding challenge for all standards of player, with interesting water hazards and well maintained greens. Hone your skills here and then play some of the great courses of the world nearby. We specialise in looking after golfers. We know what you need – and provide it.

Call 01995 600100 for details of our breaks

Bowgreave, Garstang, Lancashire, PR3 1YE

www.garstanghotelandgolf.co.uk

Hotel ★★★ 79% HL Bedford Hotel, 307-311 Clifton Dr South, LYTHAM ST ANNES ☎ 01253 724636 45 en suite

Lytham Green Drive Ballam Rd FY8 4LE
☎ 01253 737390 📄 01253 731350
e-mail: secretary@lythamgreendrive.co.uk
web: www.lythamgreendrive.co.uk
Green Drive provides a stern but fair challenge for even the most accomplished golfer. Tight fairways, strategically placed hazards and small tricky greens are the trademark of this testing course which meanders through pleasant countryside and is flanked by woods, pastures and meadows. The course demands accuracy in spite of the relatively flat terrain.
18 holes, 6363yds, Par 70, SSS 70, Course record 64.
Club membership 700.
Visitors Mon-Fri & BHs. Handicap certificate. Dress code. **Societies** Welcome. **Green Fees** £45 per day; £38 per round. **Prof** Andrew Lancaster **Course Designer** Steer **Facilities** ⑪ ⑩ 🍴 ⬛ 🖥 ♦ 🏌 ✔ **Conf** Corporate Hospitality Days **Location** E of town centre off B5259
Hotel ★★★ 79% HL Bedford Hotel, 307-311 Clifton Dr South, LYTHAM ST ANNES ☎ 01253 724636 45 en suite

Royal Lytham & St Annes see page 157

Hotel ★★★★ 79% HL Clifton Arms Hotel, West Beach, Lytham, LYTHAM ST ANNES ☎ 01253 739898 48 en suite

Hotel ★★★ 77% HL Chadwick Hotel, South Promenade, LYTHAM ST ANNES ☎ 01253 720061 Fax 01253 714455 75 en suite

Hotel ★★★ 79% HL Bedford Hotel, 307-311 Clifton Dr South, LYTHAM ST ANNES ☎ 01253 724636 Fax 01253 729244 45 en suite

Hotel ★★★ 74% HL Best Western Glendower Hotel, North Promenade, LYTHAM ST ANNES ☎ 01253 723241 Fax 01253 640069 60 en suite

St Annes Old Links Highbury Rd East FY8 2LD
☎ 01253 723597 📠 01253 781506
e-mail: secretary@stannesoldlinks.com
web: www.stannesoldlinks.com

Seaside links, qualifying course for Open Championship; compact and of very high standard, particularly greens. Windy, very long 5th, 17th and 18th holes. Famous hole: 9th (171yds), Par 3. Excellent club facilities.

18 holes, 6684yds, Par 72, SSS 72, Course record 63.
Club membership 750.

Visitors Mon-Fri except BHs. Booking required. Handicap certificate. Dress code. **Societies** Welcome. **Green Fees** Mon-Thu £50 per day, £45 am only, £40 pm only, Fri £65/£55/£50. **Prof** D J Webster **Course Designer** George Lowe **Facilities** ⊕ ﾊ ⌷ ⊻ ☐ ⚑ ✔ ✔ **Leisure** snooker room. **Conf** facs Corporate Hospitality Days **Location** N of town centre

Hotel ★★★ 77% HL Chadwick Hotel, South Promenade, LYTHAM ST ANNES ☎ 01253 720061 75 en suite

---

MORECAMBE   MAP 07 SD46

Morecambe Bare LA4 6AJ
☎ 01524 412841 📠 01524 400088
e-mail: secretary@morecambegolfclub.com
web: www.morecambegolfclub.com

Holiday golf at its most enjoyable. The well-maintained, wind-affected seaside parkland course is not long but full of character. Even so the panoramic views of Morecambe Bay, the Lake District and the Pennines make concentration difficult. The 4th is a testing hole.

18 holes, 5750yds, Par 67, SSS 69, Course record 69.
Club membership 850.

Visitors Mon-Sun & BHs, Booking required. Handicap certificate. Dress code. **Societies** booking required. **Green Fees** not confirmed. **Prof** Simon Fletcher **Course Designer** Dr Alister Mackenzie **Facilities** ⊕ ﾊ ﾊ ⌷ ⊻ ☐ ⚑ ✔ **Location** N of town centre on A5105

Hotel ★★★ 72% HL Elms Hotel, Bare Village, MORECAMBE ☎ 01524 411501 39 en suite

---

NELSON   MAP 07 SD83

Marsden Park Townhouse Rd BB9 8DG
☎ 01282 661912
e-mail: martin.robinson@pendleleisuretrust.co.uk
web: www.pendleleisuretrust.co.uk

A semi-parkland course offering panoramic views of surrounding countryside, set in the foothills of Pendle Marsden Park, a testing 18 holes for golfers of all abilities.

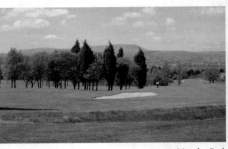

Marsden Park

18 holes, 5907yds, Par 70, SSS 68, Course record 66.
Club membership 400.

Visitors Mon-Sun & BHs. Booking required Fri-Sun & BHs. **Societies** booking required, midweek only. **Green Fees** not confirmed. **Facilities** ⊕ ﾊ ﾊ ⌷ ⊻ ☐ ⚑ ✔ ✔ **Leisure** practice nets. **Conf** facs Corporate Hospitality Days **Location** take M65 from Blackburn to end, turn right at rdbt, 2nd exit at next roundabout. left at Hour Glass Pub, signed on left

Hotel ★★★ 67% HL Sparrow Hawk Hotel, Church St, BURNLEY ☎ 01282 421551 35 en suite

Nelson King's Causeway, Brierfield BB9 0EU
☎ 01282 611834 📠 01282 611834
e-mail: secretary@nelsongolfclub.co.uk
web: www.nelsongolfclub.co.uk

Moorland course. Dr MacKenzie, who laid out the course, managed a design that does not include any wearisome climbing and created many interesting holes with wonderful panoramic views of the surrounding Pendle area.

18 holes, 6007yds, Par 70, SSS 69, Course record 64.
Club membership 580.

Visitors Tue, Wed, Fri, Sun & BHs. Booking required. Handicap certificate. Dress code. **Societies** Booking required. **Green Fees** £30 per day (£35 weekends & bank holidays). ⊛ **Prof** Neil Reeves **Course Designer** Dr Mackenzie **Facilities** ⊕ ﾊ ﾊ ⌷ ⊻ ☐ ⚑ ✔ **Conf** Corporate Hospitality Days **Location** M65 junct 12, A682 to Brierfield, left at lights onto Halifax Rd & King's Causeway

Hotel ★★★ 67% HL Sparrow Hawk Hotel, Church St, BURNLEY ☎ 01282 421551 35 en suite

---

ORMSKIRK   MAP 07 SD40

Hurlston Hall Hurlston Ln, Southport Rd, Scarisbrick L40 8HB
☎ 01704 840400 & 841120 (pro shop) 📠 01704 841404
e-mail: info@hurlstonhall.co.uk
web: www.hurlstonhall.co.uk

Designed by Donald Steel, this gently undulating course offers fine views of the Pennines and Bowland Fells. With generous fairways, large tees and greens, two streams and seven lakes, it provides a good test of golf for players of all standards.

18 holes, 6757yds, Par 72, SSS 72, Course record 66.
Club membership 650.

Visitors Mon, Tue, Thu,Fri & BHs. Booking required. Dress code. **Societies** Booking required. **Green Fees** not confirmed. **Course Designer** Donald Steel **Facilities** ⊕ ﾊ ﾊ ⌷ ⊻ ☐ ⚑ ✔ ⚑ **Leisure** heated indoor swimming pool, fishing, gymnasium. **Conf** facs Corporate Hospitality Days **Location** 2m from Ormskirk on A570

CHAMPIONSHIP COURSE

LANCASHIRE — LYTHAM ST ANNES

ROYAL LYTHAM & ST ANNES

Map 07 SD32

Links Gate FY8 3LQ
☎ **01253 724206** 🖨 **01253 780946**
e-mail: **bookings@royallytham.org**
web: **www.royallytham.org**
18 holes, 6882yds, Par 71, SSS 74,
Course record 64.
Club membership 850.
Visitors Mon-Fri & Sun. Booking
required. Handicap certificate. Dress code.
Societies Booking required.
Green Fees £180 per 36 holes, £120 per
18 holes (limited play Sun £180 per 18 holes).
All prices including lunch. **Prof** Eddie
Birchenough **Course Designer** George Lowe
Facilities ⑪ ⑩ ⓛ ⯑ ⯑ ⚥ 🖻 ◇ ⚐ ⚑
Leisure caddies available. **Conf** Corporate
Hospitality Days **Location** 0.5m E of St Annes

Founded in 1886, this huge links course
can be difficult, especially in windy
conditions. Unusually for a championship
course, it starts with a Par 3, the nearby
railway line and red-brick houses creating
distractions that add to the challenge. The
course has hosted 10 Open Championships
with some memorable victories: amateur
Bobby Jones famously won the first here
in 1926; Bobby Charles of New Zealand
became the only left-hander to win the
title; in 1969 Tony Jacklin helped to revive
British golf with his win; and the most
recent in 2001 was won by David Duval.

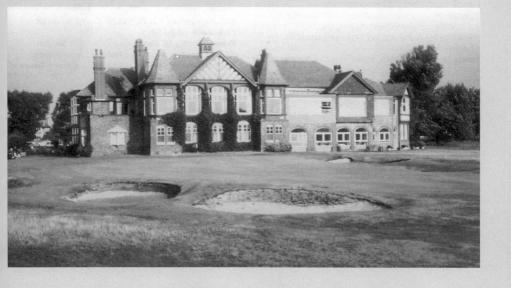

Ormskirk Cranes Ln, Lathom L40 5UJ
☎ 01695 572227 📠 01695 572227
e-mail: ormskirk@ukgolfer.org
web: www.ukgolfer.org
Pleasantly secluded, fairly flat parkland with much heath and silver birch. Accuracy from the tees will provide an interesting variety of second shots.
18 holes, 6358yds, Par 70, SSS 71, Course record 63.
Club membership 300.
Visitors Mon, Wed-Fri, Sun & BHs. Tue & Sat pm only. Booking required. Dress code. **Societies** booking required. **Green Fees** not confirmed. ⊛ **Prof** Jack Hammond **Course Designer** Harold Hilton **Facilities** ⊕ ⊦⊚⊦ ⊾ ⬚⊓ ⚌ ⛾ ✆ **Conf** Corporate Hospitality Days **Location** 1.5m NE

PLEASINGTON   MAP 07 SD62

Pleasington BB2 5JF
☎ 01254 202177 📠 01254 201028
e-mail: secretary-manager@pleasington-golf.co.uk
web: www.pleasington-golf.co.uk
Plunging and rising across lovely parkland and heathland turf, this course tests judgement of distance through the air to greens of widely differing levels. The 11th and 4th are testing holes. A regular regional qualifying course for the Open Championship.
18 holes, 6402yds, Par 71, SSS 71, Course record 65.
Club membership 700.
Visitors Mon-Fri & BHs. Booking required. Dress code. **Societies** Booking required. **Green Fees** £45 per round ⊛ **Prof** Ged Furey **Course Designer** George Lowe **Facilities** ⊕ ⊦⊚⊦ ⊾ ⬚ ⊓ ⚌ ⛾ ✆ 🜚 **Conf** facs Corporate Hospitality Days **Location** M65 junct 3, signed for Blackburn
Hotel ★★ 85% HL The Millstone at Mellor, Church Ln, Mellor, BLACKBURN ☎ 01254 813333 17 en suite 6 annexe en suite

---

POULTON-LE-FYLDE   MAP 07 SD33

Poulton-le-Fylde Breck Rd FY6 7HJ
☎ 01253 892444 & 893150
e-mail: greenwood-golf@hotmail.co.uk
A pleasant, municipal parkland course suitable for all standards of golfers although emphasis on accuracy is required.
9 holes, 2858yds, Par 35, SSS 34, Course record 66.
Club membership 300.
Visitors Mon-Sun & BHs. Booking required. **Green Fees** £15 per 18 holes, £9 per 9 holes (£18/£10 weekends). **Prof** John Greenwood **Course Designer** H Taylor **Facilities** ⊕ ⊦⊚⊦ ⊾ ⬚ ⊓ ⚌ ⛾ ✆ ⛾ ✆ **Location** M55 junct 3, A585 to Poulton, club signed
Hotel ★★ 69% HL Hotel Sheraton, 54-62 Queens Promenade, BLACKPOOL ☎ 01253 352723 104 en suite

---

PRESTON   MAP 07 SD52

Ashton & Lea Tudor Av, Lea PR4 0XA
☎ 01772 735282 📠 01772 735762
e-mail: mark@ashtonleagolfclub.co.uk
web: www.ashtonleagolfclub.co.uk
Fairly flat, well-maintained parkland course with natural water hazards, offering pleasant walks and some testing holes for golfers of all standards. Water comes into play on seven of the last nine holes. The course has three challenging Par 3s.
18 holes, 6334yds, Par 71, SSS 70, Course record 65.
Club membership 650.

Societies Booking required. ⊛ **Prof** M Greenough **Course Designer** J Steer **Facilities** ⊕ ⊦⊚⊦ ⊾ ⬚ ⊓ ⚌ ⛾ ✆ **Leisure** snooker table.
Conf facs Corporate Hospitality Days **Location** 3m W of Preston on A5085
Hotel ★★★★ 76% HL Preston Marriott Hotel, Garstang Rd, Broughton, PRESTON ☎ 01772 864087 149 en suite

Fishwick Hall Glenluce Dr, Farringdon Park PR1 5TD
☎ 01772 798300 📠 01772 704600
e-mail: fishwickhallgolfclub@supanet.com
web: www.fishwickhallgolfclub.co.uk
Meadowland course overlooking River Ribble. Natural hazards.
18 holes, 6045yds, Par 70, SSS 69, Course record 66.
Club membership 650.
Visitors Mon-Sun & BHs. Booking required. Handicap certificate. Dress code. **Societies** booking required. **Green Fees** not confirmed. **Prof** Martin Watson **Facilities** ⊕ ⊦⊚⊦ ⊾ ⬚ ⊓ ⚌ ⛾ ✆ **Conf** Corporate Hospitality Days **Location** M6 junct 31
Hotel ★★★ 75% HL Macdonald Tickled Trout, Preston New Rd, Samlesbury, PRESTON ☎ 0870 1942120 102 en suite

Ingol Tanterton Hall Rd, Ingol PR2 7BY
☎ 01772 734556 📠 01772 729815
e-mail: ingol@golfers.net
web: www.ingolgolfclub.co.uk
Championship-designed course with natural water hazards, set in 250 acres of beautiful parkland. A good test for any golfer.

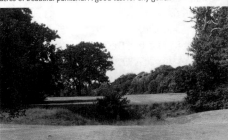

18 holes, 6294yds, Par 72, SSS 70, Course record 68.
Club membership 650.
Visitors Mon-Sun & BHs. Booking required. Dress code. **Societies** booking required. **Green Fees** not confirmed. **Prof** Ryan Grimshaw **Course Designer** Henry Cotton **Facilities** ⊕ ⊦⊚⊦ ⊾ ⬚ ⊓ ⚌ ⛾ ✆ **Leisure** squash, Snooker & Pool. **Conf** facs **Location** A5085 onto B5411, signs to Ingol
Hotel BUD Premier Travel Inn Preston East, Bluebell Way, Preston East Link Rd, Fulwood, PRESTON ☎ 08701 977215 65 en suite

Penwortham Blundell Ln, Penwortham PR1 0AX
☎ 01772 744630 📠 01772 740172
e-mail: penworthamgolfclub@supanet.com
web: www.ukgolfer.org/clubs/penwortham
18 holes, 5877yds, Par 69, SSS 69, Course record 65.
Location 1.5m W of town centre off A59
Telephone for further details
Hotel ★★★ 75% HL Macdonald Tickled Trout, Preston New Rd, Samlesbury, PRESTON ☎ 0870 1942120 102 en suite

Preston Fulwood Hall Ln, Fulwood PR2 8DD
☎ 01772 700011 📠 01772 794234
e-mail: secretary@prestongolfclub.com
web: www.prestongolfclub.com
18 holes, 6312yds, Par 71, SSS 71, Course record 68.
Course Designer James Braid **Location** 1m N of city centre on A6, right at
lights onto Watling St, left onto Fulwood Hall Ln, course 300yds on left
Telephone for further details
Hotel ★★★★ 76% HL Preston Marriott Hotel, Garstang Rd, Broughton,
PRESTON ☎ 01772 864087 149 en suite

RISHTON   MAP 07 SD73

Rishton Eachill Links, Hawthorn Dr BB1 4HG
☎ 01254 884442 📠 01254 887701
e-mail: rishtongc@onetel.net
web: www.rishtongolfclub.co.uk
Undulating moorland course with some interesting holes and fine
views of East Lancashire.
Eachill Links: 10 holes, 6097yds, Par 70, SSS 69,
Course record 68. Club membership 270.
Visitors Mon-Fri & BHs. Handicap certificate. Dress code. **Green Fees** £20.
🅰 **Course Designer** Peter Alliss/Dave Thomas **Facilities** ⑪ ⑩ 🃟 ⌺
🎱 by arrangement 🚶 **Conf** Corporate Hospitality Days **Location** M65
junct 6/7, 1m. Signed from Station Rd in Rishton
Hotel ★★★★ 74% HL Mercure Dunkenhalgh Hotel & Spa, Blackburn Rd,
Clayton-le-Moors, ACCRINGTON ☎ 0870 1942116 78 en suite 97 annexe
en suite

SILVERDALE   MAP 07 SD47

Silverdale Redbridge Ln LA5 0SP
☎ 01524 701300 📠 01524 702074
e-mail: silverdalegolfclub@ecosse.net
web: silverdalegolfclub.com
Challenging heathland course with rock outcrops, set in an Area of
Outstanding Natural Beauty with spectacular views of the Lake District
hills and Morecambe Bay. It is a course of two halves, being either
open fairways or tight hilly limestone valleys. The 13th hole has been
described as one of Britain's 100 extraordinary golf holes.
18 holes, 5526yds, Par 70, SSS 67, Course record 68.
Club membership 500.
Visitors Mon-Fri & BHs, Booking required. Handicap certificate. Dress code.
Societies Booking required. **Green Fees** £30 per day; £25 per round.
Prof Ryan Grimshaw **Facilities** ⑪ ⑩ 🃟 ⌺ 🃟 🚶 🎱 🏌 **Conf** Corporate
Hospitality Days **Location** Opp Silverdale station Moss RSPB nature reserve
Hotel ★★ 65% HL Royal Station Hotel, Market St, CARNFORTH
☎ 01524 732033 & 733636 📠 01524 720267 13 en suite

UPHOLLAND   MAP 07 SD50

Beacon Park Golf & Country Club Beacon Ln
WN8 7RU
☎ 01695 622700 📠 01695 628362
e-mail: info@beaconparkgolf.com
web: www.beaconparkgolf.com
Undulating/hilly parkland course, designed by Donald Steel, with
magnificent view of the Welsh hills. Twenty-four-bay floodlit driving
range open 9am-9pm in summer.
18 holes, 6000yds, Par 72, SSS 69, Course record 68.
Club membership 250.

Visitors Mon-Sun & BHs. Booking required. Dress code. **Societies** Booking
required. **Green Fees** £11 per 18 holes (£16 weekends & bank holidays).
Prof Colin Parkinson **Course Designer** Donald Steel **Facilities** ⑪ ⑩ 🃟
by prior arrangement 🃟 by prior arrangement ⌺ 🃟 🚶 🎱 🏌 🎱 🏌
🏌 **Conf** Corporate Hospitality Days **Location** M6 junct 26, S of Ashurst
Beacon Hill

Dean Wood Lafford Ln WN8 0QZ
☎ 01695 622219 📠 01695 622245
web: www.deanwoodgolfclub.co.uk
This parkland course has a varied terrain - flat front nine, undulating
back nine. Beware the Par 4 11th and 17th holes, which have ruined
many a card. If there were a prize for the best maintained course in
Lancashire, Dean Wood would be a strong contender.
18 holes, 6148yds, Par 71, SSS 70, Course record 65.
Club membership 730.
Visitors Mon-Fri. Booking required Tue & Wed. Handicap certificate.
Dress code. **Societies** booking required. **Green Fees** not confirmed. 🅰
Prof Stuart Danchin **Course Designer** James Braid **Facilities** ⑪ ⑩ 🃟
⌺ 🃟 🚶 🏌 **Conf** Corporate Hospitality Days **Location** M6 junct 26,
1m on A577

WHALLEY   MAP 07 SD73

Whalley Long Leese Barn, Clerk Hill Rd BB7 9DR
☎ 01254 822236
A parkland course near Pendle Hill, overlooking the Ribble Valley.
Superb views. Ninth hole over pond.
9 holes, 6258yds, Par 72, SSS 71, Course record 69.
Club membership 450.
Visitors Mon-Wed, Fri, Sun & BHs. Booking required Sun & BHs.Dress code.
Societies Booking required. **Green Fees** £25 per day (£30 Sun and bank
holidays). 🅰 **Prof** Jamie Hunt **Facilities** ⑪ ⑩ 🃟 ⌺ 🃟 🚶 🎱 🏌 **Conf**
Corporate Hospitality Days **Location** 1m SE off A671

WHITWORTH   MAP 07 SD81

Lobden Lobden Moor OL12 8XJ
☎ 01706 343228 & 345598 📠 01706 343228
Moorland course, with hard walking. Windy with superb views of
surrounding hills. Excellent greens.
9 holes, 5697yds, Par 70, SSS 68, Course record 63.
Club membership 250.
Visitors Contact club for details. Dress code. **Societies** Welcome. **Green
Fees** Phone. 🅰 **Facilities** 🚶 **Location** E of town centre off A671
Hotel ★★★★ 77% HL Mercure Norton Grange Hotel & Spa, Manchester
Rd, Castleton, ROCHDALE ☎ 0870 1942119 81 en suite

WILPSHIRE   MAP 07 SD63

Wilpshire Whalley Rd BB1 9LF
☎ 01254 248260 📠 01254 246745
18 holes, 5971yds, Par 69, SSS 69, Course record 62.
Course Designer James Braid **Location** 2m NE of Blackburn, on A666
towards Clitheroe
Telephone for further details
Hotel ★★★ 75% HL Sparth House Hotel, Whalley Rd, Clayton Le Moors,
ACCRINGTON ☎ 01254 872263 16 en suite

LEICESTERSHIRE

ASHBY-DE-LA-ZOUCH
MAP 08 SK31

Willesley Park Measham Rd LE65 2PF
☎ 01530 414596 📠 01530 564169
e-mail: info@willesleypark.com
web: www.willesleypark.com
Undulating heathland and parkland with quick-draining sandy subsoil.
18 holes, 6304yds, Par 70, SSS 70, Course record 63.
Club membership 600.
Visitors Booking required. Handicap certificate. **Societies** Welcome.
Green Fees £35 per day/round (£40 weekends and bank holidays). 🏌
Prof Ben Hill **Course Designer** J Braid **Facilities** ⑪ ⑩ 🗄 ☐ 🖤 🏌 🛆 🍴 🛒
Location SW of town centre on B5006
Hotel ★★ 67% HL Charnwood Arms Hotel, Beveridge Ln, Bardon Hill,
COALVILLE ☎ 01530 813644 34 en suite

BIRSTALL
MAP 04 SK50

Birstall Station Rd LE4 3BB
☎ 0116 267 4322 📠 0116 267 4322
e-mail: sue@birstallgolfclub.co.uk
web: www.birstallgolfclub.co.uk
Parkland with trees, shrubs, ponds and ditches, next to the Great
Central Railway Steam Train line.
18 holes, 6213yds, Par 70, SSS 70. Club membership 650.
Visitors Mon, Wed-Fri & BHs. Sat & Sun by arrangement. Handicap
certificate. Dress code. **Societies** Booking required. **Green Fees** £35
per day; £30 per round (£40 per round Sat & Sun). 🏌 **Prof** David Clark
Facilities ⑪ ⑩ 🗄 ☐ 🖤 🏌 🛆 🍴 🛒 **Leisure** billiard room. **Conf** facs
Corporate Hospitality Days **Location** 3m N of Leicester on A6
Hotel ★★★ 68% HL Rothley Court, Westfield Ln, ROTHLEY
☎ 0116 237 4141 12 en suite 18 annexe en suite

BOTCHESTON
MAP 04 SK40

Forest Hill Markfield Ln LE9 9FJ
☎ 01455 824800 📠 01455 828522
e-mail: golfadmin@foresthillgc.co.uk
Parkland course with many trees, four Par 5s, but no steep gradients.
Water features on 7 holes.
18 holes, 6600yds, Par 72, SSS 71, Course record 63.
Club membership 700.
Visitors Mon-Fri except BHs. Booking required. Handicap certificate. Dress
code. **Societies** Booking required. **Green Fees** £45 per day; £30 per
round. **Prof** Clive Fromant **Course Designer** Gaunt & Marnoch **Facilities**
⑪ ⑩ 🗄 ☐ 🖤 🏌 🛆 🍴 🛒 🚲 ⚽ 🏸 **Leisure** 9 hole Par 3 academy course.
Conf facs **Location** M1 junct 22, take A50 towards Leicester, turn right
at 1st rdbt and follow road for 4m, club on left.
Hotel ★★ 65% HL Castle Hotel & Restaurant, Main St, KIRBY MUXLOE
☎ 0116 239 5337 22 en suite

COSBY
MAP 04 SP59

Cosby Chapel Ln, Broughton Rd LE9 1RG
☎ 0116 286 4759 📠 0116 286 4484
e-mail: secretary@cosby-golf-club.co.uk
web: www.cosby-golf-club.co.uk
18 holes, 6410yds, Par 71, SSS 71, Course record 65.
Course Designer Hawtree **Location** M1 junct 21, B4114 to L-turn at BP
service station, signed Cosby

Telephone for further details
Hotel ★★★★ 79% HL Best Western Sketchley Grange Hotel, Sketchley Ln,
Burbage, HINCKLEY ☎ 01455 251133 52 en suite

EAST GOSCOTE
MAP 08 SK61

Beedles Lake 170 Broome Ln LE7 3WQ
☎ 0116 260 6759 📠 0116 260 4414
e-mail: ian@jelson.co.uk
web: www.beedleslake.co.uk
Fairly flat parkland with easy walking. Ditches, streams and rivers come
into play on many holes. Older trees and thousands of newly planted
ones give the course a mature feel. Many challenging holes where you
can ruin a good score.
18 holes, 6641yds, Par 72, SSS 72, Course record 68.
Club membership 498.
Visitors Mon-Sun & BHs. Booking required Fri-Sun & BHs. Dress code.
Societies Booking required. **Green Fees** not confirmed. **Prof** Sean Byrne
Course Designer D Tucker **Facilities** ⑪ ⑩ 🗄 ☐ 🖤 🏌 🛆 🍴 ⚽ 🛒
Leisure fishing. **Conf** facs Corporate Hospitality Days **Location** Off A607
Hotel ★★★ 68% HL Rothley Court, Westfield Ln, ROTHLEY
☎ 0116 237 4141 12 en suite 18 annexe en suite

ENDERBY
MAP 04 SP59

Enderby Mill Ln LE19 4LX
☎ 0116 284 9388 📠 0116 284 9388
An attractive gently undulating nine-hole course with various water
features. The longest hole is the 2nd at 471yds.
9 holes, 2856yds, Par 72, SSS 71, Course record 71.
Club membership 150.
Visitors Mon-Sun & BHs. **Societies** Welcome. **Green Fees** £8.20
per 18 holes, £6.70 per 9 holes. **Prof** Chris D'Araujo **Course Designer**
David Lowe **Facilities** ⑪ ⑩ 🗄 ☐ 🖤 🏌 🛆 🍴 ⚽ 🛒 **Leisure** heated
indoor swimming pool, squash, sauna, solarium, gymnasium, indoor bowls
snooker badminton. **Location** M1 junct 21, 2m S on Narborough road, right
at Toby Carvery rdbt, 0.5m on left, signed
Hotel ★★★ 68% HL Westfield House Hotel, Enderby Rd, Blaby, LEICESTER
☎ 0116 278 7898 & 0870 609 6106 📠 0116 278 1974 48 en suite

HINCKLEY
MAP 04 SP49

Hinckley Leicester Rd LE10 3DR
☎ 01455 615124 & 615014 📠 01455 890841
e-mail: proshop@hinckleygolfclub.com
web: www.hinckleygolfclub.com
Parkland course with a good variety of holes to test all abilities. Water
comes into play on a number of holes.
18 holes, 6467yds, Par 71, SSS 71, Course record 65.
Club membership 750.
Visitors Mon-Fri except BHs. Handicap certificate. Dress code.
Societies booking required. **Green Fees** not confirmed. **Prof** Richard
Jones **Course Designer** Southern Golf Ltd **Facilities** ⑪ ⑩ 🗄 ☐ 🖤
🛆 🍴 🚲 ⚽ **Leisure** snooker. **Conf** facs Corporate Hospitality Days
Location 1.5m NE on B4668
Hotel ★★★ 72% HL Best Western Weston Hall Hotel, Weston Ln,
Bulkington, NUNEATON ☎ 024 7631 2989 40 en suite

KIBWORTH
MAP 04 SP69

Kibworth Weir Rd, Beauchamp LE8 0LP
☎ 0116 279 2301 📄 0116 279 6434
e-mail: secretary@kibworthgolfclub.freeserve.co.uk
Easy walking parkland with a brook affecting a number of fairways.
Most holes are tightly bunkered.
18 holes, 6354yds, Par 71, SSS 71. Club membership 700.
Visitors Mon-Fri & BHs. Handicap certificate. Dress code **Societies** Booking
required. **Green Fees** £40 per day; £30 per round. ☻ **Prof** Mike Herbert
Facilities ⑪ �ΙΟΙ ⣐ ⣏ 🛇 ⤳ 🍴 🏌 **Location** S of village off A6
Hotel ★★★ 75% HL Best Western Three Swans Hotel, 21 High St, MARKET
HARBOROUGH ☎ 01858 466644 18 en suite 43 annexe en suite

KIRBY MUXLOE
MAP 04 SK50

Kirby Muxloe Station Rd LE9 2EP
☎ 0116 239 3457 📄 0116 238 8891
e-mail: kirbymuxloegolf@btconnect.com
web: www.kirbymuxloe-golf.co.uk
Pleasant parkland with a lake in front of the 17th green and a
short 18th.
18 holes, 6351yds, Par 71, SSS 70, Course record 62.
Club membership 870.
Visitors Booking required. Handicap certificate. **Societies** Booking required.
Green Fees £40 per day, £32 per round. ☻ **Prof** Bruce Whipham
Facilities ⑪ ΙΟΙ ⣐ ⣏ 🛇 ⤳ 🍴 🏌 **Leisure** snooker. **Conf** facs
Corporate Hospitality Days **Location** S of village off B5380
Hotel ★★ 65% HL Castle Hotel & Restaurant, Main St, KIRBY MUXLOE
☎ 0116 239 5337 22 en suite

LEICESTER
MAP 04 SK50

Humberstone Heights Gypsy Ln LE5 0TB
☎ 0116 276 3680 & 299 5570 (pro) 📄 0116 299 5569
e-mail: admin@hhmgolfclub.freeserve.co.uk
Municipal parkland course with varied layout.
18 holes, 6216yds, Par 70, SSS 70, Course record 66.
Club membership 400.
Visitors Mon-Sun & BHs. Booking required. Dress code. **Societies** Booking
required. **Green Fees** Phone. **Prof** Phil Highfield **Course Designer** Hawtry
& Sons **Facilities** ⑪ ΙΟΙ ⣐ ⣏ 🛇 ⤳ 🍴 🏌 **Leisure** 9 hole pitch
and putt course. **Location** 2.5m NE of city centre
Hotel ★★★ 85% HL Best Western Belmont House Hotel, De Montfort St,
LEICESTER ☎ 0116 254 4773 77 en suite

Leicestershire Evington Ln LE5 6DJ
☎ 0116 273 8825 📄 0116 249 8799
e-mail: enquiries@thelgc.co.uk
web: www.thelgc.co.uk
18 holes, 6134yds, Par 68, SSS 70.
Course Designer Hawtree **Location** 2m E of city off A6030
Telephone for further details
Hotel ★★★ 72% HL Regency Hotel, 360 London Rd, LEICESTER
☎ 0116 270 9634 32 en suite

Western Scudamore Rd, Braunstone Frith LE3 1UQ
☎ 0116 299 5566 📄 0116 299 5568
Pleasant, undulating parkland course with open aspect fairways in
two loops of nine holes.Not too difficult but a good test of golf off the
back tees.
18 holes, 6518yds, Par 72, SSS 71. Club membership 400.
Visitors Mon-Sun & BHs. Booking required Sat, Sun & BHs. Dress code.
I **Societies** Booking required. **Green Fees** £14.50 per 18 holes, £12
per 9 holes (£17.50/£13 Sat & Sun). **Prof** Dave Butler **Facilities** ⑪ ΙΟΙ ⣐ ⣏
🛇 ⤳ 🍴 🏌 **Location** 1.5m W of city centre off A47
Hotel ★★ 65% HL Castle Hotel & Restaurant, Main St, KIRBY MUXLOE
☎ 0116 239 5337 22 en suite

LOUGHBOROUGH
MAP 08 SK51

Longcliffe Snell's Nook Ln, Nanpantan LE11 3YA
☎ 01509 239129 📄 01509 231286
e-mail: longcliffegolf@btconnect.com
web: www.longcliffegolf.co.uk

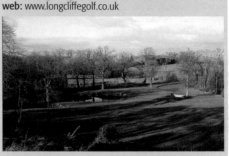

18 holes, 6625yds, Par 72, SSS 73, Course record 65.
Course Designer Williamson **Location** 1.5m from M1 junct 23 off A512
Telephone for further details
Hotel ★★★ 71% HL Quality Hotel & Suites Loughborough, New Ashby
Rd, LOUGHBOROUGH ☎ 01509 211800 94 en suite

LUTTERWORTH
MAP 04 SP58

Kilworth Springs South Kilworth Rd, North Kilworth
LE17 6HJ
☎ 01858 575082 📄 01858 575078
e-mail: kilworthsprings@ukonline.co.uk
web: www.kilworthsprings.co.uk
An 18-hole course of two loops of nine: the front nine is links style
while the back nine is in parkland with four lakes. Attractive views over
the Avon valley. Greens to USGA specifications.
18 holes, 6718yds, Par 72, SSS 71, Course record 65.
Club membership 850.
Visitors Mon-Sun & BHs. Booking required. Dress code. **Societies** Booking
required. **Green Fees** £24 (£27 Sat & Sun). **Prof** Anders Mankert **Course
Designer** Ray Baldwin **Facilities** ⑪ ΙΟΙ ⣐ ⣏ 🛇 ⤳ 🍴 🏌
Leisure half way house on course. **Conf** facs Corporate Hospitality Days
Location M1 junct 20, 4m E A4304 towards Market Harborough between
villages of North & South Kilworth
Hotel ★★★ 77% HL BW Ullesthorpe Court Country Hotel& Golf Club,
Frolesworth Rd, ULLESTHORPE ☎ 01455 209023 72 en suite

England

Lutterworth Rugby Rd LE17 4HN
☎ 01455 552532 📠 01455 553586
e-mail: sec@lutterworthgc.co.uk
web: www.lutterworthgc.co.uk
Hilly course with the River Swift running through.
18 holes, 6226yds, Par 70, SSS 70. Club membership 700.
Visitors Mon-Fri except BHs. Booking required. Handicap certificate.
Dress code. **Societies** Booking required. **Green Fees** £36 per day, £28
per 18 holes. ⊛ **Prof** Lee Challinor **Facilities** ⑪ ⑩ 🗟 🖵 🖤 🎿 🏤 ⛳ 🏌
🏌 **Conf** Corporate Hospitality Days **Location** M1 junct 20, 0.25m
Hotel ★★★ 68% HL Brownsover Hall Hotel, Brownsover Ln, Old
Brownsover, RUGBY ☎ 0870 609 6104 & 01788 546100 📠 01788 579241 27
en suite 20 annexe en suite

Market Harborough Oxendon Rd LE16 8NF
☎ 01858 463684 📠 01858 432906
e-mail: proshop@mhgolf.co.uk
web: www.mhgolf.co.uk
A parkland course close to the town. Undulating and in parts hilly.
There are wide-ranging views over the surrounding countryside. Lakes
feature on four holes; challenging last three holes.
18 holes, 6086yds, Par 70, SSS 69, Course record 61.
Club membership 650.
Visitors Mon-Fri except BHs. Handicap certificate. Dress code. **Societies**
Booking required. **Green Fees** £30 per round. ⊛ **Prof** Frazer Baxter
Course Designer H Swan **Facilities** ⑪ ⑩ 🗟 🖵 🖤 🎿 🏤 🏌
Conf Corporate Hospitality Days **Location** 1m S on A508
Hotel ★★★ 75% HL Best Western Three Swans Hotel, 21 High St, MARKET
HARBOROUGH ☎ 01858 466644 18 en suite 43 annexe en suite

Stoke Albany Ashley Rd, Stoke Albany LE16 8PL
☎ 01858 535208 📠 01858 535505
e-mail: info@stokealbanygolfclub.co.uk
web: www.stokealbanygolfclub.co.uk
A parkland course in the picturesque Welland valley. Affording good
views, the course should appeal to the mid-handicap golfer, and
provide an interesting test to the more experienced player. There
are several water features and the greens are individually contoured,
adding to the golfing challenge.
18 holes, 6175yds, Par 71, SSS 70, Course record 65.
Club membership 500.
Visitors Mon-Sun & BHs. Dress code. **Societies** Booking required.
Green Fees £21 per 18 holes (£23 Sat, Sun & BHs). **Prof** Adrian Clifford
Course Designer Hawtree **Facilities** ⑪ ⑩ 🗟 🖵 🖤 🎿 🏤 🏌
Conf facs Corporate Hospitality Days **Location** N off A427 Market
Harborough-Corby road, follow Stoke Albany 500yds towards Ashley
Hotel ★★★ 75% HL Best Western Three Swans Hotel, 21 High St, MARKET
HARBOROUGH ☎ 01858 466644 18 en suite 43 annexe en suite

Melton Mowbray Waltham Rd, Thorpe Arnold LE14 4SD
☎ 01664 562118 📠 01664 562118
e-mail: meltonmowbraygc@btconnect.com
web: www.mmgc.org
Easy walking heathland course with undulating fairways. Deceptively
challenging.

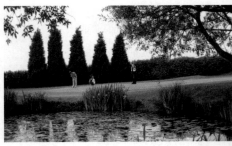
Melton Mowbray

18 holes, 6222yds, Par 70, SSS 70, Course record 65.
Club membership 650.
Visitors Mon-Fri, Sun & BHs. Booking required. Dress code. **Societies**
Booking required. **Green Fees** £35 per day, £25 per round (£30 per round
Sun and bank holidays). **Prof** Neil Curtis **Facilities** ⑪ ⑩ 🗟 🖵 🖤 🎿 🏤
🏌 🏌 **Conf** Corporate Hospitality Days **Location** 2m NE of Melton
Mowbray on A607
Hotel ★★★ 75% HL Sysonby Knoll Hotel, Asfordby Rd, MELTON
MOWBRAY ☎ 01664 563563 23 en suite 7 annexe en suite

Stapleford Park Stapleford LE14 2EF
☎ 01572 787000 & 787044 📠 01572 787001
e-mail: clubs@stapleford.com
web: www.staplefordpark.com
Set in 500 acres of parkland, lake and woods. Reminiscent of some
Scottish links, the course wraps around the heart of the estate in two
extended loops. Never more than two holes wide, the whole course is
spacious and tranquil. The beauty of the surrounding countryside is the
perfect backdrop.
18 holes, 6944yds, Par 73, SSS 73. Club membership 310.
Visitors Mon-Fri & BHs. Sat & Sun after 11am. Booking required. Handicap
certificate. Dress code. **Societies** Booking required. **Green Fees** £75 per
day, £50 per 18 holes. **Prof** Richard Alderson **Course Designer** Donald
Steel **Facilities** ⑪ ⑩ 🗟 🖵 🖤 🎿 🏤 ⛳ ◇ 🏌 🏤 🏌 🏌 **Leisure** hard
tennis courts, heated indoor swimming pool, fishing, sauna, gymnasium,
shooting, falconry, offroading, horseriding, archery. **Conf** facs Corporate
Hospitality Days **Location** 4m E of Melton Mowbray off B676
Hotel ★★★★ HL Stapleford Park, Stapleford, MELTON MOWBRAY
☎ 01572 787000 48 en suite 7 annexe en suite

Glen Gorse Glen Rd LE2 4RF
☎ 0116 271 4159 📠 0116 271 4159
e-mail: secretary@gggc.org
web: www.gggc.org
Attractive mature parkland course with strategically placed trees
encountered on every hole, rewarding the straight hitter. The long
approaches and narrow greens require the very best short game.
However, a premium is placed on accuracy and length, and no more
so than over the closing three holes, considered to be one of the finest
finishes in the county.
18 holes, 6648yds, Par 72, SSS 72, Course record 64.
Club membership 818.
Visitors Mon-Fri except BHs. Booking required. Handicap certificate. Dress
code. **Societies** Booking required. **Green Fees** Phone. ⊛ **Prof** Dominic
Fitzpatrick **Facilities** ⑪ ⑩ 🗟 🖵 🖤 🎿 🏤 🏌 🏤 🏌 **Leisure** snooker room.

Continued

Conf Corporate Hospitality Days **Location** On A6 between Oadby Glen, 5m S of Leicester
Hotel ★★★ 72% HL Regency Hotel, 360 London Rd, LEICESTER
☎ 0116 270 9634 32 en suite

Oadby Leicester Rd LE2 4AJ
☎ 0116 270 9052
e-mail: oadbygolf@supanet.com
web: www.oadbygolfclub.co.uk
18 holes, 6376yds, Par 72, SSS 70, Course record 69.
Location W of Oadby off A6
Telephone for further details
Hotel ★★★ 72% HL Regency Hotel, 360 London Rd, LEICESTER
☎ 0116 270 9634 32 en suite

ROTHLEY   MAP 08 SK51

Rothley Park Westfield Ln LE7 7LH
☎ 0116 230 2809 📄 0116 230 2809
e-mail: secretary@rothleypark.co.uk
web: www.rothleypark.com
A picturesque parkland course.
18 holes, 6477yds, Par 71, SSS 71, Course record 67.
Club membership 600.
Visitors Mon, Wed-Fri. Sat/Sun & BHs by arrangement. Handicap certificate. Dress code. **Societies** Welcome. **Green Fees** Phone. ⊛ **Prof** D Spillane
Facilities ⑪ ⥽◎ ⯑ 🍴 🏌 🛒 ♂ 🥤 **Conf** Corporate Hospitality Days
Location N of Leicester, W off A6
Hotel ★★★ 68% HL Rothley Court, Westfield Ln, ROTHLEY
☎ 0116 237 4141 12 en suite 18 annexe en suite

SCRAPTOFT   MAP 04 SK60

Scraptoft Beeby Rd LE7 9SJ
☎ 0116 241 9000 📄 0116 241 9000
e-mail: secretary@scraptoft-golf.co.uk
web: www.scraptoft-golf.co.uk
A well wooded and beautiful parkland course demanding accuracy.
18 holes, 6166yds, Par 70, SSS 70. Club membership 650.
Visitors Mon-Fri & BHs. Handicap certificate. Dress code. **Societies** Booking required. **Green Fees** £40 per day; £30 per round. **Prof** Simon Wood
Facilities ⑪ ⥽◎ ⯑ 🍴 🏌 🛒 ♀ 🥤 **Location** 1m NE
Hotel ★★★ 85% HL Best Western Belmont House Hotel, De Montfort St, LEICESTER ☎ 0116 254 4773 77 en suite

SEAGRAVE   MAP 08 SK61

Park Hill Park Hill LE12 7NG
☎ 01509 815454 📄 01509 816062
e-mail: mail@parkhillgolf.co.uk
web: www.parkhillgolf.co.uk
Nestled in the heart of Leicestershire, overlooking the Charnwood Forest and beyond, Park Hill Golf Club has an 18-hole championship length course that uses the land's natural features to ensure that no two holes are the same. The combination of water features and precisely positioned bunkers provide for a challenging, yet enjoyable course, with excellent playing conditions all year round.
18 holes, 7219yds, Par 73, SSS 75, Course record 71.
Club membership 500.
Visitors Mon-Sun & BHs. Dress code. **Societies** welcome.
Green Fees £25 (£30 weekends & bank holidays). **Prof** Matthew Ulyett

Facilities ⑪ ⥽◎ ⯑ 🍴 🏌 🛒 ♂ 🥤 🍽 ♂ 🥤 **Conf** facs Corporate Hospitality Days **Location** 3m N of Leicester off A46, signs to Seagrave
Hotel ★★★ 71% HL Quality Hotel & Suites Loughborough, New Ashby Rd, LOUGHBOROUGH ☎ 01509 211800 94 en suite

SIX HILLS   MAP 08 SK62

Six Hills Six Hills Rd LE14 3PR
☎ 01509 881225 📄 01509 881846
18 holes, 5758yds, SSS 69.
Location On B676 between Melton Mowbray
Telephone for further details
Hotel BUD Travelodge Leicester Thrussington, THRUSSINGTON
☎ 08700 850 950 32 en suite

ULLESTHORPE   MAP 04 SP58

Ullesthorpe Court Country Hotel & Golf Club
Frolesworth Rd LE17 5BZ
☎ 01455 209023 📄 01455 202537
e-mail: bookings@ullesthorpecourt.co.uk
web: www.bw-ullesthorpe.co.uk
Set in 120 acres of parkland surrounding a 17th-century manor house, this championship length course can be very demanding and offers a challenge to both beginners and professionals. Excellent leisure facilities. Water plays a part on three holes.

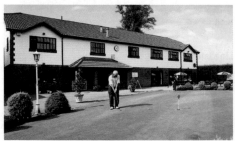

18 holes, 6662yds, Par 72, SSS 72, Course record 67.
Club membership 650.
Visitors Mon-Fri except BHs. Booking required. Dress code.
Societies booking required. **Green Fees** not confirmed. **Prof** David Bowring **Facilities** ⑪ ⥽◎ ⯑ 🍴 🏌 🛒 ◇ ♂ 🥤 ♂ **Leisure** hard tennis courts, heated indoor swimming pool, sauna, solarium, gymnasium.
Conf facs Corporate Hospitality Days **Location** M1 junct 20, 5m
Hotel ★★★ 77% HL BW Ullesthorpe Court Country Hotel& Golf Club, Frolesworth Rd, ULLESTHORPE ☎ 01455 209023 72 en suite

WHETSTONE   MAP 04 SP59

Whetstone Cambridge Rd, Cosby LE9 1SJ
☎ 0116 286 1424 📄 0116 286 1424
18 holes, 5795yds, Par 68, SSS 68, Course record 63.
Course Designer E Calloway **Location** 1m S of village
Telephone for further details
Hotel ★★★ 68% HL Westfield House Hotel, Enderby Rd, Blaby, LEICESTER
☎ 0116 278 7898 & 0870 609 6106 📄 0116 278 1974 48 en suite

WILSON MAP 08 SK42

Breedon Priory Green Ln DE73 1AT
☎ 01332 863081 📠 01332 865319
web: www.breedongolf.co.uk
18 holes, 5777yds, Par 69, SSS 68, Course record 67.
Course Designer David Snell **Location** Off A453 into Breedon
Telephone for further details
Hotel ★★★★ 78% HL The Priest House on the River, Kings Mills, CASTLE
DONINGTON ☎ 01332 810649 24 en suite 18 annexe en suite

WOODHOUSE EAVES MAP 08 SK51

Charnwood Forest Breakback Rd LE12 8TA
☎ 01509 890259
e-mail: secretary@charnwoodforestgc.co.uk
web: www.charnwoodforestgc.co.uk
Hilly heathland course with hard walking, but no bunkers. Play is round
volcanic rock giving panoramic views over the Charnwood Forest area.
9 holes, 5972yds, Par 69, SSS 69, Course record 65.
Club membership 360.
Visitors Mon, Wed-Sun except BHs. Booking required Sat & Sun. Handicap
certificate. Dress code. **Societies** Booking required. **Green Fees** £30
per 36 holes, £25 per 18 holes, £17 per 9 holes (£30 per 18 holes, £20
per 9 holes Sat & Sun). ☻ **Course Designer** James Braid **Facilities** ⊕ ⑪
🍴 ⌷ ☂ ⚐ **Conf** facs Corporate Hospitality Days **Location** M1 junct 23,
take A512 towards Loughborough. After 0.5m turn right into Snells Nook
Lane. Club 3m on left.
Hotel ★★★★ 74% HL Quorn Country Hotel, Charnwood House, 66
Leicester Rd, QUORN ☎ 01509 415050 30 en suite

Lingdale Joe Moore's Ln LE12 8TF
☎ 01509 890703
web: www.lingdale-golf-club.com
Parkland in Charnwood Forest with some hard walking at some holes.
The Par 3 3rd and Par 5 8th are testing holes. Several holes have water
hazards and the blend of strategic holes requires good club selection.
18 holes, 6545yds, Par 71, SSS 71, Course record 68.
Club membership 659.
Visitors Mon-Fri & BHs. Booking required BHs. Handicap certificate. Dress
code. **Societies** Booking required **Green Fees** Phone. ☻ **Prof** Peter
Sellears **Course Designer** David Tucker **Facilities** ⊕ ⑪ 🍴 ⌷ ☂ ⚐
⚑ **Location** 1.5m S off B5330
Hotel ★★★★ 74% HL Quorn Country Hotel, Charnwood House, 66
Leicester Rd, QUORN ☎ 01509 415050 30 en suite

LINCOLNSHIRE

BELTON MAP 08 SK93

De Vere Belton Woods Hotel NG32 2LN
☎ 01476 593200 📠 01476 574547
e-mail: belton.woods@devere-hotels.com
web: www.devereonline.co.uk
The Lakes Course: 18 holes, 6831yds, Par 72, SSS 73,
Course record 66.
The Woodside Course: 18 holes, 6623yds, Par 73, SSS 72,
Course record 67.
Red Arrows: 9 holes, 1010yds, Par 27, SSS 27.
Location On A607 2m N of Grantham
Telephone for further details
Hotel ★★★★ 77% HL De Vere Belton Woods, BELTON ☎ 01476 593200
136 en suite

BLANKNEY MAP 08 TF06

Blankney LN4 3AZ
☎ 01526 320202 📠 01526 322521
web: www.blankneygolf.co.uk
Parkland in pleasant surroundings, with mature trees and testing
greens offering a challenging test of golf. Set in the Blankney estate
and 2004 was the centenary year.
18 holes, 6634yds, Par 72, SSS 73, Course record 69.
Club membership 700.
Visitors Mon-Fri & BHs. Booking required. Dress code. **Societies** Welcome.
Green Fees Phone. **Prof** Graham Bradley **Course Designer** C Sinclair
Facilities ⊕ ⑪ 🍴 🍴 ⌷ ☂ ⚐ ⚑ **Leisure** snooker. **Conf** facs
Corporate Hospitality Days **Location** 10m SW on B1188
Hotel ★★★ 73% CHH Branston Hall Hotel, Branston Park, Branston,
LINCOLN ☎ 01522 793305 43 en suite 7 annexe en suite

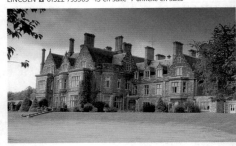

BOSTON MAP 08 TF34

Boston Cowbridge, Horncastle Rd PE22 7EL
☎ 01205 350589 📠 01205 367526
e-mail: steveshaw@bostongc.co.uk
web: www.bostongc.co.uk
Parkland with water coming into play on a number of holes. Renowned
for the quality of the greens.
18 holes, 6415yds, Par 72, SSS 71, Course record 65.
Club membership 650.
Visitors Mon, Wed-Sun & BHs. Booking required Sat, Sun & BHs. Dress
code. **Societies** Booking required. **Green Fees** £30 per day/round. ☻
Prof Nick Hiom **Facilities** ⊕ ⑪ 🍴 ⌷ ☂ ⚐ ⚑ **Conf**
Corporate Hospitality Days **Location** 2m N of Boston on B1183
Hotel ★★ 68% HL Comfort Inn, Donnington Rd, Bicker Bar Roundabout,
BOSTON ☎ 01205 820118 55 en suite

Boston West Golf Centre Hubbert's Bridge PE20 3QX
☎ 01205 290670 📠 01205 290725
e-mail: info@bostonwestgolfclub.co.uk
web: www.bostonwestgolfclub.co.uk
A well maintained maturing golf course, nestled in the Lincolnshire
countryside featuring excellent greens, well positioned lakes and
bunkers. Good test of golf for all levels of golfer.
18 holes, 6411yards, Par 72, SSS 71, Course record 63.
Club membership 650.
Visitors Mon-Sun & BHs. Dress code. **Societies** Welcome.
Green Fees £20 per 18 holes (£25 Sat, Sun & BHs). **Prof** Simon
Collingwood **Course Designer** Michael Zara **Facilities** ⊕ ⑪ 🍴 ⌷ ☂
⚐ ⚑ ⚐ ⚑ **Leisure** 6 hole academy course. **Conf** facs Corporate
Hospitality Days **Location** 2m W of Boston on A1121-B1192 x-rds
Hotel ★★★ 67% HL Golf Hotel, The Broadway, WOODHALL SPA
☎ 01526 353535 50 en suite

Kirton Holme Holme Rd, Kirton Holme PE20 1SY
☎ 01205 290669
web: www.kirtonholmegolfclub.co.uk
A young parkland course designed for mid to high handicappers. It is flat but has 2500 young trees, two natural water courses plus water hazards. The 2nd is a challenging, 386yd Par 4 dog-leg.
9 holes, 5778yds, Par 70, SSS 68, Course record 66.
Club membership 320.
Visitors Mon-Sun & BHs. Booking required Sat, Sun & BHs. Dress code.
Societies Booking required. **Green Fees** £11 per 18 holes, £7 per 9 holes (£12/£8 Sat, Sun & BHs). ● **Prof** Alison Johns **Course Designer** D W Welberry **Facilities** ⊕ ⓦ ⓑ ⌶ ╬ 丸 ♈ ⓥ **Conf** Corporate Hospitality Days **Location** 4m W of Boston off A52
Hotel ★★ 68% HL Comfort Inn, Donnington Rd, Bicker Bar Roundabout, BOSTON ☎ 01205 820118 55 en suite

---

BOURNE   **MAP 08 TF02**

Toft Hotel Toft PE10 0JT
☎ 01778 590616 📄 01778 590264

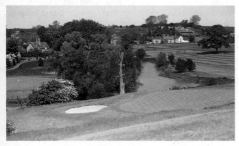

18 holes, 6486yds, Par 72, SSS 71, Course record 63.
Course Designer Roger Fitton **Location** On A6121 Bourne-Stamford road
Telephone for further details
Hotel ★★★ 85% HL The George of Stamford, 71 St Martins, STAMFORD ☎ 01780 750750 & 750700 (Res) 📄 01780 750701 47 en suite

---

CLEETHORPES   **MAP 08 TA30**

Cleethorpes Kings Rd DN35 0PN
☎ 01472 816110 📄 01472 814060
e-mail: secretary@cleethorpesgolfclub.co.uk
web: www.cleethorpesgolf club.co.uk
A mature coastal course founded in 1894. Slight undulations give variety but the flat landscape makes for easy walking. Fine putting surfaces. The course provides a challenge to all levels of player, especially when the wind blows.

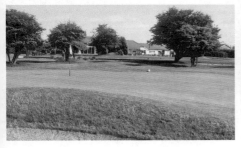

18 holes, 6272yds, Par 70, SSS 71, Course record 65.
Club membership 650.
Visitors Mon-Sun & BHs. Booking required BHs. Dress code. **Societies** Booking required. **Green Fees** £35 per day, £25 per round (£40/£30 Sun and bank holidays). ● **Prof** Paul Davies **Course Designer** Harry Vardon **Facilities** ⊕ ⓦ ⓑ ⌶ ╬ 丸 ⓢ ♈ ⓥ **Location** 2m SE of Cleethorpes near theme park
Hotel ★★★ 77% HL Kingsway Hotel, Kingsway, CLEETHORPES ☎ 01472 601122 49 en suite

Tetney Station Rd, Tetney DN36 5HY
☎ 01472 211644 📄 01472 211644
An 18-hole parkland course at the foot of the Lincolnshire Wolds, noted for its challenging water features.
18 holes, 6245yds, Par 71, SSS 69, Course record 65.
Club membership 300.
Visitors Mon-Sun & BHs. Booking required Sat & Sun. Dress code.
Societies Welcome. **Green Fees** £12 per 18 holes (£14 Sat, Sun & BHs).
Prof Jason Abrams **Course Designer** J S Grant **Facilities** ⊕ ⓦ ⓑ ⌶ ╬ 丸 ⓢ ♈ ⓥ ♈ **Conf** facs **Location** 1m off A16 Louth-Grimsby road
Hotel ★★★ 77% HL Kingsway Hotel, Kingsway, CLEETHORPES ☎ 01472 601122 49 en suite

---

CROWLE   **MAP 08 SE71**

The Lincolnshire DN17 4BU
☎ 01724 711619 📄 01724 711619
Traditional flat parkland course. Generous greens with discreet use of water and bunkers. Redeveloped greatly in the last few years offering a good test to all standards of golfer.
18 holes, 6283yds, Par 71, SSS 70. Club membership 420.
Visitors Mon-Sun & BHs. Booking required Sat/Sun & BHs. Dress code.
Societies booking required. **Green Fees** not confirmed. **Course Designer** Stubley/Byrne **Facilities** ⊕ ⓦ ⓑ ⌶ ╬ 丸 ⓢ ♈ ⓥ **Conf** Corporate Hospitality Days **Location** M180 junct 2, 0.5m on Crowle road

---

ELSHAM   **MAP 08 TA01**

Elsham Barton Rd DN20 0LS
☎ 01652 680291 (Sec) 📄 01652 680308
e-mail: manager@elshamgolfclub.co.uk
web: www.elshamgolfclub.co.uk
Gently undulating, mature parkland and heathland course in a rural setting with a variety of wildlife, including many pheasants. Each hole is different and has its own challenge. Very secluded with easy walking and a reservoir to maintain irrigation.

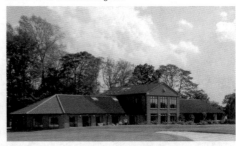

18 holes, 6426yds, Par 71, SSS 71, Course record 65.
Club membership 650.

Continued

Visitors Mon-Wed & Fri except BHs. Thu am only. Booking required. Handicap certificate. Dress code. **Societies** Welcome. **Green Fees** £37 per 36 holes, £27 per 18 holes. ⊕ **Prof** Stuart Brewer **Course Designer** Various **Facilities** ⑪ ⑩ ⬚ ☐ ⬚ ⬚ ⬚ ⬚ **Conf** facs Corporate Hospitality Days **Location** 2m NE of Brigg on B1206
Hotel ★★★ 73% HL Wortley House Hotel, Rowland Rd, SCUNTHORPE
☎ 01724 842223 38 en suite 4 annexe en suite

GAINSBOROUGH   MAP 08 SK88

Gainsborough Thonock DN21 1PZ
☎ 01427 613088 📄 01427 810172
e-mail: gainsboroughgc.co.uk
Thonock Park: 18 holes, 6266yds, Par 70, SSS 70,
Course record 63.
Karsten Lakes: 18 holes, 6721yds, Par 72, SSS 72,
Course record 65.
Course Designer Neil Coles **Location** 1m N off A159. Signed off A631
Telephone for further details
Hotel ★★★ 72% HL Best Western The West Retford Hotel, 24 North Rd,
RETFORD ☎ 01777 706333 & 0870 609 6162 📄 01777 709951 63 en suite

GEDNEY HILL   MAP 08 TF31

Gedney Hill West Drove PE12 0NT
☎ 01406 330922 📄 01406 330323
e-mail: n.venters@btinternet.com
Flat parkland course similar to a links course. Made testing by Fen winds and small greens. Also a 10-bay driving range.
18 holes, 5493yds, Par 70, SSS 66, Course record 66.
Club membership 200.
Visitors Mon-Sun & BHs. **Societies** Welcome. **Green Fees** Phone. ⊕ **Prof** N Venters **Course Designer** Monkwise Ltd **Facilities** ⑪ ⑩ ⬚ ☐ ⑪ ⬚ ⬚ ⬚ ⬚ ⬚ **Location** 5m SE of Spalding
Hotel ★★★ 73% HL Elme Hall Hotel, Elm High Rd, WISBECH
☎ 01945 475566 7 en suite

GRANTHAM   MAP 08 SK93

Belton Park Belton Ln, Londonthorpe Rd NG31 9SH
☎ 01476 567399 📄 01476 592078
e-mail: greatgolf@beltonpark
web: www.beltonpark.co.uk
Three nine-hole courses set in classic mature parkland of Lord Brownlow's country seat, Belton House. Gently undulating with streams, ponds, plenty of trees and beautiful scenery, including a deer park. Famous holes: 5th, 12th, 16th and 18th. Combine any of the three courses for a testing 18-hole round.

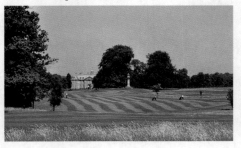

Brownlow: 18 holes, 6472yds, Par 71, SSS 71,
Course record 64.
Ancaster: 18 holes, 6325yds, Par 70, SSS 70.
Belmont: 18 holes, 6075yds, Par 69, SSS 69.
Club membership 850.
Visitors Mon-Fri, Sun & BHs. Booking required. Handicap certificate. Dress code. **Societies** Welcome. **Green Fees** £40 per day, £35 per round (£50/£40 Sun & BHs). **Prof** Simon Williams **Course Designer** Williamson/Allis **Facilities** ⑪ ⑩ ⬚ ☐ ⑪ ⬚ ⬚ ⬚ ⬚ ⬚ **Conf** facs Corporate Hospitality Days **Location** 1.5m NE of Grantham
Hotel ★★★ 72% Best Western Kings Hotel, North Pde, GRANTHAM
☎ 01476 590800 21 en suite

Sudbrook Moor Charity St, Carlton Scroop NG32 3AT
☎ 01400 250796
web: www.sudbrookmoor.co.uk
A testing nine-hole parkland and meadowland course in a picturesque valley setting with easy walking.
9 holes, 4811yds, Par 66, SSS 64, Course record 64.
Club membership 600.
Visitors Mon-Sun & BHs. Booking required. **Green Fees** £7-£9 per day (£9-£12 weekends and bank holidays). **Prof** Tim Hutton **Course Designer** Tim Hutton **Facilities** ⑪ ⬚ ☐ ⬚ ⬚ ⬚ ⬚ **Location** 6m NE of Grantham on A607
Hotel ★★★ 72% Best Western Kings Hotel, North Pde, GRANTHAM
☎ 01476 590800 21 en suite

GRIMSBY   MAP 08 TA21

Grimsby Littlecoates Rd DN34 4LU
☎ 01472 342630 📄 01472 342630
e-mail: secretary@grimsby.fsnet.co.uk
Mature undulating parkland course, not particularly long, but demanding and a good test of golf. The Par 3s are all feature holes, not a common feature on most courses. The summer greens are fast and quite small.
18 holes, 6057yds, Par 70, SSS 69, Course record 65.
Club membership 730.
Visitors Mon-Fri except BHs. Booking required Mon & Fri. Handicap certificate. Dress code. **Societies** Welcome. **Green Fees** £25 per day. ⊕ **Prof** Richard Smith **Course Designer** Colt **Facilities** ⑪ ⑩ ⬚ ☐ ⑪ ⬚ ⬚ ⬚ ⬚ **Conf** Corporate Hospitality Days **Location** 1m from A180. 1m from A46
Hotel ★★★ 72% HL Hotel Elizabeth Grimsby, Littlecoates Rd, GRIMSBY
☎ 01472 240024 & 0870 1162716 📄 01472 241354 52 en suite

Waltham Windmill Cheapside, Waltham DN37 0HT
☎ 01472 824109 📄 01472 828391
web: www.walthamgolf.co.uk
Nestling in 125 acres of Lincolnshire countryside, the natural springs have been used to great effect giving individuality and challenge to every shot. The course has a mixture of long Par 5s and water comes into play on nine holes.
18 holes, 6442yds, Par 71, SSS 71, Course record 64.
Club membership 680.
Visitors Mon-Fri except BHs.Handicap certificate. Dress code. **Societies** Booking required. **Green Fees** £26 per round. Reduced winter rates.
Prof S Bennett/M Stephenson **Course Designer** J Payne **Facilities** ⑪ ⑩ ⬚ ☐ ⑪ ⬚ ⬚ ⬚ ⬚ ⬚ ⬚ **Conf** facs Corporate Hospitality Days **Location** 1m off A16
Hotel ★★★ 73% HL Beeches Hotel, 42 Waltham Rd, Scartho, GRIMSBY
☎ 01472 278830 18 en suite

England

HORNCASTLE
MAP 08 TF26

Horncastle West Ashby LN9 5PP
☎ 01507 526800
e-mail: info@horncastlegolfclub.com
web: www.horncastlegolfclub.com
Parkland course with many water hazards and bunkers; very challenging. There is a 25-bay floodlit driving range.
18 holes, 5717yds, Par 70, SSS 68, Course record 71.
Club membership 200.
Visitors Mon-Sun & BHs. Booking required Sat, Sun & BHs. Dress code.
Societies Booking required. **Green Fees** £30 per day; £20 per round.
Prof Richard Croome **Course Designer** E C Wright **Facilities** ⊕ ⓘ ⌁ ⌑
🏌 ⌁ ⊶ ◊ ✆ **Leisure** fishing. **Conf** facs Corporate Hospitality Days
Location Off A153/A158 at West Ashby
Hotel ★★★ 70% HL Best Western Admiral Rodney Hotel, North St,
HORNCASTLE ☎ 01507 523131 31 en suite

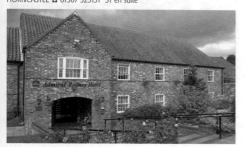

Canwick Park Golf Club
Washingborough Road, Lincoln, LN4 1EF

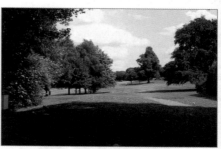

An attractive parkland course of 6,148 yards (SSS 69). Located 2 miles east of Lincoln City Centre on the B1190, with panoramic views of Lincoln Cathedral. The 5th and 13th holes are testing Par 3s. Between April to October bar facilities are available from 11am to 11pm with catering 7 days a week. Society packages are also available Monday to Friday and can be tailored to meet the needs of visiting golfers.
Great golf all year round.

Manager: tel 01522 542912
Clubhouse: tel 01522 522166
Website: www.canwickpark.org
Email: manager@canwickpark.org

IMMINGHAM
MAP 08 TA11

Immingham St Andrews Ln, off Church Ln DN40 2EU
☎ 01469 575298 🖷 01469 577636
e-mail: admin@immgc.force9.co.uk
web: www.immgc.com
18 holes, 6215yds, Par 71, SSS 70, Course record 69.
Course Designer Hawtree & Son **Location** 7m NW of Grimsby
Telephone for further details
Hotel ★★★ 72% HL Hotel Elizabeth Grimsby, Littlecoates Rd, GRIMSBY
☎ 01472 240024 & 0870 1162716 🖷 01472 241354 52 en suite

LACEBY
MAP 08 TA20

Manor 34 Worcester Rd WR14 4AA
☎ 01684 568890 🖷 01884 577530
e-mail: ragella@bredonhouse.co.uk
web: www.bredonhouse.co.uk
The first seven holes played as a parkland course lined with mature trees. The second nine are more open fairways with water courses running alongside and through the holes. The 16th hole green is surrounded by water. holes 17 and 18 are tree-lined like the first seven holes.
18 holes, 6354yds, Par 71, SSS 70. Club membership 550.
Visitors Mon-Sun & BHs. Booking required. **Societies** booking required.
Green Fees not confirmed. **Prof** Neil Laybourne **Facilities** ⊕ ⓘ⊙ ⌁ ⌑
🏌 ⌁ ⌂ ✆ **Leisure** fishing. **Conf** facs Corporate Hospitality Days
Location A18 Laceby-Louth
Hotel ★★★ 72% HL Hotel Elizabeth Grimsby, Littlecoates Rd, GRIMSBY
☎ 01472 240024 & 0870 1162716 🖷 01472 241354 52 en suite

LINCOLN
MAP 08 SK97

Canwick Park Canwick Park, Washingborough Rd
LN4 1EF
☎ 01522 542912 🖷 01522 526997
e-mail: manager@canwickpark.org
web: www.canwickpark.org
Parkland with fine views of Lincoln Cathedral. The 5th and 13th holes are testing Par 3s both nearly 200yds in length.

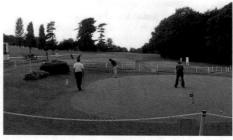

18 holes, 6160yds, Par 70, SSS 69, Course record 65.
Club membership 650.
Visitors Mon-Fri & BHs. Sat & Sun after 2.30pm. Dress code. **Societies**
Booking required. **Green Fees** £30 per day, £16 per round (£25 per round Sat & Sun). **Prof** S Williamson **Course Designer** Hawtree & Sons
Facilities ⊕ ⓘ⊙ ⌁ ⌑🏌 ⌁ ✆ ⌂ **Conf** Corporate Hospitality Days
Location 2m E of city centre on B1190
Hotel ★★★ 72% HL The Lincoln Hotel, Eastgate, LINCOLN
☎ 01522 520348 72 en suite

See advert on this page

Carholme Carholme Rd LN1 1SE

☎ 01522 523725 📄 01522 533733
e-mail: info@carholme-golf-club.co.uk
web: www.carholme-golf-club.co.uk
Parkland where prevailing west winds can add interest. Good views.
First hole out of bounds left and right of fairway, pond in front of
bunkered green at 5th, lateral water hazards across several fairways.
18 holes, 6215yds, Par 71, SSS 70, Course record 67.
Club membership 500.
Visitors Mon-Sun & BHs. Booking required Sat, Sun & BHs. Dress code.
Societies Booking required. **Green Fees** £24 per day; £20 per round.
◉ **Course Designer** Willie Park Jnr **Facilities** ⊕ 🍴 🏐 ⊡ 🖶 🏋 ♟
Conf Corporate Hospitality Days **Location** 1m W of city centre on A57
Hotel ★★★ 68% HL The White Hart, Bailgate, LINCOLN ☎ 01522 526222
50 en suite

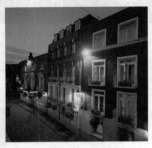

LOUTH — MAP 08 TF38

Kenwick Park Kenwick Park LN11 8NY

☎ 01507 605134 📄 01507 606556
e-mail: secretary@kenwickparkgolf.co.uk
web: www.kenwickparkgolf.co.uk
Situated on the edge of the Lincolnshire Wolds with panoramic
views. Course features a mixture of parkland and woodland holes,
complemented by a network of lakes.
18 holes, 6782yds, Par 72, SSS 73, Course record 71.
Club membership 520.
Visitors Mon-Sun & BHs. Booking required. Handicap certificate. Dress
code. **Societies** Booking required. **Green Fees** £35 per 18 holes (£45
Sat, Sun & BHs). **Prof** P Spence/M Langford **Course Designer** Patrick
Tallack **Facilities** ⊕ 🍴 by prior arrangement 🏐 ⊡ 🖶 🏋 🍴 ♟
Conf Corporate Hospitality Days **Location** 2m S of Louth on A157 (Louth
bypass)
Hotel ★★★ 75% HL Best Western Kenwick Park Hotel, Kenwick Park
Estate, LOUTH ☎ 01507 608806 29 en suite 5 annexe en suite

Louth Crowtree Ln LN11 9LJ

☎ 01507 603681 📄 01507 608501
e-mail: louthgolfclub@btconnect.com
web: www.louthgolfclub.com
Undulating parkland, fine views in an Area of Outstanding Natural
Beauty. No winter greens, offering quality golf throughout the year.
18 holes, 6430yds, Par 72, SSS 71, Course record 66.
Club membership 700.
Visitors Mon-Fri & BHs. Sun after 11am. Booking required. Handicap
certificate. Dress code. **Societies** Welcome. **Green Fees** £30 per day, £25 per
round (£36/£30 Sun & BHs). **Prof** A Blundell **Facilities** ⊕ 🍴 🏐 ⊡ 🖶 🍴
🏐 ♟ 🍴 ♟ **Leisure** squash. **Conf** facs Corporate Hospitality Days **Location**
from A157/A16 rdbt take B1521 to Louth, 1st right up Love Lane to top.

Hotel ★★★ 70% HL Beaumont Hotel, 66 Victoria Rd, LOUTH
☎ 01507 605005 16 en suite

MARKET RASEN — MAP 08 TF18

Market Rasen & District Legsby Rd LN8 3DZ

☎ 01673 842319 📄 01673 849245
e-mail: marketrasengolf@onetel.net
web: www.marketrasengolfclub.co.uk
Picturesque, well-wooded heathland course, easy walking, breezy with
becks forming natural hazards. Good views of Lincolnshire Wolds.

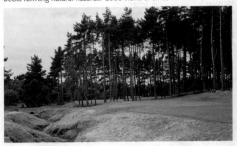

18 holes, 6239yds, Par 71, SSS 70, Course record 65.
Club membership 600.
Visitors Mon-Fri except BHs. Booking required. Handicap certificate. Dress
code. **Societies** Booking required. **Green Fees** £35 per day, £25 per round.
Prof A M Chester **Course Designer** Hawtree Ltd **Facilities** ⊕ 🍴 🏐 ⊡
🍴 🏋 🖶 ♟ 🍴 ♟ **Conf** Corporate Hospitality Days **Location** 1m E, A46
onto A631
Hotel ★★★ 70% HL Beaumont Hotel, 66 Victoria Rd, LOUTH
☎ 01507 605005 16 en suite

Market Rasen Race Course (Golf Course) Legsby Rd LN8 3EA

☎ 01673 843434 📄 01673 844532
e-mail: marketrasen@jockeyclubracecourses.com
web: www.marketrasenraces.co.uk
This is a public course set within the bounds of Market Rasen race
course - the entire racing area is out of bounds. The longest hole is
the 4th at 454yds with the race course providing a hazard over the
whole length of the drive.
9 holes, 2532yds, Par 32.
Visitors Mon-Sun & BHs. **Societies** Welcome. **Green Fees** £6 per 9 holes
(£7 Sat, Sun & BHs). ◉ **Course Designer** Edward Stenton **Facilities** ⛳ ♟
Leisure caravan site. **Conf** facs **Location** 1m E of Market Rasen
Hotel ★★★ 70% HL Beaumont Hotel, 66 Victoria Rd, LOUTH
☎ 01507 605005 16 en suite

NORMANBY — MAP 08 SE81

Normanby Hall Normanby Park DN15 9HU

☎ 01724 720226 (Pro shop)
18 holes, 6561yds, Par 72, SSS 71, Course record 66.
Course Designer Hawtree & Son **Location** 3m N of Scunthorpe on B1130
next to Normanby Hall
Telephone for further details
Hotel ★★★ 73% HL Wortley House Hotel, Rowland Rd, SCUNTHORPE
☎ 01724 842223 38 en suite 4 annexe en suite

SCUNTHORPE   MAP 08 SE81

Ashby Decoy Burringham Rd DN17 2AB
☎ 01724 866561 📠 01724 271708
e-mail: info@ashbydecoygolfclub.co.uk
web: www.ashbydecoy.co.uk
Pleasant, flat parkland course to satisfy all tastes, yet test the experienced golfer.
18 holes, 6281yds, Par 71, SSS 71, Course record 66.
Club membership 650.
Visitors Mon, Wed-Fri except BHs, Tue after 2pm. **Societies** Booking required. **Green Fees** £30 per day; £25 per round. ⊜ **Prof** A Miller
Facilities ⑪ ⑩ ⬚ ⬚ ⬚ ⬚ ⬚ ⬚ ⬚ **Conf** facs Corporate Hospitality Days **Location** 2.5m SW on B1450 near Asda store
Hotel ★★★ 73% HL Wortley House Hotel, Rowland Rd, SCUNTHORPE
☎ 01724 842223   38 en suite   4 annexe en suite

Forest Pines Hotel Ermine St, Broughton DN20 0AQ
☎ 01652 650770 📠 01652 650495
e-mail: forestpines@qhotels.co.uk
web: www.qhotels.co.uk

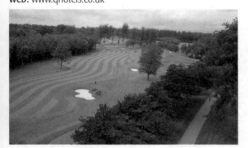

Forest Course: 9 holes, 3291yds, Par 36, SSS 36.
Pines Course: 9 holes, 3568yds, Par 37, SSS 37.
Beeches: 9 holes, 3291yds, Par 36, SSS 36.
Course Designer John Morgan **Location** M180 junct 4, 200yds
Telephone for further details
Hotel ★★★★ 77% HL Forest Pines Hotel, Ermine St, Broughton, SCUNTHORPE ☎ 01652 650770   188 en suite

See advert on this page

Grange Park Butterwick Rd, Messingham DN17 3PP
☎ 01724 762945 📠 01724 762945
e-mail: info@grangepark.com
web: www.grangepark.com
Parkland with challenging water hazards and impressive stone raised teeing areas.
18 holes, 6146yds, Par 70, SSS 69, Course record 64.
Club membership 320.
Visitors Mon-Sun & BHs. Dress code. **Societies** Booking required. **Green Fees** £16 per 18 holes (£18 Sat, Sun & BHs). **Prof** Jonathan Drury **Course Designer** R Price **Facilities** ⑪ ⑩ ⬚ ⬚ ⬚ ⬚ ⬚ ⬚ ⬚ ⬚ **Leisure** hard tennis courts, fishing, 9 hole Par 3 course. **Conf** facs Corporate Hospitality Days **Location** 1.5m W of Messingham towards East Butterwick
Hotel ★★★ 73% HL Wortley House Hotel, Rowland Rd, SCUNTHORPE
☎ 01724 842223   38 en suite   4 annexe en suite

Forest Pines Golf Club

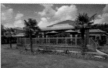
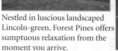
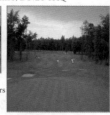

Holme Hall Holme Ln, Bottesford DN16 3RF
☎ 01724 862078 📠 01724 862081
e-mail: secretary@holmehallgolf.co.uk
web: www.holmehallgolf.co.uk
Natural heathland course with gorse and heather and sandy subsoil. Easy walking. Tight driving holes and good greens.
18 holes, 6413yds, Par 71, SSS 71, Course record 64.
Club membership 650.
Visitors Mon-Fri except BHs. Booking required. Handicap certificate. Dress code. **Societies** Booking required. **Green Fees** not confirmed. **Prof** Richard McKiernan **Facilities** ⑪ ⑩ ⬚ ⬚ ⬚ ⬚ ⬚ ⬚ ⬚ ⬚ **Conf** Corporate Hospitality Days **Location** M180 junct 4, 4m SE of Scunthorpe
Hotel ★★★ 73% HL Wortley House Hotel, Rowland Rd, SCUNTHORPE
☎ 01724 842223   38 en suite   4 annexe en suite

SKEGNESS   MAP 09 TF56

North Shore Hotel & Golf Club North Shore Rd
PE25 1DN
☎ 01754 763298 🖹 01754 761902
e-mail: golf@north-shore.co.uk
web: www.north-shore.co.uk
Part links, part parkland, with two of the nine holes situated next to the sea. A challenging course which starts and finishes outside the hotel bar.

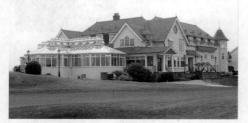

18 holes, 6200yds, Par 71, SSS 71, Course record 68.
Club membership 400.
Visitors Mon-Sun & BHs. Booking required. Handicap certificate. Dress code. **Societies** booking required. **Green Fees** not confirmed. **Prof** J Cornelius **Course Designer** James Braid **Facilities** ⊕ ⌾ ⊑ ⌷ ⋈ ⋈ ⏁ ⋒ ❖ ⛤ ∂ **Leisure** snooker. **Conf** facs Corporate Hospitality Days **Location** 1m N of town centre off A52, opp North Shore Holiday Centre **Hotel** ★★ 71% HL North Shore Hotel & Golf Course, North Shore Rd, SKEGNESS ☎ 01754 763298 33 en suite 3 annexe en suite

Seacroft Drummond Rd, Seacroft PE25 3AU
☎ 01754 763020 🖹 01754 763020
e-mail: enquiries@seacroft-golfclub.co.uk
web: www.seacroft-golfclub.co.uk
A championship seaside links traditionally laid out with tight undulations and hogsback fairways. Adjacent to Gibraltar Point Nature Reserve, overlooking the Wash.

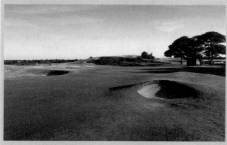

18 holes, 6492yds, Par 71, SSS 71, Course record 65.
Club membership 590.
Visitors Mon-Sun & BHs. Booking required. Handicap certificate. Dress code. **Societies** Booking required. **Green Fees** Phone. **Prof** Robin Lawie **Course Designer** Tom Dunn/Willie Fernie **Facilities** ⊕ ⌾ ⊑ ⌷ ⋈ ⏁ ⋒ ❖ ⛤ ∂ **Conf** Corporate Hospitality Days **Location** S of town centre towards Gibralter Point Nature Reserve **Hotel** ★★★ 68% HL Crown Hotel, Drummond Rd, SKEGNESS ☎ 01754 610760 29 en suite

SLEAFORD   MAP 08 TF04

Sleaford Willoughby Rd, Greylees NG34 8PL
☎ 01529 488273 🖹 01529 488644
e-mail: sleafordgolfclub@btinternet.com
web: www.sleafordgolfclub.co.uk
Inland links-type course, moderately wooded and fairly flat with sandy well-draining soil, which supports a variety of trees and shrubs. While the lowest index hole is the awkward dog-leg 4th, the 2nd hole requires two mighty hits to be reached. The feature hole is the 12th, where the green is totally protected by a copse of pine trees. A stream running through the course provides water hazards on several holes.
18 holes, 6503yds, Par 72, SSS 71, Course record 64.
Club membership 630.
Visitors Mon-Sun except BHs. Booking required Mon-Fri. Handicap certificate. Dress code. **Societies** Booking required. **Green Fees** £34 per day; £27 per round (£36 Sat & Sun). ⊕ **Prof** Nigel Pearce **Course Designer** T Williamson **Facilities** ⊕ ⌾ ⊑ ⌷ ⋈ ⏁ ⋒ ❖ ∂ **Conf** Corporate Hospitality Days **Location** 2m W of Sleaford off A153 **Hotel** ★★★ 72% Best Western Kings Hotel, North Pde, GRANTHAM ☎ 01476 590800 21 en suite

SOUTH KYME   MAP 08 TF14

South Kyme Skinners Ln LN4 4AT
☎ 01526 861113 🖹 01526 861113
e-mail: southkymegc@hotmail.com
web: www.skgc.co.uk
A challenging fenland course in a tranquil location, described as an inland links with water hazards, trees and fairway hazards.
18 holes, 6556yds, Par 72, SSS 71, Course record 67.
Club membership 400.
Visitors Mon-Sun & BHs. Dress code. **Societies** Welcome. **Green Fees** £20 per round, £10 per 9 holes (£24/£12 Sat, Sun & BHs). **Prof** Peter Chamberlain **Facilities** ⊕ ⌾ ⊑ ⌷ ⋈ ⏁ ⋒ ❖ ⛤ ∂ **Leisure** 6 hole short course. **Conf** Corporate Hospitality Days **Location** Off B1395 into South Kyme **Hotel** BUD Travelodge Sleaford, Holdingham, SLEAFORD ☎ 08700 850 950 40 en suite

SPALDING   MAP 08 TF22

Spalding Surfleet PE11 4EA
☎ 01775 680386 (office) & 680474 (pro) 🖹 01775 680988
e-mail: spaldinggc@btconnect.com
web: www.spaldinggolfclub.co.uk

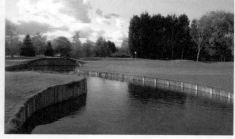

A pretty, well-laid out course in a fenland area. The River Glen runs beside the 1st, 2nd and 4th holes, and ponds and lakes are very much

Continued

CHAMPIONSHIP COURSE

LINCOLNSHIRE — WOODHALL SPA

THE NATIONAL GOLF CENTRE

Map 08 TF16

The Broadway LN10 6PU
☎ 01526 352511 📠 01526 351817
e-mail: booking@englishgolfunion.org
web: www.woodhallspagolf.com
The Hotchkin: 18 holes, 7080yds, Par 73, SSS 75, Course record 66.
The Bracken: 18 holes, 6735yds, Par 72, SSS 74, Course record 68.
Club membership 520.
Visitors Mon-Sun & BHs. Booking required. Handicap certificate. Dress code. **Societies** Booking required. **Green Fees** Hotchkin £100 per day, £65 per round. Bracken £75 per day, £50 round. £90 per day playing both courses. **Prof** A Hare **Course Designer** Col S V Hotchkin **Facilities** ⑪ 🍽 🍺 🖥 🏌 👜 🛍 ◇ 🛒 ✐ 🏇 **Leisure** pitch & putt 9 hole course. **Conf** Corporate Hospitality Days **Location** Exit A1 onto B6403 to Ancaster. Turn right onto A153 to Coningsby and then left onto B1192.

The Championship Course at Woodhall Spa, now known as the Hotchkin, is considered to be the best inland course in the UK . This classic course has cavernous bunkers and heather-lined fairways. Golf has been played here for over a century and the Hotchkin has hosted most of the top national and international amateur events. The English Golf Union acquired Woodhall Spa in 1995 to create a centre of excellence. A second course, the Bracken, has been built, along with extensive practice facilities including one of Europe's finest short-game practice areas. The English Golf Union actively encourages visitors to the National Golf Centre throughout the year, to experience the facilities and to enjoy the unique ambience.

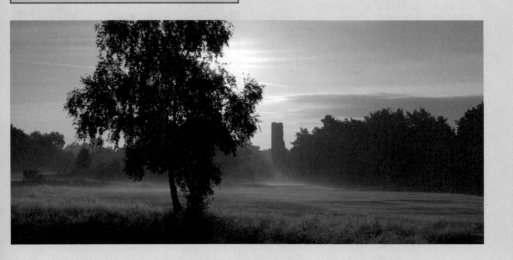

in play on the 9th, 10th and 11th holes. Challenging holes include the river dominated 2nd and the 17th where a good drive is needed for the right hand side of the fairway to leave a challenging second shot to a well protected green, bunkered in front and right with out of bounds on the left.

18 holes, 6478yds, Par 72, SSS 71, Course record 62.
Club membership 750.
Visitors Mon-Sun & BHs. Booking required. Handicap certificate. Dress code. **Societies** Booking required. **Green Fees** £35 per day; £30 per round (£40 per round Sat, Sun & BHs). ❀ **Prof** John Spencer/Chris Huggins **Course Designer** Price/Spencer/Ward **Facilities** ⊕ ⊙ ⑥ ⚑ ☐ ⚐ ☐ ⚒ ☐
⚒ ☎ ⚒ ⚓ **Conf** Corporate Hospitality Days **Location** 4m N of Spalding next to A16
Hotel ★★ 75% SHL Cley Hall Hotel, 22 High St, SPALDING
☎ 01775 725157 4 en suite 11 annexe en suite

STAMFORD MAP 04 TF00

Burghley Park St Martins PE9 3JX
☎ 01780 753789 🗎 01780 753789
e-mail: burghley.golf@lineone.net
web: www.burghleygolf.org.uk
A compact parkland layout. Tree planting, the introduction of sand and water hazards and the maintenance of fair but punishing rough, have made the course a real challenge. Free draining fairways and greens give first class playing all year.

18 holes, 6236yds, Par 70, SSS 70, Course record 65.
Club membership 775.
Visitors may play Mon-Fri. Advance booking required Mon & Fri. Handicap certificate required. Dress code. **Societies** advance booking required.
Green Fees not confirmed. ❀ **Prof** Glenn Davies **Facilities** ⊕ ⚑ ⚐ ☐ ⚒ ⚓ **Conf** Corporate Hospitality Days **Location** 1m S of town on B1081, take roundabout from A1 S of Stamford
Hotel ★★★ 85% HL The George of Stamford, 71 St Martins, STAMFORD
☎ 01780 750750 & 750700 (Res) 🗎 01780 750701 47 en suite

STOKE ROCHFORD MAP 08 SK92

Stoke Rochford NG33 5EW
☎ 01476 530275 🗎 01476 530237
web: stokerochfordgolfclub.co.uk
Parkland course designed by C Turnor and extended in 1936 to 18 holes by Major Hotchkin.

18 holes, 6252yds, Par 70, SSS 70, Course record 65.
Club membership 525.
Visitors Mon, Tue & Fri except BHs. Booking required. Handicap certificate. Dress code. **Societies** Booking required. **Green Fees** Phone. **Prof** Angus Dow **Course Designer** Major Hotchkin **Facilities** ⊕ ⊙ ⚑ ⚐ ☐ ⚒ ☐
⚒ ☎ ⚒ **Location** 5m S of Grantham off A1 southbound signed Stoke Rochford, onto A1 northbound, enter club via BP service station
Hotel ★★★ 72% Best Western Kings Hotel, North Pde, GRANTHAM
☎ 01476 590800 21 en suite

SUTTON BRIDGE MAP 09 TF42

Sutton Bridge New Rd PE12 9RQ
☎ 01406 350323
web: www.club-noticeboard.co.uk/suttonbridge
Established in 1914, the nine holes are played along, over and in a Victorian dock basin which was abandoned as a dock in 1881. The original walls of the dock are still intact and help to make the course one of the most interesting courses in the region. The greens are recognised as among the best in Lincolnshire.

9 holes, 5724yds, Par 70, SSS 68, Course record 64.
Club membership 350.
Visitors Mon, Tue & Fri. Wed & Thu pm only. Dress code.
Societies Welcome. **Green Fees** Apr-Sep £30 per day, Oct-Mar £15. ❀
Prof Antony Lowther **Facilities** ⊕ ⊙ ⚑ ⚐ ☐ ⚒ ☐ ⚒ ⚓
Conf Corporate Hospitality Days **Location** E of village off A17
Hotel BUD Travelodge Kings Lynn Long Sutton, Wisbech Rd, LONG SUTTON ☎ 08700 850 950 40 en suite

---

SUTTON ON SEA MAP 09 TF58

Sandilands Roman Bank LN12 2RJ
☎ 01507 441432 🗎 01507 441617
e-mail: andrew.myers@alliancegolf.co.uk
Well-manicured links course next to the sea, renowned for the standard of its greens. Playable all year and easy walking due to the subtle undulations. The variety of holes and bunker placement will require the use of every club in the bag

18 holes, 6021yds, Par 70, SSS 69, Course record 64.
Club membership 300.
Visitors Mon-Sun & BHs. Booking required. Dress code. **Societies** Booking required. **Green Fees** £30 per day; £20 per round (£35/£25 Sat, Sun & BHs). Reduced winter rates. **Prof** Andrew Myers **Facilities** ⊕ ⚑ ⚐ ☐ ⚒ ☐ ⚓ ◇ ⚒ ⚒ **Leisure** hard and grass tennis courts, gymnasium.
Conf facs **Location** 1.5m S off A52
Hotel ★★★ 71% HL The Grange & Links Hotel, Sea Ln, Sandilands, SUTTON-ON-SEA ☎ 01507 441334 23 en suite

---

TORKSEY MAP 08 SK87

Lincoln LN1 2EG
☎ 01427 718721 🗎 01427 718721
e-mail: info@lincolngc.co.uk
web: www.lincolngc.co.uk
A mature championship standard course offering a variety of holes, links style to parkland.

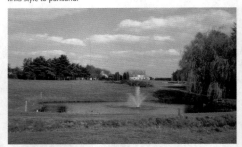

18 holes, 6438yds, Par 71, SSS 71, Course record 65.
Club membership 750.
Visitors Mon-Sun except BHs. Handicap certificate. Dress code.
Societies Booking required **Green Fees** £45 per day; £35 per round (£55/£45 Sat, Sun & BHs). ❀ **Prof** Ashley Carter **Course Designer** J H Taylor **Facilities** ⊕ ⊙ ⚑ ⚐ ☐ ⚒ ☐ ⚒ ◇ ⚒ ⚒ **Leisure** 3 hole practice course. **Conf** facs Corporate Hospitality Days **Location** NE of village off A156
Hotel ★★★ 68% HL The White Hart, Bailgate, LINCOLN ☎ 01522 526222 50 en suite

Millfield Laughterton LN1 2LB
☎ 01427 718255 📠 01427 718473
e-mail: secretary@millfieldgolfclub.fsnet.co.uk
18 holes, 6004yds, Par 72, SSS 69, Course record 68.
The Grenville Green: 18 holes, 4485yds, Par 65.
Course Designer C W Watson **Location** On A1133 1m N of A57
Telephone for further details
Hotel ★★★ 68% HL The White Hart, Bailgate, LINCOLN ☎ 01522 526222
50 en suite

WOODHALL SPA   MAP 08 TF16

The National Golf Centre see page 171

Hotel ★★★ 74% HL Petwood Hotel, Stixwould Rd, WOODHALL SPA
☎ 01526 352411 56 en suite
Hotel ★★★ 67% HL Golf Hotel, The Broadway, WOODHALL SPA
☎ 01526 353535 Fax 01526 353096 50 en suite

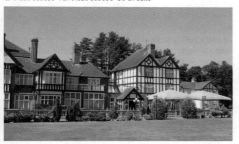

Hotel ★★★ 71% HL The Woodhall Spa Hotel, The Broadway, WOODHALL
SPA ☎ 01526 353231 Fax 01526 352797 25 en suite

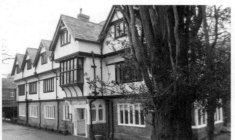

See advert on this page

WOODTHORPE   MAP 09 TF48

Woodthorpe Hall LN13 0DD
☎ 01507 450000 📠 01507 450000
e-mail: secretary@woodthorpehallgolfclub.fsnet.co.uk
web: www.woodthorpehallleisure.co.uk
Parkland course.
18 holes, 5140yds, Par 67, SSS 65, Course record 68.
Club membership 300.
Visitors Contact club for details. **Societies** Booking required **Green Fees**
£12 per round (£15 Sat, Sun & BHs). **Facilities** ⑪ ❍ 🖺 🖵 ⅋🏌 ♤ ♦ 🏌
Leisure fishing. **Conf** facs **Location** 3m N of Alford on B1373
Hotel ★★★ 71% HL The Grange & Links Hotel, Sea Ln, Sandilands,
SUTTON-ON-SEA ☎ 01507 441334 23 en suite

The Woodhall Spa Hotel

The Broadway
Woodhall Spa
Lincolnshire LN10 6ST
Tel: 01526 353 231
Fax: 01526 352 797
reception@woodhallspahotel.co.uk
www.woodhallspahotel.co.uk

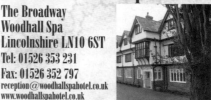

The Woodhall Spa Hotel has been recently totally
renovated and is only 500 metres from the National
Golf Centre. The hotel offers contemporary public
rooms and beautifully equipped en-suite bedrooms each
with its own 42″ plasma television and broadband. The
Lodge Restaurant serves high quality food whilst the
bar will remind you that the hotel was once one of the
drinking haunts of the famous Dambusters Squadron.

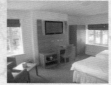
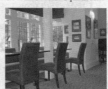

LONDON

Courses within the London Postal District area (ie those
that have London Postcodes - W1, SW1 etc) are listed
here in postal district order commencing East then North,
South and West. Courses outside the London Postal area,
but within Greater London are to be found listed under
the county of **Greater London** in the gazetteer (see
page 98).

E4 CHINGFORD

Royal Epping Forest Forest Approach, Chingford E4 7AZ
☎ 020 8529 2195 📠 020 8559 4664
e-mail: office@refgc.co.uk
web: www.refgc.co.uk
Woodland course. Red garments must be worn.
18 holes, 6281yds, Par 71, SSS 70, Course record 64.
Club membership 400.
Visitors Mon-Sun & BHs. Booking required. Dress code. **Societies** Booking
required. **Green Fees** £16 (£20 Sat & Sun). **Prof** A Traynor **Course
Designer** J G Gibson **Facilities** ⑪ by prior arrangement ❍ by prior
arrangement 🖺 by prior arrangement 🖵 ⅋🏌 ♤ 🏌 ♦ 🏌 **Conf** facs
Location 300yds E of Chingford station on Chingford Plain
Hotel ★★ 62% SHL Ridgeway Hotel, 115/117 The Ridgeway, North
Chingford, LONDON ☎ 020 8529 1964 20 en suite

West Essex Bury Rd, Sewardstonebury, Chingford E4 7QL
☎ 020 8529 7558 📄 020 8524 7870
e-mail: sec@westessexgolfclub.co.uk
web: www.westessexgolfclub.co.uk
Testing parkland course within Epping Forest with spectacular views over Essex and Middlesex. Created by James Braid in 1900 and designed to make full use of the landscape's natural attributes. The front nine is the shorter of the two and provides a test of accuracy with tree-lined fairways that meander through the undulating countryside. The back nine is equally challenging although slightly longer and requiring more long iron play.
18 holes, 6289yds, Par 71, SSS 70, Course record 63.
Club membership 710.
Visitors Mon-Fri. Handicap certificate. Dress code. **Societies** Booking required. **Green Fees** £45. ⊛ **Prof** Robert Joyce **Course Designer** James Braid **Facilities** ⊕ ⍩ ⓘ ⓛ ☷ ⎁ ⎘ ⌕ ⌕ ⬚ ⌕ **Leisure** halfway house, snooker. **Conf** facs Corporate Hospitality Days **Location** M25 junct 26, 1.5m N of Chingford station

E11 LEYTONSTONE & WANSTEAD

Wanstead Overton Dr, Wanstead E11 2LW
☎ 020 8989 3938 📄 020 8532 9138
e-mail: wgclub@aol.com
web: www.wansteadgolf.org
Flat, picturesque parkland with many trees and shrubs and easy walking. The Par 3 16th involves driving across a lake.
18 holes, 6015yds, Par 69, SSS 69, Course record 62.
Club membership 600.
Visitors Mon-Fri except BHs. Booking required. Handicap certificate. Dress code. **Societies** booking required. **Green Fees** not confirmed. **Prof** David Hawkins **Course Designer** James Braid **Facilities** �ⳑ ⎁ ⌕ **Leisure** fishing. **Conf** facs Corporate Hospitality Days **Location** Off A12 in Wanstead
Hotel ★★★★★ 87% HL Great Eastern Hotel, Liverpool St, LONDON ☎ 020 7618 5000 267 en suite

N2 EAST FINCHLEY

Hampstead Winnington Rd N2 0TU
☎ 020 8455 0203 📄 020 8731 6194
e-mail: golf@hgc.uk.com
Undulating parkland with many mature trees.
9 holes, 5822yds, Par 68, SSS 68, Course record 64.
Club membership 526.
Visitors Mon, Wed-Fri & Sun except BHs. Dress code. **Green Fees** £30 per 18 holes (£35 Sun). ⊛ **Prof** Peter Brown **Course Designer** Tom Dunn **Facilities** ⊕ �ⳑ ⎁ ⌕ ⬚ ⎘ ⌕ **Location** Off Hampstead Ln
Guesthouse ★★★★ GA Langorf Hotel & Apartments, 20 Frognal, Hampstead, LONDON ☎ 020 7794 4483 31 en suite

N6 HIGHGATE

Highgate Denewood Rd N6 4AH
☎ 020 8340 3745 📄 020 8348 9152
e-mail: nigel@highgategc.co.uk
web: www.highgategc.co.uk
18 holes, 5985yds, Par 69, SSS 69, Course record 66.
Course Designer Cuthbert Butchart **Location** Off B519 Hampstead Ln
Telephone for further details
Hotel ★★★★ 78% HL London Marriott Hotel Regents Park, 128 King Henry's Rd, LONDON ☎ 0870 400 7240 303 en suite

N9 LOWER EDMONTON

Lee Valley Leisure Lee Valley Leisure Complex, Meridian Way, Edmonton N9 0AS
☎ 020 8803 3611 📄 020 8884 4975
e-mail: rgarvey@leevalleypark.org.uk
Testing parkland course with a large lake and the river Lea providing natural hazards. Good quality greens all year round.
18 holes, 5204yds, Par 67, SSS 65, Course record 66.
Club membership 200.
Visitors Mon-Sun & BHs. Booking required Sat/Sun & BHs. Dress code. **Societies** booking required. **Green Fees** not confirmed. **Prof** R Gerken **Course Designer** John Jacobs **Facilities** ⊕ ⍩ ⓘ ⓛ ☷ ⎁ ⌕ ⬚ ⎘ ⌕

N14 SOUTHGATE

Trent Park Bramley Rd, Oakwood N14 4XS
☎ 020 8367 4653 📄 020 8366 4581
e-mail: trentpark@americangolf.uk.com
web: americangolf.com
18 holes, 6381yds, Par 70, SSS 69, Course record 64.
Course Designer D McGibbon **Location** Opp Oakwood tube station
Telephone for further details
Hotel ★★★★ 77% HL West Lodge Park Hotel, Cockfosters Rd, HADLEY WOOD ☎ 020 8216 3900 46 en suite 13 annexe en suite

N20 WHETSTONE

North Middlesex The Manor House, Friern Barnet Ln, Whetstone N20 0NL
☎ 020 8445 1604 & 020 8445 3060 📄 020 8445 5023
e-mail: manager@northmiddlesexgc.co.uk
web: www.northmiddlesexgc.co.uk
Short parkland course renowned for its tricky greens and a spectacular final hole.
18 holes, 5594yds, Par 69, SSS 67, Course record 64.
Club membership 520.
Visitors Mon-Fri. Sat, Sun & BHs restricted. Booking required. Dress code. **Societies** Booking required. **Green Fees** £29 (£34 Sat, Sun & BHs). Winter £22/£27. **Prof** Freddy George **Course Designer** Willie Park Jnr **Facilities** ⊕ ⍩ ⓘ ⓛ ☷ ⎁ ⌕ ⬚ ⌕ **Conf** facs Corporate Hospitality Days **Location** M25 junct 23, 5m S
Hotel ★★★ 73% HL Corus hotel Elstree, Barnet Ln, ELSTREE ☎ 0870 609 6151 47 en suite

South Herts Links Dr, Totteridge N20 8QU
☎ 020 8445 2035 📄 020 8445 7569
e-mail: secretary@southhertsgolfclub.co.uk
web: www.southhertsgolfclub.co.uk
An open undulating parkland course perhaps most famous for the fact that two of the greatest of all British professionals, Harry Vardon and Dai Rees CBE, were professionals at the club. The course is testing, over rolling fairways, especially in the prevailing south-west wind.
18 holes, 6432yds, Par 72, SSS 71, Course record 63.
Club membership 850.
Visitors may play Mon-Fri. Advance booking required. Handicap certificate required. Dress code. **Societies** advance booking required. **Green Fees** not confirmed. ⊛ **Prof** Bobby Mitchell **Course Designer** Harry Vardon **Facilities** ⊕ ⍩ by prior arrangement ⳑ ⎁ ⌕ ⬚ ⎘ ⌕ ⌕ **Conf** Corporate Hospitality Days **Location** 2m E of A1 at Apex Corner
Hotel BUD Innkeeper's Lodge London Southgate, 22 The Green, Southgate, LONDON ☎ 0845 112 6123 19 en suite

England

N21 WINCHMORE HILL

Bush Hill Park Bush Hill, Winchmore Hill N21 2BU
☎ 020 8360 5738 📠 020 8360 5583
e-mail: info@bushhillparkgolfclub.co.uk
web: www.bushhillparkgolfclub.co.uk
Pleasant parkland course in a tranquil setting. The holes set a challenge due to the vast array of mature trees, which make it an enjoyable course to play. The premium is on accuracy rather than length off the tee. The six Par threes are all visually stunning and along with the remodelled 17th contribute to an enjoyable round of golf for all levels of golfer.
18 holes, 5809yds, Par 70, SSS 68, Course record 59.
Club membership 700.
Visitors Mon-Sun & BHs. Booking required. Dress code. **Societies** Booking required. **Green Fees** £29 per round. Twilight £19. ☻ **Prof** Lee Fickling **Course Designer** Harry Vardon **Facilities** ⓑ ⚐ 🍴 ♨ ♨ 🏌 ♨ ♨
Conf Corporate Hospitality Days **Location** 1m S of Enfield off A105
Hotel ★★★ 83% HL Royal Chace Hotel, The Ridgeway, ENFIELD
☎ 020 8884 8181 92 en suite

N22 WOOD GREEN

Muswell Hill Rhodes Av, Wood Green N22 7UT
☎ 020 8888 1764 📠 020 8889 9380
e-mail: mhgcclubsecretary@btconnect.com
web: www.muswellhillgolf.org.uk
Undulating parkland course with a brook running through the centre, set in 87 acres.
18 holes, 6438yds, Par 71, SSS 71, Course record 65.
Club membership 560.
Visitors Mon-Sun & BHs. Booking required Sat, Sun & BHs. Handicap certificate. Dress code. **Societies** Welcome. **Green Fees** £30 per round (£35 Sat & Sun). ☻ **Prof** David Wilton **Course Designer** Braid/Wilson **Facilities** ⓑ 🍴 ⓑ ⚐ 🍴 ♨ 🏌 ♨ **Conf** facs Corporate Hospitality Days **Location** Off N Circular Rd near Bounds Green
Hotel ★★★ 68% HL Days Hotel London North, Welcome Break Service Area, LONDON ☎ 020 8906 7000 200 en suite

NW4 HENDON   MAP 04 TQ28

The Metro Golf Centre Barnet Copthall Sports Centre, Gt North Way NW4 1PS
☎ 020 8202 1202 📠 020 8203 1203
e-mail: golf@metrogolf.btinternet.com
web: www.metro-golf.co.uk
9 holes, 898yds, Par 27, SSS 27, Course record 24.
Course Designer Cousells **Location** M1 junct 2, off A41/A1, in Barnet Copthall sports complex
Telephone for further details
Hotel ★★★★ 78% HL London Marriott Hotel Regents Park, 128 King Henry's Rd, LONDON ☎ 0870 400 7240 303 en suite

NW7 MILL HILL

Finchley Nether Court, Frith Ln, Mill Hill NW7 1PU
☎ 020 8346 2436 📠 020 8343 4205
e-mail: secretary@finchleygolfclub.co.uk
web: www.finchleygolfclub.co.uk
Compact course with rolling parkland. Tree-lined fairways and heavily contoured greens.

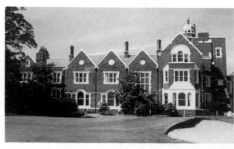
Finchley

18 holes, 6411yds, Par 72, SSS 71. Club membership 500.
Visitors may play Mon, Wed , & Fri except BHs. Sat & Sun after noon. Booking required. Handicap certificate. **Green Fees** £45 per day, £35 per 18 holes (£55/£45 Sat, Sun & BHs). **Prof** David Brown **Course Designer** James Braid **Facilities** ⓑ 🍴 by prior arrangement ⓑ ⚐ 🍴 ♨ 🏠 ♨ 🏌 ♨ ♨ **Conf** facs Corporate Hospitality Days **Location** Near Mill Hill East Tube Station
Hotel ★★★ 73% HL Corus hotel Elstree, Barnet Ln, ELSTREE
☎ 0870 609 6151 47 en suite

Hendon Ashley Walk, Devonshire Rd, Mill Hill NW7 1DG
☎ 020 8346 6023 📠 020 8343 1974
e-mail: hendongolfclub@globalnet.co.uk
web: www.hendongolfclub.co.uk
Easy walking parkland course with a good variety of trees, and providing testing golf.
18 holes, 6289yds, Par 70, SSS 70, Course record 63.
Club membership 560.
Visitors Mon-Sun except BHs. Booking required Sat & Sun. Handicap certificate. Dress code. **Societies** Booking required. **Green Fees** £35 (£40 per round Sat & Sun). Winter £25/£33. **Prof** Matt Deal **Course Designer** H S Colt **Facilities** ⓑ 🍴 ⓑ ⚐ 🍴 ♨ 🏠 ♨ 🏌 ♨ ♨ **Conf** facs Corporate Hospitality Days **Location** M1 junct 2 southbound
Hotel ★★★ 73% HL Corus hotel Elstree, Barnet Ln, ELSTREE
☎ 0870 609 6151 47 en suite

Mill Hill 100 Barnet Way, Mill Hill NW7 3AL
☎ 020 8959 2339 📠 020 8906 0731
e-mail: office@millhillgc.co.uk
web: www.millhillgc.co.uk
A mature course set in 145 acres of parkland. The 18 holes are all individually designed with many bordered by ancient oaks. Lake features on the 2nd, 9th, 10th and 17th holes.

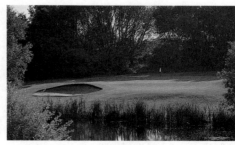

18 holes, 6247yds, Par 70, SSS 70, Course record 68.
Club membership 550.

Continued

Visitors Mon-Sun except BHs. Dress code. **Societies** Booking required. **Green Fees** £30 per round (£37 Sat & Sun). **Prof** David Beal **Course Designer** J F Abercrombie/H S Colt **Facilities** ⓘ ⊢◎ ﹗⊾ ♥ ﹗⏛ ⏛ ⏛ ✆ ⏛ ✆ ✆ **Leisure** snooker. **Conf** facs Corporate Hospitality Days **Location** M1 junct 4, take A41 towards central London. At Apex rdbt turn left and immediately right onto A5109, 3rd turn left into Hawkins Lane. From M25 exit junct 23 onto A1, 2nd exit at Stirming rdbt, A1 on left.
Hotel ★★★ 73% HL Corus hotel Elstree, Barnet Ln, ELSTREE ☎ 0870 609 6151 47 en suite

SE9 ELTHAM

Eltham Warren Bexley Rd, Eltham SE9 2PE
☎ 020 8850 4477
e-mail: secretary@elthamwarren.idps.co.uk
web: www.elthamwarrengolfclub.co.uk
Parkland with narrow tree-lined fairways, all tree lined, and small greens.
9 holes, 5874yds, Par 69, SSS 68, Course record 62.
Club membership 440.
Visitors Booking required. Handicap certificate. Dress code. **Societies** Booking required. **Green Fees** £28 per day. ⊛ **Prof** Gary Brett **Course Designer** James Braid **Facilities** ⏛ ⏛ ✆ **Leisure** snooker. **Location** 0.5m from Eltham station on A210
Hotel ★★★ 77% HL Best Western Bromley Court Hotel, Bromley Hill, BROMLEY ☎ 020 8461 8600 114 en suite

Royal Blackheath Court Rd SE9 5AF
☎ 020 8850 1795 🖷 020 8859 0150
e-mail: info@rbgc.com
web: www.royalblackheath.com
A pleasant, parkland course of great character, with many great trees and two ponds. The 18th requires a pitch to the green over a thick clipped hedge, which also crosses the front of the 1st tee. The clubhouse dates from the 17th century, and you may wish to visit the club's fine museum of golf.
18 holes, 6147yds, Par 70, SSS 70, Course record 65.
Club membership 720.
Visitors Mon-Fri except BHs. Handicap certificate. Dress code. **Societies** Booking required. **Green Fees** £70 per day; £50 per round. **Prof** Richard Harrison **Course Designer** James Braid **Facilities** ⓘ ⊢◎ ﹗⊾ ♥ ﹗⏛ ⏛ ⏛ ✆ ✆ **Leisure** golf museum. **Conf** facs Corporate Hospitality Days **Location** M25 junct 3, A20 towards London, 2nd lights right, club 500yds on right
Hotel ★★★ 77% HL Best Western Bromley Court Hotel, Bromley Hill, BROMLEY ☎ 020 8461 8600 114 en suite

SE18 WOOLWICH

Shooters Hill Eaglesfield Rd, Shooters Hill SE18 3DA
☎ 020 8854 6368 🖷 020 8854 0469
e-mail: secretary@shootershillgc.co.uk
web: www.shootershillgc.co.uk
Hilly and wooded parkland with good views and natural hazards.
18 holes, 5721yds, Par 69, SSS 68, Course record 63.
Club membership 900.
Visitors Mon-Fri except BHs. Handicap certificate. Dress code. **Societies** Booking required. **Green Fees** £35 per day, £28 per round. ⊛ **Prof** David Brotherton **Course Designer** Willie Park **Facilities** ⓘ ⊾ ♥ ﹗⏛ ⏛ ✆ **Conf** Corporate Hospitality Days **Location** Shooters Hill road from Blackheath

SE21 DULWICH

Dulwich & Sydenham Hill Grange Ln, College Rd SE21 7LH
☎ 020 8693 3961 🖷 020 8693 2481
e-mail: secretary@dulwichgolf.co.uk
web: www.dulwichgolf.co.uk
Parkland course set among mature oaks on the slopes of Sydenham Hill, overlooking Dulwich College. Demanding Par 4's and challenging Par 3's are interspersed with reachable but testing Par 5's. Tree-lined fairways off the tees, hazards and cannily placed bunkers await the approach shot. Having made the green, the golfer is then faced with tricky but true greens.
18 holes, 6079yds, Par 69, SSS 69, Course record 63.
Club membership 850.
Visitors Mon-Fri except BHs. Dress code. **Societies** Booking required. **Green Fees** £55 per day, £40 per round. Winter £30 per round. **Prof** David Baillie **Course Designer** H Colt **Facilities** ⓘ ⊢◎ ﹗⊾ ♥ ﹗⏛ ⏛ ⏛ ✆ ✆ **Conf** facs Corporate Hospitality Days **Location** 0.5m from Dulwich College off A205 (south circular)
Hotel ★★★ 77% HL Best Western Bromley Court Hotel, Bromley Hill, BROMLEY ☎ 020 8461 8600 114 en suite

SE28 WOOLWICH

Thamesview Fairway Dr, Summerton Way, Thamesmead SE28 8PP
☎ 020 8310 7975
e-mail: enquiries@thamesview-golf.fsnet.co.uk
9 holes, 5462yds, Par 70, SSS 66.
Course Designer Heffernan **Location** Off A2 near Woolwich ferry
Telephone for further details

SW15 PUTNEY

Richmond Park Roehampton Gate, Priory Ln SW15 5JR
☎ 020 8876 1795 🖷 020 8878 1354
e-mail: richmondpark@glendale-services.co.uk
web: www.gcmgolf.com
Two public parkland courses.
Princes Course: 18 holes, 5868yds, Par 69, SSS 67.
Dukes Course: 18 holes, 6036yds, Par 69, SSS 68.
Visitors Mon-Sun & BHs. Booking required Sat, Sun & BHs. Dress code. **Societies** Booking required. **Green Fees** £19 per 18 holes; (£23 weekends). **Prof** Stuart Hill & David Bown **Course Designer** Fred Hawtree **Facilities** ⓘ ⊾ ♥ ﹗⏛ ⏛ ✆ ✆ ⏛ ✆ **Conf** Corporate Hospitality Days **Location** Inside Richmond Park, entrance via Roehampton Gate
Hotel ★★★★ 71% HL Richmond Hill Hotel, Richmond Hill, RICHMOND UPON THAMES ☎ 020 8940 2247 138 en suite

SW17 WANDSWORTH

Central London Golf Centre Burntwood Ln, Wandsworth SW17 0AT
☎ 020 8871 2468 🖷 020 8874 7447
e-mail: golf@clgc.co.uk
web: www.clgc.co.uk
Attractive flat parkland course in the middle of London. The longest drive is the 430 yard 3rd to one of the course's superb greens. Well placed bunkers trap the careless shot and the course rewards the accurate player.   *Continued*

9 holes, 2277yds, Par 62, SSS 62. Club membership 200.
Visitors Mon-Sun & BHs. Booking required. **Societies** welcome. **Green Fees** not confirmed. **Prof** Jon Woodroffe/Gary Clements **Course Designer** Patrick Tallack **Facilities** ⊕ ⓑ ▯ ▯ 🏌 🏕 ☎ ✦ ♨ ⏴ **Leisure** short game area. **Conf** facs Corporate Hospitality Days **Location** Between Garatt Ln and Trinity Rd
Hotel ★★★★ 74% CHH Cannizaro House, West Side, Wimbledon Common, LONDON ☎ 020 8879 1464 45 en suite

SW19 WIMBLEDON

London Scottish Windmill Enclosure, Wimbledon Common SW19 5NQ
☎ 020 8788 0135 & 8789 1207 📄 020 8789 7517
e-mail: secretary.lsgc@virgin.net
web: www.londonscottishgolfclub.co.uk
Heathland course. The original course was seven holes around the windmill, laid out by 'Old' Willie Dunn of Musselburgh. His son, Tom Dunn, was the first professional to the club and laid out the 18-hole course.
18 holes, 5458yds, Par 68, SSS 66, Course record 61.
Club membership 300.
Visitors Mon-Fri except BHs. Dress code. **Societies** booking required.
Green Fees not confirmed. ⊛ **Prof** Steve Barr **Course Designer** Tom Dunn **Facilities** ⊕ ⓘⓞⓘ ⓑ ▯ ▯ 🏌 🏕 ☎ ✦
Hotel BUD Premier Travel Inn London Wimbledon South, Merantum Way, Merton, LONDON POSTAL DISTRICTS ☎ 0870 990 6342

Royal Wimbledon 29 Camp Rd SW19 4UW
☎ 020 8946 2125 📄 020 8944 8652
e-mail: secretary@rwgc.co.uk
web: www.rwgc.co.uk
The third-oldest club in England, established in 1865 and steeped in the history of the game. Mainly heathland with trees and heather, a good test of golf with many fine holes, the 12th being rated as the best.
18 holes, 6350yds, Par 70, SSS 71, Course record 66.
Club membership 1050.
Visitors may play Mon-Thu except BHs. Advance booking required.
Handicap certificate. Dress code. **Societies** Booking required.
Green Fees £95 per day, £70 per round. **Prof** David Jones
Course Designer H Colt **Facilities** ⊕ ⓑ ▯ ▯ 🏌 🏕 ☎ ✦ ♨ ⏴ ⏴
Conf Corporate Hospitality Days **Location** 1m from Tibbatt's Corner roundabout on A3 off Wimbledon Park before war memorial in village
Hotel BUD Premier Travel Inn London Wimbledon South, Merantum Way, Merton, LONDON POSTAL DISTRICTS ☎ 0870 990 6342

Wimbledon Common 19 Camp Rd SW19 4UW
☎ 020 8946 0294 (Pro shop) 📄 020 8947 8697
e-mail: secretary@wcgc.co.uk
web: www.wcgc.co.uk
Quick-drying course on Wimbledon Common. Well wooded, with tight fairways, challenging short holes but no bunkers.
18 holes, 5438yds, Par 68, SSS 66, Course record 63.
Club membership 290.
Visitors Mon-Fri except BHs. Dress code. **Societies** booking required.
Green Fees not confirmed. **Prof** J S Jukes **Course Designer** Tom & Willie Dunn **Facilities** ⊕ ⓘⓞⓘ ⓑ ▯ ▯ 🏌 🏕 ☎ ✦ **Leisure** snooker room. **Conf** facs Corporate Hospitality Days **Location** 0.5m N of Wimbledon Village
Hotel BUD Premier Travel Inn London Wimbledon South, Merantum Way, Merton, LONDON POSTAL DISTRICTS ☎ 0870 990 6342

Wimbledon Park Home Park Rd, Wimbledon SW19 7HR
☎ 020 8946 1250 📄 020 8944 8688
e-mail: secretary@wpgc.co.uk
web: www.wpgc.co.uk
Easy walking parkland. Sheltered lake provides hazard on three holes.

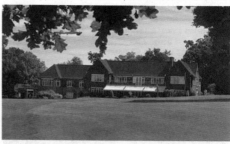

18 holes, 5483yds, Par 66, SSS 66, Course record 59.
Club membership 800.
Visitors Mon-Fri except BHs. Handicap certificate. Dress code.
Societies booking required. **Green Fees** not confirmed. **Prof** Dean Wingrove **Course Designer** Willie Park Jnr **Facilities** ⊕ ⓘⓞⓘ ⓑ ▯ ▯ 🏌 🏕 ✦ ♨ ⏴ **Leisure** sauna. **Conf** facs Corporate Hospitality Days **Location** 400yds from Wimbledon Park station
Hotel ★★★★ 71% HL Richmond Hill Hotel, Richmond Hill, RICHMOND UPON THAMES ☎ 020 8940 2247 138 en suite

W7 HANWELL

Brent Valley 138 Church Rd, Hanwell W7 3BE
☎ 020 8567 1287
18 holes, 5426yds, Par 67, SSS 66.
Telephone for further details
Hotel ★★ 67% HL Best Western Master Robert Hotel, 366 Great West Rd, HOUNSLOW ☎ 020 8570 6261 96 annexe en suite

MERSEYSIDE

BEBINGTON   MAP 07 SJ38

Brackenwood Brackenwood Golf Course, Bracken Ln CH63 2LY
☎ 0151 608 3093
Municipal parkland course with easy walking, a very testing but fair course in a fine rural setting, usually in very good condition.
18 holes, 6285yds, Par 70, SSS 70, Course record 66.
Club membership 320.
Visitors Mon-Sun & BHs. Booking required Sat/Sun. **Societies** booking required. **Green Fees** not confirmed. ⊛ **Prof** Ken Lamb **Facilities** ▯ 🏕 ⏴ ✦ **Location** M53 junct 4, 0.75m N on B5151
Hotel ★★★★ 77% HL Thornton Hall Hotel and Health Club, Neston Rd, THORNTON HOUGH ☎ 0151 336 3938 63 en suite

BIRKENHEAD   MAP 07 SJ38

Arrowe Park Woodchurch CH49 5LW
☎ 0151 677 1527
18 holes, 6435yds, Par 72, SSS 71, Course record 66.
Location M53 junct 3, 1m on A551
Telephone for further details
Hotel ★★★ 79% HL Riverhill Hotel, Talbot Rd, Prenton, BIRKENHEAD ☎ 0151 653 3773 15 en suite

Prenton Golf Links Rd, Prenton CH42 8LW
☎ 0151 609 3426 🖹 0151 609 3421
e-mail: nigel.browne@prentongolfclub.co.uk
web: www.prentongolfclub.co.uk
Parkland with easy walking and views of Welsh hills.
18 holes, 6429yds, Par 71, SSS 71. Club membership 610.
Visitors Mon-Fri, Sun & BHs. Booking required. Handicap certificate. Dress
code. **Societies** Booking required. **Green Fees** Phone. ● **Prof** Robin
Thompson **Course Designer** James Braid **Facilities** ⑪ ⑩ ⓘ ⬚ ▱ ☜ 🍴 ⛛ ⧄
⛳ **Location** M53 junct 3, off A552 towards Birkenhead
Hotel ★★★ 79% HL Riverhill Hotel, Talbot Rd, Prenton, BIRKENHEAD
☎ 0151 653 3773 15 en suite

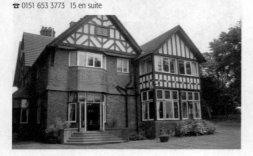

Wirral Ladies 93 Bidston Rd CH43 6TS
☎ 0151 652 1255 🖹 0151 651 3775
e-mail: sue.headford@virgin.net
Compact heathland course with heather and birch, requiring accurate
shots.
18 holes, 5185yds, Par 68, SSS 65. Club membership 590.
Visitors Mon-Sun except BHs. Handicap certificate. Dress code.
Societies Booking required. **Green Fees** £25.50 per round. ● **Prof** Angus
Law **Facilities** ⑪ ⬚ ▱ 🍴 ⧄ ☜ 🍴 ⛳ **Leisure** indoor training suite.
Conf Corporate Hospitality Days **Location** W of town centre on B5151
Hotel ★★★ 79% HL Riverhill Hotel, Talbot Rd, Prenton, BIRKENHEAD
☎ 0151 653 3773 15 en suite

BLUNDELLSANDS MAP 07 SJ39

West Lancashire Hall Rd West L23 8SZ
☎ 0151 924 1076 🖹 0151 931 4448
e-mail: golf@westlancashiregolf.co.uk
web: www.westlancashiregolf.co.uk
Challenging, traditional links with sandy subsoil overlooking the
Mersey estuary. The course provides excellent golf throughout the
year. The four short holes are very fine.
18 holes, 6763yds, Par 72, SSS 73, Course record 66.
Club membership 650.
Visitors Mon, Wed-Fri, Sun & BHs. Booking required. Dress code.
Societies Booking required. **Green Fees** £80 per day; £65 per round
(£100/£85 Sun). **Prof** Gary Edge **Course Designer** C K Cotton
Facilities ⑪ ⑩ ⓘ ⬚ ▱ 🍴 ⧄ ☜ 🍴 ⛛ ⛳ 🍴 **Conf** Corporate Hospitality
Days **Location** N of village, next to Hall Road station

BOOTLE MAP 07 SJ39

Bootle 2 Dunnings Bridge Rd L30 2PP
☎ 0151 928 1371 🖹 0151 949 1815
e-mail: bootlegolfcourse@btconnect.com
18 holes, 6362yds, Par 70, SSS 70, Course record 64.
Location 2m NE on A5036
Telephone for further details
Hotel BUD Premier Travel Inn Liverpool North, Northern Perimiter Rd,
Bootle, LIVERPOOL ☎ 08701 977158 63 en suite

BROMBOROUGH MAP 07 SJ38

Bromborough Raby Hall Rd CH63 0NW
☎ 0151 334 2155 🖹 0151 334 7300
e-mail: enquiries@bromboroughgolfclub.org.uk
web: www.bromboroughgolfclub.org.uk
Parkland course.
18 holes, 6650yds, Par 72, SSS 72, Course record 65.
Club membership 800.
Visitors Mon-Fri & Sun except BHs. Booking required. Handicap certificate.
Dress code. **Societies** Welcome. **Green Fees** Phone. ● **Prof** Geoff Berry
Course Designer J Hassall/Hawtree & Son **Facilities** ⑪ ⑩ ⓘ ⬚ ▱ 🍴 ⧄
☜ ⛛ ⛳ **Conf** Corporate Hospitality Days **Location** 0.5m W of Station
Hotel ★★★★ 77% HL Thornton Hall Hotel and Health Club, Neston Rd,
THORNTON HOUGH ☎ 0151 336 3938 63 en suite

CALDY MAP 07 SJ28

Caldy Links Hey Rd CH48 1NB
☎ 0151 625 5660 🖹 0151 625 7394
e-mail: secretarycaldygc@btconnect.com
web: www.caldygolfclub.co.uk
A heathland and clifftop links course situated on the estuary of the
River Dee with many of the fairways running parallel to the river. Of
championship length, the course offers excellent golf all year, but is
subject to variable winds that noticeably alter the day-to-day playing
of each hole. There are excellent views of the Welsh Hills.
18 holes, 6133metres, Par 72, SSS 72, Course record 65.
Club membership 900.
Visitors Mon & Thu-Fri. Booking required. Handicap certificate. Dress
code. **Societies** Booking required. **Green Fees** £70 per day, £60 per
round. ● **Prof** A Gibbons **Course Designer** J Braid **Facilities** ⑪ ⑩ ⓘ
⬚ ▱ 🍴 ⧄ ☜ 🍴 ⛳ **Leisure** ball hire & collection. **Conf** Corporate
Hospitality Days **Location** Signed from Caldy A540 rdbt to Caldy
Hotel ★★★★ 77% HL Thornton Hall Hotel and Health Club, Neston Rd,
THORNTON HOUGH ☎ 0151 336 3938 63 en suite

EASTHAM MAP 07 SJ38

Eastham Lodge 117 Ferry Rd CH62 0AP
☎ 0151 327 3003 🖹 0151 327 7574
e-mail: easthamlodge.g.c@btinternet.com
web: www.easthamlodgegolfclub.co.uk
A parkland course with many mature trees, recently upgraded
to 18 holes. Most holes have a subtle dog-leg to left or right. The 1st
hole requires an accurate drive to open up the green which is guarded
on the right by a stand of pine trees.
18 holes, 5436yds, Par 68, SSS 68. Club membership 800.
Visitors Mon-Fri except BHs. Booking required Sat/Sun. Dress code.
Societies Booking required. **Green Fees** £24.50 per day, £19.50 per round.

Continued

⊜ **Prof** N Sargent **Course Designer** Hawtree/D Hemstock **Facilities** ⑪
⎸◎⏦ ☖ ⫐⑂ ⚑ ⚔ ☖ ⚐⑂ **Leisure** snooker. **Conf** Corporate Hospitality
Days **Location** 1.5m N, off A41 to Wirral Metropolitan College Country Park
Hotel ★★★ 75% HL Quality Hotel Chester, Berwick Rd, Little Sutton,
ELLESMERE PORT ☎ 0151 339 5121 75 en suite

FORMBY   MAP 07 SD30

Formby Golf Rd L37 1LQ
☎ 01704 872164 📄 01704 833028
e-mail: info@formbygolfclub.co.uk
web: www.formbygolfclub.co.uk
Championship seaside links through sandhills and pine trees. Partly
sheltered from the wind by high dunes it features firm, springy turf,
fast seaside greens and natural sandy bunkers. Well drained it plays
well throughout the year.

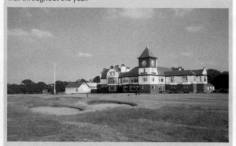

18 holes, 6701yds, Par 72, SSS 72, Course record 65.
Club membership 700.
Visitors Mon-Sun & BHs. Booking required. **Green Fees** £95 per day/round (£105 Sat & Sun).
Prof Gary Butler **Course Designer** Park/Colt **Facilities** ⑪ ⎸◎⏦ ☖ ⫐⑂
⚑ ☖ ⚐ ☖ ⚔ ⚑ **Conf** facs Corporate Hospitality Days **Location** N of
town next to Freshfield railway station

Formby Hall Resort & Spa Southport Old Rd L37 0AB
☎ 01704 875699 📄 01704 832134
e-mail: proshop@formby-hall-co-uk
web: www.formbyhallgolfclub.co.uk
A spectacular parkland course with links style bunkers. American style
design with water on 16 holes. Generous sized fairways with large
undulating greens, many of which are protected by water.
18 holes, 7048yds, Par 72, SSS 74, Course record 69.
Club membership 600.
Visitors Mon-Sun. Booking required. Handicap certificate. Dress
code. **Societies** Booking required. **Green Fees** £60 per 27 holes,
£45 per 18 holes (£55 per 18 holes Sat & Sun). **Prof** Bill Fletcher
Course Designer Alan Higgens **Facilities** ⑪ ⎸◎⏦ ☖ ⫐⑂ ⚑ ☖ ⚐⑂ ⚔ ⚔
☖ ⚔ ⚑ **Leisure** heated indoor swimming pool, fishing, sauna, solarium,
gymnasium, 9 hole Par 3 course, clay pigeon shooting, paintball, archery.
Conf facs Corporate Hospitality Days **Location** 0.5m off A565 Formby
bypass, opp RAF Woodvale

Formby Ladies Golf Rd L37 1YH
☎ 01704 873493 📄 01704 834654
e-mail: secretary@formbyladiesgolfclub.co.uk
web: www.formbyladiesgolfclub.co.uk
Seaside links - one of the few independent ladies' clubs in the country.
The course has contrasting hard-hitting holes in flat country and
tricky holes in sandhills and woods.

18 holes, 5374yds, Par 71, SSS 72, Course record 60.
Club membership 570.
Visitors Mon-Wed, Fri-Sun except BHs. Booking required. Dress code.
Societies Booking required. **Green Fees** £45 per day (£50 Sat & Sun).
⊜ **Prof** Gary Butler **Facilities** ⑪ ⎸ ☖ ⫐⑂ ⚑ ☖ ⚔ **Conf** Corporate
Hospitality Days **Location** N of town centre

HESWALL   MAP 07 SJ28

Heswall Cottage Ln CH60 8PB
☎ 0151 342 1237 📄 0151 342 6140
e-mail: dawn@heswallgolfclub.com
web: www.heswallgolfclub.com
Pleasant parkland in soft undulating country overlooking the Dee
estuary. There are excellent views of the Welsh hills and coastline,
and a good test of golf.

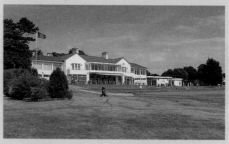

18 holes, 6556yds, Par 72, SSS 72, Course record 62.
Club membership 940.
Visitors Mon, Wed, Fri, Sun except BHs. Booking required. Handicap
certificate. Dress code. **Societies** booking required. **Green Fees** not
confirmed. **Prof** Alan Thompson **Course Designer** McKenzie/Ebert
Facilities ⑪ ☖ ⫐⑂ ⚐⑂ ⚑ ☖ ⚔ **Conf** Corporate Hospitality Days
Location 1m S off A540
Hotel ★★★★ 77% HL Thornton Hall Hotel and Health Club, Neston Rd,
THORNTON HOUGH ☎ 0151 336 3938 63 en suite

HOYLAKE   MAP 07 SJ28

Hoylake Carr Ln, Municipal Links CH47 4BG
☎ 0151 632 2956
18 holes, 6313yds, Par 70, SSS 70, Course record 67.
Course Designer James Braid **Location** SW of town off A540
Telephone for further details
Hotel ★★★ 75% HL Leasowe Castle Hotel, Leasowe Rd, MORETON
☎ 0151 606 9191 47 en suite

Royal Liverpool see page 181

Hotel ★★★ 75% HL Kings Gap Court Hotel, HOYLAKE ☎ 0151 632 2073
30 en suite
Hotel ★★★ 75% HL Leasowe Castle Hotel, Leasowe Rd, MORETON
☎ 0151 606 9191 Fax 0151 678 5551 47 en suite
Hotel ★★★ 79% HL Riverhill Hotel, Talbot Rd, Prenton, BIRKENHEAD
☎ 0151 653 3773 Fax 0151 653 7162 15 en suite

HUYTON
MAP 07 SJ49

Bowring Park Roby Rd L36 4HD
☎ 0151 443 0424 & 489 1901
e-mail: bowringpark@knowsley.gov.uk
18 holes, 6082yds, Par 70.
Location M62 junct 5, on A5080
Telephone for further details
Hotel BUD Premier Travel Inn Liverpool (Roby), Roby Rd, Huyton,
LIVERPOOL ☎ 0870 9906596 53 en suite

Huyton & Prescot Hurst Park, Huyton Ln L36 1UA
☎ 0151 489 3948 📄 0151 489 0797

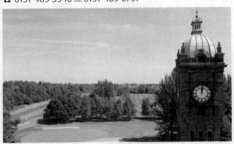

18 holes, 5779yds, Par 68, SSS 68, Course record 65.
Location 1.5m NE off B5199
Telephone for further details
Hotel BUD Premier Travel Inn Liverpool (Tarbock), Wilson Rd, Tarbock,
LIVERPOOL ☎ 08701 977159 40 en suite

LIVERPOOL
MAP 07 SJ39

Allerton Park Allerton Manor Golf Estate, Allerton Rd
L18 3JT
☎ 0151 428 7490 📄 0151 428 7490
Parkland course.
18 holes, 5494yds, Par 67, SSS 66.
Visitors contact club for details. **Societies** booking required. **Green Fees**
not confirmed. ⊛ **Prof** Barry Large **Facilities** ⓑ ⌷ ☷ 🏐 🛆 ☆ ♂ **Leisure** 9
hole Par 3 course. **Location** 5.5m SE of city centre off A562
Hotel ★★★ 80% HL The Royal Hotel, Marine Ter, Waterloo, LIVERPOOL
☎ 0151 928 2332 25 en suite

The Childwall Naylors Rd, Gateacre L27 2YB
☎ 0151 487 0654 📄 0151 487 0654
e-mail: office@childwallgolfclub.co.uk
web: www.childwallgolfclub.co.uk
Parkland golf is played here over a testing course, where accuracy
from the tee is well-rewarded. The course is very popular with
visiting societies for the clubhouse has many amenities. Course
designed by James Braid.
18 holes, 6425yds, Par 72, SSS 71, Course record 66.
Club membership 650.
Visitors Mon, Wed-Sun except BHs. Booking required. Handicap
certificate. Dress code. **Societies** booking required. **Green Fees**
not confirmed. **Prof** Nigel M Parr **Course Designer** James Braid
Facilities ⓑ 🍽 by prior arrangement ☷ ⌷ ☷ 🛆 🏐 ☆ ♂ **Conf** facs
Corporate Hospitality Days **Location** 7m E of city centre off B5178
Hotel BUD Premier Travel Inn Liverpool (Roby), Roby Rd, Huyton,
LIVERPOOL ☎ 0870 9906596 53 en suite

Kirkby-Liverpool Municipal Ingoe Ln, Kirkby L32 4SS
☎ 0151 546 5435
18 holes, 6704yds, Par 72, SSS 72, Course record 68.
Location 7.5m NE of city centre on A506
Telephone for further details
Hotel ★★★ 80% HL The Royal Hotel, Marine Ter, Waterloo, LIVERPOOL
☎ 0151 928 2332 25 en suite

Lee Park Childwall Valley Rd L27 3YA
☎ 0151 487 3882 📄 0151 498 4666
e-mail: lee.park@virgin.net
web: www.leepark.co.uk
Easy walking parkland with plenty of trees, water features and dog legs.
A test for the short game; being in the right position to attack the pins
is a premium.

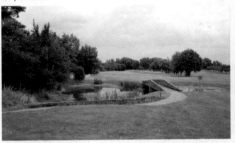

18 holes, 5959yds, Par 70, SSS 69, Course record 66.
Club membership 600.
Visitors Mon-Sun & BHs. Booking required. Dress code. **Societies** Booking
required. **Green Fees** £30 per day (£40 Sat, Sun & BHs). ⊛ **Prof** Chris
Crowder **Course Designer** G Cotton **Facilities** ⓑ 🍽 ☷ ⌷ ☷ 🛆 ♂
Leisure snooker room. **Conf** Corporate Hospitality Days **Location** M62
junct 6/M57 junct 1, take A5080 towards Huyton. Turn left at 2nd set of
lights into Wheathill Rd. After 1m turn left at 1st set of lights into Childwall
Valley Rd, club on left.
Hotel BUD Premier Travel Inn Liverpool (Roby), Roby Rd, Huyton,
LIVERPOOL ☎ 0870 9906596 53 en suite

West Derby Yew Tree Ln, West Derby L12 9HQ
☎ 0151 254 1034 📄 0151 259 0505
e-mail: pmilne@westderbygc.freeserve.co.uk
A parkland course always in first-class condition, and so giving easy
walking. The fairways are well-wooded. Care must be taken on the
first nine holes to avoid the brook which guards many of the greens.
18 holes, 6275yds, Par 72, SSS 70, Course record 65.
Club membership 550.
Visitors Mon, Wed-Fri except BHs. Booking required. Dress code.
Societies Booking required. **Green Fees** £35 per day. ⊛ **Prof** Andrew
Witherup **Facilities** ⓑ 🍽 ☷ ⌷ ☷ 🛆 ♂ **Conf** facs Corporate
Hospitality Days **Location** 4.5m E of city centre off A57
Hotel ★★★ 80% HL The Royal Hotel, Marine Ter, Waterloo, LIVERPOOL
☎ 0151 928 2332 25 en suite

Woolton Doe Park, Speke Rd, Woolton L25 7TZ
☎ 0151 486 2298 📄 0151 486 1664
e-mail: golf@wooltongolf.co.uk
web: www.wooltongolf.co.uk
18 holes, 5717yds, Par 69, SSS 68, Course record 63.
Location 7m SE of city centre off A562, near Liverpool airport
Telephone for further details
Hotel ★★★ 80% HL The Royal Hotel, Marine Ter, Waterloo, LIVERPOOL
☎ 0151 928 2332 25 en suite

CHAMPIONSHIP COURSE

MERSEYSIDE — HOYLAKE

ROYAL LIVERPOOL

Map 07 SJ28

Meols Dr CH47 4AL
☎ 0151 632 3101 & 632 3102
🖹 0151 632 6737
e-mail: secretary@royal-liverpool-golf.com
web: www.royal-liverpool-golf.com
18 holes, 6440yds, Par 72, SSS 71.
Club membership 950.
Visitors Mon-Fri except BHs. Booking required. Handicap certificate. Dress code.
Societies Booking required. **Green Fees** £135 per round inc lunch. **Prof** John Heggarty
Course Designer R Chambers/G Morris/D Steel
Facilities ⑪ ⓑ ⬛ ⬚⬚ ⚓ ⬚⬚ ⬚⬚ ⬚⬚ ⬚⬚
Conf Corporate Hospitality Days **Location** SW side of town on A540

Built in 1869 on the site of a former racecourse, this world-famous championship course was one of the first seaside courses to be established in England. In 1921 Hoylake was the scene of the first international match between the US and Britain, now known as the Walker Cup. Over the years, golfing enthusiasts have come to Hoylake to witness 18 amateur championships and 11 Open Championships, which the club hosted again in 2006. Visitors playing on this historic course can expect a challenging match, with crosswinds, deep bunkers and hollows, all set against the backdrop of stunning Welsh hills. Watch out for the 8th hole, which saw the great Bobby Jones take an 8 on this Par 5 on the way to his famous Grand Slam in 1930.

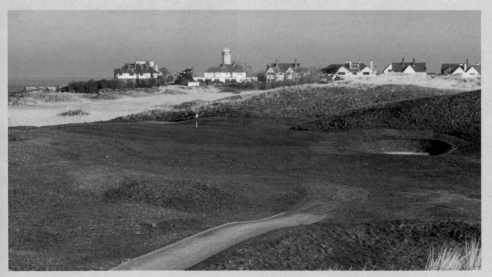

NEWTON-LE-WILLOWS   ·   MAP 07 SJ59

Haydock Park Newton Ln WA12 0HX
☎ 01925 228525 📠 01925 224984
e-mail: secretary@haydockparkgc.co.uk
web: www.haydockparkgc.co.uk
A well-wooded parkland course, close to the well-known racecourse, and always in excellent condition. The pleasant undulating fairways offer some very interesting golf and the 6th, 9th, 11th and 13th holes are particularly testing.
18 holes, 6058yds, Par 70, SSS 69, Course record 65.
Club membership 630.
Visitors Mon-Sun except BHs. Booking required. Handicap certificate. Dress code. **Societies** Booking required. **Green Fees** £35 per day, £30 per round. ☻ **Prof** Peter Kenwright **Course Designer** James Braid **Facilities** ⑪ ⑩ ⑤ 🖵 🏌 ⌂ 👜 ✔ **Location** 0.75m NE off A49
Hotel ★★ 62% HL Kirkfield Hotel, 2/4 Church St, NEWTON LE WILLOWS ☎ 01925 228196   17 en suite

RAINHILL   MAP 07 SJ49

Blundells Hill Blundells Ln L35 6NA
☎ 0151 4309551 (secretary) & 4300100 (pro)
📠 0151 4265256
e-mail: information@blundellshill.co.uk
web: www.blundellshill.co.uk
18 holes, 6256yds, Par 71, SSS 70, Course record 69.
Course Designer Steve Marnoch **Location** M62 junct 7, A57 towards Prescot, left after garage, 2nd left onto Blundells Ln
Telephone for further details
Hotel BUD Premier Travel Inn Liverpool (Rainhill), 804 Warrington Rd, Rainhill, LIVERPOOL ☎ 0870 9906446   34 en suite

Eccleston Park Rainhill Rd L35 4PG
☎ 0151 493 0033 📠 0151 493 0044
e-mail: ecclestonpark-sales@crown-golf.co.uk
web: www.crown-golf.co.uk
A tough parkland course designed to test all golfing abilities. Strategically placed water features, bunkers and mounding enhance the beauty and difficulty of this manicured course.
18 holes, 6296yds, Par 70, SSS 72. Club membership 850.
Visitors Mon-Sun & BHs. Dress code. **Societies** Welcome. **Green Fees** £20 per 18 holes, £10 per 9 holes (£25/£12 Sat, Sun & BHs). **Prof** Chris Crowder **Facilities** ⑪ ⑩ ⑤ 🖵 🖵 🏌 ⌂ 👜 ✔ **Conf** facs Corporate Hospitality Days **Location** M62 junct 7, A57 to Prescot, at hump bridge right at lights, course 1m on left
Hotel BUD Premier Travel Inn Liverpool (Rainhill), 804 Warrington Rd, Rainhill, LIVERPOOL ☎ 0870 9906446   34 en suite

ST HELENS   MAP 07 SJ59

Grange Park Prescot Rd WA10 3AD
☎ 01744 26318 📠 01744 26318
e-mail: secretary@grangeparkgolfclub.co.uk
web: www.grangeparkgolfclub.co.uk
Possibly one of the finest tests of inland golf in the northwest, set in 150 acres only a short distance from the centre of town. While not too long, the contours of the fairways, small greens and penal rough demand the best from players. A wide shot making repertoire is required to gain the best score possible.

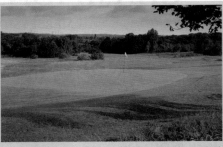

Grange Park

18 holes, 6446yds, Par 72, SSS 71, Course record 65.
Club membership 730.
Visitors Mon, Wed-Fri, Sun & BHs. Booking required. Handicap certificate. Dress code. **Societies** booking required. **Green Fees** not confirmed. ☻ **Prof** Paul Roberts **Course Designer** James Braid **Facilities** ⑪ ⑩ ⑤ 🖵 🏌 ⌂ 👜 ✔ **Conf** facs Corporate Hospitality Days **Location** 1.5m SW on A58
Hotel ★★ 62% HL Kirkfield Hotel, 2/4 Church St, NEWTON LE WILLOWS ☎ 01925 228196   17 en suite

Houghwood Golf Billinge Hill, Crank Rd, Crank WA11 8RL
☎ 01744 894444 & 894754 📠 01744 894754
e-mail: houghwoodgolf@btinternet.com
web: www.houghwoodgolfclub.co.uk
From the course's highest point, the 12th tee, there are panoramic views over the Lancashire plain to the Welsh hills. All greens built to USGA specification with a permanent track around the entire course for buggies and trolleys.

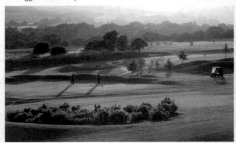

18 holes, 6268yds, Par 70, SSS 69, Course record 67.
Club membership 580.
Visitors Mon-Sun & BHs. Booking required. Dress code. **Societies** Booking required. **Green Fees** £30 per round; (£40 Sat, Sun & BHs). **Prof** Paul Dickenson **Course Designer** Neville Pearson **Facilities** ⑪ ⑩ ⑤ 🖵 🖵 🏌 ⌂ 👜 ✔ **Leisure** snooker table. **Conf** facs Corporate Hospitality Days **Location** 3.5m N of St Helens off B5205
Hotel BUD Travelodge Haydock St Helens, Piele Rd, HAYDOCK ☎ 08700 850 950   62 en suite

Sherdley Park Sherdley Rd WA9 5DE
☎ 01744 813149 📠 01744 817967
web: www.sthelens.gov.uk
Fairly hilly, challenging, pay and play parkland course with ponds in places. Excellent greens.

Continued

CHAMPIONSHIP COURSE

MERSEYSIDE — SOUTHPORT

ROYAL BIRKDALE

Map 07 SD31

Waterloo Rd, Birkdale PR8 2LX
☎ 01704 567920 🖷 01704 562327
e-mail: secretary@royalbirkdale.com
web: www.royalbirkdale.com
18 holes, 6726yds, Par 72, SSS 73.
Club membership 800.
Visitors Mon-Fri, Sun except BHs. Booking
required. Handicap certificate. Dress
code. **Societies** Booking required.
Green Fees May-Sep £165 per round (£195
per round Sun). Oct/Nov £120 per round
including soup and sandwiches (£150 Sun).
Dec-Feb £80 per round soup and sandwiches
(£105 Sun). **Prof** Brian Hodgkinson
Course Designer Hawtree **Facilities** ⑪ ⑩ by
prior arrangement ⓑ ☐ ⚲ △ ⚐ ⚘ ✦ ✦
Conf Corporate Hospitality Days **Location** 1.75m
S of town centre on A565

Founded in 1889, the Royal Birkdale is
considered by many to be the ultimate
championship venue, having hosted every
major event in the game including eight Open
Championships, two Ryder Cup matches, the
Walker Cup, the Curtis Cup and many amateur
events. The 1st hole provides an immediate
taste of what is to come, requiring a well-placed
drive to avoid a bunker, water hazard and out-
of-bounds and leave a reasonably clear view of
the green. The 10th, the first of the inward nine
is unique in that it is the only hole to display
the significant fairway undulations one would
expect from a classic links course. The 12th is
the most spectacular of the short holes on the
course, and is considered by Tom Watson to
be one of the best Par 3s in the world; tucked
away in the sand hills it continues to claim its
fair share of disasters. The approach on the
final hole is arguably the most recognisable in
golf with the distinctive clubhouse designed to
appear like an ocean cruise liner rising out of
the sand hills. It's a Par 5 for mere mortals, and
played as a Par 4 in the Open, but it will provide
a memorable finish to any round of golf.

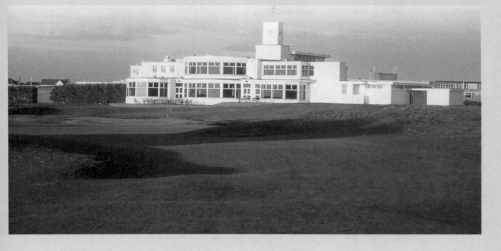

18 holes, 5974yds, Par 71, SSS 69.
Visitors Mon-Sun & BHs. Booking required. **Societies** Welcome. **Green Fees** £13.65 per 18 holes (£15.75 Sat, Sun & BHs). **Prof** Danny Jones **Facilities** ⑪ ⓑ ⌨ ▢ ❄ 🛆 ➔ ⚐ 🏌 **Conf** Corporate Hospitality Days **Location** 2m S of St Helens off A570
Hotel ★★ 62% HL Kirkfield Hotel, 2/4 Church St, NEWTON LE WILLOWS ☎ 01925 228196 17 en suite

---

SOUTHPORT   MAP 07 SD31

The Hesketh Cockle Dick's Ln, off Cambridge Rd PR9 9QQ
☎ 01704 536897 🖹 01704 539250
e-mail: secretary@heskethgolfclub.co.uk
web: www.heskethgolfclub.co.uk
The Hesketh is the oldest of the six clubs in Southport, founded in 1885. Set at the northern end of south-west Lancashire's dune system, the course sets a unique challenge with half of the holes threaded through tall dunes while the other holes border the Ribble estuary. The course is next to a renowned bird reserve and across the estuary are fine views of the mountains of Lancashire, Cumbria and Yorkshire. Used as a final qualifying course for the Open Championship.
18 holes, 6655yds, Par 72, SSS 72, Course record 67.
Club membership 600.
Visitors Mon, Wed-Fri, Sun & BHs. Tue & Sat pm only. Booking required. Handicap certificate. Dress code. **Societies** Welcome. **Green Fees** £70 per day; £55 per round (£70 per round Sat, Sun & BHs). **Prof** Scott Astin **Course Designer** J F Morris **Facilities** ⑪ ⍾ ⓑ ⌨ ▢ ❄ 🛆 ➔ ⚐ ✎ **Leisure** snooker. **Conf** Corporate Hospitality Days **Location** 1m NE of town centre off A565
Hotel ★★★ 75% HL Best Western Stutelea Hotel & Leisure Club, Alexandra Rd, SOUTHPORT ☎ 01704 544220 22 en suite

Hillside Hastings Rd, Hillside PR8 2LU
☎ 01704 567169 🖹 01704 563192
e-mail: secretary@hillside-golfclub.co.uk
web: www.hillside-golfclub.co.uk
Championship links course with natural hazards open to strong wind.
18 holes, 6850yds, Par 72, SSS 74, Course record 65.
Club membership 700.
Visitors Contact club for details. **Societies** Welcome. **Green Fees** £95 per day, £75 per round (£95 per round Sun). **Prof** Brian Seddon **Course Designer** Hawtree/Steel **Facilities** ⑪ ⍾ ⓑ ⌨ ▢ ❄ 🛆 ➔ ⚐ ✎ 🏌 **Conf** Corporate Hospitality Days **Location** 3m S of town centre on A565
Hotel ★★★ 77% HL Scarisbrick Hotel, Lord St, SOUTHPORT ☎ 01704 543000 88 en suite

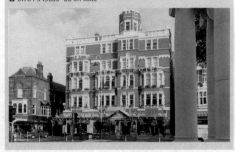

Royal Birkdale see page 183
Hotel ★★★ 77% HL Scarisbrick Hotel, Lord St, SOUTHPORT ☎ 01704 543000 88 en suite
Hotel ★★★ 75% HL Best Western Stutelea Hotel & Leisure Club, Alexandra Rd, SOUTHPORT ☎ 01704 544220 Fax 01704 500232 22 en suite
Hotel ★★★ 73% HL Best Western Royal Clifton Hotel, Promenade, SOUTHPORT ☎ 01704 533771 Fax 01704 500657 120 en suite
Hotel ★★ 71% HL Balmoral Lodge Hotel, 41 Queens Rd, SOUTHPORT ☎ 01704 544298 & 530751 Fax 01704 501224 15 rms (11 en suite)

Southport & Ainsdale Bradshaws Ln, Ainsdale PR8 3LG
☎ 01704 578000 🖹 01704 570896
e-mail: secretary@sandagolfclub.co.uk
web: www.sandagolfclub.co.uk
S and A, as it is known in the north, is another of the fine championship courses for which this part of the country is famed. The club has staged many important events and offers golf of the highest order.
18 holes, 6705yds, Par 72, SSS 73, Course record 62.
Club membership 815.
Visitors Mon-Sun & BHs. Booking required. Handicap certificate. Dress code. **Societies** Booking required. **Green Fees** £65 per 18 holes; £90 per 36 holes (£90 per 18 holes weekends). **Prof** Jim Payne **Course Designer** James Braid **Facilities** ⑪ ⍾ ⓑ ⌨ ▢ ❄ 🛆 ➔ ⚐ ✎ **Conf** facs Corporate Hospitality Days **Location** 3m S off A565
Hotel ★★★ 73% HL Best Western Royal Clifton Hotel, Promenade, SOUTHPORT ☎ 01704 533771 120 en suite

Southport Municipal Park Rd West PR9 0JR
☎ 01704 535286
18 holes, 6400yds, Par 70, SSS 69, Course record 67.
Location N of town centre off A565
Telephone for further details
Hotel ★★★ 73% HL Best Western Royal Clifton Hotel, Promenade, SOUTHPORT ☎ 01704 533771 120 en suite

Southport Old Links Moss Ln, Churchtown PR9 7QS
☎ 01704 228207 🖹 01704 505353
e-mail: secretary@solgc.freeserve.co.uk
web: www.solgc.freeserve.co.uk
Seaside course with tree-lined fairways and easy walking. One of the oldest courses in Southport, Harry Vardon won the Leeds Cup here in 1922.
9 holes, 6450yds, Par 72, SSS 71, Course record 70.
Club membership 450.
Visitors Mon, Tue, Thu-Sat except BHs. Booking required.Handicap certificate. Dress code. **Societies** Booking required. **Green Fees** £25 per 18 holes (£30 Sat). ⊛ **Prof** Gary Copeman **Facilities** ⑪ ⍾ ⓑ ⌨ ▢ 🛆 ➔ ⚐ ✎ **Conf** Corporate Hospitality Days **Location** NW of town centre off A5267
Hotel ★★ 74% HL Bold Hotel, 585 Lord St, SOUTHPORT ☎ 01704 532578 23 en suite

WALLASEY
MAP 07 SJ29

Bidston Bidston Link Rd CH44 2HR
☎ 0151 638 3412
e-mail: linda@bidstongolf.co.uk
web: www.bidstongolf.co.uk
Flat, easy walking parkland with westerly winds.
18 holes, 6233yds, Par 70, SSS 70. Club membership 600.
Visitors Mon-Fri except BHs. Handicap certificate. Dress code. **Societies**
Booking required. **Green Fees** £30 per 18 holes. ◉ **Prof** Alan Norwood
Facilities ⑪ ⑩ ⬛ ⬜ ✣⬛ 🖃 ⚐ ✂ **Location** M53 junct 1, 0.5m W
off A551
Hotel ★★★ 75% HL Leasowe Castle Hotel, Leasowe Rd, MORETON
☎ 0151 606 9191 47 en suite

Leasowe Moreton CH46 3RD
☎ 0151 677 5852 🖹 0151 641 8519
e-mail: secretary@leasowegolfclub.co.uk
web: www.leasowegolfclub.co.uk
A semi-links, seaside course which has recently undergone landscaping
on the first five holes, new mounds removing the former rather flat
appearance.
18 holes, 6151yds, Par 71, SSS 70. Club membership 637.
Visitors Tue, Thu, Fri, Sun except BHs. Booking required. Dress code.
Societies Welcome. **Green Fees** £30.50 (£35.50 Sun). **Prof** Andrew Ayre
Course Designer John Ball Jnr **Facilities** ⑪ ⑩ ⬛ ⬜ ✣⬛ 🖃 ⚐ ✂
Conf Corporate Hospitality Days **Location** M53 junct 1, 2m W on A551
Hotel ★★★ 75% HL Leasowe Castle Hotel, Leasowe Rd, MORETON
☎ 0151 606 9191 47 en suite

Wallasey Bayswater Rd CH45 8LA
☎ 0151 691 1024 🖹 0151 638 8988
e-mail: wallaseygc@aol.com
web: wallaseygolf.com
A well-established links course, adjacent to the Irish Sea. A true test
of golf due in part to the prevailing westerly winds and the natural
undulating terrain. Spectacular views across Liverpool Bay and the
Welsh hills.
18 holes, 6503yds, Par 72, SSS 72, Course record 65.
Club membership 650.
Visitors Mon-Fri & Sun. Restricted Sat & BHs. Booking required. Dress
code. **Societies** Welcome. **Green Fees** £80 per day, £70 per round
(£95/£85 Sun & BHs). **Prof** Mike Adams **Course Designer** Tom Morris
Facilities ⑪ ⑩ by prior arrangement ⬛ ⬜ ✣ 🖃 ✂ **Location** N of
town centre off A554
Hotel ★★★ 78% HL Grove House Hotel, Grove Rd, WALLASEY
☎ 0151 639 3947 & 0151 630 4558 🖹 0151 639 0028 14 en suite

Warren Grove Rd CH45 0JA
☎ 0151 639 8323
e-mail: golfer@warrengc.freeserve.co.uk
web: www.warrengc.freeserve.co.uk
9 holes, 5854yds, Par 72, SSS 68, Course record 68.
Location N of town centre off A554
Telephone for further details
Hotel ★★★ 75% HL Leasowe Castle Hotel, Leasowe Rd, MORETON
☎ 0151 606 9191 47 en suite

NORFOLK

BARNHAM BROOM
MAP 05 TG00

Barnham Broom Hotel, Golf, Conference, Leisure
Honingham Rd NR9 4DD
☎ 01603 759552 & 759393 🖹 01603 758224
e-mail: golfmanager@barnham-broom.co.uk
web: www.barnham-broom.co.uk
Course meanders through the Yare valley, parkland and mature
trees. Hill course has wide fairways, heavily guarded greens and
spectacular views.
Valley Course: 18 holes, 6483yds, Par 72, SSS 71.
Hill Course: 18 holes, 6495yds, Par 71, SSS 71.
Club membership 500.
Visitors Contact club for details. Handicap certificate. Dress code.
Societies Welcome. **Green Fees** Valley £40, Hill £35. **Prof** Ian Rollett
Course Designer Frank Pennink **Facilities** ⑪ ⑩ ⬛ ⬜ ✣⬛ 🖃 ⚐ ◇
✂ 🖙 ✂ ✦ **Leisure** hard tennis courts, heated indoor swimming pool,
squash, sauna, solarium, gymnasium, 3 academy holes. Golf school.
Squash tuition. **Conf** facs Corporate Hospitality Days **Location** Off A47
at Honingham
Hotel ★★★ 83% HL Barnham Broom Hotel, Golf & Restaurant,
BARNHAM BROOM ☎ 01603 759393 52 en suite

BAWBURGH
MAP 05 TG10

Bawburgh Glen Lodge, Marlingford Rd NR9 3LU
☎ 01603 740404 🖹 01603 740403
e-mail: info@bawburgh.com
web: www.bawburgh.com
Undulating course, mixture of parkland and heathland. The main
feature is a large hollow that meanders down to the River Yare creating
many interesting tee and green locations. Excellent 18th hole to finish
requiring a long accurate second shot to clear the lake in front of the
elevated green.
18 holes, 6209yds, Par 70, SSS 70, Course record 64.
Club membership 650.
Visitors Mon-Sun & BHs. Booking required. Dress code. **Societies** Booking
required. **Green Fees** Phone. **Prof** Chris Potter **Course Designer** John
Barnard **Facilities** ⑪ ⑩ ⬛ ⬜ ✣⬛ 🖃 🖙 ✂ ✦ **Conf** facs Corporate
Hospitality Days **Location** S of Royal Norfolk Showground, off A47 to
Bawburgh
Hotel ★★★ 82% HL Park Farm Hotel, HETHERSETT ☎ 01603 810264
3 en suite 39 annexe en suite

BRANCASTER
MAP 09 TF74

Royal West Norfolk PE31 8AX
☎ 01485 210223 🖹 01485 210087
A fine links laid out in grand manner characterised by sleepered
greens, superb cross bunkers and salt marshes. The tranquil
surroundings include a harbour, the sea, farmland and marshland,
inhabited by many rare birds. A great part of the year the club is cut
off by tidal flooding that restricts the amount of play.
18 holes, 6428yds, Par 71, SSS 71, Course record 65.
Club membership 898.
Visitors Mon-Sun except BHs. Booking required. Handicap certificate.
Societies Booking required. **Green Fees** Phone. **Prof** S Rayner
Course Designer Holcombe-Ingleby **Facilities** ⑪ ⑩ by prior arrangement
⬛ ⬜ ✣⬛ 🖃 ⚐ ✂ **Location** Off A149 in Brancaster 1m to seafront
Hotel ★★ 82% HL The White Horse, BRANCASTER STAITHE
☎ 01485 210262 7 en suite 8 annexe en suite

England

CROMER
MAP 09 TG24

Royal Cromer 145 Overstrand Rd NR27 0JH
☎ 01263 512884 📄 01263 512430
e-mail: general.manager@royal-cromer.com
web: www.royalcromergolfclub.com
Challenging course with spectacular views out to sea and
overlooking the town. Strong sea breezes affect the clifftop holes, the
most famous being the 14th (the Lighthouse) which has a green in
the shadow of a lighthouse.
18 holes, 6508yds, Par 72, SSS 72, Course record 67.
Club membership 700.
Visitors Mon-Sun & BHs. Booking required. Handicap certificate. Dress
code. **Societies** Booking required. **Green Fees** £45 per day (£55 Sat, Sun
& BHs). **Prof** Lee Patterson **Course Designer** J H Taylor
Facilities ⑪ 🍴 🐄 🖭 🌭 🏖 🖭 🌾 🖭 ⚽ **Conf** Corporate Hospitality
Days **Location** 1m E on B1159
Hotel ★★ 76% HL Red Lion, Brook St, CROMER ☎ 01263 514964
12 en suite

DENVER
MAP 05 TF60

Ryston Park PE38 0HH
☎ 01366 382133 📄 01366 383834
e-mail: rystonparkgc@tiscali.co.uk
web: www.club-noticeboard.co.uk
Parkland course with two challenging Par 4s to open. Water comes
into play on holes 5, 6 and 7. The course is well wooded with an
abundance of wildlife.
9 holes, 6310yds, Par 70, SSS 70, Course record 66.
Club membership 330.
Visitors Mon-Fri except BHs. Handicap certificate. Dress code.
Societies Booking required. **Green Fees** £30 per day; £20 per round. 🅰
Course Designer James Braid **Facilities** ⑪ 🍴 by prior arrangement 🐄 🖭
🖭 🌭 ⚽ **Conf** facs Corporate Hospitality Days **Location** 0.5m S on A10
Hotel ★★ 78% HL Castle Hotel, High St, DOWNHAM MARKET
☎ 01366 384311 12 en suite

DEREHAM
MAP 09 TF91

Dereham Quebec Rd NR19 2DS
☎ 01362 695900 📄 01362 695904
e-mail: derehamgolfclub@dgolfclub.freeserve.co.uk
web: derehamgolfclub.com
9 hole parkland course with 17 tees.
9 holes, 6194yds, Par 71, SSS 70, Course record 64.
Club membership 480.
Visitors contact club for details. Handicap certificate. Dress code.
Societies booking required. **Green Fees** not confirmed. 🅰 **Prof** Neil
Allsebrook **Facilities** ⑪ 🍴 🐄 🖭 🌭 🏖 🖭 ⚽ **Conf** Corporate
Hospitality Days **Location** N of town centre off B1110
Hotel ★★★ 83% HL Barnham Broom Hotel, Golf & Restaurant, BARNHAM
BROOM ☎ 01603 759393 52 en suite

The Norfolk Golf & Country Club Hingham Rd,
Reymerston NR9 4QQ
☎ 01362 850297 📄 01362 850614
e-mail: norfolkgolfsec@ukonline.co.uk
web: www.club-noticeboard.co.uk
The course meanders through more than 200 acres of rolling Norfolk
countryside, including ancient ditches, hedges and woodland. Large
greens built to USGA specification.

18 holes, 6609yds, Par 72, SSS 72, Course record 69.
Club membership 500.
Visitors Mon-Sun & BHs. Booking required. Dress code.
Societies Welcome. **Green Fees** £22 (£27 Sat & Sun). **Prof** Tony Varney
Facilities 🐄 🖭 🌭 ⚽ 🖭 ⚽ 🖭 **Leisure** heated indoor swimming pool,
sauna, solarium, gymnasium, pitch & putt. **Conf** facs Corporate Hospitality
Days **Location** Off B1135
Hotel ★★★ 83% HL Barnham Broom Hotel, Golf & Restaurant, BARNHAM
BROOM ☎ 01603 759393 52 en suite

FAKENHAM
MAP 09 TF92

Fakenham Gallow Sports Centre, The Race Course
NR21 7NY
☎ 01328 863534
9 holes, 6174yds, Par 71, SSS 70, Course record 65.
Course Designer Cotton(UK)
Telephone for further details

FRITTON
MAP 05 TG40

Caldecott Hall Golf & Leisure Caldecott Hall, Beccles
Rd NR31 9EY
☎ 01493 488488 📄 01493 488561
web: www.caldecotthall.co.uk
Facilities at Caldecott Hall include an 18-hole course with testing
dog-leg fairways

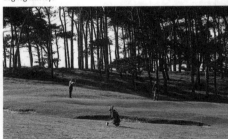

Main Course: 18 holes, 6685yards, Par 73, SSS 72.
Club membership 500.
Visitors Contact hotel for details. **Societies** Welcome. **Green Fees** £20 per
day (£26 Sat & Sun). **Prof** Syer Shulver **Facilities** ⑪ 🍴 🐄 🖭 🌭 🏖 🖭
🌊 🖭 ⚽ 🖭 **Leisure** heated indoor swimming pool, fishing, gymnasium, 18
hole Par 3 course. **Conf** facs Corporate Hospitality Days **Location** On A143
Hotel ★★★ 77% HL Caldecott Hall Golf & Leisure, Caldecott Hall, Beccles
Rd, FRITTON ☎ 01493 488488 8 en suite

GORLESTON ON SEA
MAP 05 TG50

Gorleston Warren Rd NR31 6JT
☎ 01493 661911 📄 01493 661911
e-mail: manager@gorlestongolfclub.co.uk
web: www.gorlestongolfclub.co.uk
Clifftop course, the most easterly in the British Isles. One of the
outstanding features of the course is the 7th hole, which was rescued
from cliff erosion about 20 years ago. The green, only 8yds from the
cliff edge, is at the mercy of the prevailing winds so club selection is
critical.

Continued

18 holes, 6391yds, Par 71, SSS 71, Course record 68.
Club membership 800.
Visitors Mon, Tue, Thu & Fri. Wed pm only. Booking required. Handicap certificate. Dress code. **Societies** Welcome. **Green Fees** £35 per day, £25 per 18 holes. **Prof** Nick Brown **Course Designer** J H Taylor **Facilities** ⊕ ⏱️ by prior arrangement ⓛ ⌂ ⏱ ⌂ ✆ ✦ **Conf** Corporate Hospitality Days **Location** Between Gt Yarmouth and Lowestoft, signed from A12
Hotel ★★★ 74% HL Best Western Cliff Hotel, Cliff Hill, Gorleston, GREAT YARMOUTH ☎ 01493 662179 36 en suite

GREAT YARMOUTH   MAP 05 TG50

Great Yarmouth & Caister Beach House, Caister-on-Sea NR30 5TD
☎ 01493 728699 📠 01493 728831
e-mail: office@caistergolf.co.uk
web: www.caistergolf.co.uk
A traditional links-style course played over tight and undulating fairways and partly set amongst sand dunes with gorse and marram grass. Well drained with excellent greens. A challenge for golfers of all abilities.
18 holes, 6330yds, Par 70, SSS 70, Course record 65.
Club membership 720.
Visitors Mon-Fri except BHs.Handicap certificate. Dress code.
Societies Booking required. **Green Fees** £35 per day; £25 after noon.
Prof Martyn Clarke **Course Designer** H Colt **Facilities** ⊕ ⏱️ ⓛ ⌂ ⏱ ⌂ ⏱ ✆ **Leisure** snooker. **Location** 0.5m N off A149, at S end of Caister
Hotel ★★ 72% HL Burlington Palm Court Hotel, 11 North Dr, GREAT YARMOUTH ☎ 01493 844568 & 842095 📠 01493 331848 70 en suite

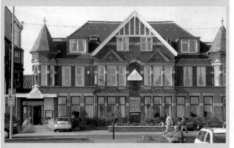

HUNSTANTON   MAP 09 TF64

Hunstanton Golf Course Rd PE36 6JQ
☎ 01485 532811 📠 01485 532319
e-mail: hunstanton.golf@eidosnet.co.uk
web: www.hunstantongolfclub.com
A championship links course set among some of the natural golfing country in East Anglia. Keep out of the numerous bunkers and master the fast greens to play to your handicap - then you only have the wind to contend with. Good playing conditions all year round.
18 holes, 6759yds, Par 72, SSS 73. Club membership 675.
Visitors Mon-Sun except BHs. Booking required. Handicap certificate.
Dress code. **Societies** welcome. **Green Fees** not confirmed. **Prof** James Dodds **Course Designer** James Braid **Facilities** ⊕ ⓛ ⌂ ⏱ ⌂ ⏱ ✆ ⌂ ✆ **Location** Off A149 in Old Hunstanton, signed
Hotel ★★★ 81% HL Best Western Le Strange Arms Hotel, Golf Course Rd, Old Hunstanton, HUNSTANTON ☎ 01485 534411 36 en suite

Searles Leisure Resort South Beach Rd PE36 5BB
☎ 01485 536010 📠 01485 533815
e-mail: golf@searles.co.uk
web: www.searles.co.uk
This nine-hole Par 34 course is designed in a links style and provides generous fairways with good greens. A river runs through the 3rd and 4th holes and the Par 5 8th follows the ancient reed bed to finish with the lake-sided Par 3 9th in front of the clubhouse. Good views of Hunstanton and the surrounding countryside and a challenge for all standards of golfer.

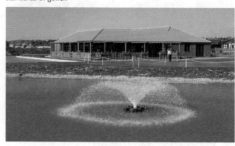

9 holes, 2773yds, Par 34. Club membership 200.
Visitors Mon-Sun & BHs. Dress code. **Societies** Booking required. **Green Fees** 18 holes £16, 9 holes £10 (£17.50/£11 Sat, Sun & BHs). **Course Designer** Paul Searle **Facilities** ⊕ ⓛ ⌂ ⏱ ⌂ ⏱ ✆ ◆ ✆ ⌂ ✆ ⏱ **Leisure** hard tennis courts, outdoor and indoor heated swimming pools, fishing, sauna, solarium, gymnasium, bowls green. **Conf** facs Corporate Hospitality Days **Location** A149 N to Hunstanton, 2nd left at rdbt, over minirdbt, 1st left signed Sports and Country Club
Hotel ★★★ 81% HL Best Western Le Strange Arms Hotel, Golf Course Rd, Old Hunstanton, HUNSTANTON ☎ 01485 534411 36 en suite

KING'S LYNN   MAP 09 TF62

Eagles 39 School Rd, Tilney All Saints PE34 4RS
☎ 01553 827147 📠 01553 829777
e-mail: shop@eagles-golf-tennis.co.uk
web: www.eagles-golf-tennis.co.uk
Parkland with a variety of trees and shrubs lining the fairways. A large area of water comes into play on several holes.
9 holes, 4284yds, Par 64, SSS 61, Course record 64.
Club membership 200.
Visitors Mon-Sun & BHs. Dress code. **Societies** Welcome. **Green Fees** 18 holes £16; 9 holes £11 (£18/£12 Sat, Sun & BHs). **Prof** Nigel Pickerell **Course Designer** D W Horn **Facilities** ⊕ by prior arrangement ⏱ ⓛ ⌂ ⏱ ⌂ ⏱ ✆ ✆ ⏱ **Leisure** hard tennis courts, Par 3 course. **Conf** Corporate Hospitality Days **Location** Off A47 at rdbt to Tilney All Saints, between Kings Lynn
Hotel BUD Premier Travel Inn King's Lynn, Freebridge Farm, KING'S LYNN ☎ 08701 977149 40 en suite

King's Lynn Castle Rising PE31 6BD
☎ 01553 631654 📄 01553 631036
e-mail: secretary@kingslynngc.co.uk
web: www.club-noticeboard.co.uk
The course is set among silver birch and fir woodland and benefits, especially in the winter, from well-drained sandy soil.

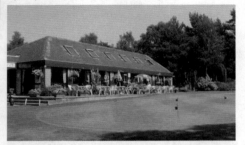

18 holes, 6609yds, Par 72, SSS 73, Course record 64.
Club membership 910.
Visitors Mon-Sun & BHs. Booking required. Handicap certificate. Dress code. **Societies** Booking required. **Green Fees** £45 per day (£50 Sat & Sun). 🌐 **Prof** John Reynolds **Course Designer** Thomas & Alliss **Facilities** ⊕ 🍴 🏐 💤 🎿 🏊 🍴 ✦ **Leisure** Snooker. **Conf** facs Corporate Hospitality Days **Location** 4m NE off A149
Hotel ★★★ 78% HL Best Western Knights Hill Hotel, Knights Hill Village, South Wootton, KING'S LYNN ☎ 01553 675566 65 en suite 12 annexe en suite

---

MATTISHALL   MAP 09 TG01

Mattishall South Green NR20 3JZ
☎ 01362 850111
Mattishall has the distinction of having the longest hole in Norfolk at a very demanding 638 yd Par 5.
9 holes, 3099yds, Par 36, SSS 35. Club membership 120.
Visitors Mon-Sun & BHs. Dress code. **Societies** Booking required.
Green Fees £20 per day, £14 per 18 holes, £10 per 9 holes. 🌐
Course Designer B Todd **Facilities** 💤 🎿 🏊 🏐 ✦ **Location** 0.75m S of Mattishall Church
Hotel ★★★ 83% HL Barnham Broom Hotel, Golf & Restaurant, BARNHAM BROOM ☎ 01603 759393 52 en suite

---

MIDDLETON   MAP 09 TF61

Middleton Hall Hall Orchards PE32 1RH
☎ 01553 841800 & 841801 📄 01553 841800
e-mail: middleton-hall@btclick.com
web: www.middletonhall.co.uk
Natural undulations and mature specimen trees offer a most attractive environment for golf. The architecturally designed course provides a challenge for the competent golfer; there is also a covered floodlit driving range and practice putting green.
18 holes, 5392yds, Par 71, SSS 67. Club membership 600.
Visitors Mon-Sun except BHs. Dress code. **Societies** Booking required.
Green Fees £40 per day; £25 per round (£40/£30 Sat, Sun & BHs). **Prof** Steve White **Course Designer** D Scott **Facilities** ⊕ 🍴 🏐 💤 🎿 🏊 🏐 🍴 ✦ ✦ **Conf** Corporate Hospitality Days **Location** 4m from King's Lynn on A47 towards Norwich
Hotel ★★★ HL Congham Hall Country House Hotel, Lynn Rd, GRIMSTON ☎ 01485 600250 14 en suite

---

MUNDESLEY   MAP 09 TG33

Mundesley Links Rd NR11 8ES
☎ 01263 720095 📄 01263 722849
e-mail: manager@mundesleygolfclub.co.uk
web: www.mundesleygolfclub.co.uk
Downland course, undulating with panoramic views. Small fast greens, tight fairways, one mile from the sea.
9 holes, 5377yds, Par 68, SSS 66, Course record 64.
Club membership 500.
Visitors Mon-Sun & BHs. Booking required Wed, Sat, Sun & BHs. Handicap certificate. Dress code. **Societies** Booking required. **Green Fees** £25 per round (£30 Sat, Sun & BHs). 🌐 **Prof** T G Symmons **Course Designer** Harry Vardon **Facilities** ⊕ 🍴 by prior arrangement 🏐 💤 🎿 🏊 🏐 ✦ ✦ **Conf** Corporate Hospitality Days **Location** W of village off B1159
Hotel ★★ 76% HL Red Lion, Brook St, CROMER ☎ 01263 514964 12 en suite

---

NORWICH   MAP 05 TG20

Costessey Park Old Costessey NR8 5AL
☎ 01603 746333 & 747085 📄 01603 746185
e-mail: cpgc@ljgroup.com
web: www.costesseypark.com
The course lies in the gently contoured Tud valley, providing players with a number of holes that bring the river and man-made lakes into play. The 1st hole starts a round with a Par 3 that requires an accurate drive across the river, to land the ball on a sculptured green beside a reed fringed lake. To end the round at the 18th hole, you need to make a straight drive past the ruined belfry to allow a second shot back over the river to land the ball on a recessed green.
18 holes, 5881yds, Par 71, SSS 69, Course record 65.
Club membership 600.
Visitors Contact course for details. **Societies** Welcome. **Green Fees** £35 per day, £20 per round. **Prof** Andrew Young **Facilities** ⊕ 🍴 🏐 💤 🎿 🏊 🏐 ✦ ✦ **Conf** Corporate Hospitality Days **Location** 4.5m NW of Norwich. A1074 onto Longwater Ln, left onto West End, club on left
Hotel ★★★ 68% HL Quality Hotel Norwich, 2 Barnard Rd, Bowthorpe, NORWICH ☎ 01603 741161 80 en suite

---

De Vere Dunston Hall Hotel Ipswich Rd NR14 8PQ
☎ 01508 470444 📄 01508 471499
e-mail: dhreception@devere-hotels.com
web: www.devereonline.co.uk
Parkland course with water features at many holes. Varied and challenging woodland setting. Floodlit driving range.
18 holes, 6300yds, Par 71, SSS 70, Course record 68.
Visitors Mon-Sun & BHs. Booking required. Dress code. **Societies** Booking required. **Green Fees** from £25. **Prof** Peter Briggs **Course Designer** M Shaw **Facilities** ⊕ 🍴 🏐 💤 🎿 🏊 🏐 ✦ ✦ **Leisure** heated indoor swimming pool, sauna, solarium, gymnasium. **Conf** facs Corporate Hospitality Days **Location** On A140
Hotel ★★★★ 78% HL De Vere Dunston Hall, Ipswich Rd, NORWICH ☎ 01508 470444 169 en suite

---

Eaton Newmarket Rd NR4 6SF
☎ 01603 451686 📄 01603 457539
e-mail: administrator@eatongc.co.uk
web: www.eatongc.co.uk
An undulating, tree-lined parkland course. Easy opening Par 5 followed by an intimidating Par 3 that is well bunkered with deep rough on both

Continued

sides. The challenging 17th hole is uphill to a small hidden green and always needs more club than expected.

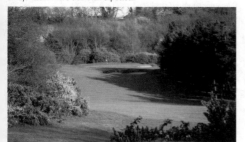

Eaton

18 holes, 6118yds, Par 70, SSS 70, Course record 64. Club membership 800.
Visitors Mon-Sun & BHs. Booking required. Handicap certificate. Dress code. **Societies** booking required. **Green Fees** not confirmed. **Prof** Mark Allen **Facilities** ⑪ ㊙ ㋡ ⌂ 仆 ⚘ ⓪ ✔ **Location** 1.5m SW of city centre off A11

Hotel ★★★ 82% HL Park Farm Hotel, HETHERSETT ☎ 01603 810264 3 en suite 39 annexe en suite

Marriott Sprowston Manor Hotel & Country Club
Wroxham Rd NR7 8RP
☎ 01603 254290 🖹 01603 788884
e-mail: ryan.oconnor@marriotthotels.com
web: www.marriottsprowstonmanor.co.uk
Set in 100 acres of parkland, including an impressive collection of oak trees that provide a backdrop to many holes. The course benefits from USGA specification tees and greens.
18 holes, 6543yds, Par 71, SSS 71, Course record 70. Club membership 500.
Visitors Mon-Sun & BHs. Booking required. Dress code. **Societies** Booking required. **Green Fees** £30 per round (£35 Sat & Sun). **Prof** Guy D Ireson **Course Designer** Ross McMurray **Facilities** ⑪ ㊙ ㋡ ⌂ 仆 ㊙ ⌂ ◇ ✔ ㊙ ✔ **Leisure** heated indoor swimming pool, sauna, gymnasium. **Conf** facs Corporate Hospitality Days **Location** 4m NE from city centre on A1151
Hotel ★★ SHL The Old Rectory, 103 Yarmouth Rd, Thorpe St Andrew, NORWICH ☎ 01603 700772 5 en suite 3 annexe en suite

Royal Norwich Drayton High Rd, Hellesdon NR6 5AH
☎ 01603 429928 & 408459 🖹 01603 417945
e-mail: mail@royalnorwichgolf.co.uk
web: www.royalnorwichgolf.co.uk
Undulating mature parkland course complimented with gorse. Largely unchanged since the alterations carried out by James Braid in 1924. A challenging test of golf.
18 holes, 6506yds, Par 72, SSS 72, Course record 65. Club membership 640.
Visitors Mon-Sun except BHs. Booking required. Handicap certificate. Dress code. **Societies** Booking required. **Green Fees** £40 per day; £25 per round. **Prof** Simon Youd **Course Designer** James Braid **Facilities** ⑪ ㊙ by prior arrangement ㊙ ㋡ 仆 ⌂ ㊙ ✔ **Conf** Corporate Hospitality Days **Location** 2.5m NW of city centre on A1067
Hotel ★★★ 68% HL Quality Hotel Norwich, 2 Barnard Rd, Bowthorpe, NORWICH ☎ 01603 741161 80 en suite

Wensum Valley Hotel, Golf & Country Club Beech
Av, Taverham NR8 6HP
☎ 01603 261012 🖹 01603 261664
e-mail: enqs@wensumvalleyhotel.co.uk
web: www.wensumvalleyhotel.co.uk
Two picturesque and contrasting courses set in 350 acres of the attractive Wensum Valley. The Valley course tests accuracy off the tee and skill on the large undulating greens. The Wensum course has smaller well protected greens requiring length and accuracy off the tee to score well.
Valley Course: 18 holes, 6223yds, Par 72, SSS 70, Course record 72.
Wensum Course: 18 holes, 6922yds, Par 72, SSS 73, Course record 64. Club membership 900.
Visitors Mon-Sun & BHs. Dress code. **Societies** Booking required. **Green Fees** £25 per day inc bar meal. Twilight £15. **Prof** Darren Game **Course Designer** B Todd **Facilities** ⑪ ㊙ ㋡ ㊙ ㋡ 仆 ⌂ ㊙ ㊙ ◇ ㊙ ✔ **Leisure** heated indoor swimming pool, fishing, sauna, solarium, gymnasium. **Conf** facs Corporate Hospitality Days **Location** 5m N of Norwich off A1067
Hotel ★★ 80% HL Wensum Valley Hotel Golf & Country Club, Beech Av, Taverham, NORWICH ☎ 01603 261012 84 en suite

SHERINGHAM	MAP 09 TG14

Sheringham Weybourne Rd NR26 8HG
☎ 01263 823488 🖹 01263 826129
e-mail: info@sheringhamgolfclub.co.uk
web: www.sheringhamgolfclub.co.uk
The course is laid out along a rolling, gorse-clad cliff top from where the sea is visible on every hole. The Par 4 holes are outstanding with a fine view along the cliffs from the 5th tee.
18 holes, 6456yds, Par 70, SSS 71, Course record 64. Club membership 760.
Visitors Mon-Sun & BHs. Booking required. Handicap certificate. Dress code. **Societies** booking required **Green Fees** not confirmed. **Prof** M W Jubb **Course Designer** Tom Dunn **Facilities** ⑪ ㊙ ㋡ ㊙ 仆 ⌂ ㊙ ◇ ✔ **Conf** Corporate Hospitality Days **Location** W of town centre on A149
Hotel ★★ 75% HL Beaumaris Hotel, South St, SHERINGHAM ☎ 01263 822370 21 en suite

SWAFFHAM	MAP 05 TF80

Swaffham Cley Rd PE37 8AE
☎ 01760 721621 🖹 01760 721621
e-mail: swaffamgc@supanet.com
web: www.club-noticeboard.co.uk
Heathland course and designated wildlife site in the heart of breckland country. Excellent drainage.
18 holes, 6544yds, Par 71, SSS 71. Club membership 500.
Visitors Contact club for details. Handicap certificate. Dress code. **Societies** Welcome. **Green Fees** £40 for 36 holes, £35 for 27 holes, £30 for 18 holes. ㊙ **Prof** Peter Field **Course Designer** Jonathan Gaunt **Facilities** ⑪ ㊙ ㋡ ㊙ ㋡ 仆 ⌂ ㊙ ㊙ ✔ **Conf** facs Corporate Hospitality Days **Location** 1.5m SW of town centre
Hotel ★★★ 72% HL Best Western George Hotel, Station Rd, SWAFFHAM ☎ 01760 721238 29 en suite

THETFORD · MAP 05 TL88

Feltwell Thor Ave (off Wilton Rd), Feltwell IP26 4AY
☎ 01842 827644 ▤ 01842 829065
e-mail: secretary.feltwellgc@virgin.net
web: www.club-noticeboard.co.uk/feltwell
In spite of being an inland links, this nine-hole course is still open and windy.
9 holes, 6488yds, Par 72, SSS 71, Course record 71.
Club membership 370.
Visitors Contact club for details. **Societies** Booking required. **Green Fees** £16 per day (£25 Sat, Sun & BHs). ⊕ **Prof** Tom Ball **Facilities** ⊕ ⚐ ⮕ ▭ ⛳ 🖪 ⚐ ⏚ ⌂ ✦ ⚑ **Conf** Corporate Hospitality Days **Location** On B1112 next to RAF Feltwell
Hotel ★★ 68% HL The Thomas Paine Hotel, White Hart St, THETFORD
☎ 01842 755631   13 en suite

Thetford Brandon Rd IP24 3NE
☎ 01842 752169 ▤ 01842 766212
e-mail: sally@thetfordgolfclub.co.uk
web: www.club-noticeboard.co.uk
18 holes, 6849yds, Par 72, SSS 73, Course record 66.
Course Designer James Braid **Location** 2m W of Thetford on B1107
Telephone for further details
Hotel ★★ 68% HL The Thomas Paine Hotel, White Hart St, THETFORD
☎ 01842 755631   13 en suite

WATTON · MAP 05 TF90

Richmond Park Saham Rd IP25 6EA
☎ 01953 881803 ▤ 01953 881817
e-mail: info@richmondpark.co.uk
web: www.richmondpark.co.uk
Compact parkland course with mature and young trees set around the Little Wissey river and spread over 100 acres of Norfolk countryside. The river and other water hazards create an interesting but not daunting challenge.

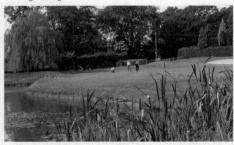

18 holes, 6258yds, Par 71, SSS 70, Course record 69.
Club membership 600.
Visitors Mon-Sun & BHs. Booking required. Dress code. **Societies** Welcome. **Green Fees** £35 per day, £24 per round (£35 per round Sat & Sun). **Prof** Alan Hemsley **Course Designer** D Jessup/D Scott **Facilities** ⊕ ⚐ ⮕ ▭ ⛳ 🖪 ⚐ ⏚ ⌂ ⚲ ⌀ ⛳ ✦ ⚑ **Leisure** gymnasium. **Conf** Corporate Hospitality Days **Location** 500yds NW of town centre
Hotel ★★★ 72% HL Best Western George Hotel, Station Rd, SWAFFHAM
☎ 01760 721238   29 en suite

WESTON LONGVILLE · MAP 09 TG11

Weston Park NR9 5JW
☎ 01603 872363 ▤ 01603 873040
e-mail: golf@weston-park.co.uk
web: www.weston-park.co.uk
Superb, challenging course, set in 200 acres of magnificent, mature woodland and parkland.
18 holes, 6648yds, Par 72, SSS 72, Course record 68.
Club membership 580.
Visitors Mon-Sun & BHs. Booking required. Handicap certificate. Dress code. **Societies** Booking required. **Green Fees** £45 per day, £37 per 18 holes (£55/£47 Sat & Sun). **Prof** Michael Few **Course Designer** Golf Technology **Facilities** ⊕ ⮕ ▭ ⛳ 🖪 ⌂ ✦ ⚑ **Leisure** hard tennis courts, croquet lawn. **Conf** facs Corporate Hospitality Days **Location** Brown tourist signs off A1067 or A47
Hotel ★★★ 68% HL Quality Hotel Norwich, 2 Barnard Rd, Bowthorpe, NORWICH ☎ 01603 741161   80 en suite

---

WEST RUNTON · MAP 09 TG14

Links Country Park Hotel & Golf Club NR27 9QH
☎ 01263 838215 ▤ 01263 838264
e-mail: proshop@links-hotel.co.uk
web: www.links-hotel.co.uk
Parkland course 500yds from the sea, with superb views overlooking West Runton. The hotel offers extensive leisure facilities.
9 holes, 4842yds, Par 66, SSS 64. Club membership 250.
Visitors Mon-Sun & BHs. Booking required. Dress code. **Societies** booking required. **Green Fees** not confirmed. **Prof** Nick Catchpole **Course Designer** J.H Taylor **Facilities** ⊕ ⚐ ⮕ ▭ ⛳ 🖪 ⏚ ⌂ ♦ ⚲ ⛳ ✦ ⚑ **Leisure** hard tennis courts, heated indoor swimming pool, sauna, solarium, gymnasium. **Conf** facs Corporate Hospitality Days **Location** S of village off A149
Hotel ★★ 75% HL Beaumaris Hotel, South St, SHERINGHAM
☎ 01263 822370   21 en suite

NORTHAMPTONSHIRE

CHACOMBE · MAP 04 SP44

Cherwell Edge OX17 2EN
☎ 01295 711591 ▤ 01295 713674
e-mail: enquiries@cherwelledgegolfclub.co.uk
web: www.cegc.co.uk
Parkland course over chalk giving good drainage. The back nine is short and tight with mature trees. The front nine is longer and more open. The course is well bunkered with three holes where water can catch the wayward golfer.
18 holes, 6092yds, Par 70, SSS 69, Course record 64.
Club membership 500.
Visitors Mon-Sun & BHs. Booking required. Dress code. **Societies** Welcome. **Green Fees** Mon-Fri £20 per 18 holes (£30 Sat & Sun). **Prof** Jason Newman **Course Designer** R Davies **Facilities** ⊕ ⚐ ⮕ ▭ ⛳ 🖪 ⏚ ⌂ ⚲ ⛳ ✦ ⚑ **Conf** facs Corporate Hospitality Days **Location** M40 junct 11, 0.5m S off B4525, 2m from Banbury
Hotel ★★★ 79% HL Whately Hall, Banbury Cross, BANBURY
☎ 0870 400 8104   69 en suite

COLD ASHBY
MAP 04 SP67

Cold Ashby Stanford Rd NN6 6EP
☎ 01604 740548 📄 01604 740548
e-mail: info@coldashbygolfclub.com
web: www.coldashbygolfclub.com
Undulating parkland course, nicely matured, with superb views.
The 27 holes consist of three loops of nine, which can be interlinked
with each other. All three loops have their own challenge and any
combination of two loops will give an excellent course. The start of
the Elkington loop offers five holes of scenic beauty and testing golf
and the 3rd on the Winwick loop is a 200yd Par 3 from a magnificent
plateau tee.
Ashby-Elkington: 18 holes, 6308yds, Par 72, SSS 71,
Course record 68.
Elkington-Winwick: 18 holes, 6293yds, Par 70, SSS 71,
Course record 69.
Winwick-Ashby: 18 holes, 6047yds, Par 70, SSS 70,
Course record 65. Club membership 600.
Visitors Mon-Sun & BHs. Booking required Sat, Sun & BHs. Dress code.
Societies Booking required **Green Fees** £18 per round (£23 Sat & Sun).
Prof Shane Rose **Course Designer** David Croxton **Facilities** ⑪ 🍴 ♨
🖵 🍴 👗 🛎 ⛳ ⚙ 🏌 ⚙ 🏌 **Conf** facs Corporate Hospitality Days
Location M1 junct 18 or A14 junct 1
Hotel BUD Hotel Ibis Rugby East, Parklands, CRICK ☎ 01788 824331
111 en suite

COLLINGTREE
MAP 04 SP75

Collingtree Park Windingbrook Ln NN4 0XN
☎ 01604 700000 & 701202 📄 01604 702600
e-mail: info@collingtreeparkgolf.com
web: www.collingtreeparkgolf.com
An 18-hole resort course designed by former US and British Open
champion Johnny Miller. The American-style course has water
hazards on 10 holes with a spectacular Par 5 18th Island Green.

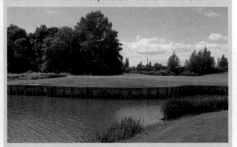

18 holes, 6776yds, Par 72, SSS 72, Course record 66.
Club membership 660.
Visitors Mon-Sun & BHs. Booking required. Handicap certificate. Dress
code. **Societies** welcome. **Green Fees** not confirmed. **Prof** G.Pook/
A.Carter **Course Designer** Johnny Miller **Facilities** ⑪ 🍴 ♨ 🖵 🍴
👗 🛎 ⛳ ⚙ 🏌 **Leisure** fishing, Golf Academy. **Conf** facs Corporate
Hospitality Days **Location** M1 junct 15, on A508 to Northampton
Hotel ★★★★ 73% HL Northampton Marriott Hotel, Eagle Dr,
NORTHAMPTON ☎ 01604 768700 120 en suite

CORBY
MAP 04 SP88

Corby Public Stamford Rd, Weldon NN17 3JH
☎ 01536 260756 📄 01536 260756
web: www.corbygolfcourse.co.uk
Parkland course with generous fairways, mature trees and 58 bunkers.
18 holes, 6677yds, Par 72, SSS 72, Course record 68.
Club membership 600.
Visitors Mon-Sun & BHs. **Societies** Booking required. **Green Fees** £15
for 18 holes (£19.50 Sat & Sun). **Prof** Jeff Bradbrook **Course Designer** F
Hawtree **Facilities** ⑪ 🍴 ♨ 🖵 🍴 👗 🛎 ⛳ ⚙ 🏌 ⚙ **Location** 4m NE
on A43

DAVENTRY
MAP 04 SP56

Daventry & District Norton Rd NN11 5LS
☎ 01327 702829
e-mail: ms@teltec.com
web: www.ddgc.co.uk
An undulatory course providing panoramic views and whose tight
fairways and small fast greens with large borrows provide a good test
of golf.
9 holes, 5812yds, Par 69, SSS 68, Course record 62.
Club membership 285.
Visitors Mon-Sat & BHs, Sun pm only. Dress code. **Societies** Booking
required. **Green Fees** £15 per day (£20 Sat & Sun). ⊛ **Facilities** 🖵 🍴 👗
🛎 **Conf** facs Corporate Hospitality Days **Location** 0.5m E of Daventry
Hotel ★★★★ 69% HL The Paramount Daventry Hotel, Sedgemoor Way,
DAVENTRY ☎ 01327 307000 138 en suite

FARTHINGSTONE
MAP 04 SP65

Farthingstone Hotel & Golf Course Everdon Rd
NN12 8HA
☎ 01327 361291 📄 01327 361645
e-mail: info@farthingstone.co.uk
web: www.farthingstone.co.uk
A mature and challenging course set in picturesque countryside.

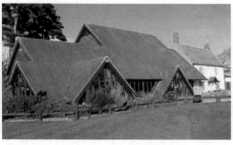

18 holes, 6299yds, Par 70, SSS 70, Course record 68.
Club membership 350.
Visitors Mon-Sun & BHs. Dress code. **Societies** Welcome.
Green Fees Phone. **Prof** Mike Gallagher **Course Designer** Don
Donaldson **Facilities** ⑪ 🍴 ♨ 🖵 🍴 👗 🛎 ⛳ ♦ ⚙ 🛎 ⚙ 🏌
Leisure squash, Snooker room. **Conf** facs Corporate Hospitality Days
Location M1 junct 16, W near Farthingstone
Hotel BUD Premier Travel Inn Daventry, High St, WEEDON
☎ 0870 9906364 46 en suite

England

HELLIDON
MAP 04 SP55

Hellidon Lakes Hotel & Country Club NN11 6GG
☎ 01327 262550 📠 01327 262559
e-mail: hellidonlakes@qhotels.co.uk
web: www.qhotels.co.uk
18 holes, 6691yds, Par 72, SSS 72.
Course Designer D Snell **Location** Off A361 into Hellidon, 2nd right
Telephone for further details
Hotel ★★★★ 78% HL Hellidon Lakes, HELLIDON ☎ 01327 262550
110 en suite

KETTERING
MAP 04 SP87

Kettering Headlands NN15 6XA
☎ 01536 511104 📠 01536 511104
e-mail: secretary@kettering-golf.co.uk
web: www.kettering-golf.co.uk
A mature woodland course with gentle slopes.
18 holes, 6081yds, Par 69, SSS 69, Course record 63.
Club membership 700.
Visitors Mon-Fri except BHs. Handicap certificate required. Dress code.
Societies Booking required. **Green Fees** £29 per round. **Prof** Kevin
Theobald **Course Designer** Tom Morris **Facilities** ⑪ ⑩ 🍴 🍺 ☐ 🖙 🎱 ♨
♞ ✆ **Conf** Corporate Hospitality Days **Location** S of town centre
Hotel ★★★★ 79% HL Kettering Park Hotel & Spa, Kettering Parkway,
KETTERING ☎ 01536 416666 119 en suite

Pytchley Golf Lodge Kettering Rd, Pytchley NN14 1EY
☎ 01536 511527 📠 01536 790266
e-mail: info@pytchleygolflodgekettering.co.uk
web: www.pytchleygolflodgekettering.co.uk
Academy nine-hole pay and play course, offering a challenge to both
experienced and novice players.
9 holes, 2574yards, Par 34, SSS 65, Course record 70.
Club membership 200.
Visitors Mon-Sun & BHs. Dress code. **Societies** Booking required.
Green Fees £13 per 18 holes, £7 per 9 holes (£17/£9 weekends and bank
holidays). Winter £13 per 18 holes, £7 per 9 holes. **Prof** Peter Machin
Course Designer Roger Griffiths Associates **Facilities** ⑪ 🍺 ☐ 🖙 🎱 ♨
♞ ✆ ♞ **Location** A14 junct 9, A509 towards Kettering signed
Hotel ★★★★ 79% HL Kettering Park Hotel & Spa, Kettering Parkway,
KETTERING ☎ 01536 416666 119 en suite

NORTHAMPTON
MAP 04 SP76

Brampton Heath Sandy Ln, Church Brampton NN6 8AX
☎ 01604 843939 📠 01604 843885
e-mail: crose@bhgc.co.uk
web: www.bhgc.co.uk
Appealing to both the novice and experienced golfer, this beautiful,
well drained heathland course affords panoramic views over
Northampton. It plays like an inland links in the summer - fast
running fairways, true rolling greens with the wind always providing a
challenge. Excellent play all year round.
18 holes, 6533yds, Par 72, SSS 71, Course record 66.
Club membership 500.
Visitors Mon-Sun & BHs. Booking required. Dress code. **Societies** Booking
required. **Green Fees** £18 per round, £12 for 9 holes (£23/£14 Sat, Sun &
BHs). **Course Designer** D Snell **Facilities** ⑪ ⑩ 🍺 ☐ 🖙 🎱 ♨ 🖙 ✆ 🍺
✆ ♞ **Conf** facs Corporate Hospitality Days **Location** Signed off A5199 2m
N of Kingsthorpe

Hotel ★★★ 71% HL Best Western Lime Trees Hotel, 8 Langham Place,
Barrack Rd, NORTHAMPTON ☎ 01604 632188 20 en suite 8 annexe
en suite

Delapre Golf Complex Eagle Dr, Nene Valley Way
NN4 7DU
☎ 01604 764036 📠 01604 706378
e-mail: delapre@jbgolf.co.uk
web: www.jackbarker.com
Rolling parkland course, part of a municipal golf complex, which
includes two nine-hole Par 3 courses, pitch and putt, and a 40-bay
floodlit driving range.
*The Oaks: 18 holes, 6269yds, Par 70, SSS 70,
Course record 66.*
Hardingstone Course: 9 holes, 2109yds, Par 32, SSS 32.
Club membership 500.
Visitors Mon-Sun & BHs. Dress code. **Societies** booking required.
Green Fees not confirmed. **Prof** John Cuddihy **Course Designer** John
Jacobs/John Corby **Facilities** ⑪ ⑩ 🍺 ☐ 🖙 🎱 ♨ 🖙 ✆ ♞ **Leisure**
Par 3 courses. **Conf** facs Corporate Hospitality Days **Location** M1 junct 15,
3m on A508/A45
Hotel ★★★ 63% HL Quality Hotel Northampton, Ashley Way, Weston
Favell, NORTHAMPTON ☎ 01604 739955 33 en suite 38 annexe en suite

Kingsthorpe Kingsley Rd NN2 7BU
☎ 01604 710610 📠 01604 710610
e-mail: secretary@kingsthorpe-golf.co.uk
web: www.kingsthorpe-golf.co.uk
A compact, undulating parkland course set within the town boundary.
Not a long course but the undulating terrain provides a suitable
challenge for golfers of all standards. The 18th hole is claimed to be the
longest 400yds in the county when played into wind the and is among
the finest finishing holes in the area. New clubhouse.
18 holes, 5903yds, Par 69, SSS 69, Course record 63.
Club membership 650.
Visitors Mon-Fri except BHs. Dress code. **Societies** Booking required.
Green Fees £40 per day, £305 per round. £25 per round winter. **Prof** Paul
Armstrong **Course Designer** Mr Alison/ H Colt **Facilities** ⑪ ⑩ 🍺 ☐ 🖙
🎱 ♨ 🖙 ✆ **Conf** facs Corporate Hospitality Days **Location** N of town centre
on A5095 between Kingsthorpe and racecourse
Hotel ★★★ 63% HL Quality Hotel Northampton, Ashley Way, Weston
Favell, NORTHAMPTON ☎ 01604 739955 33 en suite 38 annexe en suite

Northampton Harlestone NN7 4EF
☎ 01604 845155 📠 01604 820262
e-mail: golf@northamptongolfclub.co.uk
web: www.northamptongolfclub.co.uk
Parkland with water in play on four holes.
18 holes, 6615yds, Par 72, SSS 72, Course record 63.
Club membership 750.
Visitors Mon, Tue, Thu, Fri except BHs. Handicap certificate. Dress code.
Societies booking required. **Green Fees** not confirmed. **Prof** Barry Randall
Course Designer Sinclair Steel **Facilities** ⑪ ⑩ by prior arrangement 🍺
☐ 🖙 🎱 ♨ 🖙 ✆ 🍺 ✆ **Conf** facs Corporate Hospitality Days **Location** NW
of town centre on A428
Hotel ★★★ 71% HL Best Western Lime Trees Hotel, 8 Langham Place,
Barrack Rd, NORTHAMPTON ☎ 01604 632188 20 en suite 8 annexe
en suite

Northamptonshire County Golf Ln, Church Brampton NN6 8AZ

☎ 01604 843025 📄 01604 843463
e-mail: secretary@countrygolfclub.org.uk
web: www.countygolfclub.org
A fine, traditional championship course situated on undulating heathland with areas of gorse, heather and extensive coniferous and deciduous woodland. A river and a railway line pass through the course and there is a great variety of holes. Current improvements to the course will be completed for the club centenary in 2009.
18 holes, 6505yds, Par 70, SSS 72, Course record 65.
Club membership 750.
Visitors Contact club for details. **Societies** Booking required. **Green Fees** £55 per 27/36 holes, £45 per 18 holes. Winter £40/£35. **Course Designer** H S Colt **Facilities** ⑪ ⑩ 🍴 ☐ 🍴 🔨 🏆 🔨 🏌 🏆 **Conf** Corporate Hospitality Days **Location** 5m NW of Northampton off A5199
Hotel ★★★ 63% HL Quality Hotel Northampton, Ashley Way, Weston Favell, NORTHAMPTON ☎ 01604 739955 33 en suite 38 annexe en suite

Overstone Park Billing Ln NN6 0AS

☎ 01604 647666 📄 01604 642635
e-mail: enquiries@overstonepark.com
web: www.overstonepark.com
A testing parkland course, gently undulating within panoramic views of local stately home. Excellent drainage and fine greens make the course great all year round. Water comes into play on three holes.

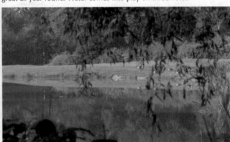

18 holes, 6472yds, Par 72, SSS 72, Course record 69.
Club membership 500.
Visitors Mon-Sun & BHs. Booking required Sat/Sun & BHs. Dress code. **Societies** booking required. **Green Fees** not confirmed. **Prof** Brain Mudge **Course Designer** Donald Steel **Facilities** ⑪ ⑩ 🍴 ☐ 🍴 🔨 🏆 🔨 🏌
🏌 **Leisure** hard tennis courts, heated indoor swimming pool, fishing, sauna, solarium, gymnasium. **Conf** facs Corporate Hospitality Days **Location** M1 junct 15, A45 to Billing Aquadrome turn off, course 2m off A5076 Gt Billing Way
Hotel ★★★ 71% HL Best Western Lime Trees Hotel, 8 Langham Place, Barrack Rd, NORTHAMPTON ☎ 01604 632188 20 en suite 8 annexe en suite

---

OUNDLE   MAP 04 TL08

Oundle Benefield Rd PE8 4EZ

☎ 01832 273267 📄 01832 273267
e-mail: office@oundlegolfclub.com
web: www.oundlegolfclub.com
Undulating parkland in countryside. Stream running through course in play on nine holes. Small greens demand careful placement from tees and accurate iron play.

18 holes, 6265yds, Par 72, SSS 70, Course record 63.
Club membership 650.
Visitors Mon-Sun & BHs. Booking required for Sat, Sun & BHs. Handicap certificate required. Dress code. **Societies** Booking required. **Green Fees** £34 per day; £25.50 per round (£44 per day/round Sat & Sun). **Prof** Richard Keys **Facilities** ⑪ ⑩ 🍴 ☐ 🍴 🔨 🏆 🔨 **Leisure** Short game practice area.
Conf facs Corporate Hospitality Days **Location** 1m W on A427

STAVERTON   MAP 04 SP56

Staverton Park Staverton Park NN11 6JT

☎ 01327 302000
18 holes, 6661yds, Par 71, SSS 72, Course record 65.
Course Designer Cmdr John Harris **Location** 0.75m NE on A425
Telephone for further details
Hotel ★★★★ 69% HL The Paramount Daventry Hotel, Sedgemoor Way, DAVENTRY ☎ 01327 307000 138 en suite

---

WELLINGBOROUGH   MAP 04 SP86

Rushden Kimbolton Rd, Chelveston NN9 6AN

☎ 01933 418511 📄 01933 418511
web: www.rushdengolfclub.org
Undulating parkland with a brook bisecting the course.
10 holes, 6249yds, Par 71, SSS 70, Course record 68.
Club membership 400.
Visitors Mon, Tue, Thu, Fri. Booking required Tue & Fri. Dress code. **Societies** telephone in advance. **Green Fees** not confirmed. ⊛ **Facilities** ⑪ ⑩ 🍴 ☐ 🍴 🔨 **Location** 6m E of Wellingborough off B645
Hotel BUD Travelodge Wellingborough Rushden, Saunders Lodge, RUSHDEN ☎ 08700 850 950 40 en suite

Wellingborough Great Harrowden Hall NN9 5AD

☎ 01933 677234 📄 01933 679379
e-mail: info@wellingboroughgolfclub.com
web: www.wellingboroughgolfclub.com
Undulating parkland with many trees. The 514yd 14th is a testing hole. The clubhouse is a stately home and the 18th is the signature hole.

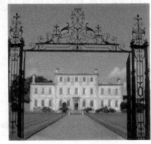

18 holes, 6711yds, Par 72, SSS 72, Course record 68.
Club membership 820.
Visitors Mon, Wed-Fri except BHs. Booking required. Handicap certificate. Dress code. **Societies** Welcome. **Green Fees** £48 per day. ⊛ **Prof** David Clifford **Course Designer** Hawtree **Facilities** ⑪ ⑩ 🍴 ☐ 🍴 🔨 🏆 🔨 🏌
🏌 **Leisure** outdoor swimming pool. **Conf** facs Corporate Hospitality Days **Location** 2m N of Wellingborough on A509
Hotel BUD Travelodge Wellingborough Rushden, Saunders Lodge, RUSHDEN ☎ 08700 850 950 40 en suite

England

WHITTLEBURY
MAP 04 SP64

Whittlebury Park Golf & Country Club NN12 8WP
☎ 01327 850000 📄 01327 850001
e-mail: enquiries@whittlebury.com
web: www.whittlebury.com
The 36 holes incorporate three loops of tournament-standard nines
plus a short course. The 1905 course is a reconstruction of the original
parkland course built at the turn of the century, the Royal Whittlewood
is a lakeland course playing around copses and the Grand Prix, next
to Silverstone Circuit, has a strong links feel playing over gently
undulating grassland with many challenging features.

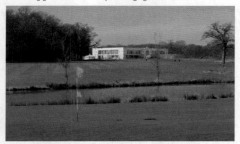

Grand Prix: 9 holes, 3339yds, Par 36, SSS 36.
Royal Whittlewood: 9 holes, 3323yds, Par 36, SSS 36.
1905: 9 holes, 3256yds, Par 36, SSS 36.
Club membership 350.
Visitors Mon-Sun & BHs. Booking required. Dress code.
Societies booking required. **Green Fees** not confirmed. **Prof** Mark Booth
Course Designer Cameron Sinclair **Facilities** ⑪ ⓞ 🏐 ⌷ 🍴 ⅃ ⚲ 🍷
◇ ✦ 🚶 ⚿ 𝄞 **Leisure** heated indoor swimming pool, sauna, solarium,
shooting, archery, falconry, karting. **Conf** facs Corporate Hospitality Days
Location M1 junct 15a, on A413 Buckingham Road
Hotel ★★★★ 80% HL Whittlebury Hall Hotel and Spa, WHITTLEBURY
☎ 01327 857857 211 en suite

NORTHUMBERLAND

ALLENDALE
MAP 12 NY85

Allendale High Studdon, Allenheads Rd NE47 9DH
☎ 07005 808246
web: www.allendale-golf.co.uk
Challenging and hilly parkland course set 1000ft above sea level with
superb views of East Allen valley.
9 holes, 4541yds, Par 66, SSS 64, Course record 62.
Club membership 130.
Visitors Mon-Sun & BHs. **Societies** Booking required. **Green Fees** £12 per
day (£15 weekends). ⊛ **Facilities** ⌷ ⅃ **Conf** Corporate Hospitality Days
Location 1m S of Allendale on B6295
Hotel ★★★ 75% HL Best Western Beaumont Hotel, Beaumont St,
HEXHAM ☎ 01434 602331 25 en suite

ALNMOUTH
MAP 12 NU21

Alnmouth Foxton Hall NE66 3BE
☎ 01665 830231 📄 01665 830922
e-mail: secretary@alnmouthgolfclub.com
web: www.alnmouthgolfclub.com
The original course, situated on the Northumberland coast, was
established in 1869, being the fourth oldest in England. The existing
course, created in 1930, provides a testing and enjoyable challenge.
18 holes, 6429yds, Par 71, SSS 71, Course record 64.
Club membership 800.
Visitors Mon-Sun & BHs. Booking required. Handicap certificate. Dress
code. **Societies** Welcome. **Green Fees** £40 per day; £30 per round
(£35 per round Sat & Sun). **Prof** Linzi Hardy **Course Designer** H S
Colt **Facilities** ⑪ ⓞ 🏐 ⌷ 🍴 ⅃ ⚲ ◇ 🚶 ⚿ **Leisure** snooker room.
Conf Corporate Hospitality Days **Location** 1m NE of Alnmouth
Hotel ★★★ 67% HL White Swan Hotel, Bondgate Within, ALNWICK
☎ 01665 602109 56 en suite

Alnmouth Village Marine Rd NE66 2RZ
☎ 01665 830370
web: www.ukgolfer.com
Seaside course with part coastal view. The oldest 9 hole course in
England.
9 holes, 6090yds, Par 70, SSS 70, Course record 63.
Club membership 480.
Visitors Contact club for details. **Societies** Booking required. **Green
Fees** 18 holes £16 (£20 Sat, Sun & BHs). Weekly ticket £60. ⊛ **Course
Designer** Mungo Park **Facilities** ⑪ ⓞ 🏐 ⌷ 🍴 ⅃ **Location** E of village
Hotel ★★★ 67% HL White Swan Hotel, Bondgate Within, ALNWICK
☎ 01665 602109 56 en suite

ALNWICK
MAP 12 NU11

Alnwick Swansfield Park NE66 1AB
☎ 01665 602632
web: www.alnwickgolfclub.co.uk
A mixture of mature parkland, open grassland and gorse bushes with
panoramic views out to sea 5m away. Offers a fair test of golf.
18 holes, 6284yds, Par 70, SSS 70, Course record 66.
Club membership 400.
Visitors Mon-Sun & BHs. Booking required. Dress code. **Societies**
Welcome. **Green Fees** £25 per day; £20 per round. **Course Designer**
Rochester, Rae **Facilities** ⑪ ⓞ 🏐 ⌷ 🍴 ⅃ ⚲ 🚶 ⚿ **Leisure** small practice
area. **Location** S of town centre off B6341
Hotel ★★★ 67% HL White Swan Hotel, Bondgate Within, ALNWICK
☎ 01665 602109 56 en suite

BAMBURGH
MAP 12 NU13

Bamburgh Castle The Club House, 40 The Wynding
NE69 7DE
☎ 01668 214378 (club) & 214321 (sec) 📄 01668 214607
e-mail: sec@bamburghcastlegolfclub.co.uk
web: www.bamburghcastlegolfclub.co.uk
Superb coastal course with excellent greens that are both fast
and true; natural hazards of heather and whin bushes abound.
Magnificent views of the Farne Islands, Holy Island, Lindisfarne
Castle, Bamburgh Castle and the Cheviot Hills.
18 holes, 5621yds, Par 68, SSS 67, Course record 64.
Club membership 785.

Continued

Visitors Mon-Fri & Sun except BHs. Booking required. Handicap certificate. Dress code. **Societies** Booking required. **Green Fees** £45 per day, £33 per round (£50/£38 Sun). **Course Designer** George Rochester **Facilities** ⑪ ⌘ ≞ ⌷ ⌺ ⚐ ⚑ ☰ ✧ **Conf** Corporate Hospitality Days **Location** 6m E of A1 via B1341 or B1342 **Hotel** ★★ 72% HL The Lord Crewe, Front St, BAMBURGH ☎ 01668 214243 18 rms (17 en suite)

BEDLINGTON   MAP 12 NZ28

Bedlingtonshire Acorn Bank NE22 6AA
☎ 01670 822457 📄 01670 823048
e-mail: secretary@bedlingtongolfclub.com
web: www.bedlingtongolfclub.com
Meadowland and parkland with easy walking. Under certain conditions the wind can be a distinct hazard.

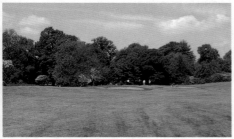

18 holes, 6813yards, Par 73, SSS 73, Course record 64.
Club membership 800.
Visitors Mon-Sun & BHs. Booking required. Dress code. **Societies** Booking required. **Green Fees** £35 per day; £25 per round (£40/£32 Sat, Sun & BHs). ⚐ **Prof** Marcus Webb **Course Designer** Frank Pennink **Facilities** ⑪ ⌘ by prior arrangement ≞ ⌷ ⌺ ☰ ⚑ ✦ ✧ **Conf** Corporate Hospitality Days **Location** 1m SW on A1068 **Hotel** ★★★ 80% HL Holiday Inn Newcastle upon Tyne, Great North Rd, Seaton Burn, NEWCASTLE UPON TYNE ☎ 0191 201 9988 & 0870 787 3291 📄 0191 236 8091 154 en suite

BELFORD   MAP 12 NU13

Belford South Rd NE70 7DP
☎ 01668 213232 & 07764582427 📄 01668 213282
web: www.thebelford.co.uk
A coastal parkland course recently in new ownership. Many new trees have been added and nine new tee boxes, allowing golfers to play each hole from two different angles for a full 18 holes. The course is overlooked by the 18th-century Belford Hall and has fine views of Holy Island.
9 holes, 3227yds, Par 71, SSS 71. Club membership 200.
Visitors Mon-Sun & BHs. **Societies** Welcome. **Green Fees** £19 per 18 holes; £13 per 9 holes (£22/£16 Sat, Sun & BHs). **Prof** Simon Whitaker **Course Designer** Nigel Williams **Facilities** ⑪ ⌘ ≞ ⌷ ⌺ ☰ ⚑ ✦ ☰ ✧ ✦ **Conf** Corporate Hospitality Days **Location** Off A1 between Alnwick on Tweed
Hotel ★★ 69% HL Purdy Lodge, Adderstone Services, BELFORD ☎ 01668 213000 20 en suite

BELLINGHAM   MAP 12 NY88

Bellingham Boggle Hole NE48 2DT
☎ 01434 220530 (Secretary)
e-mail: admin@bellinghamgolfclub.com
web: www.bellinghamgolfclub.com
Rolling parkland with many natural hazards. This highly regarded 18-hole course lies between Hadrian's Wall and the Scottish border. There is a mixture of testing Par 3s, long Par 5s and tricky Par 4s.

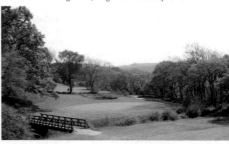

18 holes, 6093yds, Par 70, SSS 70, Course record 65.
Club membership 500.
Visitors Mon-Sun & BHs. Dress code. **Societies** Booking required. **Green Fees** £24 per day/round (£30 per round weekends). **Course Designer** E Johnson/I Wilson **Facilities** ⑪ ⌘ ≞ ⌷ ⌺ ☰ ⚑ ✦ ✧ **Location** N of village on B6320 **Hotel** ★★★ 72% HL The Otterburn Tower Hotel, OTTERBURN ☎ 01830 520620 18 en suite

BERWICK-UPON-TWEED   MAP 12 NT95

Berwick-upon-Tweed (Goswick) Goswick TD15 2RW
☎ 01289 387256 📄 01289 387334
e-mail: goswickgc@btconnect.com
web: www.goswicklinksgc.co.uk
Natural seaside links course, with undulating fairways, elevated tees and good greens. Qualifying course for the Open Championship from 2008.
18 holes, 6686yds, Par 72, SSS 72, Course record 69.
Club membership 700.
Visitors Mon-Sun & BHs. Booking required. Dress code. **Societies** Booking required. **Green Fees** contact for details. **Prof** Paul Terras **Course Designer** James Braid **Facilities** ⑪ ⌘ ≞ ⌷ ⌺ ☰ ⚑ ✦ ☰ ✦ **Conf** Corporate Hospitality Days **Location** 6m S of Berwick off A1 **Hotel** ★★★ 72% HL Marshall Meadows Country House Hotel, BERWICK-UPON-TWEED ☎ 01289 331133 19 en suite

Magdalene Fields Magdalene Fields TD15 1NE
☎ 01289 306130 📄 01289 306384
e-mail: mail@magdalene-fields.co.uk
web: www.magdalene-fields.co.uk
Seaside course on a clifftop with natural hazards formed by bays. All holes open to winds. Testing 8th hole over bay (Par 3). Scenic views to Holy Island and north to Scotland.
18 holes, 6407yds, Par 72, SSS 71, Course record 65.
Club membership 350.
Visitors Mon-Sun & BHs. Booking required Fri-Sun & BHs. Dress code. **Societies** Booking required. **Green Fees** £22 per round (£24 Sat & Sun). **Course Designer** Willie Park **Facilities** ⑪ ⌘ ≞ ⌷ ⌺ ☰ ⚑ ✦ ✧ **Conf** Corporate Hospitality Days **Location** 0.5m E of town centre **Hotel** ★★★ 83% HL Tillmouth Park Country House Hotel, CORNHILL-ON-TWEED ☎ 01890 882255 12 en suite 2 annexe en suite

England

BLYTH
MAP 12 NZ38

Blyth New Delaval, Newsham NE24 4DB
☎ 01670 540110 (sec) & 356514 (pro) 🖥 01670 540134
e-mail: clubmanager@blythgolf.co.uk
web: www.blythgolf.co.uk
Course built over old colliery. Parkland with water hazards. Superb greens.
18 holes, 6424yds, Par 72, SSS 71, Course record 63.
Club membership 860.
Visitors Mon-Sun & BHs. Booking required. Dress code. **Societies** Booking required. **Green Fees** £32 per day; £22.50 per round (£38/£25 per round Sat & Sun). **Prof** Andrew Brown **Course Designer** Hamilton Stutt **Facilities** ⑪ ▯ 🖭 ➷ ◫ ➹ 👜 🍴 ⚴ 🏌 **Location** 1m S of town centre
Hotel ★★★ 71% HL Windsor Hotel, South Pde, WHITLEY BAY ☎ 0191 251 8888 0191 232 3158 🖥 0191 297 0272 69 en suite

CRAMLINGTON
MAP 12 NZ27

Arcot Hall NE23 7QP
☎ 0191 236 2794 🖥 0191 217 0370
e-mail: arcothall@tiscali.co.uk
web: www.arcothallgolfclub.com
Wooded parkland, reasonably flat.
18 holes, 6329yds, Par 70, SSS 70, Course record 60.
Club membership 695.
Visitors Mon-Fri. Restricted Sat, Sun & BHs. Handicap certificate. Dress code. **Societies** Booking required. **Green Fees** £28 per day; £23 after 3pm summer (£32 per round Sat & Sun). **Prof** John Metcalfe **Course Designer** James Braid **Facilities** ⑪ �🍴 ▯ 🖭 ➷ ◫ ➹ 👜 🍴 ⚴ **Conf** facs **Location** 2m SW off A1
Hotel BUD Innkeeper's Lodge Cramlington, Blagdon Ln, CRAMLINGTON ☎ 0845 112 6013 18 rms

EMBLETON
MAP 12 NU22

Dunstanburgh Castle NE66 3XQ
☎ 01665 576562 🖥 01665 576562
e-mail: enquiries@dunstanburgh.com
web: www.dunstanburgh.com
Rolling links designed by James Braid, adjacent to the beautiful Embleton Bay. Historic Dunstansburgh Castle is at one end of the course and a National Trust lake and bird sanctuary at the other. Superb views.
18 holes, 6298yds, Par 70, SSS 69, Course record 69.
Club membership 376.
Visitors Mon-Sun & BHs. Booking required Sat & Sun. **Societies** Welcome. **Green Fees** £24 per day (£35 per day; £28 per round Sat, Sun & BHs).
🌐 **Course Designer** James Braid **Facilities** ⑪ �🍴 ▯ 🖭 ➷ ◫ ➹ 👜 🍴 ⚴ **Conf** facs **Location** 7m NE of Alnwick off A1
Hotel ★★ 76% HL Dunstanburgh Castle Hotel, EMBLETON ☎ 01665 576111 20 en suite

FELTON
MAP 12 NU10

Burgham Park NE65 9QP
☎ 01670 787898 (office) & 787978 (pro shop)
🖥 01670 787164
e-mail: info@burghampark.co.uk
web: www.burghampark.co.uk
PGA associates designed course, making the most of the gentle rolling landscape with views to the sea and the Northumbrian hills.

18 holes, 6804yards, Par 72, SSS 72, Course record 67.
Club membership 560.
Visitors Mon-Sun & BHs. Booking required. Dress code.
Societies Welcome. **Green Fees** Phone. **Prof** David Mather
Course Designer Andrew Mair **Facilities** ⑪ �🍴 ▯ 🖭 ➷ ◫ ➹ 👜 🍴 ⚴ 🏌 **Leisure** Par 3 course. **Conf** Corporate Hospitality Days **Location** 5m N of Morpeth, 0.5m off A1
Hotel ★★★★ 82% HL Macdonald Linden Hall, Golf & Country Club, LONGHORSLEY ☎ 01670 500 000 50 en suite

GREENHEAD
MAP 12 NY66

Haltwhistle Wallend Farm CA6 7HN
☎ 016977 47367 🖥 01434 344311
18 holes, 5522yds, Par 69, SSS 67, Course record 70.
Location N on A69 past Haltwhistle on Gilsland Road
Telephone for further details
Hotel ★★★ HL Farlam Hall Hotel, BRAMPTON ☎ 016977 46234 11 en suite 1 annexe en suite

HEXHAM
MAP 12 NY96

De Vere Slaley Hall, Golf Resort & Spa Slaley NE47 0BY
☎ 01434 673154 🖥 01434 673152
e-mail: slaley.hall@devere-hotels.com
web: www.deveregolf.co.uk
Measuring 7073yds from the championship tees, this Dave Thomas course incorporates forest, parkland and moorland with an abundance of lakes and streams. The challenging Par 4 9th (452yds) is played over water through a narrow avenue of towering trees and dense rhododendrons. The Priestman Course designed by Neil Coles is of equal length and standard as the Hunting Course. Opened in spring 1999, the club is situated in 280 acres on the western side of the estate, giving panoramic views over the Tyne valley.
Hunting Course: 18 holes, 7088yds, Par 72, SSS 74, Course record 63.
Priestman Course: 18 holes, 6951yds, Par 72, SSS 72, Course record 63. Club membership 350.
Visitors Booking required. **Societies** Booking required. **Green Fees** Phone. **Prof** Gordon Robinson **Course Designer** Dave Thomas/Neil Coles **Facilities** ⑪ �🍴 ▯ 🖭 ➷ ◫ ➹ 👜 🍴 ⚴ 🏌 **Leisure** heated indoor swimming pool, fishing, sauna, solarium, gymnasium. **Conf** facs **Location** 8m S of Hexham off A68
Hotel ★★★★ 78% HL De Vere Slaley Hall, Slaley, HEXHAM ☎ 01434 673350 139 en suite

Hexham Spital Park NE46 3RZ
☎ 01434 603072 🖥 01434 601865
e-mail: info@hexhamgolf.co.uk
web: www.hexhamgolf.co.uk
A very pretty, well-drained course with interesting natural contours. Exquisite views from parts of the course of the Tyne valley below. As good a parkland course as any in the north of England.
18 holes, 6294yds, Par 70, SSS 70, Course record 61.
Club membership 700.
Visitors Mon-Sun & BHs. Booking required. Dress code. **Societies** Booking required. **Green Fees** £30 per round (£40 Sat, Sun & BHs).
Prof Ben West **Course Designer** Vardon/Caird **Facilities** ⑪ �🍴 ▯ 🖭 ◫ ➹ 👜 🍴 ⚴ **Leisure** squash, squash courts. **Conf** facs Corporate Hospitality Days **Location** 1m NW on B6531
Hotel ★★★ 75% HL Best Western Beaumont Hotel, Beaumont St, HEXHAM ☎ 01434 602331 25 en suite

LONGHORSLEY
MAP 12 NZ19

Linden Hall NE65 8XF
☎ 01670 500011 📄 01670 500001
e-mail: golf.lindenhall@macdonald-hotels.co.uk
web: www.macdonaldhotels.co.uk/lindenhall
Set within the picturesque Linden Hall Estate on a mixture of mature woodland and parkland, established lakes and burns provide interesting water features to match the peaceful surroundings. This award-winning course is a pleasure to play for all standards of golfer.

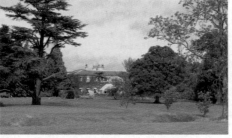

18 holes, 6846yds, Par 72, SSS 73. Club membership 350.
Visitors Mon-Sun & BHs. Booking required. Dress code. **Societies** Booking required. **Green Fees** £45 per day; £30 per round (£50/£35 Sat & Sun).
Prof David Curry **Course Designer** Jonathan Gaunt **Facilities** ⊕ ⊚ ⅃
⬜ ⌂ ⌯ ⚑ ♥ ◔ 🏌 ♥ 🏊 **Leisure** hard tennis courts, heated indoor swimming pool, sauna, solarium, gymnasium, chipping green. **Conf** facs Corporate Hospitality Days **Location** from A1 take A697, 0.5m from village. of Longhorsley
Hotel ★★★★ 82% HL Macdonald Linden Hall, Golf & Country Club,
LONGHORSLEY ☎ 01670 500 000 50 en suite

MATFEN
MAP 12 NZ07

Matfen Hall NE20 0RH
☎ 01661 886400 📄 01661 886055
e-mail: golf@matfenhall.com
web: www.matfenhall.com
An 18-hole parkland course set in beautiful countryside with many natural and man-made hazards. The course is an enjoyable test for players of all abilities but it does incorporate challenging water features in the shape of a large lake and a fast flowing river. The dry stone wall presents a unique obstacle on several holes. The 4th, 9th, 12th and 14th holes are particularly testing Par 4s, the dog-leg 16th is the pick of the Par 5s but Matfen's signature hole is the long Par 3 17th with its narrow green teasingly sited just over the river. New 9 holes open from June 2007.
18 holes, 6700yds, Par 72, SSS 72, Course record 63.
Club membership 500.
Visitors Mon-Sun & BHs. Booking required. Dress code. **Societies** Booking required. **Green Fees** £45 per 36/27 holes; £35 per 18 holes (£50/£40 Sat & Sun). **Prof** John Harrison **Course Designer** Mair/James/Gaunt
Facilities ⊕ ⊚ ⅃ ⬜ ⌯ ⌂ ⚑ ◔ ♥ 🏌 **Leisure** heated indoor swimming pool, sauna, gymnasium, 9 hole Par 3 course. Leisure complex & health spa. **Conf** facs Corporate Hospitality Days **Location** Off B6318
Hotel ★★★★ 81% HL Matfen Hall, MATFEN ☎ 01661 886500 855708
📄 01661 886055 53 en suite

MORPETH
MAP 12 NZ28

Morpeth The Clubhouse NE61 2BT
☎ 01670 504942 📄 01670 504918
18 holes, 6206yds, Par 71, SSS 69, Course record 65.
Course Designer Harry Vardon **Location** S of town centre on A197
Telephone for further details
Hotel ★★★★ 82% HL Macdonald Linden Hall, Golf & Country Club,
LONGHORSLEY ☎ 01670 500 000 50 en suite

NEWBIGGIN-BY-THE-SEA
MAP 12 NZ38

Newbiggin-by-the-Sea Prospect Place NE64 6DW
☎ 01670 817344
e-mail: info@newbiggingolfclub.co.uk
web: www.newbiggingolfclub.co.uk
Seaside-links course.
18 holes, 6452yds, Par 72, SSS 71, Course record 65.
Club membership 694.
Visitors Mon-Sun & BHs. Booking required Sat & Sun. Dress code.
Societies Booking required. **Green Fees** £25 per day, £18 per round
(£35/£25 Sat, Sun & BHs). ☻ **Prof** James Kerr **Course Designer** Willie Park **Facilities** ⊕ ⊚ ⅃ ⬜ ⌯ ⌂ ♥ 🏌 **Leisure** snooker. **Conf** facs
Corporate Hospitality Days **Location** N of town centre
Hotel ★★★★ 82% HL Macdonald Linden Hall, Golf & Country Club,
LONGHORSLEY ☎ 01670 500 000 50 en suite

PONTELAND
MAP 12 NZ17

Ponteland 53 Bell Villas NE20 9BD
☎ 01661 822689 📄 01661 860077
e-mail: secretary@thepontelandgolfclub.co.uk
web: www.thepontelandgolfclub.co.uk
Open parkland course offering testing golf and good views.
18 holes, 6587yds, Par 72, SSS 72, Course record 65.
Club membership 720.
Visitors Mon-Fri, Sun & BHs. Booking required. Handicap certificate. Dress code. **Societies** Booking required. **Green Fees** Phone. **Prof** Alan Robson-Crosby **Course Designer** Harry Fernie **Facilities** ⊕ ⊚ ⅃ ⬜ ⌯ ⌂ ♥
🏌 ♥ **Conf** Corporate Hospitality Days **Location** 0.5m E on A696
Hotel ★★★ 74% HL Novotel Newcastle, Ponteland Rd, Kenton,
NEWCASTLE UPON TYNE ☎ 0191 214 0303 126 en suite

PRUDHOE
MAP 12 NZ06

Prudhoe Eastwood Park NE42 5DX
☎ 01661 832466 📄 01661 830710
e-mail: secretary@prudhoegolfclub.co.uk
18 holes, 5812yds, Par 69, SSS 69, Course record 60.
Location E of town centre off A695
Telephone for further details
Hotel ★★★ 70% HL Gibside Hotel, Front St, WHICKHAM
☎ 0191 488 9292 45 en suite

England

ROTHBURY MAP 12 NU00

Rothbury Whitton Rd NE65 7RX
☎ 01669 621271
e-mail: secretary@rothburygolfclub.com
web: www.rothburygolfclub.com
Scenic, flat parkland course set alongside the River Coquet, surrounded by Simonside hills and Cragside Hall.
18 holes, 6102yds, Par 70. Club membership 306.
Visitors Mon-Sun & BHs. Booking required Sat & Sun. Dress code.
Societies Booking required. **Green Fees** £30 per day, £20 per 18 holes (£35/£25 Sat, Sun & BHs). **Course Designer** J Radcliffe **Facilities** ⑪ ⑩ ▮ ☐ ♉ ☒ ⚒ ✦ **Conf** Corporate Hospitality Days **Location** SW of town off B6342
Hotel ★★★★ 82% HL Macdonald Linden Hall, Golf & Country Club, LONGHORSLEY ☎ 01670 500 000 50 en suite

SEAHOUSES MAP 12 NU23

Seahouses Beadnell Rd NE68 7XT
☎ 01665 720794 📄 01665 721994
e-mail: secretary@seahousesgolf.co.uk
web: www.seahousesgolf.co.uk
Traditional links course with many hazards. Signature holes are the famous Par 3 10th hole, Logans Loch, water hole and the Par 3 15th, nominated as one of the most difficult holes in the world. Spectacular views of the coastline to the Farne Islands and Lindisfarne.
18 holes, 5542yds, Par 67, SSS 67, Course record 63.
Club membership 550.
Visitors Mon-Sun & BHs. Booking required Sat, Sun & BHs. Dress code.
Societies Booking required **Green Fees** £27 per day; £20 per round (£32/£27 Sat, Sun & BHs). ⊛ **Facilities** ⑪ ⑩ ▮ ☐ ♉ ☒ ✦ **Conf** Corporate Hospitality Days **Location** S of village on B1340, 5m E of A1
Hotel ★★★ 72% HL Bamburgh Castle Hotel, SEAHOUSES
☎ 01665 720283 20 en suite

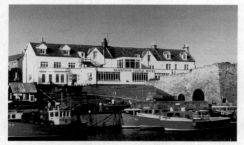

STOCKSFIELD MAP 12 NZ06

Stocksfield New Ridley Rd NE43 7RE
☎ 01661 843041 📄 01661 843046
e-mail: info@sgcgolf.co.uk
web: www.sgcgolf.co.uk
Challenging course: parkland (nine holes), woodland (nine holes). Some elevated greens, giving fine views, and water hazards.
18 holes, 5991yds, Par 70, SSS 69, Course record 61.
Club membership 550.
Visitors Mon, Tue, Thu, Fri, Sun & BHs. Wed pm only. Booking required. Dress code. **Societies** Welcome. **Green Fees** £25 per day; £20 per round (£25 Sun and BHs). **Prof** Steven Harrison **Course Designer** Pennick **Facilities** ⑪ ⑩ ▮ ▮ ☐ ♉ ☒ ☰ ☜ ⚒ ✦ **Leisure** snooker. **Conf** Corporate Hospitality Days **Location** 1.5m S off A695
Hotel ★★★ 75% HL Best Western Beaumont Hotel, Beaumont St, HEXHAM ☎ 01434 602331 25 en suite

SWARLAND MAP 12 NU10

Swarland Hall Coast View NE65 9JG
☎ 01670 787010
e-mail: info@swarlandgolf
web: www.swarlandgolf.co.uk
18 holes, 6335yds, Par 72, SSS 72.
Location 1m W of A1
Telephone for further details
Hotel ★★★★ 82% HL Macdonald Linden Hall, Golf & Country Club, LONGHORSLEY ☎ 01670 500 000 50 en suite

WOOLER MAP 12 NT92

Wooler Dod Law, Doddington NE71 6EA
☎ 01668 282135
web: www.woolergolf.co.uk
9 holes, 6411yds, Par 72, SSS 71, Course record 69.
Location At Doddington on B6525
Telephone for further details
Hotel ★★ 69% HL Purdy Lodge, Adderstone Services, BELFORD
☎ 01668 213000 20 en suite

NOTTINGHAMSHIRE

CALVERTON MAP 08 SK64

Ramsdale Park Golf Centre Oxton Rd NG14 6NU
☎ 0115 965 5600 📄 0115 965 4105
e-mail: info@ramsdaleparkgc.co.uk
web: www.ramsdaleparkgc.co.uk
The Seely Course is a challenging and comprehensive test for any standard of golf. A relatively flat front nine is followed by an undulating back nine that is renowned as one of the best in the county. The Lee Course is an 18-hole Par 3 course which is gaining a similar reputation.
Seely Course: 18 holes, 6546yds, Par 71, SSS 71, Course record 70.
Lee Course: 18 holes, 2844yds, Par 54, SSS 54.
Club membership 400.
Visitors Mon-Sun & BHs. Booking required. Dress code. **Societies** Booking required. **Green Fees** Seely Course £20.50 per 18 holes (£26 Sat & Sun). Lee Course £10.50 per 18 holes. **Prof** Robert Macey **Course Designer**

Continued

Hawtree **Facilities** ⓦ ⓘ⊙ ⓛ 🖵 🏴 ⚎ 🏌 ⚏ ⚑ ✔ ⚑ 🏌 **Leisure** fishing.
Conf facs Corporate Hospitality Days **Location** 8m NE of Nottingham off B6386
Hotel ★★★ 70% HL Best Western Bestwood Lodge, Bestwood Country Park, Arnold, NOTTINGHAM ☎ 0115 920 3011 39 en suite

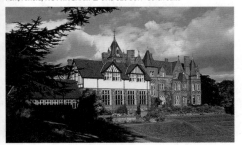

Ramsdale Park Golf Centre

Springwater Moor Ln NG14 6FZ
☎ 0115 965 2129 (pro shop) & 965 4946 🖹 0115 965 4957
e-mail: springwater@rapidial.co.uk
web: www.springwatergolfclub.co.uk
This attractive course set in rolling countryside overlooking the Trent valley, offers an interesting and challenging game of golf to players of all handicaps. The 18th hole is particularly noteworthy, a 183yd Par 3 over two ponds

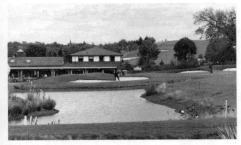

18 holes, 6262yds, Par 71, SSS 71, Course record 68.
Club membership 440.
Visitors Mon-Sun & BHs. Booking required. Dress code. **Societies** Booking required. **Green Fees** £22 per round (£27 weekends & bank holidays). **Prof** Paul Drew **Course Designer** Neil Footitt/Paul Wharmsby **Facilities** ⓦ ⓘ⊙ ⓛ 🖵 🏴 ⚎ 🏌 ⚏ ⚑ ✔ ⚑ 🏌 **Leisure** short game academy. **Conf** facs Corporate Hospitality Days **Location** Off A6097 to Calverton, 600yds on left
Hotel ★★★ 73% HL Best Western Westminster Hotel, 312 Mansfield Rd, Carrington, NOTTINGHAM ☎ 0115 955 5000 73 en suite

EAST LEAKE   MAP 08 SK52

Rushcliffe Stocking Ln LE12 5RL
☎ 01509 852959 🖹 01509 852688
e-mail: secretary.rushcliffegc@btopenworld.com
Hilly, tree-lined and picturesque parkland.
18 holes, 6013yds, Par 70, SSS 69, Course record 63.
Club membership 750.
Visitors Contact club for details. **Societies** Welcome. **Green Fees** Phone.
⚑ **Prof** Chris Hall **Facilities** 🏴 ⚎ 🏌 ⚏ **Location** M1 junct 24
Hotel ★★★★ 76% HL Best Western Premier Yew Lodge Hotel, Packington Hill, KEGWORTH ☎ 01509 672518 87 en suite

HUCKNALL   MAP 08 SK54

Hucknall Golf Centre Wigwam Ln NG15 7TA
☎ 0115 964 2037 🖹 0115 964 2724
e-mail: leen@jbgolf.co.uk
web: www.jackbarker.com
A course on two different levels. Upper level has a links feel while the lower level with its ponds, streams and ditches has a parkland feel. A relatively short course but still a challenge for all abilities.
18 holes, 6026yds, Par 70, SSS 70. Club membership 250.
Visitors Mon-Sun & BHs. **Societies** Welcome. **Green Fees** £10 per round (£13 Sat & Sun). **Prof** Cyril Jepson **Course Designer** Tom Hodgetts **Facilities** ⓦ ⓘ⊙ ⓛ 🖵 🏴 ⚎ 🏌 ⚏ ⚑ ✔ ⚑ 🏌 **Conf** facs Corporate Hospitality Days **Location** 0.5m from town centre, signs for railway station, right onto Wigwam Ln
Hotel BUD Premier Travel Inn Nottingham North West, Nottingham Rd, HUCKNALL ☎ 0870 9906518 35 en suite

KEYWORTH   MAP 08 SK63

Stanton on the Wolds Golf Course Rd, Stanton-on-the-Wolds NG12 5BH
☎ 0115 937 4885 🖹 0115 937 1652
e-mail: swgc@zoom.co.uk
Fairly flat parkland with a stream running through four holes. Physically not demanding but challenging to score well.
18 holes, 6369yds, Par 73, SSS 71, Course record 67.
Club membership 705.
Visitors Mon-Fri except BHs. Booking required. Handicap certificate required. Dress code. **Societies** booking required. **Green Fees** not confirmed. ⚑ **Prof** Nick Hernon **Course Designer** Tom Williamson **Facilities** ⓦ ⓘ⊙ 🖵 🏴 ⚎ 🏌 ⚏ ⚑ ✔ **Location** E side of village off A606
Hotel BUD Premier Travel Inn Nottingham South, Loughborough Rd, Ruddington, NOTTINGHAM ☎ 0870 9906422 42 en suite

KIRKBY IN ASHFIELD   MAP 08 SK55

Notts Derby Rd NG17 7QR
☎ 01623 753225 🖹 01623 753655
e-mail: office@nottsgolfclub.co.uk
web: www.nottsgolfclub.co.uk
Undulating heathland championship course.
18 holes, 7213yds, Par 72, SSS 75, Course record 64.
Club membership 450.
Visitors Mon-Fri except BHs. Booking required. Handicap certificate.
Societies Welcome. **Green Fees** £99 per day; £66 per round. **Prof** Mike Bradley **Course Designer** Willie Park **Facilities** ⓦ ⓘ⊙ ⓛ 🖵 🏴 ⚎ 🏌 ⚏ ⚑ ✔ ⚑ 🏌 **Conf** facs **Location** 2m SE of Mansfield off A611
Hotel ★★★★ 77% HL Renaissance Derby/Nottingham Hotel, Carter Ln East, SOUTH NORMANTON ☎ 01773 812000 & 0870 4007262 🖹 01773 580032 & 0870 4007362 158 en suite

MANSFIELD   MAP 08 SK56

Sherwood Forest Eakring Rd NG18 3EW
☎ 01623 627403 🖹 01623 420412
e-mail: sherwood@forest43.freeserve.co.uk
As the name suggests, the forest is the main feature of this natural heathland course with its heather, silver birch and pine trees. The homeward nine holes are particularly testing. The 11th to the 14th are notable Par 4 holes on this well-bunkered course.

Continued

18 holes, 6289yds, Par 71, SSS 71. Club membership 750.
Visitors Mon, Wed-Fri except BHs, Tue pm only. Booking required.
Handicap certificate. Dress code. **Societies** booking required. **Green
Fees** not confirmed. **Prof** Ken Hall **Course Designer** H S Colt/James
Braid **Facilities** ⑪ ⓍⓌ ℉ 🍴 ♨ 🍷 🍺 ✔ ♣ **Leisure** snooker.
Conf facs Corporate Hospitality Days **Location** E of Mansfield
Hotel ★★ 69% HL Pine Lodge Hotel, 281-283 Nottingham Rd,
MANSFIELD ☎ 01623 622308 20 en suite

NEWARK-ON-TRENT   MAP 08 SK75

Newark Coddington NG24 2QX
☎ 01636 626282 📠 01636 626497
e-mail: secretary@newark-golf-club.co.uk
web: www.newark-golf-club.co.uk
Wooded parkland in a secluded position with easy walking.
18 holes, 6458yds, Par 71, SSS 71, Course record 66.
Club membership 650.
Visitors Mon-Fri except BHs. Booking required. Handicap certificate. Dress
code. **Societies** Booking required. **Green Fees** not confirmed. **Prof** P A
Lockley **Course Designer** T Williamson **Facilities** ⑪ ⓍⓌ ℉ 🍴 ♨ 🍷
🍺 ✔ ♣ **Leisure** snooker. **Conf** Corporate Hospitality Days **Location** 4m E
of Newark on Sleaford road
Hotel ★★★ 80% HL The Grange Hotel, 73 London Rd, NEWARK
☎ 01636 703399 10 en suite 9 annexe en suite

NOTTINGHAM   MAP 08 SK53

Beeston Fields Old Dr, Wollaton Rd, Beeston NG9 3DD
☎ 0115 925 7062 📠 0115 925 4280
e-mail: beestonfields@btconnect.com
web: www.beestonfields.co.uk
Parkland course with sandy subsoil and wide, tree-lined fairways. The
Par 3 14th has an elevated tee and a small bunker-guarded green.

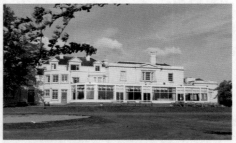

18 holes, 6402yds, Par 71, SSS 71, Course record 64.
Club membership 600.
Visitors Mon, Wed, Fri & Sun except BHs. Booking required. Handicap
certificate. Dress code. **Societies** Booking required. **Green Fees** £43
per day, £33 per round (£39 per round Sun). **Prof** Alun Wardle **Course
Designer** Tom Williamson **Facilities** ⑪ ⓍⓌ by prior arrangement 🍺 🍷 ℉
♨ 🍴 🏤 ✔ **Conf** facs Corporate Hospitality Days **Location** 400yds SW
off A52 Nottingham-Derby road
Hotel BUD Travelodge Nottingham Trowell (M1), TROWELL
☎ 08700 850 950 35 en suite

Bulwell Forest Hucknall Rd, Bulwell NG6 9LQ
☎ 0115 976 3172 (pro shop) 📠 0115 967 1734
e-mail: david@dnehra.co.uk
Municipal heathland course with many natural hazards. Very tight
fairways and subject to wind. Five challenging Par 3s. Excellent
drainage.
18 holes, 5667yds, Par 68, SSS 67, Course record 62.
Club membership 350.
Visitors Mon-Sun & BHs. Booking required. **Societies** Booking required.
Green Fees £13 per round (£16 Sat, Sun & BHs). **Course Designer** John
Doleman **Facilities** ⑪ 🍺 ℉ 🍴 ♨ 🏤 ♣ ✔ **Leisure** hard tennis courts,
children's playground. **Location** 4m NW of city on A611
Hotel ★★★ 70% HL Best Western Bestwood Lodge, Bestwood Country
Park, Arnold, NOTTINGHAM ☎ 0115 920 3011 39 en suite

Chilwell Manor Meadow Ln, Chilwell NG9 5AE
☎ 0115 925 8958 📠 0115 922 0575
e-mail: chilwellmanorgolfclub@barbox.net
18 holes, 6255yds, Par 70, SSS 71, Course record 66.
Course Designer Tom Williamson **Location** 4m SW on A6005
Telephone for further details

Edwalton Municipal Wellin Ln, Edwalton NG12 4AS
☎ 0115 923 4775 📠 0115 923 1647
e-mail: edwalton@glendale-services.co.uk
web: www.glendale-golf.com
Gently sloping nine-hole parkland course. Also a nine-hole Par 3 and
large practice ground.
9 holes, 3336yds, Par 72, SSS 72, Course record 71.
Club membership 650.
Visitors Mon-Sun & BHs. Booking required. **Societies** Welcome. **Green
Fees** Phone. **Prof** Lee Rawlings **Facilities** ⑪ ⓍⓌ by prior arrangement 🍺
℉ 🍴 ♨ ✔ ♣ **Leisure** Par 3 course. **Conf** facs Corporate
Hospitality Days **Location** S of Nottingham off A606
Hotel BUD Premier Travel Inn Nottingham South, Loughborough Rd,
Ruddington, NOTTINGHAM ☎ 0870 9906422 42 en suite

Mapperley Central Av, Plains Rd, Mapperley NG3 6RH
☎ 0115 955 6673 (pro) & 955 6672 (sec)
📠 0115 955 6670
e-mail: house@mapperleygolfclub.org
web: www.mapperleygolfclub.org
Hilly meadowland course but with easy walking.
18 holes, 6307yds, Par 71, SSS 70, Course record 65.
Club membership 700.
Visitors Mon-Fri, Sun & BHs. Booking required BHs. Dress code.
Societies Booking required. **Green Fees** £25 per day/round (£27.50 Sun
& bank holidays). **Prof** John Newham **Course Designer** John Mason
Facilities ⑪ ⓍⓌ ℉ 🍴 ♨ 🏤 🍷 ✔ **Leisure** pool room. **Location** 3m
NE of city centre off B684
Hotel BUD Travelodge Nottingham Trowell (M1), TROWELL
☎ 08700 850 950 35 en suite

England

Nottingham City Sandhurst Rd, Bulwell Hall Park NG6 8LF

☎ 0115 927 2767 (pro) & 07740 688694
e-mail: garyandkate1@talktalk.net
web: www.nottinghamcitygolfclub.co.uk
A pleasant municipal parkland course on the city outskirts.
18 holes, 6218yds, Par 69, SSS 70, Course record 63.
Club membership 250.
Visitors Mon-Sun & BHs. Booking required. **Societies** Welcome. **Green
Fees** Phone. **Course Designer** H Braid **Facilities** ⚒ 🍴 ☕ 🏌 🛈 ✆ **Conf**
facs Corporate Hospitality Days **Location** 4m NW of city centre off A6002
Hotel ★★★ 70% HL Best Western Bestwood Lodge, Bestwood Country
Park, Arnold, NOTTINGHAM ☎ 0115 920 3011 39 en suite

Wollaton Park Limetree Av, Wollaton Park NG8 1BT

☎ 0115 978 7574 📄 0115 970 0736
e-mail: wollatonparkgc@aol.com
web: www.wollatonparkgolfclub.com
A traditional parkland course on slightly undulating land, winding
through historic woodland and set in a historic deer park. Fine views
of 16th-century Wollaton Hall.
18 holes, 6445yds, Par 71, SSS 71, Course record 64.
Club membership 700.
Visitors Mon, Tue, Thu, Fri, Sun & BHs. Dress code. **Societies** Booking
required. **Green Fees** £48 per day; £35 per round (£55/£40 Sun & BHs).
Prof John Lower **Course Designer** T Williamson **Facilities** ⚒ 🍴 ☕ 🖥
🛈 🏌 ☕ ✆ **Conf** Corporate Hospitality Days **Location** 2.5m W of city
centre off ring road junct A52
Hotel ★★★ 68% HL Swans Hotel & Restaurant, 84-90 Radcliffe Rd,
West Bridgford, NOTTINGHAM ☎ 0115 981 4042 30 en suite

OLLERTON   MAP 08 SK66

Rufford Park Golf & Country Club Rufford Ln, Rufford NG22 9DG

☎ 01623 825253 📄 01623 825254
e-mail: enquiries@ruffordpark.co.uk
web: www.ruffordpark.co.uk
Set in the heart of Sherwood Forest, Rufford Park is noted for its
picturesque 18 holes with its especially challenging Par 3s. From
the unique 175yd Par 3 17th over water to the riverside 641yd 13th,
the course offers everything the golfer needs from beginner to
professional.
18 holes, 6368yds, Par 70, SSS 70, Course record 66.
Club membership 600.
Visitors Mon-Fri & BHs. Sat & Sun after 12.30pm. Dress code. **Societies**
Booking required. **Green Fees** £22 per 18 holes (£28 Sat & Sun). **Prof** John
Vaughan/James Thompson **Course Designer** David Hemstock/Ken Brown
Facilities ⚒ 🍴 ☕ 🖥 🛈 🏌 ☕ ✆ **Conf** facs Corporate
Hospitality Days **Location** S of Ollerton, off A614 for Rufford Mill
Hotel ★★★ 70% HL Clumber Park Hotel, Clumber Park, WORKSOP
☎ 0870 609 6158 48 en suite

OXTON   MAP 08 SK65

Oakmere Park Oaks Ln NG25 0RH

☎ 0115 965 3545 📄 0115 965 5628
e-mail: enquiries@oakmerepark.co.uk
web: www.oakmerepark.co.uk
Twenty-seven holes set in rolling heathland in the heart of picturesque
Robin Hood country. The Par 4 16th and Par 5 1st are notable, as are
the all weather playing qualities.

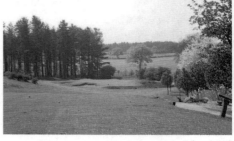

Oakmere Park

Admirals: *18 holes, 6617yds, Par 73, SSS 72,
Course record 64.*
Commanders: *9 holes, 6407yds, Par 72, SSS 72.*
Club membership 900.
Visitors Mon-Sun & BHs. Dress code. **Societies** Welcome.
Green Fees Admirals £20 per 18 holes (£28 weekends). Commanders
£12/£16. **Prof** Daryl St-John Jones **Course Designer** Frank Pennick
Facilities ⚒ 🍴 ☕ 🖥 🛈 🏌 ☕ ✆ **Conf** facs Corporate
Hospitality Days **Location** 1m NW of Oxton off A6097 or A614
Hotel ★★★ 73% HL Best Western Westminster Hotel, 312 Mansfield Rd,
Carrington, NOTTINGHAM ☎ 0115 955 5000 73 en suite

RADCLIFFE ON TRENT   MAP 08 SK63

Cotgrave Place Golf Club Stragglethorpe, Nr Cotgrave Village NG12 3HB

☎ 0115 933 3344 📄 0115 933 4567
e-mail: cotgrave@americangolf.com
web: www.americangolf.com
Masters: *18 holes, 5933yds, Par 70, SSS 69,
Course record 66.*
Open: *18 holes, 6302yds, Par 71, SSS 68, Course record 69.*
Course Designer Peter Aliss/John Small **Location** 2m SW of Radcliffe
off A52
Telephone for further details
Hotel ★★★ 79% HL Langar Hall, LANGAR ☎ 01949 860559 12 en suite

Radcliffe-on-Trent Dewberry Ln, Cropwell Rd NG12 2JH

☎ 0115 933 3000 📄 0115 911 6991
e-mail: les.wake@radcliffeontrentgc.co.uk
web: www.radcliffeontrentgc.co.uk
Fairly flat, parkland course with three good finishing holes: 16th (423
yds) Par 4; 17th (174 yds) through spinney, Par 3; 18th (336 yds) dog-
leg Par 4. Excellent views.
18 holes, 6374yds, Par 70, SSS 71, Course record 64.
Club membership 700.
Visitors Mon-Sun except BHs. Booking required Sat & Sun. Handicap
certificate. Dress code **Societies** Booking required. **Green Fees** £36
per day, £26 per 18 holes. **Prof** Craig George **Course Designer** Tom
Williamson **Facilities** ⚒ 🍴 ☕ 🖥 🛈 🏌 ☕ ✆ **Conf** Corporate
Hospitality Days **Location** 0.5m SE of town centre off A52
Hotel ★★★ 68% HL Swans Hotel & Restaurant, 84-90 Radcliffe Rd, West
Bridgford, NOTTINGHAM ☎ 0115 981 4042 30 en suite

RETFORD   MAP 08 SK78

Retford Brecks Rd, Ordsall DN22 7UA
☎ 01777 711188 (Secretary) 🖹 01777 710412
Wooded parkland.
18 holes, 6446yds, Par 72, SSS 72, Course record 67.
Club membership 700.
Visitors Mon, Wed & Fri. Sat, Sun & BHs by arrangement. Booking required.
i **Societies** Welcome. **Green Fees** £35 per day; £28 per round (£28 per round Sat & Sun). ⊕ **Prof** Craig Morris **Course Designer** Tom Williamson
Facilities ⊕ ⦿ 🍴 🖿 ⬚ 🏌 🛈 ♿ ⛳ **Location** 1.5m S A620, between Worksop & Gainsborough
Hotel ★★★ 72% HL Best Western The West Retford Hotel, 24 North Rd, RETFORD ☎ 01777 706333 & 0870 609 6162 🖹 01777 709951 63 en suite

RUDDINGTON   MAP 08 SK53

Ruddington Grange Wilford Rd NG11 6NB
☎ 0115 921 1951 (pro shop) & 984 6141 🖹 0115 940 5165
e-mail: info@ruddingtongrange.com
web: www.ruddingtongrange.com
18 holes, 6543yds, Par 72, SSS 72, Course record 69.
Course Designer E MacAusland/J Small **Location** 1m N of town centre on B680
Telephone for further details
Hotel ★★★ 68% HL Swans Hotel & Restaurant, 84-90 Radcliffe Rd, West Bridgford, NOTTINGHAM ☎ 0115 981 4042 30 en suite

SERLBY   MAP 08 SK68

Serlby Park DN10 6BA
☎ 01777 818268
e-mail: kjcrook@onetel.com
Peaceful, picturesque setting on well-drained areas of woodland, parkland and farmland on the Serlby Hall Estate. Easy walking.
11 holes, 5404yds, Par 66, SSS 66, Course record 63.
Club membership 260.
Visitors Mon, Wed-Sun & BHs. Booking required. Handicap certificate. Dress code. **Societies** Booking required. **Green Fees** £20 per round (£25 Sat, Sun & BHs). ⊕ **Course Designer** Tom Williamson **Facilities** ⊕ ⦿ 🍴 ⬚ 🏌 🛈 **Location** E of village off A638
Hotel ★★★ 85% HL Best Western Charnwood Hotel, Sheffield Rd, BLYTH ☎ 01909 591610 47 en suite

SOUTHWELL   MAP 08 SK65

Norwood Park Norwood Park NG25 0PF
☎ 01636 816626
e-mail: golf@norwood park.co.uk
web: www.norwoodpark.co.uk
A parkland course that blends perfectly with the historic setting of Norwood Park and highlights its natural features. Built to USGA standards, the course will appeal to all golfers, who will appreciate the well-shaped fairways, large undulating greens, natural and man-made water hazards, and fine views over the surrounding countryside.
18 holes, 6805yds, Par 72, SSS 72, Course record 68.
Club membership 600.
Visitors Mon-Sun & BHs. Booking required. **Societies** Welcome. **Green Fees** £20 per 18 holes, £24 Fri, £28 Sat, Sun & BHs. **Prof** Paul Thornton
Course Designer Clyde B Johnston **Facilities** ⊕ ⦿ 🍴 ⬚ 🏌 🛈 🍴 ♿ ⛳ 🛈 ⛳ **Leisure** Par 3 academy course opens 2008. **Conf** facs Corporate

Hospitality Days **Location** Off A617 Newark to Mansfield road. Take turning to Southwell in Kirklington, golf course 5m on right.
Hotel ★★★ 73% HL Saracens Head Hotel, Market Place, SOUTHWELL ☎ 01636 812701 27 en suite

SUTTON IN ASHFIELD   MAP 08 SK45

Coxmoor Coxmoor Rd NG17 5LF
☎ 01623 557359 🖹 01623 557435
e-mail: coxmoorgc@btconnect.com
web: www.coxmoor.freeuk.com
Undulating moorland and heathland course with easy walking and excellent views. The clubhouse is traditional with a well-equipped games room. The course lies adjacent to Forestry Commission land over which there are several footpaths and extensive views.
18 holes, 6577yds, Par 73, SSS 72, Course record 65.
Club membership 700.
Visitors Mon, Wed-Fri except BHs. Booking required. Handicap certificate. Dress code. **Societies** Booking required. **Green Fees** £55 per day; £40 per round. **Prof** Craig Wright **Facilities** ⊕ ⦿ 🍴 ⬚ 🏌 🛈 ♿ **Leisure** snooker. **Conf** Corporate Hospitality Days **Location** 2m SE off A611
Hotel ★★★★ 77% HL Renaissance Derby/Nottingham Hotel, Carter Ln East, SOUTH NORMANTON ☎ 01773 812000 & 0870 4007262 🖹 01773 580032 & 0870 4007362 158 en suite

WORKSOP   MAP 08 SK57

Bondhay Golf & Country Club Bondhay Ln, Whitwell S80 3EH
☎ 01909 723608 🖹 01909 720226
e-mail: enquiries@bondhay.com
web: www.bondhay.com
The wind usually plays quite an active role in making this flat championship course testing. Signature holes are the 10th which requires a second shot over water into a basin of trees; the 11th comes back over the same expanse of water and requires a mid to short iron to a long, narrow green; the 18th is a Par 5 with a lake - the dilemma is whether to lay up short or go for the carry. The Par 3s are generally island-like in design, requiring accuracy to avoid the many protective bunker features.
Devonshire Course: 18 holes, 6807yds, Par 72, SSS 73, Course record 67. Club membership 450.
Visitors Mon-Sun & BHs. Booking required. Dress code. **Societies** Booking required. **Green Fees** 18 holes Mon-Tues £16, Wed-Fri £19; Sat-Sun £25. Par 3 course £5. **Prof** Michael Ramsden **Course Designer** Donald Steel **Facilities** ⊕ ⦿ 🍴 ⬚ 🏌 🛈 ♿ ⛳ 🛈 ⛳ **Leisure** fishing, Par 3 family course. **Conf** facs Corporate Hospitality Days **Location** M1 junct 30, 5m W of Worksop off A619
Hotel ★★★ 70% HL Sitwell Arms Hotel, Station Rd, RENISHAW ☎ 01246 435226 & 437327 🖹 01246 433915 30 en suite

College Pines Worksop College Dr S80 3AL
☎ 01909 501431 🖹 01909 481227
e-mail: snelljunior@btinternet.com
web: www.collegepinesgolfclub.co.uk
This course was opened in 1994 and the Par 73 layout covers 150 acres of well-drained land with heathland characteristics. It is club policy to remain open on full tees and greens all year round.
18 holes, 6801yards, Par 73, SSS 73, Course record 67.
Club membership 500.

Continued

Visitors Mon-Sun & BHs. Booking required. Dress code. **Societies** Booking required. **Green Fees** £22 per day, £15 per round (£30/£21 Sat, Sun & BHs). ❷ **Prof** Charles Snell **Course Designer** David Snell **Facilities** ⓣ ⓦ ⓐ 🖢 ⓛ ⓨ 🕱 ⓔ ❢ ❢ **Conf** Corporate Hospitality Days **Location** M1 junct 30/31, S of Worksop on B6034 Edwinstowe road
Hotel ★★★ 70% HL Clumber Park Hotel, Clumber Park, WORKSOP
☎ 0870 609 6158 48 en suite

Kilton Forest Blyth Rd S81 0TL
☎ 01909 486563
18 holes, 6424yds, Par 72, SSS 71, Course record 66.
Location 1m NE of town centre on B6045
Telephone for further details
Hotel ★★★ 78% HL Best Western Lion Hotel, 112 Bridge St, WORKSOP
☎ 01909 477925 45 en suite

Lindrick Lindrick Common S81 8BH
☎ 01909 475282 ▤ 01909 488685
e-mail: lgc@ansbronze.com
web: www.lindrickgolfclub.co.uk
Heathland course with some trees and masses of gorse which has hosted many major golf tournaments including the Ryder Cup.
18 holes, 6486yds, Par 71, SSS 71, Course record 63.
Club membership 510.
Visitors Mon, Wed-Fr & Sun except BHs. Booking required. Handicap certificate. Dress code. **Societies** Booking required. **Green Fees** £65 per day, £50 per 18 holes. Reduced winter rate. **Prof** John R King **Facilities** ⓣ ⓦ ⓛ ⓓ ⓣⓛ ⓐ 🖢 ⓨ **Leisure** buggies for disabled only. **Conf** Corporate Hospitality Days **Location** M1 junct 31, 4m NW of Worksop on A57
Hotel ★★★ 78% HL Best Western Lion Hotel, 112 Bridge St, WORKSOP
☎ 01909 477925 45 en suite

Worksop Windmill Ln S80 2SQ
☎ 01909 477731 ▤ 01909 530917
e-mail: thesecretary@worksopgolfclub.co.uk
web: www.worksopgolfclub.com
Adjacent to Clumber Park, this course has heathland terrain, with gorse, broom, oak and birch trees. Fast, true greens, dry all year round.
18 holes, 6660yds, Par 72, SSS 72. Club membership 600.
Visitors Mon, Wed & Fri except BHs. Dress code. **Societies** Welcome.
Green Fees £55 per day, £40 per 18 holes. **Prof** K Crossland **Course Designer** Tom Williamson **Facilities** ⓣ ⓦ ⓛ ⓓ ⓣⓛ ⓐ 🖢 ⓨ 🕱 ⓨ
Leisure snooker. **Conf** facs Corporate Hospitality Days **Location** A57 ring road onto B6034 to Edwinstowe
Hotel ★★★ 70% HL Clumber Park Hotel, Clumber Park, WORKSOP
☎ 0870 609 6158 48 en suite

OXFORDSHIRE

ABINGDON   MAP 04 SU49

Drayton Park Steventon Rd, Drayton OX14 4LA
☎ 01235 550607 (Pro Shop) ▤ 01235 525731

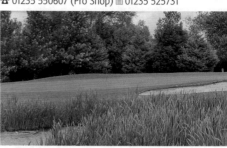

18 holes, 6030yds, Par 67, SSS 67, Course record 60.
Course Designer Hawtree **Location** Off A34 at Didcot
Telephone for further details
Hotel ★★★ 74% HL Abingdon Four Pillars Hotel, Marcham Rd,
ABINGDON ☎ 0800 374 692 & 01235 553456 ▤ 01235 554117 63 en suite

BANBURY   MAP 04 SP44

Banbury Aynho Rd, Adderbury OX17 3NT
☎ 01295 810419 & 812880 ▤ 01295 810056
e-mail: office@banburygolfcentre.co.uk
Undulating wooded course with water features and USGA specification greens.
Red & Yellow: 18 holes, 6557yds, Par 71, SSS 71.
Yellow & Blue: 18 holes, 6603yds, Par 71, SSS 71.
Red & Blue: 18 holes, 6746yds, Par 72, SSS 72.
Club membership 300.
Visitors Mon-Sun & BHs. Booking required Sat, Sun & BHs. **Societies** Booking required. **Green Fees** £23 per 18 holes (£29 Sat & Sun). **Prof** Mark McGeehan **Course Designer** Reed/Payn **Facilities** ⓣ ⓦ ⓛ ⓓ ⓣⓛ ⓐ 🖢 ⓨⓣ ⓨ ⓨ **Conf** Corporate Hospitality Days **Location** Off B4100 between Adderbury
Hotel BUD Premier Travel Inn Banbury, Warwick Rd, Warmington,
BANBURY ☎ 0870 9906512 39 en suite

Rye Hill Milcombe OX15 4RU
☎ 01295 721818 ▤ 01295 720089
e-mail: info@ryehill.co.uk
web: www.ryehill.co.uk
Well-drained course, set in 200 acres of rolling countryside, with both parkland and heathland features, including wide fairways, large undulating greens, dramatic lakes, and fine views of the surrounding countryside.
18 holes, 6919yds, Par 72, SSS 73, Course record 62.
Club membership 575.
Visitors Mon-Sun & BHs. **Societies** tbooking required. **Green Fees** not confirmed. **Prof** Tony Pennock **Facilities** ⓣ ⓦ ⓛ by prior arrangement ⓛ ⓓ ⓣⓛ ⓐ 🖢 ⓨ 🕱 ⓨ **Leisure** fishing, pitch & putt course, tri-golf 9 hole family course. **Conf** facs Corporate Hospitality Days **Location** M40 junct 11, A361 towards Chipping Norton, signed 1m out of Bloxham
Hotel ★★★ 70% HL Best Western Wroxton House Hotel, Wroxton St Mary,
BANBURY ☎ 01295 730777 32 en suite

England

England

BURFORD
MAP 04 SP21

Burford Swindon Rd OX18 4JG
☎ 01993 822583 ▤ 01993 822801
e-mail: secretary@burfordgc.co.uk
web: www.burfordgolfclub.co.uk
Parkland with mature, tree-lined fairways and high quality greens.
18 holes, 6401yds, Par 71, SSS 71, Course record 64.
Club membership 770.
Visitors may play Mon-Sun except BHs. Booking required. Dress code.
Societies Booking required. **Green Fees** £40 per day. **Prof** Michael Ridge
Course Designer John H Turner **Facilities** ⑪ ⦿⍟ ➚ ♨ ⏱ ⚐ ♠ ⚑ ✦
Location 0.5m S off A361
Hotel ★★★ 73% HL Cotswold Gateway Hotel, Cheltenham Rd, BURFORD
☎ 01993 822695 13 en suite 8 annexe en suite

CHESTERTON
MAP 04 SP52

Bicester Golf & Country Club OX26 1TE
☎ 01869 242023 ▤ 01869 240754
e-mail: bicestergolf@ukonline.co.uk
18 holes, 6600yds, Par 71, SSS 70, Course record 68.
Course Designer R Stagg **Location** 0.5m W off A4095
Telephone for further details
Hotel ★★ 75% HL Best Western Jersey Arms Hotel, BICESTER
☎ 01869 343234 6 en suite 14 annexe en suite

CHIPPING NORTON
MAP 04 SP32

Chipping Norton Southcombe OX7 5QH
☎ 01608 642383 ▤ 01608 645422
e-mail: chipping.nortongc@virgin.net
Downland course situated at 800ft above sea level, its undulations
providing a good walk. On a limestone base, the course dries quickly
in wet conditions. The opening few holes provide a good test of golf
made more difficult when the prevailing wind makes the player use the
extremes of the course.

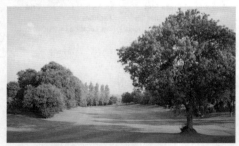

18 holes, 6241yds, Par 71, SSS 70, Course record 62.
Club membership 900.
Visitors Mon-Fri except BHs. Handicap certificate. Dress code.
Societies Welcome. **Green Fees** £32 per day. ⚉ **Prof** Neil Rowlands
Facilities ⑪ ⦿⍟ ➚ ♨ ⏱ ⚑ ⚐ ⛳ ✦ **Location** 1.5m E on A44
Hotel ★★★ 79% HL The Mill House Hotel & Restaurant, KINGHAM
☎ 01608 658188 21 en suite 2 annexe en suite

Wychwood Lyneham OX7 6QQ
☎ 01993 831841 ▤ 01993 831775
e-mail: wychwoodgolfclub@btconnect.com
Wychwood was designed to use the natural features of its location. It
is set in 170 acres on the fringe of the Cotswolds and blends superbly

with its surroundings. Lakes and streams enhance the challenge of the
course with water coming into play on eight of the 18 holes. All greens
are sand based, built to USGA specification.
18 holes, 6844yds, Par 72, SSS 72, Course record 67.
Club membership 750.
Visitors may play Mon-Sun except BHs. Advance booking required. Dress
code. **Societies** advance booking required. **Green Fees** not confirmed.
Prof James Fincher **Facilities** ⑪ ⦿⍟ ➚ ♨ ⏱ ⚑ ⚐ ⛳ ✦ ✦
Leisure fishing. **Conf** facs Corporate Hospitality Days **Location** Off A361
between Burford & Norton
Hotel ★★★ 79% HL The Mill House Hotel & Restaurant, KINGHAM
☎ 01608 658188 21 en suite 2 annexe en suite

DIDCOT
MAP 04 SU59

Hadden Hill Wallingford Rd OX11 9BJ
☎ 01235 510410 ▤ 01235 511260
e-mail: info@haddenhillgolf.co.uk
web: www.haddenhillgolf.co.uk
A challenging course on undulating terrain with excellent drainage.
Superb greens and fairways.
18 holes, 6563yds, Par 71, SSS 71, Course record 65.
Club membership 400.
Visitors Mon-Sun & BHs. Booking required. Dress code. **Societies** Booking
required. **Green Fees** £19 per 18 holes; £11.50 per 9 holes (£24/£14.50
Sat & Sun). ⚉ **Prof** Ian Mitchell **Course Designer** Michael V Morley
Facilities ⑪ ⦿⍟ by prior arrangement ➚ ♨ ⏱ ⚑ ⚐ ♠ ⚑ ⛳ ✦ ✦
Leisure teaching academy. **Conf** Corporate Hospitality Days **Location**
A34 Milton interchange, follow A4130, Course located 1m E of Didcot on
Wallingford Road
Hotel ★★★ 74% HL Abingdon Four Pillars Hotel, Marcham Rd,
ABINGDON ☎ 0800 374 692 & 01235 553456 ▤ 01235 554117 63 en suite

FARINGDON
MAP 04 SU29

Carswell Carswell SN7 8PU
☎ 01367 870422
e-mail: info@carswellgolfandcountryclub.co.uk
web: www.carswellgolfandcountryclub.co.uk
An attractive course set in undulating wooded countryside close
to Faringdon. Mature trees, five lakes and well-placed bunkers add
interest to the course. Floodlit driving range.

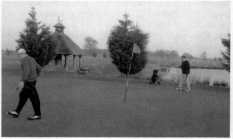

18 holes, 6183yds, Par 72, SSS 70. Club membership 520.
Visitors Mon-Sun & BHs. Booking required. Dress code. **Societies** Booking
required. **Green Fees** £20 per 18 holes (£28 Sat, Sun & BHs). **Prof** Jamie
Clutterbuck **Course Designer** J & E Ely **Facilities** ⑪ ⦿⍟ ➚ ♨ ⏱ ⚑ ⚐
♠ ✦ ⛳ ✦ ✦ **Leisure** sauna, solarium, gymnasium. **Conf** Corporate
Hospitality Days **Location** Off A420
Hotel ★★★ 75% HL BW Sudbury House Hotel & Conference Centre,
London St, FARINGDON ☎ 01367 241272 49 en suite

FRILFORD
MAP 04 SU49

Frilford Heath OX13 5NW
☎ 01865 390864 📠 01865 390823
e-mail: secretary@frilfordheath.co.uk
web: www.frilfordheath.co.uk
Fifty-four holes in three layouts of differing character. The Green course is a fully mature heathland course of some 6006yds. The Red Course is of championship length at 6884yds with a parkland flavour and a marked degree of challenge. The Blue Course is of modern design, and at 6728yds, it incorporates water hazards and large shallow sand traps.
Red Course: 18 holes, 6884yds, Par 73, SSS 73, Course record 66.
Green Course: 18 holes, 6006yds, Par 69, SSS 69, Course record 67.
Blue Course: 18 holes, 6728yds, Par 72, SSS 72, Course record 63. Club membership 1300.
Visitors may play Mon-Sun & BHs. Handicap certificate. Dress code. **Societies** Booking required. **Green Fees** £65 per day (£80 Sat & Sun). **Prof** Derek Craik **Course Designer** J Taylor/D Cotton/S Gidman **Facilities** ⑪ ⑩ ⅃ ⅃ ⅃ ⅃ ⅃ ⅃ ⅃ ⅃ **Conf** facs Corporate Hospitality Days **Location** 0.5m N of Frilford off A338
Hotel ★★★ 74% HL Abingdon Four Pillars Hotel, Marcham Rd, ABINGDON ☎ 0800 374 692 & 01235 553456 📠 01235 554117 63 en suite

HENLEY-ON-THAMES
MAP 04 SU78

Badgemore Park Badgemore RG9 4NR
☎ 01491 637300 📠 01491 576899
e-mail: info@badgemorepark.com
web: www.badgemorepark.com
Formerly a country estate, Badgemore Park was transformed in 1971 into a beautiful 18 hole parkland golf course, cleverly designed to challenge golfers of all standards.

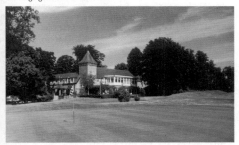

18 holes, 6129yds, Par 69, SSS 69, Course record 64.
Club membership 700.
Visitors Mon-Sun & BHs. Booking required Fri-Sun & BHs. Dress code. **Societies** Booking required. **Green Fees** £29 per round (£38 Sat, Sun & BHs). **Prof** Jonathan Dunn **Course Designer** Robert Sandow **Facilities** ⑪ ⅃ ⅃ ⅃ ⅃ ⅃ ⅃ ⅃ ⅃ **Conf** facs Corporate Hospitality Days **Location** N from Henley towards Rotherfield Greys, 1.5m on right
Hotel ★★★ 72% HL The White Hart Nettlebed, High St, Nettlebed, HENLEY-ON-THAMES ☎ 01491 641245 6 en suite 6 annexe en suite

Henley Harpsden RG9 4HG
☎ 01491 575742 📠 01491 412179
e-mail: admin@henleygc.com
web: www.henleygc.com
Designed by James Braid in 1907, the course retains many of his classic features, while being a challenge for all golfers even with modern technology. The first four holes are considered the hardest opening holes of any course in Oxfordshire and possibly the UK. The club celebrated its centenary in 2007.
18 holes, 6329yds, Par 70, SSS 70, Course record 62.
Club membership 700.
Visitors Mon-Fri. Handicap certificate required. Dress code. **Societies** Booking required. **Green Fees** £55 per day, £45 per round, £35 after 4pm. **Prof** Mark Howell **Course Designer** James Braid **Facilities** ⑪ ⑩ ⅃ ⅃ ⅃ ⅃ ⅃ ⅃ ⅃ **Conf** Corporate Hospitality Days **Location** 1.25m S off A4155

HORTON-CUM-STUDLEY
MAP 04 SP51

Studley Wood The Straight Mile OX33 1BF
☎ 01865 351122 & 351144 📠 01865 351166
e-mail: admin@swgc.co.uk.
web: www.studleywoodgolf.co.uk.
Gently undulating woodland course set in a former deer park. Tranquil setting with an abundance of wildlife. USGA specification tees and greens, with lakes coming into play on nine holes.
18 holes, 6811yds, Par 73, SSS 72, Course record 65.
Club membership 700.
Visitors Mon-Fri. Sat, Sun & BHs pm only. Booking required. Dress code. **Societies** Booking required. **Green Fees** £36 per round (£46 per round Sat & Sun). **Prof** Tony Williams **Course Designer** Simon Gidman **Facilities** ⑪ ⑩ ⅃ ⅃ ⅃ ⅃ ⅃ ⅃ ⅃ **Leisure** teaching studio with video facilities. **Conf** facs Corporate Hospitality Days **Location** 6m NE of Oxford, off B4027 to Horton
Hotel ★★★★ 76% HL The Paramount Oxford Hotel, Godstow Rd, Wolvercote Roundabout, OXFORD ☎ 01865 489988 168 en suite

KIRTLINGTON
MAP 04 SP41

Kirtlington OX5 3JY
☎ 01869 351133 📠 01869 351143
e-mail: info@kirtlingtongolfclub.com
web: www.kirtlingtongolfclub.com
An inland links-type course with challenging greens. The course incorporates many natural features and has 102 bunkers and a 110yd Par 3 19th when an extra hole is required to determine a winner. The 9 hole course has three Par 4's and six Par 3's with all year round buggy track.
18 holes, 6107yds, Par 70, SSS 69, Course record 68.
Academy Course: 9 holes, 1535yds, Par 30, SSS 53.
Club membership 400.
Visitors Mon-Sun & BHs. Booking required. Dress code. Must contact in advance. **Societies** Booking required. **Green Fees** £24 per 18 holes, £10 per 9 holes (£29/£12 Sat, Sun & BHs). **Prof** Andy Taylor **Course Designer** Graham Webster **Facilities** ⑪ ⅃ ⅃ ⅃ ⅃ ⅃ ⅃ ⅃ ⅃ **Leisure** 9 hole academy course. **Conf** facs Corporate Hospitality Days **Location** M40 junct 9, on A4095 outside Kirtlington
Hotel ★★★ 78% HL Weston Manor Hotel, WESTON-ON-THE-GREEN ☎ 01869 350621 15 en suite 20 annexe en suite

MILTON COMMON   MAP 04 SP60

The Oxfordshire Rycote Ln OX9 2PU
☎ 01844 278300 📠 01844 278003
e-mail: info@theoxfordshiregolfclub.com
web: www.theoxfordshiregolfclub.com
Designed by Rees Jones, The Oxfordshire is considered to be one of the most exciting courses in the country. The strategically contoured holes blend naturally into the surrounding countryside to provide a challenging game of golf. With four lakes and 135 bunkers, the course makes full use of the terrain and the natural elements to provide characteristics similar to those of a links course.

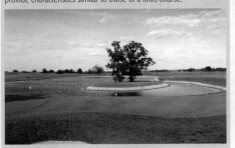

18 holes, 7192yds, Par 72, SSS 75, Course record 64.
Club membership 456.
Visitors Mon-Fri. Sat, Sun & BHs pm only. Booking required. Handicap certificate. Dress code. **Societies** Booking required. **Green Fees** Summer: £90 per 18 holes (£110 Sat, Sun & BHs). Winter: £65/£75.
Prof Stephen Gibson **Course Designer** Rees Jones **Facilities** ⑪ ⑩ by prior arrangement ▲ ☑ 𝄡 ⚐ 🏠 ☞ ⚒ ⚒ ⚐ **Leisure** Japanese ofuro baths, halfway house. **Conf** facs Corporate Hospitality Days
Location M40 junct 7, 1.5m on A329
Hotel ★★★ 82% HL Spread Eagle Hotel, Cornmarket, THAME
☎ 01844 213661 33 en suite

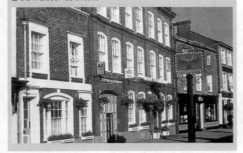

NUFFIELD   MAP 04 SU68

Huntercombe RG9 5SL
☎ 01491 641207 📠 01491 642060
e-mail: office@huntercombegolfclub.co.uk
web: www.huntercombegolfclub.co.uk
This heathland and woodland course overlooks the Oxfordshire plain and has many attractive and interesting fairways and fair true greens. Walking is easy after the 3rd which is a notable hole. The course is subject to wind and grass pot bunkers are interesting hazards.

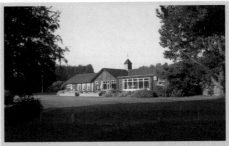

Huntercombe

18 holes, 6271yds, Par 70, SSS 70, Course record 63.
Club membership 800.
Visitors Mon-Sun & BHs. **Societies** Welcome. **Green Fees** £60 per day; £45 per round (£75/£60 per round Sat, Sun & BHs). **Prof** Ian Roberts
Course Designer Willie Park jnr **Facilities** ⑪ ⑩ ▲ ☑ 𝄡 ⚐ 🏠 ☞ ⚒
🏠 ⚒ **Location** Off A4130 at Nuffield
Hotel ★★★ 74% HL Shillingford Bridge Hotel, Shillingford, WALLINGFORD ☎ 01865 858567 32 en suite 8 annexe en suite

OXFORD   MAP 04 SP50

Hinksey Heights South Hinksey OX1 5AB
☎ 01865 327775 📠 01865 736930
e-mail: play@oxford-golf.co.uk
web: www.oxford-golf.co.uk
Set in an Area of Outstanding Natural Beauty, overlooking the incomparable Dreaming Spires of Oxford and the Thames Valley. The course has a heathland or links feel with several fairways running along the bottom of valleys created by the use of natural and man-made features.
18 holes, 6936yds, Par 72, SSS 73.
9 holes, 2547yds, Par 70, SSS 65. Club membership 600.
Visitors Mon-Sun & BHs. Booking required Mon & Tue. Dress code.
Societies Booking required. **Green Fees** £25 Mon-Thu, £28 Fri, £31 Sat & Sun. **Prof** Dean Davis **Course Designer** David Heads **Facilities** ⑪ ⑩ ▲
☑ 𝄡 ⚐ 🏠 ☞ ⚒ ⚒ **Leisure** 9 hole Par 3 course. **Conf** facs Corporate Hospitality Days **Location** On A34 Oxford bypass between Hinksey Hill and Botley Junct, signed
Hotel ★★★ 74% HL Hawkwell House, Church Way, Iffley Village, OXFORD ☎ 01865 749988 66 en suite

North Oxford Banbury Rd OX2 8EZ
☎ 01865 554924 📠 01865 515921
e-mail: manager@nogc.co.uk
web: www.nogc.co.uk
Gently undulating parkland.
18 holes, 5736yds, Par 67, SSS 67, Course record 62.
Club membership 600.
Visitors Mon-Sun & BHs. **Societies** booking required. **Green Fees** not confirmed. **Prof** Robert Harris **Facilities** ⑪ ⑩ ▲ ☑ 𝄡 ⚐ 🏠 ☞ ⚒
Conf Corporate Hospitality Days **Location** 3m N of city centre on A4165
Hotel ★★★★ 76% HL The Paramount Oxford Hotel, Godstow Rd, Wolvercote Roundabout, OXFORD ☎ 01865 489988 168 en suite

Southfield Hill Top Rd OX4 1PF
☎ 01865 242158 📠 01865 250023
e-mail: sgcltd@btopenworld.com
web: www.southfieldgolf.com
Home of the City, University and Ladies Clubs, and well-known to
graduates throughout the world. A challenging course, in a varied
parkland setting, providing a real test for players.

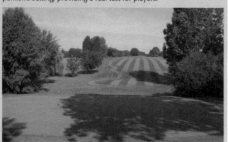

18 holes, 6325yds, Par 70, SSS 70, Course record 61.
Club membership 740.
Visitors Mon-Sun & BHs. Booking required Sat, Sun & BHs. Dress code.
Societies Welcome. **Green Fees** £40 per day/round. **Prof** Tony Rees
Course Designer H S Colt **Facilities** ⊕ ⏸ ▮ ☕ ☞ ⚬ ⛿ ☟ ▦ ▦
⚌ **Conf** Corporate Hospitality Days **Location** 1.5m SE of city centre
off B480
Hotel ★★★ 77% HL Westwood Country Hotel, Hinksey Hill, Boars Hill,
OXFORD ☎ 01865 735408 23 en suite

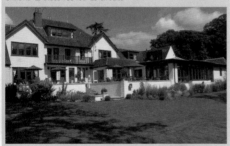

SHRIVENHAM   MAP 04 SU28

Shrivenham Park Penny Hooks Ln SN6 8EX
☎ 01793 783853
e-mail: info@shrivenhampark.com
web: www.shrivenhampark.com
A flat, mature parkland course with excellent drainage. A good
challenge for all standards of golfer.
18 holes, 5769yds, Par 69, SSS 69, Course record 64.
Club membership 150.
Visitors Mon & BHs. Booking required Sat, Sun & BHs. Dress code.
Societies Welcome. **Green Fees** £16 per 18 holes £10 per 9 holes (£21/£12
Sat, Sun & BHs). **Prof** Richard Jefferies **Course Designer** Gordon Cox
Facilities ⊕ ⏸ ▮ ☕ ☞ ⚬ ☟ ▦ ⚬ **Conf** Corporate Hospitality Days
Location 0.5m NE of town centre on A420 towards Oxford
Hotel ★★★ 75% HL BW Sudbury House Hotel & Conference Centre,
London St, FARINGDON ☎ 01367 241272 49 en suite

TADMARTON   MAP 04 SP33

Tadmarton Heath OX15 5HL
☎ 01608 737278 📠 01608 730548
e-mail: thgc@btinternet.com
web: ww.thgc.btinternet.co.uk
A mixture of heath and sandy land on a plateau in the Cotswolds.
The course opens gently before reaching the scenic 7th hole across
a trout stream close to the clubhouse. The course then progressively
tightens through the gorse before a challenging 430yd dog-leg
completes the round.
18 holes, 5936yds, Par 69, SSS 69, Course record 62.
Club membership 650.
Visitors Mon-Wed, Fri-Sun & BHs. Booking required. Handicap certificate.
Dress code. **Societies** Booking required. **Green Fees** £45 per day,
£40 after 10am (£50 Sat & Sun, £40 after 12pm). Reduced winter rates.
Prof Tom Jones **Course Designer** Col C K Hutchison **Facilities** ⊕ ⏸
by prior arrangement ▮ ☕ ☞ ⚬ ☟ ▦ ▦ ⚬ **Leisure** fishing.
Conf facs Corporate Hospitality Days **Location** 1m SW of Lower
Tadmarton off B4035, 6m from Banbury
Hotel ★★★ 77% HL Best Western Banbury House, Oxford Rd,
BANBURY ☎ 01295 259361 64 en suite

WALLINGFORD   MAP 04 SU68

The Springs Hotel & Golf Club Wallingford Rd, North
Stoke OX10 6BE
☎ 01491 827310 📠 01491 827312
e-mail: proshop@thespringshotel.com
web: www.thespringshotel.com
The 133 acres of parkland are bordered by the River Thames, within
which lie three lakes and challenging wetland areas. The course has
traditional features like a double green and sleepered bunker with
sleepered lake edges of typical American design.
18 holes, 6470yds, Par 72, SSS 71, Course record 67.
Club membership 610.
Visitors Mon-Sun & BHs. Booking required. Dress code. **Societies** Booking
required. **Green Fees** £29 per 18 holes (£35 Sat, Sun & BHs). **Prof** David
Boyce **Course Designer** Brian Hugget **Facilities** ⊕ ⏸ ▮ ☕ ☞ ⚬ ☟ ▦
⚬ ▦ ⚬ **Leisure** heated outdoor swimming pool, fishing, sauna, croquet
lawn. **Conf** facs Corporate Hospitality Days **Location** 2m SE of town centre
over River Thames
Hotel ★★★ 78% HL The Springs Hotel & Golf Club, Wallingford Rd, North
Stoke, WALLINGFORD ☎ 01491 836687 32 en suite

WATERSTOCK   MAP 04 SP60

Waterstock Thame Rd OX33 1HT
☎ 01844 338093 📠 01844 338036
e-mail: wgc_oxfordgolf@btinternet.com
web: www.waterstockgolf.co.uk
A 6500yd course designed by Donald Steel with USGA greens and
tees fully computer irrigated. Four Par 3s facing north, south, east and
west. A brook and hidden lake affect six holes, with dog-legs being 4th
and 10th holes. Five Par 5s on the course, making it a challenge for
players of all standards.
18 holes, 6535yds, Par 72, SSS 72, Course record 69.
Club membership 500.
Visitors Mon-Sun & BHs. Booking required. Dress code. **Societies** Booking
required. **Green Fees** £39 per day, £22 per round, £16 twilight, £12
for 9 holes (£46.50/£27/£18.50/£14.50 Sat. Sun & BHs). **Prof** Paul Bryant

Continued

Course Designer Donald Steel Facilities ⑪ ⦿ 🍴 ⛳ 🏌 ☂ 🏕 🎯 🏌 🛥
🏌 🎣 Leisure fishing. Conf facs Corporate Hospitality Days Location M40
junct 8/8A, E of Oxford near Wheatley
Hotel ★★★ 82% HL Spread Eagle Hotel, Cornmarket, THAME
☎ 01844 213661 33 en suite

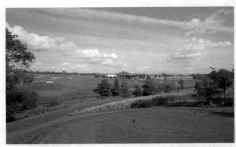

WITNEY   MAP 04 SP31

Witney Lakes Downs Rd OX29 0SY
☎ 01993 893011 📠 01993 778866
e-mail: golf@witney-lakes.co.uk
web: www.witney-lakes.co.uk
Five large lakes come into play on eight holes. An excellent test of golf
that will use every club in your bag.
18 holes, 6700yds, Par 71, Course record 67.
Club membership 450.
Visitors Mon-Sun & BHs. Dress code. Societies Welcome.
Green Fees £20 per 18 holes (£29 Sat & Sun). Course Designer Simon
Gidman Facilities ⑪ ⦿ 🍴 ⛳ 🏌 ☂ 🏕 🎯 🏌 🎣 Leisure outdoor
and indoor heated swimming pools, sauna, solarium, gymnasium, trim
trail. Conf facs Corporate Hospitality Days Location 2m W of Witney town
centre, off B4047 Witney/Burford road
Hotel ★★★ 75% HL Witney Four Pillars Hotel, Ducklington Ln, WITNEY
☎ 0800 374 692 & 01993 779777 📠 01993 703467 86 en suite

RUTLAND

GREAT CASTERTON   MAP 04 TF00

Rutland County PE9 4AQ
☎ 01780 460330 📠 01780 460437
e-mail: info@rutlandcountygolf.co.uk
web: www.rutlandcountygolf.co.uk
Inland links-style course with gently rolling fairways, large tees and
greens. Playable all year round due to good drainage.
18 holes, 6425yds, Par 71, SSS 71, Course record 64.
Club membership 740.
Visitors Mon-Sun & BHs. Booking required. Dress code. Societies
Welcome. Green Fees £30 per day, £25 per round (£40/£30 Sat & Sun).
Prof Ian Melville Course Designer Cameron Sinclair Facilities ⑪ ⦿ 🍴 ⛳
🏌 ☂ 🏕 🎯 🏌 🎣 Leisure Par 3 course. Conf facs Corporate
Hospitality Days Location 2m N of Stamford on A1
Hotel ★★ 74% HL The White Horse Inn, Main St, EMPINGHAM
☎ 01780 460221 4 en suite 9 annexe en suite

GREETHAM   MAP 08 SK91

Greetham Valley Wood Ln LE15 7NP
☎ 01780 460444 📠 01780 460623
e-mail: info@greethamvalley.co.uk
web: www.greethamvalley.co.uk
Set in 267 acres of attractive undulating countryside. Both courses
feature numerous water hazards including ponds, lakes and the
meandering North Brook. Renowned for hand cut greens which are
fast and true.

Greetham Valley

Lakes: 18 holes, 6764yds, Par 72, SSS 72, Course record 65.
Valley: 18 holes, 5595yds, Par 68, SSS 67,
Course record 64. Club membership 1100.
Visitors Mon-Sun & BHs. Booking required. Dress code. Societies Booking
required. Green Fees £50 per day. Prof Neil Evans Course Designer
F E Hinch/B Stephens Facilities ⑪ ⦿ 🍴 ⛳ 🏌 ☂ 🏕 🎯 🏌 🎣
🎣 Leisure fishing, bowls green, 9 hole Par 3, quad biking. Conf facs
Corporate Hospitality Days Location A1 onto B668 Oakham road, course
signed
Hotel ★★★ 74% HL Greetham Valley, Wood Ln, GREETHAM
☎ 01780 460444 35 en suite

KETTON   MAP 04 SK90

Luffenham Heath PE9 3UU
☎ 01780 720205 📠 01780 722146
e-mail: jringleby@theluffenhamheathgc.co.uk
web: www.luffenhamheath.co.uk
A James Braid course with firm driving fairways framed by swaying
fescue, cross bunkers, grassy wastes and subtly undulating
greens, hemmed in by sculpted traps. Many outstanding and
challenging holes, placing a premium on accuracy. The 17th Par 3
signature hole is downhill over a tangle of mounds and studded with
tricky bunkers.

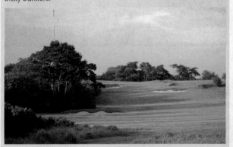

18 holes, 6563yds, Par 70, SSS 72, Course record 64.
Club membership 550.
Visitors Mon, Wed-Sun & BHs. Booking required Sat, Sun & BHs.
Handicap certificate. Dress code. Societies Booking required.
Green Fees Phone. Prof Ian Burnett Course Designer James Braid
Facilities ⑪ ⦿ 🍴 ⛳ 🏌 ☂ 🏕 🎯 Conf Corporate Hospitality Days
Location 1.5m SW of Ketton on A6121 by Foster's Bridge
Hotel ★★★ 85% HL The George of Stamford, 71 St Martins, STAMFORD
☎ 01780 750750 & 750700 (Res) 📠 01780 750701 47 en suite

England

SHROPSHIRE

BRIDGNORTH
MAP 07 SO79

Bridgnorth Stanley Ln WV16 4SF
☎ 01746 763315 📠 01746 763315
e-mail: secretary.bgc@tiscali.co.uk
web: www.bridgnorthgolfclub.co.uk
Pleasant parkland by the River Severn.
18 holes, 6582yds, Par 73, SSS 72, Course record 68.
Club membership 725.
Visitors Mon.Tue, Thu, Fri, Sun & BHs. Booking required Sat. Dress code.
Societies Booking required. **Green Fees** £35 per day, £28 per round
(£45/£35 Sat, Sun & BHs). ⊕ **Prof** Paul Hinton **Facilities** ⑪ ⑩ ☕ ☁ ☉
⚲ ☎ ✓ ☎ ✓ **Leisure** fishing, sauna. **Conf** Corporate Hospitality Days
Location 1m N off B4373

CHURCH STRETTON
MAP 07 SO49

Church Stretton Trevor Hill SY6 6JH
☎ 01694 722281 📠 01743 861918
e-mail: secretary@churchstrettongolfclub.co.uk
web: www.churchstrettongolfclub.co.uk
Hillside course designed by James Braid on the lower slopes of the
Long Mynd, with magnificent views and well-drained turf. One of the
highest courses in Britain.
18 holes, 5020yds, Par 66, SSS 65, Course record 58.
Club membership 450.
Visitors Contact club for details. Dress code. **Societies** Welcome.
Green Fees £20 (£25 weekends & bank holidays). **Prof** J Townsend
Course Designer James Braid **Facilities** ⑪ ⑩ ☕ ☁ ☉ ⚲ ☎ ☓ ✓
Location W of town. From Cardington Valley up steep Trevor Hill

CLEOBURY MORTIMER
MAP 07 SO67

Cleobury Mortimer Wyre Common DY14 8HQ
☎ 01299 271112 📠 01299 271468
e-mail: secretary@cleoburygolfclub.com
web: www.cleoburygolfclub.com
Well-designed 27-hole parkland course set in undulating countryside
with fine views from all holes. An interesting challenge to golfers of
all abilities.

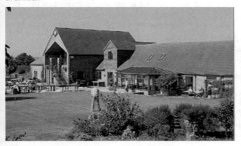

Foxes Run: 9 holes, 2980yds, Par 34, SSS 34.
Badgers Sett: 9 holes, 3271yds, Par 36, SSS 36.
Deer Park: 9 holes, 3167yds, Par 35, SSS 35.
Club membership 650.
Visitors Mon-Sun & BHs. Booking required. Dress code. **Societies** Booking
required. **Green Fees** £30 per day, £24 per 18 holes (£40/£32 Sat & Sun).
Prof Jon Jones/Martin Payne **Course Designer** E.G.U **Facilities** ⑪ ⑩

☕ ☁ ☉ ⚲ ☎ ✓ ☎ ✓ **Leisure** fishing, snooker table. **Conf** facs
Corporate Hospitality Days **Location** On A4117 1m N of Cleobury Mortimer
Inn ★★★★ INN The Crown Inn, Hopton Wafers, CLEOBURY MORTIMER
☎ 01299 270372 18 rms

LILLESHALL
MAP 07 SJ71

Lilleshall Hall TF10 9AS
☎ 01952 603840 & 604776 📠 01952 604776
18 holes, 5906yds, Par 68, SSS 68, Course record 65.
Course Designer H S Colt **Location** 3m SE
Telephone for further details
Hotel ★★★ 78% HL Hadley Park House, Hadley Park, TELFORD
☎ 01952 677269 12 en suite

LUDLOW
MAP 07 SO57

Ludlow Bromfield SY8 2BT
☎ 01584 856366 📠 01584 856366
e-mail: secretary@ludlowgolfclub.com
web: www.ludlowgolfclub.com
A long-established heathland course in the middle of the racecourse.
Very flat, quick drying, with broom and gorse-lined fairways.
18 holes, 6277yds, Par 70, SSS 70, Course record 65.
Club membership 700.
Visitors Mon-Sun & BHs. Handicap certificate. Dress code. **Societies**
Booking required. **Green Fees** £28 per round/£35 per day (£35 per round
Sat, Sun & BHs). ⊕ **Prof** Russell Price **Facilities** ⑪ ⑩ ☕ ☁ ☉ ⚲ ☎ ✓
✓ **Conf** Corporate Hospitality Days **Location** 1m N of Ludlow off A49
Hotel ★★★ 79% HL The Feathers Hotel, The Bull Ring, LUDLOW
☎ 01584 875261 40 en suite

MARKET DRAYTON
MAP 07 SJ63

Market Drayton Sutton Ln TF9 2HX
☎ 01630 652266 📠 01630 656564
e-mail: market.draytongc@btconnect.com
web: www.marketdraytongolfclub.co.uk
Undulating parkland course with two steep banks in quiet, picturesque
surroundings, providing a good test of golf.
18 holes, 6290yds, Par 71, SSS 71, Course record 67.
Club membership 600.
Visitors Mon, Wed-Fri except BHs. Booking required. Handicap certificate.
Dress code. **Societies** Welcome. **Green Fees** Summer £28 per round;
Winter £22. ⊕ **Prof** Russell Clewes **Facilities** ⑪ ⑩ ☕ ☁ ☉ ⚲ ☎ ◇ ☎
✓ **Conf** Corporate Hospitality Days **Location** 1m S off A41/A529
Hotel ★★★ 82% HL Goldstone Hall, Goldstone, MARKET DRAYTON
☎ 01630 661202 11 en suite

NEWPORT
MAP 07 SJ72

Aqualate Golf Centre Stafford Rd TF10 9DB
☎ 01952 811699
9 holes, 5659yds, Par 69, SSS 67, Course record 67.
Location 2m E of town centre on A518, 400yds from junct A41
Telephone for further details
Hotel ★★★ 78% HL Hadley Park House, Hadley Park, TELFORD
☎ 01952 677269 12 en suite

OSWESTRY

MAP 07 SJ22

Mile End Mile End, Old Shrewsbury Rd SY11 4JF
☎ 01691 671246 📄 01691 670580
e-mail: info@mileendgolfclub.co.uk
web: www.mileendgolfclub.co.uk
A gently undulating parkland-type course covering over 135 acres and including a number of water features, notably the 3rd, 8th and 17th holes, which have greens protected by large pools. The longest hole is the Par 5, 542yd 14th, complete with its two tiered green.
18 holes, 6233yds, Par 71, SSS 70, Course record 66.
Club membership 700.
Visitors Mon-Sun & BHs. Dress code. **Societies** Booking required.
Green Fees £17 per round, Fri £19, £26 Sat, Sun & BHs). **Prof** Scott Carpenter **Course Designer** Price/Gough **Facilities** ⑪ ⓑ ⌨ ⅋ ⏛ ⌚ ⌂ ⌇ ⌁ **Conf** Corporate Hospitality Days **Location** 1m SE of Oswestry, signposted off A5/A483
Hotel ★★★ 87% HL Best Western Wynnstay Hotel, Church St, OSWESTRY ☎ 01691 655261 29 en suite

Oswestry Aston Park, Queens Head SY11 4JJ
☎ 01691 610535 📄 01691 610535
e-mail: secretary@oswestrygolfclub.co.uk
web: www.oswestrygolfclub.co.uk
Gently undulating mature parkland course set in splendid Shropshire countryside. Free draining soils make Oswestry an ideal year round test of golf.
18 holes, 6038yds, Par 70, SSS 69, Course record 61.
Club membership 960.
Visitors Mon-Sun & BHs. Booking required. Handicap certificate. Dress code. **Societies** Booking required. **Green Fees** £35 per day, £28 per round (£38/£32 Sat & Sun). **Prof** D Skelton/J Davies **Course Designer** James Braid **Facilities** ⑪ ⍥ ⓑ ⌨ ⅋ ⏛ ⌚ ⌂ ⌇ ⌁ **Conf** Corporate Hospitality Days **Location** 2m SE on A5
Hotel ★★★ 87% HL Best Western Wynnstay Hotel, Church St, OSWESTRY ☎ 01691 655261 29 en suite

PANT

MAP 07 SJ22

Llanymynech SY10 8LB
☎ 01691 830983 & 830542 📄 01691 839184
e-mail: secretary.llanygc@btinternet.com
web: www.llanymynechgolfclub.co.uk
Upland course on the site of a prehistoric hill fort with far-reaching views. With 15 holes in Wales and three in England, drive off in Wales and putt out in England on 4th hole. A quality mature course with a tremendous variety of holes.
18 holes, 6114yds, Par 70, SSS 69, Course record 64.
Club membership 750.
Visitors Mon-Fri & BHs. Booking required. Dress code. **Societies** booking required. **Green Fees** £38 per day, £28 per round (£35 BHs). ⓔ **Prof** Andrew P Griffiths **Facilities** ⑪ ⍥ ⓑ ⌨ ⅋ ⏛ ⌚ ⌂ ⌁ **Conf** Corporate Hospitality Days **Location** 6m S of Oswestry, off A483 in Pant at Cross Guns Inn
Hotel ★★★ 87% HL Best Western Wynnstay Hotel, Church St, OSWESTRY ☎ 01691 655261 29 en suite

SHIFNAL

MAP 07 SJ70

Shifnal Decker Hill TF11 8QL
☎ 01952 460330 📄 01952 460330
e-mail: secretary@shifnalgolfclub.co.uk
web: www.shifnalgolfclub.co.uk
Well-wooded parkland. Walking is easy and an attractive country mansion serves as the clubhouse.
18 holes, 6468yds, Par 71, SSS 71, Course record 65.
Club membership 700.
Visitors Mon-Fri except BHs. Booking required. Handicap certificate.
Dress code. **Societies** Booking required. **Green Fees** £40 per day, £30 per 18 holes. **Prof** David Ashton **Course Designer** Pennick **Facilities** ⑪ ⍥ ⓑ ⌨ ⅋ ⏛ ⌚ ⌂ ⌁ **Conf** Corporate Hospitality Days **Location** 1m N off B4379
Hotel ★★★★ 75% HL Park House Hotel, Park St, SHIFNAL
☎ 01952 460128 38 en suite 16 annexe en suite

SHREWSBURY

MAP 07 SJ41

Arscott Arscott, Pontesbury SY5 0XP
☎ 01743 860114 📄 01743 860881
e-mail: golf@arscott.dydirect.net
web: www.arscottgolfclub.co.uk
At 365ft above sea level, the views from Arscott Golf Club of the hills of south Shropshire and Wales are superb. Arscott is set in mature parkland with water features and holes demanding all sorts of club choice. A challenge to all golfers both high and low handicap.
18 holes, 6178yds, Par 70, SSS 69, Course record 66.
Club membership 550.
Visitors Mon-Sun & BHs. Booking required. Dress code. **Societies** Booking required. **Green Fees** £20 per round (£25 Sat, Sun & BHs). ⓔ **Prof** Glyn Sadd **Course Designer** M Hamer **Facilities** ⑪ ⍥ ⓑ ⌨ ⅋ ⏛ ⌚ ⌂ ⌁ **Leisure** fishing, sports injury treatment, massage. **Conf** facs **Location** Off A488 S of town
Hotel The Lion Hotel, Wyle Cop, SHREWSBURY ☎ 01743 353107 59 en suite

Shrewsbury Condover SY5 7BL
☎ 01743 872977 📄 01743 872977
e-mail: info@shrewsbury-golf-club.co.uk
web: www.club-noticeboard.co.uk/shrewsbury
Parkland course. First nine flat, second undulating with good views of the Long Mynd. Several holes with water features. Fast putting surfaces.
18 holes, 6300yds, Par 70, SSS 70. Club membership 872.
Visitors Mon & Fri. Booking required. Handicap certificate. Dress code.
Societies Booking required. **Green Fees** Phone. ⓔ **Prof** Peter Seal **Facilities** ⑪ ⍥ ⓑ ⌨ ⅋ ⏛ ⌚ ⌂ ⌇ ⌁ **Location** 4m S off A49
Hotel ★★★ 82% HL Prince Rupert Hotel, Butcher Row, SHREWSBURY ☎ 01743 499955 70 en suite

TELFORD
MAP 07 SJ60

Shropshire Golf Centre Granville Park, Muxton TF2 8PQ
☎ 01952 677800 📠 01952 677622
e-mail: sales@theshropshire.co.uk
web: www.theshropshire.co.uk
This 27-hole course is set in rolling countryside. The three loops of nine make the most of the natural undulations and provide a challenge for golfer of all abilities. Ample stretches of water and bullrush lined ditches, wide countered fairways and rolling greens guarded by mature trees, hummocks and vast bunkers. Several elevated tees with spectacular views.
Blue: 9 holes, 3286yds, Par 35, SSS 35.
Silver: 9 holes, 3303yds, Par 36, SSS 36.
Gold: 9 holes, 3334yds, Par 36, SSS 36.
Club membership 495.
Visitors Mon-Sun & BHs. Booking required. Dress code. **Societies** Booking required. **Green Fees** £25 per 27 holes, £18 per 18 holes, £12 per 9 holes (£30/£22/£14 Sat, Sun & BHs). **Prof** Rob Grier **Course Designer** Martin Hawtree **Facilities** ⊕ �️🍴 ⅃ ⬜ ⏚ ⚐ ⅄ ⌂ ✔ ✔ 🏌 ⌁ **Leisure** Par 3 14 hole academy course. **Conf** facs Corporate Hospitality Days **Location** M54/A5 onto B5060 towards Donnington, 3rd exit at Granville rdbt
Hotel ★★★ 78% HL Hadley Park House, Hadley Park, TELFORD
☎ 01952 677269 12 en suite

Telford Golf & Country Club Great Hay Dr, Sutton Heights TF7 4DT
☎ 01952 429977 📠 01952 586602
18 holes, 6761yds, Par 72, SSS 72, Course record 66.
Course Designer Harris/Griffiths **Location** 4m S of town off A442
Telephone for further details
Hotel ★★★ 78% HL Hadley Park House, Hadley Park, TELFORD
☎ 01952 677269 12 en suite

WELLINGTON
MAP 07 SJ61

Wrekin Ercall Woods, Golf Links Ln TF6 5BX
☎ 01952 244032 📠 01952 252906
e-mail: wrekingolfclub@btconnect.com
Downland course with some hard walking but superb views.

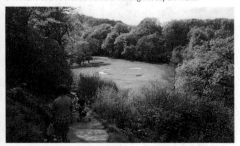

18 holes, 5570yds, Par 67, SSS 66, Course record 62.
Club membership 675.
Visitors Mon, Wed-Sun & BHs. Tue pm only. Booking required. Dress code.
Societies Booking required. **Green Fees** £30 per day, £22 per round (£30 per round Sat, Sun & BHs). ⊛ **Prof** K Housden **Facilities** ⊕ ⊍🍴 ⅃ ⬜ ⏚
⌂ ⚐ ✔ **Location** M54 junct 7, 1.25m S off B5061
Hotel ★★★ 78% HL Hadley Park House, Hadley Park, TELFORD
☎ 01952 677269 12 en suite

WESTON-UNDER-REDCASTLE
MAP 07 SJ52

Hawkstone Park Hotel SY4 5UY
☎ 01939 200611 📠 01939 200335
e-mail: info@hawkstone.co.uk
web: www.hawkstone.co.uk
Hawkstone Course: 18 holes, 6491yds, Par 72, SSS 71, Course record 65.
Windmill Course: 18 holes, 6476yds, Par 72, SSS 72, Course record 64.
Academy Course: 6 holes, 741yds, Par 18, SSS 18.
Course Designer J Braid **Location** Off A49/A442
Telephone for further details

WHITCHURCH
MAP 07 SJ54

Hill Valley Terrick Rd SY13 4JZ
☎ 01948 663584 & 667788 📠 01948 665927
e-mail: info@hillvalley.co.uk
web: www.hill-valley.co.uk
Emerald: 18 holes, 6628yds, Par 73, SSS 72, Course record 64.
Sapphire: 18 holes, 4800yds, Par 66, SSS 64.
Course Designer Peter Alliss/Dave Thomas **Location** 1m N. Follow signs from Bypass
Telephone for further details
Hotel ★★ 71% HL Best Western Crown Hotel & Restaurant, High St, NANTWICH ☎ 01270 625283 18 en suite

WORFIELD
MAP 07 SO79

Chesterton Valley Chesterton WV15 5NX
☎ 01746 783682
Dry course built on sandy soil giving excellent drainage. No temporary greens and no trolley ban.
18 holes, 5938yards, SSS 69. Club membership 450.
Visitors may play Mon-Sun & BHs. Advance booking required. Dress code.
Societies telephone in advance. **Green Fees** not confirmed. ⊛
Prof Philip HInton **Course Designer** Len Vanes **Facilities** ⬜ ⏚ ⅃ ⌂ ✔
⌁ ✔ **Location** On B4176
Hotel ★★★ HL Old Vicarage Hotel, Worfield, BRIDGNORTH
☎ 01746 716497 10 en suite 4 annexe en suite

Worfield Roughton WV15 5HE
☎ 01746 716372 📠 01746 716302
e-mail: enquiries@worfieldgolf.co.uk
web: www.worfieldgolf.co.uk
A parkland links mix with three large lakes, many bunkers and large trees giving a challenge to golfers. Superb views and drainage which allows play on full greens and tees all year. Water comes into play on four holes, including the short Par 4 18th where it lies in front of the green.
18 holes, 6545yds, Par 73, SSS 72, Course record 68.
Club membership 600.
Visitors Mon-Fri & BHs. Sat & Sun pm only. Booking required. Dress code.
Societies Booking required. **Green Fees** £20 per round. **Prof** Steve Russell
Course Designer T Williams **Facilities** ⊕ ⊍🍴 ⅃ ⬜ ⏚ ⅄ ⌂ ⚐ ✔
Conf facs Corporate Hospitality Days **Location** 3m W of off A454
Hotel ★★★ HL Old Vicarage Hotel, Worfield, BRIDGNORTH
☎ 01746 716497 10 en suite 4 annexe en suite

SOMERSET

BACKWELL
MAP 03 ST46

Tall Pines Cooks Bridle Path, Downside BS48 3DJ
☎ 01275 472076 🖹 01275 474869
e-mail: terry.murray3@btinternet.com
web: www.tallpinesgolfclub.co.uk
Free draining parkland with views over the Bristol Channel.
18 holes, 6049yds, Par 70, SSS 70, Course record 65.
Club membership 500.
Visitors Mon–Sun & BHs. Booking required Sat & Sun. Dress code.
Societies Welcome. **Green Fees** £20 per round. ⊜ **Prof** Alex Murray
Course Designer T Murray **Facilities** ⊕ ⊺⊙⊦ ⅃ ℡ ⊑ ⊀⅃ ♨ ☎ ♦ ⍾ ⏖ ⌖
Conf Corporate Hospitality Days **Location** Next to Bristol Airport, 1m off
A38/A370
Hotel ★★★ 70% HL Beachlands Hotel, 17 Uphill Rd North, WESTON-
SUPER-MARE ☎ 01934 621401 23 en suite

BATH
MAP 03 ST76

Bath Sham Castle, North Rd BA2 6JG
☎ 01225 463834 🖹 01225 331027
e-mail: enquiries@bathgolfclub.org.uk
web: www.bathgolfclub.org.uk
Considered to be one of the finest courses in the west, this is the
site of Bath's oldest golf club. Situated on high ground overlooking
the city and with splendid views over the surrounding countryside.
The rocky ground supports good quality turf and there are many
good holes. The 17th is a dog-leg right past, or over the corner of an
out of bounds wall, and then on to an undulating green.
18 holes, 6442yds, Par 71, SSS 71, Course record 66.
Club membership 750.
Visitors Mon–Sun & BHs. Handicap certificate. Dress code. **Societies**
Booking required. **Green Fees** £36 per 18 holes (£40 Sat, Sun & BHs).
Prof Peter J Hancox **Course Designer** Colt & others **Facilities** ⊕ ⊺⊙⊦ ℡
⊑ ⊀⅃ ♨ ☎ ♈ ♦ ⌖ **Conf** Corporate Hospitality Days **Location** 1.5m
SE city centre off A36
Hotel ★★★ 72% HL Mercure Francis Hotel, Queen Square, BATH
☎ 0870 400 8223 95 en suite

Entry Hill BA2 5NA
☎ 01225 834248
e-mail: timtapley@aol.com
web: www.bathpublicgolf.co.uk
Opened in 1984, this is a short but interesting 9 hole public pay and
play facility within a mile of the city centre. With its picturesque settings
and stunning views across Bath, the course provides enjoyment for
golfers of all standard.
9 holes, 2065yds, Par 33, SSS 30. Club membership 250.
Visitors Mon–Sun & BHs. Booking required Sat/Sun & BHs. **Societies**
booking required. **Green Fees** not confirmed. **Prof** Tim Tapley **Facilities** ⊕
℡ ⊑ ⊀ ☎ ♈ ♦ **Location** Off A367

Lansdown Lansdown BA1 9BT
☎ 01225 422138 🖹 01225 339252
e-mail: admin@lansdowngolfclub.co.uk
web: www.lansdowngolfclub.co.uk
A level parkland course situated 800ft above sea level, providing a
challenge to both low and high handicap golfers. Stunning views from
the 5th and 14th holes.

18 holes, 6428yds, Par 71, SSS 70, Course record 67.
Club membership 700.
Visitors Contact club for details. **Societies** Booking required.
Green Fees £40 per day, £30 per round, 9 holes £15. **Prof** Terry Mercer
Course Designer C A Whitcombe **Facilities** ⊕ ⊺⊙⊦ ℡ ⊑ ⊀⅃ ♨ ☎ ♙
♦ **Conf** facs Corporate Hospitality Days **Location** M4 junct 18, 6m SW by
Bath racecourse
Hotel ★★★ 73% HL Pratt's Hotel, South Pde, BATH ☎ 01225 460441
46 en suite

BRIDGWATER
MAP 03 ST23

Cannington Cannington Centre for, Land Based Studies,
Cannington TA5 2LS
☎ 01278 655050 🖹 01278 655055
e-mail: macrowr@bridgwater.ac.uk
Nine-hole links-style course with 18 tees. The 4th hole is a
challenging 464 yd Par 4, slightly uphill and into the prevailing wind.
9 holes, 6072yds, Par 68, SSS 70, Course record 64.
Club membership 300.
Visitors Mon–Sun & BHs. Booking required Sat, Sun & BHs. Dress code.
Societies Booking required. **Green Fees** 9 holes £10 (£13 per 9 holes,
£18.50 per 18 holes Sat & Sun). ⊜ **Prof** Ron Macrow **Course Designer**
Martin Hawtree **Facilities** ℡ ⊑ ⊀ ☎ ♈ ♦ ♈ **Location** 4m NW off A39
Hotel ★★ 79% HL Combe House Hotel, HOLFORD ☎ 01278 741382
17 en suite 1 annexe en suite

BURNHAM-ON-SEA
MAP 03 ST34

Brean Coast Rd, Brean Sands TA8 2QY
☎ 01278 752111(pro shop) 🖹 01278 752111
e-mail: proshop@brean.com
web: www.breangolfclub.co.uk

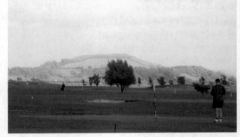

18 holes, 5715yds, Par 69, SSS 68, Course record 66.
Course Designer In House **Location** M5 junct 22, 4m on coast road
Telephone for further details
Hotel ★★ 72% HL Batch Country Hotel, Batch Ln, LYMPSHAM
☎ 01934 750371 10 en suite

Burnham & Berrow St Christopher's Way TA8 2PE
☎ 01278 785760 🖹 01278 795440
e-mail: secretary@burnhamandberrow.plus.com
web: www.burnhamandberrowgolfclub.co.uk
Natural championship links course with panoramic views of the
Somerset hills and the Bristol Channel. A true test of golf suitable
only for players with a handicap of 22 or better.

Continued

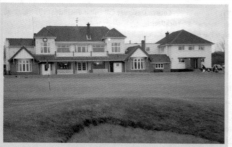

Burnham & Berrow

Championship Course: *18 holes, 6393yds, Par 71, SSS 71, Course record 64.*
Channel Course: *9 holes, 6120yds, Par 70, SSS 69.*
Club membership 900.
Visitors Mon-Fri & Sun except BHs. Handicap certificate required. Dress code. **Societies** Booking required. **Green Fees** Championship Course: £63 per day, £50 per round (£63 per round Sat, Sun & BHs). **Prof** Mark Crowther-Smith **Course Designer** H S Colt **Facilities** ⑪ ⑩↑ 🏐 ☐ 🏋 🏌 🏖 ⛳♥ ✦ **Location** 1m N of town on B3140
Hotel ★★ 71% HL Battleborough Grange Country Hotel, Bristol Rd - A38, BRENT KNOLL ☎ 01278 760208 22 en suite

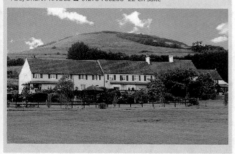

CHARD   MAP 03 ST30

Windwhistle Cricket St Thomas TA20 4DG
☎ 01460 30231 📄 01460 30055
e-mail: info@windwhistlegolfclub.co.uk
web: www.windwhistlegolf.co.uk
Parkland course at 735ft above sea level with outstanding views over the Somerset Levels to the Bristol Channel and south Wales.
East/West Course: *18 holes, 6176yds, Par 72, SSS 70, Course record 69. Club membership 500.*
Visitors Mon-Sun & BHs. Booking required. Dress code. **Societies** Booking required. **Green Fees** Phone. **Prof** Paul Deeprose **Course Designer** Braid & Taylor/Fisher **Facilities** ⑪ 🏐 ☐ 🏋 🏌 🏖 ⛳♥ ✦ **Leisure** squash.
Conf facs Corporate Hospitality Days **Location** 3m E on A30
Hotel ★★★ 77% HL Best Western Shrubbery Hotel, ILMINSTER ☎ 01460 52108 21 en suite

CLEVEDON   MAP 03 ST47

Clevedon Castle Rd, Walton St Mary BS21 7AA
☎ 01275 874057 📄 01275 341228
e-mail: secretary@clevedongolfclub.co.uk
web: clevedongolfclub.co.uk
Situated on the cliff overlooking the Severn estuary with distant views of the Welsh coast. Excellent parkland course in first-class condition. Magnificent scenery and some tremendous drop holes.
18 holes, 6557yds, Par 72, SSS 72, Course record 68.
Club membership 750.
Visitors Mon-Sun & BHs. Booking required. Handicap certificate. Dress code. **Societies** Booking required. **Green Fees** £32 per day (£40 Sat & Sun). ❀ **Prof** Robert Scanlan **Course Designer** S Herd **Facilities** ⑪ ⑩↑ 🏐 ☐ 🏋 🏌 🏖 ⛳ **Conf** facs Corporate Hospitality Days **Location** M5 junct 20, 1m NE of town centre
Hotel ★★★ 71% HL Best Western Walton Park Hotel, Wellington Ter, CLEVEDON ☎ 01275 874253 40 en suite

CONGRESBURY   MAP 03 ST46

Mendip Spring Honeyhall Ln BS49 5JT
☎ 01934 852322 📄 01934 853021
e-mail: info@mendipspringgolfclub.com
web: www.mendipspring.co.uk
Set in peaceful countryside with the Mendip Hills as a backdrop, this 18-hole course includes lakes and numerous water hazards covering some 12 acres of the course. The 12th is an island green surrounded by water and there are long drives on the 7th and 13th. The nine-hole Lakeside course is easy walking, mainly Par 4. Floodlit driving range.
Brinsea Course: *18 holes, 6352yds, Par 71, SSS 70, Course record 64.*
Lakeside: *9 holes, 2392yds, Par 34, SSS 66.*
Club membership 500.
Visitors Mon-Sun & BHs. Booking required for Brinsea course. Handicap certificate. Dress code. **Societies** Booking required. **Green Fees** Brinsea £28 (£38 Sat & Sun). Lakeside: £9.50/£10. **Prof** John Blackburn & Robert Moss **Facilities** ⑪ ⑩↑ 🏐 ☐ 🏋 🏌 🏖 ⛳♥ ✦ 🏖 ⛳ 🏌 **Conf** facs Corporate Hospitality Days **Location** 2m S between A370

ENMORE   MAP 03 ST23

Enmore Park TA5 2AN
☎ 01278 672100 (office) & 672102 (pro) 📄 01278 672101
e-mail: golfclub@enmore.fsnet.co.uk
web: www.enmorepark.co.uk
A parkland course on the foothills of the Quantocks, with water features. Wooded countryside and views of the Mendips; 1st and 10th are testing holes.
18 holes, 6406yds, Par 71, SSS 71, Course record 64.
Club membership 700.
Visitors Mon, Tue, Thu, Fri & BHs. Booking required. Dress code. **Societies** Booking required. **Green Fees** £32 per round. **Prof** Nigel Wixon **Course Designer** Hawtree **Facilities** ⑪ ⑩↑ 🏐 ☐ 🏋 🏌 🏖 ⛳♥ ✦ **Conf** Corporate Hospitality Days **Location** 0.5m E of village, 3.5m SW of Bridgewater
Hotel ★★ 79% HL Combe House Hotel, HOLFORD ☎ 01278 741382 17 en suite 1 annexe en suite

FARRINGTON GURNEY   MAP 03 ST65

Farrington Golf & Country Club Marsh Ln BS39 6TS
☎ 01761 451596 📠 01761 451021
e-mail: info@farringtongolfclub.net
web: www.farringtongolfclub.net
Main Course: 18 holes, 6335yds, Par 72, SSS 71,
Course record 66.
Course Designer Peter Thompson **Location** SE of village off A37
Telephone for further details
Hotel ★★★ 78% HL Centurion Hotel, Charlton Ln, MIDSOMER NORTON
☎ 01761 417711   44 en suite

FROME   MAP 03 ST74

Frome Golf Centre Critchill Manor BA11 4LJ
☎ 01373 453410
e-mail: fromegolfclub@yahoo.co.uk
web: www.fromegolfclub.fsnet.co.uk
Attractive parkland course, founded in 1992, situated in a picturesque
valley just outside the town, complete with practice areas and a driving
range.
18 holes, 5527yds, Par 69, SSS 67, Course record 64.
Club membership 500.
Visitors Mon-Sun & BHs. Booking required Sat, Sun & BHs. Dress code.
Societies Booking required. **Green Fees** £26 per day, £22 per 18 holes;
£15.50 per 9 holes (£29.50/£25.50/£18.50 Sat, Sun & BHs). ⊛ **Prof**
Lawrence Wilkin **Facilities** ⊕ ⅃ ☐ ⅊⅃ ⅄ 📷 ⅊ ⅊ ⅊ **Location** 1m SW
of town centre
Hotel ★★ 67% HL The George at Nunney, 11 Church St, NUNNEY
☎ 01373 836458 9 rms (8 en suite)

Orchardleigh BA11 2PH
☎ 01373 454200 📠 01373 454202
e-mail: info@orchardleighgolf.co.uk
web: www.orchardleighgolf.co.uk
An 18-hole parkland course set amid Somerset countryside routed
through mature trees with water coming into play on seven holes.
18 holes, 6824yds, Par 72, SSS 73, Course record 67.
Club membership 550.
Visitors Mon-Sun & BHs. Booking required. Handicap certificate. Dress
code. **Societies** Booking required. **Green Fees** £35 per round (£37.50 Sat,
Sun & BHs). **Prof** Ian Ridsdale **Course Designer** Brian Huggett **Facilities**
⊕ ⅃⊙⅃ ⅃ ☐ ⅊⅃ ⅄ 📷 ⅊ ⅊ ⅊ **Leisure** fishing. **Conf** facs   Corporate
Hospitality Days **Location** On A362 Frome to Radstock road near village of
Buckland Dinham
Hotel ★★ 67% HL The George at Nunney, 11 Church St, NUNNEY
☎ 01373 836458 9 rms (8 en suite)

GURNEY SLADE   MAP 03 ST64

Mendip BA3 4UT
☎ 01749 840570 📠 01749 841439
e-mail: secretary@mendipgolfclub.com
web: www.mendipgolfclub.com
Undulating downland course offering an interesting test of golf on
superb fairways and extensive views over the surrounding countryside.
18 holes, 6383yds, Par 71, SSS 71, Course record 65.
Club membership 900.
Visitors Contact club for details. Handicap certificate. Dress code.
Societies Boooking required. **Green Fees** £27 per round (£38 Sat & Sun).

Prof Adrian Marsh **Course Designer** C K Cotton **Facilities** ⊕ ⅃⊙⅃ ⅃ ☐ ⅊⅃
⅄ 📷 ⅊ ⅊ ⅊ **Location** 1.5m S off A37
Hotel ★★★ 78% HL Centurion Hotel, Charlton Ln, MIDSOMER NORTON
☎ 01761 417711   44 en suite

KEYNSHAM   MAP 03 ST66

Stockwood Vale Stockwood Ln BS31 2ER
☎ 0117 986 6505 📠 0117 986 8974
e-mail: stockwoodvalegc@netscapeonline.co.uk
web: www.stockwoodvale.com
18 holes, 6031yds, Par 71, SSS 69.
Location Off Hicks Gate on junct A4
Telephone for further details
Guesthouse ★★★★ GH Grasmere Court, 22-24 Bath Rd, KEYNSHAM
☎ 0117 986 2662   16 en suite

LONG ASHTON   MAP 03 ST57

Long Ashton The Clubhouse, Clarken Coombe
BS41 9DW
☎ 01275 392229 📠 01275 394395
e-mail: secretary@longashtongolfclub.co.uk
web: www.longashtongolfclub.co.uk
Wooded parkland course with fine turf, wonderful views of Bristol and
surrounding areas, and a spacious practice area. Good testing holes,
especially the back nine, in prevailing south-west wind. Good drainage
ensures pleasant winter golf.

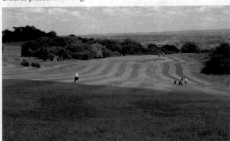

18 holes, 6400yds, Par 71, SSS 71. Club membership 700.
Visitors contact club for details. Dress code. **Societies** booking required.
Green Fees not confirmed. **Prof** Mike Hart **Course Designer** J H Taylor
Facilities ⊕ ⅃⊙⅃ by prior arrangement ⅃ ☐ ⅊⅃ ⅄ 📷 ⅊ **Conf** Corporate
Hospitality Days **Location** 0.5m N on B3128
Hotel ★★★ 70% HL Redwood Hotel & Country Club, Beggar Bush Ln,
Failand, BRISTOL ☎ 0870 609 6144   112 en suite

Woodspring Golf & Country Club Yanley Ln BS41 9LR
☎ 01275 394378 📠 01275 394473
e-mail: info@woodspring-golf.com
web: www.woodspring-golf.com
Set in 245 acres of undulating Somerset countryside, featuring superb
natural water hazards, protected greens and a rising landscape.
Designed by Peter Alliss and Clive Clark and laid out by Donald Steel,
the course has three individual nine-hole courses, the Avon, Severn
and Brunel. The 9th hole on the Brunel Course is a feature hole,
with an elevated tee shot over a natural gorge. In undulating hills

Continued

south of Bristol, long carries to tight fairways, elevated island tees and challenging approaches to greens make the most of the 27 holes.
Avon Course: 9 holes, 2960yds, Par 35, SSS 34.
Brunel Course: 9 holes, 3320yds, Par 37, SSS 35.
Severn Course: 9 holes, 3267yds, Par 36, SSS 35.
Club membership 400.
Visitors Mon-Sun & BHs. Dress code. **Societies** Booking required.
Green Fees £30 per 18 holes (£34 Sat, Sun & BHs). **Prof** Kevin Pitts
Course Designer Clarke/Alliss/Steel **Facilities** ⊕ ⚑ ⛾ ⚏ ⛗ ⊡ 🏌 ⚑
⚑ ⚑ 🏌 ⚑ ⛳ **Conf** facs Corporate Hospitality Days **Location** Off A38 Bridgwater Road
Hotel ★★★ 70% HL Redwood Hotel & Country Club, Beggar Bush Ln, Failand, BRISTOL ☎ 0870 609 6144 112 en suite

MIDSOMER NORTON   MAP 03 ST65

Fosseway Golf Course Charlton Ln BA3 4BD
☎ 01761 412214 📄 01761 418357
e-mail: centurion@centurionhotel.co.uk
web: www.centurionhotel.co.uk
9 holes, 4565yds, Par 67, SSS 61.
Course Designer C K Cotton/F Pennink **Location** SE of town centre off A367
Telephone for further details
Hotel ★★★ 78% HL Centurion Hotel, Charlton Ln, MIDSOMER NORTON ☎ 01761 417711 44 en suite

MINEHEAD   MAP 03 SS94

Minehead & West Somerset The Warren TA24 5SJ
☎ 01643 702057 📄 01643 705095
e-mail: secretary@mineheadgolf.co.uk
web: www.mineheadgolf.co.uk
Flat seaside links, very exposed to wind, with good turf set on a shingle bank. The last five holes adjacent to the beach are testing. The 215yd 18th is wedged between the beach and the club buildings and provides a good finish.
18 holes, 6228yds, Par 71, SSS 69, Course record 65.
Club membership 620.
Visitors Mon-Sun & BHs. Dress code. **Societies** Booking required. **Green Fees** £35 per day (£40 Sat & Sun). **Prof** Ian Read
Facilities ⊕ ⚑ ⛾ ⚏ ⛗ ⊡ 🏌 ⚑ 🏌 **Conf** Corporate Hospitality Days
Location E end of esplanade
Hotel ★★ 80% HL Channel House Hotel, Church Path, MINEHEAD ☎ 01643 703229 8 en suite

SALTFORD   MAP 03 ST66

Saltford Golf Club Ln BS31 3AA
☎ 01225 873513 📄 01225 873525
18 holes, 6081yds, Par 71, SSS 71.
Course Designer Harry Vardon **Location** S of village
Telephone for further details
Hotel ★★★ 82% CHH Hunstrete House Hotel, HUNSTRETE ☎ 01761 490490 25 en suite

SOMERTON   MAP 03 ST42

Long Sutton Long Sutton TA10 9JU
☎ 01458 241017 📄 01458 241022
e-mail: reservations@longsuttongolf.com
web: www.longsuttongolf.com
Gentle, undulating, but testing parkland course. Pay and play course.

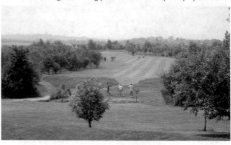

18 holes, 6369yds, Par 71, SSS 70, Course record 64.
Club membership 750.
Visitors Mon-Sun & BHs. Booking required Fri-Sun & BHs. Dress code.
Societies Booking required. **Green Fees** £30 per day, £20 per 18 holes, £10 per 9 holes (£35/£25/£12.50 Sat & Sun). **Prof** Andrew Hayes
Course Designer Patrick Dawson **Facilities** ⊕ ⚑ ⛾ ⚏ ⛗ ⊡ 🏌 ⚑ 🏌 ⚑
⚑ ⛳ **Conf** facs Corporate Hospitality Days **Location** 3.5m E of Langport, 0.5m S of Long Sutton on B3165
Hotel ★★★ 74% HL The Hollies, Bower Hinton, MARTOCK ☎ 01935 822232 44 annexe en suite

Wheathill Wheathill TA11 7HG
☎ 01963 240667 📄 01963 240230
e-mail: wheathill@wheathill.fsnet.co.uk
web: www.foremostonline.com/wheathill
A Par 68 parkland course with nice views in quiet countryside. It is flat lying with the 13th hole along the river. There is an academy course and a massive practice area.
18 holes, 5839yds, Par 68, SSS 66, Course record 61.
Club membership 550.
Visitors Mon-Sun & BHs. Booking required Fri-Sun & BHs. Dress code.
Societies Booking required. **Green Fees** £20 per round. **Prof** A England
Course Designer J Pain **Facilities** ⊕ ⚑ ⛾ ⚏ ⛗ ⊡ 🏌 ⚑ 🏌 ⚑
Leisure 8 hole academy course. **Conf** facs Corporate Hospitality Days
Location 5m E of Somerton off B3153
Hotel ★★ 65% HL Wessex Hotel, High St, STREET ☎ 01458 443383 49 en suite

TAUNTON   MAP 03 ST22

Oake Manor Oake TA4 1BA
☎ 01823 461993 📄 01823 461995
e-mail: russell@oakemanor.com
web: www.oakemanor.com
A parkland and lakeland course situated in breathtaking Somerset countryside with views of the Quantock, Blackdown and Brendon hills. Ten holes feature water hazards such as lakes, cascades and a trout stream. The 15th hole (Par 5, 476yds) is bounded by water all down

Continued

England

the left with a carry over another lake on to an island green. The course is challenging yet great fun for all standards of golfer.

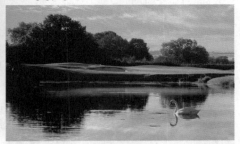

Oake Manor

18 holes, 6109yds, Par 70, SSS 70, Course record 65.
Club membership 600.
Visitors Mon-Sun & BHs. Booking required. **Societies** Booking required. **Green Fees** £23 per 18 holes, £28 Fri, £30 Sat & Sun. **Prof** R Gardner/J Smallacombe **Course Designer** Adrian Stiff **Facilities** ⑨ ⑩ ♨ ⌷ ⛴ ⚒ **Leisure** 2 hole academy course, short game area. **Conf** facs Corporate Hospitality Days **Location** M5 junct 26, A38 towards Taunton. Signed at World's End pub
Hotel ★★★ 80% HL Best Western Rumwell Manor Hotel, Rumwell, TAUNTON ☎ 01823 461902 10 en suite 10 annexe en suite

Taunton & Pickeridge Corfe TA3 7BY
☎ 01823 421537 📄 01823 421742
e-mail: admin@tauntongolf.co.uk
web: www.taunton-golf.co.uk
Downland course established in 1892 with extensive views of the Quantock and Mendip hills. Renowned for its excellent greens.
18 holes, 6056yds, Par 69, SSS 69, Course record 66.
Club membership 800.
Visitors Mon-Fri, Sun & BHs.Handicap certificate. Dress code. **Societies** Welcome. **Green Fees** £32 per day; £26 per round (£40 Sat & Sun). **Prof** Simon Stevenson **Facilities** ⑨ ⑩ ♨ ⌷ ⛴ ⚒ **Conf** facs Corporate Hospitality Days **Location** 4m S off B3170
Hotel ★★★ 78% HL The Mount Somerset Hotel, Lower Henlade, TAUNTON ☎ 01823 442500 11 en suite

Taunton Vale Creech Heathfield TA3 5EY
☎ 01823 412220 📄 01823 413583
e-mail: tvgc@gotadsl.co.uk
web: www.tauntonvalegolf.co.uk
An 18-hole and a nine-hole course in a parkland complex occupying 156 acres in the Vale of Taunton. Floodlit driving range.

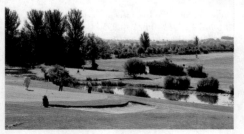

Charlton Course: 18 holes, 6218yds, Par 70, SSS 70.
Durston Course: 9 holes, 2004yds, Par 32.
Club membership 800.
Visitors Mon-Sun & BHs. Booking required. Dress code. **Societies** Booking required. **Green Fees** 18 hole course £23 per round (£28 Sat , Sun & BHs). 9 hole course £10 per round (£12 Sat & Sun). **Prof** Martin Keitch **Course Designer** John Payne **Facilities** ⑨ ⑩ by prior arrangement ♨ ⌷ ⛴ ⚒ 🏠 ⚒ **Conf** facs Corporate Hospitality Days **Location** M5 junct 24 or 25, off A38
Hotel ★★★ 78% HL The Mount Somerset Hotel, Lower Henlade, TAUNTON ☎ 01823 442500 11 en suite

See advert on opposite page

Vivary Park Municipal Fons George TA1 3JU
☎ 01823 333875 📄 01823 352713
e-mail: vivary.golf.course@tauntondeane.gov.uk
18 holes, 4620yds, Par 63, SSS 63, Course record 59.
Course Designer W H Fowler **Location** S of town centre off A38
Telephone for further details
Hotel ★★★ 72% HL Corner House Hotel, Park St, TAUNTON ☎ 01823 284683 28 en suite

---

WEDMORE   MAP 03 ST44

Isle of Wedmore Lineage BS28 4QT
☎ 01934 712452 (Pro-Shop) 📄 01934 713554
e-mail: wedmoregolfclub@supanet.com
web: www.wedmoregolfclub.com
Gently undulating course designed to maintain natural environment. Existing woodland and hedgerow enhanced by new planting. Magnificent panoramic views of Cheddar valley and Glastonbury Tor from the back nine. The course design provides two loops of nine holes both starting and finishing at the clubhouse.
18 holes, 6057yds, Par 70, SSS 69, Course record 67.
Club membership 680.
Visitors Mon-Sun & BHs. Dress code. **Societies** Booking required. **Green Fees** £32 per day, £24 per round. Reduced winter rates. **Prof** Nick Pope **Course Designer** Terry Murray **Facilities** ⑨ ⑩ ♨ ⌷ 🏠 ⚒ ⚒ **Leisure** indoor teaching studio & custom fitting centre. **Conf** facs Corporate Hospitality Days **Location** 0.5m N of Wedmore
Hotel ★★★ 85% HL Best Western Swan Hotel, Sadler St, WELLS ☎ 01749 836300 49 en suite

---

WELLS   MAP 03 ST54

Wells (Somerset) Blackheath Lne, East Horrington BA5 3DS
☎ 01749 675005 📄 01749 683170
e-mail: secretary@wellsgolfclub.co.uk
web: www.wellsgolfclub.co.uk
Beautiful wooded course with wonderful views. The prevailing SW wind complicates the 448yd 3rd. Good drainage and paths for trolleys are being constructed all round the course.
18 holes, 6053yds, Par 70, SSS 69, Course record 66.
Club membership 670.
Visitors Mon-Sun & BHs. Dress code. **Societies** Welcome. **Green Fees** £30 per 18 holes (£35 Sat, Sun & BHs). **Prof** Adrian Bishop **Facilities** ⑨ ♨ ⌷ 🏠 ⚒ ⚒ ⚒ **Conf** Corporate Hospitality Days **Location** 1.5m E off B3139
Hotel ★★ 67% HL Ancient Gate House Hotel, 20 Sadler St, WELLS ☎ 01749 672029 8 en suite

WESTON-SUPER-MARE MAP 03 ST36

Weston-Super-Mare Uphill Rd North BS23 4NQ
☎ 01934 626968 & 633360(pro) 📠 01934 621360
e-mail: wsmgolfclub@eurotelbroadband.com
web: www.westonsupermaregolfclub.com
A compact and interesting layout with the opening hole adjacent to the beach. The sandy, links-type course is slightly undulating and has beautifully maintained turf and greens. The 15th is a testing 455yd Par 4. Superb views across the Bristol Channel to Cardiff.

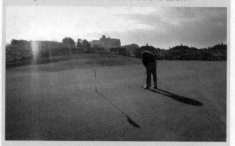

18 holes, 6245yds, Par 70, SSS 70, Course record 65. Club membership 750.
Visitors Mon-Sun & BHs. Handicap certificate. Dress code.
Societies Booking required. **Green Fees** £48 per day, £36 per round.
Prof Mike Laband **Course Designer** T Dunne/Dr Mackenzie
Facilities ⊕ 🏌 🏌 🏌 🏌 🏌 **Location** S of town centre off A370
Hotel ★★★ 70% HL Beachlands Hotel, 17 Uphill Rd North, WESTON-SUPER-MARE ☎ 01934 621401 23 en suite

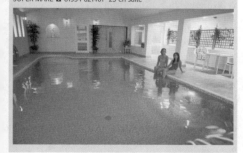

Worlebury Monks Hill BS22 9SX
☎ 01934 625789 📠 01934 621935
e-mail: secretary@worleburygc.co.uk
web: www.worleburygc.co.uk
Parkland course on the ridge of Worlebury Hill, with fairly easy walking and extensive views of the Severn estuary and Wales.
18 holes, 5963yds, Par 70, SSS 68, Course record 66. Club membership 650.
Visitors Mon-Sun & BHs. Booking required. Handicap certificate. Dress code. **Societies** Booking required. **Green Fees** Phone. **Prof** Gary Marks **Course Designer** H Vardon **Facilities** ⊕ 🏌 🏌 🏌 🏌 🏌 🏌
Location 2m NE off A370
Hotel ★★★ 70% HL Beachlands Hotel, 17 Uphill Rd North, WESTON-SUPER-MARE ☎ 01934 621401 23 en suite

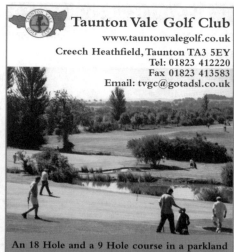

Taunton Vale Golf Club
www.tauntonvalegolf.co.uk
Creech Heathfield, Taunton TA3 5EY
Tel: 01823 412220
Fax 01823 413583
Email: tvgc@gotadsl.co.uk

An 18 Hole and a 9 Hole course in a parkland complex occupying 156 acres in the Vale of Taunton with Floodlit Driving Range.
Charlton Course: 18 Holes, 6234 yds, par 70
Durston Course: 9 Holes, 2004 yds, par 32
Green Fees: 18 Holes—£23, £28 Sat & Sun
9 Holes—£10, £12 Sat & Sun
Visitors & Societies Welcome

YEOVIL MAP 03 ST51

Yeovil Sherborne Rd BA21 5BW
☎ 01935 422965 📠 01935 411283
e-mail: office@yeovilgolfclub.com
web: www. yeovilgolfclub.com
On the Old Course the opener lies by the River Yeo before the gentle climb to high downs with good views. The outstanding 14th and 15th holes present a challenge, being below the player with a deep railway cutting on the left of the green. The 1st on the Newton Course is played over the river which then leads to a challenging but scenic course.
Old Course: 18 holes, 6150yds, Par 71, SSS 70, Course record 64.
Newton Course: 9 holes, 4905yds, Par 68, SSS 65, Course record 63. Club membership 1000.
Visitors Mon-Sun & BHs. Booking required. Handicap certificate for Old Course. Dress code. **Societies** Booking required. **Green Fees** Old Course Apr-Oct: £35 (£45 Sat, Sun & BHs) Nov-Mar: £25 (£30). Newton Course £20. **Prof** Geoff Kite **Course Designer** Fowler & Allison **Facilities** ⊕ 🏌
🏌 🏌 🏌 🏌 🏌 🏌 **Location** 1m E on A30
Hotel ★★★ 75% HL The Yeovil Court Hotel & Restaurant, West Coker Rd, YEOVIL ☎ 01935 863746 18 en suite 12 annexe en suite

STAFFORDSHIRE

BROCTON — MAP 07 SJ91

Brocton Hall ST17 0TH
☎ 01785 661901 🖷 01785 661591
e-mail: broctonsec@aol.com
web: www.broctonhall.com
18 holes, 6064yds, Par 69, SSS 69, Course record 66.
Course Designer Harry Vardon **Location** NW of village off A34
Telephone for further details
Hotel ★★★★ 82% HL The Moat House, Lower Penkridge Rd, Acton Trussell, STAFFORD ☎ 01785 712217 41 en suite

BURTON UPON TRENT — MAP 08 SK22

Belmont Tutbury Rd, Needwood DE13 9PH
☎ 01283 814381 🖷 01283 814381
A nine-hole course with five Par 4s, the longest hole being 430yds. The course comprises trees, bunkers, some water and great views.
9 holes, 2201yds, Par 32, Course record 31.
Visitors Mon-Sun & BHs. Dress code. **Societies** welcome. **Green Fees** not confirmed. ● **Prof** R Coy **Facilities** ⌂🖥🕯✔ **Leisure** fishing, archery. **Conf** Corporate Hospitality Days **Location** 3m NW of Tutbury, off B5017 towards Tutbury
Hotel ★★ 72% HL Riverside Hotel, Riverside Dr, Branston, BURTON UPON TRENT ☎ 01283 511234 22 en suite

Branston Burton Rd, Branston DE14 3DP
☎ 01283 512211 🖷 01283 566984
e-mail: info@branston-golf-club.co.uk
web: www.branston-golf-club.co.uk
Semi-parkland course on undulating ground next to the River Trent. Natural water hazards on 13 holes. A nine-hole course has recently been opened.

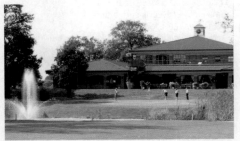

18 holes, 6697yds, Par 72, SSS 72, Course record 65.
Club membership 800.
Visitors Mon-Sun & BHs. Booking required. **Societies** Booking required.
Green Fees £36 per 18 holes (£44 Fri-Sun). **Prof** Iain Ross **Course Designer** G Ramshall **Facilities** ⊕🍴🖥🕯✔ **Leisure** heated indoor swimming pool, sauna, solarium, gymnasium, 9 hole course.
Conf facs Corporate Hospitality Days **Location** 1.5m SW on A5121
Hotel ★★ 72% HL Riverside Hotel, Riverside Dr, Branston, BURTON UPON TRENT ☎ 01283 511234 22 en suite

Burton-upon-Trent 43 Ashby Rd East DE15 0PS
☎ 01283 544551 (sec) & 562240 (pro) 🖷 01283 544551
e-mail: TheSecretary@BurtonGolfClub.co.uk
web: www.burtongolfclub.co.uk
Undulating parkland course with notable trees and water features on two holes. Testing Par 3s at 10th and 12th.

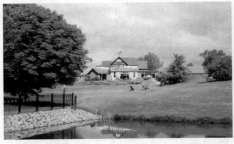

18 holes, 6579yds, Par 71, SSS 71, Course record 63.
Club membership 700.
Visitors Contact club for details. Handicap certificate. Dress code. **Societies** Booking required. **Green Fees** £50 per day; £38 per round (£57/£44 Sat, Sun & BHs). ● **Prof** Gary Stafford **Course Designer** H S Colt **Facilities** ⌂🖥🕯✔ **Conf** Corporate Hospitality Days **Location** 3m E of Burton on A511
Guesthouse ★★★★ GH The Edgecote, 179 Ashby Rd, BURTON UPON TRENT ☎ 01283 568966 11 rms (5 en suite)

Craythorne Craythorne Rd, Rolleston on Dove DE13 0AZ
☎ 01283 564329 🖷 01283 511908
e-mail: admin@craythorne.co.uk
web: www.craythorne.co.uk
A relatively short and challenging parkland course with tight fairways and views of the Trent valley. Excellent greens giving all year play. Suits all standards but particularly good for society players. The course is now settled and in good condition after major refurbishment.
18 holes, 5645yds, Par 68, SSS 68, Course record 66.
Club membership 500.
Visitors Mon-Sun & BHs. Booking required. Dress code. **Societies** Booking required. **Green Fees** £25 per day, £20 per round. **Prof** Steve Hadfield **Course Designer** A A Wright **Facilities** ⊕🍴🖥🕯✔ **Conf** facs Corporate Hospitality Days **Location** Off A38 through Stretton, tourist signs
Guesthouse ★★★★ GH The Edgecote, 179 Ashby Rd, BURTON UPON TRENT ☎ 01283 568966 11 rms (5 en suite)

Hoar Cross Hall Health Spa Golf Academy
Hoar Cross DE13 8QS
☎ 01283 575671 🖷 01283 575652
e-mail: info@hoarcross.co.uk
web: www.hoarcross.co.uk
9 holes, Par 27.
Course Designer Geoffrey Collins
Telephone for further details
Hotel BUD Travelodge Rugeley, Western Springs Rd, RUGELEY ☎ 08700 850 950 32 en suite

CANNOCK — MAP 07 SJ91

Beau Desert Rugeley Rd, Hazelslade WS12 0PJ
☎ 01543 422626 ▤ 01543 451137
e-mail: bdgc@btconnect.com
web: www.bdgc.co.uk
A moorland course with firm and fast fairways and greens, used on many occasions as an Open qualifier course. The course has many varied and testing holes ranging from the 1st over a pit, the 10th over a ravine, to the 18th with a second shot across gorse traversing the fairway.
18 holes, 6310yds, Par 70, SSS 71, Course record 64.
Club membership 650.
Visitors Mon-Sun & BHs. Booking required Sat, Sun & BHs. Handicap certificate. Dress code. **Societies** Booking required. **Green Fees** £55 per day, £45 per round (£65 Sat, Sun & BHs). ● **Prof** Barrie Stevens **Course Designer** Herbert Fowler **Facilities** ⊕ ⊚ ⓛ ☐ ⊞ ⊿ ☎ ☜ ◈ ✔ ⌐ ✔ ⌐ **Conf** facs Corporate Hospitality Days **Location** Off A460 NE of Hednesford

Cannock Park Stafford Rd WS11 2AL
☎ 01543 578850 ▤ 01543 578850
e-mail: seccpgc@yahoo.co.uk
Part of a large leisure centre, this parkland-type course plays alongside Cannock Chase. Severe slopes on some greens. Good drainage, open all year.
18 holes, 5200yds, Par 67, SSS 65. Club membership 150.
Visitors Mon-Sun except BHs. Booking required Sat, Sun & BHs. Dress code. **Societies** Booking required. **Green Fees** £11.80 per round (£14.90 Sat & Sun). **Prof** Jonathan Craddock **Course Designer** John Mainland **Facilities** ⊕ ⊚ ⓛ ☐ ⊞ ⊿ ☎ ✔ **Leisure** hard tennis courts, heated indoor swimming pool, sauna, solarium, gymnasium. **Location** 0.5m N of town centre on A34

ENVILLE — MAP 07 SO88

Enville Highgate Common DY7 5BN
☎ 01384 872074 (Office) ▤ 01384 873396
e-mail: secretary@envillegolfclub.com
web: www.envillegolfclub.com
Easy walking on two fairly flat woodland and heathland courses. Qualifying course for the Open Championship.
Highgate Course: 18 holes, 6556yds, Par 72, SSS 72, Course record 65.
Lodge Course: 18 holes, 6290yds, Par 70, SSS 70, Course record 66. Club membership 900.
Visitors Mon-Fri except BHs. Dress code. **Societies** Welcome. **Green Fees** £50 per day; £40 per 18 holes. ● **Prof** Sean Power **Facilities** ⊕ ⊚ ⓛ ☐ ⊞ ⊿ ☎ ✔ **Conf** Corporate Hospitality Days **Location** 2m NE of Enville off A458
Hotel ★★★★ 78% HL Mill Hotel & Restaurant, ALVELEY ☎ 01746 780437 41 en suite

GOLDENHILL — MAP 07 SJ85

Goldenhill Mobberley Rd ST6 5SS
☎ 01782 787678 ▤ 01782 787678
web: www.jackbarker.com
Rolling parkland with two Par 3's holes surrounded by water and water in play on 6 of the back 9 holes.
18 holes, 5957yds, Par 71, SSS 69. Club membership 300.

Visitors Mon-Sun & BHs. **Societies** booking required. **Green Fees** not confirmed. **Facilities** ⊕ ⊚ ⓛ ☐ ⊞ ⊿ ☎ ✔ ◈ ✔ ⌐ **Location** On A50 4m N of Stoke
Hotel ★★★ 82% HL Best Western Manor House Hotel, Audley Rd, ALSAGER ☎ 01270 884000 57 en suite

HIMLEY — MAP 07 SO89

Himley Hall Golf Centre Log Cabin, Himley Hall Park DY3 4DF
☎ 01902 895207
9 holes, 6215yds, Par 72, SSS 70, Course record 65.
Course Designer A Baker **Location** 0.5m E on B4176
Telephone for further details
Hotel ★★★ 66% HL Himley Country Hotel, School Rd, HIMLEY ☎ 01902 896716 71 en suite

LEEK — MAP 07 SJ95

Leek Birchall, Cheddleton Rd ST13 5RE
☎ 01538 384779 & 384767 (pro) ▤ 01538 384535
e-mail: secretary@leekgolfclub.fsnet.co.uk
web: www.leekgolfclub.co.uk
Undulating, challenging, mainly parkland course, reputedly one of the best in the area. In its early years the course was typical moorland with sparse tree growth but its development since the 1960s has produced tree-lined fairways which are much appeciated by golfers for their lush playing qualities.
18 holes, 6218yds, Par 70, SSS 70, Course record 63.
Club membership 825.
Visitors Mon-Sun & BHs. Booking required. Handicap certificate. Dress code. **Societies** Booking required. **Green Fees** £26 per day (£32 weekends). ● **Prof** Paul Toyer **Facilities** ⊕ ⊚ ⓛ ☐ ⊞ ⊿ ☎ ☜ ✔ **Leisure** snooker. **Conf** facs Corporate Hospitality Days **Location** 0.75m S on A520
Hotel ★★★ 79% HL Three Horseshoes Inn & Country Hotel, Buxton Rd, Blackshaw Moor, LEEK ☎ 01538 300296 26 en suite

Westwood (Leek) Newcastle Rd ST13 7AA
☎ 01538 398385 ▤ 01538 382485
A challenging moorland and parkland course set in beautiful open countryside with an undulating front nine. The back nine is more open and longer with the River Churnet coming into play on several holes.
18 holes, 6207yds, Par 70, SSS 69, Course record 66.
Club membership 700.
Visitors Mon-Fri except BHs. Handicap certificate. Dress code. **Societies** Welcome. **Green Fees** Phone. **Prof** Darren Squire **Facilities** ⊕ ⓛ ☐ ⊞ ⊿ ☎ ✔ **Conf** facs Corporate Hospitality Days **Location** On A53 S of Leek
Hotel ★★★ 79% HL Three Horseshoes Inn & Country Hotel, Buxton Rd, Blackshaw Moor, LEEK ☎ 01538 300296 26 en suite

LICHFIELD — MAP 07 SK10

Seedy Mill Elmhurst WS13 8HE
☎ 01543 417333 ▤ 01543 418098
e-mail: gtreadwell@theclubcompany.com
web: www.theclubcompany.com
A 27-hole course in picturesque parkland scenery. Numerous holes crossed by meandering mill streams. Undulating greens defended by hazards lie in wait for the practised approach.
Mill Course: 18 holes, 6042yds, Par 72, SSS 70, Course record 67. Club membership 1200. *Continued*

Visitors Mon-Fr. Sat, Sun & BHs after noon. Booking required. Dress code. **Societies** Booking required. **Green Fees** Mill course £35 per 18 holes (£40 Sat & Sun), 9 holes: £9.50. **Prof** Simon Joyce **Course Designer** Hawtree & Son **Facilities** ⊕ ⚲ ⌕ 🍴 ⌂ ⌕ 🍴 ⌂ ♣ ⚐ **Leisure** 9 hole Par 3 course. **Conf** facs Corporate Hospitality Days **Location** 3m N of Lichfield off B5014
Hotel ★★★ 74% HL Little Barrow Hotel, 62 Beacon St, LICHFIELD ☎ 01543 414500 32 en suite

Whittington Heath Tamworth Rd WS14 9PW
☎ 01543 432317 📠 01543 433962
e-mail: info@whittingtonheathgc.co.uk
web: www.whittingtonheathgc.co.uk
The 18 magnificent holes wind through heathland and trees, presenting a good test for the serious golfer. Leaving the fairway can be severely punished. The dog-legs are most tempting, inviting the golfer to chance his arm. Local knowledge is a definite advantage. Clear views of the famous three spires of Lichfield Cathedral.
18 holes, 6490yds, Par 70, SSS 71, Course record 64.
Club membership 660.
Visitors Mon-Fri except BHs. Booking required. Handicap certificate. Dress code. **Societies** Booking required. **Green Fees** £55 per 36 holes; £48 per 27 holes; £40 per 18 holes. **Prof** Adrian Sadler **Course Designer** Colt **Facilities** ⊕ ⚲ ⌕ 🍴 ⌂ **Conf** Corporate Hospitality Days **Location** 2.5m SE on A51
Hotel ★★★ 74% HL Little Barrow Hotel, 62 Beacon St, LICHFIELD ☎ 01543 414500 32 en suite

---

NEWCASTLE-UNDER-LYME   MAP 07 SJ84

Keele Golf Centre Newcastle Rd, Keele ST5 5AB
☎ 01782 627596 📠 01782 714555
e-mail: jackbarker_keelegolfcentreltd@hotmail.com
web: www.jackbarker.com
Parkland with mature trees and great views of Stoke-on-Trent and the surrounding area.

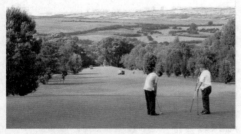

18 holes, 6396yds, Par 71, SSS 70, Course record 64.
Club membership 400.
Visitors Mon-Sun & BHs. **Societies** Welcome. **Green Fees** £10.50 per round, £13 Fri, £15.50 Sat & Sun. **Course Designer** Hawtree **Facilities** ⊕ ⚲ ⌕ 🍴 ⌂ ♣ ⚐ **Leisure** 9 hole Par 3 course. **Location** 2m W on A525 opp Keele University
Hotel ★★ 62% HL Stop Inn Newcastle-under-Lyme, Liverpool Rd, Cross Heath, NEWCASTLE-UNDER-LYME ☎ 01782 717000 43 rms (42 en suite) 24 annexe en suite

Newcastle-Under-Lyme Whitmore Rd ST5 2QB
☎ 01782 617006 📠 01782 617531
e-mail: info@newcastlegolfclub.co.uk
web: www.newcastlegolfclub.co.uk
Parkland course.
18 holes, 6395yds, Par 72, SSS 71, Course record 66.
Club membership 600.
Visitors Mon, Wed-Fri except BHs. Handicap certificate. Dress code. **Societies** Booking required. **Green Fees** £35 per day, £25 per round. 🌐 **Prof** Ashley Salt **Facilities** ⊕ ⚲ ⌕ 🍴 ⌂ **Conf** Corporate Hospitality Days **Location** 1m SW on A53
Hotel ★★ 62% HL Stop Inn Newcastle-under-Lyme, Liverpool Rd, Cross Heath, NEWCASTLE-UNDER-LYME ☎ 01782 717000 43 rms (42 en suite) 24 annexe en suite

Wolstanton Dimsdale Old Hall, Hassam Pde, Wolstanton ST5 9DR
☎ 01782 622413 (Sec)
A challenging undulating suburban course incorporating six difficult Par 3 holes. The 6th hole (Par 3) is 233yds from the Medal Tee.

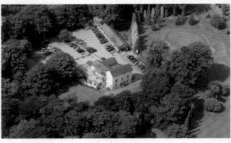

18 holes, 5533yds, Par 68, SSS 68, Course record 63.
Club membership 700.
Visitors Mon-Fri. Booking required. Handicap certificate. Dress code. **Societies** Booking required. **Green Fees** £27.50 per 18 holes. **Prof** Simon Arnold **Facilities** ⊕ ⚲ ⌕ 🍴 ⌂ **Conf** facs Corporate Hospitality Days **Location** 1.5m from town centre. Turn off A34 at MacDonalds
Hotel ★★ 62% HL Stop Inn Newcastle-under-Lyme, Liverpool Rd, Cross Heath, NEWCASTLE-UNDER-LYME ☎ 01782 717000 43 rms (42 en suite) 24 annexe en suite

---

ONNELEY   MAP 07 SJ74

Onneley CW3 5QF
☎ 01782 750577 & 846759
e-mail: all@onneleygolf.co.uk
web: www.onneleygolf.co.uk
Parkland having panoramic views to the Welsh hills.
18 holes, 5728yds, Par 70, SSS 68. Club membership 410.
Visitors Contact club for details. **Societies** booking required. **Green Fees** not confirmed. 🌐 **Course Designer** A Benson/G Marks **Facilities** ⊕ ⌕ 🍴 ⌂ **Location** 2m from Woore on A525
Hotel ★★ 62% HL Stop Inn Newcastle-under-Lyme, Liverpool Rd, Cross Heath, NEWCASTLE-UNDER-LYME ☎ 01782 717000 43 rms (42 en suite) 24 annexe en suite

PATTINGHAM
MAP 07 SO89

Patshull Park Hotel Golf & Country Club WV6 7HR
☎ 01902 700100 🖹 01902 700874
e-mail: sales@patshull-park.co.uk
web: www.patshull-park.co.uk
Picturesque course set in 280 acres of glorious 'Capability' Brown
landscaped parkland. Designed by John Jacobs, the course meanders
alongside trout fishing lakes. Water comes into play alongside
the 3rd hole and there is a challenging drive over water on the 13th.
Wellingtonia and cedar trees prove an obstacle to wayward drives off
several holes. The 12th is the toughest hole on the course and the tee
shot is vital, anything wayward and the trees block out the second to
the green.

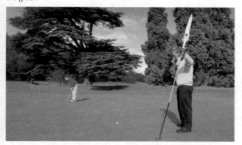

18 holes, 6400yds, Par 72, SSS 71, Course record 64.
Club membership 345.
Visitors Mon-Sun & BHs, Booking required. Handicap certificate. Dress
code. **Societies** Booking required. **Green Fees** £40 per round. **Prof** Richard
Bissell **Course Designer** John Jacobs **Facilities** ⑪ ⑨ 🏌 ♥ 🏋 🍴 ♨ 🏌
♡ ✔ 🍴 ✔ **Leisure** heated indoor swimming pool, fishing, sauna, solarium,
gymnasium. **Conf** facs Corporate Hospitality Days **Location** 1.5m W of
Pattingham at Pattingham Church take the Patshull Rd, Golf club on right
Hotel ★★★ 77% HL Patshull Park Hotel Golf & Country Club, Patshull
Park, PATTINGHAM ☎ 01902 700100 49 en suite

PENKRIDGE
MAP 07 SJ91

The Chase Pottal Pool Rd ST19 5RN
☎ 01785 712888 🖹 01785 712191
e-mail: tcgc@crown-golf.co.uk
web: www.crown-golf.co.uk
18 holes, 6707yds, Par 72, SSS 74.
Location 2m E off B5012
Telephone for further details
Hotel ★★★ 71% HL Quality Hotel Stafford, Pinfold Ln, PENKRIDGE
☎ 01785 712459 47 en suite

PERTON
MAP 07 SO89

Perton Park Wrottesley Park Rd WV6 7HL
☎ 01902 380073 🖹 01902 326219
e-mail: admin@pertongolfclub.co.uk
web: www.pertongolfclub.co.uk
Challenging inland links style course set in picturesque Staffordshire
countryside.
18 holes, 6520yds, Par 72, SSS 72, Course record 61.
Club membership 500.
Visitors Mon-Sun & BHs. Booking required Sat, Sun & BHs. Dress code.
Societies Booking required **Green Fees** £18 per round (£23 Sat, Sun &

BHs). **Prof** Jeremy Harrold **Facilities** ⑪ ⑨ 🏌 ♥ 🏋 🍴 ♨ 🏌 ✔ 🏌
Leisure hard tennis courts, bowling greens. **Location** SE of Perton off A454

RUGELEY
MAP 07 SK01

St Thomas's Priory Armitage Ln WS15 1ED
☎ 01543 492096 🖹 01543 492096
e-mail: rohanlonpro@aol.com
Parkland with undulating fairways. Excellent drainage facilitates golf all
year round. A good test of golf for both pro and amateur players.
18 holes, 5969yds, Par 70, SSS 70, Course record 64.
Club membership 400.
Visitors Mon-Sun & BHs. Booking required. **Societies** booking
required. **Green Fees** not confirmed. **Prof** Richard O'Hanlon **Course
Designer** P I Mulholland **Facilities** ⑪ ⑨ 🏌 ♥ 🏋 🍴 ♨ ✔ 🏌 ✔ **Leisure**
fishing. **Conf** facs **Location** A51 onto A513
Hotel BUD Travelodge Rugeley, Western Springs Rd, RUGELEY
☎ 08700 850 950 32 en suite

STAFFORD
MAP 07 SJ92

Stafford Castle Newport Rd ST16 1BP
☎ 01785 223821 🖹 01785 223821
e-mail: staffordcastle.golfclub@globaluk.net
Undulating parkland-type course built around Stafford Castle.
9 holes, 6383yds, Par 71, SSS 70, Course record 68.
Club membership 400.
Visitors Mon-Sat except BHs. Booking required Sat. Dress code. **Societies**
Booking required. **Green Fees** £18 per day (£22 Sat). ♨ **Facilities** ⑪ 🏌
🍴 🏋 🏌 **Conf** Corporate Hospitality Days **Location** SW of town centre
off A518
Hotel ★★★ 81% HL The Swan Hotel, 46 Greengate St, STAFFORD
☎ 01785 258142 31 en suite

STOKE-ON-TRENT
MAP 07 SJ84

Burslem Wood Farm, High Ln, Tunstall ST6 7JT
☎ 01782 837006
e-mail: alanporterburslemgc@yahoo.co.uk
On the outskirts of Tunstall, a moorland course with hard walking.
9 holes, 5354yds, Par 66, SSS 66, Course record 66.
Club membership 250.
Visitors Mon-Fri except BHs. Booking required. Handicap certificate. Dress
code. **Societies** Booking required. **Green Fees** Phone. ♨ **Facilities** ⑪ by
prior arrangement ⑨ by prior arrangement 🏌 by prior arrangement 🍴 🏌
Location 4m N of city centre on B5049
Hotel ★★★ 67% HL Quality Hotel, 66 Trinity St, Hanley, STOKE-ON-TRENT
☎ 01782 202361 128 en suite 8 annexe en suite

Greenway Hall Stanley Rd, Stockton Brook ST9 9LJ
☎ 01782 503158 🖹 01782 504691
e-mail: greenway@jackbarker.com
web: www.jackbarker.com
Moorland course with fine views of the Pennines.
18 holes, 5678yds, Par 68, SSS 67, Course record 65.
Club membership 300.
Visitors Mon-Sun & BHs. Booking required. Dress code. **Societies** Booking
required. **Green Fees** £10 (£15 Sat & Sun). **Facilities** ⑪ ⑨ 🏌 🍴 🏌 🏋
🍴 🏌 ✔ 🍴 ✔ **Conf** Corporate Hospitality Days **Location** 5m NE off A53
Hotel ★★★ 67% HL Quality Hotel, 66 Trinity St, Hanley, STOKE-ON-TRENT
☎ 01782 202361 128 en suite 8 annexe en suite

Trentham 14 Barlaston Old Rd, Trentham ST4 8HB
☎ 01782 658109 📠 01782 644024
e-mail: secretary@trenthamgolf.org
web: www.trenthamgolf.org
Parkland course. The Par 3 4th is a testing hole reached through a copse of trees.

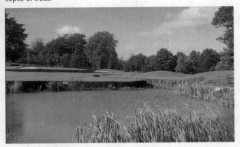

18 holes, 6644yds, Par 72, SSS 72, Course record 67.
Club membership 600.
Visitors Mon-Fri except BHs. Booking required. Handicap certificate. Dress code. **Societies** Booking required. **Green Fees** £40. **Prof** Sandy Wilson **Course Designer** Colt & Alison **Facilities** ⊕ ⭘⭐ ⭐ ⊑ ⭐⭐ ⭐ ⭐ ⭐ ⭐ **Leisure** squash. **Conf** Corporate Hospitality Days **Location** Off A5035 in Trentham
Hotel ★★★ 70% HL Haydon House Hotel, Haydon St, Basford, STOKE-ON-TRENT ☎ 01782 711311 17 en suite 6 annexe en suite

Trentham Park Trentham Park ST4 8AE
☎ 01782 658800 📠 01782 658800
e-mail: trevor-berrisford@barbox.net
18 holes, 6425yds, Par 71, SSS 71, Course record 67.
Location M6 junct 15, 1m E. 3m SW of Stoke off A34
Telephone for further details
Hotel ★★★ 70% HL Haydon House Hotel, Haydon St, Basford, STOKE-ON-TRENT ☎ 01782 711311 17 en suite 6 annexe en suite

STONE · MAP 07 SJ93

Barlaston Meaford Rd ST15 8UX
☎ 01782 372795 & 372867 📠 01782 372867
e-mail: barlaston.gc@virgin.net
web: www.bgc.everplay.net
Picturesque parkland course designed by Peter Alliss. A number of water features come into play on several holes.
18 holes, 5800yds, Par 69, SSS 68, Course record 65.
Club membership 600.
Visitors Mon-Sun & BHs. Booking required. Handicap certificate. Dress code. **Societies** booking required. **Green Fees** not confirmed. ⊛ **Prof** Ian Rogers **Course Designer** Peter Alliss **Facilities** ⊕ ⭘⭐ ⭐ ⊑ ⭐⭐ ⭐ ⭐ ⭐ **Conf** Corporate Hospitality Days **Location** M6 junct 15, 5m S
Hotel ★★★ 74% HL The Crown Hotel, 38 High St, STONE
☎ 01785 813535 9 en suite 16 annexe en suite

Izaak Walton Eccleshall Rd, Cold Norton ST15 0NS
☎ 01785 760900 (sec) & 760808 (pro)
e-mail: secretary @izaakwaltongolfclub.co.uk
web: www.izaakwaltongolfclub.co.uk
A gently undulating meadowland course with streams and ponds as features.

18 holes, 6370yds, Par 72, SSS 72, Course record 66.
Club membership 450.
Visitors Mon-Sun & BHs. Booking required Sat & Sun. Dress code.
Societies Booking required. **Green Fees** £25 per day, £20 per round (£35/£25 Sat, Sun & BHs). ⊛ **Prof** Paul Brunt **Facilities** ⊕ ⭘⭐ ⭐ ⊑ ⭐⭐ ⭐ ⭐ **Location** On B5026 between Stone & Eccleshall
Hotel ★★★ 74% HL The Crown Hotel, 38 High St, STONE
☎ 01785 813535 9 en suite 16 annexe en suite

Stone Filleybrooks ST15 0NB
☎ 01785 813103
e-mail: enquiries@stonegolfclub.co.uk
web: www.stonegolfclub.co.uk
Nine-hole parkland course with easy walking and 18 different tees.
9 holes, 6299yds, Par 71, SSS 70, Course record 67.
Club membership 310.
Visitors Mon-Fri except BHs. Handicap certificate. Dress code. **Societies** Booking required. **Green Fees** £20 per day or round. ⊛ **Facilities** ⊕ ⭘⭐ ⭐ ⊑ ⭐⭐ ⭐ ⭐ **Location** 0.5m W on A34
Hotel ★★★ 74% HL The Crown Hotel, 38 High St, STONE
☎ 01785 813535 9 en suite 16 annexe en suite

TAMWORTH · MAP 07 SK20

Drayton Park Drayton Park, Fazeley B78 3TN
☎ 01827 251139 📠 01827 284035
e-mail: draytonparkgc.co.uk
web: www.draytonparkgc.co.uk
18 holes, 6439yds, Par 71, SSS 71, Course record 62.
Course Designer James Braid **Location** 2m S on A4091, next to Drayton Manor Leisure Park
Telephone for further details
Hotel ★★★★ 80% HL The De Vere Belfry, WISHAW ☎ 0870 900 0066 324 en suite

Tamworth Municipal Eagle Dr, Amington B77 4EG
☎ 01827 709303 📠 01827 709305
e-mail: david-warburton@tamworth.gov.uk
web: www.tamworth.gov.uk
First-class municipal parkland course and a good test of golf.
18 holes, 6488yds, Par 73, SSS 72, Course record 63.
Club membership 460.
Visitors Mon-Sun & BHs. Booking required. **Societies** booking required.
Green Fees not confirmed. **Prof** Wayne Alcock **Course Designer** Hawtree & Son **Facilities** ⊕ ⭐ ⊑ ⭐⭐ ⭐ ⭐ ⭐ **Conf** facs Corporate Hospitality Days **Location** 2.5m E off B5000
Hotel ★★ 61% HL Angel Croft Hotel, Beacon St, LICHFIELD
☎ 01543 258737 10 rms (8 en suite) 8 annexe en suite

UTTOXETER · MAP 07 SK03

Manor Leese Hill, Kingstone ST14 8QT
☎ 01889 563234 📠 01889 563234
e-mail: manorgc@btinternet.com
web: www.manorgolfclub.co.uk
A short but tough course set in the heart of the Staffordshire countryside with fine views of the surrounding area.
18 holes, 6060yds, Par 71, SSS 69, Course record 67.
Club membership 400.
Visitors Mon-Sun & BHs. Booking required Sat/Sun. Dress code. **Societies** booking required. **Green Fees** not confirmed. **Prof** Chris Miller **Course**

Continued

Designer Various **Facilities** ⑪ ❘❍❙ 🟦 🖵 🍴❙ 🏊 ✐ 🛢 ✐ 🍴 **Leisure** fishing. **Conf** Corporate Hospitality Days **Location** 2m from Uttoxeter on A518 towards Stafford
Hotel ★★★ 73% HL The Boars Head Hotel, Lichfield Rd, SUDBURY
☎ 01283 820344 22 en suite 1 annexe en suite

Uttoxeter Wood Ln ST14 8JR
☎ 01889 564884 (Pro) & 566552 (Office)
🖨 01889 567501
web: uttoxetergolfclub.com
18 holes, 5801yds, Par 70, SSS 69, Course record 64.
Course Designer G Rothera **Location** Near A50, 0.5m beyond main entrance to racecourse
Telephone for further details
Hotel ★★★ 73% HL The Boars Head Hotel, Lichfield Rd, SUDBURY
☎ 01283 820344 22 en suite 1 annexe en suite

WESTON   MAP 07 SJ92

Ingestre Park ST18 0RE
☎ 01889 270845 🖨 01889 271434
e-mail: office@ingestregolf.co.uk
web: www.ingestregolf.co.uk
Parkland course set in the grounds of Ingestre Hall, former home of the Earl of Shrewsbury, with mature trees and pleasant views.
18 holes, 6352yds, Par 70, SSS 70, Course record 67.
Club membership 750.
Visitors Mon-Fri except BHs. Handicap certificate. Dress code. **Societies** Booking required. **Green Fees** £40 per day; £30 per round. 🌑 **Prof** Danny Scullion **Course Designer** Hawtree **Facilities** ⑪ ❘❍❙ 🟦 🖵 🍴❙ 🏊 🛢 ✐ 🛢 ✐ **Conf** Corporate Hospitality Days **Location** 2m SE off A51
Hotel ★★★ 81% HL The Swan Hotel, 46 Greengate St, STAFFORD
☎ 01785 258142 31 en suite

WHISTON   MAP 07 SK04

Whiston Hall Mansion Court Hotel ST10 2HZ
☎ 01538 266260 🖨 01538 266820
e-mail: enquiries@whistonhall.com
web: www.whistonhall.com
A challenging 18-hole course in scenic countryside 2m fro Alton Towers, incorporating many natural obstacles and providing a test for all golfing abilities.
18 holes, 5742yds, Par 71, SSS 69, Course record 70.
Club membership 400.
Visitors Mon-Sun & BHs. **Societies** Booking required. **Green Fees** £10 per round. **Course Designer** T Cooper **Facilities** ⑪ ❘❍❙ 🟦 🖵 🍴❙ 🏊 ◇ 🛢 ✐
Leisure fishing, snooker. **Conf** facs Corporate Hospitality Days **Location** E of village centre off A52

SUFFOLK

ALDEBURGH   MAP 05 TM45

Aldeburgh Saxmundham Rd IP15 5PE
☎ 01728 452890 🖨 01728 452937
e-mail: info@aldeburghgolfclub.co.uk
web: www.aldeburghgolfclub.co.uk
Good natural drainage provides year round golf in links-type conditions. Accuracy is the first challenge on well-bunkered, gorse-lined holes. Fine views over an Area of Outstanding Natural Beauty.

18 holes, 6349yds, Par 68, SSS 71, Course record 65.
River Course: 9 holes, 4228yds, Par 64, SSS 61,
Course record 900.
Visitors Contact club for details. Handicap certificate. Dress code.
Societies Booking required. **Green Fees** £55 per day; £45 after 12 noon (weekends £60/£50). **Prof** Keith Preston **Course Designer** Thompson, Fernie, Taylor, Park. **Facilities** ⑪ 🟦 🖵 🍴❙ 🏊 🛢 ✐ 🛢 ✐ **Location** 1m W on A1094
Hotel ★★★ 86% HL Wentworth Hotel, Wentworth Rd, ALDEBURGH
☎ 01728 452312 28 en suite 7 annexe en suite

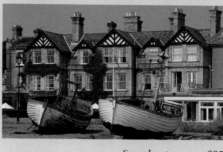

See advert on page 225

BECCLES   MAP 05 TM48

Beccles The Common NR34 9YN
☎ 01502 712244
e-mail: alan@ereira.wanadoo.co.uk
Commons course with gorse bushes, no water hazards or bunkers.
9 holes, 5566yds, Par 68, SSS 67, Course record 66.
Club membership 50.
Visitors Mon-Sun & BHs. **Societies** Welcome. **Green Fees** £5 per day (£10 Sat & Sun). 🌑 **Facilities** 🟦 🖵 🍴❙ 🏊 ✐ **Location** NE of town centre
Hotel ★★★ 72% HL Hotel Hatfield, The Esplanade, LOWESTOFT
☎ 01502 565337 33 en suite

BUNGAY   MAP 05 TM38

Bungay & Waveney Valley Outney Common NR35 1DS
☎ 01986 892337 🖨 01986 892222
e-mail: golfclub@onetel.com
web: www.club-noticeboard.co.uk
Heathland course, lined with fir trees and gorse. Excellent greens all-year-round, easy walking.
18 holes, 6044yds, Par 69, SSS 69, Course record 64.
Club membership 730.
Visitors may play Mon-Fri. Advance booking required. Dress code.
Societies advance booking required. **Green Fees** not confirmed. 🌑
Prof Andrew Collison **Course Designer** James Braid **Facilities** ⑪ ❘❍❙ 🟦 🖵 🍴❙ 🏊 🛢 🛢 ✐ **Conf** Corporate Hospitality Days **Location** 0.5m NW on A143 at junct with A144
Hotel ★★★ 72% HL Hotel Hatfield, The Esplanade, LOWESTOFT
☎ 01502 565337 33 en suite

BURY ST EDMUNDS MAP 05 TL86

Bury St Edmunds Tut Hill IP28 6LG
☎ 01284 755979 📠 01284 763288
e-mail: info@burygolf.co.uk
web: www.clubnoticeboard.co.uk/burystedmunds
A mature, undulating course, full of character with some challenging holes. The nine-hole pay and play course consists of five Par 3s and four Par 4s with modern construction greens.
18 holes, 6675yds, Par 72, SSS 72, Course record 65.
9 holes, 2217yds, Par 62, SSS 62. Club membership 850.
Visitors 18 hole course Mon-Fri except BHs, 9 hole course Mon-Sun & BHs. Handicap certificate. Dress code. **Societies** Booking required. **Green Fees** 18 hole course £45 per day, £35 per round, 9 hole course £15 per round (£17 Sat & Sun). **Prof** Mark Jillings **Course Designer** Ted Ray **Facilities** ⑪ ⦿ by prior arrangement ♨ ⚲ 🏌 ♨ 🍴 ✦ 🏌 **Conf** Corporate Hospitality Days **Location** A14 junct 42, 0.5m NW on B1106
Hotel ★★★ 87% HL Angel Hotel, Angel Hill, BURY ST EDMUNDS ☎ 01284 714000 76 en suite

Swallow Suffolk Hotel Golf & Country Club Fornham St Genevieve IP28 6JQ
☎ 01284 706801 📠 01284 706721
e-mail: golfreservations.suffolk@swallowhotels.com
web: www.swallowhotels.com
A classic parkland course with the River Lark running through it. Criss-crossed by ponds and streams with rich fairways. Considerable upgrading of the course in recent years and the three finishing holes are particularly challenging.
The Genevieve Course: 18 holes, 6376yds, Par 72, SSS 71, Course record 69. Club membership 600.
Visitors Mon-Sun & BHs. Advance booking required. Dress code. **Societies** advance booking required. **Green Fees** not confirmed. **Prof** Steve Hall **Facilities** ⑪ ⦿ ♨ ⚲ 🏌 ♨ 🍴 ◈ 🏌 ♨ 🏌 **Leisure** heated indoor swimming pool, sauna, solarium, gymnasium. **Conf** facs Corporate Hospitality Days **Location** Off A14 at Bury St Edmunds, W onto B1106 towards Brandon, club 2.5m on right
Hotel ★★★ 87% HL Angel Hotel, Angel Hill, BURY ST EDMUNDS ☎ 01284 714000 76 en suite

CRETINGHAM MAP 05 TM26

Cretingham IP13 7BA
☎ 01728 685275 📠 01728 685488
e-mail: cretinghamgolfclub@hotmail.co.uk
web: www.club-noticeboard.co.uk/cretingham
Parkland course, tree-lined with numerous water features, including the River Deben which runs through part of the course.
18 holes, 4968yds, Par 68, SSS 66. Club membership 350.
Visitors Mon-Sun & BHs. Booking required. **Societies** Booking required. **Green Fees** £18 per 18 holes, £10 per 9 holes. **Prof** Neil Jackson/Tim Johnson **Course Designer** J Austin **Facilities** ⑪ ⦿ ♨ ⚲ 🏌 ♨ 🏌 ◈ 🏌 ✦ 🏌 **Leisure** hard tennis courts, outdoor swimming pool, fishing, pitch & putt, 9 hole course. **Conf** facs Corporate Hospitality Days **Location** NE of village off A1120
Hotel ★★ 76% HL Cedars Hotel, Needham Rd, STOWMARKET ☎ 01449 612668 25 en suite

FELIXSTOWE MAP 05 TM33

Felixstowe Ferry Ferry Rd IP11 9RY
☎ 01394 286834 📠 01394 273679
e-mail: secretary@felixstowegolf.co.uk
web: www.felixstowegolf.co.uk
An 18-hole seaside links with pleasant views, easy walking. Nine-hole pay and play course, a good test of golf.
Martello Course: 18 holes, 6166yds, Par 72, SSS 70, Course record 66.
Kingsfleet: 9 holes, 2941yds, Par 35, SSS 35.
Club membership 900.
Visitors Mon-Wed & Fri. Thu, Sat, Sun & BHs pm only. Booking required. Handicap certificate & dress code for 18 hole course. **Societies** Welcome. **Green Fees** Martello £37.50 per day (£27.50 after 1pm), £40 Sat, Sun & BHs. Kingsflee £11 (£13.50 Sat, Sun & BHs). ◉ **Prof** Ian MacPherson **Course Designer** Henry Cotton **Facilities** ⑪ ⦿ ♨ ⚲ 🏌 ♨ 🍴 🏌 **Conf** facs Corporate Hospitality Days **Location** NE of town centre, signed from A14
Hotel ★★★ 78% HL Elizabeth Orwell Hotel, Hamilton Rd, FELIXSTOWE ☎ 01394 285511 60 en suite

FLEMPTON MAP 05 TL86

Flempton IP28 6EQ
☎ 01284 728291 📠 01284 728468
e-mail: flemptongolfclub@freebie.net
Breckland course with gorse and wooded areas. Very little water but surrounded by woodland and Suffolk Wildlife Trust lakes.
9 holes, 6240yds, Par 70, SSS 70, Course record 67.
Club membership 250.
Visitors Mon-Sun except BHs. Booking required. Handicap certificate. Dress code. **Green Fees** £35 per day, £30 per 18 holes. ◉ **Prof** Chris Aldred **Course Designer** J H Taylor **Facilities** ⑪ ♨ ⚲ 🏌 ♨ 🍴 🏌 **Location** 0.5m W on A1101
Hotel ★★★ 79% HL Best Western Priory Hotel, Milden Hall Rd, BURY ST EDMUNDS ☎ 01284 766181 9 en suite 30 annexe en suite

HALESWORTH MAP 05 TM37

Halesworth Bramfield Rd IP19 9XA
☎ 01986 875567 📠 01986 874565
e-mail: info@halesworthgc.co.uk
web: www.club-noticeboard.co.uk/halesworth
18 holes, 6580yds, Par 72, SSS 72, Course record 71.
9 holes, 2398yds, Par 33, SSS 33.
Course Designer J W Johnson **Location** 0.75m S of town, signed off A144 to Bramfield
Telephone for further details
Hotel ★★★ 80% HL Swan Hotel, Market Place, SOUTHWOLD ☎ 01502 722186 25 en suite 17 annexe en suite

HAVERHILL
MAP 05 TL64

Haverhill Coupals Rd CB9 7UW
☎ 01440 761951 📄 01440 761951
e-mail: haverhillgolf@coupalsroad.fsnet.co.uk
web: www.club-noticeboard.co.uk
An 18-hole course lying across two valleys in pleasant parkland. The front nine with undulating fairways is complemented by a saucer-shape back nine, bisected by the River Stour, presenting a challenge to golfers of all standards.
18 holes, 5967yds, Par 70, SSS 69, Course record 64.
Club membership 750.
Visitors Mon-Sun & BHs. Dress code. **Societies** Welcome. **Green Fees** Phone. **Prof** Nick Duc **Course Designer** P Pilgrem/C Lawrie **Facilities** ⑪
🍴 🛒 🖵 🗑 ⌔ 🏌 🏪 ⚲ **Leisure** chipping green. **Conf** facs Corporate Hospitality Days **Location** 1m SE off A1017
Hotel ★★★ 82% HL Swynford Paddocks Hotel, SIX MILE BOTTOM
☎ 01638 570234 15 en suite

HINTLESHAM
MAP 05 TM04

Hintlesham IP8 3JG
☎ 01473 652761 📄 01473 652750
e-mail: office@hintleshamgolfclub.com
web: www.hintleshamgolfclub.com
Magnificent championship length course blending harmoniously with the ancient parkland surrounding the hotel. Opened in 1991 but seeded two years beforehand, this parkland course has reached a level maturity that allows it to be rivalled in the area only by a few ancient courses. The signature holes are the 4th and 17th, both featuring water at very inconvenient interludes.
18 holes, 6638yds, Par 72, SSS 72, Course record 63.
Club membership 470.
Visitors Mon-Sun & BHs. Booking required. Dress code.
Societies Welcome. **Green Fees** £36 per round (£44 Sat, Sun & BHs).
Prof Henry Roblin **Course Designer** Hawtree & Sons **Facilities** ⑪
🍴 🛒 🖵 🗑 ⌔ 🏌 ◇ ⚲ 🏪 ⚲ **Leisure** hard tennis courts, heated outdoor swimming pool, sauna, gymnasium, spa bath. **Conf** Corporate Hospitality Days **Location** In village on A1071
Hotel ★★★★ HL Hintlesham Hall Hotel, George St, HINTLESHAM
☎ 01473 652334 33 en suite

IPSWICH
MAP 05 TM14

Alnesbourne Priory Priory Park IP10 0JT
☎ 01473 727393 📄 01473 278372
e-mail: golf@priory-park.com
web: www.priory-park.com
A fabulous outlook facing due south across the River Orwell is one of the many good features of this course set in woodland. All holes run among trees with some fairways requiring straight shots. The 8th green is on saltings by the river.
9 holes, 1700yds, Par 29. Club membership 30.
Visitors Mon-Sun & BHs. Dress code. **Societies** Booking required.
Green Fees £10 (£15 Sat, Sun & BHs). 🌐 **Facilities** ⑪ 🍴 🛒 🖵 🗑 ⌔
🏁 **Leisure** practice net. **Conf** facs Corporate Hospitality Days **Location** 3m SE off A14

Fynn Valley IP6 9JA
☎ 01473 785267 📄 01473 785632
e-mail: enquiries@fynn-valley.co.uk
web: www.fynn-valley.co.uk.
Undulating parkland alongside a protected river valley. The course has matured into an excellent test of golf enhanced by more than 100 bunkers and protected greens that have tricky slopes and contours.

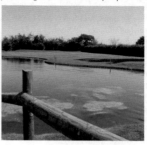

18 holes, 6371yds, Par 70, SSS 71, Course record 65.
Club membership 680.
Visitors Mon-Fri & BHs. Sat & Sun after 10.30am. Dress code. **Societies** Booking required. **Green Fees** £36 per day, £26 per 18 holes (£40/£32 Sat, Sun & BHs). **Prof** S Dainty/D Barton **Course Designer** Antonio Primavera **Facilities** ⑪ 🍴 🛒 🖵 🗑 ⌔ 🏌 🏪 ⚲ 🏁 **Leisure** 9 hole Par 3 course, practice bunker. **Conf** facs Corporate Hospitality Days **Location** 2m N of Ipswich on B1077
Hotel ★★★ 72% HL Novotel Ipswich Centre, Greyfriars Rd, IPSWICH
☎ 01473 232400 101 en suite

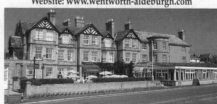

Ipswich Purdis Heath IP3 8UQ

☎ 01473 728941 📠 01473 715236
e-mail: neill@ipswichgolfclub.com
web: www.ipswichgolfclub.com
Many golfers are surprised when they hear that Ipswich has, at
Purdis Heath, a first-class course. In some ways it resembles some of
Surrey's better courses; a beautiful heathland course with two lakes
and easy walking.
Purdis Heath: 18 holes, 6439yds, Par 71, SSS 71,
Course record 64. 9 holes, 1930yds, Par 31.
Club membership 885.
Visitors Mon-Sun except BHs. Booking required for main course.
Handicap certificate.for main course. Dress code. **Societies** Booking
required. **Green Fees** 18 hole course £45 per day; £35 per round pm
(£50/£40 Sat, Sun & BHs), 9 hole course £10 per day (£12.50 Sat, Sun &
BHs). **Course Designer** James Braid **Facilities** ⑪ ⑩I 🍴 🍽 🖥 🛒 🏌 🏖 ✇
Location 3m E of town centre off A1156

Rushmere Rushmere Heath IP4 5QQ

☎ 01473 725648 📠 01473 273852
e-mail: rushmeregolfclub@btconnect.com
web: www.club-noticeboard.co.uk/rushmere
Heathland course with gorse and prevailing winds. A good test of golf.
18 holes, 6262yds, Par 70, SSS 70, Course record 66.
Club membership 700.
Visitors Mon-Fri except BHs. Dress code. **Societies** Booking required.
Green Fees £40 per day. **Prof** K. Vince **Course Designer** James Braid
Facilities ⑪ ⑩I 🍴 🍽 🖥 🛒 🏌 🏖 ✇ **Conf** facs Corporate Hospitality Days
Location On A1214 Woodbridge road near hospital, signed
Hotel ★★★ 74% HL The Hotel Elizabeth, Old London Rd, Copdock,
IPSWICH ☎ 01473 209988 76 en suite

LOWESTOFT   MAP 05 TM59

Rookery Park Beccles Rd, Carlton Colville NR33 8HJ

☎ 01502 509190 📠 01502 509191
e-mail: office@rookeryparkgolfclub.co.uk
web: www.club-noticeboard.co.uk
Mature tree lined parkland course over gently undulating ground. The
Par 3 course is a smaller version of the main course in every respect.
18 holes, 6714yds, Par 71, SSS 71. Club membership 1000.
Visitors Mon-Sun except BHs. Handicap cerificate. Dress code. **Societies**
Booking required. **Green Fees** £29.50 (£35 Sat, Sun & BHs). **Prof** Martin
Elsworthy **Course Designer** C D Lawrie **Facilities** ⑪ ⑩I 🍴 🍽 🖥 🛒 🏌
🏖 ✇ 🏌 **Leisure** 9 hole Par 3 course. **Conf** Corporate Hospitality Days
Location 3.5m SW of Lowestoft on A146
Hotel ★★★ 72% HL Hotel Hatfield, The Esplanade, LOWESTOFT
☎ 01502 565337 33 en suite

MILDENHALL   MAP 05 TL77

West Suffolk Golf Centre New Drove, Beck Row
IP28 8DS

☎ 01638 718972 📠 01353 675447
web: www.club-noticeboard.co.uk
This course has been gradually improved to provide a unique
opportunity to play an inland course in all weather conditions. Situated
on the edge of the Breckland, the dry nature of the course makes for
easy walking with rare flora and fauna.

18 holes, 6461yds, Par 71, SSS 71.
Visitors Mon-Sun & BHs. Dress code. **Societies** Booking required.
Green Fees £10.50 per day (£14 Sat, Sun & BHs). **Prof** Duncan Abbott
Facilities ⑪ 🍴 🍽 🛒 🏌 🏖 🛒 🏌 ✇ 🏌 **Leisure** fishing, pitch and putt
practice course. **Conf** Corporate Hospitality Days **Location** A1101 from
Mildenhall to Beck Row, 1st left after Beck Row signed to West Row/Golf
Centre, 0.5m on right
Hotel ★★★★ 80% HL Bedford Lodge Hotel, Bury Rd, NEWMARKET
☎ 01638 663175 55 en suite

NEWMARKET   MAP 05 TL66

Links Cambridge Rd CB8 0TG

☎ 01638 663000 📠 01638 661476
e-mail: secretary@linksgc.fsbusiness.co.uk
web: www.clubnoticeboard.co.uk/newmarket
Gently undulating parkland.
18 holes, 6582yds, Par 72, SSS 72, Course record 66 or ,
Par 72. Club membership 780.
Visitors Mon-Sun & BHs. Booking required. Handicap certificate. Dress code.
Societies Welcome. **Green Fees** £34 per day, £26 per round (£38/£30 Sat
& Sun). 🏌 **Prof** John Sharkey **Course Designer** Col. Hotchkin **Facilities** ⑪
⑩I 🍴 🍽 🖥 🛒 🏌 ✇ **Location** 1m SW on A1034
Hotel ★★★ 78% HL Best Western Heath Court Hotel, Moulton Rd,
NEWMARKET ☎ 01638 667171 41 en suite

NEWTON   MAP 05 TL94

Newton Green Newton Green CO10 0QN

☎ 01787 377217 & 377501 📠 01787 377549
e-mail: info@newtongreengolfclub.co.uk
web: www.newtongreengolfclub.co.uk
Flat 18-hole course with pond. First nine holes are open with bunkers
and trees. Second nine holes are tight with ditches and gorse.
18 holes, 5960yds, Par 69, SSS 68. Club membership 570.
Visitors Mon & Wed-Fri. Sat, Sun & BHs pm only. Dress code. **Societies**
Booking required. **Green Fees** £23 per round (£27 Sat & Sun). **Prof** Tim
Cooper **Facilities** ⑪ ⑩I 🍴 🍽 🖥 🛒 🏌 ✇ **Location** W of village on A134
Hotel ★★★ 75% HL The Bull, Hall St, LONG MELFORD ☎ 01787 378494
25 en suite

RAYDON   MAP 05 TM03

Brett Vale Noakes Rd IP7 5LR

☎ 01473 310718
e-mail: info@brettvalegolf.co.uk
web: www.brettvalegolf.co.uk
Brett Vale course takes you through a nature reserve and on lakeside
walks, affording views over Dedham Vale. The excellent fairways
demand an accurate tee and good approach shots; 1, 2, 3, 8, 10
and 15 are all affected by crosswinds, but once in the valley it is
much more sheltered. Although only 5864yds the course is testing
and interesting at all levels of golf.
18 holes, 5864yds, Par 70, SSS 69, Course record 65.
Club membership 600.
Visitors Mon-Sun & BHs. Dress code. **Societies** Booking required.
Green Fees £22.50 per 18 holes (£28 Sat, Sun & BHs). **Prof** Paul Bate
Course Designer Howard Swan **Facilities** ⑪ ⑩I 🍴 🍽 🖥 🛒 🏌 🏖 🛒 ✇
🏖 ✇ 🏌 **Leisure** fishing, gymnasium. **Conf** facs Corporate Hospitality
Days **Location** A12 onto B1070 towards Hadleigh, left at Raydon, by
water tower
Hotel ★★★ CHH Maison Talbooth, Stratford Rd, DEDHAM
☎ 01206 322367 10 en suite

SOUTHWOLD
MAP 05 TM57

Southwold The Common IP18 6TB
☎ 01502 723234
Commonland course with fine greens and panoramic views of the sea.
9 holes, 6052yds, Par 70, SSS 69, Course record 67.
Club membership 350.
Visitors Contact club for details. **Societies** Booking required **Green Fees**
£26 per 18 holes; £13 per 9 holes (£28/£14 Sat & Sun). Reduced rate pm. ●
Prof Brian Allen **Course Designer** J Braid **Facilities** ⑪ ⓑ ▭ ⑪ ⌂ ☖ ☂
⌀ **Conf** Corporate Hospitality Days **Location** S of town off A1095
Hotel ★★★ 80% HL Swan Hotel, Market Place, SOUTHWOLD
☎ 01502 722186   25 en suite   17 annexe en suite

STOWMARKET
MAP 05 TM05

Stowmarket Lower Rd, Onehouse IP14 3DA
☎ 01449 736473 ▤ 01449 736826
e-mail: mail@stowmarketgolfclub.co.uk
web: www.club-noticeboard.co.uk
Parkland course in rolling countryside with river in play on three holes.
Many majestic trees and fine views of the Suffolk countryside.
18 holes, 6107yds, Par 69, SSS 69, Course record 65.
Club membership 630.
Visitors Mon, Tue, Thu-Sun except BHs. Booking required. Handicap
certificate. Dress code **Societies** Booking required. **Green Fees** £40 per
day, £32 per round (£50/£40 Sat & Sun). **Prof** Duncan Burl **Facilities** ⌂
☖ ☂ ⌀ ⌀ ⌀ **Conf** Corporate Hospitality Days **Location** 2.5m SW
off B1115
Hotel ★★ 76% HL Cedars Hotel, Needham Rd, STOWMARKET
☎ 01449 612668   25 en suite

STUSTON
MAP 05 TM17

Diss Stuston IP21 4AA
☎ 01379 641025 ▤ 01379 644586
e-mail: sec.dissgolf@virgin.net
web: www.club-noticeboard.co.uk
An inland commonland course with the river Waveney coming into
play on the 6th hole and having a part parkland, part links feel with
small tight greens. Well bunkered with easy walking. Depending on the
direction of the wind, the golfer can find the last three holes a pleasure
or a pain. The signature hole is the long Par 4 13th, a test on any day -
the drive must be long to give any chance of reaching the green in two.
18 holes, 6206yds, Par 70, SSS 70, Course record 67.
Club membership 750.
Visitors Mon-Sun & BHs. Booking required. Dress code. **Societies** Welcome.
Green Fees £36 per day; £28 per 18 holes, £14 per 9 holes. **Prof** N J Taylor
Facilities ⑪ ⓘ ⓑ ▭ ⑪ ⌂ ☖ ⌀ ☖ ⌀ **Leisure** driving nets. **Conf** facs
Corporate Hospitality Days **Location** 1.5m SE on B1118
Inn ★★★★ INN The White Horse Inn, Stoke Ash, EYE ☎ 01379 678222
11 annexe en suite

THORPENESS
MAP 05 TM45

Thorpeness Golf Club & Hotel Lakeside Av IP16 4NH
☎ 01728 452176 ▤ 01728 453868
e-mail: info@thorpeness.co.uk
web: www.thorpeness.co.uk
A 6271yd coastal heathland course, designed in 1923 by James Braid.
The quality of his design combined with modern green keeping
techniques has resulted in an extremely challenging course for
golfers at all levels. It is also one of the driest courses in the region.

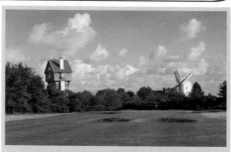
Thorpeness Golf Club & Hotel

18 holes, 6271yds, Par 69, SSS 71, Course record 66.
Club membership 700.
Visitors Mon-Sun & BHs. Booking required. Handicap certificate. Dress
code. **Societies** Booking required. **Green Fees** £37 per day/round (£42
Sat, Sun & BHs), £25 after 3pm. **Prof** Frank Hill **Course Designer** James
Braid **Facilities** ⑪ ⓘ ⓑ ▭ ⑪ ⌂ ☖ ⌀ ☖ ⌀ **Leisure** hard and grass
tennis courts, fishing, snooker room. **Conf** facs Corporate Hospitality
Days **Location** Off A1094 to Aldeburgh, signed
Hotel ★★★ 77% HL Thorpeness Hotel, Lakeside Av, THORPENESS
☎ 01728 452176   30 annexe en suite

WALDRINGFIELD
MAP 05 TM24

Waldringfield Heath Newbourne Rd IP12 4PT
☎ 01473 736768 ▤ 01473 736793
e-mail: patgolf1@aol.com
Easy walking heathland course with long drives on 1st and 13th
(590yds) and some ponds.
18 holes, 6057yds, Par 70, SSS 69, Course record 69.
Club membership 550.
Visitors may play Mon-Fri except BHs Sat & Sun after noon. Booking
required. Dress code. **Societies** Welcome. **Green Fees** 18 holes £24
(£28 Sat, Sun & BHs). **Prof** Tim Huffer **Course Designer** Phillip Pilgrem
Facilities ⑪ ⓘ ⓑ ▭ ⑪ ⌂ ☖ ⌀ ☖ ⌀ **Conf** facs **Location** 1m W of
village off A12
Hotel ★★★ 78% CHH Seckford Hall Hotel, WOODBRIDGE
☎ 01394 385678   22 en suite   10 annexe en suite

WOODBRIDGE
MAP 05 TM24

Best Western Ufford Park Hotel Golf & Leisure
Yarmouth Rd, Ufford IP12 1QW
☎ 0844 4773737 ▤ 0844 4773727
e-mail: mail@uffordpark.co.uk
web: www.uffordpark.co.uk
The 18-hole Par 71 course is set in 120 acres of ancient parkland
with 12 water features and voted one of the best British winter courses.
The course enjoys excellent natural drainage and a large reservoir
supplements a spring feed pond to ensure ample water for irrigation.
The course is host to the Sky Sports PGA Europro Tour.
18 holes, 6312yds, Par 71, SSS 71, Course record 61.
Club membership 350.
Visitors Mon-Sun & BHs. Booking required. Handicap certificate. Dress
code. **Societies** Booking required. **Green Fees** £30 per day (£40 Sat &
Sun). **Prof** Stuart Robertson **Course Designer** Phil Pilgrim **Facilities** ⑪
ⓘ ⓑ ▭ ⑪ ⌂ ☖ ☂ ◇ ☖ ⌀ ⌀ **Leisure** heated indoor swimming pool,
sauna, solarium, gymnasium, golf academy, health club & spa. **Conf** facs
Corporate Hospitality Days **Location** A12 onto B1438
Hotel ★★★ 77% HL Best Western Ufford Park Hotel Golf & Leisure,
Yarmouth Rd, Ufford, WOODBRIDGE ☎ 0844 4773737   87 en suite

Seckford Seckford Hall Rd, Great Bealings IP13 6NT
☎ 01394 388000 🖹 01394 382818
e-mail: info@seckfordgolf.co.uk
web: www.seckfordgolf.co.uk
A challenging course interspersed with young tree plantations,
numerous bunkers, water hazards and undulating fairways, providing
a tough test for all levels of golfer. The testing 18th is almost completely
surrounded by water.
18 holes, 5303yds, Par 68, SSS 66, Course record 62.
Club membership 400.
Visitors Booking required. **Societies** booking required. **Green Fees** not
confirmed. **Prof** Simon Jay **Course Designer** J Johnson **Facilities** ⑪ ⑩ℂ
ᕮ ♉⑪ 🏌 🛏 ℘ ◇ ₼ ℐ **Leisure** heated indoor swimming pool,
fishing, gymnasium. **Conf** Corporate Hospitality Days **Location** 1m W of
Woodbridge 0ff A12, next to Seckford Hall Hotel
Hotel ★★★ 78% CHH Seckford Hall Hotel, WOODBRIDGE
☎ 01394 385678 22 en suite 10 annexe en suite

Woodbridge Bromeswell Heath IP12 2PF
☎ 01394 382038 🖹 01394 382392
e-mail: woodbridgegc@anglianet.co.uk
web: www.woodbridgegolfclub.com
Main Course: 18 holes, 6299yds, Par 70, SSS 70,
Course record 64.
Forest Course: 9 holes, 3191yds, Par 70, SSS 70.
Course Designer Davie Grant **Location** 2.5m NE off A1152
Telephone for further details
Hotel ★★★ 78% CHH Seckford Hall Hotel, WOODBRIDGE
☎ 01394 385678 22 en suite 10 annexe en suite

WORLINGTON   MAP 05 TL67

Royal Worlington & Newmarket Golf Links Rd
IP28 8SD
☎ 01638 712216 & 717787 🖹 01638 717787
web: www.royalworlington.co.uk
Inland links course, renowned as one of the best nine-hole courses
in the world. Well drained, giving excellent winter playing conditions.
9 holes, 3123yds, Par 35, SSS 70, Course record 65.
Club membership 325.
Visitors Mon-Sun & BHs. Booking required. Handicap certificate. Dress
code. **Societies** Booking required. **Green Fees** £60 per day (reductions
after 2 pm). ⊛ **Prof** Steve Barker **Course Designer** Tom Dunn
Facilities ⑪ by prior arrangement ᕮ ♉⑪ 🏌 🛏 ℘ ℐ **Location** 0.5m
SE of Worlington near Mildenhall
Hotel ★★★★ 80% HL Bedford Lodge Hotel, Bury Rd, NEWMARKET
☎ 01638 663175 55 en suite

SURREY

ADDLESTONE   MAP 04 TQ06

New Zealand Woodham Ln KT15 3QD
☎ 01932 345049 🖹 01932 342891
e-mail: roger.marrett@nzgc.org
18 holes, 6073yds, Par 68, SSS 69, Course record 66.
Course Designer Muir Fergusson/Simpson **Location** 1.5m E of Woking
Telephone for further details
Hotel ★★★ 71% HL The Ship Hotel, Monument Green, WEYBRIDGE
☎ 01932 848364 77 en suite

ASHFORD   MAP 04 TQ07

Ashford Manor Fordbridge Rd TW15 3RT
☎ 01784 424644 🖹 01784 424649
e-mail: secretary@amgc.co.uk
web: www.amgc.co.uk
Tree-lined parkland course is built on gravel and drains well, never
needing temporary tees or greens. A heavy investment in fairway
irrigation and an extensive woodland management programme
over the past few years have formed a strong future for this course,
originally built over a 100 years ago.
18 holes, 6352yds, Par 70, SSS 71, Course record 65.
Club membership 700.
Visitors Mon-Fri except BHs. Booking required. Handicap certificate. Dress
code. **Societies** Booking required. **Green Fees** £50 per day, £40 per round.
⊛ **Prof** Ian Campbell **Course Designer** Tom Hogg **Facilities** ⑪ ᕮ ♉⑪
🛏 ℐ **Conf** Corporate Hospitality Days **Location** 2m E of Staines via
A308 Staines bypass
Hotel ★★★ 74% HL Mercure Thames Lodge, Thames St, STAINES
☎ 0870 400 8121 & 01784 464433 🖹 01784 454858 78 en suite

BAGSHOT   MAP 04 SU96

Pennyhill Park Hotel & Country Club London Rd
GU19 5EU
☎ 01276 471774 🖹 01276 473217
e-mail: enquiries@pennyhillpark.co.uk
web: www.exclusivehotels.co.uk
A nine-hole course set in 11 acres of beautiful parkland. It is
challenging to even the most experienced golfer.
9 holes, 2055yds, Par 32, SSS 32. Club membership 100.
Visitors contact hotel for details. Dress code. **Green Fees** not confirmed.
Facilities ⑪ ⑩ℂ ᕮ ♉⑪ 🏌 ℘ ◇ ℐ **Leisure** hard tennis courts, outdoor
and indoor heated swimming pools, sauna, gymnasium. **Conf** facs **Location**
Off A30 between Camberley
Hotel ★★★★★ HL Pennyhill Park Hotel & The Spa, London Rd,
BAGSHOT ☎ 01276 471774 26 en suite 97 annexe en suite

Windlesham Grove End GU19 5HY
☎ 01276 452220 🖹 01276 452290
e-mail: admin@windleshamgolf.com
web: www.windleshamgolf.com
A parkland course with many demanding Par 4 holes over 400 yards.
Thoughtfully designed by Tommy Horton.
18 holes, 6650yds, Par 72, SSS 72, Course record 69.
Club membership 800.
Visitors Mon-Fri, Sat/Sun & BHs pm only. Dress code. **Societies** booking
required. **Green Fees** not confirmed. **Prof** Lee Mucklow **Course Designer**
Tommy Horton **Facilities** ⑪ ⑩ℂ ᕮ ♉⑪ 🏌 🛏 ℘ ✤ ℐ ℱ **Conf** facs
Corporate Hospitality Days **Location** Junct A30
Hotel ★★★★★ HL Pennyhill Park Hotel & The Spa, London Rd,
BAGSHOT ☎ 01276 471774 26 en suite 97 annexe en suite

BANSTEAD   MAP 04 TQ25

Banstead Downs Burdon Ln, Belmont, Sutton SM2 7DD
☎ 020 8642 2284 🖷 020 8642 5252
e-mail: secretary@bansteaddowns.com
A natural downland course set on a site of botanic interest. A
challenging 18 holes with narrow fairways and tight lies.
18 holes, 6192yds, Par 69, SSS 69, Course record 64.
Club membership 902.
Visitors Mon-Thu except BHs. Handicap certificate. Dress code. **Societies**
Welcome. **Green Fees** £45 before noon. £35 after noon. 🅟 **Prof** Ian
Golding **Course Designer** J H Taylor/James Braid **Facilities** 🅟 🍽 by
prior arrangement 🏌 🖵 🎱 ⚒ 🏌 **Conf** Corporate Hospitality Days
Location M25 junct 8, A217 N for 6m
Hotel ★★ 58% HL Thatched House Hotel, 135 Cheam Rd, Sutton
☎ 020 8642 3131 32 rms (29 en suite)

Cuddington Banstead Rd SM7 1RD
☎ 020 8393 0952 🖷 020 8786 7025
e-mail: ds@cuddingtongc.co.uk
18 holes, 6614yds, Par 71, SSS 71, Course record 64.
Course Designer H S Colt **Location** N of Banstead station on A2022
Telephone for further details
Hotel ★★ 58% HL Thatched House Hotel, 135 Cheam Rd, Sutton
☎ 020 8642 3131 32 rms (29 en suite)

BLETCHINGLEY   MAP 05 TQ35

Bletchingley Church Ln RH1 4LP
☎ 01883 744666 🖷 01883 744284
e-mail: info@bletchingleygolf.co.uk
web: www.bletchingleygolf.co.uk
Panoramic views create a perfect backdrop for this course, constructed
on rich sandy loam and playable all year round. The course design has
made best use of the interesting and undulating land features with a
variety of mixed and mature trees providing essential course definition.
A mature stream creates several interesting water features.
18 holes, 6169yds, Par 72, SSS 69. Club membership 500.
Visitors Mon-Sun & BHs. Booking required. Dress code. **Societies** booking
required. **Green Fees** not confirmed. **Prof** Alasdair Dyer **Facilities** 🅟 🍽
by prior arrangement 🏌 🖵 🎱 ⚒ 🏌 **Conf** facs Corporate
Hospitality Days **Location** A25 onto Church Ln in Bletchingley
Hotel ★★★★ 80% HL Nutfield Priory, Nutfield, REDHILL
☎ 01737 824400 60 en suite

BRAMLEY   MAP 04 TQ04

Bramley GU5 0AL
☎ 01483 892696 🖷 01483 894673
e-mail: secretary@bramleygolfclub.co.uk
Parkland course. From the high ground picturesque views of the Wey
valley on one side and the Hog's Back. Full on course irrigation system
with three reservoirs on the course.
18 holes, 5990yds, Par 69, SSS 68, Course record 61.
Club membership 850.
Visitors Mon-Fri except BHs. Dress code. **Societies** booking required.
Green Fees not confirmed. **Prof** Gary Peddie **Course Designer** Charles
Mayo/James Braid **Facilities** 🅟 🍽 🏌 🖵 🎱 🏌 ⚒ ⚒ 🏌 ⚒
Location 3m S of Guildford on A281
Hotel BUD Innkeeper's Lodge Godalming, Ockford Rd, GODALMING
☎ 0845 112 6102 19 rms

BROOKWOOD   MAP 04 SU95

West Hill Bagshot Rd GU24 0BH
☎ 01483 474365 🖷 01483 474252
e-mail: secretary@westhill-golfclub.co.uk
web: www.westhill-golfclub.co.uk
A challenging course with fairways lined with heather and tall pines,
one of Surrey's finest courses. Demands every club in the bag to
be played.
18 holes, 6343yds, Par 69, SSS 70, Course record 62.
Club membership 500.
Visitors Mon-Fri except BHs. Booking required. Handicap certificate.
Dress code. **Societies** Booking required. **Green Fees** £85 per
day, £65 per round. £45 per round winter. **Prof** Guy Shoesmith
Course Designer C Butchart/W Parke **Facilities** 🅟 🍽 by prior
arrangement 🏌 🖵 🎱 ⚒ ⚒ 🏌 **Leisure** halfway hut.
Conf facs Corporate Hospitality Days **Location** E of village on A322
Hotel ★★★★★ HL Pennyhill Park Hotel & The Spa, London Rd,
BAGSHOT ☎ 01276 471774 26 en suite 97 annexe en suite

CAMBERLEY   MAP 04 SU86

Camberley Heath Golf Dr GU15 1JG
☎ 01276 23258 🖷 01276 692505
e-mail: info@camberleyheathgolfclub.co.uk
web: www.camberleyheathgolfclub.co.uk
Set in attractive Surrey countryside, a challenging golf course that
features an abundance of pine and heather. A true classic heathland
course with many assets, including the mature fairways.

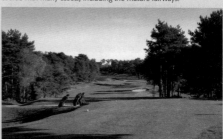

18 holes, 6147yds, Par 72, SSS 70, Course record 65.
Club membership 600.
Visitors Mon-Thu except BHs. Booking required. Handicap certificate.
Dress code. **Societies** Booking required. **Green Fees** £74 per 36 holes,
£57 per 18 holes. **Prof** Glenn Ralph **Course Designer** Harry S Colt
Facilities 🅟 🍽 🏌 🖵 🎱 🏌 ⚒ ⚒ 🏌 **Conf** facs Corporate
Hospitality Days **Location** 1.25m SE of town centre off A325
Hotel ★★★★★ HL Pennyhill Park Hotel & The Spa, London Rd,
BAGSHOT ☎ 01276 471774 26 en suite 97 annexe en suite

Pine Ridge Old Bisley Rd, Frimley GU16 9NX
☎ 01276 675444 & 20770 🖷 01276 678837
e-mail: enquiry@pineridgegolf.co.uk
web: www.pineridgegolf.co.uk
18 holes, 6458yds, Par 72, SSS 71, Course record 65.
Course Designer Clive D Smith **Location** Off B3015, near A30
Telephone for further details
Hotel ★★★★ 80% HL Macdonald Frimley Hall Hotel & Spa, Lime Av,
CAMBERLEY ☎ 0870 400 8224 98 en suite

CATERHAM
MAP 05 TQ35

Surrey National Rook Ln, Chaldon CR3 5AA
☎ 01883 344555 📧 01883 344422
e-mail: caroline@surreynational.co.uk
web: www.surreynational.co.uk
Opened in April 1999, this American-style course is set in beautiful
countryside and features fully irrigated greens and fairways. The setting
is dramatic with rolling countryside, thousands of mature trees and
water features. The chalk based sub-soil, computerised irrigation and
buggy paths combine to make the course enjoyable to play at any
time of year.

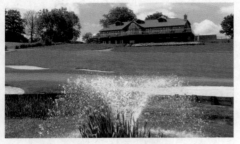

18 holes, 6612yds, Par 72, SSS 73, Course record 64.
Club membership 750.
Visitors Mon-Sun & BHs. Booking required. Dress code. **Societies** Booking
required **Green Fees** £30 per round (£32 Sat & Sun). **Prof** David Kent/
Matthew Stock **Course Designer** David Williams **Facilities** ⑪ ⑩ by prior
arrangement 🍴 ⊞ 🖭 🏌 🛋 🛒 ✂ 🏇 **Conf** facs Corporate Hospitality
Days **Location** M25 junct 7, A23/M25 junct 6, A22
Hotel ★★★★ 73% HL Coulsdon Manor Hotel, Coulsdon Court Rd,
Coulsdon, CROYDON ☎ 020 8668 0414 35 en suite

CHERTSEY
MAP 04 TQ06

Laleham Laleham Reach KT16 8RP
☎ 01932 564211 📧 01932 564448
e-mail: manager@laleham-golf.co.uk
web: www.laleham-golf.co.uk
Well-bunkered parkland and meadowland course. The prevailing wind
and strategic placement of hazards makes it a fair but testing challenge.
Natural drainage due to the underlying gravel.
18 holes, 6291yds, Par 70, SSS 70, Course record 65.
Club membership 600.
Visitors Mon-Sun & BHs. Dress code. **Societies** Booking required **Green
Fees** £30 per round (£32 Sat & Sun). **Prof** Hogan Stott **Course Designer**
Jack White **Facilities** ⑪ 🍴 ⊞ 🖭 🏌 🛋 🛒 ✂ **Conf** facs Corporate
Hospitality Days **Location** M25 junct 11, A320 to Thorpe Park rdbt, exit
Penton Marina, signed
Hotel ★★★ 74% HL Mercure Thames Lodge, Thames St, STAINES
☎ 0870 400 8121 & 01784 464433 📧 01784 454858 78 en suite

CHIDDINGFOLD
MAP 04 SU93

Chiddingfold Petworth Rd GU8 4SL
☎ 01428 685888 📧 01428 685939
e-mail: chiddingfoldgolf@btconnect.com
web: www.chiddingfoldgc.co.uk
With panoramic views across the Surrey hills, this challenging course
offers a unique combination of lakes, mature woodland and wildlife.
18 holes, 5568yds, Par 70, SSS 67. Club membership 250.
Visitors Mon-Sun except BHs. Booking required. Dress code. **Societies**
Booking required. **Green Fees** Phone. **Prof** John Wells **Course Designer**
Johnathan Gaunt **Facilities** ⊞ 🖭 🏌 🛋 🛒 ✂ 🛒 ✂ 🏇 **Conf** facs
Location Off A283
Hotel ★★★★ 77% HL Lythe Hill Hotel & Spa, Petworth Rd, HASLEMERE
☎ 01428 651251 41 en suite

CHIPSTEAD
MAP 04 TQ25

Chipstead How Ln CR5 3LN
☎ 01737 555781 📧 01737 555404
e-mail: office@chipsteadgolf.co.uk
web: www.chipsteadgolf.co.uk
Testing downland course with good views.
18 holes, 5504yds, Par 68, SSS 67, Course record 61.
Club membership 475.
Visitors Mon-Fri except BHs. booking required. Dress code. **Societies**
Booking required. **Green Fees** £40 per day, £30 per round. **Prof** Gary
Torbett **Facilities** ⑪ 🍴 🏌 🛋 🛒 ✂ 🛒 ✂ **Conf** facs Corporate
Hospitality Days **Location** 0.5m N of village
Hotel ★★★★ 73% HL Selsdon Park Hotel & Golf Club, Addington Rd,
Sanderstead, CROYDON ☎ 020 8657 8811 204 en suite

CHOBHAM
MAP 04 SU96

Chobham Chobham Rd, Knaphill GU21 2TZ
☎ 01276 855584 📧 01276 855663
e-mail: info@chobhamgolfclub.co.uk
web: www.chobhamgolfclub.co.uk
Designed by Peter Allis and Clive Clark, Chobham course sits among
mature oaks and tree nurseries offering tree-lined fairways, together
with six man-made lakes.
18 holes, 5959yds, Par 69, SSS 69, Course record 67.
Club membership 750.
Visitors Mon-Thu except BHs. Booking required. Handicap certificate.
Dress code. **Societies** booking required. **Green Fees** not confirmed.
Prof Tim Coombes **Course Designer** Peter Alliss/Clive Clark **Facilities** ⑪
🍴 by prior arrangement 🍴 ⊞ 🖭 🏌 🛋 🛒 ✂ 🛒 ✂ **Conf** facs Corporate
Hospitality Days **Location** on Chobham road between Chobham and
Knaphill
Hotel ★★★ 67% HL Falcon Hotel, 68 Farnborough Rd, FARNBOROUGH
☎ 01252 545378 30 en suite

England

COBHAM
MAP 04 TQ16

Silvermere Redhill Rd KT11 1EF
☎ 01932 584300 🖹 01932 584301
e-mail: sales@silvermere-golf.co.uk
web: www.silvermere-golf.co.uk
A mixture of light heathland on the first six holes and parkland on holes 7-16, then two signature water holes at the 17th and 18th, played over the Silvermere Lake.

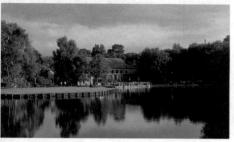

18 holes, 6430yds, Par 71. Club membership 500.
Visitors Mon-Sun & BHs. Booking required. Dress code. **Societies** Welcome. **Green Fees** £24 per 18 holes (£37.50 Sat & Sun). **Prof** Doug McClelland **Course Designer** Neil Coles **Facilities** ⑪ 🍴 🍺 🍷 🏌️ ⚒️ 🏌️ ⛳ 🚶 **Leisure** fishing. **Conf** facs Corporate Hospitality Days **Location** 0.5m from M25 junct 10, off A245
Hotel ★★★★ 84% HL Woodlands Park Hotel, Woodlands Ln, STOKE D'ABERNON ☎ 01372 843933 57 en suite

CRANLEIGH
MAP 04 TQ03

Cranleigh Golf and Leisure Club Barhatch Ln GU6 7NG
☎ 01483 268855 🖹 01483 267251
e-mail: info@cranleighgolfandleisure.co.uk
web: www.cranleighgolfandleisure.co.uk
Scenic woodland and parkland at the base of the Surrey hills, easy walking. The golfer should not be deceived by the length of the course. Clubhouse in 400-year-old barn.
18 holes, 5263yds, Par 68, SSS 65, Course record 62.
Club membership 1400.
Visitors Mon-Sun & BHs. Booking required. Dress code **Societies** booking required. **Green Fees** not confirmed. **Prof** Trevor Longmuir **Facilities** ⑪ 🍺 🍷 🏌️ 🏌️ ⚒️ 🏌️ ⛳ **Leisure** hard tennis courts, heated indoor swimming pool, sauna, solarium, gymnasium, steam room, spa bath. **Conf** Corporate Hospitality Days **Location** 0.5m N of town centre
Hotel ★★★ 73% HL Gatton Manor Hotel & Golf Club, Standon Ln, OCKLEY ☎ 01306 627555 18 en suite

Wildwood Golf & Country Club Horsham Rd, Alfold GU6 8JE
☎ 01403 753255 🖹 01403 752005
e-mail: info@wildwoodgolf.co.uk
web: www.wildwoodgolf.co.uk
Parkland with stands of old oaks dominating several holes, a stream fed by a natural spring winds through a series of lakes and ponds. The greens are smooth, undulating and large. Course consists of three loops of nine holes with a signature hole on each.
27 holes, 6655yds, Par 72, SSS 73, Course record 65.
Club membership 600.

Visitors Mon-Sun & BHs.Booking required. Dress code. **Societies** Booking required. **Green Fees** Phone. **Prof** Phil Harrison **Course Designer** Hawtree & Sons **Facilities** ⑪ 🍴 🍺 🍷 🏌️ 🏌️ ⚒️ 🏌️ ⛳ **Leisure** gymnasium, Par 3 course. **Conf** facs Corporate Hospitality Days **Location** Off A281 3m SW of Cranleigh
Hotel ★★ 68% HL Hurtwood Inn Hotel, Walking Bottom, PEASLAKE ☎ 01306 730851 15 en suite 6 annexe en suite

CROYDON

For other golf courses in the area, please see **Greater London.**

DORKING
MAP 04 TQ14

Betchworth Park Reigate Rd RH4 1NZ
☎ 01306 882052 🖹 01306 877462
e-mail: manager@betchworthparkgc.co.uk
web: www.betchworthparkgc.co.uk
Established parkland course with beautiful views, on the southern side of the North Downs near Boxhill.
18 holes, 6307yds, Par 69, SSS 70, Course record 64.
Club membership 725.
Visitors Mon-Fri except BHs. Dress code. **Societies** Booking required. **Green Fees** £40 per day. **Prof** Andy Tocher **Course Designer** Harry Colt **Facilities** ⑪ 🍺 🍷 🏌️ 🏌️ ⚒️ 🏌️ ⛳ **Conf** Corporate Hospitality Days **Location** 1m E of Dorking on A25 towards Reigate
Hotel ★★★ 68% HL Mercure White Horse Hotel, High St, DORKING ☎ 0870 400 8282 37 en suite 41 annexe en suite

Dorking Chart Park, Deepdene Av RH5 4BX
☎ 01306 886917
e-mail: info@dorkinggolfclub.co.uk
web: www.dorkinggolfclub.co.uk
Undulating parkland, easy slopes, wind sheltered. Testing holes: 5th Tom's Puddle (Par 4); 7th Rest and Be Thankful (Par 4); 9th Double Decker (Par 4).
9 holes, 5120yds, Par 66, SSS 65, Course record 62.
Club membership 392.
Visitors Tue, Thu & Fri. Mon, Wed, Sat, Sun & BHs pm only. Dress code. **Societies** booking advance. **Green Fees** not confirmed. **Prof** Allan Smeal **Course Designer** J Braid/Others **Facilities** ⑪ 🍺 🍷 🏌️ 🏌️ ⚒️ 🏌️ ⛳ **Location** 1m S on A24
Hotel ★★★★ 81% HL Mercure Burford Bridge Hotel, Burford Bridge, Box Hill, DORKING ☎ 0870 400 8283 57 en suite

EAST HORSLEY
MAP 04 TQ05

Drift The Drift, Off Forest Rd KT24 5HD
☎ 01483 284641 & 284772(shop) 🖹 01483 284642
e-mail: info@driftgolfclub.com
web: www.driftgolfclub.com
18 holes, 6425yds, Par 73, SSS 72, Course record 65.
Course Designer Sir Henry Cotton/Robert Sandow **Location** 0.5m N of East Horsley off B2039
Telephone for further details
Hotel ★★ 67% HL Bookham Grange Hotel, Little Bookham Common, Bookham, LEATHERHEAD ☎ 01372 452742 27 en suite

EFFINGHAM
MAP 04 TQ15

Effingham Guildford Rd KT24 5PZ
☎ 01372 452203 📠 01372 459959
e-mail: secretary@effinghamgolfclub.com
web: www.effinghamgolfclub.com
Easy-walking downland course laid out on 270 acres with tree-lined fairways. It is one of the longest of the Surrey courses with wide subtle greens that provide a provocative but by no means exhausting challenge. Fine views of the London skyline.
18 holes, 6554yds, Par 71, SSS 71, Course record 64.
Club membership 800.
Visitors may play Mon-Sun except BHs. Handicap certificate. Dress code. **Societies** Booking required. **Green Fees** £60 per day, £45 per round, £25 after 3.30pm. ♿ **Prof** Steve Hoatson **Course Designer** H S Colt **Facilities** ⊕ ⏵ by prior arrangement 🏌 ♨ 🍴 🎯 🥎 💺 🏆 ♿ 🏌 **Leisure** hard tennis courts, snooker table. **Conf** facs Corporate Hospitality Days **Location** W of village on A246
Hotel ★★ 67% HL Bookham Grange Hotel, Little Bookham Common, Bookham, LEATHERHEAD ☎ 01372 452742 27 en suite

ENTON GREEN
MAP 04 SU94

West Surrey GU8 5AF
☎ 01483 421275 📠 01483 415419
e-mail: office@wsgc.co.uk
web: www.wsgc.co.uk
An attractive downland course with tree-lined fairways and contrasting views of the Surrey landscape. The course winds slowly upwards towards its highest point 440ft above sea level.
18 holes, 6482yds, Par 71, SSS 71, Course record 65.
Club membership 600.
Visitors Mon-Sun & BHs. Booking required. Handicap certificate. Dress code. **Societies** Booking required. **Green Fees** £60 per day; £40 per round (£70/£50 Sat, Sun & BHs). ♿ **Prof** Alister Tawse
Course Designer Herbert Fowler **Facilities** ⊕ ⏵ 🏌 ♨ 🍴 🎯 🥎 💺 ♿ 🏆 **Leisure** hard tennis courts. **Conf** Corporate Hospitality Days **Location** S of village
Hotel ★★★ 78% HL Mercure Bush Hotel, The Borough, FARNHAM ☎ 0870 400 8225 & 01252 715237 📠 01252 733530 83 en suite

EPSOM
MAP 04 TQ26

Epsom Longdown Ln South KT17 4JR
☎ 01372 721666 📠 01372 817183
e-mail: secretary@epsomgolfclub.co.uk
web: www.epsomgolfclub.co.uk
Traditional downland course with many mature trees and fast undulating greens. Thought must be given to every shot to play to one's handicap.
18 holes, 5656yds, Par 69, SSS 67, Course record 63.
Club membership 770.
Visitors Mon, Wed-Fri & BHs. Sat/Sun pm only. Booking required. Dress code. **Societies** booking required. **Green Fees** not confirmed. **Prof** Ron Goudie **Course Designer** Willie Dunne **Facilities** ⊕ ⏵ 🏌 ♨ 🍴 💺 ♿ 🏆 🥎 ♿ **Conf** facs Corporate Hospitality Days **Location** SE of town centre on B288
Hotel ★★★★ 84% HL Woodlands Park Hotel, Woodlands Ln, STOKE D'ABERNON ☎ 01372 843933 57 en suite

Horton Park Golf & Country Club Hook Rd KT19 8QG
☎ 020 8393 8400 & 8394 2626 📠 020 8394 1369
e-mail: hortonparkgc@aol.com

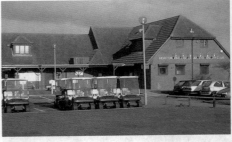

Millennium: 18 holes, 6257yds, Par 71, SSS 70.
Course Designer Dr Peter Nicholson
Telephone for further details
Hotel ★★★★ 84% HL Woodlands Park Hotel, Woodlands Ln, STOKE D'ABERNON ☎ 01372 843933 57 en suite

ESHER
MAP 04 TQ16

Moore Place Portsmouth Rd KT10 9LN
☎ 01372 463533
web: www.moore-place.co.uk
9 holes, 2078yds, Par 33, SSS 30, Course record 27.
Course Designer H Vardon/D Allen/N Gadd **Location** 0.5m from town centre on A307
Telephone for further details
Hotel ★★★ 71% HL The Ship Hotel, Monument Green, WEYBRIDGE ☎ 01932 848364 77 en suite

Thames Ditton & Esher Portsmouth Rd KT10 9AL
☎ 020 8398 1551
web: www.tdandegc.co.uk
18 holes, 5149yds, Par 66, SSS 65, Course record 63.
Location 1m NE on A307, next to Marquis of Granby pub
Telephone for further details
Hotel BUD Premier Travel Inn Cobham, Portsmouth Rd, Fairmile, COBHAM ☎ 0870 9906358 48 en suite

FARLEIGH
MAP 05 TQ36

Farleigh Court Farleigh Common CR6 9PE
☎ 01883 627711 📠 01883 627722
e-mail: enquiry.farleigh@ohiml.com
web: www.farleighcourtgolf.com
The course occupies 350 acres of land and is surrounded by a bird sanctuary and natural woodlands. The course designer has instinctively utilised two valleys to make the course interesting and challenging.
Members: 18 holes, 6409yds, Par 72, SSS 70,
Course record 67.
9 holes, 3281yds, Par 36. Club membership 550.
Visitors Mon-Sun & BHs. Booking required Sat, Sun & BHs. Dress code. **Societies** Welcome **Green Fees** Phone. **Prof** S Graham **Course Designer** John Jacobs **Facilities** ⊕ ⏵ 🏌 ♨ 🍴 🎯 💺 ♿ 🏆 🥎 ♿ 🏌 **Leisure** sauna. **Conf** facs Corporate Hospitality Days **Location** 1.5m from Selsdon
Hotel ★★★★ 73% HL Selsdon Park Hotel & Golf Club, Addington Rd, Sanderstead, CROYDON ☎ 020 8657 8811 204 en suite

FARNHAM
MAP 04 SU84

Blacknest Binsted GU34 4QL
☎ 01420 22888 📄 01420 22001
Privately owned pay and play golf centre catering for all ages and levels of ability. Facilities include a 15-bay driving range, gymnasium and a challenging 18-hole course featuring water on 14 holes.
18 holes, 5938yds, Par 69, SSS 69, Course record 64.
Club membership 450.
Visitors Contact club for details. **Societies** Booking required. **Green Fees** £20 per round (£25 Sat & Sun). **Prof** Darren Burgess **Course Designer** Mr Nicholson **Facilities** ⑪ 🍴 ⛳ ▭ ⊪ ⛳ 🏋 🚗 🛒 ⛳ 🛒 **Leisure** sauna, solarium, gymnasium. **Conf** facs **Location** 5m SW of Farnham off A325

Farnham The Sands GU10 1PX
☎ 01252 782109 📄 01252 781185
e-mail: farnhamgolfclub@tiscali.co.uk
web: www.farnhamgolfclub.co.uk
A mixture of meadowland and heath with quick drying sandy subsoil. Several of the earlier holes have interesting features.
18 holes, 6447yds, Par 72, SSS 71, Course record 66.
Club membership 700.
Visitors Mon-Fri except BHs. Handicap certificate. Dress code **Societies** Welcome. **Green Fees** £50 per day; £45 per round. **Prof** Grahame Cowlishaw **Course Designer** Donald Steel **Facilities** ⑪ 🍴 by prior arrangement ⊪ ▭ 🍴 ▭ 🏋 ⛳ **Conf** Corporate Hospitality Days **Location** 3m E off A31
Hotel ★★★ 78% HL Mercure Bush Hotel, The Borough, FARNHAM
☎ 0870 400 8225 & 01252 715237 📄 01252 733530 83 en suite

Farnham Park Folly Hill, Farnham Park GU9 0AU
☎ 01252 715216
Pay & Play parkland course in Farnham Park. Challenging and scenic.
9 holes, 1163yds, Par 27, SSS 48, Course record 48.
Club membership 70.
Visitors Mon-Sun & BHs. Dress code. **Societies** Booking required. **Green Fees** £11 per 18 holes, £6 per 9 holes (£7/£13 Sat & Sun). **Prof** N Ogilvy **Course Designer** Henry Cotton **Facilities** ⑪ 🍴 ⊪ ▭ 🍴 ▭ 🏋 ⛳ **Location** N of town centre on A287, next to Farnham Castle
Hotel ★★★ 78% HL Mercure Bush Hotel, The Borough, FARNHAM
☎ 0870 400 8225 & 01252 715237 📄 01252 733530 83 en suite

GODALMING
MAP 04 SU94

Broadwater Park Guildford Rd, Farncombe GU7 3BU
☎ 01483 429955 📄 01483 429955
A Par 3 public course with floodlit driving range.
9 holes, 1287yds, Par 54, SSS 50. Club membership 160.
Visitors contact club for details. **Societies** welcome. **Green Fees** not confirmed. **Prof** Kevin D Milton/Nick English **Course Designer** Kevin Milton **Facilities** ⊪ ▭ 🍴 ▭ 🏋 ⛳ **Conf** Corporate Hospitality Days **Location** NE of Godalming on A3100

Hurtmore Hurtmore Rd, Hurtmore GU7 2RN
☎ 01483 426492 📄 01483 426121
web: www.hurtmore-golf.co.uk
A Peter Alliss and Clive Clark pay and play course with seven lakes and 85 bunkers. The 15th hole is the longest at 537yds. Played mainly into the wind there are 10 bunkers to negotiate. The 3rd hole at 448yds stroke Index 1 is a real test. A dog-leg right around a lake and nine bunkers makes this hole worthy of its stroke index.
18 holes, 5254yds, Par 70. Club membership 200.

Visitors Mon-Sun & BHs. Booking required. Dress code. **Societies** Welcome. **Green Fees** £14.50 per 18 holes, £11 per 9 holes (£20.50/£13 Sat & Sun). Twilight £11 (£13 Sat & Sun). **Prof** Maxine Burton **Course Designer** Peter Alliss/Clive Clark **Facilities** ⑪ 🍴 ⊪ ▭ 🍴 ▭ 🏋 ⛳ **Leisure** practice nets. **Conf** Corporate Hospitality Days **Location** 2m NW of Godalming off A3

GUILDFORD
MAP 04 SU94

Guildford High Path Rd, Merrow GU1 2HL
☎ 01483 563941 📄 01483 453228
e-mail: secretary@guildfordgolfclub.co.uk
web: www.guildfordgolfclub.co.uk
The course is on Surrey downland bordered by attractive woodlands. Situated on chalk, it is acknowledged to be one of the best all-weather courses in the area, and the oldest course in Surrey. Although not a long course, the prevailing winds across the open downs make low scoring difficult. It is possible to see four counties on a clear day.

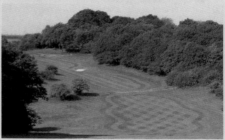

18 holes, 6090yds, Par 69, SSS 69, Course record 64.
Club membership 700.
Visitors Mon, Tue, Thu, Fri except BHs. Wed pm only.
Societies welcome. **Green Fees** not confirmed. 🏌 **Prof** P G Hollington **Course Designer** J H Taylor/Hawtree **Facilities** 🏋 ▭ ⛳ ⛳ **Conf** facs Corporate Hospitality Days **Location** E of town centre off A246

Merrist Wood Coombe Ln, Worplesdon GU3 3PE
☎ 01483 238890 📄 01483 238896
e-mail: mwgc@merristwood-golfclub.co.uk
web: merristwood-golfclub.co.uk
18 holes, 6600yds, Par 72, SSS 71, Course record 69.
Course Designer David Williams **Location** 3m from Guildford on A323 to Aldershot
Telephone for further details

Milford Station Ln, Milford GU8 5HS
☎ 01483 419200 📄 01483 419199
e-mail: milford-sales@crown-golf.co.uk
web: www.crowngolf.com/milford
The design has cleverly incorporated a demanding course within existing woodland and meadow.
18 holes, 5960yds, Par 69, SSS 68, Course record 64.
Club membership 650.
Visitors Mon-Fri. Sat, Sun & BHs pm only. Booking required. Dress code. **Societies** Booking required. **Green Fees** £26 per 18 holes (£33 Fri-Sun). **Prof** Paul Creamer **Course Designer** Peter Allis **Facilities** ⑪ 🍴 ⊪ ▭ 🍴 ▭ 🏋 ⛳ 🏋 ⛳ **Conf** facs Corporate Hospitality Days **Location** 6m SW Guildford. Off A3 into Milford, E towards station

Roker Park Rokers Farm, Aldershot Rd GU3 3PB
☎ 01483 236677 📄 01483 232324
A pay and play nine-hole parkland course. A challenging course with two Par 5 holes.
9 holes, 3037yds, Par 36, SSS 72. Club membership 200.
Visitors contact course for details. Dress code. **Societies** booking required.
Green Fees not confirmed. **Prof** Adrian Carter **Course Designer** W V
Roker **Facilities** ⑪ ⓑ ☑ ⅋ ⌲ ⚑ ⚏ ✔ ⚏ ✔ ☂ **Location** 3m NW of
Guildford on A323

HINDHEAD   MAP 04 SU83

Hindhead Churt Rd GU26 6HX
☎ 01428 604614 📄 01428 608508
e-mail: secretary@the-hindhead-golf-club.co.uk
web: www.hindhead-golfclub.co.uk
A picturesque Surrey heathland course. The front nine holes follow heather lined valleys which give the players a very remote and secluded feel. For the back nine play moves on to a plateau which offers a more traditional game before the tough challenge of the final two finishing holes.
18 holes, 6356yds, Par 70, SSS 70, Course record 63.
Club membership 610.
Visitors Mon-Sun & BHs. Booking required. Handicap certificate. Dress code. **Societies** Booking required. **Green Fees** £60 per day; £50 per round (£70/£60 Sat, Sun & BHs). **Prof** Ian Benson **Course Designer** J H Taylor **Facilities** ⑪ ⓑ ☑ ⅋ ⌲ ⚑ ⚏ ✔ ☂ **Leisure** snooker. **Conf** Corporate Hospitality Days **Location** 1.5m NW of Hindhead on A287
Hotel ★★★★ 77% HL Lythe Hill Hotel & Spa, Petworth Rd, HASLEMERE ☎ 01428 651251 41 en suite

---

KINGSWOOD   MAP 04 TQ25

Kingswood Golf and Country House Sandy Ln KT20 6NE
☎ 01737 832188 📄 01737 833920
e-mail: sales@kingswood-golf.co.uk
web: www.kingswood-golf.co.uk
Mature parkland course sited on a plateau with delightful views of the Chipstead valley. The course features lush, shaped fairways, testing bunkers positions and true greens. Recent improvements ensure it plays every inch of its 6900yds.
18 holes, 6904yds, Par 72, SSS 73. Club membership 700.
Visitors Mon-Fri. Sat, Sun & BHs after 11am. Booking required. Dress code. **Societies** Booking required. **Green Fees** Phone. **Prof** Terry Sims
Course Designer James Braid **Facilities** ⓑ ☑ ⅋ ⌲ ⚑ ⚏ ✔ ☂
Leisure squash, 3 snooker tables. **Conf** facs Corporate Hospitality Days
Location 0.5m S of village off A217
Hotel ★★★ 72% HL Best Western Reigate Manor Hotel, Reigate Hill, REIGATE ☎ 01737 240125 50 en suite

Surrey Downs Outwood Ln KT20 6JS
☎ 01737 839090 📄 01737 839080
e-mail: booking@surreydownsgc.co.uk
web: www.surreydownsgc.co.uk
A new course on a 200 acre site with spectacular views over the North Downs and home to rabbits, foxes, deer and herons.
18 holes, 6303yards, Par 71, SSS 70, Course record 64.
Club membership 652.
Visitors Mon-Sun & BHs. Booking required. Dress code. **Societies** Booking required **Green Fees** £25 per round (£35 Sat & Sun). **Prof** Stephen

---

Blacklee **Course Designer** Aliss/Clarke **Facilities** ⌲ ⚑ ⚏ ✔ ☂ **Leisure** sauna. **Conf** facs Corporate Hospitality Days **Location** Off A217 E onto B2032 at Kingswood for 1m, club on right after Eyhurst Park
Hotel BUD Premier Travel Inn Epsom South, Brighton Rd, Burgh Heath, TADWORTH ☎ 0870 9906442 78 en suite

---

LEATHERHEAD   MAP 04 TQ15

Leatherhead Kingston Rd KT22 0EE
☎ 01372 843966 & 843956 📄 01372 842241
e-mail: secretary@lgc-golf.co.uk
web: www.lgc-golf.co.uk
Undulating, 100-year-old parkland course with tree-lined fairways and strategically placed bunkers. Easy walking.
18 holes, 5795yds, Par 70, SSS 68. Club membership 630.
Visitors Mon, Tue, Thu & Fri except BHs. Booking required. Dress code.
Societies booking required. **Green Fees** not confirmed. **Prof** Simon Norman **Facilities** ⑪ ⚏ ⓑ ☑ ⅋ ⌲ ⚑ ⚏ ✔ **Conf** facs Corporate Hospitality Days **Location** 0.25m from junct 9 of M25, on A243
Hotel ★★ 67% HL Bookham Grange Hotel, Little Bookham Common, Bookham, LEATHERHEAD ☎ 01372 452742 27 en suite

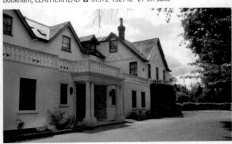

See advert on opposite page

Pachesham Park Golf Complex Oaklawn Rd KT22 0BT
☎ 01372 843453
e-mail: enquiries@pacheshamgolf.co.uk
web: www.pacheshamgolf.co.uk
An undulating parkland course starting with five shorter but tight holes on one side of the road, followed by four longer more open but testing holes to finish.
9 holes, 2805yds, Par 70, SSS 67, Course record 67.
Club membership 150.
Visitors Mon-Sun & BHs. Booking required Sat, Sun & BHs.
Societies Booking required. **Green Fees** £18 per 18 holes; £10 per 9 holes (£20/£14 Sat, Sun & BHs). **Prof** Philip Taylor **Course Designer** Phil Taylor **Facilities** ⑪ ⓑ ☑ ⅋ ⌲ ⚑ ⚏ ✔ ☂ **Leisure** fitting centre. **Conf** facs Corporate Hospitality Days **Location** M25 junct 9, 0.5m off A244 or A245
Hotel ★★★★ 84% HL Woodlands Park Hotel, Woodlands Ln, STOKE D'ABERNON ☎ 01372 843933 57 en suite

Tyrrells Wood The Drive KT22 8QP
☎ 01372 376025 📄 01372 360836
e-mail: general.manager@tyrrellswoodgolfclub.com
web: www.tyrrellswoodgolfclub.com
Easy walking course set in276 acres of parkland with fine views and a
Grade 2 listed clubhouse.
18 holes, 6282yds, Par 71, SSS 70, Course record 65.
Club membership 700.
Visitors Mon-Fri except BHs. Booking required. Handicap certificate. Dress
code. **Societies** Booking required. **Green Fees** £42 per round. **Prof** Simon
Defoy **Course Designer** James Braid **Facilities** ⑪ ⑩ ⓛ ☐ 🗲 🍴 🏌 🍴 🏌
🍴 ✂ **Conf** facs Corporate Hospitality Days **Location** M25 junct 9, 2m SE
of town off A24
Hotel ★★★★ 81% HL Mercure Burford Bridge Hotel, Burford Bridge, Box
Hill, DORKING ☎ 0870 400 8283 57 en suite

LIMPSFIELD   MAP 05 TQ45

Limpsfield Chart Westerham Rd RH8 0SL
☎ 01883 723405 & 722106
Attractive heathland course on National Trust land, easy walking with
tree lined fairways.
9 holes, 5718yds, Par 70, SSS 68, Course record 64.
Club membership 300.
Visitors Mon-Wed & Fri. Thu after 2.30pm. Booking required Sat & Sun.
Dress code. **Societies** Welcome. **Green Fees** Phone. ⊛ **Prof** Mike McLean
Facilities ⓛ ⚘ **Conf** Corporate Hospitality Days **Location** M25 junct 6,
1m E on A25
Hotel ★★★ 75% HL Best Western Donnington Manor, London Rd,
Dunton Green, SEVENOAKS ☎ 01732 462681 60 en suite

LINGFIELD   MAP 05 TQ34

Lingfield Park Lingfield Rd, Racecourse Rd RH7 6PQ
☎ 01342 832659 📄 01342 836077
e-mail: cmorley@lingfieldpark.co.uk
web: www.lingfieldpark.co.uk
18 holes, 6473yds, Par 71, SSS 72, Course record 65.
Location M25 junct 6, signs to racecourse
Telephone for further details
Hotel BUD Premier Travel Inn East Grinstead, London Rd, Felbridge, EAST
GRINSTEAD ☎ 08701 977088 41 en suite

NEWDIGATE   MAP 04 TQ14

Rusper Rusper Rd RH5 5BX
☎ 01293 871871 (shop) 📄 01293 871456
e-mail: jill@ruspergolfclub.co.uk
web: www.ruspergolfclub.co.uk
The 18-hole course is set in countryside and offers golfers of all abilities
a fair and challenging test. After a gentle start the holes wind through
picturesque scenery, tree-lined fairways and natural water hazards.
18 holes, 6724yds, Par 72, SSS 72. Club membership 350.
Visitors Mon-Sun & BHs. Booking required. Dress code. **Societies** Booking
required. **Green Fees** £20 (£28 Sat, Sun & BHs). **Prof** Janice Arnold
Course Designer A Blunden **Facilities** ⑪ ⑩ ⓛ ☐ 🗲 ⚘ 🏌 🍴 ✂ 🍴 ✂
🍴 **Conf** Corporate Hospitality Days **Location** Off A24 between Newdigate
and Rusper
Hotel ★★★★ 81% HL Mercure Burford Bridge Hotel, Burford Bridge, Box
Hill, DORKING ☎ 0870 400 8283 57 en suite

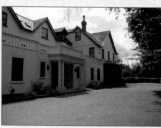

OCKLEY   MAP 04 TQ14

Gatton Manor Hotel Standon Ln RH5 5PQ
☎ 01306 627555 📄 01306 627713
e-mail: info@gattonmanor.co.uk
web: www.gattonmanor.co.uk
A mature woodland course, formerly part of the Abinger estate. The
challenging course makes imaginative use of the various streams,
lakes and woodlands. A good scorecard can be suddenly ruined if the
individual challenges each hole presents are not carefully considered.
18 holes, 6563yds, Par 72, SSS 72, Course record 68.
Club membership 300.
Visitors Mon-Sat & BHs. Sun pm only. Booking required. Dress code.
Societies Booking required **Green Fees** £28 (£38 Sat & Sun). Winter
£20/£30. **Prof** Rob Humphrey **Course Designer** John D Harris **Facilities**
⑪ ⑩ ⓛ ☐ 🗲 ⚘ 🏌 ◇ ✂ 🍴 ✂ 🍴 **Leisure** fishing, gymnasium. **Conf**
facs Corporate Hospitality Days **Location** 1.5m SW off A29
Hotel ★★★ 73% HL Gatton Manor Hotel & Golf Club, Standon Ln,
OCKLEY ☎ 01306 627555 18 en suite

OTTERSHAW
MAP 04 TQ06

Foxhills Club and Resort Stonehill Rd KT16 0EL
☎ 01932 872050 📄 01932 875200
e-mail: events@foxhills.co.uk
web: www.foxhills.co.uk
The Bernard Hunt Course: 18 holes, 6770yds, Par 73, SSS 72, Course record 65.
Longcross Course: 18 holes, 6453yds, Par 72, SSS 71, Course record 70.
Course Designer F W Hawtree **Location** 1m NW of Ottershaw
Telephone for further details
Hotel ★★★★ 79% HL Foxhills Club & Resort, Stonehill Rd,
OTTERSHAW ☎ 01932 872050 70 en suite

PIRBRIGHT
MAP 04 SU95

Goal Farm Gole Rd GU24 0PZ
☎ 01483 473183 📄 01483 473205
e-mail: secretary@gfgc.co.uk
web: www.gfgc.co.uk
Beautiful landscaped parkland pay and play course with excellent greens. A range of enjoyable yet demanding holes over trees and over water with plenty of bunkers to swallow up tee shots.
9 holes, 1273yds, Par 54, SSS 48, Course record 50.
Club membership 350.
Visitors Mon-Wed, Fri, Sun & BHs. Dress code. **Societies** booking required.
Green Fees not confirmed. **Prof** Peter Fuller **Course Designer** Bill Cox
Facilities 🏌 🖵 🍴 **Location** 1.5m NW on B3012
Hotel ★★★ 67% HL Falcon Hotel, 68 Farnborough Rd, FARNBOROUGH
☎ 01252 545378 30 en suite

PUTTENHAM
MAP 04 SU94

Puttenham Heath Rd GU3 1AL
☎ 01483 810498 📄 01483 810988
e-mail: enquiries@puttenhamgolfclub.co.uk
web: www.puttenhamgolfclub.co.uk
Mixture of heathland and woodland - undulating layout with stunning views across the Hog's Back and towards the South Downs. Sandy subsoil provides free drainage for year round play.
18 holes, 6220yds, Par 71, SSS 70. Club membership 650.
Visitors Mon-Fri except BHs. Booking required. Handicap certificate. Dress code. **Societies** Booking required, **Green Fees** £50 per day; £35 per round. **Prof** Dean Lintott **Facilities** ⑪ ⑩ by prior arrangement 🏌 🖵 🍴 🏌 🍴 🍴 **Conf** Corporate Hospitality Days **Location** 1m SE on B3000
Hotel ★★★ 78% HL Mercure Bush Hotel, The Borough, FARNHAM
☎ 0870 400 8225 & 01252 715237 📄 01252 733530 83 en suite

REDHILL
MAP 04 TQ25

Redhill & Reigate Clarence Rd, Pendelton Rd RH1 6LB
☎ 01737 244433 📄 01737 242117
e-mail: mail@rrgc.net
web: www.rrgc.net
Flat picturesque tree-lined course, well over 100 years old.
18 holes, 5272yds, Par 68, SSS 66, Course record 65.
Club membership 600.
Visitors Mon-Sun except BHs. Booking required Sat, Sun & BHs. Dress code. **Societies** Welcome. **Green Fees** £21 per 18 holes. **Prof** Warren Pike
Course Designer James Braid **Facilities** ⑪ ⑩ by prior arrangement 🖵 🍴 🏌 🍴 🍴 **Conf** facs Corporate Hospitality Days **Location** 1m S on A23
Hotel ★★★ 72% HL Best Western Reigate Manor Hotel, Reigate Hill,
REIGATE ☎ 01737 240125 50 en suite

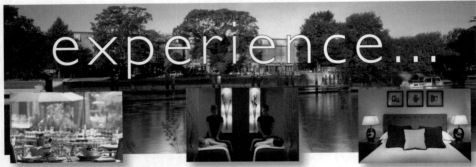

experience...

...the perfect setting

A privately owned 4 star hotel set on the banks of the River Thames in Egham, Surrey, 5 miles from Royal Windsor and just minutes from the M25 & Heathrow Airport and Wentworth Club. The hotel features 180 guestrooms, two riverside restaurants and an extensive Spa including: an indoor pool, 5 tennis courts, gymnasium, saunas, eucalyptus steam room and a deluxe day package suite perfect for relaxing after a day on the greens. The Runnymede is also perfectly located for exploring the wealth of tourist attractions in the area.

Please call reservations on 01784 220980 for more details.

Runnymede hotel&spa
Windsor Road, Egham, Surrey, TW20 0AG
t: 01784 436171   f: 01784 436340
www.runnymedehotel.com   e: info@runnymedehotel.com

CHAMPIONSHIP COURSE

SURREY — VIRGINIA WATER

WENTWORTH

Map 04 TQ06

Wentworth Dr GU25 4LS
☎ 01344 842201 🖷 01344 842804
e-mail: reception@wentworthclub.com
web: www.wentworthclub.com
West Course: 18 holes, 7301yds, Par 73, SSS 74, Course record 63.
East Course: 18 holes, 6201yds, Par 68, SSS 70, Course record 62.
Edinburgh Course: 18 holes, 7004yds, Par 72, SSS 74, Course record 67.
Visitors Mon-Fri except BHs. Booking required. Handicap certificate. Dress code.
Societies booking required. **Green Fees** West Course: from £100-£285; Edinburgh Course: from £80-£160; East Course: from £75-£130.
Prof Jason Macniven **Course Designer** Colt/Jacobs/Gallacher/Player **Facilities** ⑪ ⑩ 🍴 🕭 ⊡
🏌 🛋 📷 ⛵ ♢ 🏌 🛒 ♂ 🏌 **Leisure** hard and grass tennis courts, outdoor and indoor heated pools, fishing, sauna, solarium, gym, spa with 6 treatment rooms. **Conf** Corporate Hospitality Days **Location** Main gate directly opposite turning for A329 on A30

Wentworth Club, the home of the PGA and World Match Play championships, is a very special venue for any sporting, business or social occasion. The West Course is familiar to millions of television viewers who have followed the championships here. There are two other courses, the East Course and the Edinburgh Course, and a nine-hole Par 3 executive course. The courses cross Surrey heathland with woods of pine, oak and birch. The Club is renowned for its fine food, and the health and leisure facilities include a holistic spa, 13 outdoor tennis courts (with four different playing surfaces) and a 25-metre indoor swimming pool.

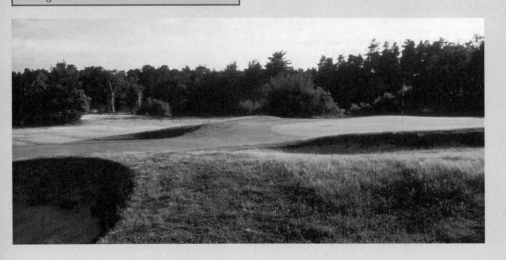

REIGATE
MAP 04 TQ25

Reigate Heath Flanchford Rd RH2 8QR
☎ 01737 242610 & 226793 📄 01737 249226
e-mail: reigateheath@surreygolf.co.uk
web: www.reigateheathgolfclub.co.uk
Gorse, heather, pine and birch trees abound on this popular nine-hole heathland course. The course is short by modern standards but is a good test of golf. Playing 18 holes from nine greens, the second nine is quite different with changes of angle as well as length.
9 holes, 5658yds, Par 67, SSS 67, Course record 65.
Club membership 550.
Visitors Mon-Fri. Handicap certificate. Dress code. **Societies** Booking required. **Green Fees** £33 per round. Reduced twilight rate. **Prof** Richard Arnold **Facilities** ⑪ by prior arrangement ⬛ ⬜ ✦⬛ ⬛ ✦ **Conf** facs Corporate Hospitality Days **Location** 1.5m W off A25
Hotel ★★★ 72% HL Best Western Reigate Manor Hotel, Reigate Hill, REIGATE ☎ 01737 240125 50 en suite

Reigate Hill Gatton Bottom RH2 0TU
☎ 01737 645577 📄 01737 642650
e-mail: info@reigatehillgolfclub.co.uk
web: www.reigatehillgolfclub.co.uk
Championship standard course with fully irrigated tees and greens. Feature holes include the 5th which is divided by four bunkers and the Par 5 14th involving a tricky second shot across a lake. Very good short holes at 8th and 12th with panoramic views from the tees.
18 holes, 6175yds, Par 72, SSS 70, Course record 63.
Club membership 450.
Visitors Mon-Sun & BHs. Dress code. **Societies** Booking required. **Green Fees** £40 (£50 Sat & Sun). **Prof** Stephen Dundas **Course Designer** David Williams **Facilities** ⑪ ⦿ ⬛ ⬜ ✦⬛ ⬛ ⭳ ✦ ✦ ✦ **Conf** facs Corporate Hospitality Days **Location** M25 junct 8, 1m
Hotel ★★★ 72% HL Best Western Reigate Manor Hotel, Reigate Hill, REIGATE ☎ 01737 240125 50 en suite

SHEPPERTON
MAP 04 TQ06

Sunbury Golf Centre Charlton Ln TW17 8QA
☎ 01932 771414 📄 01932 789300
e-mail: sunbury@crown-golf.co.uk
web: www.crown-golf.co.uk
Twenty-seven holes for all standards of golfer and a 32 bay floodlit driving range. Easy walking.
18 holes, 5103yds, Par 68, SSS 65, Course record 60.
Academy: 9 holes, 2444yds, Par 33, SSS 32.
Club membership 400.
Visitors Mon-Sun & BHs. **Societies** Booking required. **Green Fees** £18.50 per 18 holes; £10 per 9 holes (£23/£12 Sat & Sun). **Prof** Adrian McColgan **Course Designer** Peter Alliss **Facilities** ⑪ ⦿ ⬛ ⬜ ✦⬛ ⬛ ⭳ ✦ ✦ **Conf** facs Corporate Hospitality Days **Location** M3, junct 1, 1m N off A244
Hotel ★★★ 74% HL Mercure Thames Lodge, Thames St, STAINES ☎ 0870 400 8121 & 01784 464433 📄 01784 454858 78 en suite

SOUTH GODSTONE
MAP 05 TQ34

Home Park Croydon Barn Ln, Horne RH9 8JP
☎ 01342 844443 📄 01342 841828
e-mail: info@homepark.co.uk
web: www.homepark.co.uk
Set in attractive Surrey countryside with water coming into play in 5 holes. Relatively flat for easy walking. A different set of tees pose an intriguing second 9 holes.
9 holes, 5436yds, Par 68, SSS 66, Course record 62.
Club membership 350.
Visitors Mon-Sun & BHs. Booking required Sat/Sun & BHs. Dress code. **Societies** booking required. **Green Fees** not confirmed. **Prof** Neil Burke **Course Designer** Howard Swan **Facilities** ⑪ ⦿ by prior arrangement ⬛ ⬜ ✦⬛ ⬛ 🛋 ✦ ✦ ✦ **Leisure** caddies available, swing analysis system, teaching academy. **Location** A22, signposted 3m N of East Grinstead
Hotel BUD Premier Travel Inn East Grinstead, London Rd, Felbridge, EAST GRINSTEAD ☎ 08701 977088 41 en suite

SUTTON GREEN
MAP 04 TQ05

Sutton Green New Ln GU4 7QF
☎ 01483 747898 📄 01483 750289
e-mail: admin@suttongreengc.co.uk
web: www.suttongreengc.co.uk
Set in the Surrey countryside, a challenging course with many water features. Excellent year round conditions with fairway watering. Many testing holes with water surrounding greens and fairways, making accuracy a premium.
18 holes, 6350yds, Par 71, SSS 70, Course record 64.
Club membership 600.
Visitors Mon-Fri except BHs. Dress code. **Societies** Booking required. **Green Fees** Phone. **Prof** Paul Tedder **Course Designer** David Walker/ Laura Davies **Facilities** ⑪ ⦿ ⬛ ⬜ ✦⬛ ⬛ 🛋 ✦ ✦ ✦ **Conf** facs Corporate Hospitality Days **Location** Off A320 between Woking & Guildford
Hotel ★★★★★ HL Pennyhill Park Hotel & The Spa, London Rd, BAGSHOT ☎ 01276 471774 26 en suite 97 annexe en suite

TANDRIDGE
MAP 05 TQ35

Tandridge RH8 9NQ
☎ 01883 712274 📄 01883 730537
e-mail: secretary@tandridgegolfclub.com
web: www.tandridgegolfclub.com
A parkland course with two loops of nine holes from the clubhouse. The first nine are relatively flat. The second nine undulate with outstanding views of the North Downs.
18 holes, 6277yds, Par 70, SSS 70, Course record 66.
Club membership 750.
Visitors Mon, Wed & Thu except BHs. Booking required. Handicap certificate. Dress code. **Societies** Booking required. **Green Fees** £65 per day, £45 after noon. Winter:£35 per round. **Prof** Chris Evans **Course Designer** H S Colt **Facilities** ⑪ ⬛ ⬜ ✦⬛ ⬛ 🛋 ✦ ✦ **Conf** Corporate Hospitality Days **Location** M25 junct 6, 2m SE on A25
Hotel ★★★★ 80% HL Nutfield Priory, Nutfield, REDHILL ☎ 01737 824400 60 en suite

TILFORD   MAP 04 SU84

Hankley Common The Club House GU10 2DD
☎ 01252 792493 📠 01252 795699
web: hankley.co.uk
A natural heathland course subject to wind. Greens are first rate.
The 18th, a long Par 4, is most challenging, the green being beyond
a deep chasm which traps any but the perfect second shot. The 7th
is a spectacular one-shotter.
18 holes, 6702yds, Par 72, SSS 72, Course record 62.
Club membership 700.
Visitors Mon-Sun except BHs. Booking required. Handicap certificate.
Dress code. **Societies** Booking required. **Green Fees** £85 per
day, £70 per round (£85 per round Sat & Sun). **Prof** Peter Stow
Course Designer James Braid **Facilities** ⑪ 🍴 ⌷ 🖫 ⌷ 🏌 🛆 🏊 🚲 ✔
Location 0.75m SE of Tilford
Hotel ★★★ 78% HL Mercure Bush Hotel, The Borough, FARNHAM
☎ 0870 400 8225 & 01252 715237 📠 01252 733530 83 en suite

VIRGINIA WATER   MAP 04 TQ06

Wentworth see page 237

Hotel ★★ 79% HL The Wheatsheaf, London Rd, VIRGINIA WATER
☎ 01344 842057 17 en suite
Hotel ★★★★ 77% HL Runnymede Hotel & Spa, Windsor Rd, EGHAM
☎ 01784 436171 Fax 01784 436340 180 en suite

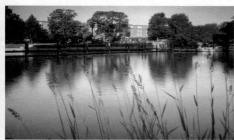

Hotel ★★★★ 78% HL Macdonald Berystede Hotel & Spa, Bagshot Rd,
Sunninghill, ASCOT ☎ 0870 400 8111 Fax 01344 872301 126 en suite
Hotel ★★★★ 77% HL The Royal Berkshire Ramada Plaza, London Rd,
Sunninghill, ASCOT ☎ 01344 623322 Fax 01344 627100 63 en suite

See advert on page 236

WALTON-ON-THAMES   MAP 04 TQ16

Burhill Burwood Rd KT12 4BL
☎ 01932 227345 📠 01932 267159
e-mail: info@burhillgolf-club.co.uk
web: www.burhillgolf-club.co.uk
The Old Course is a mature tree-lined parkland course with some
of the finest greens in Surrey. The New Course, opened in 2001, is a
modern course built to USGA specifications has many bunkers and
water hazards, including the River Mole.
Old Course: 18 holes, 6479yds, Par 70, SSS 71,
Course record 65. New Course: 18 holes, 6597yds,
Par 72, SSS 71. Club membership 1100.
Visitors Mon-Fri except Bhs. Booking required. Dress code.
Societies Booking required. **Green Fees** £85 per day, £65 per 18 holes.
Course Designer Willie Park/Simon Gidman **Facilities** ⑪ 🍴 🖫 ⌷ 🏌

🛆 🏠 ⌂ 🚲 🛆 🏌 ✔ ✔ **Conf** facs Corporate Hospitality Days
Location M25 junct 10 on to A3 towards London, 1st exit(Painshill junct
Hotel ★★★ 71% HL The Ship Hotel, Monument Green, WEYBRIDGE
☎ 01932 848364 77 en suite

WALTON-ON-THE-HILL   MAP 04 TQ25

Walton Heath see page 241

Hotel ★★ 67% HL Bookham Grange Hotel, Little Bookham Common,
Bookham, LEATHERHEAD ☎ 01372 452742 27 en suite
Hotel ★★★ 77% HL Chalk Lane Hotel, Chalk Ln, Woodcote End, EPSOM
☎ 01372 721179 Fax 01372 727878 22 en suite
Hotel ★★★ 72% HL Best Western Reigate Manor Hotel, Reigate Hill,
REIGATE ☎ 01737 240125 Fax 01737 223983 50 en suite
Hotel ★★★★ 81% HL Mercure Burford Bridge Hotel, Burford Bridge, Box
Hill, DORKING ☎ 0870 400 8283 Fax 01306 880386 57 en suite
Hotel ★★★ 68% HL Mercure White Horse Hotel, High St, DORKING
☎ 0870 400 8282 Fax 01306 887241 37 en suite 41 annexe en suite

WEST BYFLEET   MAP 04 TQ06

West Byfleet Sheerwater Rd KT14 6AA
☎ 01932 343433 📠 01932 340667
e-mail: secretary@wbgc.co.uk
web: www.wbgc.co.uk
An attractive course set against a background of woodland and
gorse. The 13th is the famous pond shot with a water hazard and
two bunkers fronting the green. No less than six holes of 420yds
or more.
18 holes, 6211yds, Par 70, SSS 70. Club membership 622.
Visitors Contact club for details. **Societies** Welcome.
Green Fees £70 per day, £50 per round. **Prof** David Regan
Course Designer C S Butchart **Facilities** ⑪ 🍴 🖫 ⌷ 🏌 🛆 🏠 ⌂ 🚲 ✔
✔ 🏌 **Conf** Corporate Hospitality Days **Location** W of village on A245

WEST CLANDON   MAP 04 TQ05

Clandon Regis Epsom Rd GU4 7TT
☎ 01483 224888 📠 01483 211781
e-mail: office@clandonregis-golfclub.co.uk
web: www.clandonregis-golfclub.co.uk
High quality parkland course with challenging lake holes on the back
nine. European Tour specification tees and greens.
18 holes, 6485yds, Par 72, SSS 71, Course record 66.
Club membership 652.
Visitors Mon-Sun except BHs. Booking required Sat & Sun. Dress code.
Societies Welcome. **Green Fees** Mon-Fri £37.50 per 18 holes. £45 per day.
Prof Steve Lloyd **Course Designer** David Williams **Facilities** ⑪ 🍴 🖫 ⌷
🏌 🛆 🏠 ⌂ ✔ 🏌 **Leisure** sauna. **Conf** facs Corporate Hospitality Days
Location SE of village off A246

England

WEST END   MAP 04 SU96

Windlemere Windlesham Rd GU24 9QL
☎ 01276 858727
A parkland course, undulating in parts with natural water hazards.
There is also a floodlit driving range.
9 holes, 2673yds, Par 34, SSS 33, Course record 30.
Visitors contact club for details. **Societies** welcome.
Green Fees not confirmed. **Prof** David Thomas **Course Designer** Clive
Smith **Facilities** ⓦ ⓛ ▯ ▮ ⚑ ☂ ♥ ✦ **Leisure** pool/snooker tables.
Location N of village at junct A319
Hotel ★★★★★ HL Pennyhill Park Hotel & The Spa, London Rd,
BAGSHOT ☎ 01276 471774   26 en suite   97 annexe en suite

WEYBRIDGE   MAP 04 TQ06

St George's Hill Golf Club Rd, St George's Hill
KT13 0NL
☎ 01932 847758 🖷 01932 821564
e-mail: admin@stgeorgeshillgolfclub.co.uk
web: stgeorgeshillgolfclub.co.uk
Comparable and similar to Wentworth, a feature of this course is the
number of long and difficult Par 4s. To score well it is necessary to
place the drive - and long driving pays handsomely. Walking is hard
on this undulating, heavily wooded course with plentiful heather and
rhododendrons.
Red & Blue: 18 holes, 6513yds, Par 70, SSS 71,
Course record 64.
Green: 9 holes, 2897yds, Par 35. Club membership 600.
Visitors Wed-Fri except BHs. Booking required. Handicap certificate.
Dress code. **Societies** booking required. **Green Fees** not confirmed.
Prof A C Rattue **Course Designer** H S Colt **Facilities** ⚒ 🍴 ☂ ♥ ✦
Conf Corporate Hospitality Days **Location** 2m S off B374
Hotel ★★★ 71% HL The Ship Hotel, Monument Green, WEYBRIDGE
☎ 01932 848364   77 en suite

WOKING   MAP 04 TQ05

Hoebridge Golf Centre Old Woking Rd GU22 8JH
☎ 01483 722611 🖷 01483 740369
e-mail: info@hoebridgegc.co.uk
web: www.hoebridgegc.co.uk
The setting encompasses 200 acres of mature parkland and includes 3
golf courses containing 45 holes. The Hoebridge course has tree lined
fairways, challenging bunkers and fine views. The testing 9 hole Shey
Copse is a Par 4/Par 3 course which winds around the woodland. The
Maybury is an 18 holes Par 4 course for beginners or golfers wishing to
improve their game.

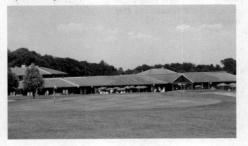

Main Course: 18 holes, 6536yds, Par 72, SSS 71.
Shey Course: 9 holes, 2294yds, Par 33.
Maybury Course: 18 holes, 2181yds, Par 54.
Club membership 1000.
Visitors Mon-Sun & BHs. Booking required. Dress code. **Societies**
Welcome. **Green Fees** Main £22 Mon-Thu, £25 Fri (£29.50 Sat & Sun) Shey
£12 (£14.50Sat & Sun) Maybury £9.50 (£12 Sat & Sun). **Prof** Rob Jones
Course Designer John Jacobs **Facilities** ⓦ 🍴 ⓛ ▯ ▮ ⚑ ☂ ♥ ✦
✦ ⚒ ✦ ✦ **Leisure** sauna, solarium, gymnasium, health & fitness club.
Conf facs   Corporate Hospitality Days **Location** M25 junct 11, follow signs
for Old Woking, then Hoebridge
Hotel ★★★★★ HL Pennyhill Park Hotel & The Spa, London Rd,
BAGSHOT ☎ 01276 471774   26 en suite   97 annexe en suite

Pyrford Warren Ln, Pyrford GU22 8XR
☎ 01483 723555 🖷 01483 729777
e-mail: pyrford@americangolf.uk.com
web: www.americangolf.com
18 holes, 6256yds, Par 72, SSS 70, Course record 64.
Course Designer Peter Allis & Clive Clark **Location** Off A3 Ripley to Pyrford
Telephone for further details
Hotel ★★★★★ HL Pennyhill Park Hotel & The Spa, London Rd,
BAGSHOT ☎ 01276 471774   26 en suite   97 annexe en suite

Traditions Pyrford Rd, Pyrford GU22 8UE
☎ 01932 350355 🖷 01932 350234
e-mail: traditions@americangolf.uk.com
18 holes, 6304yds, Par 71, SSS 70, Course record 67.
Course Designer Peter Alliss **Location** M25 junct 10, A3, signs to RHS
Garden Wisley, through Wisley to Pyford, course 0.5m
Telephone for further details
Hotel ★★★★★ HL Pennyhill Park Hotel & The Spa, London Rd,
BAGSHOT ☎ 01276 471774   26 en suite   97 annexe en suite

Woking Pond Rd, Hook Heath GU22 0JZ
☎ 01483 760053 🖷 01483 772441
e-mail: woking.golf@btconnect.com
web: www.wokinggolfclub.co.uk
An 18-hole course on Surrey heathland with few changes from the
original course designed in 1892 by Tom Dunn. Bernard Darwin, a
past captain and president, has written 'the beauty of Woking is that
there is something distinctive about every hole'.
18 holes, 6340yds, Par 70, SSS 70, Course record 65.
Club membership 600.
Visitors Mon-Fri except BHs. Handicap certificate. Dress code.
Societies booking required. **Green Fees** not confirmed. **Prof** Carl Bianco
Course Designer Tom Dunn **Facilities** ⓦ 🍴 ⓛ ▯ ▮ ⚑ ☂ ♥ ✦ ✦
✦ **Conf** Corporate Hospitality Days **Location** W of town centre in area
of St Johns Heath
Hotel ★★★★★ HL Pennyhill Park Hotel & The Spa, London Rd,
BAGSHOT ☎ 01276 471774   26 en suite   97 annexe en suite

Worplesdon Heath House Rd GU22 0RA
☎ 01483 472277
e-mail: office@worplesdongc.co.uk
The scene of the celebrated mixed-foursomes competition. Accurate
driving is essential on this heathland course. The short 10th across
a lake from tee to green is a notable hole, and the 18th provides a
wonderfully challenging Par 4 finish.
18 holes, 6431yds, Par 71, SSS 71, Course record 66.
Club membership 610.

Continued

CHAMPIONSHIP COURSE

SURREY — WALTON-ON-THE-HILL

WALTON HEATH

Map 04 TQ25

Deans Ln, Walton-on-the-Hill KT20 7TP
☎ **01737 812380** 🖹 **01737 814225**
e-mail: secretary@whgc.co.uk
web: www.whgc.co.uk
Old Course: 18 holes, 6836yds, Par 72, SSS 73,
Course record 65.
New Course: 18 holes, 6613yds, Par 72,
SSS 72, Course record 67.
Club membership 1000.
Visitors Mon-Fri. Booking required. Sat, Sun
& BHs by arrangement. Handicap certificate.
Dress code. **Societies** Booking required.
Green Fees Old Course £100; New Course
£90. Both courses £120 (Old Course £120:
New Course £100 weekends). **Prof** Ken
Macpherson **Course Designer** Herbert
Fowler **Facilities** ⑨ ⓑ 🖵 ⓥ 🎿 🖴 ⓟ ⚐
Conf Corporate Hospitality Days **Location** SE
of village off B2032

Walton Heath, a traditional member club,
has two extremely challenging courses.
Enjoying an enviable international
reputation, the club was founded in 1903.
It has played host to over 60 major
amateur and professional championships,
including the 1981 Ryder Cup and five
European Open Tournaments (1991,
1989, 1987, 1980 and 1977); among the
many prestigious amateur events, Walton
Heath hosted the English Amateur in 2002.
In recent years the club has hosted the
European qualification for the U.S. Open
Championship. The Old Course is popular
with visitors, while the New Course is very
challenging, requiring subtle shots to get
the ball near the hole. Straying from the
fairway brings gorse, bracken and heather
to test the golfer.

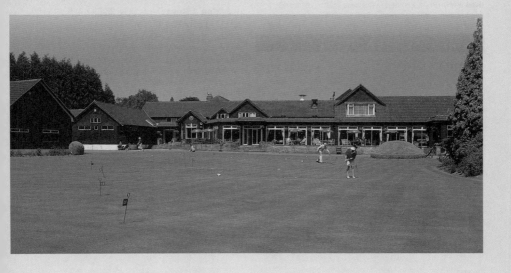

England

Visitors Mon-Fri except BHs. Booking required. Handicap certificate. Dress code. **Societies** booking required. **Green Fees** not confirmed. **Prof** J Christine **Course Designer** J F Abercromby **Facilities** ⬚ ⬚ ⬚ ⬚ ⬚ **Location** 1.5m N of village off A322
Hotel ★★★★★ HL Pennyhill Park Hotel & The Spa, London Rd, BAGSHOT ☎ 01276 471774 26 en suite 97 annexe en suite

WOLDINGHAM   MAP 05 TQ35

North Downs Northdown Rd CR3 7AA
☎ 01883 652057 📠 01883 652832
e-mail: info@northdownsgolfclub.co.uk
web: www.northdownsgolfclub.co.uk
Parkland course, 850ft above sea level, with several testing holes and magnificent views.
18 holes, 5857yds, Par 69, SSS 68, Course record 64.
Club membership 550.
Visitors Mon-Wed & Fri. Thu after noon. Sat, Sun & BHs after 3pm summer, noon winter. Booking required Thu, Sat, Sun & BHs. Handicap certificate. Dress code. **Societies** Booking required. **Green Fees** £45 per day; £35 per round (£35 per round Sat, Sun & BHs). **Prof** M Homewood **Course Designer** Pennink **Facilities** ⬚ ⬚ ⬚ ⬚ ⬚ ⬚ ⬚ ⬚ **Conf** facs Corporate Hospitality Days **Location** 0.75m S of Woldingham
Hotel ★★★ 75% HL Best Western Donnington Manor, London Rd, Dunton Green, SEVENOAKS ☎ 01732 462681 60 en suite

Woldingham Halliloo Valley Rd CR3 7HA
☎ 01883 653501 📠 01883 653502
e-mail: membership@woldingham-golfclub.co.uk
web: www.woldingham-golfclub.co.uk
Located in Halliloo Valley and designed by the American architect Bradford Benz, this pleasant course utilises all the contours and features of the valley.
18 holes, 6393yds, Par 71, SSS 70, Course record 64.
Club membership 695.
Visitors Mon-Sun & BHs, Booking required Sat/Sun & BHs. Dress code. **Societies** booking required. **Green Fees** not confirmed. **Prof** James Hillen **Course Designer** Bradford Benz **Facilities** ⬚ ⬚ ⬚ ⬚ ⬚ ⬚ ⬚ ⬚ ⬚ ⬚ **Conf** facs Corporate Hospitality Days **Location** M25 junct 6, A22 N, 1st rdbt onto Woldingham Rd Valley Rd, on left
Hotel ★★★ 75% HL Best Western Donnington Manor, London Rd, Dunton Green, SEVENOAKS ☎ 01732 462681 60 en suite

SUSSEX, EAST

BEXHILL   MAP 05 TQ70

Cooden Beach Cooden Sea Rd TN39 4TR
☎ 01424 842040 & 843938 (Pro Shop) 📠 01424 842040
e-mail: enquiries@coodenbeachgc.com
web: www.coodenbeachgc.com
The course is close by the sea, but is not real links. Despite that, it is dry and plays well throughout the year. There are some excellent holes such as the 4th, played to a built-up green, the short 12th, and three good holes to finish. There are added ponds which make the player think more about tee shots and shots to the green.

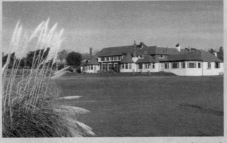

Cooden Beach

18 holes, 6504yds, Par 72, SSS 71, Course record 67.
Club membership 850.
Visitors Mon-Fri excep& BHs. Sat after 1pm, Sun after 11am. Booking required. Handicap certificate. Dress code. **Societies** Booking required. **Green Fees** £43 per day, £37 per round (£46/£49 weekends). **Prof** Jeffrey Sim **Course Designer** W Herbert Fowler **Facilities** ⬚ ⬚ ⬚ ⬚ ⬚ ⬚ ⬚ ⬚ ⬚ ⬚ **Leisure** indoor practice facility. **Conf** facs Corporate Hospitality Days **Location** 2m W on A259
Hotel ★★★ 79% HL Powder Mills Hotel, Powdermill Ln, BATTLE ☎ 01424 775511 30 en suite 10 annexe en suite

Highwoods Ellerslie Ln TN39 4LJ
☎ 01424 212625 📠 01424 216866
e-mail: highwoods@btconnect.com
web: www.highwoodsgolfclub.co.uk
Undulating parkland with water on six holes.
18 holes, 6218yds, Par 70, SSS 70, Course record 63.
Club membership 750.
Visitors Mon-Sun except BHs. booking required. Handicap certificate. Dress code. **Societies** Welcome. **Green Fees** £32 per 18 holes (£35 Sat & Sun). **Prof** Mike Andrews **Course Designer** J H Taylor **Facilities** ⬚ ⬚ ⬚ ⬚ ⬚ ⬚ **Location** 1.5m NW
Hotel ★★★ 72% HL Best Western Royal Victoria Hotel, Marina, St Leonards-on-Sea, HASTINGS ☎ 01424 445544 50 en suite

BRIGHTON & HOVE   MAP 04 TQ30

Brighton & Hove Devils Dyke Rd BN1 8YJ
☎ 01273 556482 📠 01273 554247
e-mail: phil@bhgc68.fsnet.co.uk
web: www.brightonandhovegolfclub.co.uk
Testing nine-hole course with glorious views over the Downs and the sea. Famous Par 3 6th hole considered to be one of the most extraordinary holes in golf.
9 holes, 5704yds, Par 68, SSS 67, Course record 64.
Club membership 400.
Visitors Mon-Sun & BHs. Booking required Sat, Sun & BHs. Dress code. **Societies** Booking required **Green Fees** £20 per 18 holes; £12 per 9 holes (£25/£15 Sat & Sun). **Prof** Phil Bonsall **Course Designer** James Braid **Facilities** ⬚ ⬚ ⬚ ⬚ ⬚ ⬚ ⬚ ⬚ ⬚ ⬚ **Conf** facs Corporate Hospitality Days **Location** 4m NW of Brighton, 1m from A27 & A23
Hotel ★★★ 72% HL Best Western Old Tollgate Restaurant & Hotel, The Street, BRAMBER ☎ 01903 879494 12 en suite 28 annexe en suite

Dyke Devils Dyke, Dyke Rd BN1 8YJ
☎ 01273 857296(office) & 857260(pro shop)
📠 01273 857078
e-mail: dykegolfclub@btconnect.com
web: www.dykegolf.com
Easy drasining downland course has some glorious views both towards the sea and inland. The signature hole on the course is probably the 17th; it is one of those tough Par 3s of just over 200yds, and is played across a gully to a well protected green. Greens are small,fast and true.
18 holes, 6627yds, Par 72, SSS 72, Course record 66. Club membership 800.
Visitors Mon, Wed-Sun & BHs. Booking required. Dress code.
Societies Booking required. **Green Fees** £35 per round (£45 Sat & Sun).
Prof Richard Arnold **Course Designer** Fred Hawtree
Facilities ⊕ ⏸ ↳ ⌨ ⚑ ⚐ ↥ 🕭 ⚑ 🏌 🏌 **Conf** facs Corporate
Hospitality Days **Location** 4m N of Brighton, between A23 & A27
Hotel ★★★ 72% HL Best Western Old Tollgate Restaurant & Hotel, The Street, BRAMBER ☎ 01903 879494 12 en suite 28 annexe en suite

Hollingbury Park Ditchling Rd BN1 7HS
☎ 01273 552010 (sec) & 500086 (pro) 📠 01273 552010/6
e-mail: graemecrompton@sussexgolfcentre.fsnet.co.uk
web: www.hollingburygolfclub.co.uk
Municipal course in hilly situation on the South Downs, overlooking the sea.
18 holes, 6500yds, Par 72, SSS 71, Course record 65. Club membership 240.
Visitors Mon-Sun & BHs. Booking required. Dress code. **Societies** Welcome. **Green Fees** £17 per 18 holes (£23 Sat & Sun). **Prof** Graeme Crompton **Facilities** ⊕ ⌨ ⚑ ↥ 🕭 🏌 **Location** 2m N of town centre
Hotel ★★★ 64% HL Quality Hotel Brighton, West St, BRIGHTON
☎ 01273 220033 140 en suite

Waterhall Saddlescombe Rd BN1 8YN
☎ 01273 508658
18 holes, 5773yds, Par 69, SSS 68, Course record 66.
Location 2m NE from A27
Telephone for further details
Hotel ★★★ 72% HL Best Western Old Tollgate Restaurant & Hotel, The Street, BRAMBER ☎ 01903 879494 12 en suite 28 annexe en suite

West Hove Badgers Way, Hangleton BN3 8EX
☎ 01273 419738 & 413494 (pro) 📠 01273 439988
e-mail: info@westhovegolf.co.uk
web: www.westhovegolfclub.info
A challenging downland course with good drainage due to its chalk based location.
18 holes, 6226yds, Par 71, SSS 70, Course record 62. Club membership 600.
Visitors Mon-Sun & BHs. Booking required. Dress code. **Societies** Booking required. **Green Fees** £25 per 18 holes (£30 Sat & Sun). **Prof** Darren Cook **Course Designer** Hawtree & Sons **Facilities** ⊕ ⏸ ↳ ⌨ ⚑ ↥ 🕭 🏌 ↥ 🏌 ⚐ **Conf** facs Corporate Hospitality Days **Location** Off A27 N of Brighton
Hotel ★★★ 68% HL The Courtlands, 15-27 The Drive, HOVE
☎ 01273 731055 60 en suite 7 annexe en suite

CROWBOROUGH   MAP 05 TQ53

Crowborough Beacon Beacon Rd TN6 1UJ
☎ 01892 661511 📠 01892 611988
e-mail: secretary@cbgc.co.uk
web: www.cbgc.co.uk
Standing some 800ft above sea level, this is a testing heathland course where accuracy off the tee rather than distance is paramount. Panoramic views of the South Downs, Eastbourne and even the sea on a clear day.

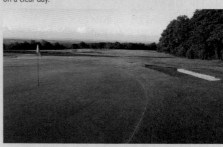

18 holes, 6031yds, Par 71, SSS 69, Course record 66. Club membership 700.
Visitors Mon-Fri. Sat, Sun & BHs after 2.30pm. Booking required. Handicap certificate. Dress code. **Societies** Booking required. **Green Fees** £50 per round, £60 per day (£60 per round Sat, Sun & BHs). **Prof** Mr D C Newnham **Facilities** ⊕ ⏸ by prior arrangement ↳ ⌨ ⚑ ↥ 🕭 ⚑ 🏌 **Conf** Corporate Hospitality Days **Location** 9m S of Tunbridge Wells on A26
Hotel ★★★★ 74% HL The Spa Hotel, Mount Ephraim, TUNBRIDGE WELLS ☎ 01892 520331 69 en suite

Dewlands Manor Cottage Hill, Rotherfield TN6 3JN
☎ 01892 852266 📠 01892 853015
A meadowland course built on land surrounding a 15th-century manor. The short Par 4 4th can be played by the brave by launching a driver over the trees; the 7th requires accurate driving on a tight fairway; and the final two holes are sweeping Par 5s travelling parallel to each other, a small stream guarding the front of the 9th green.
9 holes, 3186yds, Par 36, SSS 70. Club membership 400.
Visitors Mon-Sun & BHs. Booking required. Dress code. **Societies** Booking required. **Green Fees** t£18.50 per 18 holes, £16.50 per 9 holes (£32/£18.50 Sat, Sun & BHs). **Prof** Nick Godin **Course Designer** R M & N M Godin **Facilities** ⊕ ↳ ⌨ ⚑ ↥ 🕭 ⚑ 🏌 **Leisure** indoor teaching facilities with computer analysis. **Conf** facs Corporate Hospitality Days **Location** 0.5m S of Rotherfield

DITCHLING   MAP 05 TQ31

Mid Sussex Spatham Ln BN6 8XJ
☎ 01273 846567 📠 01273 847815
e-mail: admin@midsussexgolfclub.co.uk
web: www.midsussexgolfclub.co.uk
Mature parkland course with many trees, water hazards, strategically placed bunkers and superbly contoured greens. The 14th hole, a spectacular Par 5, demands accurate shotmaking to avoid the various hazards along its length.

Continued

18 holes, 6462yds, Par 71, SSS 71, Course record 65.
Club membership 650.
Visitors Mon-Fri. Sat/Sun & BHs pm only. Dress code. **Societies** booking
required. **Green Fees** not confirmed. **Prof** Neil Plimmer **Course Designer**
David Williams **Facilities** ⑪ ⑩ ⑥ ⑯ ⑨ ⑨ ⑥ ⑨ ⑨ ⑥ **Conf** facs
Corporate Hospitality Days **Location** 1m E of Ditchling
Hotel ★★★ 79% HL Shelleys Hotel, High St, LEWES ☎ 01273 472361
19 en suite

EASTBOURNE   MAP 05 TV69

Eastbourne Downs East Dean Rd BN20 8ES
☎ 01323 720827 📄 01323 412506
e-mail: tony.reeves@btconnect.com
This downland course has spectacular views over the South Downs
and Channel. Situated in an Area of Outstanding Natural Beauty 1m
behind Beachy Head. The club celebrates its centenary in 2008.
18 holes, 6601yds, Par 72, SSS 71, Course record 69.
Club membership 600.
Visitors Mon-Sun & BHs. Booking required Sat, Sun & BHs. Handicap
certificate weekends. **Societies** Welcome. **Green Fees** £25 per day, £20
per round (£32/£28 Sat, Sun & BHs). **Prof** T Marshall **Course Designer** J H
Taylor **Facilities** ⑪ ⑩ ⑥ ⑯ ⑨ ⑨ ⑥ ⑨ **Conf** Corporate Hospitality
Days **Location** 0.5m W of town centre on A259
Hotel ★★★ 75% HL Best Western Lansdowne Hotel, King Edward's Pde,
EASTBOURNE ☎ 01323 725174 101 en suite

Royal Eastbourne Paradise Dr BN20 8BP
☎ 01323 729738 📄 01323 744048
e-mail: sec@regc.co.uk
web: www.regc.co.uk
A famous club which celebrated its centenary in 1987. The course
plays longer than it measures. Testing holes are the 8th, a Par 3
played to a high green and the 16th, a Par 5 righthand dog-leg.
Devonshire Course: 18 holes, 6077yds, Par 70, SSS 69,
Course record 62.
Hartington Course: 9 holes, 2147yds, Par 64, SSS 61.
Club membership 800.
Visitors Mon-Sun & BHs. Booking required Mon, Sat, Sun & BHs.
Handicap certificate. Dress code. **Societies** Booking required.
Green Fees Devonshire £33 per round (£39 Sat, Sun & BHs),
Hartington £19 per day. **Prof** Alan Harrison **Course Designer** Arthur
Mayhewe **Facilities** ⑪ ⑩ by prior arrangement ⑥ ⑨ ⑨ ⑥ ⑨ ⑥
⑨ ⑥ ⑨ **Leisure** snooker table. **Conf** facs Corporate Hospitality Days
Location 0.5m W of town centre
Hotel ★★★ 75% HL Best Western Lansdowne Hotel, King Edward's
Pde, EASTBOURNE ☎ 01323 725174 101 en suite

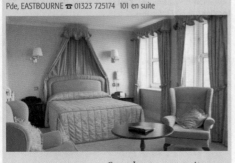

See advert on opposite page

Willingdon Southdown Rd, Willingdon BN20 9AA
☎ 01323 410981 📄 01323 411510
e-mail: secretary@willingdongolfclub.co.uk
web: www.willingdongolfclub.co.uk
Unique downland course set in an oyster-shaped amphitheatre.
18 holes, 6118yds, Par 69, SSS 69. Club membership 610.
Visitors Mon-Sun & BHs. Dress code. **Societies** Booking required.
Green Fees £30 per day, £24 per round (£37/£32 Sat & Sun). **Prof** Troy
Moore **Course Designer** J Taylor/Dr Mackenzie **Facilities** ⑥ ⑨ ⑨ ⑥
⑨ ⑥ **Location** 0.5m N of town centre off A22
Hotel ★★★ 78% HL Hydro Hotel, Mount Rd, EASTBOURNE
☎ 01323 720643 84 rms (83 en suite)

FOREST ROW   MAP 05 TQ43

Royal Ashdown Forest Chapel Ln RH18 5LR
☎ 01342 822018 📄 01342 825211
e-mail: office@royalashdown.co.uk
web: www.royalashdown.co.uk
Old Course is on undulating heathland with no bunkers. Long carries
off the tees and magnificent views over the Forest. Not a course for
the high handicapper. West Course on natural heathland with no
bunkers. Less demanding than Old Course although accuracy is at
a premium.

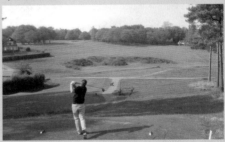

Old Course: 18 holes, 6502yds, Par 72, SSS 71,
Course record 67.
West Course: 18 holes, 5606yds, Par 68, SSS 67,
Course record 65. Club membership 450.
Visitors Mon-Sun & BHs. Booking required. Dress code.
Societies Booking required. **Green Fees** Old Course £55 per round
(£75 Sat & Sun). West Course £28 per round (£33 Sat & Sun). Reduced
winter rates. **Prof** Martyn Landsborough **Course Designer** Archdeacon
Scott **Facilities** ⑪ ⑩ by prior arrangement ⑥ ⑨ ⑨ ⑥ ⑨ ⑨ ⑥ ⑨
Location On B2110 in Forest Row
Hotel ★★★★ HL Ashdown Park Hotel and Country Club, Wych Cross,
FOREST ROW ☎ 01342 824988 106 en suite

HAILSHAM   MAP 05 TQ50

Wellshurst Golf & Country Club North St, Hellingly
BN27 4EE
☎ 01435 813456 (pro shop) 📄 01435 812444
e-mail: info@wellshurst.com
web: www.wellshurst.com
There are outstanding views of the South Downs and the Weald from
this well-manicured, undulating 18-hole course. There are varied
features and some water hazards. A practice sand bunker, putting

Continued

green and driving range are available to improve your golf. The clubhouse and leisure facilities are open to visitors.
18 holes, 5992yds, Par 70, SSS 68, Course record 64.
Club membership 450.
Visitors Mon-Sun & BHs. Dress code. **Societies** Welcome. **Green Fees** £20 per 18 holes (£24 Sat & Sun). **Prof** Mark Jarvis **Course Designer** The Golf Corporation **Facilities** ⊕ ⏐⊙⏐ ⓑ ⊑ ⊤⏐ ⌄ ♤ ☞ ✆ ♥ ⌁ ♠ **Leisure** sauna, solarium, gymnasium, spa bath. **Conf** facs Corporate Hospitality Days **Location** 2.5m N off A22 junct at Hailsham, on A267
Hotel ★★ 75% HL The Olde Forge Hotel & Restaurant, Magham Down, HAILSHAM ☎ 01323 842893 7 en suite

---

HASTINGS & ST LEONARDS   MAP 05 TQ80

Beauport Battle Rd TN37 7BP
☎ 01424 854243 ▤ 01424 854244
Played over Hastings Public Course. Undulating parkland with stream and fine views.
18 holes, 6248yds, Par 71, SSS 70, Course record 70.
Club membership 400.
Visitors Mon-Fri & BHs. Sat & Sun after 11am. Handicap certificate. Dress code. **Societies** Booking required. **Green Fees** not confirmed. **Prof** Charles Giddins **Facilities** ⊕ ⏐⊙⏐ ⓑ ⊑ ⊤⏐ ⌄ ♤ ☞ ✆ ♥ ⌁ **Leisure** hard tennis courts, outdoor swimming pool. **Location** 3m N of Hastings on A2100
Hotel ★★★ 72% HL Beauport Park Hotel, Battle Rd, HASTINGS
☎ 01424 851222 25 en suite

HEATHFIELD   MAP 05 TQ52

Horam Park Chiddingly Rd, Horam TN21 0JJ
☎ 01435 813477 ▤ 01435 813677
e-mail: angie@horamgolf.freeserve.co.uk
web: www.horamparkgolf.co.uk
A pretty, woodland course with lakes and quality fast-running greens.
9 holes, 6128yds, Par 70, SSS 70, Course record 64.
Club membership 350.
Visitors Mon-Sun & BHs. Dress code. **Societies** Booking required. **Green Fees** £18 per 18 holes; £12 per 9 holes (£20/£13 Sat & Sun). Twilight £11. **Prof** Giles Velvick **Course Designer** Glen Johnson **Facilities** ⊕ ⏐⊙⏐ ⓑ ⊑ ⊤⏐ ⌄ ♤ ☞ ✆ ♥ ⌁ **Leisure** pitch & putt, video swingbay on range, digital coaching room. **Conf** Corporate Hospitality Days **Location** Off A267 Hailsham to Heathfield
Hotel ★★★★ 74% HL Boship Farm Hotel, Lower Dicker, HAILSHAM
☎ 01323 844826 & 442600 ▤ 01323 843945 47 en suite

HOLTYE   MAP 05 TQ43

Holtye TN8 7ED
☎ 01342 850635 & 850576 ▤ 01342 851139
e-mail: secretary@holtye.com
web: www.holtye.com
Undulating forest and heathland course with tree-lined fairways providing testing golf. Different tees on the back nine.
9 holes, 5325yds, Par 66, SSS 66, Course record 62.
Club membership 265.
Visitors Mon-Sun & BHs. Booking required Wed, Thu, Sat, Sun & BHs. Dress code. **Societies** Booking required. **Green Fees** £16 per 18 holes, £10 per 9 holes (£20/£13 Sat & Sun). **Prof** Kevin Hinton **Facilities** ⊕ ⓑ ⊑ ⊤⏐ ⌄ ♤ ☞ ✆ ♥ **Location** 4m E of East Grinstead on A264
Hotel BUD Premier Travel Inn East Grinstead, London Rd, Felbridge, EAST GRINSTEAD ☎ 08701 977088 41 en suite

---

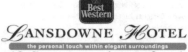

*L*ANSDOWNE *H*OTEL
the personal touch within elegant surroundings
13 Courses to choose from!
Any 2 days – 18th January–31st December 2008
Extra days pro rata. Your break includes 2 days'
golf (up to 36 holes each day on the same course),
en suite accommodation, full English Breakfast,
light Lunch at the golf club and a 4 course Dinner
at the Hotel. For prices, dates, etc., please contact
Reservations for our Golfing Breaks brochure.

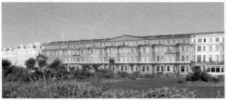

King Edward's Parade
Eastbourne, East Sussex BN21 4EE
Tel: 01323 725 174   Fax: 01323 739 721
Website: www.bw-lansdownehotel.co.uk
E-mail: reception@lansdowne-hotel.co.uk

AA
★★★
Hotel

LEWES   MAP 05 TQ41

Lewes Chapel Hill BN7 2BB
☎ 01273 473245 ▤ 01273 483474
e-mail: secretary@lewesgolfclub.co.uk
web: www.lewesgolfclub.co.uk
Downland course with undulating fairways. Fine views. Proper greens all-year-round.
18 holes, 6190yds, Par 71, SSS 70, Course record 64.
Club membership 568.
Visitors Mon-Sun & BHs. Dress code. **Societies** Booking required. **Green Fees** £34 per round, £14 Mon, £13 Twilight. **Prof** Paul Dobson **Course Designer** Jack Rowe **Facilities** ⊕ ⏐⊙⏐ by prior arrangement ⓑ ⊑ ⊤⏐ ⌄ ♤ ☞ **Conf** Corporate Hospitality Days **Location** E of town centre
Hotel ★★★ 80% HL Deans Place, Seaford Rd, ALFRISTON
☎ 01323 870248 36 en suite

NEWHAVEN   MAP 05 TQ40

Peacehaven Brighton Rd BN9 9UH
☎ 01273 512571 ▤ 01273 512571
e-mail: peacehavengolfclub@tiscali.co.uk
Downland course, sometimes windy. Testing holes: 1st (Par 3), 4th (Par 4), 9th (Par 3). Attractive views over the South Downs, the River Ouse and Newhaven Harbour.
9 holes, 5488yds, Par 70, SSS 66, Course record 65.
Club membership 270.

Continued

Visitors Contact club for details. **Societies** Welcome. **Green Fees** £17 per 18 holes, £11 per 9 holes (£23/£15 Sat & Sun). ⊛ **Prof** Alan Tyson **Course Designer** James Braid **Facilities** ⓑ ▯ 𝔃 ☖ 🛆 🗇 ✔ **Location** 0.75m W on A259

Hotel ★★★ 70% HL The Star Inn, ALFRISTON ☎ 01323 870495 37 en suite

RYE   MAP 05 TQ92

Rye New Lydd Rd, Camber TN31 7QS
☎ 01797 225241 📄 01797 225460
e-mail: links@ryegolfclub.co.uk
web: www.ryegolfclub.co.uk

Unique links course with superb undulating greens set among ridges of sand dunes alongside Rye Harbour. Fine views over Romney Marsh and towards Fairlight and Dungeness.

Old Course: 18 holes, 6317yds, Par 68, SSS 71,
Course record 64.
Jubilee Course: 18 holes, 5848yds, Par 69, SSS 69,
Course record 71. Club membership 1200.

Visitors Mon-Sun & BHs. Booking required. Handicap certificate. Dress code. **Green Fees** Phone. **Prof** Michael Lee **Course Designer** H S Colt **Facilities** ⓘ ⓑ ▯ 𝔃 🛆 🗇 ◇ ✔ **Location** 2.75m SE off A259
Hotel ★★★★ 80% HL The George in Rye, 98 High St, RYE
☎ 01797 222114 24 en suite

SEAFORD   MAP 05 TV49

Seaford Firle Rd BN25 2JD
☎ 01323 892442 📄 01323 894113
e-mail: secretary@seafordgolfclub.co.uk
web: www.seafordgolfclub.co.uk

The great H Taylor did not perhaps design as many courses as his friend and rival, James Braid, but Seaford's original design was Taylor's. It is a splendid downland course with magnificent views and some fine holes.

18 holes, 6546yds, Par 69, SSS 71. Club membership 600.

Visitors Mon-Sat except BHs. Handicap certificate. Dress code. **Societies** Booking required. **Green Fees** £40 per 18 holes (£30 winter). **Prof** David Mills/Clay Morris **Course Designer** J H Taylor **Facilities** ⓘ 🍴 by prior arrangement ⓑ ▯ 𝔃 🛆 🗇 ◇ ✔ 🏌 🛒 **Conf** Corporate Hospitality Days **Location** Turn inland off A259 at war memorial

Hotel ★★★ 70% HL The Star Inn, ALFRISTON ☎ 01323 870495 37 en suite

Seaford Head Southdown Rd BN25 4JS
☎ 01323 890139 📄 01323 894491
e-mail: fraser1974@mac.com
web: www.seafordheadgolfcourse.co.uk

A links type course situated on the cliff edge giving exception views over the Seven Sisters and coastline. The upper level is reached via a short hole with elevated green - known as the 'Hell Hole' and the 18th Par 5 tee is on the 'Head' being 300 feet above sea level.

18 holes, 5848yds, Par 71, SSS 68, Course record 62.
Club membership 450.

Visitors Mon-Sun & BHs. Booking required. Dress code. **Societies** Booking required. **Green Fees** £20 (£23 Sat & Sun). **Prof** Fraser Morley **Facilities** ⓘ 🍴 ⓑ ▯ 𝔃 🛆 🗇 ◇ ✔ ✔ **Location** E of Seaford on A259
Hotel ★★★ 80% HL Deans Place, Seaford Rd, ALFRISTON
☎ 01323 870248 36 en suite

SEDLESCOMBE   MAP 05 TQ71

Sedlescombe Kent St TN33 0SD
☎ 01424 871700 📄 01424 871712
e-mail: golf@golfschool.co.uk
web: www.golfschool.co.uk
18 holes, 6269yds, Par 72, SSS 70.
Location 4m N of Hastings on A21
Telephone for further details
Hotel ★★★ 75% HL Brickwall Hotel, The Green, Sedlescombe, BATTLE ☎ 01424 870253 & 870339 📄 01424 870785 25 en suite

TICEHURST   MAP 05 TQ63

Dale Hill Hotel & Golf Club TN5 7DQ
☎ 01580 200112 📄 01580 201249
e-mail: info@dalehill.co.uk
web: www.dalehill.co.uk

Dale Hill is set in over 350 acres, high on the Weald in an Area of Outstanding Natural Beauty. Offering two 18-hole courses, one of which has been designed by Ian Woosnam to USGA specifications.

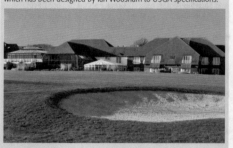

Dale Hill: 18 holes, 6106yds, Par 70, SSS 69.
Ian Woosnam: 18 holes, 6512yds, Par 71, SSS 71,
Course record 64. Club membership 850.

Visitors Mon-Sun & BHs. Dress code. **Societies** Welcome. **Green Fees** Dale Hill: £25 (£35 weekends). Ian Woosnam (including buggy) £60 (£70 Sat & Sun). **Prof** Mark Wood **Course Designer** Ian Woosnam **Facilities** ⓘ 🍴 ⓑ ▯ 𝔃 🛆 🗇 ◇ ✔ 🏌 ✔ 🛒 **Leisure** heated indoor swimming pool, sauna, gymnasium. **Conf** facs Corporate Hospitality Days **Location** M25 junct 5,A21, B2087 left after 1 mile

Hotel ★★★★ 80% HL Dale Hill Hotel & Golf Club, TICEHURST ☎ 01580 200112 35 en suite

UCKFIELD   MAP 05 TQ42

East Sussex National see page 247

Hotel ★★★★ 87% HL Buxted Park Country House Hotel, Buxted, UCKFIELD ☎ 01825 733333 44 en suite
Hotel ★★★ HL Horsted Place, Little Horsted, UCKFIELD ☎ 01825 750581 Fax 01825 750459 17 en suite 3 annexe en suite
Hotel ★★★ HL Newick Park Hotel & Country Estate, NEWICK ☎ 01825 723633 Fax 01825 723969 13 en suite 3 annexe en suite

CHAMPIONSHIP COURSE

EAST SUSSEX — UCKFIELD

EAST SUSSEX NATIONAL GOLF RESORT AND SPA

Map 05 TQ42

Little Horsted TN22 5ES
☎ 01825 880088 📄 01825 880066
e-mail: golf@eastsussexnational.co.uk
web: www.eastsussexnational.co.uk
East Course: 18 holes, 7138yds, Par 72, SSS 74, Course record 63.
West Course: 18 holes, 7154yds, Par 72, SSS 74.
Club membership 650.
Visitors Mon-Sun & BHs. Booking required. Dress code. **Societies** booking required.
Green Fees £50 per 18 holes (£60 weekends).
Prof Sarah Maclennan/Mike Clark
Course Designer Bob Cupp **Facilities** ⑨ 🍴 🍺 🍷 🐚 🏌 🎣 🛒 🛥 🏇 **Leisure** hard tennis courts, heated indoor swimming pool, fishing, sauna, solarium, health club and spa, gymnasium, golf academy shop. **Conf** Corporate Hospitality Days **Location** 2m S of Uckfield on A22

East Sussex National offers two huge courses ideal for big-hitting professionals. The European Open has been staged here and it is home to the European Headquarters of the David Leadbetter Golf Academy, with indoor and outdoor video analysis. Bob Cupp designed the courses using 'bent' grass from tee to green, resulting in an American-style course to test everyone. The greens on both courses are immaculately maintained. The West Course, with stadium design and chosen for major events, is reserved for members and their guests; visitors are welcome on the East Course, also with stadium design, and which was the venue for the 1993 and 1994 European Open. The complex features a new 104-bedroom hotel and a bespoke conference centre capable of seating up to 600 delegates.

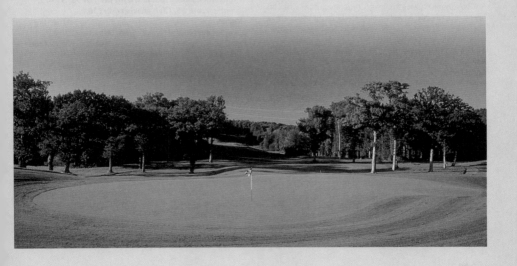

England

Piltdown Piltdown TN22 3XB
☎ 01825 722033 📠 01825 724192
e-mail: info@piltdowngolfclub.co.uk
web: www.piltdowngolfclub.co.uk
A relatively short, but difficult heather and gorse course built on Sussex clay. No bunkers, easy walking, fine views.
18 holes, 6076yds, Par 68, SSS 69, Course record 64.
Club membership 400.
Visitors Mon, Wed, Fri, Sat & Sun. Tue, Thu & BHs pm only. Booking required. Handicap certificate. Dress code. **Societies** Booking required.
Green Fees £50 per day , £35 per round, £30 after 1.30pm, £18 after 4pm.
🏌 **Prof** Jason Partridge **Facilities** ⑪ ▙ ⌴ ▜ 🖥 🛦 🍴 ✔ ✔ 🏌
Location 2m W of Uckfield off A272, club signed
Hotel ★★★ HL Horsted Place, Little Horsted, UCKFIELD ☎ 01825 750581
17 en suite 3 annexe en suite

SUSSEX, WEST

ANGMERING   MAP 04 TQ00

Ham Manor West Dr BN16 4JE
☎ 01903 783288 📠 01903 850886
e-mail: secretary@hammanor.co.uk
web: www.hammanor.co.uk
Two miles from the sea, this parkland course has fine springy turf and provides an interesting test in two loops of nine holes each.
18 holes, 6267yds, Par 70, SSS 70, Course record 64.
Club membership 780.
Visitors Mon-Sun & BHs. Handicap certificate. Dress code. **Societies** Welcome. **Green Fees** £35 (£50 Sat & Sun). **Prof** Simon Buckley **Course Designer** Harry Colt **Facilities** ⑪ ⑩ ▙ ⌴ ▜ 🛦 🖥 🍴 ✔ **Conf** Corporate Hospitality Days **Location** Off A259
Guesthouse ★★★★ GA Kenmore Guest House, Claigmar Rd, RUSTINGTON ☎ 01903 784634 7 rms (6 en suite)

ARUNDEL   MAP 04 TQ00

Avisford Park Yapton Ln, Walberton BN18 0LS
☎ 01243 554611 📠 01243 555580
e-mail: avisfordparkgolf@aol.com
A 18 hole course enjoying a country hotel complex setting which has recently been redesigned and lengthened. The course opens with a real challenge as there is out of bounds water and tree hazards the whole length of the 414yard drive.
18 holes, 5703yds, Par 68, SSS 66. Club membership 300.
Visitors Mon-Sun & BHs. Dress code. **Societies** Booking required.
Green Fees £16.50 per 18 holes, £12 per 9 holes (£20/£12 Sat, Sun & BHs).
Prof K Mann **Facilities** ⑪ ▙ ⌴ ▜ 🛦 🖥 ⚲ ✔ ✔ **Leisure** hard tennis courts, outdoor and indoor heated swimming pools. **Location** Off A27 towards Yapton
Hotel ★★★ 71% HL Norfolk Arms Hotel, High St, ARUNDEL
☎ 01903 882101 21 en suite 13 annexe en suite

BOGNOR REGIS   MAP 04 SZ99

Bognor Regis Downview Rd, Felpham PO22 8JD
☎ 01243 821929 (Secretary) 📠 01243 860719
e-mail: sec@bognorgolfclub.co.uk
web: www.bognorgolfclub.co.uk
This flattish, well tree-lined, parkland course has more variety than is to be found on some other south coast courses. The course is open

to the prevailing wind and the River Rife and many water ditches need negotiation.
18 holes, 6238yds, Par 70, SSS 70, Course record 64.
Club membership 700.
Visitors Mon, Wed-Fri except BHs. Tue pm only. Handicap certificate.
Dress code. **Societies** Booking required. **Green Fees** £30. 🏌 **Prof** Matthew Kirby **Course Designer** James Braid **Facilities** ⑪ ⑩ ▙ ⌴ ▜ 🛦 🖥 ✔ 🖥 ✔ **Conf** facs **Location** 0.5m N at Felpham lights on A259
Hotel ★★ 71% HL Beachcroft Hotel, Clyde Rd, Felpham Village,
BOGNOR REGIS ☎ 01243 827142 35 en suite

BURGESS HILL   MAP 04 TQ31

Burgess Hill Cuckfield Rd RH15 8RE
☎ 01444 258585 📠 01444 247318
e-mail: enquiries@burgesshillgolfcentre.co.uk
Very challenging nine-hole course. Gently undulating layout with trees and water. Used for PGA short course championships
9 holes, 1250yds, Par 27.
Visitors Mon-Fri except BHs. **Societies** Welcome. **Green Fees** £10 per 9 holes. **Prof** Mark Collins **Course Designer** Donald Steel **Facilities** ⑪ ⑩ ▙ ⌴ ▜ 🛦 🖥 ✔ 🏌 **Leisure** pitching & chipping green. **Conf** facs Corporate Hospitality Days **Location** N of town on B2036
Hotel ★★ 72% HL Hilton Park Hotel, Tylers Green, CUCKFIELD
☎ 01444 454555 11 en suite

CHICHESTER   MAP 04 SU80

Chichester Hunston Village PO20 1AX
☎ 01243 533833 📠 01243 539922
e-mail: enquiries@chichestergolf.com
web: www.chichestergolf.co.uk
The front nine of the Cathedral course has a 601yd Par 5 that will challenge the best golfer. This is sandwiched between two formidable Par 3s over water. The back nine is more subtle with two Par 5s that can be reached in two by the most adventurous and the short but deceptive 15th, framed with 300 Portland stones and surrounded by sand.
Tower Course: 18 holes, 6175yds, Par 72, SSS 69,
Course record 67.
Cathedral Course: 18 holes, 6461yds, Par 72, SSS 71,
Course record 65. Club membership 750.
Visitors Mon-Sun & BHs. Booking required. Handicap certificate. Dress code. **Societies** Booking required. **Green Fees** Tower £17.50 (£21.50 weekend). Cathedral £22 (£30 weekends). **Prof** James Willmott **Course Designer** Philip Saunders **Facilities** ⑪ ⑩ by prior arrangement ▙ ⌴ ▜ 🛦 🖥 🍴 ✔ 🏌 **Leisure** mini golf and Par 3 course. **Conf** facs Corporate Hospitality Days **Location** 3m S of Chichester on B2145

COPTHORNE   MAP 05 TQ33

Copthorne Borers Arms Rd RH10 3LL
☎ 01342 712033 & 712508 📠 01342 717682
e-mail: info@copthornegolfclub.co.uk
web: www.copthornegolfclub.co.uk
Despite it having been in existence since 1892, this club remains one of the lesser known Sussex courses. It is hard to know why because it is most attractive with plenty of trees and much variety.
18 holes, 6435yds, Par 71, SSS 71, Course record 66.
Club membership 550.

Continued

Visitors Mon-Fri except BHs. Handicap certificate. Dress code. **Societies** Welcome. **Green Fees** £38. **Prof** Joe Burrell **Course Designer** James Braid **Facilities** 🏌 🍴 ⚐ ✓ **Conf** Corporate Hospitality Days **Location** M23 junct 10, E of village off A264
Hotel ★★★★ 71% HL Copthorne Hotel London Gatwick, Copthorne Way, COPTHORNE ☎ 01342 348800 & 348888 📄 01342 348833 227 en suite

Effingham Park The Copthorne Effingham Park, Hotel, West Park Rd RH10 3EU
☎ 01342 716528 📄 0870 8900 215
web: efgcecrownpartsplc.com
Parkland course.

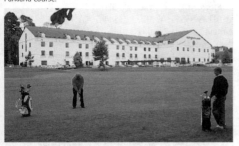

9 holes, 1822yds, Par 30, SSS 57, Course record 28.
Club membership 230.
Visitors contact club for details. **Societies** welcome. **Green Fees** not confirmed. **Prof** Mark Root **Course Designer** Francisco Escario **Facilities** 🏌 🍴 ⚐ ✓ ✓ **Leisure** hard tennis courts, heated indoor swimming pool, sauna, solarium, gymnasium. **Conf** facs Corporate Hospitality Days **Location** 2m E on B2028
Hotel ★★★★ 74% HL Copthorne Hotel and Resort Effingham Park, West Park Rd, Copthorne, ☎ 01342 714994 122 en suite

---

CRAWLEY   MAP 04 TQ23

Cottesmore Buchan Hill, Pease Pottage RH11 9AT
☎ 01293 528256 (reception) & 861777 (shop)
📄 01293 522819
e-mail: cottesmore-pro@crown-golf.co.uk
web: www.crown-golf.co.uk
Founded in 1974, the Griffin course is a fine test of golfing skill with fairways lined by silver birch, pine, oak and rhododendrons. The natural lakes play a major part in the score. The Phoenix course is easier though still weaving through the same terrain.

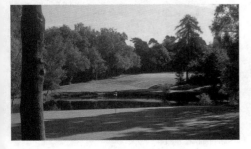

Griffin: 18 holes, 6248yds, Par 71, SSS 70,
Course record 67.
Phoenix: 18 holes, 5600yds, Par 69, SSS 66.
Visitors Mon-Sun & BHs. Booking required. Dress code. **Societies** Booking required. **Green Fees** Griffin Mon-Thu £29 per round (Fri-Sun £33). Phoenix £16/£20. **Prof** Calum J Callan **Course Designer** Michael J Rogerson **Facilities** 🏌 🍴 ⚐ 🍴 ✓ ⚐ ◇ 🍴 ✓ **Leisure** hard tennis courts, heated indoor swimming pool, sauna, solarium, gymnasium. **Conf** facs Corporate Hospitality Days **Location** M23 junct 11, through village of Pease Pottage, 2m on right
Hotel ★★★★ HL Alexander House Hotel & Utopia Spa, East St, TURNERS HILL ☎ 01342 714914 32 en suite

Ifield Golf & Country Club Rusper Rd, Ifield RH11 0LN
☎ 01293 520222 📄 01293 612973
e-mail: gfielding.igcc@btconnect.com
Parkland course.
18 holes, 6330yds, Par 70, SSS 70, Course record 64.
Club membership 750.
Visitors Mon-Fri except BHs. Booking required. Handicap certificate. Dress code. **Societies** Welcome. **Green Fees** £50 per day; £40 per round. **Prof** Jonathan Earl **Course Designer** Hawtree & Taylor **Facilities** 🏌 🍴 🍴 ⚐ 🍴 ✓ ⚐ ✓ 🍴 **Location** 1m W side of town centre off A23
Hotel ★★★★ HL Alexander House Hotel & Utopia Spa, East St, TURNERS HILL ☎ 01342 714914 32 en suite

Tilgate Forest Golf Centre Titmus Dr RH10 5EU
☎ 01293 530103 📄 01293 523478
e-mail: tilgate@glendale-services.co.uk
Designed by former Ryder Cup players Neil Coles and Brian Huggett, the course has been carefully cut through a silver birch and pine forest. It is possibly one of the most beautiful public courses in the country. The 17th is a treacherous Par 5 demanding an uphill third shot to a green surrounded by rhododendrons.
18 holes, 6359yds, Par 71, SSS 70, Course record 69.
Club membership 200.
Visitors Mon-Sun & BHs. Booking required. Dress code. **Societies** booking required. **Green Fees** not confirmed. **Prof** Sean Trussell **Course Designer** Neil Coles/Brian Huggett **Facilities** 🏌 🍴 🍴 ⚐ 🍴 ✓ ⚐ 🍴 🍴 ✓ 🍴 **Leisure** Par 3 nine hole course. **Conf** Corporate Hospitality Days **Location** 2m E of town centre
Hotel ★★★★ HL Alexander House Hotel & Utopia Spa, East St, TURNERS HILL ☎ 01342 714914 32 en suite

---

EAST GRINSTEAD   MAP 05 TQ33

Chartham Park Felcourt Rd, Felcourt RH19 2JT
☎ 01342 870340 & 870008 (pro shop) 📄 01342 870719
e-mail: charthampk.retail@theclubcompany.com
web: www.theclubcompany.com
Mature parkland course.
18 holes, 6680yards, Par 72, SSS 72, Course record 64.
Club membership 740.
Visitors Contact course for details. Dress code. **Societies** Booking required. **Green Fees** Phone. **Prof** Ben Knight **Course Designer** Neil Coles **Facilities** 🏌 🍴 🍴 ⚐ 🍴 ✓ ⚐ 🍴 🍴 ✓ 🍴 **Conf** Corporate Hospitality Days **Location** 2m N from town centre towards Felcourt, on right
Hotel ★★★ HL Gravetye Manor Hotel, EAST GRINSTEAD ☎ 01342 810567 18 en suite

HASSOCKS
MAP 04 TQ31

Hassocks London Rd BN6 9NA
☎ 01273 846630 & 846990 📠 01273 846070
e-mail: hassocksgolfclub@btconnect.com
web: www.hassocksgolfclub.co.uk
Set against the backdrop of the South Downs, Hassocks is an 18-hole Par 70 course designed and contoured to blend naturally with the surrounding countryside. A friendly and relaxed course, appealing to golfers of all ages and abilities.
18 holes, 5703yds, Par 70, SSS 67, Course record 66.
Club membership 400.
Visitors Mon-Sun & BHs. Booking required. Dress code. **Societies** Booking required. **Green Fees** £18 per 18 holes (£24.50 Sat, Sun & BHs). **Prof** Charles Ledger **Course Designer** Paul Wright **Facilities** ⑪ ⑩ ⅃ ⊑ ⊡ ⅊ ⌁ 🖢 🕏 ⌁ 🥄 ⅀ **Conf** facs Corporate Hospitality Days **Location** On A273 between Burgess Hill and Hassocks

HAYWARDS HEATH
MAP 05 TQ32

Haywards Heath High Beech Ln RH16 1SL
☎ 01444 414457 📠 01444 458319
e-mail: info@haywardsheathgolfclub.co.uk
web: www.haywardsheathgolfclub.co.uk
Pleasant undulating parkland course with easy walking. Several challenging Par 4s and 3s.
18 holes, 6216yds, Par 71, SSS 70, Course record 65.
Club membership 770.
Visitors Booking required Mon-Wed, Sat, Sun & BHs. Handicap certificate. Dress code. **Societies** Booking required. **Green Fees** £30 per 18 holes (£40 Sat, Sun & BHs). **Prof** Michael Henning **Course Designer** James Braid **Facilities** ⑪ ⑩ ⅃ ⊑ ⊡ ⅊ 🖢 🕏 ⌁ **Conf** Corporate Hospitality Days **Location** 1.25m N of Haywards Heath off B2028
Hotel ★★★ 75% HL Best Western The Birch Hotel, Lewes Rd, HAYWARDS HEATH ☎ 01444 451565 51 en suite

Paxhill Park East Mascalls Ln, Lindfield RH16 2QN
☎ 01444 484467 📠 01444 482709
e-mail: mail@paxhill.co.uk
web: www.paxhillpark.co.uk
An easy downland course in two loops of nine in an Area of Outstanding Natural Beauty. Water hazards on 5th, 13th and 14th holes.
18 holes, 5981yds, Par 70, SSS 69, Course record 67.
Club membership 320.
Visitors Mon-Sun & BHs. Booking required. Dress code. **Societies** Bernard Firkins **Green Fees** not confirmed. **Course Designer** P Tallack **Facilities** ⑪ ⑩ ⅃ ⊑ ⊡ ⅊ 🖢 🕏 ⌁ **Leisure** snooker. **Conf** facs Corporate Hospitality Days **Location** 2m NE of Haywards Heath, E of Lindfield off B2011
Hotel ★★★ 75% HL Best Western The Birch Hotel, Lewes Rd, HAYWARDS HEATH ☎ 01444 451565 51 en suite

HORSHAM
MAP 04 TQ13

See Slinfold

Horsham Worthing Rd RH13 7AX
☎ 01403 271525 📠 01403 274528
e-mail: golf@horshamgolfandfitness.co.uk
web: www.horshamgolfandfitness.co.uk
A short but challenging course, with six Par 4s and three Par 3s, two of which are played across water. Designed for beginners and intermediates but also challenges better players with a standard scratch of six below par.
9 holes, 4122yds, Par 33, SSS 30, Course record 55.
Club membership 280.
Visitors Mon-Sun & BHs. Dress code. **Societies** Welcome. **Green Fees** £11 for 18 holes, £8 for 9 holes (£13/£9 Sat & Sun). **Prof** Warren Pritchard **Facilities** ⑪ ⑩ ⅃ ⊑ ⊡ ⅊ 🖢 🕏 ⌁ **Leisure** solarium, gymnasium. **Conf** Corporate Hospitality Days **Location** A24 rdbt onto B2237, by garage **Hotel** ★★★★ CHH South Lodge Hotel, Brighton Rd, LOWER BEEDING ☎ 01403 891711 45 en suite

HURSTPIERPOINT
MAP 04 TQ21

Singing Hills Albourne BN6 9EB
☎ 01273 835353 📠 01273 835444
e-mail: info@singinghills.co.uk
web: www.singinghills.co.uk

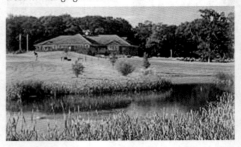

Lake: 9 holes, 3253yds, Par 35, SSS 35.
River: 9 holes, 2861yds, Par 34, SSS 34.
Valley: 9 holes, 3362yds, Par 36, SSS 34.
Course Designer M R M Sandow **Location** A23 onto B2117
Telephone for further details

LITTLEHAMPTON
MAP 04 TQ00

Littlehampton 170 Rope Walk, Riverside West BN17 5DL
☎ 01903 717170 📠 01903 726629
e-mail: lgc@talk21.com
web: www.littlehamptongolf.co.uk
A delightful seaside links in an equally delightful setting - and the only links course in the area.

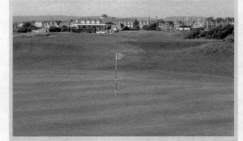

18 holes, 6226yds, Par 70, SSS 70, Course record 61.
Club membership 600.

Continued

Visitors Mon-Sun & BHs. Dress code. **Societies** Booking required.
Green Fees Phone. **Prof** Stuart Fallow **Course Designer** Hawtree
Facilities ⑪ ⑩ ㅑ ☐ ⌀ ⚐ ⤬ ⚑ ⌀ **Conf** facs Corporate Hospitality
Days **Location** 1m W off A259
Hotel BUD Travelodge Littlehampton Rustington, Worthing Rd,
RUSTINGTON ☎ 08700 850 950 36 en suite

LOWER BEEDING   MAP 04 TQ22

Mannings Heath Hotel Winterpit Ln RH13 6LY
☎ 01403 891191 🖹 01403 891499
e-mail: info@manningsheathhotel.com
web: www.manningsheathhotel.com
A nine-hole, 18-tee course with three Par 4s set in glorious countryside.
9 holes, 1529yds, Par 31. Club membership 150.
Visitors Mon-Thu, Sun & BHs. Dress code. **Societies** Welcome. **Green
Fees** £7.50 per 18 holes. **Prof** Terry Betts **Facilities** ⑪ ⑩ ㅑ ☐ ⚐ ⤬ ⚑
Leisure fishing. **Conf** facs Corporate Hospitality Days **Location** Off A281
S of Horsham
Hotel ★★★★ CHH South Lodge Hotel, Brighton Rd, LOWER BEEDING
☎ 01403 891711 45 en suite

MANNINGS HEATH   MAP 04 TQ22

Mannings Heath Fullers, Hammerpond Rd RH13 6PG
☎ 01403 210228 🖹 01403 270974
e-mail: enquiries@manningsheath.com
web: www.manningsheath.com
The Waterfall is a downhill, parkland, part heathland, championship
course with streams and trees in abundance. It has three spectacular
Par 3s but all the holes are memorably unique. The Kingfisher
course is a modern design with a lake which comes into play. It is
more open and forgiving but not to be underestimated.
*Waterfall: 18 holes, 6483yds, Par 72, SSS 71,
Course record 63.
Kingfisher: 18 holes, 6217yds, Par 70, SSS 70,
Course record 66. Club membership 700.*
Visitors Mon-Sun & BHs. Booking required Fri-Sun & BHs. Dress code.
Societies welcome. **Green Fees** not confirmed. **Prof** Neil Darnell
Course Designer David Williams **Facilities** ⑪ ⑩ ㅑ ☐ ⚐ ⤬ ⚑ ⚐ ⚑
⤬ ⚑ ⤬ **Leisure** hard tennis courts, fishing, sauna, chipping practice
area. **Conf** facs Corporate Hospitality Days **Location** Off A281 on N side
of village
Hotel ★★★★ CHH South Lodge Hotel, Brighton Rd, LOWER BEEDING
☎ 01403 891711 45 en suite

MIDHURST   MAP 04 SU82

Cowdray Park Petworth Rd GU29 0BB
☎ 01730 813599 🖹 01730 815900
e-mail: enquiries@cowdraygolf.co.uk
web: www.cowdraygolf.co.uk
Undulating parkland with scenic views of the surrounding countryside,
including Elizabethan ruins. The course is in a park designed by
'Capability' Brown in the 18th century.

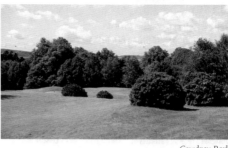

Cowdray Park

*18 holes, 6212yds, Par 70, SSS 70, Course record 65.
Club membership 720.*
Visitors Mon-Sun & BHs. Booking required. Handicap certificate. Dress
code. **Societies** Booking required. **Green Fees** £45 per 18 holes. **Prof**
Scott Brown **Course Designer** Jack White **Facilities** ⑪ ⑩ ㅑ ☐ ⚐ ⤬ ⚑
⚐ ⚑ ⤬ ⚑ ⤬ ⚑ **Conf** facs Corporate Hospitality Days **Location** 1m E of
Midhurst on A272
Hotel ★★★ 80% HL Spread Eagle Hotel and Spa, South St, MIDHURST
☎ 01730 816911 35 en suite 4 annexe en suite

PULBOROUGH   MAP 04 TQ01

West Sussex Golf Club Ln, Wiggonholt RH20 2EN
☎ 01798 872563 🖹 01798 872033
e-mail: secretary@westsussexgolf.co.uk
web: www.westsussexgolf.co.uk
An outstanding beautiful heathland course occupying an oasis of
sand, heather and pine in the middle of attractive countryside,
which is predominately clay and marsh. The 6th and 13th holes are
particularly notable.
*18 holes, 6264yds, Par 68, SSS 70, Course record 61.
Club membership 850.*
Visitors Mon, Wed, Thu. Tue pm only. Sat & Sun by arrangement.
Booking required. Handicap certificate. Dress code. **Societies** Booking
required. **Green Fees** £75 per day (£80 Sat & Sun). **Prof** Tim Packham
Course Designer Campbell/Hutcheson/Hotchkin **Facilities** ⑪ ㅑ ☐ ⚐ ⤬
⚐ ⚑ ⤬ ⚑ ⤬ ⚑ **Location** 1.5m E of Pulborough off A283
Hotel ★★★ 75% HL Best Western Roundabout Hotel, Monkmead Ln,
WEST CHILTINGTON ☎ 01798 813838 23 en suite

PYECOMBE   MAP 04 TQ21

Pyecombe Clayton Hill BN45 7FF
☎ 01273 845372 🖹 01273 843338
e-mail: info@pyecombegolfclub.com
web: www.pyecombegolfclub.com
Typical downland course on the inland side of the South Downs with
panoramic views of the Weald.
*18 holes, 6278yds, Par 71, SSS 70, Course record 65.
Club membership 525.*
Visitors Mon-Sun & BHs. Dress code. **Societies** booking required.
Green Fees not confirmed. **Prof** C R White **Course Designer** James Braid
Facilities ⑪ by prior arrangement ⑩ by prior arrangement ㅑ ☐ ⚐ ⤬ ⚐
⚑ ⤬ ⚑ **Location** E of village on A273
Hotel ★★★ 68% HL The Courtlands, 15-27 The Drive, HOVE
☎ 01273 731055 60 en suite 7 annexe en suite

SELSEY
MAP 04 SZ89

Selsey Golf Links Ln PO20 9DR
☎ 01243 608935 📠 01243 607101
e-mail: secretary@selseygolfclub.co.uk
web: www.selseygolfclub.co.uk
Fairly difficult links type seaside course, exposed to wind and has
natural ditches.
9 holes, 5834yds, Par 68, SSS 68, Course record 64.
Club membership 360.
Visitors Mon-Sun & BHs. Booking required Mon, Wed, Sat & Sun. **Societies**
Booking required. **Green Fees** Phone. **Prof** Peter Grindley **Course**
Designer J H Taylor **Facilities** ⊕ ⚑ ⛳ ▣ 🛢 🏌 ▲ 🎯 🏌 **Leisure** hard
tennis courts. **Location** 1m N off B2145

SLINFOLD
MAP 04 TQ13

Slinfold Park Golf & Country Club Stane St RH13 7RE
☎ 01403 791555 📠 01403 791465
e-mail: info@slinfoldpark.co.uk
web: www.slinfoldpark.co.uk

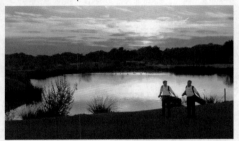

Championship Course: 18 holes, 6407yds, Par 72, SSS 71,
Course record 64.
Academy Course: 9 holes, 1315yds, Par 28.
Course Designer John Fortune **Location** 4m W on A29
Telephone for further details
Hotel ★★ 68% HL Hurtwood Inn Hotel, Walking Bottom, PEASLAKE
☎ 01306 730851 15 en suite 6 annexe en suite

WEST CHILTINGTON
MAP 04 TQ01

West Chiltington Broadford Bridge Rd RH20 2YA
☎ 01798 812115 (bookings) & 813574 📠 01798 812631
e-mail: richard@westchiltgolf.co.uk
web: www.westchiltgolf.co.uk
Set in an area of outstanding natural beauty with panoramic views
of the Sussex Downs. The Main Course has well-drained greens and,
although quite short, is in places extremely tight. Three large double
greens provide an interesting feature to this course. Also a 9-hole short
course.
Windmill: 18 holes, 5866yds, Par 70, SSS 69,
Course record 66. 9 holes, 1360yds, Par 28.
Club membership 500.
Visitors Mon-Sun & BHs. Booking required. Dress code. **Societies** Booking
required **Green Fees** 18 hole course: £25 per round, £15 twilight (£30 per
round Sat & Sun) 9 hole course: £7.50. **Prof** Lorraine Cousins **Course**
Designer Brian Barnes **Facilities** ⊕ ⚑ ⛳ ▣ 🛢 🏌 ▲ 🎯 🏌 🍴 🏌 **Conf**
facs Corporate Hospitality Days **Location** N of village
Hotel ★★★ 75% HL Best Western Roundabout Hotel, Monkmead Ln,
WEST CHILTINGTON ☎ 01798 813838 23 en suite

WORTHING
MAP 04 TQ10

Hill Barn Hill Barn Ln BN14 9QF
☎ 01903 237301 📠 01903 217613
e-mail: info@hillbarngolf.com
web: www.hillbarngolf.com
Downland course with views of both Isle of Wight and Brighton.
18 holes, 6224yds, Par 70, SSS 70, Course record 64.
Club membership 500.
Visitors Mon-Sun & BHs. Booking required. Dress code. **Societies**
Booking required. **Green Fees** £17.50 per 18 holes (weekends £21.50).
Prof Tony Westwood **Course Designer** Fred Hawtree **Facilities** ⊕ 🍴
by prior arrangement ⚑ ▣ 🛢 🏌 ▲ 🎯 🏌 **Leisure** croquet. **Conf**
facs Corporate Hospitality Days **Location** Signposted from Grove Lodge
roundabout by Norwich Union on A27
Hotel ★★★ 67% HL Findon Manor Hotel, High St, Findon, WORTHING
☎ 01903 872733 11 en suite

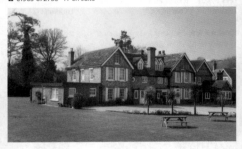

Worthing Links Rd BN14 9QZ
☎ 01903 260801 📠 01903 694664
e-mail: enquiries@worthinggolf.com
web: www.worthinggolf.co.uk
The Upper Course, short and tricky with entrancing views, will
provide good entertainment. Lower Course is considered to be one
of the best downland courses in the country.
Lower Course: 18 holes, 6505yds, Par 71, SSS 71,
Course record 62.
Upper Course: 18 holes, 5211yds, Par 66, SSS 65.
Club membership 1200.
Visitors Mon, Thu & Fri. Booking required. Handicap certificate. Dress
code. **Societies** Booking required. **Green Fees** Phone. 🅿 **Prof** Stephen
Rolley **Course Designer** H S Colt **Facilities** ⊕ ⚑ ▣ 🛢 🏌 ▲ 🎯 🏌 🍴
🏌 **Location** N of town centre off A27
Hotel ★★★ 77% HL Ardington Hotel, Steyne Gardens, WORTHING
☎ 01903 230451 45 en suite

TYNE & WEAR

BACKWORTH
MAP 12 NZ37

Backworth The Hall NE27 0AH
☎ 0191 268 1048
9 holes, 5930yds, Par 71, SSS 69, Course record 63.
Location W of town on B1322
Telephone for further details
Hotel BUD Premier Travel Inn Newcastle (Holystone), Holystone
Roundabout, NEWCASTLE ☎ 08701 977189 40 en suite

England

BIRTLEY
MAP 12 NZ25

Birtley Birtley Ln DH3 2LR
☎ 0191 410 2207
e-mail: birtleygolfclub@aol.com
web: www.birtleyportobellogolfclub.co.uk
A nine-hole parkland course. Good test of golf with challenging Par 3 and Par 4 holes.
9 holes, 5729yds, Par 67, SSS 67, Course record 63.
Club membership 350.
Visitors Mon-Fri except BHs. Dress code. **Societies** Booking required.
Green Fees £15 per 18 holes. ⊛ **Facilities** by prior arrangement ⏛ ⩘
Conf Corporate Hospitality Days
Hotel BUD Travelodge Washington A1 North bound, Motorway Service Area, Portobello, BIRTLEY ☎ 08700 850 950 31 en suite

BOLDON
MAP 12 NZ36

Boldon Dipe Ln, East Boldon NE36 0PQ
☎ 0191 536 5360 & 0191 536 4182 📄 0191 537 2270
e-mail: info@boldongolfclub.co.uk
web: www.boldongolfclub.co.uk
Parkland links course, easy walking, distant sea views.
18 holes, 6362yds, Par 72, SSS 70, Course record 67.
Club membership 700.
Visitors Mon-Sun & BHs. Booking required. Dress code. **Societies** Booking required. **Green Fees** £20 per day (£23 Sat, Sun & BHs). ⊛ **Prof** S Richardson **Course Designer** Harry Varden **Facilities** ⏀ ⍾⃝ ⍳ ⏛ ⊀⍭
⩘ ⎐⍧ ⍧ ⛿ ⍧ 🏴 **Leisure** snooker. **Conf** Corporate Hospitality Days
Location S of village off A184
Hotel ★★★ 74% HL Quality Hotel Sunderland, Witney Way, Boldon, SUNDERLAND ☎ 0191 519 1999 82 en suite

CHOPWELL
MAP 12 NZ15

Garesfield NE17 7AP
☎ 01207 561309 📄 01207 561309
e-mail: office@garesfieldgc.fsnet.co.uk
web: www.garesfieldgolf.com
18 holes, 6458yds, Par 72, SSS 70, Course record 68.
Course Designer Harry Fernie **Location** Off B6315 in High Spen at Bute Arms for Chopwell
Telephone for further details
Hotel ★★★ 68% HL Quality Hotel Newcastle upon Tyne, Newgate St, NEWCASTLE UPON TYNE ☎ 0191 232 5025 93 en suite

FELLING
MAP 12 NZ26

Heworth Gingling Gate, Heworth NE10 8XY
☎ 0191 469 4424 📄 0191 469 9898
18 holes, 6422yds, Par 71, SSS 71.
Location On A195, 0.5m NW of junc with A1(M)
Telephone for further details
Hotel BUD Travelodge Newcastle Whitemare Pool, Wardley, Whitemare Pool, WARDLEY ☎ 08700 850 950 71 en suite

GATESHEAD
MAP 12 NZ26

Ravensworth Angel View, Longbank, Wrekenton NE9 7NE
☎ 0191 487 6014 📄 0191 487 6014
e-mail: ravensworth.golfclub@virgin.net
web: www.ravensworthgolfclub.co.uk
18 holes, 5966yds, Par 69, SSS 69.
Course Designer J W Fraser **Location** leave A1(M) at Junction for A167 (Angel of the North) take A1295 for 300 yds
Telephone for further details
Hotel ★★★ 77% HL Eslington Villa Hotel, 8 Station Rd, Low Fell, GATESHEAD ☎ 0191 487 6017 & 420 0666 📄 0191 420 0667 17 en suite

GOSFORTH
MAP 12 NZ26

Gosforth Broadway East NE3 5ER
☎ 0191 285 3495 & 285 6710(catering) 📄 0191 284 6274
e-mail: gosforth.golf@virgin.net
web: www.gosforthgolfclub.co.uk
Easy walking parkland with natural water hazards.
18 holes, 6024yds, Par 69, SSS 68, Course record 62.
Club membership 500.
Visitors Mon-Sun & BHs. Dress code. **Societies** Booking required. **Green Fees** £30 per day, £25 per round (£32/£28 Sat & Sun). **Prof** G Garland
Facilities ⏀ ⍾⃝ ⍳ ⏛ ⊀⍭ ⩘ ⍧ ⛿ ⍧ **Conf** Corporate Hospitality Days
Location N of town centre off A6125
Hotel ★★★★ 76% HL Newcastle Marriott Hotel Gosforth Park, High Gosforth Park, Gosforth, NEWCASTLE UPON TYNE ☎ 0191 236 4111 178 en suite

Parklands Gosforth Park Golfing Complex, High Gosforth Park NE3 5HQ
☎ 0191 236 4480 📄 0191 236 3322
18 holes, 6013yds, Par 71, SSS 69, Course record 66.
Location 3m N at end A1 western bypass
Telephone for further details
Hotel ★★★★ 76% HL Newcastle Marriott Hotel Gosforth Park, High Gosforth Park, Gosforth, NEWCASTLE UPON TYNE ☎ 0191 236 4111 178 en suite

HOUGHTON-LE-SPRING
MAP 12 NZ34

Elemore Elemore Ln, Hetton-le-Hole DH5 0QB
☎ 0191 517 3061 📄 0191 517 3054
18 holes, 5947yds, Par 69, SSS 68.
Course Designer J Gaunt **Location** 4m S of Houghton-le-Spring on A182
Telephone for further details
Hotel ★★ 71% HL Chilton Country Pub & Hotel, Black Boy Rd, Chilton Moor, Fencehouses, HOUGHTON-LE-SPRING ☎ 0191 385 2694 25 en suite

Houghton-le-Spring Copt Hill DH5 8LU
☎ 0191 584 1198 & 584 7421 📄 0191 584 7421
e-mail: houghton.golf@ntlworld.com
web: www.houghtongolfclub.co.uk
Hilly, downland course with natural slope hazards and excellent greens.
18 holes, 6381yds, Par 72, SSS 71, Course record 64.
Club membership 680.
Visitors Mon-Sat & BHs, Sun after 3pm. Booking required. Dress code.
Societies booking required. **Green Fees** not confirmed. **Prof** Kevin Gow
Facilities ⏀ ⍾⃝ ⍳ ⏛ ⊀⍭ ⩘ ⍧ ⛿ ⍧ **Location** 0.5m E on B1404
Hotel ★★ 71% HL Chilton Country Pub & Hotel, Black Boy Rd, Chilton Moor, Fencehouses, HOUGHTON-LE-SPRING ☎ 0191 385 2694 25 en suite

England

NEWCASTLE UPON TYNE · MAP 12 NZ26

City of Newcastle Three Mile Bridge NE3 2DR
☎ 0191 285 1775 🗎 0191 284 0700
e-mail: info@cityofnewcastlegolfclub.com
web: www.cityofnewcastlegolfclub.com
A well-manicured parkland course in the Newcastle suburbs.
18 holes, 6528yds, Par 72, SSS 71, Course record 64.
Club membership 600.
Visitors Mon-Sun & BHs. Dress code. **Societies** Booking required. **Green
Fees** £34 per day; £28 per round (£25 per round Sun). ☻ **Prof** Steve
McKenna **Course Designer** Harry Vardon **Facilities** ⑪ 🍴 ⊾ ⤳ ☇ ☖ ⚑ ☄
⚑ ☄ **Conf** Corporate Hospitality Days **Location** 3m N on B1318
Hotel ★★★ 72% HL The Caledonian Hotel, Newcastle, 64 Osborne Rd,
Jesmond, NEWCASTLE UPON TYNE ☎ 0191 281 7881 89 en suite

Newcastle United Ponteland Rd, Cowgate NE5 3JW
☎ 0191 286 9998
e-mail: info@www.nugc.co.uk
web: www.nugc.co.uk
18 holes, 6617yds, Par 72, SSS 72, Course record 66.
Course Designer Various **Location** 1.25m NW of city centre off A6127
Telephone for further details
Hotel ★★★ 72% HL The Caledonian Hotel, Newcastle, 64 Osborne Rd,
Jesmond, NEWCASTLE UPON TYNE ☎ 0191 281 7881 89 en suite

Northumberland High Gosforth Park NE3 5HT
☎ 0191 236 2498 🗎 0191 236 2036
e-mail: sec@thengc.co.uk
Predominatly a level heathland style course, the firm, fast greens are
a particular feature.
18 holes, 6683yds, Par 72, SSS 72, Course record 65.
Club membership 580.
Visitors Mon-Sun & BHs. Booking required Sat/Sun & BHs. Handicap
certificate. Dress code. **Societies** booking required. **Green Fees** not
confirmed. ☻ **Course Designer** Colt/Braid **Facilities** ⑪ 🍴 ⊾ ⤳ ☇
⚑ ☄ **Conf** Corporate Hospitality Days **Location** 4m N of city centre
off A1
Hotel ★★★★ 76% HL Newcastle Marriott Hotel Gosforth Park, High
Gosforth Park, Gosforth, NEWCASTLE UPON TYNE ☎ 0191 236 4111
178 en suite

Westerhope Whorlton Grance, Westerhope NE5 1PP
☎ 0191 286 7636 🗎 0191 2146287
e-mail: wgc@btconnect.com
Attractive, easy walking parkland with tree-lined fairways. Good open
views towards the airport.
18 holes, 6444yds, Par 72, SSS 71, Course record 64.
Club membership 778.
Visitors Mon-Fri except BHs. Booking required. Handicap certificate. Dress
code. **Societies** Welcome, **Green Fees** £26 per round. **Prof** Michael Nesbit
Facilities ⑪ 🍴 ⊾ ⤳ ☇ ⚑ ☖ ⚑ ☄ **Location** 4.5m NW of city centre
off B6324
Hotel ★★★★ 76% HL Newcastle Marriott Hotel Gosforth Park, High
Gosforth Park, Gosforth, NEWCASTLE UPON TYNE ☎ 0191 236 4111
178 en suite

RYTON · MAP 12 NZ16

Ryton Clara Vale NE40 3TD
☎ 0191 413 3253 🗎 0191 413 1642
e-mail: secretary@rytongolfclub.co.uk
web: www.rytongolf.org
Parkland course.
18 holes, 6014yds, Par 70, SSS 69, Course record 67.
Club membership 600.
Visitors Mon-Fri & BHs. Booking required Tue, Wed & BHs. Handicap
certificate. Dress code. **Societies** Booking required. **Green Fees** £26 per
day; £20 per round. ☻ **Facilities** ⑪ 🍴 ⊾ ⤳ ☇ ⚑ **Conf** Corporate
Hospitality Days **Location** NW of town centre off A695
Hotel ★★★ 70% HL Gibside Hotel, Front St, WHICKHAM
☎ 0191 488 9292 45 en suite

Tyneside Westfield Ln NE40 3QE
☎ 0191 413 2742 🗎 0191 413 0199
web: www.tynesidegolfclub.co.uk
Open, part hilly parkland course with a water hazard.
18 holes, 6009yds, Par 70, SSS 69, Course record 65.
Club membership 641.
Visitors Mon-Fri, Sun & BHs. Handicap certificate. Dress code. **Societies**
Booking required. **Green Fees** £35 per day, £25 per round. **Prof** Geoff
Dixon **Course Designer** H S Colt **Facilities** ⑪ 🍴 ⊾ ⤳ ☇ ⚑ ☖ ☄ ☄ ☄
☄ **Conf** Corporate Hospitality Days **Location** NW of town centre off A695
Hotel ★★★ 70% HL Gibside Hotel, Front St, WHICKHAM
☎ 0191 488 9292 45 en suite

SOUTH SHIELDS · MAP 12 NZ36

South Shields Cleadon Hills NE34 8EG
☎ 0191 456 8942 🗎 0191 456 8942
e-mail: thesecretary@south-shields-golf.freeserve.co.uk
web: www.ssgc.co.uk
A slightly undulating downland course on a limestone base ensuring
good conditions underfoot. Open to strong winds, the course is testing
but fair. There are fine views of the coastline.
18 holes, 6174yds, Par 71, SSS 70, Course record 64.
Club membership 700.
Visitors Mon-Sun & BHs. Booking required except Thu. Handicap certificate.
Dress code. **Societies** Welcome. **Green Fees** £32-40 per day; £22-28 per
round. ☻ **Prof** Glyn Jones **Course Designer** McKenzie-Braid **Facilities** ⑪
🍴 ⊾ ⤳ ☇ ⚑ ☄ **Conf** facs Corporate Hospitality Days **Location** SE
of town centre off A1300
Hotel ★★★ 71% HL Best Western Sea Hotel, Sea Rd, SOUTH SHIELDS
☎ 0191 427 0999 32 en suite 5 annexe en suite

Whitburn Lizard Ln NE34 7AF
☎ 0191 529 4944 (Sec) 🗎 0191 529 4944
e-mail: wgsec@ukonline.co.uk
web: golf-whitburn.co.uk
Parkland with sea views. Situated on limestone making it rarely
unplayable.
18 holes, 5899yds, Par 70, SSS 68, Course record 67.
Club membership 700.
Visitors Mon-Fri except BHs. Booking required Sat & BHs. Handicap
certificate. Dress code. **Societies** Booking required. **Green Fees** £22 (£27
Sat & Sun). **Prof** Neil Whinham **Course Designer** Colt, Alison & Morrison
Facilities ⑪ 🍴 ⊾ ⤳ ☇ ⚑ ☖ ☄ ⚑ ☄ **Conf** Corporate Hospitality Days
Location 2.5m SE off A183
Hotel ★★★★ 75% HL Sunderland Marriott Hotel, Queen's Pde, Seaburn,
SUNDERLAND ☎ 0191 529 2041 82 en suite

SUNDERLAND   MAP 12 NZ35

Wearside Coxgreen SR4 9JT
☎ 0191 534 2518 🖩 0191 534 6186
web: wearsidegolfclub.com
Open, undulating parkland rolling down to the River Wear beneath
the shadow of the famous Penshaw Monument. Built on the lines of
a Greek temple it is a well-known landmark. Two ravines cross the
course presenting a variety of challenging holes.
18 holes, 6373yds, Par 71, SSS 74, Course record 63.
Club membership 648.
Visitors Contact club for details. **Societies** Welcome. **Green Fees**
Phone. **Prof** Doug Brolls **Facilities** ⓘ ⓞ 🛒 🖳 🎯 👕 ⚒ 🏌 **Conf**
Corporate Hospitality Days **Location** 3.5m W off A183
Hotel ★★★★ 75% HL Sunderland Marriott Hotel, Queen's Pde,
Seaburn, SUNDERLAND ☎ 0191 529 2041   82 en suite

TYNEMOUTH   MAP 12 NZ36

Tynemouth Spital Dene NE30 2ER
☎ 0191 257 4578 🖩 0191 259 5193
e-mail: secretary@tynemouthgolfclub.com
web: www.tynemouthgolfclub.com
Well-drained parkland course, not physically demanding but providing
a strong challenge to both low and high handicap players.
18 holes, 6359yds, Par 70, SSS 70, Course record 66.
Club membership 850.
Visitors Mon, Wed-Fri except BHs. Tue pm only. Dress code. **Societies**
Welcome. **Green Fees** £22.50 per 18 holes; £25 per day. **Prof** J P McKenna
Course Designer Willie Park **Facilities** ⓘ ⓞ 🛒 🖳 🎯 👕 ⚒ 🏌
Location 0.5m W
Hotel ★★★ 77% HL Grand Hotel, Grand Pde, TYNEMOUTH
☎ 0191 293 6666   40 en suite   4 annexe en suite

WALLSEND   MAP 12 NZ26

Wallsend Rheydt Av, Bigges Main NE28 8SU
☎ 0191 262 1973
Parkland course.
18 holes, 6031yds, Par 70, SSS 69, Course record 64.
Club membership 655.
Visitors Mon-Sun & BHs. **Societies** Booking required. **Green Fees** £20.40
per round (£24 Sat, Sun & BHs). **Prof** Ken Phillips **Course Designer**
A Snowball **Facilities** 🛒 🖳 🎯 ⚒ 🏌 **Location** NW of town centre
off A193
Hotel ★★★ 72% HL The Caledonian Hotel, Newcastle, 64 Osborne Rd,
Jesmond, NEWCASTLE UPON TYNE ☎ 0191 281 7881   89 en suite

WASHINGTON   MAP 12 NZ25

George Washington Golf & Country Club Stone
Cellar Rd, High Usworth NE37 1PH
☎ 0191 417 8346 🖩 0191 415 1166
e-mail: reservations@georgewashington.co.uk
web: www.georgewashington.co.uk
The course is set in 150 acres of rolling parkland. Wide generous
fairways and large greens. Trees feature on most holes, penalising the
wayward shot.

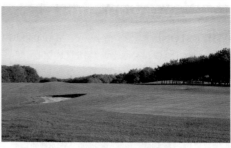

George Washington Golf & Country Club
18 holes, 6604yds, Par 73, SSS 71, Course record 68.
Club membership 550.
Visitors Mon-Sun & BHs. Booking required. Dress code. **Societies** book
in advance. **Green Fees** not confirmed. **Prof** Graeme Robinson **Course
Designer** Eric Watson **Facilities** ⓘ ⓞ 🛒 🖳 🎯 👕 ⚒ 🏌 🎯 ⚒ 🏌
Leisure heated indoor swimming pool, sauna, solarium, gymnasium, 9 hole
Par 3 course, hair & beauty salon. **Conf** facs Corporate Hospitality Days
Location From A195 signed Washington North take last exit on rdbt, then
right at mini-rdbt
Hotel ★★★ 74% HL George Washington Golf & Country Club, Stone
Cellar Rd, High Usworth, WASHINGTON ☎ 0191 402 9988   103 en suite

WHICKHAM   MAP 12 NZ26

Whickham Hollinside Park, Fellside Rd NE16 5BA
☎ 0191 488 1576 🖩 0191 488 1577
e-mail: enquiries@whickhamgolfclub.co.uk
web: www.whickhamgolfclub.co.uk
Undulating parkland in the beautiful Derwent valley. Its undulating
fairways and subtly contoured greens create an interesting challenge
for players of all abilities.
18 holes, 6542yds, Par 71, SSS 71. Club membership 680.
Visitors Mon-Fri, Sun & BHs. Handicap certificate. Dress code. **Societies**
Booking required. **Green Fees** £25 (£30 Sun & BHs). **Prof** Simon
Williamson **Facilities** ⓘ ⓞ 🛒 🖳 🎯 👕 ⚒ 🏌 **Conf** Corporate
Hospitality Days **Location** exit A1 for Whickham. Club is 1m from junct off
Front St signed Burnopfield
Hotel ★★★ 70% HL Gibside Hotel, Front St, WHICKHAM
☎ 0191 488 9292   45 en suite

WHITLEY BAY   MAP 12 NZ37

Whitley Bay Claremont Rd NE26 3UF
☎ 0191 252 0180 🖩 0191 297 0030
e-mail: secretary@whitleybaygolfclub.co.uk
web: www.whitleybaygolfclub.co.uk
An 18-hole links type course, close to the sea, with a stream running
through the undulating terrain.
18 holes, 6579yds, Par 71, SSS 71, Course record 66.
Club membership 800.
Visitors Mon, Wed-Fri, Sun &BHs. Booking required. Dress code. **Societies**
Booking required. **Green Fees** £40 per day; £30 per round. **Prof** Gary
Shipley **Facilities** ⓘ ⓞ 🛒 🖳 🎯 👕 ⚒ 🏌 **Location** NW of town
centre off A1148
Hotel ★★★ 71% HL Windsor Hotel, South Pde, WHITLEY BAY ☎ 0191 251
8888 0191 232 3158 🖩 0191 297 0272   69 en suite

WARWICKSHIRE

ATHERSTONE
MAP 04 SP39

Atherstone The Outwoods, Coleshill Rd CV9 2RL
☎ 01827 713110 📠 01827 715686
Scenic parkland course, established in 1894 and laid out on hilly ground. Interesting challenge on every hole.
18 holes, 6006yds, Par 72, SSS 70, Course record 68.
Club membership 450.
Visitors Mon-Fri except BHs. Dress code. **Societies** Welcome. **Green Fees** £30 per day. ⊛ **Course Designer** Hawtree & Gaunt Mornoch **Facilities** ⊕ ⍾ ⌷ ≜ ⊕ ⬥ ⩘ ⚲ **Conf** Corporate Hospitality Days **Location** 0.5m S, A5 onto B4116
Hotel BUD Travelodge Tamworth (M42), Green L, TAMWORTH
☎ 08700 850 950 & 0800 850950 📠 01827 260145 62 en suite

BIDFORD-ON-AVON
MAP 04 SP15

Bidford Grange Stratford Rd B50 4LY
☎ 01789 490319 📠 01789 490998
web: www.golfinghotel.com
18 holes, 7233yds, Par 72, SSS 74, Course record 66.
Location E of village off B439
Telephone for further details

BRANDON
MAP 04 SP47

City of Coventry-Brandon Wood Brandon Ln, Wolston CV8 3GQ
☎ 024 7654 3141 📠 024 7654 5108
18 holes, 6610yds, Par 72, SSS 71, Course record 68.
Location Off A45 S
Telephone for further details
Hotel ★★★★ 72% HL Mercure Brandon Hall Hotel & Spa, Main St, BRANDON ☎ 0870 400 8105 60 en suite 60 annexe en suite

COLESHILL
MAP 04 SP28

Maxstoke Park Castle Ln B46 2RD
☎ 01675 466743 📠 01675 466185
e-mail: maxstokepark@btinternet.com
Parkland with easy walking. Numerous trees and a lake form natural hazards.
18 holes, 6442yds, Par 71, SSS 71, Course record 64.
Club membership 720.
Visitors Mon-Fr except BHs. Booking required Tue & Thu. Handicap certificate. Dress code. **Societies** booking required. **Green Fees** not confirmed. ⊛ **Prof** Neil McEwan **Course Designer** various **Facilities** ⊕ ⍾ ⌷ ≜ ⊕ ⬥ ⩘ ⚲ **Conf** Corporate Hospitality Days **Location** 3m E of Coleshill, off B4114 for Maxstoke
Hotel ★★★ 71% HL Grimstock Country House Hotel, Gilson Rd, Gilson, COLESHILL ☎ 01675 462121 & 462161 📠 01675 467646 44 en suite

HENLEY-IN-ARDEN
MAP 04 SP16

Henley Golf & Country Club Birmingham Rd B95 5QA
☎ 01564 793715 📠 01564 795754
e-mail: enquiries@henleygcc.co.uk
web: www.henleygcc.co.uk
Attractive course in peaceful rural location which can be played off 4 different tee positions allowing golfers to play the course at varying length to suit different playing and physical abilities.
18 holes, 6933yds, Par 73, SSS 73. Club membership 500.
Visitors Mon-Sun & BHs. Booking required. Dress code. **Societies** welcome. **Green Fees** not confirmed. **Prof** Neale Hyde **Course Designer** N Selwyn Smith **Facilities** ⊕ ⍾ ⌷ ≜ ⊕ ⬥ ⩘ ⚲ 𝄐 **Leisure** hard tennis courts, 9 hole Par 3 course, beauty salon. **Conf** facs Corporate Hospitality Days **Location** On A3400 just N of Henley-in-Arden
Hotel ★★★ 66% HL Quality Hotel Redditch, Pool Bank, Southcrest, REDDITCH ☎ 01527 541511 73 en suite

KENILWORTH
MAP 04 SP27

Kenilworth Crewe Ln CV8 2EA
☎ 01926 858517 📠 01926 864453
e-mail: secretary@kenilworthgolfclub.co.uk
web: www.kenilworthgolfclub.co.uk
Parkland course in an open hilly location. Club founded in 1889.
18 holes, 6400yds, Par 72, SSS 71, Course record 66.
Club membership 755.
Visitors Mon-Sun & BHs. Booking required Wed. Dress code. **Societies** Booking required. **Green Fees** £35 per day (£45 Sat & Sun). **Prof** Steve Yates **Course Designer** Hawtree **Facilities** ⊕ ⍾ ⌷ ≜ ⊕ ⬥ ⩘ ⚲ **Leisure** Par 3 chipping green. **Conf** facs Corporate Hospitality Days **Location** 0.5m NE
Hotel ★★★★ 71% HL Chesford Grange Hotel, Chesford Bridge, KENILWORTH ☎ 01926 859331 209 en suite

LEA MARSTON
MAP 04 SP29

Lea Marston Hotel & Leisure Complex Haunch Ln B76 0BY
☎ 01675 470468 📠 01675 470871
e-mail: info@leamarstonhotel.co.uk
web: www.leamarstonhotel.co.uk
The Marston Lakes course was opened in April 2001. The layout includes many water and sand hazards through undulating parkland. While short by modern standards, it is a good test for even low handicap players, requiring virtually everything in the bag. Tees and greens have been built to championship course specifications.

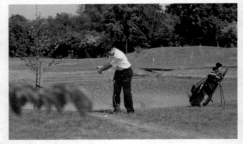

Marston Lakes: 9 holes, 2054yds, Par 31, SSS 30.
Club membership 330. *Continued*

Visitors Mon-Sun & BHs. Booking required. Dress code. **Societies** booking required. **Green Fees** not confirmed. **Prof** Darren Lewis **Course Designer** Contour Golf **Facilities** ⊕ ⑩ ⌕ ⌾ ♫ ☐ ⚲ ☎ ⚑ ♦ ✔ ⛟ ⛳
Leisure hard tennis courts, heated indoor swimming pool, sauna, solarium, gymnasium, golf simulator. **Conf** facs Corporate Hospitality Days **Location** M42 junct 9, A4097 towards Kingsbury, 1m right
Hotel ★★★ 75% HL BW Lea Marston Hotel & Leisure Complex, Haunch Ln, LEA MARSTON ☎ 01675 470468 80 en suite

LEAMINGTON SPA — MAP 04 SP36

Leamington & County Golf Ln, Whitnash CV31 2QA
☎ 01926 425961 🖶 01926 425961
e-mail: secretary@leamingtongolf.co.uk
web: www.leamingtongolf.co.uk
Undulating parkland with extensive views.
18 holes, 6418yds, Par 72, SSS 71, Course record 65.
Club membership 854.
Visitors Mon-Sun & BHs. Handicap certificate. Dress code. **Societies** booking required. **Green Fees** not confirmed. **Prof** Julian Mellor **Course Designer** H S Colt **Facilities** ⊕ ⑩ ⌕ ⌾ ♫ ☐ ⚲ ☎ ✔ ✔ **Leisure** snooker. **Conf** Corporate Hospitality Days **Location** S of town centre
Hotel ★★★ 70% HL Courtyard by Marriott Leamington Spa, Olympus Av, Tachbrook Park, ROYAL LEAMINGTON SPA ☎ 01926 425522 91 en suite

Newbold Comyn Newbold Ter East CV32 4EW
☎ 01926 421157
e-mail: colin@newcomyngc-70.wanadoo.co.uk
Municipal parkland course with a hilly front nine. The Par 4 9th is a 467yd testing hole. The back nine is rather flat but include two Par 5s. Presently undergoing extensive upgrade.
18 holes, 6315yds, Par 70, SSS 70, Course record 69.
Club membership 280.
Visitors Mon-Sun & BHs. Booking required. **Societies** welcome. **Green Fees** not confirmed. **Facilities** ⊕ ⑩ ⌕ ⌾ ♫ ☐ ⚲ ☎ ✔ **Leisure** heated indoor swimming pool, gymnasium. **Location** 0.75m E of town centre off B4099
Hotel ★★★ 67% HL Episode - Leamington, 64 Upper Holly Walk, LEAMINGTON SPA ☎ 01926 883777 32 en suite

LEEK WOOTTON — MAP 04 SP26

The Warwickshire CV35 7QT
☎ 01926 409409 🖶 01926 408409
e-mail: ptaylor@theclubcompany.com
web: www.theclubcompany.com
Two courses, the Kings which is an American style course with lots of water and the Earls, which is mainly a woodland course.
Kings: 18 holes, 7000yds, Par 72, SSS 72, Course record 68.
Earls: 18 holes, 7421yds, Par 74, SSS 73, Course record 70.
Club membership 1500.
Visitors Mon-Sun & BHs. Booking required. Handicap certificate. Dress code. **Societies** booking required. **Green Fees** not confirmed. **Prof** Mark Dulson **Course Designer** Karl Litten **Facilities** ⊕ ⑩ ⌕ ⌾ ♫ ☐ ⚲ ☎ ⚑ ✔ ⛟ **Leisure** heated indoor swimming pool, sauna, solarium, gymnasium, health club. **Conf** facs Corporate Hospitality Days **Location** S of village off A46
Hotel ★★★★ 71% HL Chesford Grange Hotel, Chesford Bridge, KENILWORTH ☎ 01926 859331 209 en suite

LOWER BRAILES — MAP 04 SP33

Brailes Sutton Ln, Lower Brailes OX15 5BB
☎ 01608 685633 🖶 01608 685205
e-mail: office@brailesgolfclub.co.uk
web: www.brailesgolfclub.co.uk
Undulating meadowland on 105 acres of Cotswold countryside. Sutton Brook passes through the course and must be crossed five times. The Par 5 17th offers the most spectacular view of three counties from the tee. Challenging Par 3 short holes. Suitable for golfers of all standards.
18 holes, 6304yds, Par 71, SSS 70, Course record 67.
Club membership 600.
Visitors Mon-Sun & BHs. Booking required. Handicap certificate. Dress code. **Societies** Booking required **Green Fees** £40 per day, £25 per round, £35 Sat & Sun (Winter: £18/£25/£25). **Prof** Mark McGeehan **Course Designer** R Baldwin **Facilities** ⊕ ⑩ ⌕ ⌾ ♫ ☐ ⚲ ☎ ✔ ⛟ ⛳ **Conf** facs Corporate Hospitality Days **Location** S of Lower Brailes off B4035
Inn ★★★★ INN The Red Lion, Main St, Long Compton, SHIPSTON ON STOUR ☎ 01608 684221 5 en suite

NUNEATON — MAP 04 SP39

Nuneaton Golf Dr, Whitestone CV11 6QF
☎ 024 7634 7810 🖶 024 7632 7563
e-mail: nuneatongolfclub@btconnect.com
18 holes, 6429yds, Par 71, SSS 71.
Location 2m SE off B4114
Telephone for further details
Hotel ★★★ 72% HL Best Western Weston Hall Hotel, Weston Ln, Bulkington, NUNEATON ☎ 024 7631 2989 40 en suite

Oakridge Arley Ln, Ansley Village CV10 9PH
☎ 01676 541389 & 540542 🖶 01676 542709
e-mail: admin@oakridgegolf.fsnet.co.uk
web: www.oakridgegolf.fsnet.co.uk
The water hazards on the back nine add to the natural beauty of the countryside. The undulating course is affected by winter cross winds on several holes. Overall it will certainly test golfing skills.
18 holes, 6208yds, Par 71, SSS 71. Club membership 500.
Visitors Mon-Sun & BHs. Booking required. Dress code. **Societies** Booking required. **Green Fees** £18 per day. **Course Designer** Algy Jayes **Facilities** ⊕ ⑩ ⌕ ⌾ ♫ ☐ ⚲ ☎ ⚑ ✔ ⛟ **Conf** Corporate Hospitality Days **Location** 4m W
Hotel ★★★ 72% HL Best Western Weston Hall Hotel, Weston Ln, Bulkington, NUNEATON ☎ 024 7631 2989 40 en suite

Purley Chase Pipers Ln, Ridge Ln CV10 0RB
☎ 024 7639 3118 🖶 024 7639 8015
e-mail: enquiries@purley-chase.co.uk
web: www.purley-chase.co.uk
18 holes, 6772yds, Par 72, SSS 72, Course record 64.
Location 2m NW off B4114
Telephone for further details
Hotel ★★★ 72% HL Best Western Weston Hall Hotel, Weston Ln, Bulkington, NUNEATON ☎ 024 7631 2989 40 en suite

RUGBY MAP 04 SP57

Rugby Clifton Rd CV21 3RD
☎ 01788 542306 (Sec) & 575134 (Pro) 🖹 01788 542306
e-mail: rugbygolfclub@tiscali.co.uk
web: www.rugbygc.co.uk
A short parkland course across the undulating Clifton valley. Clifton brook runs through the lower level of the course and comes into play on seven holes. Accuracy is the prime requirement for a good score.
18 holes, 5457yds, Par 68, SSS 67, Course record 60.
Club membership 700.
Visitors Mon-Fri. Booking required. Handicap certificate. Dress code.
Societies Booking required. **Green Fees** £25 per day, £50 per week. ⊛
Prof David Quinn **Facilities** ⊕ ⏃ 🍴 🖢 ☐ 🏐 ⚐ 🏌 **Leisure** snooker room. **Conf** Corporate Hospitality Days **Location** 1m NE on B5414

Whitefields Hotel Golf & Country Club London Rd, Thurlaston CV23 9LF
☎ 01788 521800 🖹 01788 521695
e-mail: mail@draycotehotel.co.uk
web: www.draycotehotel.co.uk
Whitefields has superb natural drainage. There are many water features and the 13th has a stunning dog-leg 442yd Par 4 with a superb view across Draycote Water. The 16th is completely surrounded by water and is particularly difficult.

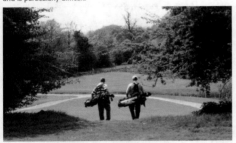

18 holes, 6289yds, Par 71, SSS 70, Course record 64.
Club membership 400.
Visitors contact course for details. **Societies** booking required. **Green Fees** not confirmed. **Course Designer** Reg Mason **Facilities** ⊕ ⏃ 🍴 🖢 ☐ 🏐 🖢 ⚐ 🏌 🏐 **Leisure** gymnasium. **Conf** facs Corporate Hospitality Days **Location** M45 junct 1, 0.5m on A45, on left. W of Dunchurch
Hotel ★★★ 74% HL The Golden Lion Hotel, Easenhall, RUGBY
☎ 01788 833577 & 832265 🖹 01788 832878 21 en suite

STONELEIGH MAP 04 SP37

Stoneleigh Deer Park The Clubhouse, The Old Deer Park, Coventry Rd CV8 3DR
☎ 024 7663 9991 & 7663 9912 🖹 024 7651 1533
e-mail: stoneleighdeerpark@ukgateway.net
Parkland course in old deer park with many mature trees. The River Avon meanders through the course and comes into play on four holes. Also a nine-hole Par 3 course.
Tantara Course: 18 holes, 6056yds, Par 71, SSS 69, Course record 67.
Avon Course: 9 holes, 1251yds, Par 27.
Club membership 750.
Visitors Mon-Sun & BHs. Booking required. Handicap certificate. Dress code. **Societies** Booking required. **Green Fees** £20 (£22 Fri, £30 Sat, Sun

& BHs). **Prof** Matt McGuire & Paul Preston **Facilities** ⊕ ⏃ 🍴 🖢 ☐ 🏐 ⚐ **Conf** facs Corporate Hospitality Days **Location** 3m NE of Kenilworth
Hotel ★★★ 74% HL Macdonald De Montfort Hotel, Abbey End, KENILWORTH ☎ 0870 1942127 108 en suite

STRATFORD-UPON-AVON MAP 04 SP25

Ingon Manor Golf & Country Ingon Ln, Snitterfield CV37 0QE
☎ 01789 731857 🖹 01789 731657
e-mail: info@ingonmanor.co.uk
web: www.ingonmanor.co.uk
Nestling in the Welcombe Hills, a short distance from the town. The Manor, dating back to the 14th century, lies within 171 acres of land. The championship course is open all year round and has been designed to test all standards of golfers with a variety of challenging holes.
18 holes, 6623yds, Par 72. Club membership 400.
Visitors Mon-Sun & BHs. Booking required. Dress code. **Societies** welcome. **Green Fees** not confirmed. **Prof** Niel Evans **Facilities** ⊕ ⏃ 🍴 🖢 ☐ 🏐 🖢 ◇ ⚐ 🏌 **Leisure** caddies available. **Conf** facs Corporate Hospitality Days
Hotel ★★★ 79% HL Best Western Grosvenor Hotel, Warwick Rd, STRATFORD-UPON-AVON ☎ 01789 269213 73 en suite

Menzies Welcombe Hotel, Spa & Golf Club Warwick Rd CV37 0NR
☎ 01789 295252 🖹 01789 414666
e-mail: welcombe.golfpro@menzies-hotels.co.uk
web: www.bookmenzies.com
Wooded parkland course of great character and boasting superb views of the River Avon and Stratford. Set within the hotel's 157-acre estate, it has two lakes and other water features.
18 holes, 6288yds, Par 70, SSS 69, Course record 64.
Club membership 450.
Visitors Mon-Sun & BHs. Booking required. **Societies** Booking required **Green Fees** Phone. **Prof** Matt Nixon **Course Designer** Thomas Macauley **Facilities** ⊕ ⏃ 🍴 🖢 ☐ 🏐 🖢 ⚐ ◇ ⚐ 🏌 **Leisure** hard tennis courts, heated indoor swimming pool, fishing, solarium, gymnasium, golf lessons for individual/groups/company days. **Conf** facs Corporate Hospitality Days **Location** 1.5m NE off A46
Hotel ★★★★ 77% HL Billesley Manor Hotel, Billesley, Alcester, STRATFORD-UPON-AVON ☎ 01789 279955 43 en suite 29 annexe en suite

Stratford Oaks Bearley Rd, Snitterfield CV37 0EZ
☎ 01789 731980 🖹 01789 731981
e-mail: admin@stratfordoaks.co.uk
web: www.stratfordoaks.co.uk
American-style, level parkland course with some water features designed by Howard Swan.
18 holes, 6135yds, Par 71, SSS 69, Course record 61.
Club membership 700.
Visitors Mon-Sun & BHs. Booking required. Dress code.
Societies welcome. **Green Fees** not confirmed. **Prof** Andrew Dunbar **Course Designer** H Swann **Facilities** ⊕ ⏃ 🍴 🖢 ☐ 🏐 🖢 ⚐ ◇ 🏌 **Leisure** gymnasium, massage and physiotherapy facility. **Conf** Corporate Hospitality Days **Location** 4m N of Stratford-upon-Avon
Hotel ★★★★ 80% HL Stratford Manor, Warwick Rd, STRATFORD-UPON-AVON ☎ 01789 731173 104 en suite

CHAMPIONSHIP COURSE

WARWICKSHIRE — WISHAW

THE BELFRY

Map 07 SP19

Wishaw B76 9PR
☎ **01675 470301** 📄 **01675 470178**
e-mail: enquiries@thebelfry.com
web: www.devereonline.co.uk
The Brabazon: 18 holes, 6724yds, Par 72, SSS 71.
PGA National: 18 holes, 6639yds, Par 71, SSS 70.
The Derby: 18 holes, 6057yds, Par 69, SSS 69.
Club membership 450.
Visitors booking required for non-residents.
Handicap certificate. **Societies** booking required.
Green Fees Brabazon: £140, PGA: £75,
Derby: £40. Reduced winter rates. **Prof** Simon
Wordsworth **Course Designer** Dave Thomas/
Peter Alliss **Facilities** ⑪ †◎↓ 🛏 ⊑🖥🗍 人 🗎🎁
◇ 🚗 🚗 🚗 ☘ **Leisure** hard tennis courts, heated
indoor swimming pool, squash, sauna, solarium,
gymnasium, PGA National Golf Academy.
Conf facs Corporate Hospitality Days
Location M42 junct 9, 4m E on A446

The Belfry is unique as the only venue
to have staged the biggest golf event
in the world, the Ryder Cup matches,
an unprecedented four times, most
recently in 2002. The Brabazon is
regarded throughout the world as a great
championship course with some of the
most demanding holes in golf; the 10th
(Ballesteros's Hole) and the 18th, with
its dangerous lakes and its amphitheatre
around the final green, are world famous.
Alternatively, you can pit your wits against
a new legend in the making, the PGA
National Course. The Dave Thomas and
Peter Alliss designed course has been used
for professional competition and is one of
Britain's leading courses. For those who like
their golf a little easier or like to get back
into the swing gently, the Derby is ideal and
can be played by golfers of any standard.

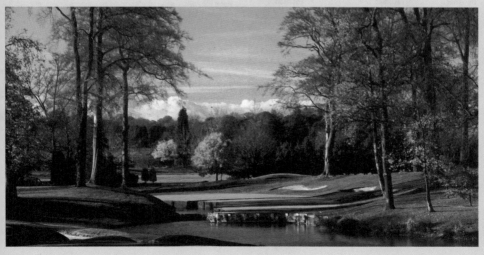

England

Stratford-upon-Avon Tiddington Rd CV37 7BA
☎ 01789 205749 📄 01789 414909
e-mail: sec@stratfordgolf.co.uk
web: www.stratfordgolf.co.uk
Beautiful parkland course. The Par 3 16th is tricky and the Par 5 17th
and 18th provide a tough end.
18 holes, 6311yds, Par 72, SSS 70, Course record 63.
Club membership 750.
Visitors contact club for details. **Societies** welcome. **Green Fees** not
confirmed. ☻ **Prof** D Sutherland **Course Designer** Taylor **Facilities** ⚄ 🍴
⛳ ♂ 🏌 ♂ **Location** 0.75m E on B4086
Hotel ★★★★ 80% HL Macdonald Alveston Manor, Clopton Bridge,
STRATFORD-UPON-AVON ☎ 0870 400 8181   113 en suite

TANWORTH IN ARDEN   MAP 07 SP17

Ladbrook Park Poolhead Ln B94 5ED
☎ 01564 742264 📄 01564 742909
e-mail: secretary@ladbrookparkgolf.co.uk
Parkland course lined with trees.
18 holes, 6427yds, Par 71, SSS 71, Course record 65.
Club membership 700.
Visitors Mon-Fri except BHs. Booking required. Handicap certificate. Dress
code. **Societies** Booking required. **Green Fees** £45 per 36 holes, £40
per 28 holes, £35 per 18 holes. **Prof** Richard Mountford **Course Designer**
H S Colt **Facilities** ⚄ 🍴 🛒 🍴 ⚄ 🍴 ♂ ♂ **Location** M42 junct 3,
2.5m SE
Hotel ★★★ 86% HL Nuthurst Grange Country House Hotel and
Restaurant, Nuthurst Grange Ln, HOCKLEY HEATH ☎ 01564 783972
15 en suite

WARWICK   MAP 04 SP26

Warwick The Racecourse CV34 6HW
☎ 01926 494316
Easy walking parkland. Driving range with floodlit bays.
9 holes, 2682yds, Par 34, SSS 66, Course record 67.
Club membership 150.
Visitors Mon-Sat & BHs. Booking required. **Societies** Booking required.
Green Fees £6.50 per 9 holes (£7 Sat & Sun). ☻ **Prof** Mario Luca **Course
Designer** D G Dunkley **Facilities** 🛒 🍴 ⚄ 🍴 ⛳ ♂ 🏌 **Location** W of
town centre
Hotel ★★★★ 79% HL Ardencote Manor Hotel, Country Club & Spa, Lye
Green Rd, Claverdon, WARWICK ☎ 01926 843111   75 en suite

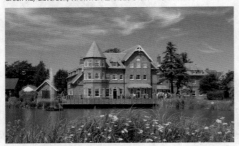

WISHAW   MAP 07 SP19

The Belfry see page 259
Hotel ★★★★ 80% HL The De Vere Belfry, WISHAW ☎ 0870 900 0066
324 en suite
Hotel ★★★★ 75% HL BW Lea Marston Hotel & Leisure Complex, Haunch
Ln, LEA MARSTON ☎ 01675 470468 Fax 01675 470871   80 en suite
Hotel ★★★★ 74% HL Best Western Premier Moor Hall Hotel &
Spa, Moor Hall Dr, Four Oaks, SUTTON COLDFIELD ☎ 0121 308 3751
Fax 0121 308 8974   82 en suite

WEST MIDLANDS

ALDRIDGE   MAP 07 SK00

Druids Heath Stonnall Rd WS9 8JZ
☎ 01922 455595 (Office) 📄 01922 452887
e-mail: dhgcadmin@uku.co.uk
web: www.druidsheathgc.co.uk
Testing, undulating heathland course. Large greens with subtle slopes.
18 holes, 6661yds, Par 72, SSS 73, Course record 68.
Club membership 660.
Visitors Mon-Fri except BHs. Sat & Sun pm only. Handicap certificate. Dress
code. **Societies** Booking required **Green Fees** £35 per day (£43 Sat and
Sun). ☻ **Prof** Glenn Williams **Facilities** ⚄ 🍴 🛒 🍴 ⚄ ♂ **Leisure**
snooker. **Conf** Corporate Hospitality Days **Location** NE of town centre
off A454
Hotel ★★★ 85% HL Fairlawns Hotel & Spa, 178 Little Aston Rd, ALDRIDGE
☎ 01922 455122   59 en suite

BIRMINGHAM   MAP 07 SP08

Alison Nicholas Golf Academy Host Centre, Queslett
Park, Great Barr B42 2RG
☎ 0121 360 7600 📄 0121 360 7603
e-mail: info@ the hostcorporation.com
web: www.thehostcorporation.com
9 holes, 905yds, Par 27, SSS 27, Course record 21.
Course Designer Alison Nicholas/Francis Colella **Location** M6 junct 7
Telephone for further details
Hotel BUD Innkeeper's Lodge Birmingham Sutton Coldfield, Chester Rd,
Streetley, SUTTON COLDFIELD ☎ 0845 112 6065   7 en suite 59 annexe
en suite

Cocks Moors Woods Alcester Rd South, Kings Heath
B14 4ER
☎ 0121 464 3584 📄 0121 441 1305
18 holes, 5769yds, Par 69, SSS 68.
Location M42 junct 3, 4m N on A435
Telephone for further details
Hotel ★★★ 71% HL Corus hotel Solihull, Stratford Rd, Shirley, SOLIHULL
☎ 0870 609 6133   111 en suite

Edgbaston Church Rd, Edgbaston B15 3TB
☎ 0121 454 1736 📠 0121 454 2395
e-mail: secretary@edgbastongc.co.uk
web: www.edgbastongc.co.uk
Set in 144 acres of woodland, lake and parkland, 2m from the centre of Birmingham, this delightful course utilises the wealth of natural features to provide a series of testing and adventurous holes set in the traditional double loop that starts directly in front of the clubhouse, an imposing Georgian mansion.
18 holes, 6106yds, Par 69, SSS 69, Course record 63.
Club membership 970.
Visitors Mon-Sun except BHs. Booking required Sat & Sun. Handicap certificate. Dress code. **Societies** Booking required **Green Fees** Phone. **Prof** Jamie Cundy **Course Designer** H S Colt **Facilities** ⑪ ⑨ 🍴 ⬛ 🗜 🏌 ⬥ 🍴 🛒 ⬥ **Conf** facs Corporate Hospitality Days **Location** 2m S of city centre on B4217, off A38
Hotel ★★★ 73% HL Thistle Birmingham Edgbaston, 225 Hagley Rd, Edgbaston, BIRMINGHAM ☎ 0870 333 9127 151 en suite

Great Barr Chapel Ln, Great Barr B43 7BA
☎ 0121 358 4376 📠 0121 358 4376
e-mail: info@greatbarrgolfclub.co.uk
web: www.greatbarrgolfclub.co.uk
Eeasy walking parkland with views of Barr Beacon Park.
18 holes, 6523yds, Par 72, SSS 72, Course record 67.
Club membership 600.
Visitors Mon-Fri except BHs. Handicap certificate. **Societies** Booking required **Green Fees** Phone. ⑨ **Prof** Richard Spragg **Facilities** ⑪ ⑨ 🍴 🗜 🍴 ⬥ **Conf** Corporate Hospitality Days **Location** 6m N of city centre off A 34
Hotel BUD Innkeeper's Lodge Birmingham Sutton Coldfield, Chester Rd, Streetley, SUTTON COLDFIELD ☎ 0845 112 6065 7 en suite 59 annexe en suite

Handsworth 11 Sunningdale Close, Handsworth Wood B20 1NP
☎ 0121 554 3387 📠 0121 554 6144
e-mail: info@handsworthgolfclub.net
Undulating parkland with some tight fairways and strategic bunkering with a number of well-placed water features.
18 holes, 6289yds, Par 70, SSS 71, Course record 64.
Club membership 730.
Visitors Mon-Fri except BHs. Handicap certificate. Dress code. **Societies** Booking required. **Green Fees** £40 per day. ⑨ **Prof** Lee Bashford **Course Designer** H. S. Colt **Facilities** ⑪ ⑨ 🍴 ⬛ 🗜 🍴 🏌 ⬛ 🛒 ⬥ **Leisure** squash. **Conf** Corporate Hospitality Days **Location** 3.5m NW of city centre off A4040
Hotel BUD Premier Travel Inn West Bromwich, New Gas St, WEST BROMWICH ☎ 08701 977264 40 en suite

Harborne 40 Tennal Rd, Harborne B32 2JE
☎ 0121 427 3058 📠 0121 427 4039
e-mail: harborne@hgolf.fsnet.co.uk
web: www.harbornegolfclub.co.uk
Parkland course in a hilly location, with a brook running through.
18 holes, 6230yds, Par 70, SSS 70, Course record 65.
Club membership 600.
Visitors Mon, Wed-Fri except BHs. Booking required. Handicap certificate. Dress code. **Societies** Booking required. **Green Fees** £30 per day. ⑨ **Prof** Paul Johnson **Course Designer** Harry Colt **Facilities** ⑪ ⑨ 🍴 ⬛ 🗜 🍴 🛒 ⬥ **Conf** facs Corporate Hospitality Days **Location** 3.5 m SW of city centre off A4040
Hotel ★★★ 73% HL Thistle Birmingham Edgbaston, 225 Hagley Rd, Edgbaston, BIRMINGHAM ☎ 0870 333 9127 151 en suite

Harborne Church Farm Vicarage Rd, Harborne B17 0SN
☎ 0121 427 1204 📠 0121 428 3126
Parkland with two brooks running through. Course is small but tight.
9 holes, 2441yds, Par 66, SSS 64, Course record 62.
Club membership 115.
Visitors Mon-Sun & BHs. Booking required. **Societies** booking required. **Green Fees** not confirmed. **Prof** Paul Johnson **Facilities** ⑪ ⑨ 🗜 🏌 🏌 **Leisure** practice net. **Location** 3.5m SW of city centre off A4040
Hotel ★★★ 73% HL Thistle Birmingham Edgbaston, 225 Hagley Rd, Edgbaston, BIRMINGHAM ☎ 0870 333 9127 151 en suite

Hatchford Brook Coventry Rd, Sheldon B26 3PY
☎ 0121 743 9821 📠 0121 743 3420
e-mail: idt@hbgc.freeserve.co.uk
web: golfpro-direct.co.uk
18 holes, 6155yds, Par 69, SSS 70.
Location 6m E of city centre on A45
Telephone for further details
Hotel ★★★ 74% HL Novotel Birmingham Airport, BIRMINGHAM AIRPORT ☎ 0121 782 7000 & 782 4111 📠 0121 782 0445 195 en suite

Hilltop Park Ln, Handsworth B21 8LJ
☎ 0121 554 4463
A good test of golf with interesting layout, undulating fairways and large greens, located in the Sandwell Valley conservation area.
18 holes, 6208yds, Par 71, SSS 70, Course record 65.
Club membership 400.
Visitors Mon-Sun & BHs. Booking required. **Societies** Booking required. **Green Fees** 18 holes: £11, 9 holes: £6.50 (£13/£7.50 Sat, Sun & BHs). **Prof** Kevin Highfield **Course Designer** Hawtree **Facilities** ⑪ ⑨ 🍴 ⬛ 🗜 🍴 🏌 ⬛ 🛒 ⬥ **Conf** facs Corporate Hospitality Days **Location** M5 junct 1, 1m on A41
Hotel BUD Premier Travel Inn West Bromwich, New Gas St, WEST BROMWICH ☎ 08701 977264 40 en suite

Lickey Hills Rosehill, Rednal B45 8RR
☎ 0121 453 3159 📠 0121 457 8779
Hilly municipal course overlooking the city, set in National Trust land.
Rose Hill: 18 holes, 5835yds, Par 68, SSS 68.
Club membership 300.
Visitors Mon-Sun & BHs. Booking required. Dress code. **Societies** booking required. **Green Fees** not confirmed. **Prof** Mark Toombs **Facilities** ⑪ 🍴 🗜 🏌 🛒 🏌 ⬥ **Leisure** hard tennis courts. **Conf** facs Corporate Hospitality Days **Location** 10m SW of city centre on B4096

Moseley Springfield Rd, Kings Heath B14 7DX
☎ 0121 444 4957 🖷 0121 441 4662
e-mail: admin@mosgolf.freeserve.co.uk
web: www.moseleygolfclub.co.uk
Parkland with a lake, pond and a stream providing natural hazards. The Par 3 4th goes through a cutting in woodland to a tree and garden-lined amphitheatre, and the Par 4 5th entails a drive over a lake to a dog-leg fairway.

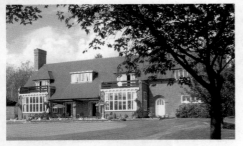

18 holes, 6300yds, Par 70, SSS 71, Course record 63.
Club membership 600.
Visitors Mon-Fri except BHs. Booking required. Handicap certificate. Dress code. **Societies** booking required. **Green Fees** not confirmed. ☻ **Prof** Martin Griffin **Course Designer** H S Colt with others **Facilities** ⑪ ⑩ ⑥ ♨ 🖫 ⌖ 🏌 🛴 🍴 🏌 **Conf** Corporate Hospitality Days **Location** 4m S of city centre on B4146

North Worcestershire Frankley Beeches Rd, Northfield
B31 5LP
☎ 0121 475 1047 🖷 0121 476 8681
Designed by James Braid and established in 1907, this is a mature parkland course. Tree plantations rather than heavy rough are the main hazards.
18 holes, 5959yds, Par 69, SSS 68, Course record 64.
Club membership 600.
Visitors Mon-Fri except BHs. Booking required. Handicap certificate. Dress code. **Societies** booking required. **Green Fees** not confirmed. ☻ **Prof** Dan Cummins **Course Designer** James Braid **Facilities** ⑪ ⑩ ⑥ 🖫 ⌖ 🏌 🛴 🍴 🏌 **Location** 7m SW of Birmingham city centre, off A38

Warley Woods The Pavilion, Lightswood Hill, Warley
B67 5ED
☎ 0121 429 2440 & 686 2619(secretary) 🖷 0121 434 4430
web: Warleygolfclub.co.uk
9 holes, 5346yds, Par 68, SSS 66, Course record 64.
Location 4m W of city centre off A456
Telephone for further details
Hotel ★★ 68% HL Fountain Court Hotel, 339-343 Hagley Rd, EDGBASTON
☎ 0121 429 1754 23 en suite

COVENTRY   MAP 04 SP37

Ansty Golf Centre Brinklow Rd, Ansty CV7 9JH
☎ 024 7662 1341 🖷 024 7660 2568
web: www.coventry.co.uk/ansty/
18 holes, 6079yds, Par 71, SSS 68, Course record 66.
Course Designer David Morgan **Location** M6/M69 junct 2, 1m
Telephone for further details
Hotel ★★★ 71% HL Novotel Coventry, Wilsons Ln, COVENTRY
☎ 024 7636 5000 98 en suite

Coventry St Martins Rd, Finham Park CV3 6RJ
☎ 024 7641 4152 🖷 024 7669 0131
e-mail: coventrygolfclub@hotmail.com
web: www.coventrygolfcourse.co.uk
The scene of several major professional events, this undulating parkland course has a great deal of quality. More than that, it usually plays its length, and thus scoring is never easy, as many professionals have found to their cost.
18 holes, 6601yds, Par 73, SSS 73, Course record 66.
Club membership 500.
Visitors Mon-Fri except BHs. Handicap certificate. Dress code. **Societies** Booking required **Green Fees** £40 per day. **Prof** Philip Weaver **Course Designer** Vardon Bros/Hawtree **Facilities** ⑪ ⑩ ⑥ 🖫 ⌖ 🏌 🛴 🍴 🏌 **Conf** Corporate Hospitality Days **Location** 3m S of city centre on B4113
Hotel ★★★ 66% HL Hylands Hotel, Warwick Rd, COVENTRY
☎ 024 7650 1600 61 en suite

Coventry Hearsall Beechwood Av CV5 6DF
☎ 024 7671 3470 🖷 024 7669 1534
18 holes, 6005yds, Par 70, SSS 69.
Location 1.5m SW of city centre off A429
Telephone for further details
Hotel ★★★ 66% HL Hylands Hotel, Warwick Rd, COVENTRY
☎ 024 7650 1600 61 en suite

Windmill Village Hotel Golf & Leisure Club
Birmingham Rd, Allesley CV5 9AL
☎ 024 7640 4041 🖷 024 7640 4042
e-mail: leisure@windmillvillagehotel.co.uk
web: www.windmillvillagehotel.co.uk
An attractive 18-hole course over rolling parkland with plenty of trees and two lakes that demand shots over open water. Four challenging Par 5 holes.
18 holes, 5184yds, Par 70, SSS 66, Course record 63.
Club membership 600.
Visitors Mon-Sun & BHs. Booking required. Dress code. **Societies** Booking required. **Green Fees** Phone. **Prof** Robert Hunter **Course Designer** Robert Hunter **Facilities** ⑪ ⑩ ⑥ 🖫 ⌖ 🏌 🛴 🍴 ♡ 🏌 🏌 **Leisure** hard tennis courts, heated indoor swimming pool, sauna, solarium, gymnasium, practice nets. **Conf** facs Corporate Hospitality Days **Location** 3m W of Coventry on A45
Hotel ★★★ 70% HL Brooklands Grange Hotel & Restaurant, Holyhead Rd, COVENTRY ☎ 024 7660 1601 31 en suite

---

DUDLEY   MAP 07 SO99

Dudley Turner's Hill, Rowley Regis B65 9DP
☎ 01384 233877 🖷 01384 233877
e-mail: secretary@dudleygolfclub.com
web: www.dudleygolfclub.com
Fairly hilly parkland course.
18 holes, 5714yds, Par 69, SSS 68. Club membership 350.
Visitors Mon-Fri & BHs. Booking required. **Societies** Booking required **Green Fees** Phone. **Prof** Gary Kilmister **Facilities** ⑪ ⑩ ⑥ 🖫 ⌖ 🏌 🛴 🍴 🏌 **Location** 2m S of town centre off B4171
Hotel ★★★ 66% HL Himley Country Hotel, School Rd, HIMLEY
☎ 01902 896716 71 en suite

CHAMPIONSHIP COURSE

WEST MIDLANDS — MERIDEN

MARRIOTT FOREST OF ARDEN

Map 04 SP28

Maxstoke Ln CV7 7HR
☎ **0870 400 7272** 🖨 **0870 400 7372**
web: www.marriotthotels.com/cvtgs
Arden Course: 18 holes, 6707yds, Par 72, SSS 73, Course record 63.
Aylesford Course: 18 holes, 5801yds, Par 69, SSS 68.
Club membership 800.
Visitors Mon-Sun & BHs. Booking required. Handicap certificate. Dress code.
Societies booking required. **Green Fees** Arden £100 (£110 Fri-Sun). Aylesford £45/£55.
Prof Philip Hoye **Course Designer** Donald Steele **Facilities** ⚒ 🏠 ♈ ◇ ✦ 🏌 ✦ ✦
Leisure hard tennis courts, heated indoor pool, fishing, sauna, solarium, gym, croquet lawn, steam room, jacuzzi, aerobics studio.
Conf Corporate Hospitality Days
Location 1m SW on B4102

This is one of the finest golf destinations in the UK, with a range of facilities to impress every golfer. The jewel in the crown is the Arden championship parkland course, set in 10,000 acres of the Packington Estate. Designed by Donald Steel, it presents one of the country's most spectacular challenges and has hosted a succession of international tournaments, including the British Masters and English Open. Beware the 18th hole, which is enough to stretch the nerves of any golfer. The shorter Aylesford Course offers a varied and enjoyable challenge, which golfers of all abilities will find rewarding. Golf events are a speciality, and there is a golf academy and extensive leisure facilities.

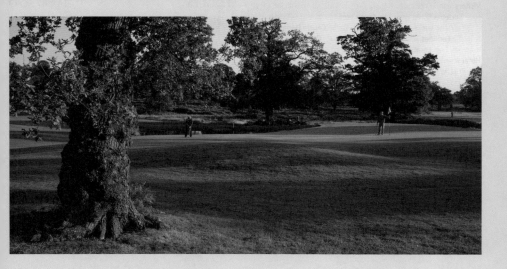

Swindon Bridgnorth Rd, Swindon DY3 4PU
☎ 01902 897031 📠 01902 326219
e-mail: admin@swindongolfclub.co.uk
web: www.swindongolfclub.co.uk
Attractive, undulating woodland and parkland with spectacular views.
Old Course: 18 holes, 6121yds, Par 71, SSS 70.
Club membership 700.
Visitors Mon-Sun & BHs. Booking required Sat, Sun & BHs **Societies**
Booking required **Green Fees** £20 per round (£30 Sat, Sun & BHs).
Facilities ⊕ ⊚ ⅃ ⅃ ⊡ ⅃ ⅃ 🖥 🖥 🖉 🏌 **Leisure** fishing, Par 3 9-hole
course. **Location** 4m W of Dudley on B4176
Hotel ★★★ 66% HL Himley Country Hotel, School Rd, HIMLEY
☎ 01902 896716 71 en suite

HALESOWEN   MAP 07 SO98

Halesowen The Leasowes, Leasowes Ln B62 8QF
☎ 0121 501 3606 📠 0121 501 3606
e-mail: halesowengolfclub@btconnect.com
web: www.halesowengolfclub.com
Parkland course within the only Grade I listed park in the Midlands.
18 holes, 5754yds, Par 69, SSS 69, Course record 64.
Club membership 625.
Visitors Mon-Sun & BHs. Booking required Sat, Sun & BHs. Dress code.
Societies Booking required. **Green Fees** £34 per day, £28 per round. ⊜
Prof Jon Nicholas **Facilities** ⊕ ⊚ ⅃ ⅃ ⊡ ⅃ ⅃ 🖥 🖉 🖉 🖉 **Conf** facs
Corporate Hospitality Days **Location** M5 junct 3, 1m E, off Manor Ln
Hotel ★★★ 68% HL Quality Hotel Dudley, Birmingham Rd, DUDLEY
☎ 01384 458070 72 en suite

KNOWLE   MAP 07 SP17

Copt Heath 1220 Warwick Rd B93 9LN
☎ 01564 772650 & 731620 📠 01564 771022/731621
e-mail: golf@copt-heath.co.uk
web: coptheathgolf.co.uk
Flat heathland and parkland course designed by H Vardon.
18 holes, 6522yds, Par 71, SSS 71, Course record 64.
Club membership 700.
Visitors Mon-Sun except BHs. Booking required. Handicap certificate. Dress
code. **Societies** Booking required. **Green Fees** £55 per day, £45 per round
(£50 per round weekends). ⊜ **Prof** Brian J Barton **Course Designer**
H Vardon **Facilities** ⊕ ⊚ ⅃ ⅃ ⊡ ⅃ ⅃ 🖥 🖉 🖉 🖉 **Conf** Corporate
Hospitality Days **Location** M42 junct 5, 0.5m S on A4141
Hotel ★★★★ 77% HL Renaissance Solihull Hotel, 651 Warwick Rd,
SOLIHULL ☎ 0121 711 3000 179 en suite

MERIDEN   MAP 04 SP28

**Marriott Forest of Arden Golf & Country
Club see page 263**
Hotel ★★★★ 81% HL Marriott Forest of Arden Hotel & Country Club,
Maxstoke Ln, MERIDEN ☎ 0870 400 7272 214 en suite
Hotel ★★★ 81% HL Manor Hotel, Main Rd, MERIDEN ☎ 01676 522735
Fax 01676 522186 110 en suite

North Warwickshire Hampton Ln CV7 7LL
☎ 01676 522259 (shop) & 522915 (sec) 📠 01676 523004
9 holes, 6390yds, Par 72, SSS 71, Course record 65.
Location 1m SW on B4102
Telephone for further details
Hotel ★★★ 81% HL Manor Hotel, Main Rd, MERIDEN ☎ 01676 522735
110 en suite

Stonebridge Golf Centre Somers Rd CV7 7PL
☎ 01676 522442 📠 01676 522447
e-mail: golf.shop@stonebridgegolf.co.uk
web: www.stonebridgegolf.co.uk
A parkland course set in 170 acres with towering oak trees, lakes, and
the River Blythe on its borders.
18 holes, 6240yds, Par 70, SSS 70, Course record 67.
Club membership 400.
Visitors Mon-Sun & BHs. Booking required. Dress code. **Societies** Booking
required. **Green Fees** £19 per 18 holes (£20 Fri, £25 Sat, Sun & BHs).
Prof Darren Murphey **Course Designer** Mark Jones **Facilities** ⊕ ⊚
⅃ ⊡ ⅃ ⅃ 🖥 🖉 🖉 🖉 **Leisure** fishing, golf academy. **Conf** facs
Corporate Hospitality Days **Location** M42 junct 6, 3m
Hotel ★★★ 71% HL Best Western Stade Court, West Pde, HYTHE
☎ 01303 268263 42 en suite
Hotel ★★★ 71% HL Arden Hotel & Leisure Club, Coventry Rd, Bickenhill,
SOLIHULL ☎ 01675 443221 Fax 01675 445604 216 en suite

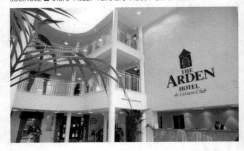

SEDGLEY   MAP 07 SO99

Sedgley Golf Centre Sandyfields Rd DY3 3DL
☎ 01902 880503
e-mail: info@sedgleygolf.co.uk
Public pay and play course. Undulating contours and mature trees with
extensive views over surrounding countryside.
9 holes, 3147yds, Par 72, SSS 70. Club membership 100.
Visitors Mon-Sun & BHs. **Societies** Booking required. **Green Fees** £10.50
per 18 holes, £8 per 9 holes. ⊜ **Prof** Garry Mercer **Course Designer** W G
Cox **Facilities** ⊡ ⅃ 🖉 🏌 **Location** 0.5m from town centre off A463
Hotel ★★★ 66% HL Himley Country Hotel, School Rd, HIMLEY
☎ 01902 896716 71 en suite

SOLIHULL   MAP 07 SP17

Olton Mirfield Rd B91 1JH
☎ 0121 704 1936 📠 0121 711 2010
e-mail: mailbox@oltongolfclub.fsnet.co.uk
web: www.oltongolf.co.uk
Parkland course, over 100 years old, with prevailing south-west wind.
18 holes, 6265yds, Par 69, SSS 70, Course record 63.
Club membership 600.   *Continued*

Visitors Mon-Fri except BHs. Handicap certficate. Dress code. **Societies** Booking required. **Green Fees** £50 per 36 holes, £45 per 27 holes, £40 per 18 holes. ☻ **Prof** Charles Haynes **Course Designer** J H Taylor **Facilities** ⊕ ⓘ◎ ⓑ ⌱ ⅌ ⌇ ⅄ ☞ ⅌ ✔ ☞ **Leisure** snooker. **Conf** Corporate Hospitality Days **Location** M42 junct 5, A41 for 1.5m **Hotel** ★★★★ 77% HL Renaissance Solihull Hotel, 651 Warwick Rd, SOLIHULL ☎ 0121 711 3000 179 en suite

Robin Hood St Bernards Rd B92 7DJ
☎ 0121 706 0061 📋 0121 700 7502
e-mail: robin.hood.golf.club@dial.pipex.com
Pleasant parkland with easy walking and good views. Tree-lined fairways and varied holes, culminating in two excellent finishing holes.
18 holes, 6635yds, Par 72, SSS 72, Course record 68. Club membership 650.
Visitors Mon, Thu & Fri except BHs. Handicap certificate. Dress code. **Societies** Booking required. **Green Fees** £30 per day. ☻ **Prof** Alan Harvey **Course Designer** H S Colt **Facilities** ⊕ ⓘ◎ ⓑ ⌱ ⅌ ⅄ ☞ ⅌ ✔ **Conf** Corporate Hospitality Days **Location** 2m W off B4025 **Hotel** ★★★★ 77% HL Renaissance Solihull Hotel, 651 Warwick Rd, SOLIHULL ☎ 0121 711 3000 179 en suite

Shirley Stratford Rd, Monkspath, Shirley B90 4EW
☎ 0121 744 6001 📋 0121 746 5645
e-mail: shirleygolfclub@btclick.com
Undulating parkland with water features.
18 holes, 6510yds, Par 72, SSS 71. Club membership 600.
Visitors Mon-Fri except BHs. Handicap certificate. Dress code. **Green Fees** not confirmed. ☻ **Prof** S Bottrill **Facilities** ⊕ ⓘ◎ ⓑ ⌱ ⅌ ⅄ ☞ ✔ **Conf** facs Corporate Hospitality Days **Location** M42 junct 4, 0.5m N on A34 **Hotel** ★★★ 71% HL Corus hotel Solihull, Stratford Rd, Shirley, SOLIHULL ☎ 0870 609 6133 111 en suite

West Midlands Marsh House Farm Ln, Barston B92 0LB
☎ 01675 444890 📋 01675 444891
e-mail: westmidlandsgc@aol.com
web: www.wmgc.co.uk
18 holes, 6624yds, Par 72, SSS 72.
Course Designer Nigel & Mark Harrhy/David Griffith **Location** From NEC A45 towards Coventry for 0.5m, onto A452 towards Leamington, club on right
Telephone for further details
Hotel ★★★ 71% HL Arden Hotel & Leisure Club, Coventry Rd, Bickenhill, SOLIHULL ☎ 01675 443221 216 en suite

Widney Manor Saintbury Dr, Widney Manor B91 3SZ
☎ 0121 704 0704 📋 0121 704 7999
web: www.wmgc.co.uk
18 holes, 5654yards, Par 71, SSS 66.
Course Designer Nigel & Mark Harrhy **Location** M42 junct 4, signs to Monkspath Manor
Telephone for further details
Hotel ★★★★ 77% HL Renaissance Solihull Hotel, 651 Warwick Rd, SOLIHULL ☎ 0121 711 3000 179 en suite

STOURBRIDGE — MAP 07 SO88

Hagley Golf & Country Club Wassell Grove Ln, Hagley DY9 9JW
☎ 01562 883701 📋 01562 887518
e-mail: manager@hagleygcc.freeserve.co.uk
web: www.hagleygolfandcountryclub.co.uk
Undulating parkland beneath the Clent Hills. Superb views. Testing 15th, Par 5, 559yds, named Monster under Clent Hills.
18 holes, 6353yds, Par 72, SSS 72, Course record 66. Club membership 700.
Visitors Mon-Fri except BHs. Booking required. Handicap certificate. Dress code. **Societies** Booking required. **Green Fees** £36 per day, £31 per 18 holes. **Prof** Iain Clark **Course Designer** Garratt & Co **Facilities** ⊕ ⓘ◎ ⓑ ⌱ ⅌ ⅄ ✔ ✔ **Leisure** squash. **Conf** facs Corporate Hospitality Days **Location** 1m E of Hagley off A456. 2m from junct 3 on M5 **Hotel** BUD Premier Travel Inn Hagley, Birmingham Rd, HAGLEY ☎ 08701 977123 40 en suite

Stourbridge Worcester Ln, Pedmore DY8 2RB
☎ 01384 395566 📋 01384 444660
e-mail: secretary@stourbridge-golf-club.co.uk
web: www.stourbridge-golf-club.co.uk
Parkland course.
18 holes, 6231yds, Par 70, SSS 69, Course record 67. Club membership 705.
Visitors Mon-Fri except BHs. Handicap certificate. Dress code **Societies** Booking required. **Green Fees** £30 per 18 holes, £37.50 per day. ☻ **Prof** M Male **Facilities** ⊕ ⓘ◎ ⓑ ⌱ ⅌ ⅄ ☞ ✔ **Conf** Corporate Hospitality Days **Location** 2m S from town centre **Hotel** BUD Premier Travel Inn Hagley, Birmingham Rd, HAGLEY ☎ 08701 977123 40 en suite

SUTTON COLDFIELD — MAP 07 SP19

Boldmere Monmouth Dr B73 6JL
☎ 0121 354 3379 📋 0121 355 4534
18 holes, 4493yds, Par 63, SSS 62, Course record 57.
Location Next to Sutton Park
Telephone for further details
Hotel ★★★★ 74% HL Best Western Premier Moor Hall Hotel & Spa, Moor Hall Dr, Four Oaks, SUTTON COLDFIELD ☎ 0121 308 3751 82 en suite

Little Aston Roman Rd, Streetly B74 3AN
☎ 0121 353 2942 📋 0121 580 8387
e-mail: manager@littleastongolf.co.uk
web: www.littleastongolf.co.uk
This parkland course is set in the rolling countryside of the former Little Aston Hall and there is a wide variety of mature trees. There are three Par 3 holes and three Par 5 holes and although the fairways are not unduly narrow there are rewards for accuracy - especially from the tee. The course features two lakes. At the Par 5 12th the lake cuts into the green and at the Par 4 17th the lake is also adjacent to the green.
18 holes, 6670yds, Par 72, SSS 73, Course record 63. Club membership 350.
Visitors Mon-Wed, Fri, Sun & BHs. Booking required. Handicap certificate. Dress code. **Societies** Booking required. **Green Fees** £95 per day, £75 per round. **Prof** Brian Rimmer **Course Designer** H Vardon **Facilities** ⊕ ⓘ◎ ⓑ ⌱ ⅌ ⅄ ☞ ✔ ✔ ☞ **Location** 3.5m NW of Sutton Coldfield off A454 **Hotel** ★★★★ 74% HL Best Western Premier Moor Hall Hotel & Spa, Moor Hall Dr, Four Oaks, SUTTON COLDFIELD ☎ 0121 308 3751 82 en suite

Moor Hall Moor Hall Dr B75 6LN

☎ 0121 308 6130 📄 0121 308 9560
e-mail: secretary@moorhallgolfclub.co.uk
Outstanding parkland course with mature trees lining the fairways. The 14th hole is notable and is part of a challenging finish to the round.
18 holes, 6293yds, Par 70, SSS 70, Course record 64.
Club membership 600.
Visitors Mon-Wed, Thu pm only. Booking required. Dress code. **Societies** Booking required. **Green Fees** £60 per day, £45 per round. **Prof** Cameron Clark **Course Designer** Hawtree & Taylor **Facilities** ⊕ ⏻ ⌗ ☷ ▱ ▜ ⚘ ⌸ **Conf** Corporate Hospitality Days **Location** 2.5m N of town centre off A453
Hotel ★★★★ 74% HL Best Western Premier Moor Hall Hotel & Spa, Moor Hall Dr, Four Oaks, SUTTON COLDFIELD ☎ 0121 308 3751 82 en suite

Pype Hayes Eachel Hurst Rd, Walmley B76 1EP

☎ 0121 351 1014 📄 0121 313 0206
e-mail: colinmarson@btinternet.com
Attractive, fairly flat course with excellent greens.
18 holes, 5927yds, Par 71, SSS 69, Course record 65.
Club membership 240.
Visitors Mon-Sun & BHs. Booking required. **Societies** booking required **Green Fees** not confirmed. **Prof** Joe Kelly **Course Designer** Bobby Jones **Facilities** ⊕ ▱ ⌸ ▜ ⚘ **Location** 2.5m S off B4148
Hotel ★★★★ 74% HL Best Western Premier Moor Hall Hotel & Spa, Moor Hall Dr, Four Oaks, SUTTON COLDFIELD ☎ 0121 308 3751 82 en suite

Sutton Coldfield 110 Thornhill Rd, Streetly B74 3ER

☎ 0121 580 7878 📄 0121 353 5503
e-mail: admin@suttoncoldfieldgc.com
web: www.suttoncoldfieldgc.com
A fine natural, all-weather, heathland course, with tight fairways, gorse, heather and trees. A good challenge for all standards of golfer.
18 holes, 6541yds, Par 72, SSS 71, Course record 65.
Club membership 600.
Visitors Mon-Sun & BHs. Booking required. Dress code. **Societies** Booking required. **Green Fees** £44 per day, £33 per round (£44 Sat & Sun). ⊜ **Prof** Jerry Hayes **Course Designer** Dr A McKenzie **Facilities** ⊕ ⏻ ☷ ▱ ▜ ⌸ ⚘ **Conf** facs Corporate Hospitality Days **Location** M6 junct 7, A34 towards Birmingham, 1st lights left onto A4041 Queslett Rd Thornhill Rd, entrance after 4th left
Hotel ★★★★ 74% HL Best Western Premier Moor Hall Hotel & Spa, Moor Hall Dr, Four Oaks, SUTTON COLDFIELD ☎ 0121 308 3751 82 en suite

Walmley Brooks Rd, Wylde Green B72 1HR

☎ 0121 373 0029 📄 0121 377 7272
e-mail: walmleygolfclub@aol.com
web: www.walmleygolfclub.co.uk
Pleasant parkland with many trees. The hazards are not difficult.
18 holes, 6585yds, Par 72, SSS 72, Course record 67.
Club membership 700.
Visitors Mon, Wed-Fri except BHs. Booking required. Handicap certificate. Dress code. **Societies** booking required. **Green Fees** not confirmed. ⊜ **Prof** C J Wicketts **Facilities** ⊕ ⏻ ☷ ▱ ▜ ⌸ ⚘ **Conf** Corporate Hospitality Days **Location** 2m S off A5127
Hotel ★★★★ 74% HL Best Western Premier Moor Hall Hotel & Spa, Moor Hall Dr, Four Oaks, SUTTON COLDFIELD ☎ 0121 308 3751 82 en suite

Wishaw Bulls Ln, Wishaw B76 9QW

☎ 0121 313 2110 📄 0121 351 7498
Parkland with one hill on the course at the 9th and 18th holes. Well drained with irrigation on tees and greens.
18 holes, 5729yards, Par 70, SSS 68, Course record 67.
Club membership 338.
Visitors Mon-Fri, Sun & BHs. Dress code. **Societies** Booking required. **Green Fees** not confirmed. **Prof** Alan Partridge **Course Designer** R. Wallis **Facilities** ⊕ ⏻ ☷ ▱ ▜ ⌸ ⚘ **Conf** facs Corporate Hospitality Days **Location** W of village off A4097
Hotel ★★★★ 80% HL The De Vere Belfry, WISHAW ☎ 0870 900 0066 324 en suite
Hotel ★★★★ 75% HL BW Lea Marston Hotel & Leisure Complex, Haunch Ln, LEA MARSTON ☎ 01675 470468 Fax 01675 470871 80 en suite

WALSALL

MAP 07 SP09

Bloxwich Stafford Rd, Bloxwich WS3 3PQ

☎ 01922 47659 📄 01922 493449
e-mail: secretary@bloxwichgolfclub.com
web: www.bloxwichgolfclub.com
Undulating parkland with natural hazards and subject to strong north wind.
18 holes, 6257yds, Par 71, SSS 71, Course record 68.
Club membership 680.
Visitors Mon-Fri except BHs. Booking required. Handicap certificate. Dress code. **Societies** Booking required. **Green Fees** Phone. **Prof** Richard J Dance **Facilities** ⊕ ☷ ▱ ▜ ⌸ ⚘ **Conf** facs Corporate Hospitality Days **Location** M 6 junct 11/M6 (toll) T7, 3m N of town centre on A34
Hotel ★★★ 85% HL Fairlawns Hotel & Spa, 178 Little Aston Rd, ALDRIDGE ☎ 01922 455122 59 en suite

Calderfields Aldridge Rd WS4 2JS

☎ 01922 632243 📄 01922 640540
e-mail: calderfield@bigfoot.com
web: www.calderfieldsgolf.com
Scenic parkland in peaceful setting, enhanced by a lake and water fountain.
18 holes, 6509yds, Par 73, SSS 71. Club membership 650.
Visitors Mon-Sun & BHs. Dress code. **Societies** Booking required. **Green Fees** £18 per round (£20 Sat, Sun & BHs). **Prof** Simon Edwin **Course Designer** Roy Winter **Facilities** ⊕ ⏻ ☷ ▱ ▜ ⌸ ⚘ ▜ **Leisure** fishing. **Conf** facs Corporate Hospitality Days **Location** On A454
Hotel ★★★ 85% HL Fairlawns Hotel & Spa, 178 Little Aston Rd, ALDRIDGE ☎ 01922 455122 59 en suite

Walsall The Broadway WS1 3EY

☎ 01922 613512 📄 01922 616460
e-mail: golfclub@walsallgolf.freeserve.co.uk
web: www.walsallgolfclub.co.uk
18 holes, 6300yds, Par 70, SSS 70, Course record 65.
Course Designer McKenzie **Location** 1m S of town centre off A34
Telephone for further details
Hotel BUD Travelodge Birmingham Walsall, Birmingham Rd, WALSALL ☎ 0870 191 1823 96 en suite

WEST BROMWICH MAP 07 SP09

Dartmouth Vale St B71 4DW
☎ 0121 588 5746 & 588 2131
web: www.dartmouthgolfclub.co.uk
Very tight meadowland course with undulating but easy walking.
The 617yd Par 5 1st hole is something of a challenge.
9 holes, 6036yds, Par 71, SSS 71, Course record 66.
Club membership 250.
Visitors Mon-Fri & BHs. Sat & Sun afternoon. Handicap certificate. Dress
code. **Societies** Booking required **Green Fees** £20 per day (£25 Sat & Sun
pm). ☻ **Facilities** ⑪ ⑱ ⓔ ⓓ ✠⃝ ⚐ ⚑ **Location** E of town centre off
A4041
Hotel ★★★ 68% HL Great Barr Hotel & Conference Centre, Pear Tree Dr,
Newton Rd, Great Barr, BIRMINGHAM ☎ 0121 357 1141 105 en suite

Sandwell Park Birmingham Rd B71 4JJ
☎ 0121 553 4637 ▤ 0121 525 1651
e-mail: secretary@sandwellparkgolfclub.co.uk
web: www.sandwellparkgolfclub.co.uk
A picturesque course wandering over wooded heathland and
utilising natural features. Each hole is entirely separate, shielded
from the others by either natural banks or lines of trees. A course
that demands careful placing of shots that have been given a great
deal of thought. Natural undulating fairways create difficult and
testing approach shots to the greens.

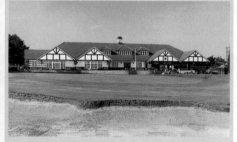

18 holes, 6204yds, Par 71, SSS 71, Course record 65.
Club membership 550.
Visitors Mon-Fri except BHs. Booking required. Handicap certificate.
Dress code. **Societies** booking required. **Green Fees** not confirmed. ☻
Prof Nigel Wylie **Course Designer** H S Colt **Facilities** ⑪ ⑱ ⓔ ⓓ ✠⃝
⚐ ⚑ ✔ **Leisure** practice chipping area. **Conf** facs Corporate Hospitality
Days **Location** M5 junct 1, 200yds on A41
Hotel ★★★ 68% HL Great Barr Hotel & Conference Centre, Pear Tree
Dr, Newton Rd, Great Barr, BIRMINGHAM ☎ 0121 357 1141 105 en suite

WOLVERHAMPTON MAP 07 SO99

Oxley Park Stafford Rd, Bushbury WV10 6DE
☎ 01902 773989 ▤ 01902 773981
e-mail: secretary@oxleyparkgolfclub.co.uk
web: www.oxleyparkgolfclub.co.uk
Rolling parkland with trees, bunkers and water hazards.
18 holes, 6226yds, Par 71, SSS 71, Course record 66.
Club membership 550.
Visitors contact club for details. **Societies** welcome. **Green Fees** not
confirmed. **Prof** Les Burlison **Course Designer** H S Colt **Facilities** ⑪
⑱ by prior arrangement ⓔ ⓓ ✠⃝ ⚐ ⚑ ✔ **Leisure** snooker. **Conf** facs
Corporate Hospitality Days **Location** M54 junct 2, 2m S

Penn Penn Common, Penn WV4 5JN
☎ 01902 341142 ▤ 01902 620504
e-mail: penn-golf.freeserve.co.uk
Heathland course just outside the town.
18 holes, 6487yds, Par 70, SSS 72, Course record 65.
Club membership 650.
Visitors Mon-Fri. Dress code. **Societies** Booking required. **Green Fees** £28
per round, £33 per day. ☻ **Prof** Guy Dean **Facilities** ⑪ ⑱ ⓔ ⓓ ✠⃝ ⚐
⚑ ✔ **Location** SW of town centre off A449
Hotel ★★★ 72% HL Quality Hotel Wolverhampton, Penn Rd,
WOLVERHAMPTON ☎ 01902 429216 66 en suite 26 annexe en suite

South Staffordshire Danescourt Rd, Tettenhall WV6 9BQ
☎ 01902 751065 ▤ 01902 751159
e-mail: suelebeau@southstaffsgc.co.uk
web: www.southstaffordshiregolfclub.co.uk
A parkland course.

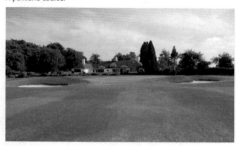

18 holes, 6531yds, Par 71, SSS 71, Course record 64.
Club membership 500.
Visitors Mon, Wed-Fri except BHs. Booking required. Handicap certificate.
Dress code. **Societies** Booking required. **Green Fees** £36 per round. ☻
Prof Peter Baker/Shaun Ball **Course Designer** Harry Vardon **Facilities**
⑪ ⑱ ⓔ ⓓ ✠⃝ ⚐ ⚑ ✔ **Conf** Corporate Hospitality Days
Location 3m NW off A41

Three Hammers Short Course Old Stafford Rd, Coven
WV10 7PP
☎ 01902 790428 ▤ 01902 791777
e-mail: info@3hammers.co.uk
web: www.3hammers.co.uk
Well maintained short course designed by Henry Cotton and providing
a unique challenge to golfers of all standards.
18 holes, 1438yds, Par 54, SSS 54, Course record 43.
Visitors Mon-Sun & BHs. **Societies** Welcome. **Green Fees** £6.50 per round
(£7.50 Sat, Sun & BHs). ☻ **Prof** Piers Ward, Andy Proudman
Course Designer Henry Cotton **Facilities** ⑪ ⑱ ⓔ ⓓ ✠⃝ ⚐ ✔
Conf Corporate Hospitality Days **Location** M54 junct 2, on A449 N

Wergs Keepers Ln, Tettenhall WV6 8UA
☎ 01902 742225 ▤ 01902 744748
e-mail: wergs.golfclub@btinternet.com
web: www.wergs.com
Gently undulating parkland with streams and ditches, a mix of
evergreen and deciduous trees and large greens.
18 holes, 6250yds, Par 72, SSS 70. Club membership 150.
Visitors Mon-Sun & BHs. Booking required Sat & Sun. Dress code.
Societies Booking required. **Green Fees** £17 per round (£22 Sat, Sun &
BHs). **Prof** Steve Weir **Course Designer** C W Moseley **Facilities** ⑪ ⑱ ⓔ ⓓ
✠⃝ ⚐ ⚑ ✔ ⚑ ✔ **Location** 3m W of Wolverhampton off A41

WIGHT, ISLE OF

COWES
MAP 04 SZ49

Cowes Crossfield Av PO31 8HN
☎ 01983 292303 (secretary) 📠 01983 292303
Fairly level, tight parkland course with difficult Par 3s and Solent views.
9 holes, 5934yds, Par 70, SSS 68, Course record 66.
Club membership 350.
Visitors Mon-Wed, Fri-Sun except BHs. Handicap certificate. Dress code.
Societies Booking required. **Green Fees** £20 (£25 Sat & Sun). 🔵
Course Designer Hamilton-Stutt **Facilities** ⑪ 🍴 🍵 🦵 ☕ 🏌 🧺 ⚲ ✍
Conf Corporate Hospitality Days **Location** NW of town centre next to
Cowes High School
Hotel ★★★ 72% HL Best Western New Holmwood Hotel, Queens Rd,
Egypt Point, COWES ☎ 01983 292508 26 en suite

EAST COWES
MAP 04 SZ59

Osborne Osborne House Estate PO32 6JX
☎ 01983 295421
e-mail: osbornegolfclub@tiscali.co.uk
web: www.osbornegolfclub.co.uk
Undulating parkland course in the grounds of Osborne House. Quiet
and peaceful situation with outstanding views.
9 holes, 6398yds, Par 70, SSS 70, Course record 69.
Club membership 450.
Visitors Mon, Thu, Fri & BHs. Tue, Sat & Sun pm only. Booking required Sat,
Sun & BHs. Handicap certificate. Dress code. **Societies** Booking required.
Green Fees £25 (£30 Sat, Sun & BHs). 🔵 **Facilities** ⑪ 🍴 🍵 🦵 ☕ 🏌 🧺
⚲ ✍ ✍ **Leisure** caddies available. **Location** E of town centre off A3021, in
Osborne House Estate
Hotel ★★★ 72% HL Best Western New Holmwood Hotel, Queens Rd,
Egypt Point, COWES ☎ 01983 292508 26 en suite

FRESHWATER
MAP 04 SZ38

Freshwater Bay Afton Down PO40 9TZ
☎ 01983 752955 📠 01983 752955
e-mail: tr.fbgc@btopenworld.com
web: www.isle-of-wight.uk.com/golf
18 holes, 5725yds, Par 69, SSS 68.
Course Designer J H Taylor **Location** 0.5m E of village off A3055
Telephone for further details
Hotel ★★★ 72% HL Sentry Mead Hotel, Madeira Rd, TOTLAND BAY
☎ 01983 753212 13 en suite

NEWPORT
MAP 04 SZ58

Newport St George's Down, Shide PO30 3BA
☎ 01983 525076
e-mail: mail@newportgolfclub.co.uk
web: www.newportgolfclub.co.uk
Challenging nine-hole course with water hazards, dog legs and fine
views.
9 holes, 5350yds, Par 68, SSS 66. Club membership 350.
Visitors Mon-Wed, Fri except BHs. Thu & Sun pm only. Booking required.
Societies booking required. **Green Fees** not confirmed. 🔵

Course Designer Guy Hunt **Facilities** ⑪ 🦵 ☕ 🏌 🧺 ⚲ 🍵 ✍
Location 1.5m S off A3020, 200yds past Newport Football Club on left
Hotel ★★★ 72% HL Best Western New Holmwood Hotel, Queens Rd,
Egypt Point, COWES ☎ 01983 292508 26 en suite

RYDE
MAP 04 SZ59

Ryde Binstead Rd PO33 3NF
☎ 01983 614809 📠 01983 567418
e-mail: ryde.golfclub@btinternet.com
web: www.rydegolf.co.uk
Downland course with wide views over the Solent. Very tight with out
of bound areas on most holes and five dog-legs.
9 holes, 5587yds, Par 70, SSS 69, Course record 65.
Club membership 500.
Visitors Mon, Tue, Thu & Fri. Wed, Sat, Sun & BHs pm only. Handicap
certificate. Dress code. **Societies** Booking required **Green Fees** 18 holes:
£20, 9 holes: £12 (£24/£16 Sat & Sun). 🔵 **Course Designer** Hamilton-Stutt
Facilities ⑪ 🍴 by prior arrangement 🦵 ☕ 🏌 🧺 ✍ **Location** 1m W
from town centre on A3054
Hotel ★★★ 72% HL Yelf's Hotel, Union St, RYDE ☎ 01983 564062
31 en suite 9 annexe en suite

SANDOWN
MAP 04 SZ58

Shanklin & Sandown The Fairway, Lake PO36 9PR
☎ 01983 403217 (office) & 404424 (pro) 📠 01983 403007
(office)/404424 (pro)
e-mail: club@ssgolfclub.com
web: www.ssgolfclub.com
An 18-hole county championship course, recognised for its natural
heathland beauty, spectacular views and challenging qualities. The
course demands respect, with accurate driving and careful club
selection the order of the day.
18 holes, 6062yds, Par 70, SSS 69, Course record 63.
Club membership 700.
Visitors Mon-Sun & BHs. Handicap certificate. Dress code. **Societies**
Booking required. **Green Fees** £32 (£40 Sat, Sun & BHs). **Prof** Peter
Hammond **Course Designer** Braid **Facilities** ⑪ 🍴 🍵 🦵 ☕ 🏌 🧺 ⚲ 🍵
✍ **Location** From Sandown towards Shanklin past Heights Leisure Centre,
200yds right into Fairway for 1m
Hotel ★★ 68% HL Cygnet Hotel, 58 Carter St, SANDOWN
☎ 01983 402930 45 en suite

VENTNOR
MAP 04 SZ57

Ventnor Steephill Down Rd PO38 1BP
☎ 01983 853326 & 853388 📠 01983 853326
e-mail: secretary@ventnorgolfclub.co.uk
web: www.ventnorgolfclub.co.uk
Downland course subject to wind. Fine seascapes.
12 holes, 5767yds, Par 70, SSS 68, Course record 64.
Club membership 297.
Visitors Mon-Sun except BHs. Dress code. **Societies** booking required.
Green Fees not confirmed. **Facilities** ⑪ 🍴 🍵 🦵 ☕ 🏌 🧺 ⚲ 🍵 ✍
Leisure practice nets. **Location** 1m NW off B3327, turn at chip shop
Hotel ★★★★ 76% HL The Royal Hotel, Belgrave Rd, VENTNOR
☎ 01983 852186 55 en suite

WILTSHIRE

BISHOPS CANNINGS
MAP 04 SU06

North Wilts SN10 2LP
☎ 01380 860627 📠 01380 860877
e-mail: secretary@northwiltsgolf.com
web: northwiltsgolf.com
Established in 1890 and one of the oldest courses in Wiltshire, North Wilts is situated high on the downlands of Wiltshire, with spectacular views over the surrounding countryside. The chalk base allows free draining and the course provides a challenge to golfers of all abilities.
18 holes, 6414yds, Par 71, SSS 71, Course record 65.
Club membership 800.
Visitors Mon-Sun & BHs. Dress code. **Societies** Booking Required **Green Fees** £32 per day (£37 per round Sat & Sun). **Prof** Graham Laing **Course Designer** H. S. Colt **Facilities** ⑪ ⑩ ⅃ ⅃ ♿ ☕ ⅃ ⌲ ⅃ ⅃ ⅃ ⅃ ⅃ **Conf** Corporate Hospitality Days **Location** 2m NW of Devizes between A4
Hotel ★★★ 72% HL Bear Hotel, Market Place, DEVIZES ☎ 01380 722444 25 en suite

BRADFORD-ON-AVON
MAP 03 ST86

Cumberwell Park BA15 2PQ
☎ 01225 863322 📠 01225 868160
e-mail: enquiries@cumberwellpark.com
web: www.cumberwellpark.com
Set within tranquil woodland, parkland, lakes and rolling countryside, this 27-hole course comprises three linked sets of nine holes. A challenge for all levels of golfer.

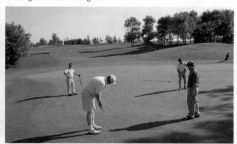

Red: 9 holes, 3296yds, Par 35.
Yellow: 9 holes, 3139yds, Par 36.
Blue: 9 holes, 3291yds, Par 36.
Orange: 9 holes, 3061yds, Par 35. Club membership 1300.
Visitors Mon-Sun & BHs. Booking required. Dress code. **Societies** Booking required. **Green Fees** £52 per 36 holes, £42 per 27 holes, £28 per 18 holes, £17 per 9 holes (£62/£52/£35/£26 Sat, Sun & BHs). **Prof** John Jacobs **Course Designer** Adrian Stiff **Facilities** ⑪ ⅃ ⅃ ♿ ☕ ⅃ ⅃ **Conf** facs Corporate Hospitality Days **Location** 1.5m N on A363
Hotel ★★★ 82% HL Woolley Grange, Woolley Green, BRADFORD-ON-AVON ☎ 01225 864705 14 en suite 12 annexe en suite

CALNE
MAP 03 ST97

Bowood Golf & Country Club Derry Hill SN11 9PQ
☎ 01249 822228 📠 01249 822218
e-mail: golfclub@bowood.org
web: www.bowood.org
This Dave Thomas designed course weaves through 200 acres of 'Capability' Brown's mature woodland with cavernous moulded bunkers, skilfully planned hillocks defining the fairways and vast rolling greens. Numerous doglegs, bunkers, tees and lakes will prove a test for any golfer.

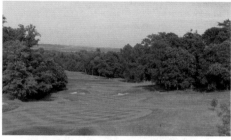

18 holes, 6890yds, Par 72, SSS 73, Course record 63.
Club membership 500.
Visitors Mon-Sun & BHs. Dress code. **Societies** Booking required. **Green Fees** £48 per round (£60 Sat & Sun). **Prof** John Hansel **Course Designer** Dave Thomas **Facilities** ⑪ ⑩ ⅃ ⅃ ♿ ☕ ⅃ ⅃ ⌲ ⅃ ⅃ ⅃ **Leisure** Bowood House and Gardens. **Conf** facs Corporate Hospitality Days **Location** 2.5m W of Calne off A4
Hotel ★★★ 72% HL Best Western Lansdowne Strand Hotel, The Strand, CALNE ☎ 01249 812488 21 en suite 5 annexe en suite

CASTLE COMBE
MAP 03 ST87

Manor House SN14 7HR
☎ 01249 782206 📠 01249 782992
e-mail: enquiries@manorhousegolfclub.com
web: www.exclusivehotels.co.uk
Set in a wonderful location within the wooded estate of the 14th-century Manor House, this course includes five Par 5s and some spectacular Par 3s. Manicured fairways and hand-cut greens, together with the River Bybrook meandering through the middle make for a picturesque and dramatic course.
The Manor House Golf Club at Castle Combe: 18 holes, 6500yds, Par 72. Club membership 450.
Visitors Mon-Sun & BHs. Booking required. Handicap certificate. Dress code. **Societies** Booking required. **Green Fees** £75 per round (£90 Fri-Sun). Spring/Autumn: £65/£80. Winter £40/$40. **Prof** Peter Green **Course Designer** Peter Alliss/Clive Clark **Facilities** ⑪ ⑩ ⅃ ⅃ ♿ ☕ ⅃ ⌲ ⅃ ⅃ ⅃ ⅃ **Leisure** hard tennis courts, fishing, sauna, croquet. **Conf** facs Corporate Hospitality Days **Location** 5m NW of Chippenham on B4039
Hotel ★★★★ CHH Manor House Hotel and Golf Club, CASTLE COMBE ☎ 01249 782206 22 en suite 26 annexe en suite

CHIPPENHAM
MAP 03 ST97

Chippenham Malmesbury Rd SN15 5LT
☎ 01249 652040 📄 01249 446681
e-mail: chippenhamgc@onetel.com
web: www.chippenhamgolfclub.co.uk
Easy walking on downland course. Testing holes at 1st and 15th.
18 holes, 5327yds, Par 69, SSS 66. Club membership 650.
Visitors Mon-Sun & BHs. Dress code. **Societies** Booking required. **Green Fees** £30 per day, £22 per round (£27 Sat & Sun). 😄 **Prof** Bill Creamer
Facilities ⊕ ⊚ ⊫ ⊑ ◨ ⊿ ⊜ ⚘ ⚔ ⏃ **Conf** Corporate Hospitality Days
Location M4 junct 17, 1m N of Chippenham by A350
Hotel ★★★★ CHH Manor House Hotel and Golf Club, CASTLE COMBE
☎ 01249 782206 22 en suite 26 annexe en suite

CRICKLADE
MAP 04 SU09

Cricklade Hotel & Country Club Common Hill
SN6 6HA
☎ 01793 750751 📄 01793 751767
e-mail: reception@crickladehotel.co.uk
web: www.crickladehotel.co.uk
A challenging nine-hole course with undulating greens and beautiful
views. Par 3 6th (128yds) signature hole from an elevated tee to a
green protected by a deep pot bunker.

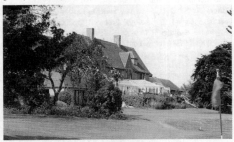

9 holes, 1830yds, Par 62, SSS 58, Course record 59.
Club membership 130.
Visitors Mon-Fri except BHs. Dress code. **Societies** Booking required.
Green Fees £25 per day, £16 for 18 holes. **Prof** Ian Bolt **Course Designer**
Ian Bolt/Colin Smith **Facilities** ⊕ ⊚ ⊫ ⊑ ◨ ⊿ ⚘ ◇ ⚔ **Leisure** hard
tennis courts, heated indoor swimming pool, solarium, gymnasium, snooker,
pool, jacuzzi, tennis, steam room. **Conf** facs **Location** On B4040 from
Cricklade towards Malmesbury
Hotel ★★★ 77% HL Cricklade Hotel, Common Hill, CRICKLADE
☎ 01793 750751 25 en suite 21 annexe en suite

ERLESTOKE
MAP 03 ST95

Erlestoke Sands SN10 5UB
☎ 01380 831069 📄 01380 831284
e-mail: info@erlestokesands.co.uk
web: www.erlestokesands.co.uk
18 holes, 6406yds, Par 73, SSS 71, Course record 66.
Course Designer Adrian Stiff **Location** On B3098 Devizes-Westbury road
Telephone for further details
Hotel ★★★ 72% HL Bear Hotel, Market Place, DEVIZES ☎ 01380 722444
25 en suite

GREAT DURNFORD
MAP 04 SU13

High Post SP4 6AT
☎ 01722 782356 📄 01722 782674
e-mail: admin@highpostgolfclub.co.uk
web: www.highpostgolfclub.co.uk
The free-draining, easy walking downland course offers summer tees
and greens all year. The opening three holes, usually played with the
wind, get you to off to a flying start, but the closing three provide a
tough finish. Peter Alliss has rated the 9th among his dream holes.
The club welcomes golfers of all abilities.

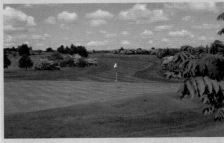

18 holes, 6305yds, Par 70, SSS 70, Course record 64.
Club membership 625.
Visitors Mon-Sun & BHs. Dress code. **Societies** Booking required.
Green Fees £50 per day; £32 per round (£50/£42 Sun & Sat). **Prof** Tony
Isaacs **Course Designer** Hawtree & Ptrs **Facilities** ⊕ ⊚ ⊫ ⊑ ◨ ⊿ ⊜
⚔ ⏃ **Conf** facs Corporate Hospitality Days **Location** On A345 between
Sailsbury and Amesbury
Hotel ★★★ 63% HL Quality Hotel Andover, Micheldever Rd, ANDOVER
☎ 01264 369111 13 en suite 36 annexe en suite

HIGHWORTH
MAP 04 SU29

Highworth Community Golf Centre Swindon Rd
SN6 7SJ
☎ 01793 766014 📄 01793 766014
9 holes, 3120yds, Par 35, SSS 35, Course record 29.
Course Designer T Watt/ B Sandry/D Lang **Location** Off A361 Swindon-
Lechlade road
Telephone for further details
Hotel ★★★ 75% HL BW Sudbury House Hotel & Conference Centre,
London St, FARINGDON ☎ 01367 241272 49 en suite

Wrag Barn Golf & Country Club Shrivenham Rd
SN6 7QQ
☎ 01793 861327 📄 01793 861325
e-mail: info@wragbarn.com
web: www.wragbarn.com
A fast maturing parkland course in an Area of Outstanding Natural
Beauty with views to the Lambourne Hills and Vale of the White Horse.
18 holes, 6633yds, Par 72, SSS 72, Course record 65.
Club membership 750.
Visitors Mon-Sun & BHs. Booking required Sat/Sun & BHs. Handicap
certificate. Dress code. **Societies** welcome. **Green Fees** not confirmed.
Prof Barry Loughrey **Course Designer** Hawtree **Facilities** ⊕ ⊚ ⊫ ⊑ ◨
⊿ ⊜ ⚘ ◇ ⚔ ⏃ **Conf** facs Corporate Hospitality Days **Location** On
B4000 from Highworth, signed
Hotel ★★★ 73% HL Stanton House Hotel, The Avenue, Stanton
Fitzwarren, SWINDON ☎ 0870 084 1388 82 en suite

England

KINGSDOWN MAP 03 ST86

Kingsdown SN13 8BS
☎ 01225 743472 📠 01225 743472
e-mail: kingsdowngc@btconnect.com
web: www.kingsdowngolfclub.co.uk
Fairly flat, open downland course with very sparse tree cover but surrounding wood. Many interesting holes with testing features.
18 holes, 6445yds, Par 72, SSS 71, Course record 64.
Club membership 750.
Visitors Mon-Fri except BHs. Dress code. **Societies** Booking required.
Green Fees £34 per day. ⊛ **Prof** Andrew Butler **Facilities** ⑪ ⓑ 🖤 🍴 🎿 ♨
🍴♟ 🏌 🏴 **Location** W of village between Corsham and Bathford
Hotel ★★★★★ CHH Lucknam Park, COLERNE ☎ 01225 742777
23 en suite 18 annexe en suite

LANDFORD MAP 04 SU21

Hamptworth Golf & Country Club Hamptworth Rd, Hamptworth SP5 2DU
☎ 01794 390155 📠 01794 390022
e-mail: info@hamptworthgolf.co.uk
web: www.hamptworthgolf.co.uk
Hamptworth enjoys ancient woodland and an abundance of wildlife in a beautiful setting on the northern edge of the New Forest. Many holes play alongside or over the Blackwater river with mature forest oaks guarding almost every fairway. Especially difficult holes are the 2nd, 5th, 7th, 9th, 11th and 14th.

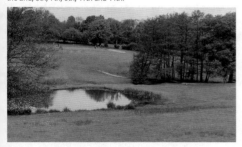

18 holes, 6448yds, Par 72, SSS 71, Course record 66.
Club membership 750.
Visitors Mon-Sun & BHs. Booking required. Dress code. **Societies** Booking required. **Green Fees** Apr-Sep: £30 per round, Oct-Mar: £25 (£40/£30 Sat & Sun). **Prof** Andy Beal **Course Designer** Philip Sanders/Brian Pierson **Facilities** ⑪ ⓞ ⓑ 🖤 🍴 🎿 🍴♟ 🏌 🏴 🏌 🏴 **Leisure** hard tennis courts, gymnasium, croquet lawns. **Conf** facs Corporate Hospitality Days **Location** 1.5m W of Landford off B3079
Hotel ★★★ 75% HL Bartley Lodge, Lyndhurst Rd, CADNAM
☎ 023 8081 2248 31 en suite

MARLBOROUGH MAP 04 SU16

Marlborough The Common SN8 1DU
☎ 01672 512147 📠 01672 513164
e-mail: contactus@marlboroughgolfclub.co.uk
web: www.marlboroughgolfclub.co.uk
Undulating downland course with extensive views over the Og valley and the Marlborough Downs.
18 holes, 6369yds, Par 72, SSS 71, Course record 61.
Club membership 900.

Visitors Mon-Sun & BHs. Booking required Sat, Sun & BHs. Dress code. **Societies** Booking required. **Green Fees** £42 per day, £30 per round (£55/£40 weekends). **Prof** S Amor **Facilities** ⑪ ⓞ ⓑ 🖤 🍴 🎿 🍴♟ 🏌 🏴 **Conf** facs Corporate Hospitality Days **Location** N of town centre on A346
Hotel ★★★ 64% HL The Castle & Ball, High St, MARLBOROUGH
☎ 01672 515201 34 en suite

OGBOURNE ST GEORGE MAP 04 SU27

Ogbourne Downs SN8 1TB
☎ 01672 841327 📠 01672 841101
web: www.ogdgc.co.uk
Downland turf and magnificent greens. Wind and slopes make this one of the most challenging courses in Wiltshire. Extensive views.
18 holes, 6363yds, Par 71, SSS 70, Course record 65.
Club membership 800.
Visitors Mon-Sun & BHs. Booking required. Dress code. **Societies** Booking required. **Green Fees** Phone. **Prof** Andrew Kirk **Course Designer** J H Taylor **Facilities** ⑪ ⓞ ⓑ 🖤 🎿 🍴♟ 🏌 🏴 **Conf** Corporate Hospitality Days **Location** N of village on A346
Hotel ★★★ 64% HL The Castle & Ball, High St, MARLBOROUGH
☎ 01672 515201 34 en suite

SALISBURY MAP 04 SU12

Salisbury & South Wilts Netherhampton SP2 8PR
☎ 01722 742645 📠 01722 742676
e-mail: mail@salisburygolf.co.uk
web: www.salisburygolf.co.uk
Gently undulating and well-drained parkland courses in country setting with panoramic views of the cathedral and surrounding countryside. Never easy with six excellent opening holes and four equally testing closing holes.
Main Course: 18 holes, 6485yds, Par 71, SSS 71, Course record 61.
Bibury Course: 9 holes, 2837yds, Par 34.
Club membership 1150.
Visitors Mon-Sun & BHs. Booking required Sat, Sun & BHs. Handicap certificate. Dress code. **Societies** Booking required. **Green Fees** Main: £36 per day, £30 per round. Bibury: £13 per 18 holes, £10 per 9 holes (£60/£45, £16/£13 Sat & Sun). ⊛ **Prof** Geraldine Teschner **Course Designer** J H Taylor/S Gidman **Facilities** ⑪ ⓞ ⓑ 🖤 🍴 🎿 🍴♟ 🏌 🏴 🏌 🏴 **Conf** facs Corporate Hospitality Days **Location** 2m SW of Salisbury on A3094
Hotel ★★★ 68% HL Grasmere House Hotel, Harnham Rd, SALISBURY
☎ 01722 338388 7 en suite 31 annexe en suite

SWINDON MAP 04 SU18

Broome Manor Golf Complex Pipers Way SN3 1RG
☎ 01793 532403 (bookings) 495761 (enquiries)
📠 01793 433255
Two courses and a 34-bay floodlit driving range. Parkland with water hazards, open fairways and short cut rough. Walking is easy on gentle slopes.
18 holes, 5989yds, Par 71, SSS 70, Course record 61.
9 holes, Par 33. Club membership 800.
Visitors Mon-Sun & BHs. Booking required. **Societies** welcome. **Green Fees** not confirmed. **Prof** Barry Sandry **Course Designer** Hawtree **Facilities** ⑪ ⓑ 🖤 🍴 🎿 🍴♟ 🏌 🏴 **Leisure** gymnasium. **Conf** facs Corporate Hospitality Days **Location** 1.75m SE of town centre off B4006
Hotel ★★★★ 76% HL Swindon Marriott Hotel, Pipers Way, SWINDON
☎ 0870 400 7281 156 en suite

TIDWORTH — MAP 04 SU24

Tidworth Garrison Bulford Rd SP9 7AF
☎ 01980 842301 ▤ 01980 842301
e-mail: tidworthgolfclub@btconnect.com
web: www.tidworthgolfclub.co.uk
A breezy, dry downland course with lovely turf, fine trees and
views over Salisbury Plain and the surrounding area. The 4th
and 12th holes are notable. The 565yd 14th, going down towards
the clubhouse, gives the big hitter a chance to let fly.
18 holes, 6320yds, Par 70, SSS 70, Course record 63.
Club membership 750.
Visitors Mon-Sun & BHs. Booking required. Handicap certificate. Dress
code. **Societies** Booking required. **Green Fees** £47 per round/day. ☺
Prof Terry Gosden **Course Designer** Donald Steel **Facilities** ⓣ ⓧ ▤
▯▯▯ ⚒ ⓹ ⓹ ⓹ **Location** W of village off A338
Hotel ★★★ 63% HL Quality Hotel Andover, Micheldever Rd, ANDOVER
☎ 01264 369111   13 en suite   36 annexe en suite

TOLLARD ROYAL — MAP 03 ST91

Rushmore SP5 5QB
☎ 01725 516326 ▤ 01725 516437
e-mail: golf@rushmoreuk.com
web: www.rushmoregolfclub.co.uk
Peaceful and testing parkland course situated on Cranborne Chase with
far-reaching views. An undulating course with avenues of trees and
well-drained greens. With water on seven out of 18 holes, it will test the
most confident of golfers.
18 holes, 6131yds, Par 71, SSS 70. Club membership 590.
Visitors Mon-Sun & BHs. Booking required. Dress code. **Societies** Booking
required. **Green Fees** £25 per round (£30 Sat & Sun). **Prof** Phil Jenkins
Course Designer David Pottage/John Jacobs Developments **Facilities** ⓣ
ⓧ by prior arrangement ▯▯ ⚒ ⓹ ⓹ ⓹ **Conf** facs Corporate
Hospitality Days **Location** N off B3081 between Sixpenny Handley & Tollard
Royal
Hotel ★★★ 71% HL Best Western Royal Chase Hotel, Royal Chase
Roundabout, SHAFTESBURY ☎ 01747 853355   33 en suite

UPAVON — MAP 04 SU15

Upavon Douglas Av SN9 6BQ
☎ 01980 630787 & 630281 ▤ 01980 635419
e-mail: play@upavongolfclub.co.uk
web: www.upavongolfclub.co.uk
Free-draining course on chalk downland with panoramic views over
the Vale of Pewsey and the Alton Barnes White Horse. A fair test of golf
with a good mixture of holes including a 602yd Par 5 and an excellent
finishing hole, a Par 3 of 169yds across a valley.
18 holes, 6402yds, Par 71, SSS 71, Course record 69.
Club membership 600.
Visitors Mon-Sun & BHs. Booking required. Dress code. **Societies** Booking
required. **Green Fees** £30 per day (£40 Sat & Sun). **Prof** Richard Blake
Course Designer Richard Blake **Facilities** ⓣ ⓧ by prior arrangement ▯
▯▯ ⚒ ⓹ ⓹ **Location** 1.5m SE of Upavon on A342
Hotel ★★★ 72% HL Bear Hotel, Market Place, DEVIZES ☎ 01380 722444
25 en suite

WARMINSTER — MAP 03 ST84

West Wilts Elm Hill BA12 0AU
☎ 01985 213133 ▤ 01985 219809
e-mail: sec@westwiltsgolfclub.co.uk
web: www.westwiltsgolfclub.co.uk
A hilltop chalk downland course among the Wiltshire downs. Free
draining, short, but a very good test of accurate iron play. Excellent
fairways and greens all year round.
18 holes, 5754yds, Par 70, SSS 68, Course record 60.
Club membership 570.
Visitors Mon-Fri, Sun & BHs. Booking required Sun. Handicap certificate.
Dress code. **Societies** Booking required. **Green Fees** £30 per day (£35
Sun & BHs). **Prof** Rob Morris **Course Designer** J H Taylor
Facilities ⓣ ⓧ by prior arrangement ▯ ▯▯ ⚒ ⓹ ⓹ ⓹
Conf Corporate Hospitality Days **Location** N of town centre off A350
Hotel ★★★★ 79% HL Bishopstrow House, WARMINSTER
☎ 01985 212312   32 en suite

WOOTTON BASSETT — MAP 04 SU08

Woodbridge Park Longmans Farm, Brinkworth
SN15 5DG
☎ 01666 510277
web: www.woodbridgepark.co.uk
Fairly long and open course with ditches and water hazards on the 2nd
and 18th holes. Several testing Par 3s with crosswinds and three long
and tricky Par 5s, notably the 4th, 8th and 14th holes.
18 holes, 5884yds, Par 70, SSS 70. Club membership 200.
Visitors Mon-Sun & BHs. **Societies** Booking required **Green Fees** £13 per
round (£17 Sat, Sun & BHs). ☺ **Course Designer** Chris Kane **Facilities**
▯▯ ⚒ ⓹ ⓹ ⓹ **Conf** facs Corporate Hospitality Days **Location** Off
B4042 between Malmesbury and Wootton Bassett
Hotel ★★★ 70% HL Marsh Farm Hotel, Coped Hall, WOOTTON BASSETT
☎ 01793 848044 & 842800 ▤ 01793 851528   11 en suite   39 annexe en suite

Wiltshire Vastern SN4 7PB
☎ 01793 849999 ▤ 01793 849988
e-mail: reception@the-wiltshire.co.uk
web: www.the-wiltshire.co.uk
A Peter Alliss and Howard Swan design set in rolling Wiltshire
downland. A number of lakes add a challenge for both low and high
handicappers.
Genevieve: 18 holes, 6519yds, Par 72, SSS 72,
Course record 67.
Garden: 9 holes, 3200yds, Par 71, SSS 71.
Club membership 450.
Visitors Mon-Sun & BHs. Booking required. Dress code. **Societies** Booking
required. **Green Fees** £25 per 18 holes (£35 Sat, Sun & BHs). **Course
Designer** Peter Allis & Howard Swan **Facilities** ⓣ ⓧ ▯ ▯▯ ⚒ ⓹ ⓹
⓹ ⓹ ⓹ **Leisure** heated indoor swimming pool, sauna, solarium,
gymnasium, creche. **Conf** facs Corporate Hospitality Days **Location** Off
A3102 SW of Wootton Bassett
Hotel ★★★ 75% HL The Wiltshire Hotel & Country Club, WOOTTON
BASSETT ☎ 01793 849999 58 rms (56 en suite)

England

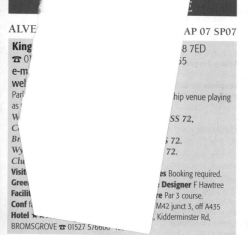

ALVE   AP 07 SP07

King   8 7ED
☎ 01   55
e-m
web
Par   hip venue playing
as
W   SS 72,
C
Br   72.
Wy   72.
Clu
Visit   es Booking required.
Gree   **Designer** F Hawtree
Facilit   e Par 3 course.
Conf f   M42 junct 3, off A435
Hotel ★   Kidderminster Rd,
BROMSGROVE ☎ 01527 576600

BEWDLEY   MAP 07 SO77

Little Lakes Golf and Country Club Lye Head
DY12 2UZ
☎ 01299 266385 ▤ 01299 266398
e-mail: mark.laing@littlelakes.co.uk
web: www.little-lakes.co.uk
A pleasant undulating 18-hole parkland course. A challenging test
of golf with stunning views of the Worcestershire countryside. Well
acclaimed for the use of natural features.
18 holes, 6298yds, Par 71, SSS 70, Course record 68.
Club membership 475.
Visitors Mon-Sun & BHs. Booking required. Dress code. **Societies** booking
required. **Green Fees** not confirmed. **Prof** Mark A Laing **Course Designer**
M Laing **Facilities** ⊕ by prior arrangement ⬤ by prior arrangement ⬤
by prior arrangement ⬚ by prior arrangement ⬚ ⬚ ⬚ ⬚ ⬚ ⬚ **Leisure**
hard tennis courts, heated outdoor swimming pool, fishing. **Conf** facs
Location 2.25m W of Bewdley off A456

Wharton Park Longbank DY12 2QW
☎ 01299 405163 ▤ 01299 405121
e-mail: enquiries@whartonpark.co.uk
web: www.whartonpark.co.uk
An 18-hole championship-standard course set in 200 acres of beautiful
Worcestershire countryside, with stunning views. Some long Par 5s
such as the 9th (594yds) as well as superb Par 3 holes at 3rd, 10th
and 15th make this a very challenging course.

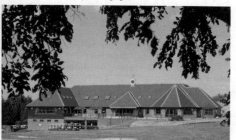

---

18 holes, 6435yds, Par 72, SSS 71, Course record 66.
Club membership 500.
Visitors Mon-Sun & BHs. Booking required. Dress code. **Societies** Booking
required. **Green Fees** Phone. **Prof** Angus Hoare **Course Designer** Howard
Swan **Facilities** ⊕ ⦿ ⬚ ⬚ ⬚ ⬚ ⬚ ⬚ ⬚ ⬚ ⬚ **Conf** facs Corporate
Hospitality Days **Location** Off A456 Bewdley bypass

BISHAMPTON   MAP 03 SO95

Vale Golf Club Hill Furze Rd WR10 2LZ
☎ 01386 462781 ▤ 01386 462597
e-mail: vale-sales@crown-golf.co.uk
web: www.crown-golf.co.uk
This course offers an American-style layout, with large greens, trees
and bunkers and several water hazards. Its rolling fairways provide a
testing round, as well as superb views of the Malvern Hills. Picturesque
and peaceful.
*International Course: 18 holes, 7174yds, Par 74, SSS 74,
Course record 67.*
Lenches Course: 9 holes, 5518yds, Par 70, SSS 66.
Club membership 800.
Visitors Mon-Sun & BHs. Booking required. Dress code. **Societies** Booking
required. **Green Fees** International: £28 per round, Lenchese: 9 holes £11
(£40/£12 Sat & Sun). **Prof** Richard Jenkins **Course Designer** Bob Sandow
Facilities ⊕ ⦿ ⬚ ⬚ ⬚ ⬚ ⬚ ⬚ ⬚ ⬚ ⬚ **Conf** facs Corporate
Hospitality Days **Hotel** ★★★ 80% HL Best Western Salford Hall Hotel, ABBOT'S SALFORD
☎ 01386 871300 & 0800 212671 ▤ 01386 871301 14 en suite 19 annexe
en suite

BROADWAY   MAP 04 SP03

Broadway Willersey Hill WR12 7LG
☎ 01386 853683 ▤ 01386 858643
e-mail: secretary@broadwaygolfclub.co.uk
web: www.broadwaygolfclub.co.uk
At the edge of the Cotswolds this downland course lies at an altitude
of 900ft above sea level, with extensive views. Natural contours
and man-made hazards mean that drives have to be placed and
approaches carefully judged. The small contour greens demand well
placed and accurate shots and a Par is by no means a certainty.
18 holes, 6228yds, Par 72, SSS 70, Course record 63.
Club membership 850.
Visitors Mon-Sun & BHs. Handicap certificate. Dress code. **Societies**
Booking required **Green Fees** £38 per day, £30 per round (£38 Sat, Sun &
BHs). **Prof** Martyn Freeman **Course Designer** James Braid **Facilities** ⊕
⦿ ⬚ ⬚ ⬚ ⬚ ⬚ ⬚ ⬚ ⬚ **Conf** facs Corporate Hospitality Days
Location 1.5m E on A44
Hotel ★★★ 83% HL Dormy House Hotel, Willersey Hill, BROADWAY
☎ 01386 852711 25 en suite 20 annexe en suite
Hotel ★★★★ 82% GH Leasow House, Laverton Meadows, BROADWAY
☎ 01386 584526 Fax 01386 584596 5 en suite 2 annexe en suite

England

BROMSGROVE MAP 07 SO97

Blackwell Agmore Rd, Blackwell B60 1PY
☎ 0121 445 1994 📠 0121 445 4911
e-mail: info@blackwellgolfclub.com
web: www.blackwellgolfclub.co.uk
Mature undulating parkland course over a 110 years old, with a variety
of trees. Laid out in two nine-hole loops.
18 holes, 6080yds, Par 70, SSS 71, Course record 61.
Club membership 355.
Visitors Mon, Wed-Fri except BHs. Tue pm only. Handicap certificate. Dress
code. **Societies** Booking required. **Green Fees** £75 per day, £65 per round.
🟢 **Prof** Finlay Clark **Course Designer** Herbert Fowler/Tom Simpson
Facilities ⑪ by prior arrangement 🍴 by prior arrangement 🧺 🖺 🏌 ⚷
🏠 ⛳ 🏌 ⚷ **Conf** Corporate Hospitality Days **Location** 2.5m NE of
Bromsgrove off B4096

Bromsgrove Golf Centre Stratford Rd B60 1LD
☎ 01527 575886 & 570505 📠 01527 570964
e-mail: enquiries@bromsgrovegolfcentre.com
web: www.bromsgrovegolfcentre.com
This gently undulating course with superb views over Worcestershire is
not to be underestimated. Creative landscaping and a selection of well-
defined bunkers ensure that the course delivers a uniquely satisfying
experience through a variety of challenging, yet enjoyable, holes.

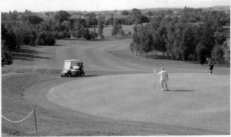

18 holes, 5969yds, Par 68, SSS 69. Club membership 900.
Visitors Mon-Sun & BHs. Dress code. **Societies** Booking required. **Green
Fees** £19.70 per 18 holes (£26.20 Sat & Sun). **Prof** Graeme Long/Danny
Wall **Course Designer** Hawtree & Son **Facilities** ⑪ 🍴 🧺 🖺 🏌 🧺 ⚷
⛳ 🏠 ⚷ 🏌 **Conf** facs Corporate Hospitality Days **Location** 1m from town
centre at junct A38A448, signed
Hotel ★★★★ 71% HL The Bromsgrove Hotel, Kidderminster Rd,
BROMSGROVE ☎ 01527 576600 109 en suite

DROITWICH MAP 03 SO86

Droitwich Golf & Country Club Ford Ln WR9 0BQ
☎ 01905 774344 📠 01905 797290
e-mail: droitwich-golf-club@tiscali.co.uk
Undulating wooded parkland with scenic views from the highest
points.
Droitwich Golf Club: 18 holes, 5976yds, Par 70, SSS 69,
Course record 62. Club membership 732.
Visitors Mon-Fri except BHs. Handicap certificate. Dress code. **Societies**
Booking required. **Green Fees** £30 per day, £25 per round. 🟢 **Prof** Phil
Gundy **Course Designer** J Braid/G Franks **Facilities** ⑪ 🍴 🧺 🖺 🏌 🧺 ⚷
⚷ **Leisure** snooker. **Conf** Corporate Hospitality Days **Location** M5 junct 5,
off A38 at Droitwich opposite Chateau Impney Hotel
Hotel ★★★★ 72% HL Raven Hotel, Victoria Square, DROITWICH SPA
☎ 01905 772224 72 en suite

Gaudet Luce Middle Ln, Hadzor WR9 7DP
☎ 01905 796375 📠 01905 797245
e-mail: info@gaudet-luce.co.uk
web: www.gaudet-luce.co.uk
18 holes, 6040yds, Par 70, SSS 68.
Course Designer M A Laing **Location** M5 junct 5, left at Tagwell Rd onto
Middle Ln, 1st driveway on left
Telephone for further details
Hotel ★★★★ 72% HL Raven Hotel, Victoria Square, DROITWICH SPA
☎ 01905 772224 72 en suite

Ombersley Bishops Wood Rd, Lineholt, Ombersley
WR9 0LE
☎ 01905 620747 📠 01905 620047
e-mail: enquiries@ombersleygolfclub
web: www.ombersleygolfclub.co.uk
Undulating course in beautiful countryside high above the edge of the
Severn valley. Covered driving range and putting green.
18 holes, 6139yds, Par 72, SSS 69, Course record 67.
Club membership 750.
Visitors Mon-Sun & BHs. Dress code. **Societies** Booking required.
Green Fees £18.95 per 18 holes, £11.40 per 9 holes (£26.90/£16.20 Sat,
Sun & BHs). **Prof** Glenister, Woodman **Course Designer** David Morgan
Facilities ⑪ 🍴 🧺 🖺 🏌 🧺 🏠 ⛳ ⚷ 🏌 ⚷ **Leisure** chipping green &
practice bunker. **Conf** facs Corporate Hospitality Days **Location** 3m W of
Droitwich off A449. At Mitre Oak pub A4025 to Stourport, signed 400yds
on left
Hotel ★★★★ 72% HL Raven Hotel, Victoria Square, DROITWICH SPA
☎ 01905 772224 72 en suite

FLADBURY MAP 03 SO94

Evesham Craycombe Links, Old Worcester Rd WR10 2QS
☎ 01386 860395 📠 01386 861356
e-mail: eveshamgolfclub@talk21.com
web: eveshamgolf.com
9 holes, 6415yds, Par 72, Course record 65.
Location 0.75m N on A4538
Telephone for further details
Hotel ★★★ 79% HL The Evesham Hotel, Coopers Ln, Off Waterside,
EVESHAM ☎ 01386 765566 & 0800 716969 (Res) 📠 01386 765443 39 en s
uite 1 annexe en suite

HOLLYWOOD MAP 07 SP07

Gay Hill Hollywood Ln B47 5PP
☎ 0121 430 8544 & 474 6001 (pro) 📠 0121 436 7796
e-mail: secretary@ghgc.org.uk
web: www.ghgc.org.uk
Parkland with some 10,000 trees and a brook running through.
18 holes, 6406yds, Par 72, SSS 72, Course record 64.
Club membership 700.
Visitors Mon-Sun except BHs. Booking required. Handicap certificate. Dress
code. **Societies** Booking required. **Green Fees** £35 per round. **Prof** Chris
Harrison **Facilities** ⑪ 🧺 🖺 🏌 🧺 🏠 ⛳ ⚷ **Location** N of village
Hotel ★★★ 71% HL Corus hotel Solihull, Stratford Rd, Shirley, SOLIHULL
☎ 0870 609 6133 111 en suite

KIDDERMINSTER
MAP 07 SO87

Churchill and Blakedown Churchill Ln, Blakedown DY10 3NB
☎ 01562 700018 📠 0871 242 2049
e-mail: cbgolfclub@tiscali.co.uk
Mature hilly course, playable all year round, with good views.
9 holes, 6488yds, Par 72, SSS 71. Club membership 410.
Visitors may play Tue,Wed, Fri & BHs. Advance booking required. Handicap certificate required. Dress code. **Societies** advance booking required.
Green Fees not confirmed. 🌐 **Prof** G. Wright **Facilities** ⑪ ⑩ 🍴 🍺 ♡ ⚑ 🏌 🎯 💰 **Conf** Corporate Hospitality Days **Location** W of village off A456
Hotel ★★★★ 78% HL Stone Manor Hotel, Stone, KIDDERMINSTER
☎ 01562 777555 52 en suite 5 annexe en suite

Habberley Low Habberley, Trimpley Rd DY11 5RF
☎ 01562 745756 📠 01562 745756
e-mail: dave.mcdermott@blueyonder.co.uk
web: www.habberleygolfclub.co.uk
Wooded, undulating parkland.
9 holes, 5401yds, Par 69, SSS 67, Course record 62. Club membership 108.
Visitors Mon-Fri & BHs. Booking required Sat & Sun. Dress code.
Societies Booking required. **Green Fees** £15 per day (£10 winter). 🌐
Facilities ⑪ ⑩ 🍺 ♡ ⚑ 🎯 **Location** 2m NW of Kidderminster
Hotel ★★★★ 78% HL Stone Manor Hotel, Stone, KIDDERMINSTER
☎ 01562 777555 52 en suite 5 annexe en suite

Kidderminster Russell Rd DY10 3HT
☎ 01562 822303 📠 01562 827866
e-mail: info@kidderminstergolfclub.com
web: www.kidderminstergolfclub.com
Pleasant wooded parkland course, mainly flat, but a good test of golf for all levels of player. Two small lakes add to the challenge.

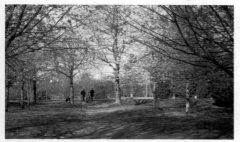

18 holes, 6422yds, Par 72, SSS 71, Course record 65. Club membership 860.
Visitors Mon & Wed-Fri except BHs. Handicap certificate. Dress code.
Societies Booking required. **Green Fees** £35 per day. **Prof** Pat Smith
Facilities ⑪ ⑩ 🍺 ♡ ⚑ 🏌 🎯 💰 🏌 💰 **Conf** facs Corporate Hospitality Days **Location** 0.5m SE of town centre, signed off A449
Hotel ★★★★ 78% HL Stone Manor Hotel, Stone, KIDDERMINSTER
☎ 01562 777555 52 en suite 5 annexe en suite

Wyre Forest Zortech Av DY11 7EX
☎ 01299 822682 📠 01299 879433
e-mail: chris@wyreforestgolf.com
web: www.wyreforestgolf.co.uk
Making full use of the existing contours, this interesting and challenging course is bounded by woodland and gives extensive views over the surrounding area. Well drained fairways and greens give an inland links style.
18 holes, 5790yds, Par 70, SSS 68, Course record 68. Club membership 397.
Visitors Mon-Sun & BHs. Booking required Sat/Sun & BHs. Dress code.
Societies booking required. **Green Fees** not confirmed. **Prof** Chris Botterill **Facilities** ⑪ ⑩ 🍴 🍺 ♡ ⚑ 🏌 🎯 🏌 💰 🎯 **Conf** Corporate Hospitality Days **Location** On A451 between Kidderminster and Stourport
Hotel ★★★ 72% HL Gainsborough House Hotel, Bewdley Hill, KIDDERMINSTER ☎ 01562 820041 42 en suite

MALVERN
MAP 03 SO74

Worcestershire Wood Farm, Wood Farm Rd WR14 4PP
☎ 01684 575992 📠 01684 893334
e-mail: secretary@worcsgolfclub.co.uk
web: www.worcsgolfclub.co.uk
Fairly easy walking on windy downland course with trees, ditches and other natural hazards. Outstanding views of the Malvern Hills and the Severn valley. The 17th hole (Par 5) is approached over small lake.
18 holes, 6455yds, Par 71, SSS 72. Club membership 750.
Visitors Mon-Fri except BHs. Booking required. Handicap certificate. Dress code. **Societies** Booking required. **Green Fees** £38 per day, £32 per round. 🌐 **Prof** Richard Lewis **Course Designer** J H Taylor **Facilities** ⑪ ⑩ 🍺 ♡ ⚑ 🎯 🏌 💰 **Leisure** indoor teaching facility. **Conf** Corporate Hospitality Days **Location** 2m S of Gt Malvern on B4209
Hotel ★★★ 83% HL The Cottage in the Wood Hotel, Holywell Rd, Malvern Wells, MALVERN ☎ 01684 575859 8 en suite 23 annexe en suite

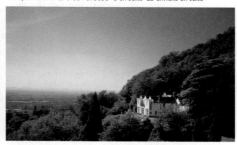

Hotel ★★ 80% HL Holdfast Cottage Hotel, Marlbank Rd, Welland, MALVERN ☎ 01684 310288 Fax 01684 311117 8 en suite

England

REDDITCH
MAP 07 SP06

Abbey Hotel Golf & Country Club Dagnell End Rd, Hither Green Ln B98 9BE
☎ 01527 406600 & 406500 📠 01527 406514
e-mail: info@theabbeyhotel.co.uk
web: www.theabbeyhotel.co.uk
Parkland with rolling fairways with trees and lakes on several holes. Course improvements have resulted in a course which requires more thought than before. Pure putting surfaces are a worthy reward for some solid iron play, allowing the golfer to make the most of a birdie.

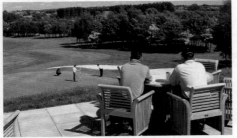

18 holes, 6561yds, Par 72, SSS 72. Club membership 397.
Visitors Mon-Sun & BHs. Booking required. Dress code. **Societies** booking required. **Green Fees** not confirmed. **Prof** R Davies **Course Designer** Donald Steele **Facilities** ⊕ ⍟ ⯊ ⬛ ➘ ⬛ ⚒ ⛿ ✦ ⬟ ✦ **Leisure** heated indoor swimming pool, fishing, sauna, solarium, gymnasium. **Conf** facs Corporate Hospitality Days **Location** A441 N from town, onto B4101 signed Beoley, right onto Hither Green Ln
Hotel ★★★★ 80% HL Best Western Abbey Hotel Golf & Country Club, Hither Green Ln, Dagnell End Rd, Bordesley, REDDITCH ☎ 01527 406600 100 en suite

See advert on this page

Pitcheroak Plymouth Rd B97 4PB
☎ 01527 541054 📠 01527 65216
Woodland course, hilly in places. There is also a putting green and a practice ground.
9 holes, 4561yds, Par 65, SSS 62. Club membership 150.
Visitors Mon-Sun & BHs. Booking required Sat/Sun & BHs. **Societies** booking required. **Green Fees** not confirmed. **Prof** David Stewart **Facilities** ⊕ ⍟ ⯊ ⬛ ➘ ⬛ ⚒ ⛿ ✦ **Location** SW of town centre off A448
Hotel ★★★ 66% HL Quality Hotel Redditch, Pool Bank, Southcrest, REDDITCH ☎ 01527 541511 73 en suite

Redditch Lower Grinsty, Green Ln, Callow Hill B97 5PJ
☎ 01527 543079 (sec) 📠 01527 547413
e-mail: lee@redditchgolfclub.com
web: www.redditchgolfclub.com
Parkland with many tree-lined fairways, excellent greens, and a particularly tough finish. The Par 3s are all long and demanding.
18 holes, 6671yds, Par 72, SSS 72, Course record 68. Club membership 650.
Visitors Mon-Fri except BHs. Booking required Tue & Thu. Handicap certificate. Dress Code. **Societies** Booking required **Green Fees** £45 per day, £35 per round. **Prof** David Down **Course Designer** F Pennick **Facilities** ⊕ ⍟ ⯊ ⬛ ➘ ⬛ ⚒ ⛿ ✦ **Location** 2m SW
Hotel ★★★ 66% HL Quality Hotel Redditch, Pool Bank, Southcrest, REDDITCH ☎ 01527 541511 73 en suite

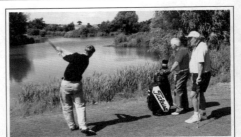

TENBURY WELLS
MAP 07 SO56

Cadmore Lodge Hotel & Country Club St Michaels, Berrington Green WR15 8TQ
☎ 01584 810044 📠 01584 810044
e-mail: info@cadmorelodge.demon.co.uk
web: www.cadmorelodge.demon.co.uk
A picturesque 9-hole course in a brook valley. Challenging holes include the 1st and 6th over the lake, 8th over the valley and 9th over hedges.

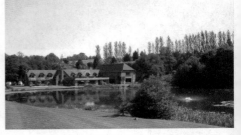

9 holes, 5132yds, Par 68, SSS 65. Club membership 200.
Visitors Mon-Fri & BHs. Booking required Wed, Fri & BHs. Dress code. **Societies** Booking required **Green Fees** £11 per day (£15 Sat & Sun). **Course Designer** G Farr, J Weston **Facilities** ⊕ ⍟ ⯊ ⬛ ➘ ⬛ ⚒ ◇ ✦ **Leisure** heated indoor swimming pool, fishing, sauna, gymnasium, pool table. **Conf** facs Corporate Hospitality Days **Location** A4112 from Tenbury to Leominster, 2m right for Berrington, 0.75m on left
Hotel ★★ 74% HL Cadmore Lodge Hotel & Country Club, Berrington Green, St Michaels, TENBURY WELLS ☎ 01584 810044 15 rms (14 en suite)

WORCESTER MAP 03 SO85

Bank House Hotel Golf & Country Club Bransford
WR6 5JD
☎ 01886 833545 📠 01886 832461
e-mail: bankhouse@brook-hotels.co.uk
web: www.bw-bankhouse.co.uk

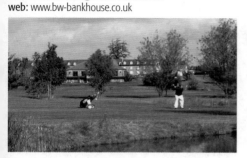

*Bransford Course: 18 holes, 6204yds, Par 72, SSS 71,
Course record 65.*
Course Designer Bob Sandow **Location** M5 junct 7, A4103 3m S of
Worcester
Telephone for further details

Perdiswell Park Bilford Rd WR3 8DX
☎ 01905 754668 & 457189
Set in 85 acres of attractive parkland and suitable for all levels of golfer.
18 holes, 5297yds, Par 68, SSS 66. Club membership 300.
Visitors Mon-Sun & BHs. Dress code. **Societies** Welcome. **Green Fees**
£10.50 per 18 holes, £7 per 9 holes (£14.25/£9 Sat & Sun). **Prof** Mark
Woodward **Facilities** ⊕ ⭐ 🍴 ⭐ 💬 🍴 🏌 🍴 ✓ **Leisure** gymnasium.
Conf facs Corporate Hospitality Days **Location** N of city centre off A30
Hotel ★★★ 81% HL Pear Tree Inn & Country Hotel, Smite, WORCESTER
☎ 01905 756565 24 en suite

Worcester Golf & Country Club Boughton Park
WR2 4EZ
☎ 01905 422555 📠 01905 749090
e-mail: worcestergcc@btconnect.com
web: www.worcestergcc.co.uk
Fine parkland course with many trees, lakes and views of the Malvern
Hills.
*18 holes, 6251yds, Par 70, SSS 70, Course record 64.
Club membership 1050.*
Visitors Mon-Fri & BHs. Booking required. Handicap certificate. Dress code.
Societies Booking required. **Green Fees** £45 per day, £35 per round.
Prof Graham Farr **Course Designer** Dr A Mackenzie **Facilities** ⊕ by
prior arrangement ⭐ by prior arrangement 🍴 💬 🍴 🏌 🍴 ✓ **Leisure**
hard and grass tennis courts, squash. **Conf** facs Corporate Hospitality Days
Location 1.5m from city centre on A4103

WYTHALL MAP 07 SP07

Fulford Heath Tanners Green Ln B47 6BH
☎ 01564 824758 📠 01564 822629
e-mail: secretary@fulfordheath.co.uk
web: www.fulfordheath.co.uk
A mature parkland course encompassing two classic Par 3s. The 11th,
a mere 149yds, shoots from an elevated tee through a channel of trees
to a well-protected green. The 16th, a 166yd Par 3, elevated green,
demands a 140yd carry over an imposing lake.

18 holes, 5959yds, Par 70, SSS 69. Club membership 850.
Visitors Mon-Fri except BHs. Handicap certificate. Dress code **Societies**
Booking required. **Green Fees** £36 per day. ⊕ **Prof** Richard Dunbar
Course Designer Braid/Hawtree **Facilities** ⊕ ⭐ 🍴 💬 🍴 🏌 🍴 ✓
Conf Corporate Hospitality Days **Location** 1m SE off A435
Hotel ★★★★ 77% HL Renaissance Solihull Hotel, 651 Warwick Rd,
SOLIHULL ☎ 0121 711 3000 179 en suite

YORKSHIRE, EAST RIDING OF

ALLERTHORPE MAP 08 SE85

Allerthorpe Park Allerthorpe Park YO42 4RL
☎ 01759 306686 📠 01759 304308
e-mail: allerthorpepark@aol.com
web: www.allerthorpeparkgolfclub.com
A picturesque parkland course, maintained to a high standard, with
many interesting features, including a meandering beck and the 18th
hole over the lake.
*18 holes, 6430yds, Par 70, SSS 70, Course record 67.
Club membership 500.*
Visitors Mon-Sun & BHs. Dress code. **Societies** Booking required **Green
Fees** £30 per day, £22 per 18 holes. **Prof** James Calam **Course Designer**
J G Hatcliffe & Partners **Facilities** ⊕ ⭐ 🍴 ⭐ 💬 by prior arrangement ⭐🍴
🏌 🍴 ✓ **Conf** facs Corporate Hospitality Days **Location** 2m SW of
Pocklington off A1079
Hotel ★★ 65% HL Feathers Hotel, 56 Market Place, POCKLINGTON
☎ 01759 303155 10 en suite 6 annexe en suite

AUGHTON MAP 08 SE73

Oaks Aughton Common YO42 4PW
☎ 01757 288577 📠 01757 288232
e-mail: sheila@theoaksgolfclub.co.uk
web: www.theoaksgolfclub.co.uk
The course is built in harmony with its natural wooded parkland
setting, near to the Derwent Ings. The wide green fairways blend and
bend with the gentle countryside. Seven lakes come into play.

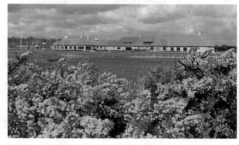

*18 holes, 6792yds, Par 72, SSS 72, Course record 65.
Club membership 700.*
Visitors Mon-Fri excluding BHs. Booking required. Dress code. **Societies**
Booking required. **Green Fees** £40 per day, £28.per round. **Prof** Graham
Walker **Course Designer** Julian Covey **Facilities** ⊕ ⭐ 🍴 🍴 💬 🍴 🏌 🍴
🏐 ◇ ✓ 🍴 🏌 **Leisure** heated indoor swimming pool, sauna, solarium,
gymnasium, small outdoor & indoor own putting greens. **Conf** facs
Corporate Hospitality Days **Location** 1m N of Bubwith on B1228
Hotel ★★★ 78% HL The Parsonage Country House Hotel, York Rd,
ESCRICK ☎ 01904 728111 12 en suite 36 annexe en suite

See advert on page 281

BEVERLEY   MAP 08 TA03

Beverley & East Riding The Westwood HU17 8RG
☎ 01482 868757 📠 01482 868757
e-mail: golf@beverleyandeastridinggolfclub.karoo.co.uk
Picturesque parkland with some hard walking and natural hazards
- trees and gorse bushes. Only two fairways adjoin. Cattle (spring to
autumn) and horse-riders are occasional early morning hazards.
Westwood: 18 holes, 6127yds, Par 69, SSS 69,
Course record 64. Club membership 530.
Visitors Mon-Sun & BHs. Booking required. Dress code. **Societies** booking
required. **Green Fees** not confirmed. ⊕ **Prof** Alex Ashby **Facilities** ⊕ ⓘⓘ
🝾 ⌨ 🍴 ⏣ 📷 ☂ ✦ **Location** 1m SW on B1230
Hotel ★★ 76% HL The Manor House, Northlands, Walkington, BEVERLEY
☎ 01482 881645   6 en suite   1 annexe en suite

BRANDESBURTON   MAP 08 TA14

Hainsworth Park Burton Holme YO25 8RT
☎ 01964 542362
18 holes, 6362yds, Par 71, SSS 71.
Location SW of village on A165
Telephone for further details
Hotel ★★ 69% HL Burton Lodge Hotel, BRANDESBURTON
☎ 01964 542847   7 en suite   2 annexe en suite

BRIDLINGTON   MAP 08 TA16

Bridlington Belvedere Rd YO15 3NA
☎ 01262 606367 📠 01262 606367
e-mail: enquiries@bridlingtongolfclub.co.uk
web: www.bridlingtongolfclub.co.uk
Parkland alongside Bridlington Bay, with tree-lined fairways and six
ponds, comprising two loops of 9 holes. Excellent putting surfaces.
18 holes, 6638yds, Par 72, SSS 72, Course record 66.
Club membership 600.
Visitors Mon-Sun & BHs. Booking required. Dress code. **Societies** Booking
required. **Green Fees** £30 per day, £23 per round (£40/£32 Sat & Sun).
Prof Anthony Howarth **Course Designer** James Braid **Facilities** 🝾 ⌨
🍴 ⏣ 📷 ☂ ✦ 🛒 ✦ **Leisure** snooker. **Conf** Corporate Hospitality Days
Location 1m S off A165
Hotel ★★★ 73% HL Revelstoke Hotel, 1-3 Flamborough Rd,
BRIDLINGTON ☎ 01262 672362   26 en suite

Bridlington Links Flamborough Rd, Marton YO15 1DW
☎ 01262 401584 📠 01262 401702
Main: 18 holes, 6719yds, Par 72, SSS 72, Course record 70.
Course Designer Swan **Location** On B1255 between Bridlington
Telephone for further details
Hotel ★★★ 74% HL Expanse Hotel, North Marine Dr, BRIDLINGTON
☎ 01262 675347   48 en suite

BROUGH   MAP 08 SE92

Brough Cave Rd HU15 1HB
☎ 01482 667291 📠 01482 669873
e-mail: gt@brough-golfclub.co.uk
web: www.brough-golfclub.co.uk
Parkland course, where accurate positioning of the tee ball is required
for good scoring. Testing for the scratch player without being too
difficult for the higher handicap.
18 holes, 6067yds, Par 68, SSS 69, Course record 62.
Club membership 680.

Visitors Mon, Tue, Thu-Sun & BHs. Booking required. Handicap certificate.
Dress code. **Societies** Booking required. **Green Fees** £50 per day, £35 per
round (£70/£55 Sat, Sun & BHs). ⊕ **Prof** Gordon Townhill **Facilities** ⊕
ⓘⓘ 🝾 ⌨ 🍴 ⏣ 📷 ☂ ✦ **Conf** Corporate Hospitality Days **Location** 8m
W of Hull off A63
Hotel ★★★ 68% HL Elizabeth Hotel Hull, Ferriby High Rd, NORTH
FERRIBY ☎ 01482 645212   95 en suite

BURSTWICK   MAP 08 TA22

Burstwick Country Golf Ellifoot Ln HU12 9EF
☎ 01964 670112 📠 01964 670116
e-mail: info@burstwickcountrygolf.co.uk
web: www.burstwickcountrygolf.co.uk
A newly designed 18 hole course with 72 bunkers, 5 lakes and 4,500
trees set in attractive countryside. Not a long course but very
challenging with well-guarded greens, exposed tee shots and sharp
dog-legs. All greens to full USGA specification.
18 holes, 6100yds, Par 70, SSS 69. Club membership 250.
Visitors Mon-Sun & BHs. Booking required Sat, Sun & BHs. Dress code.
Societies Booking required. **Green Fees** £14-£15 per 18 holes, £9-£10
per 9 holes (£18/£12 Sat & Sun). ⊕ **Prof** Steve Priestman **Course
Designer** Jonathan Gaunt **Facilities** 🝾 ⌨ 🍴 ⏣ 📷 ✦ 🌳 **Conf** Corporate
Hospitality Days **Location** 10 miles E of Hull, A63 towards Hull, then A1033
to Hedon. Follow minor roads signed for Burstwick.
Hotel ★★★ 75% HL Portland Hotel, Paragon St, HULL ☎ 01482 326462
  126 en suite

COTTINGHAM   MAP 08 TA03

Cottingham Parks Golf & Country Club Woodhill Way
HU16 5RZ
☎ 01482 846030 📠 01482 845932
e-mail: jane.wiles@cottinghamparks.co.uk
web: www.cottinghamparks.co.uk
Gently undulating parkland course incorporating many natural features,
including lateral water hazards, several ponds on the approach to
greens, and rolling fairways.

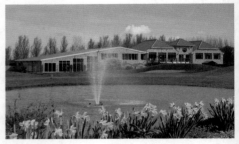

18 holes, 6453yds, Par 72, SSS 71, Course record 66.
Club membership 600.
Visitors Mon-Sun & BHs. Booking required. Dress code. **Societies** Booking
required. **Green Fees** £20 per round (£30 Sat, Sun & BHs). **Prof** Chris Gray
Course Designer Terry Litten **Facilities** ⊕ ⓘⓘ 🝾 ⌨ 🍴 ⏣ 📷 ☂ ✦
🌳 **Leisure** heated indoor swimming pool, sauna, solarium, gymnasium,
Jacuzzi, Remedial masseur, hair & beauty salon. **Conf** facs Corporate
Hospitality Days **Location** A164 onto B1233 towards Cottingham, 100yds left
onto Woodhill Way
Hotel ★★★ 79% HL Best Western Willerby Manor Hotel, Well Ln,
WILLERBY ☎ 01482 652616   51 en suite

England

DRIFFIELD (GREAT) — MAP 08 TA05

Driffield Sunderlandwick YO25 9AD
☎ 01377 253116 📠 01377 240599
e-mail: info@diffieldgolfclub.co.uk
web: www.driffieldgolf.co.uk
An easy walking, mature parkland course set within the beautiful Sunderlandwick Estate, including numerous water features, one of which is a renowned trout stream.
18 holes, 6215yds, Par 70, SSS 69, Course record 65.
Club membership 693.
Visitors Mon-Sun & BHs. Booking required. Handicap certificate. Dress code. **Societies** Booking required. **Green Fees** £35 per day, £26 per round (£45/£35 Sat & Sun). **Prof** Kenton Wright **Facilities** ⊕ ⦾ ⅃ ☜ ⬚ ⛳ 🔟 ⅃ 🏌 🚵 🚻 ☞ **Leisure** fishing. **Conf** facs Corporate Hospitality Days **Location** 0.5m S off A164
Hotel ★★★ 78% HL Best Western Bell Hotel, 46 Market Place, DRIFFIELD ☎ 01377 256661   16 en suite

FLAMBOROUGH — MAP 08 TA27

Flamborough Head Lighthouse Rd YO15 1AR
☎ 01262 850333 📠 01262 850279
e-mail: secretary@flamboroughheadgolfclub.co.uk
web: www.flamboroughheadgolfclub.co.uk
Undulating cliff top links type course on the Flamborough headland.
18 holes, 6189yds, Par 71, SSS 69, Course record 71.
Club membership 500.
Visitors Mon-Sun & BHs. Booking required Wed, Sat, Sun & BHs. Dress code. **Societies** booking required. **Green Fees** not confirmed. ⦾ **Prof** Paul Harrison **Facilities** ⊕ ☜ ⬚ 🔟 ⅃ 🏌 🚵 ☞ **Location** 2m E off B1259
Hotel ★★ 74% SHL North Star Hotel, North Marine Dr, FLAMBOROUGH ☎ 01262 850379   7 en suite

HESSLE — MAP 08 TA02

Hessle Westfield Rd, Raywell HU16 5YL
☎ 01482 650171 & 650190 (Prof) 📠 01482 652679
e-mail: secretary@hessle-golf-club.co.uk
web: www.hessle-golf-club.co.uk
Well-wooded downland course with easy walking. The greens, conforming to USGA specification, are large and undulating with excellent drainage, enabling play throughout the year.
18 holes, 6608yds, Par 72, SSS 72, Course record 65.
Club membership 720.
Visitors Mon-Sun & BHs. Booking required. Dress code. **Societies** booking required. **Green Fees** not confirmed. **Prof** Grahame Fieldsend **Course Designer** D Thomas/P Allis **Facilities** ⊕ ⦾ ☜ ⬚ 🔟 ⅃ 🏌 🚵 ⛳ **Conf** facs Corporate Hospitality Days **Location** 3m SW of Cottingham
Hotel ★★★ 68% HL Elizabeth Hotel Hull, Ferriby High Rd, NORTH FERRIBY ☎ 01482 645212   95 en suite

HORNSEA — MAP 08 TA14

Hornsea Rolston Rd HU18 1XG
☎ 01964 532020 📠 01964 532080
e-mail: hornseagolfclub@aol.com
web: www.hornseagolfclub.co.uk
Easy walking parkland course renowned for the quality of its greens.
18 holes, 6685yds, Par 72, SSS 72, Course record 66.
Club membership 600.
Visitors Mon-Sun & BHs. Booking required. Dress code. **Societies** Welcome. **Green Fees** £36 per day, £30 per round. **Prof** Stretton Wright

Course Designer Herd/Mackenzie/Braid **Facilities** ⊕ ⦾ by prior arrangement ☜ ⬚ 🔟 ⅃ 🏌 🚵 ⛳ **Conf** Corporate Hospitality Days **Location** 1m S on B1242, signs for Hornsea Freeport
Hotel ★★ 69% HL Burton Lodge Hotel, BRANDESBURTON ☎ 01964 542847   7 en suite   2 annexe en suite

HOWDEN — MAP 08 SE72

Boothferry Spaldington Ln DN14 7NG
☎ 01430 430364 📠 01430 430567
web: www.boothferrygolfclub.co.uk
Pleasant, meadowland course in the Vale of York with interesting natural dykes, creating challenges on some holes. The Par 5 9th is a test for any golfer with its dyke coming into play on the tee shot, second shot and approach.
18 holes, 6651yds, Par 73, SSS 72, Course record 64.
Eagles: 9 holes, 2700yds, Par 29, SSS 30.
Club membership 300.
Visitors Mon-Sun & BHs. Booking required Fri-Sun & BHs. Dress code. **Societies** Booking required. **Green Fees** £15 per 18 holes, £11 per 9 holes (£18/£13 Sat & Sun). Eagles: £8 per 18 holes, £5 per 9 holes. **Prof** Matthew Rumble **Course Designer** Donald Steel **Facilities** ⊕ ⦾ ☜ ⬚ 🔟 ⅃ 🏌 🚵 ⛳ ☞ **Conf** facs Corporate Hospitality Days **Location** M62 junct 37, 2.5m N of Howden off B1228
Hotel BUD Premier Travel Inn Goole, Rawcliffe Rd, Airmyn, GOOLE ☎ 08701 977 031   79 en suite

KINGSTON UPON HULL — MAP 08 TA02

Ganstead Park Longdales Ln, Coniston HU11 4LB
☎ 01482 817754 📠 01482 817754
e-mail: secretary@gansteadpark.co.uk
web: www.gansteadpark.co.uk
Easy walking parkland with water features.
18 holes, 6801yds, Par 72, SSS 73, Course record 62.
Club membership 500.
Visitors Mon-Sun except BHs. Booking required. Handicap certificate. Dress code. **Societies** Booking required. **Green Fees** £27 per day, £20 per round. ⦾ **Prof** Michael J Smee **Course Designer** P Green **Facilities** ⊕ ⦾ ☜ ⬚ 🔟 ⅃ 🏌 🚵 ⛳ **Conf** Corporate Hospitality Days **Location** A165 Hull exit, pass Ganstead right onto B1238 to Bilton, course on right
Hotel ★★★ 72% HL Quality Hotel Royal Hull, 170 Ferensway, HULL ☎ 01482 325087   155 en suite

Hull The Hall, 27 Packman Ln HU10 7TJ
☎ 01482 658919 📠 01482 658919
e-mail: info.hullgolfclub@virgin.net
web: hullgolfclub.com
Attractive mature parkland course.

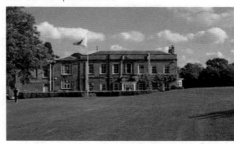

Continued

England

18 holes, 6262yds, Par 70, SSS 70, Course record 64.
Club membership 768.
Visitors Mon, Tue, Thu-Sun & BHs. Booking required. Handicap certificate.
Dress code. **Societies** Booking required. **Green Fees** Dec-Feb £20
per round; Mar-Nov £35 per day, £27.50 per round. **Prof** David Jagger
Course Designer James Braid **Facilities** ⊕ ⏱ 🍴 ⬛ ⬛ ⚘ 🛍 ✈ ⛑
✦ **Leisure** snooker. **Conf** Corporate Hospitality Days **Location** 5m W of
city off A164
Hotel ★★★ 79% HL Best Western Willerby Manor Hotel, Well Ln,
WILLERBY ☎ 01482 652616 51 en suite

See advert on this page

Springhead Park Willerby Rd HU5 5JE
☎ 01482 656309
18 holes, 6402yds, Par 71, SSS 71.
Location 5m W off A164
Telephone for further details
Hotel ★★★ 79% HL Best Western Willerby Manor Hotel, Well Ln,
WILLERBY ☎ 01482 652616 51 en suite

Sutton Park Salthouse Rd HU8 9HF
☎ 01482 374242 📠 01482 701428
18 holes, 6251yds, Par 70, SSS 69, Course record 67.
Location 3m NE on B1237, off A165
Telephone for further details
Hotel ★★★ 72% HL Quality Hotel Royal Hull, 170 Ferensway, HULL
☎ 01482 325087 155 en suite

POCKLINGTON   MAP 08 SE84

Kilnwick Percy Kilnwick Percy YO42 1UF
☎ 01759 303090 📠 01759 303090
e-mail: aaronpheasant@easy.com
web: kilnwickpercygolfclub.co.uk
This parkland course on the edge of the Wolds above Pocklington
combines a good walk with interesting golf. Undulating fairways,
mature trees, water hazards and breathtaking views from every hole.
Recent developments include increased drainage, a new bunker
programme and a new clubhouse.
18 holes, 6218yds, Par 70, SSS 70, Course record 66.
Club membership 450.
Visitors Mon-Sun & BHs. Booking required Sun & BHs. Dress code.
Societies Booking required. **Green Fees** £18 per 18 holes, £12 per 9 holes
(£20/£14 Sat, Sun & BHs). ❸ **Prof** Aaron Pheasant **Course Designer**
John Day **Facilities** ⊕ ⏱ 🍴 ⬛ ⬛ ⚘ 🛍 ✦ **Conf** Corporate
Hospitality Days **Location** 1m E of Pocklington off B1246
Hotel ★★ 65% HL Feathers Hotel, 56 Market Place, POCKLINGTON
☎ 01759 303155 10 en suite 6 annexe en suite

SOUTH CAVE   MAP 08 SE93

Cave Castle Hotel & Country Club Church Hill, South
Cave HU15 2EU
☎ 01430 426262 & 426259 📠 01430 421118
e-mail: admin@cavecastlegolf.co.uk
web: www.cavecastlegolf.co.uk
Undulating meadow and parkland at the foot of the Wolds, with
superb views.
18 holes, 6524yds, Par 72, SSS 71, Course record 68.
Club membership 410.

Hull Golf Club

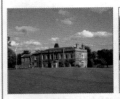
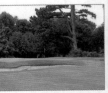

Hull Golf Club is a picturesque parkland course,
designed by James Braid over 100 years ago.

It offers a good challenge to golfers of all
abilities, and has a well-stocked bar and
excellent catering in the fine Grade II Listed
clubhouse.

A warm welcome is extended to societies
and visitors.

Contact the General Manager, David Crossley,
who will be happy to discuss your requirements.

Packman Lane, Kirk Ella, Hull HU10 7TJ
Tel: 01482 658919
Website: www.hullgolfclub.com

Visitors Mon-Sun & BHs. Booking required. Dress code.
Societies Booking required. **Green Fees** Phone. **Prof** Stephen MacKinder
Course Designer Mrs N Freling **Facilities** ⊕ ⏱ 🍴 ⬛ ⬛ ⚘ 🛍 ✦ ⛑
✦ **Leisure** heated indoor swimming pool, sauna, solarium, gymnasium.
Conf facs Corporate Hospitality Days **Location** 1m from A63
Hotel ★★★ 68% HL Elizabeth Hotel Hull, Ferriby High Rd, NORTH
FERRIBY ☎ 01482 645212 95 en suite

WITHERNSEA   MAP 08 TA32

Withernsea Chesnut Av HU19 2PG
☎ 01964 612078 & 612258 📠 01964 612078
e-mail: johnboasman@btconnect.com
Exposed seaside links with narrow, undulating fairways, bunkers and
small greens.
9 holes, 6207yds, Par 72, SSS 69. Club membership 250.
Visitors Mon-Sun & BHs. Booking required Sat/Sun. Dress code. **Societies**
Booking required **Green Fees** £15 per 18 holes. ❸ **Facilities** ⊕ ⏱ 🍴
⬛ ⬛ ⚘ **Leisure** senior/junior coaching. **Conf** facs Corporate Hospitality
Days **Location** S of town centre off A1033, signed from Victoria Av
Hotel ★★★ 72% HL Quality Hotel Royal Hull, 170 Ferensway, HULL
☎ 01482 325087 155 en suite

YORKSHIRE, NORTH

ALDWARK
MAP 08 SE46

Aldwark Manor YO61 1UF
☎ 01347 838353 📠 01347 833991
An easy walking, scenic 18-hole parkland course with holes both sides of the River Ure. The course surrounds the Victorian Aldwark Manor Golf Hotel.

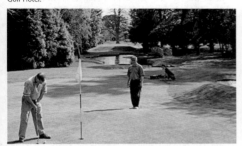

18 holes, 6187yds, Par 72, SSS 70, Course record 67.
Club membership 400.
Visitors Mon-Sun & BHs. Booking required. Dress code. **Societies** Booking required. **Green Fees** £35 per day, £25 per round (£40/£30 Sat, Sun & BHs). **Facilities** ⑪ ⑩ ⓛ ☲ ▽ ⑪ ▴ 🍴 ❖ ✔ 🛥 ✔ **Leisure** heated indoor swimming pool, fishing, sauna, gymnasium. **Conf** facs Corporate Hospitality Days **Location** 5m SE of Boroughbridge off A1
Hotel ★★★★ 85% HL Aldwark Manor, ALDWARK ☎ 01347 838146 55 en suite

BEDALE
MAP 08 SE28

Bedale Leyburn Rd DL8 1EZ
☎ 01677 422451 (sec) 📠 01677 427143
e-mail: bedalegolfclub@aol.com
web: www.bedalegolfclub.com
One of North Yorkshire's most picturesque and interesting courses. The 18-hole course is in parkland with mature trees, water hazards and strategically placed bunkers. Easy walking, no heavy climbs.

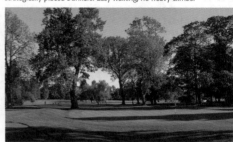

18 holes, 6610yds, Par 72, SSS 72, Course record 68.
Club membership 600.
Visitors Mon-Fri except BHs. Booking required. Handicap certificate. Dress code. **Societies** Booking required. **Green Fees** £33 per day, £27 per round (£41/£36 Sat & Sun). **Prof** Tony Johnson **Course Designer** Hawtree **Facilities** ⑪ ⑩ ⓛ ☲ ▽ ⑪ ▴ 🍴 ❖ ✔ 🛥 ✔ **Conf** facs Corporate Hospitality Days **Location** A1 onto A684 at Leeming Bar to Bedale
Hotel ★★ 64% HL The White Rose Hotel, Bedale Rd, LEEMING BAR ☎ 01677 422707 18 en suite

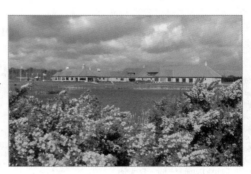

BENTHAM
MAP 07 SD66

Bentham Robin Ln LA2 7AG
☎ 015242 62470
e-mail: secretary@benthamgolfclub.co.uk
web: www.benthamgolfclub.co.uk
Moorland course with glorious views and excellent greens.
18 holes, 6005yds, Par 71, SSS 69, Course record 69.
Club membership 500.
Visitors Mon-Sun & BHs. Booking required. Dress code. **Societies** Booking
required. **Green Fees** £35 per day, £30 per round (£35 Sat & Sun). ⊕
Prof Alan Watson **Facilities** ⓘ ⓘ ⓘ ⓘ ⓘ ⓘ ⓘ ⓘ ⓘ ⓘ **Conf**
Corporate Hospitality Days **Location** N side of High Bentham

CATTERICK GARRISON
MAP 08 SE29

Catterick Leyburn Rd DL9 3QE
☎ 01748 833268 ▤ 01748 833268
e-mail: grant@catterickgolfclub.co.uk
web: www.catterickgolfclub.co.uk
18 holes, 6329yds, Par 71, SSS 71, Course record 64.
Course Designer Arthur Day **Location** 0.5m W of Catterick Garrison
Telephone for further details
Hotel ★★★ 75% HL King's Head Hotel, Market Place, RICHMOND
☎ 01748 850220 26 en suite 4 annexe en suite

COPMANTHORPE
MAP 08 SE54

Pike Hills Tadcaster Rd YO23 3UW
☎ 01904 700797 ▤ 01904 700797
e-mail: thesecretary@pikehills.fsnet.co.uk
web: www.pikehillsgolfclub.com
Parkland course surrounding a nature reserve. Level terrain.
18 holes, 6146yds, Par 71, SSS 70, Course record 63.
Club membership 750.
Visitors Mon-Fri except BHs. Booking required. Dress code. **Societies**
Booking required. **Green Fees** Phone. ⊕ **Prof** Ian Gradwell **Facilities** ⓘ
ⓘ ⓘ ⓘ ⓘ ⓘ ⓘ ⓘ ⓘ ⓘ **Conf** facs Corporate Hospitality Days
Location 3m SW of York on A64
Hotel ★★★★ 75% HL York Marriott Hotel, Tadcaster Rd, YORK
☎ 01904 701000 151 en suite

EASINGWOLD
MAP 08 SE56

Easingwold Stillington Rd YO61 3ET
☎ 01347 821964 (Pro) & 822474 (Sec) ▤ 01347 822474
e-mail: brian@easingwold-golf-club.fsnet.co.uk
web: www.easingwold-golf-club.co.uk
Parkland with easy walking. Trees are a major feature and on six holes
water hazards come into play.
18 holes, 6559yds, Par 74, SSS 72. Club membership 750.
Visitors Mon-Fri except BHs. Booking required. Dress code. **Societies**
Booking required. **Green Fees** £35 per day, £28 per round. ⊕ **Prof** John
Hughes **Course Designer** Hawtree **Facilities** ⓘ ⓘ ⓘ ⓘ ⓘ ⓘ ⓘ ⓘ ⓘ
ⓘ **Conf** Corporate Hospitality Days **Location** 1m S of Easingwold
Hotel ★★ 75% SHL George Hotel, Market Place, EASINGWOLD
☎ 01347 821698 15 en suite

FILEY
MAP 08 TA18

Filey West Av YO14 9BQ
☎ 01723 513293 ▤ 01723 514952
e-mail: secretary@fileygolfclub.com
web: www.fileygolfclub.com
Links and parkland course with good views. Stream runs through
course. Testing 9th and 13th holes.
18 holes, 6112yds, Par 70, SSS 69, Course record 64
9 holes, 1513yds, Par 30. Club membership 900.
Visitors Mon-Sun & BHs. Handicap certificate. Dress code. **Societies**
booking required. **Green Fees** not confirmed. **Prof** Gary Hutchinson
Course Designer Braid **Facilities** ⓘ ⓘ ⓘ ⓘ ⓘ ⓘ ⓘ ⓘ ⓘ ⓘ
Location 0.5m S of Filey
Hotel ★★ 76% HL Downcliffe House Hotel, 6 The Beach, FILEY
☎ 01723 513310 12 en suite

GANTON
MAP 08 SE97

Ganton YO12 4PA
☎ 01944 710329 ▤ 01944 710922
e-mail: secretary@gantongolfclub.com
web: www.gantongolfclub.com
Championship course, heathland, gorse-lined fairways and heavily
bunkered; variable winds. The opening holes make full use of the
contours of the land and the approach to the second demands the
finest touch. The 4th is considered one of the best holes on the
outward half with its shot across a valley to a plateau green, the
surrounding gorse punishing anything less than a perfect shot. The
finest hole is possibly the 18th, requiring an accurately placed drive
to give a clear shot to the sloping, well-bunkered green.
18 holes, 6753yds, Par 72, SSS 73, Course record 65.
Club membership 500.
Visitors Mon-Sun & BHs. Booking required. Handicap certificate. Dress
code. **Societies** Booking required. **Green Fees** £73 per day (£83 Sat, Sun
& BHs). **Prof** Gary Brown **Course Designer** Dunn/Vardon/Braid/Colt
Facilities ⓘ ⓘ ⓘ ⓘ ⓘ ⓘ ⓘ ⓘ ⓘ ⓘ **Conf** Corporate Hospitality
Days **Location** N of village off A64
Hotel ★★★ 68% HL East Ayton Lodge Country House, Moor Ln, Forge
Valley, EAST AYTON ☎ 01723 864227 12 en suite 14 annexe en suite

HARROGATE
MAP 08 SE35

Harrogate Forest Ln Head, Starbeck HG2 7TF
☎ 01423 862999 ▤ 01423 860073
e-mail: secretary@harrogate-gc.co.uk
web: www.harrogate-gc.co.uk
Course on fairly flat terrain with MacKenzie-style greens and tree-
lined fairways. While not a long course, the layout penalises the
golfer who strays off the fairway. Subtly placed bunkers and copses
of trees require the golfer to adopt careful thought and accuracy if
Par is be bettered. The last six holes include five Par 4s, of which four
exceed 400yds.
18 holes, 6241yds, Par 69, SSS 70, Course record 63.
Club membership 700.
Visitors Mon, Wed-Fri, Sun & BHs. Tue pm only. Handicap certificate.
Dress code. **Societies** Booking required. **Green Fees** £40 per day, £35
per round (£45 Sat & Sun). **Prof** Gary Stothard, Sam Evison
Course Designer Sandy Herd **Facilities** ⓘ ⓘ ⓘ ⓘ ⓘ ⓘ ⓘ ⓘ ⓘ ⓘ
ⓘ **Leisure** snooker. **Conf** Corporate Hospitality Days **Location** 2.25m
N on A59
Hotel ★★★ 79% HL Grants Hotel, 3-13 Swan Rd, HARROGATE
☎ 01423 560666 42 en suite

Oakdale Oakdale Glen HG1 2LN
☎ 01423 567162 📠 01423 536030
e-mail: sec@oakdale-golfclub.com
web: www.oakdale-golfclub.com
A pleasant, undulating parkland course which provides a good test of golf for the low handicap player without intimidating the less proficient. A special feature is an attractive stream which comes in to play on four holes. Excellent views from the clubhouse with good facilities.
18 holes, 6456yds, Par 71, SSS 71, Course record 61.
Club membership 975.
Visitors Mon-Sun & BHs. Booking required Sat, Sun & BHs. Handicap certificate. Dress code. **Societies** Booking required. **Green Fees** £46 for 27 holes, £39 per round (£55 Sat, Sun & BHs).
Course Designer Dr McKenzie **Facilities** ⊕ ⓘ 🍴 ↆ ⌂ ⏶ ⏶ ⏶ ⏶
⏶ **Conf** Corporate Hospitality Days **Location** N of town centre off A61
Hotel ★★★★ 75% HL Paramount Majestic Hotel, Ripon Rd, HARROGATE ☎ 01423 700300 156 en suite

Rudding Park Rudding Park, Follifoot HG3 1JH
☎ 01423 872100 📠 01423 872286
e-mail: reservations@ruddingpark.com
web: www.ruddingpark.com
The course runs through 18th century parkland and provides a challenge for the most seasoned golfer with mature trees, attractive lakes and water features.

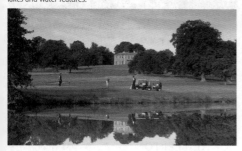

18 holes, 6883yds, Par 72, SSS 73, Course record 68.
Par 3 Short Course: 6 holes, 689yds, Par 18.
Club membership 700.
Visitors Mon-Sun & BHs. Booking required. Handicap certificate. Dress code. **Societies** Booking required. **Green Fees** £35 per 18 holes (£39.50 Fri-Sun). **Prof** M Moore/N Moore/R Hobkinson **Course Designer** Martin Hawtree **Facilities** ⊕ ⓘ 🍴 ↆ ⌂ ⏶ ⏶ ⏶ ⏶ ⏶ **Leisure** Par 3 short course. **Conf** facs Corporate Hospitality Days **Location** 2m SE of Harrogate town centre, off A658, brown tourist signs
Hotel ★★★★ HL Rudding Park Hotel & Golf, Rudding Park, Follifoot, HARROGATE ☎ 01423 871350 49 en suite

See advert on this page

KIRKBYMOORSIDE   MAP 08 SE68

Kirkbymoorside Manor Vale YO62 6EG
☎ 01751 430402 📠 01751 433190
e-mail: enqs@kirkbymoorsidegolf.co.uk
web: www.kirkbymoorsidegolf.co.uk
Hilly parkland with narrow fairways, gorse and hawthorn bushes. Beautiful views and several interesting holes.
18 holes, 6207yds, Par 69, SSS 69, Course record 65.
Club membership 650.

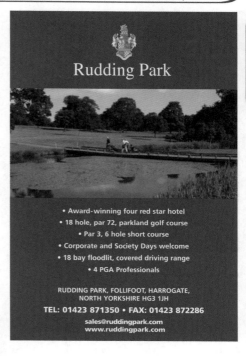

Visitors Mon-Sun except BHs. Booking required. Dress code. **Societies** Booking required. **Green Fees** £28 per day, £22 per round (£32 Sat, Sun & BHs). **Prof** John Hinchliffe **Facilities** ⊕ ⓘ 🍴 ↆ ⌂ ⏶ ⏶ ⏶ ⏶ ⏶
Leisure snooker room. **Conf** facs Corporate Hospitality Days **Location** N of village

---

KNARESBOROUGH   MAP 08 SE35

Knaresborough Boroughbridge Rd HG5 0QQ
☎ 01423 862690 📠 01423 869345
e-mail: thekgc@btconnect.com
web: www.knaresboroughgolfclub.co.uk
Pleasant and well-presented parkland course in a rural setting. The first 11 holes are tree-lined and are constantly changing direction around the clubhouse. The closing holes head out overlooking the old quarry with fine views.
18 holes, 6780yds, Par 72, SSS 72, Course record 69.
Club membership 840.
Visitors Mon-Sun & BHs. Handicap certificate. Dress code. **Societies** Booking required. **Green Fees** £40 per day, £30 per round (£35 Sat & Sun). ⊛ **Prof** Darren Tear **Course Designer** Hawtree **Facilities** ⊕ 🍴 ↆ ⌂ ⏶ ⏶ ⏶ ⏶ ⏶ ⏶ **Conf** Corporate Hospitality Days **Location** 1.25m N on A6055
Hotel ★★★ 77% HL Best Western Dower House Hotel, Bond End, KNARESBOROUGH ☎ 01423 863302 28 en suite 3 annexe en suite

England

MALTON   MAP 08 SE77

Malton & Norton Welham Park, Norton YO17 9QE
☎ 01653 697912 📠 01653 697912
e-mail: maltonandnorton@btconnect.com
web: www.maltonandnortongolfclub.co.uk
Parkland course, consisting of three nine-hole loops, with panoramic
views of the moors. Very testing 1st hole (564yd dog-leg, left) on the
Welham Course.

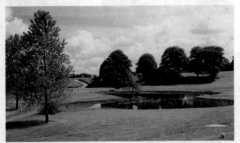

Welham Course: 18 holes, 6456yds, Par 72, SSS 71,
Course record 66.
Park Course: 18 holes, 6251yds, Par 72, SSS 70,
Course record 67.
Derwent Course: 18 holes, 6295yds, Par 72, SSS 70,
Course record 66. Club membership 880.
Visitors Mon-Sun & BHs. Dress code. **Societies** Booking required.
Green Fees £27 per round (£32 Sat, Sun & BHs). **Prof** S Robinson
Facilities ⑪ ⍟ ⍪ ⌴ ♡ 🏌 ⚐ 🛆 🍴 🥪 ✂ ☏ **Conf** Corporate Hospitality Days
Location 0.75m from Malton

See advert on opposite page

MASHAM   MAP 08 SE28

Masham Burnholme, Swinton Rd HG4 4HT
☎ 01765 688054 & 689379 📠 01765 688054
e-mail: info@mashamgolfclub.co.uk
web: www.mashamgolfclub.co.uk
Flat parkland crossed by River Burn, which comes into play on
six holes.
9 holes, 6068yds, Par 70, SSS 69, Course record 70.
Club membership 290.
Visitors Mon-Fri & BHs. Booking required Mon, Wed & Thu. Dress code.
Societies Booking required. **Green Fees** £20 per day, £17 per round. ⚐
Facilities ⍪ ⌴ ♡ 🏌 🛆 **Conf** Corporate Hospitality Days **Location** SW of
Masham centre off A6108
Hotel ★★★★ HL Swinton Park, MASHAM ☎ 01765 680900 30 en suite

MIDDLESBROUGH   MAP 08 NZ41

Middlesbrough Brass Castle Ln, Marton TS8 9EE
☎ 01642 311515 📠 01642 319607
e-mail: enquiries@middlesbroughgolfclub.co.uk
web: www.middlesbroughgolfclub.co.uk
Undulating wooded parkland affected by the wind. Testing 6th, 8th
and 12th holes.
18 holes, 6278yds, Par 70, SSS 70, Course record 63.
Club membership 1004.

Visitors Mon, Wed-Fri, Sun & BHs. Handicap certificate. Dress code.
Societies Booking required **Green Fees** £37 per round (£42 Sat & Sun).
⚐ **Prof** Don Jones **Course Designer** Baird **Facilities** ⑪ ⍟ ⍪ ⌴ ♡ 🏌 🛆
⚐ 🥪 🍴 ✂ **Leisure** snooker table. **Conf** facs Corporate Hospitality Days
Location 4m S off A172
Hotel Best Western Parkmore Hotel & Leisure Park, 636 Yarm Rd,
Eaglescliffe, STOCKTON-ON-TEES ☎ 01642 786815 55 en suite

Middlesbrough Municipal Ladgate Ln TS5 7YZ
☎ 01642 315533 📠 01642 300726
e-mail: maurice_gormley@middlesbrough.gov.uk
web: www.middlesbrough.gov.uk
Parkland course with good views. The front nine holes have wide
fairways and large, often well-guarded greens while the back nine
demand shots over tree-lined water hazards and narrow entrances to
subtly contoured greens.

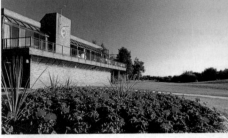

18 holes, 6333yds, Par 71, SSS 70, Course record 67.
Club membership 630.
Visitors Mon-Sun & BHs. Dress code. **Societies** Booking required **Green
Fees** £12.30 per round (£15.50 Sat & Sun). **Prof** Alan Hope **Course
Designer** Shuttleworth **Facilities** ⍪ ⌴ ♡ 🏌 🛆 ⚐ 🥪 ✂ 🍴 ☏ **Conf**
Corporate Hospitality Days **Location** 2m S of Middlesbrough on the A174
Hotel 🅤 Best Western Parkmore Hotel & Leisure Park, 636 Yarm Rd,
Eaglescliffe, STOCKTON-ON-TEES ☎ 01642 786815 55 en suite

NORTHALLERTON   MAP 08 SE39

Romanby Yafforth Rd DL7 0PE
☎ 01609 778855 📠 01609 779084
e-mail: grant@romanby.com
web: www.romanbygolf.co.uk
Set in natural undulating terrain with the River Wiske meandering
through the course, it offers a testing round of golf for all abilities.
In addition to the river, two lakes come into play on the 2nd, 5th
and 11th holes. A 12-bay floodlit driving range.
18 holes, 6663yds, Par 72, SSS 72, Course record 72.
Club membership 525.
Visitors Mon-Sun & BHs. Dress code. **Societies** booking required. **Green
Fees** not confirmed. **Prof** Richard Wood **Course Designer** Will Adamson
Facilities ⑪ ⍟ ⍪ ⌴ ♡ 🏌 🛆 ⚐ 🥪 ✂ 🍴 ☏ **Leisure** 6 hole Par 3
academy course. **Conf** facs Corporate Hospitality Days **Location** 1m W of
Northallerton on B6271
Hotel ★★★ 72% HL Solberge Hall Hotel, Newby Wiske,
NORTHALLERTON ☎ 01609 779191 24 en suite

PANNAL
MAP 08 SE35

Pannal Follifoot Rd HG3 1ES
☎ 01423 872628 🖹 01423 870043
e-mail: secretary@pannalgc.co.uk
web: www.pannalgc.co.uk
Fine championship course chosen as a regional qualifying venue for the Open Championship. Moorland turf but well-wooded with trees closely involved with play. Excellent views enhance the course.
18 holes, 6622yds, Par 72, SSS 72, Course record 62. Club membership 850.
Visitors Mon-Sun & BHs. Booking required. Handicap certificate. Dress code. **Societies** Booking required. **Green Fees** £55 per day, £45 per round (£60 Sat & Sun). **Prof** David Padgett **Course Designer** Sandy Herd **Facilities** ⑪ ⑩ ﹗ ⯑ ☐ ﹗ ⅃ ⯑ 🍴 ⚿ 🏌 **Leisure** snooker. **Conf** Corporate Hospitality Days **Location** E of village off A61

RAVENSCAR
MAP 08 NZ90

Raven Hall Hotel Golf Course YO13 0ET
☎ 01723 870353 🖹 01723 870072
e-mail: enquiries@ravenhall.co.uk
web: www.ravenhall.co.uk
Opened by the Earl of Cranbrook in 1898, this nine-hole clifftop course is sloping and with good quality small greens. Because of its clifftop position it is subject to strong winds which make it great fun to play, especially the 6th hole.
9 holes, 1894yds, Par 32, SSS 32. Club membership 120.
Visitors Mon-Sun & BHs. **Societies** Booking required **Green Fees** £8 per round. **Facilities** ⑪ ⑩ ﹗ ⯑ ☐ ﹗ ⯑ **Leisure** hard tennis courts, heated indoor swimming pool, sauna, gymnasium, croquet, bowls. **Conf** facs Corporate Hospitality Days **Location** A171 from Scarborough towards Whitby, through Cloughton, right to Ravenscar, hotel on clifftop
Hotel ★★★ 70% HL Raven Hall Country House Hotel, RAVENSCAR
☎ 01723 870353 52 en suite

REDCAR
MAP 08 NZ62

Cleveland Majuba Rd TS10 5BJ
☎ 01642 471798 🖹 01642 471798
e-mail: secretary@clevelandgolfclub.co.uk
web: www.clevelandgolfclub.co.uk
18 holes, 6696yds, Par 72, SSS 72, Course record 67.
Course Designer Donald Steel (new holes) **Location** 8m E of Middlesbrough, at N end of Redcar
Telephone for further details
Hotel ★★★ 73% HL Rushpool Hall Hotel, Saltburn Ln, SALTBURN-BY-THE-SEA ☎ 01287 624111 21 en suite

Wilton Wilton TS10 4QY
☎ 01642 465265 (Secretary) 🖹 01642 465463
e-mail: secretary@wiltongolfclub.co.uk
web: www.wiltongolfclub.co.uk
Parkland with some fine views and an abundance of trees and shrubs.
18 holes, 6540yds, Par 70, SSS 69, Course record 64. Club membership 650.
Visitors Mon-Fri, Sun & BHs. Booking required Sun. Dress code.
Societies Booking required **Green Fees** £26 per day (£32 Sat, Sun & BHs).
⭐ **Prof** P D Smillie **Facilities** ⑪ ⑩ by prior arrangement ⯑ ☐ ﹗ ⅃ ⯑ 🍴

Malton & Norton Golf Club
Welham Park, Norton Malton, North Yorkshire, YO17 9QE

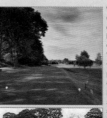

Welcome to Malton and Norton Golf Club, a twenty-seven hole course of three contrasting loops providing challenge and enjoyment for members and visitors alike.

The club is ideally situated between York and Scarborough with marvellous views of the North Yorkshire Moors. In addition to the Clubhouse Bar and catering, the excellent facilities include a driving range, short game practice facility and well stocked shop. Modern golfers demand the highest standards and these have been pursued here with singular determination.

Renowned for the quality of the course and the warmth to visitors, groups and societies.

Corporate Golf Days a speciality. No Winter Greens Guaranteed.

Tel: 01653 697912
Website: www.maltonandnortongolfclub.co.uk
Email: maltonandnorton@btconnect.com

﹗ 🍴 ⚿ 🏌 **Leisure** snooker. **Conf** Corporate Hospitality Days **Location** 3m W of Redcar on A174
Hotel ★★★ 73% HL Rushpool Hall Hotel, Saltburn Ln, SALTBURN-BY-THE-SEA ☎ 01287 624111 21 en suite

RICHMOND
MAP 07 NZ10

Richmond Bend Hagg DL10 5EX
☎ 01748 823231 (Secretary) 🖹 01748 821709
e-mail: secretary@richmondyorksgolfclub.co.uk
web: www.richmondyorksgolfclub.co.uk
Undulating parkland. Ideal to play 27 holes, not too testing but very interesting.
18 holes, 6073yds, Par 71, SSS 69, Course record 63. Club membership 600.
Visitors Mon-Sat & BHs. Booking required Sat & BHs. Handicap certificate. Dress code. **Societies** Booking required **Green Fees** £25 per day, £23 per round (£30/£25 Sat, Sun & BHs). ⭐ **Prof** James Cousins **Course Designer** F Pennink **Facilities** ⑪ ⑩ ﹗ ⯑ ☐ ﹗ ⅃ ⯑ 🍴 🏌 **Conf** facs **Location** 0.75m N
Hotel ★★★ 75% HL King's Head Hotel, Market Place, RICHMOND
☎ 01748 850220 26 en suite 4 annexe en suite

RIPON
MAP 08 SE37

Ripon City Palace Rd HG4 3HH
☎ 01765 603640 📠 01765 692880
e-mail: secretary@riponcitygolfclub.com
web: www.riponcitygolfclub.com
Moderate walking on undulating parkland course; three testing Par 3s at 5th, 7th and 14th.
18 holes, 6084yds, Par 70, SSS 69, Course record 65.
Club membership 600.
Visitors Mon-Fri, Sun & BHs. Booking required Tue & Sun. Handicap certificate. Dress code. **Societies** Booking required **Green Fees** Phone. 🅿 **Prof** S T Davis **Course Designer** H Varden **Facilities** ⊕ ⊗ ⚲ ⊑ 🖵 🎏 🍴 ⚑ ☂ 🏌 **Conf** Corporate Hospitality Days **Location** 1m NW on A6108
Hotel ★★★ 79% HL Best Western Ripon Spa Hotel, Park St, RIPON
☎ 01765 602172 40 en suite

SALTBURN-BY-THE-SEA
MAP 08 NZ62

Hunley Hall Golf Club & Hotel Ings Ln, Brotton TS12 2QQ
☎ 01287 676216 📠 01287 678250
e-mail: enquiries@hunleyhall.co.uk
web: www.hunleyhall.co.uk
A picturesque 27-hole coastal course with panoramic views of the countryside and coastline, providing a good test of golf and a rewarding game for all.

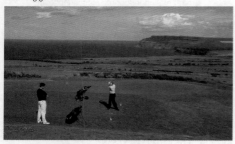

Morgans: 18 holes, 6872yds, Par 73, SSS 73, Course record 63.
Millennium: 18 holes, 5945yds, Par 68, SSS 68, Course record 67.
Jubilee: 18 holes, 6289yds, Par 71, SSS 70, Course record 65. Club membership 500.
Visitors Mon-Sun & BHs. Booking required. Dress code. **Societies** Booking required. **Green Fees** £25 per day (£35 Sat, Sun & BHs) **Prof** Andrew Brook **Course Designer** John Morgan **Facilities** ⊕ ⊗ ⚲ ⊑ 🖵 🎏 ⚑ ☂ 🍴 ◇ ⚑ 🏌 **Conf** facs Corporate Hospitality Days **Location** Off A174 in Brotton onto St Margarets Way, 700yds to club
Hotel ★★ 69% HL Hunley Hall Golf Club & Hotel, Ings Ln, Brotton, SALTBURN ☎ 01287 676216 28 en suite

Saltburn by the Sea Hob Hill, Guisborough Rd TS12 1NJ
☎ 01287 622812 📠 01287 625988
e-mail: info@saltburngolf.co.uk
web: www.saltburngolf.co.uk
Parkland course surrounded by woodland. Particularly attractive in autumn. There are fine views of the Cleveland Hills and of Tees Bay.

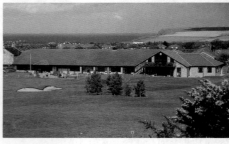

18 holes, 5846yds, Par 70, SSS 68, Course record 62.
Club membership 900.
Visitors Mon-Fri, Sun & BHs. Handicap certificate. Dress code. **Societies** Booking required. **Green Fees** £28 per round (£32 Sat & Sun). **Prof** Paul Bolton **Course Designer** J Braid **Facilities** ⊕ ⊗ ⚲ ⊑ 🖵 🎏 🍴 ⚑ ☂ 🏌 **Leisure** 2 snooker tables. **Conf** Corporate Hospitality Days **Location** 0.5m S from Saltburn
Hotel ★★★ 73% HL Rushpool Hall Hotel, Saltburn Ln, SALTBURN-BY-THE-SEA ☎ 01287 624111 21 en suite

SCARBOROUGH
MAP 08 TA08

Scarborough North Cliff North Cliff Av YO12 6PP
☎ 01723 355397 📠 01723 362134
e-mail: info@northcliffgolfclub.co.uk
web: www.northcliffgolfclub.co.uk
Seaside course beginning on clifftop overlooking North Bay and castle winding inland through parkland with stunning views of the North Yorkshire Moors.
18 holes, 6493yds, Par 72, SSS 71, Course record 65.
Club membership 850.
Visitors Mon, Wed-Sun & BHs. Tue pm only. Handicap certificate. Dress code. **Societies** Booking required. **Green Fees** £40 per day, £35 per round (£45/£40 Fri-Sun & BHs). 🅿 **Prof** Simon N Deller **Course Designer** James Braid **Facilities** ⊕ ⊗ ⚲ ⊑ 🖵 🎏 ⚑ ◇ ☂ 🏌 **Conf** Corporate Hospitality Days **Location** 2m N of town centre off A165
Hotel ★★★ 70% HL Esplanade Hotel, Belmont Rd, SCARBOROUGH ☎ 01723 360382 73 en suite

Scarborough South Cliff Deepdale Av YO11 2UE
☎ 01723 374737 📠 01723 374737
e-mail: clubsecretary.sscgc@virgin.net
web: www.scarboroughgolfclub.co.uk
Parkland and seaside course which falls into two parts, divided from one another by the main road from Scarborough to Filey. On the seaward side of the road lie holes 4 to 10. On the landward side the first three holes and the last eight are laid out along the bottom of a rolling valley, stretching southwards into the hills.
18 holes, 6405yds, Par 72, SSS 71, Course record 68.
Club membership 560.
Visitors Mon-Fri & Sun. Sat pm only. Booking required. Dress code. **Societies** booking required. **Green Fees** not confirmed. **Prof** Tony Skingle

Continued

Course Designer McKenzie **Facilities** ⓣ 🍴 🍺 ⌑ 🎎 🏋 📐 🛏 ✓ 🛥 ⚓
Location 1m S on A165
Hotel ★★★ 72% HL Palm Court Hotel, St Nicholas Cliff, SCARBOROUGH
☎ 01723 368161 40 en suite

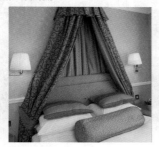

SELBY   MAP 08 SE63

Selby Mill Ln, Brayton YO8 9LD
☎ 01757 228622 📄 01757 228622
e-mail: selbygolfclub@aol.com
web: www.selbygolfclub.co.uk
Mainly flat, links-type course; prevailing south-west wind. Testing holes
including the 3rd, 7th and 16th.
18 holes, 6374yds, Par 71, SSS 71, Course record 68.
Club membership 840.
Visitors Mon, Wed-Fri & BHs. Booking required. Handicap certificate. Dress
code. **Societies** Booking required. **Green Fees** £37 per day, £32 per round.
Prof Nick Ludwell **Course Designer** J Taylor & Hawtree **Facilities** ⓣ 🍴 🍺
⌑ 🎎 📐 🛏 ⚓ ✓ 🚩 **Location** Off A63 Selby bypass
Hotel ★★★ 80% CHH Monk Fryston Hall Hotel, MONK FRYSTON
☎ 01977 682369 29 en suite

SETTLE   MAP 07 SD86

Settle Buckhaw Brow, Giggleswick BD24 0DH
☎ 01729 825288 & 823727 (sec) 📄 01729 825288
web: settlegolfclub.com
Picturesque parkland with a stream affecting play on four holes.
9 holes, 6200yds, Par 72, SSS 72, Course record 70.
Club membership 380.
Visitors Mon-Sat & BHs. Dress code. **Societies** Booking required.
Green Fees £20 per round. ⚑ **Course Designer** Tom Vardon
Facilities 📐 **Location** 1m W of Settle on Kendal Rd
Inn ★★★★ INN Golden Lion, 5 Duke St, SETTLE ☎ 01729 822203 12 rms
(10 en suite)

SKIPTON   MAP 07 SD95

Skipton Short Lee Ln BD23 3LF
☎ 01756 795657 📄 01756 796665
e-mail: enquiries@skiptongolfclub.co.uk
web: www.skiptongolfclub.co.uk
Undulating parkland with some water hazards and panoramic views.
18 holes, 6049yds, Par 70, SSS 69, Course record 66.
Club membership 800.
Visitors Mon-Sun & BHs. Booking required. Dress code. **Societies** Booking
required. **Green Fees** £30 per day, £24 per 18 holes (£26 Sat & Sun).

⚑ **Prof** Peter Robinson **Facilities** ⓣ 🍴 🍺 ⌑ 🎎 📐 🛏 ⚓ ✓ **Leisure**
snooker. **Conf** Corporate Hospitality Days **Location** 1m N of Skipton on
A59
Hotel ★★★★ HL The Devonshire Arms Country House Hotel & Spa,
BOLTON ABBEY ☎ 01756 710441 & 718111 📄 01756 710564 40 en suite

TADCASTER   MAP 08 SE44

Scarthingwell Scarthingwell LS24 9PF
☎ 01937 557864 (pro) 557878 (club) 📄 01937 557909
Testing water hazards and well-placed bunkers and trees provide a
challenging test of golf for all handicaps at this scenic parkland course.
Easy walking.
18 holes, 6771yds, Par 72, SSS 72. Club membership 500.
Visitors Mon-Fri, Sun & BHs. Booking required. Dress code.
Societies Booking required. **Green Fees** Phone. ⚑ **Prof** Simon Danby
Facilities ⓣ 🍺 ⌑ 🎎 📐 🛏 ✓ **Leisure** snooker. **Conf** facs Corporate
Hospitality Days **Location** 4m S of Tadcaster on A162 Tadcaster-Ferrybridge
road
Hotel ★★★ 83% HL Hazlewood Castle, Paradise Ln, Hazlewood,
TADCASTER ☎ 01937 535353 9 en suite 12 annexe en suite

THIRSK   MAP 08 SE48

Thirsk & Northallerton Thornton-le-Street YO7 4AB
☎ 01845 522170 & 525115 📄 01845 525115
e-mail: secretary@tngc.co.uk
web: www.tngc.co.uk
The course has good views of the nearby Hambleton Hills to the east
and Wensleydale to the west. Testing course, mainly flat.
18 holes, 6495yds, Par 72, SSS 71, Course record 66.
Club membership 500.
Visitors Mon-Sat & BHs. Booking required. Handicap certificate. Dress
code. **Societies** Booking required. **Green Fees** £32 per day, £26 per round
(£42/£32 Sat & Sun). ⚑ **Prof** Robert Garner **Course Designer** ADAS
Facilities 🍺 ⌑ 🎎 📐 🛏 ⚓ ✓ 🛥 **Location** 2m N on A168
Hotel ★★ 74% HL The Angel Inn, Long St, TOPCLIFFE ☎ 01845 577237
15 en suite

WHITBY   MAP 08 NZ81

Whitby Low Straggleton, Sandsend Rd YO21 3SR
☎ 01947 600660 📄 01947 600660
e-mail: office@whitbygolfclub.co.uk
web: www.whitbygolfclub.co.uk
Seaside course with four holes along clifftops and over ravines. Good
views and a fresh sea breeze.
18 holes, 6003yds, Par 70, SSS 69, Course record 66.
Club membership 500.
Visitors Mon-Sun & BHs. Booking required. Handicap certificate. Dress
code. **Societies** Booking required. **Green Fees** £26 per day (£32 Sat &
Sun). ⚑ **Prof** Tony Mason **Course Designer** Simon Gidman **Facilities** ⓣ
🍴 🍺 ⌑ 🎎 📐 🛏 ⚓ ✓ **Conf** Corporate Hospitality Days **Location** 1.5m
NW on A174
Hotel ★★ 70% HL White House Hotel, Upgang Ln, West Cliff, WHITBY
☎ 01947 600469 11 en suite 5 annexe en suite

England

YORK

MAP 08 SE65

Forest of Galtres Moorlands Rd, Skelton YO32 2RF

☎ 01904 766198 📄 01904 769400

e-mail: secretary@forestofgaltres.co.uk

web: www.forestofgaltres.co.uk

Level parkland in the heart of the ancient Forest of Galtres, with mature oak trees and interesting water features coming into play on the 6th, 14th and 17th holes. Views of York Minster.

18 holes, 6534yds, Par 72, SSS 71, Course record 67.
Club membership 450.

Visitors Mon-Fri, Sun & BHs. Booking required. Dress code. **Societies** Booking required. **Green Fees** £35 per day, £25 per round (£45/£35 Sun & BHs). **Prof** Phil Bradley **Course Designer** Simon Gidman **Facilities** ⊕ ⚊ by prior arrangement ⚊ ⚏ ⚊ ⚊ ⚊ ⚊ **Conf** Corporate Hospitality Days **Location** 0.5m from the York ring road B1237, just off A19 Thirsk road through the village of Skelton

Hotel ★★ 74% HL Beechwood Close Hotel, 19 Shipton Rd, Clifton, YORK ☎ 01904 658378 & 627093 📄 01904 647124 14 en suite

Forest Park Stockton-on-the-Forest YO32 9UW

☎ 01904 400425

e-mail: admin@forestparkgolfclub.co.uk

web: www.forestparkgolfclub.co.uk

Flat parkland 27-hole course with large greens and narrow tree-lined fairways. The Old Foss beck meanders through the course, creating a natural hazard on many holes.

Old Foss Course: 18 holes, 6673yds, Par 71, SSS 72, Course record 66.
The West Course: 9 holes, 3186yds, Par 70, SSS 70.
Club membership 600.

Visitors Mon-Sun & BHs. Booking required. Dress code. **Societies** booking required. **Green Fees** not confirmed. **Prof** Mark Winterburn **Facilities** ⊕ ⚊ ⚊ ⚏ ⚊ ⚊ ⚊ ⚊ **Conf** facs Corporate Hospitality Days **Location** 4m NE of York off A64 York bypass

Hotel ★★ 68% HL Jacobean Lodge Hotel, Plainville Ln, Wigginton, YORK ☎ 01904 762749 8 en suite

Fulford Heslington Ln YO10 5DY

☎ 01904 413579 📄 01904 416918

e-mail: gary@fulfordgolfclub.co.uk

web: www.fulfordgolfclub.co.uk

A flat, parkland and heathland course well-known for the superb quality of its turf, particularly the greens, and now famous as the venue for some of the best golf tournaments in the British Isles in past years.

18 holes, 6775yds, Par 72, SSS 72, Course record 62.
Club membership 700.

Visitors Mon-Fri & Sun. Booking required. Handicap certificate. Dress code. **Societies** Booking required **Green Fees** £65 per day. **Prof** Guy Wills **Course Designer** C. MacKenzie **Facilities** ⊕ ⚊ ⚊ ⚏ ⚊ ⚊ ⚊ **Conf** Corporate Hospitality Days **Location** 2m S of York off A19

Hotel ★★★★ 75% HL York Marriott Hotel, Tadcaster Rd, YORK ☎ 01904 701000 151 en suite

Hotel ★★★ 74% HL Best Western York Pavilion Hotel, 45 Main St, Fulford, YORK ☎ 01904 622099 Fax 01904 626939 57 en suite

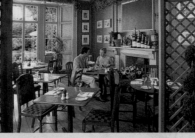

Best Western York Pavilion Hotel

Heworth Muncaster House, Muncastergate YO31 9JY

☎ 01904 422389 📄 01904 426156

e-mail: golf@heworth-gc.fsnet.co.uk

web: www.heworth-gc.co.uk

A 12-hole parkland course, easy walking. holes 3 to 7 and 9 played twice from different tees.

12 holes, 6105yds, Par 69, SSS 69, Course record 68.
Club membership 550.

Visitors Mon-Sun & BHs. Dress code. **Societies** booking required. **Green Fees** not confirmed. ⊛ **Prof** Stephen Burdett **Course Designer** B Cheal **Facilities** ⊕ by prior arrangement ⚊ by prior arrangement ⚊ by prior arrangement ⚊ ⚏ ⚊ ⚊ **Conf** Corporate Hospitality Days **Location** 1.5m NE of city centre on A1036

Hotel ★★★ 79% HL Best Western Monkbar Hotel, Monkbar, YORK ☎ 01904 638086 99 en suite

Swallow Hall Crockey Hill YO19 4SG

☎ 01904 448889 📄 01904 448219

e-mail: jtscores@hotmail.com

web: www.swallowhall.co.uk

A small 18-hole, Par 3 course with three Par 4s. Attached to a caravan park and holiday cottages.

18 holes, 3600yds, Par 57, SSS 56, Course record 58.
Club membership 100.

Visitors Mon-Sun & BHs. **Societies** Booking required. **Green Fees** £12 per round (£14 Sat & Sun). **Prof** Dan Moodie **Course Designer** Brian Henry **Facilities** ⊕ ⚊ ⚊ ⚏ ⚊ ⚊ ⚊ ⚊ **Leisure** hard tennis courts, fishing. **Conf** facs Corporate Hospitality Days **Location** Off A19 signed Wheldrake

Hotel ★★★ 74% HL Best Western York Pavilion Hotel, 45 Main St, Fulford, YORK ☎ 01904 622099 57 en suite

York Lords Moor Ln, Strensall YO32 5XF

☎ 01904 491840 (Sec) & 490304 (Pro) 📄 01904 491852

e-mail: secretary@yorkgolfclub.co.uk

web: www.yorkgolfclub.co.uk

A pleasant, well-designed, heathland course with easy walking. The course is of good length but is flat so not too tiring. The course is well bunkered with excellent greens and there are two testing pond holes.

Continued

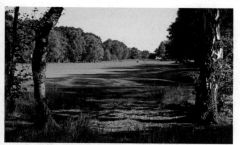

York

18 holes, 6301yds, Par 70, SSS 70, Course record 66.
Club membership 750.
Visitors Mon-Fri except BHs. Booking required. Handicap certificate. Dress code. **Societies** Booking required. **Green Fees** £50 for 36 holes, £42 for 27 holes, £36 for 18 holes. ⏺ **Prof** A P Hoyles **Course Designer** J H Taylor **Facilities** ⑪ ⑪◎ 🍴 ▯🛒 ⚑ 🏊 ✓ **Conf** Corporate Hospitality Days **Location** 6m NE of York, E of Strensall
Hotel ★★★ 85% HL Best Western Dean Court Hotel, Duncombe Place, YORK ☎ 01904 625082 37 en suite

YORKSHIRE, SOUTH

BARNSLEY   MAP 08 SE30

Barnsley Wakefield Rd, Staincross S75 6JZ
☎ 01226 382856 📠 01226 382856
e-mail: barnsleygolfclub@hotmail.com
Undulating municipal parkland course with easy walking apart from last 4 holes. Testing 8th and 18th holes.
18 holes, 5951yds, Par 69, SSS 69, Course record 64.
Club membership 450.
Visitors Mon-Sun & BHs. Booking required. **Societies** Booking required **Green Fees** £12.50 per 18 holes (£15 Sat & Sun). ⏺ **Prof** Shaun Wyke **Facilities** ⑪ by prior arrangement ◎ by prior arrangement ▯🛒 🏊 ⚑ ✓ **Location** 3m N on A61
Hotel ★★★ 78% HL Ardsley House Hotel & Health Club, Doncaster Rd, Ardsley, BARNSLEY ☎ 01226 309955 75 en suite

Sandhill Middlecliffe Ln, Little Houghton S72 0HW
☎ 01226 753444 📠 01226 753444
web: www.sandhillgolfclub.co.uk
Attractive, easy walking parkland with views of the surrounding countryside. Designed with strategically placed bunkers, the 4th hole having a deep bunker directly in front of the green.
18 holes, 6273yds, Par 71, SSS 70, Course record 69.
Club membership 450.
Visitors Mon-Sun & BHs. Booking required. Dress code. **Societies** Booking required **Green Fees** £15 per round (£20 Sat, Sun & BHs).
Course Designer John Royston **Facilities** ⑪◎ 🍴 ▯🛒 🏊 ⚑ ✓ ⚐ **Location** 5m E of Barnsley off A635
Hotel ★★★ 78% HL Ardsley House Hotel & Health Club, Doncaster Rd, Ardsley, BARNSLEY ☎ 01226 309955 75 en suite

BAWTRY   MAP 08 SK69

Bawtry Cross Ln, Austerfield DN10 6RF
☎ 01302 710841
web: www.bawtrygolfclub.co.uk
18 holes, 6994yds, Par 73, SSS 73, Course record 67.
Location 2m from Bawtry on A614
Telephone for further details
Hotel ★★★★ 77% HL Best Western Mount Pleasant Hotel, Great North Rd, DONCASTER ☎ 01302 868696 & 868219 📠 01302 865130 57 en suite

CONISBROUGH   MAP 08 SK59

Crookhill Park Municipal Carr Ln DN12 2AH
☎ 01709 862979 📠 01709 866455
Naturally sloping parkland with many holes featuring tight dog-legs and small, undulating greens. The signature hole (11th) involves a fearsome tee shot over a ditch onto a sloping fairway and final shot to an elevated green surrounded by tall trees and deep bunkers.
18 holes, 5849yds, Par 70, SSS 68, Course record 64.
Club membership 350.
Visitors Mon-Sun & BHs. Booking required. **Societies** Booking required **Green Fees** £12.75 per round (£13.95 Sat & Sun). ⏺ **Prof** Richard Swaine **Facilities** 🛒 ▯🛒 🏊 ⚑ ⚐ **Location** 1.5m SE on B6094
Hotel ★★ 65% HL Pastures Hotel, Pastures Rd, MEXBOROUGH ☎ 01709 577707 29 en suite

DONCASTER   MAP 08 SE50

Doncaster 278 Bawtry Rd, Bessacarr DN4 7PD
☎ 01302 865632 📠 01302 865994
e-mail: doncastergolf@aol.com
web: www.doncastergolfclub.org.uk
18 holes, 6220yds, Par 69, SSS 70, Course record 66.
Course Designer Mackenzie/Hawtree **Location** 4m SE on A638
Telephone for further details
Hotel ★★★★ 77% HL Best Western Mount Pleasant Hotel, Great North Rd, DONCASTER ☎ 01302 868696 & 868219 📠 01302 865130 57 en suite

Doncaster Town Moor Bawtry Rd, Belle Vue DN4 5HU
☎ 01302 535286 (pro shop) & 533778 (office)
📠 01302 533778
e-mail: dtmgc@btconnect.com
web: www.doncastertownmoorgolfclub.co.uk
Easy walking, but testing, heathland course with good true greens. Notable hole is 11th (Par 4), 464yds. Situated in centre of racecourse.
18 holes, 6072yds, Par 69, SSS 69, Course record 63.
Club membership 520.
Visitors Mon-Sun except BHs. Booking required Sat & Sun. Dress code. **Societies** Booking required. **Green Fees** £24 per round (£26 Sat & Sun).
⏺ **Prof** Steven Shaw **Facilities** ⑪◎ 🍴 ▯🛒 🏊 ⚑ ✓ **Conf** facs Corporate Hospitality Days **Location** 1.5m E at racecourse on A638
Hotel BUD Campanile, Doncaster Leisure Park, Bawtry Rd, DONCASTER ☎ 01302 370770 50 en suite

Owston Park Owston Ln, Owston DN6 8EF
☎ 01302 330821
e-mail: michael.parker@foremostgolf.com
A flat easy walking course surrounded by woodland. A lot of mature trees and a few ditches in play. A practice putting green and chipping area.
9 holes, 2866yds, Par 35, SSS 70.
Visitors no restrictions. **Societies** Booking required **Green Fees** phone. **Prof** Mike Parker **Course Designer** M Parker **Facilities** ⊒ ⚍ 🖫 ☜ 🍴 🍸 🖫 🍴 **Location** 5m N of Doncaster off A19
Hotel ★★★ 70% HL Danum Hotel, High St, DONCASTER
☎ 01302 342261 64 en suite

Thornhurst Park Holme Ln, Owston DN5 0LR
☎ 01302 337799 📠 01302 721495
e-mail: info@thornhurst.co.uk
web: www.thornhurst.co.uk
Surrounded by Owston Wood, this scenic parkland course has numerous strategically placed bunkers, and a lake comes into play at the 7th and 8th holes.
18 holes, 6490yds, Par 72, SSS 72, Course record 72.
Club membership 160.
Visitors Mon-Sun & BHs. Booking required Fri-Sun & BHs. Dress code. **Societies** Booking required. **Green Fees** £12 per 18 holes, £7 per 9 holes (£14/£8 Sat, Sun & BHs). **Prof** Kevin Pearce **Facilities** ⊕ 🍴 🍸 🖫 ⊒ 🍴 ⚍ 🖫 🍴 **Conf** facs Corporate Hospitality Days **Location** On A19 between Bentley and Askern
Hotel ★★★ 70% HL Danum Hotel, High St, DONCASTER
☎ 01302 342261 64 en suite

Wheatley Armthorpe Rd DN2 5QB
☎ 01302 831655 📠 01302 812736
e-mail: secretary@wheatleygolfclub.co.uk
Fairly flat well-bunkered, lake-holed, parkland course. Well-drained, in excellent condition all year round.
18 holes, 6405yds, Par 71, SSS 71, Course record 64.
Club membership 600.
Visitors Mon-Fri except BHs. Handicap certificate. Dress code. Must contact in advance. **Societies** Booking required **Green Fees** £30 per round (£37 Sat & Sun). **Prof** Steven Fox **Course Designer** George Duncan **Facilities** ⊕ 🍴 🍸 🖫 ⊒ 🍴 ⚍ 🖫 🍴 **Conf** Corporate Hospitality Days **Location** NE of town centre off A18
Hotel ★★★ 74% HL Regent Hotel, Regent Square, DONCASTER
☎ 01302 364180 52 en suite

HATFIELD MAP 08 SE60

Kings Wood Thorne Rd DN7 6EP
☎ 01405 741343
A flat course with ditches that come into play on several holes, especially on the testing back nine. Notable holes are the 12th Par 4, 16th and Par 5 18th. Water is a prominent feature with several large lakes strategically placed.
18 holes, 6002yds, Par 70, SSS 69, Course record 67.
Club membership 100.
Visitors Mon-Sun & BHs. Booking required. **Societies** Welcome. **Green Fees** £7.50 per 18 holes, £4.50 per 9 holes (£8.50/£5 Sat, Sun & BHs). **Prof** Mark Cunningham **Course Designer** John Hunt **Facilities** ⊒ 🖫 🍴 🍸 🖫 **Location** M180 junct 1, A614 towards Thorne, onto A1146 towards Hatfield for 0.8m

HICKLETON MAP 08 SE40

Hickleton Lidgett Ln DN5 7BE
☎ 01709 896081 📠 01709 896083
e-mail: john@hickletongolfclub.co.uk
web: www.hickletongolfclub.co.uk
Undulating, picturesque parkland course designed by Neil Coles and Brian Huggett offering a good test of golf and fine views of the eastern Pennines.
18 holes, 6434yds, Par 71, SSS 71, Course record 64.
Club membership 625.
Visitors Mon-Fri except BHs. Booking required. Dress code. **Societies** Booking required. **Green Fees** £40 per day, £32 per round. **Prof** Paul J Audsley **Course Designer** Huggett/Coles **Facilities** ⊕ 🍴 🍸 🖫 ⊒ 🍴 ⚍ 🖫 **Conf** facs Corporate Hospitality Days **Location** 3m W from A1(M) junct 37, off A635
Hotel ★★★ 70% HL Danum Hotel, High St, DONCASTER
☎ 01302 342261 64 en suite

HIGH GREEN MAP 08 SK39

Tankersley Park S35 4LG
☎ 0114 246 8247 📠 0114 245 7818
e-mail: secretary@tpgc.freeserve.co.uk
web: www.tankersleyparkgolfclub.org.uk
Rolling parkland course that demands accuracy rather than length. Lush fairways. The 18th hole considered to be one of the best last hole tests in Yorkshire.
18 holes, 6244yds, Par 70, SSS 70, Course record 64.
Club membership 634.
Visitors Mon-Fri & BHs. Booking required. Handicap certificate. Dress code. **Societies** booking required. **Green Fees** not confirmed. **Prof** Ian Kirk **Course Designer** Hawtree **Facilities** ⊕ 🍴 🍸 🖫 ⊒ 🍴 ⚍ 🖫 ☜ 🍴 🍸 **Conf** Corporate Hospitality Days **Location** A61/M1 onto A616 Stocksbridge bypass
Hotel ★★★★ 75% HL Tankersley Manor, Church Ln, TANKERSLEY
☎ 01226 744700 99 en suite

RAWMARSH MAP 08 SK49

Wath Abdy Ln S62 7SJ
☎ 01709 878609 📠 01709 877097
e-mail: golf@wathgolfclub.co.uk
Parkland course, not easy in spite of its length. Testing course with narrow fairways and small greens. Many dikes crisscross fairways, making playing for position paramount. Strategically placed copses reward the golfer who is straight off the tee. Playing over a pond into a prevailing wind on the 12th hole to a postage stamp size green, will test the most accomplished player.
18 holes, 6123yds, Par 70, SSS 69, Course record 65.
Club membership 650.
Visitors Mon-Fri except BHs. Booking required. Handicap certificate. Dress code. **Societies** Booking required. **Green Fees** £31 per day, £26 per round. 🖫 **Prof** Chris Bassett **Facilities** ⊕ 🍴 🍸 🖫 ⊒ 🍴 ⚍ 🖫 ☜ 🍴 🍸 **Conf** facs Corporate Hospitality Days **Location** 2m N of Rotherham on B6089
Hotel ★★★ 77% HL Carlton Park Hotel, 102/104 Moorgate Rd, ROTHERHAM ☎ 01709 849955 80 en suite

ROTHERHAM MAP 08 SK49

Grange Park Upper Wortley Rd S61 2SJ
☎ 01709 559497
18 holes, 6421yds, Par 71, SSS 71, Course record 65.
Course Designer Fred Hawtree **Location** 3m NW off A629
Telephone for further details
Hotel ★★★★ 75% HL Tankersley Manor, Church Ln, TANKERSLEY ☎ 01226 744700 99 en suite

Phoenix Pavilion Ln, Brinsworth S60 5PA
☎ 01709 363864 & 382624 📠 01709 363788
e-mail: secretary@phoenixgolfclub.co.uk
web: www.phoenixgolfclub.co.uk
Easy walking, slightly undulating meadowland course with excellent greens.
18 holes, 6182yds, Par 71, SSS 70, Course record 65. Club membership 930.
Visitors contact club for details. Handicap certificate. Dress code. **Societies** welcome. **Green Fees** not confirmed. **Prof** M Roberts **Course Designer** C K Cotton **Facilities** **Leisure** squash, fishing, gymnasium. **Conf** facs Corporate Hospitality Days **Location** SW of Rotherham off A630
Hotel ★★★ 77% HL Carlton Park Hotel, 102/104 Moorgate Rd, ROTHERHAM ☎ 01709 849955 80 en suite

Rotherham Golf Club Ltd Thrybergh Park, Doncaster Rd, Thrybergh S65 4NU
☎ 01709 859500 📠 01709 859517
e-mail: manager@rotherhamgolfclub.com
web: www.rotherhamgolfclub.com
Parkland with easy walking along the tree-lined fairways.
18 holes, 6324yds, Par 70, SSS 70, Course record 65. Club membership 500.
Visitors Mon-Sun & BHs. Handicap certificate. Dress code. **Societies** Booking required **Green Fees** £30 per round, £38 per 27 holes, £45 per day. **Prof** Simon Thornhill **Course Designer** Sandy Herd **Facilities** **Location** 3.5m E on A630
Hotel ★★★ 77% HL Best Western Elton Hotel, Main St, Bramley, ROTHERHAM ☎ 01709 545681 13 en suite 16 annexe en suite

Sitwell Park Shrogswood Rd S60 4BY
☎ 01709 541046 📠 01709 703637
e-mail: secretary@sitwellgolf.co.uk
Undulating parkland.
18 holes, 5960yds, Par 71, SSS 69. Club membership 450.
Visitors Mon-Fri, Sun except BHs. Handicap certificate. Dress code. **Societies** booking required. **Green Fees** not confirmed. **Prof** Nic Taylor **Course Designer** A MacKenzie **Facilities** **Conf** Corporate Hospitality Days **Location** 2m SE of Rotherham centre off A631
Hotel ★★★★ 71% HL Hellaby Hall Hotel, Old Hellaby Ln, Hellaby, ROTHERHAM ☎ 01709 702701 90 en suite

SHEFFIELD MAP 08 SK38

Abbeydale Twentywell Ln, Dore S17 4QA
☎ 0114 236 0763 📠 0114 236 0762
e-mail: abbeygolf@btconnect.com
web: www.abbeydalegolf.co.uk
Undulating parkland course set in the Beauchief Estate with fine views over Sheffield and the Derbyshire hills.
18 holes, 6261yds, Par 71, SSS 70, Course record 64. Club membership 711.
Visitors Mon, Tue, Fri, Sun & BHs. Wed pm Only. Booking required. Handicap certificate. Dress code. **Societies** Booking required **Green Fees** £45 per day, £35 per round (£45 Sat & Sun, £35 after 2.30pm). **Prof** Nigel Perry **Course Designer** Herbert Fowler **Facilities** **Leisure** snooker. **Conf** facs Corporate Hospitality Days **Location** 4m SW of city off A621
Hotel ★★★ 72% HL The Beauchief Hotel, 161 Abbeydale Rd South, SHEFFIELD ☎ 0114 262 0500 50 en suite

Beauchief Public Abbey Ln S8 0DB
☎ 0114 236 7274
18 holes, 5469yds, Par 67, SSS 66, Course record 65.
Location 4m SW of city off A621
Telephone for further details
Hotel ★★★ 72% HL The Beauchief Hotel, 161 Abbeydale Rd South, SHEFFIELD ☎ 0114 262 0500 50 en suite

Birley Wood Birley Ln S12 3BP
☎ 0114 264 7262
e-mail: birley@sivltd.com
web: www.birleywood.com
Undulating meadowland course with well-varied features, easy walking and good views.
Fairway course: 18 holes, 5734yds, Par 69, SSS 67, Course record 64.
Birley Course: 18 holes, 5037, Par 66, SSS 65.
Club membership 278.
Visitors Mon-Sun & BHs. **Societies** booking required. **Green Fees** not confirmed. **Prof** Peter Ball **Facilities** **Location** 4.5m SE of city off A616
Hotel ★★★ 77% HL Best Western Mosborough Hall Hotel, High St, Mosborough, SHEFFIELD ☎ 0114 248 4353 47 en suite

Concord Park Shiregreen Ln S5 6AE
☎ 0114 257 7378
Hilly municipal parkland course with some fairways wood-flanked, good views, often windy. Seven Par 3 holes.
18 holes, 4872yds, Par 67, SSS 64, Course record 57. Club membership 220.
Visitors contact club for details. **Societies** welcome. **Green Fees** not confirmed. **Prof** W Allcroft **Facilities** **Leisure** hard tennis courts, heated indoor swimming pool, squash, sauna, solarium, gymnasium. **Conf** Corporate Hospitality Days **Location** 3.5m N of city on B6086, off A6135
Hotel BUD Premier Travel Inn Sheffield (Meadowhall), Sheffield Rd, Meadowhall, SHEFFIELD ☎ 0870 9906440 103 en suite

Dore & Totley Bradway Rd, Bradway S17 4QR
☎ 0114 2366 844 ▤ 0114 2366 844
e-mail: dtgc@lineone.net
web: www.doreandtotleygolf.co.uk
Flat parkland course recently upgraded with the addition of 5
new holes making the course 500 yards longer.
18 holes, 6763yds, Par 72, SSS 72, Course record 66.
Club membership 580.
Visitors Mon-Fri, Sun & BHs. Booking required. Dress code. **Societies**
Booking required. **Green Fees** £37 per day, £32 per round (£36 Sun). ⊕
Prof Gregg Roberts **Facilities** ⓦ ⍟ ⓛ ⎚ ⌀ ⏚ ⚑ ✎ ✦ ✎ **Leisure**
snooker. **Conf** facs Corporate Hospitality Days **Location** 7m S of city on
B6054, off A61
Hotel ★★★ 72% HL The Beauchief Hotel, 161 Abbeydale Rd South,
SHEFFIELD ☎ 0114 262 0500 50 en suite

Hallamshire Golf Club Ltd Sandygate S10 4LA
☎ 0114 230 2153 ▤ 0114 230 5413
e-mail: secretary@hallamshiregolfclub.co.uk
web: www.hallamshiregolfclub.co.uk
Situated on a shelf of land at a height of 850ft. Magnificent views
to the west. Moorland turf, long carries over ravine and small and
quick greens.
18 holes, 6346yds, Par 71, SSS 71, Course record 65.
Club membership 600.
Visitors Mon-Fri except BHs. Booking required. Handicap certificate.
Dress code. **Societies** Booking required. **Green Fees** £45 per day. **Prof**
G R Tickell **Course Designer** Various **Facilities** ⓦ ⍟ ⓛ ⎚ ⌀ ⏚ ⚑
⚑ ✎ **Conf** Corporate Hospitality Days **Location** Off A57 at Crosspool
onto Sandygate Rd, clubhouse 0.75m on right
Hotel ★★★★ 76% HL Sheffield Marriott, Kenwood Rd, SHEFFIELD
☎ 0114 258 3811 114 en suite

Hillsborough Worrall Rd S6 4BE
☎ 0114 234 9151 (Sec) ▤ 0114 229 4105
e-mail: admin@hillsboroughgolfclub.co.uk
web: www.hillsboroughgolfclub.co.uk
Beautiful moorland and woodland course 500ft above sea level,
reasonable walking. Challenging first four holes into a prevailing wind
and a tight, testing 14th hole.
18 holes, 6345yards, Par 71, SSS 70, Course record 63.
Club membership 650.
Visitors Mon-Fri except BHs. Sun pm only. Booking required. Dress code.
Societies Booking required. **Green Fees** Phone. ⊕ **Prof** Lewis Horsman
Facilities ⓦ ⍟ ⓛ ⎚ ⌀ ⏚ ⚑ ⚑ ✦ **Conf** Corporate Hospitality
Days **Location** 3m NW of city off A616
Hotel ★★★★ 75% HL Tankersley Manor, Church Ln, TANKERSLEY
☎ 01226 744700 99 en suite

Lees Hall Hemsworth Rd, Norton S8 8LL
☎ 0114 250 7868
18 holes, 6171yds, Par 71, SSS 70, Course record 63.
Location 3.5m S of city off A6102
Telephone for further details
Hotel ★★★★ 76% HL Sheffield Marriott, Kenwood Rd, SHEFFIELD
☎ 0114 258 3811 114 en suite

Rother Valley Golf Centre Mansfield Rd, Wales Bar
S26 5PQ
☎ 0114 247 3000 ▤ 0114 247 6000
e-mail: rother-jackbarker@btinternet.com
web: www.jackbarker.com
The challenging Blue Monster parkland course features a variety of
water hazards. Notable holes include the 7th, with its island green
fronted by water and dominated by bunkers to the rear. Lookout for
the water on the Par 5 18th.
18 holes, 6602yds, Par 72, SSS 72, Course record 70.
Club membership 500.
Visitors Mon-Sun & BHs. Booking required Fri-Sun & BHs. Dress code.
Societies booking required. **Green Fees** not confirmed. **Prof** Jason Ripley
Course Designer Michael Shattock & Mark Roe **Facilities** ⓦ ⍟ ⓛ ⎚ ⌀ ⏚
⏚ ⚑ ⚑ ✦ ✎ ✦ ⚑ **Conf** facs Corporate Hospitality Days **Location** M1
junct 31, signs to Rother Valley Country Park
Hotel ★★★ 77% HL Best Western Mosborough Hall Hotel, High St,
Mosborough, SHEFFIELD ☎ 0114 248 4353 47 en suite

Tinsley Park Municipal Golf High Hazels Park, Darnall
S9 4PE
☎ 0114 244 8974
Undulating parkland with plenty of trees and rough. Easy walking. The
signature hole is the Par 3 17th.
18 holes, 6064yds, Par 70, SSS 68, Course record 66.
Club membership 239.
Visitors Mon-Sun & BHs. Booking required Fri-Sun. Dress code. **Societies**
Booking required. **Green Fees** £10.40 per round (£13 Fri-Sun). **Prof** W
Yellott **Facilities** ⎚ ⏚ ⚑ ⚑ ✦ **Location** 4m E of city off A630
Hotel ★★★ 77% HL Best Western Mosborough Hall Hotel, High St,
Mosborough, SHEFFIELD ☎ 0114 248 4353 47 en suite

SILKSTONE   MAP 08 SE20

Silkstone Field Head, Elmhirst Ln S75 4LD
☎ 01226 790328 ▤ 01226 794902
e-mail: silkstonegolf@hotmail.co.uk
web: www.silkstone-golf-club.co.uk
Parkland and downland course, fine views over the Pennines. Testing
golf.
18 holes, 6069yds, Par 70, SSS 70, Course record 64.
Club membership 530.
Visitors Mon-Fri except BHs. Booking required. Dress code. **Societies**
Booking required. **Green Fees** £36 per day, £28 per round. ⊕ **Prof** Kevin
Guy **Facilities** ⓦ ⍟ ⓛ ⎚ ⌀ ⏚ ⚑ ✦ ✦ **Conf** Corporate Hospitality
Days **Location** M1, junct 37, 1m E off A628
Hotel ★★★ 78% HL Ardsley House Hotel & Health Club, Doncaster Rd,
Ardsley, BARNSLEY ☎ 01226 309955 75 en suite

STOCKSBRIDGE   MAP 08 SK29

Stocksbridge & District Royd Ln, Deepcar S36 2RZ
☎ 0114 288 2003 (office) ▤ 0114 283 1460
e-mail: secretary@stocksbridgeanddistrictgolfclub.com
web: www.stocksbridgeanddistrictgolfclub.com
18 holes, 5200yds, Par 65, SSS 65, Course record 60.
Course Designer Dave Thomas **Location** S of town centre
Telephone for further details
Hotel ★★★ 74% HL Whitley Hall Hotel, Elliott Ln, Grenoside, SHEFFIELD
☎ 0114 245 4444 20 en suite

THORNE — MAP 08 SE61

Thorne Kirton Ln DN8 5RJ
☎ 01405 812084 📠 01405 741899
web: www.thornegolf.co.uk
Picturesque parkland with 6000 newly planted trees. Water hazards on 11th, 14th and 18th holes.
18 holes, 5366yds, Par 68, SSS 66, Course record 62. Club membership 300.
Visitors Mon-Sun & BHs. **Societies** Booking required. **Green Fees** £11 per round (£12 Sat & Sun). **Prof** Edward Highfield **Course Designer** R D Highfield **Facilities** ⑪ ⑩ ⅃ ⬛ ☖ ⑪ ⅄ 🛒 ⑰ ⑰ ⑰ **Conf** facs Corporate Hospitality Days **Location** M180 Junct 1, A614 into Thorne, left onto Kirton Ln

WORTLEY — MAP 08 SK39

Wortley Hermit Hill Ln S35 7DF
☎ 0114 288 8469 📠 0114 288 8488
e-mail: wortley.golfclub@btconnect.com
Well-wooded, undulating parkland, sheltered from the prevailing wind. Excellent greens in a totally pastoral setting.

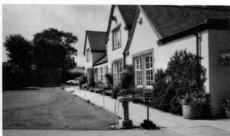

18 holes, 6028yds, Par 69, SSS 68, Course record 62. Club membership 600.
Visitors Mon-Sun & BHs. Booking required. Dress code. **Societies** Booking required **Green Fees** £30 per day (£35 per round Sat & Sun). **Prof** Ian Kirk **Facilities** ⑪ ⑩ ⅃ ⬛ ☖ ⑪ ⅄ 🛒 ⑰ ⑰ **Conf** Corporate Hospitality Days **Location** 0.5m NE of village off A629
Hotel ★★★ 74% HL Whitley Hall Hotel, Elliott Ln, Grenoside, SHEFFIELD ☎ 0114 245 4444 20 en suite

YORKSHIRE, WEST

ADDINGHAM — MAP 07 SE04

Bracken Ghyll Skipton Rd LS29 0SL
☎ 01943 831207 📠 01943 839453
e-mail: secretary@brackenghyll.co.uk
web: www.brackenghyll.co.uk
On the edge of the Yorkshire Dales, the course commands superb views over Ilkley Moor and the Wharfe valley. The demanding 18-hole layout is a test of both golfing ability and sensible course management.
18 holes, 5600yds, Par 69, SSS 67, Course record 66. Club membership 350.
Visitors Mon-Fri & BHs. Sat & Sun pm only. Booking required. Dress code. **Societies** Booking required. **Green Fees** £25 per day, £20 per round (£29/£24 Sat, Sun & BHs). **Facilities** ⑪ ⑩ ⅃ ⬛ ☖ ⑪ ⅄ 🛒 ⑰ **Conf** Corporate Hospitality Days **Location** Off A65 between Ilkley and Skipton

Hotel ★★★ 82% HL Best Western Rombalds Hotel & Restaurant, 11 West View, Wells Rd, ILKLEY ☎ 01943 603201 15 en suite

ALWOODLEY — MAP 08 SE24

Alwoodley Wigton Ln LS17 8SA
☎ 0113 268 1680
e-mail: alwoodley@btconnect.com
web: www.alwoodley.co.uk
Natural moorland course with heather, whins and shrubs. Plentifully and cunningly bunkered with undulating and interesting greens.
18 holes, 6666yds, Par 72, SSS 72. Club membership 460.
Visitors Mon-Sun except BHs. Booking required. Dress code. **Societies** Booking required **Green Fees** £70 per day (£85 Sat & Sun). £40 per 4pm. **Prof** John R Green **Course Designer** Dr Alistair MacKenzie **Facilities** ⑪ ⑩ ⅃ ⬛ ☖ ⑪ ⅄ 🛒 ⑰ **Conf** Corporate Hospitality Days **Location** 5m N off A61
Hotel ★★★ 72% HL The Merrion Hotel, Merrion Centre, LEEDS ☎ 0113 243 9191 109 en suite

BAILDON — MAP 07 SE13

Baildon Moorgate BD17 5PP
☎ 01274 584266
web: www.baildongolfclub.com
Moorland course set out in links style with the outward front nine looping back to clubhouse. Panoramic views with testing short holes in prevailing winds. The 2nd hole has been described as one of Britain's scariest.

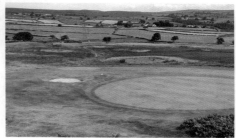

18 holes, 6225yds, Par 70, SSS 70, Course record 63. Club membership 750.
Visitors Mon-Sun & BHs. Booking required Tue, Sat & Sun. Handicap certificate. Dress code. **Societies** Booking required. **Green Fees** 18 holes £26 (£30 Sat & Sun). ⑨ **Prof** Richard Masters **Course Designer** Tom Morris/James Braid **Facilities** ⑪ ⑩ ⅃ ⬛ ☖ ⑪ ⅄ 🛒 ⑰ **Leisure** snooker tables. **Conf** facs Corporate Hospitality Days **Location** 3m N of Bradford off A6038 at Shipley
Hotel ★★★★ 78% HL Marriott Hollins Hall Hotel & Country Club, Hollins Hill, Baildon, SHIPLEY ☎ 0870 400 7227 122 en suite

England

BINGLEY

MAP 07 SE13

Bingley St Ives Golf Club House, St Ives Estate, Harden BD16 1AT

☎ 01274 562436 🖹 01274 511788

e-mail: secretary@bingleystivesgc.co.uk

web: www.bingleystivesgc.co.uk

Parkland and moorland course.

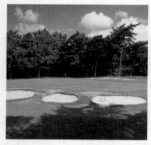

18 holes, 6485yds, Par 71, SSS 71, Course record 69.
Club membership 450.
Visitors Mon-Fri, Sun & BHs. Booking required. Handicap certificate. Dress code. **Societies** Booking required **Green Fees** Phone. **Prof** Nigel Barber **Course Designer** Alastair Mackenzie **Facilities** ⑪ ⑩ ⒧ ☐ ⊤ℐ ⌣ 🖻 🎿 ⚐ 🏌 **Conf** facs Corporate Hospitality Days **Location** 0.75m W off B6429
Hotel ★★ 70% HL Dalesgate Hotel, 406 Skipton Rd, Utley, KEIGHLEY
☎ 01535 664930 20 en suite

Shipley Beckfoot Ln BD16 1LX

☎ 01274 568652 (Secretary) 🖹 01274 567739

e-mail: office@shipleygc.co.uk

web: www.shipleygc.co.uk

Well-established parkland course, founded in 1922, featuring six good Par 3s.
18 holes, 6209yds, Par 71, SSS 70, Course record 66.
Club membership 600.
Visitors Mon, Wed-Fri, Sun & BHs. Tue & Sat pm only. Dress code.
Societies Booking required. **Green Fees** £42 per day, £35 per round (£49/£40 Sun & BHs). **Prof** J R Parry **Course Designer** Colt, Allison, Mackenzie, Braid **Facilities** ⑪ ⑩ ⒧ ☐ ⊤ℐ ⌣ 🖻 ⚐ 🏌 **Conf** facs Corporate Hospitality Days **Location** 6m N of Bradford on A650
Hotel ★★ 70% HL Dalesgate Hotel, 406 Skipton Rd, Utley, KEIGHLEY
☎ 01535 664930 20 en suite

BRADFORD

MAP 07 SE13

Bradford Moor Scarr Hall, Pollard Ln BD2 4RW

☎ 01274 771716 & 771693

Moorland course with tricky undulating greens.
9 holes, 5900yds, Par 70, SSS 68, Course record 65.
Club membership 330.
Visitors Mon-Fr & BHs. Booking required BHs. Dress code. **Societies** booking required. **Green Fees** not confirmed. ⚐ **Facilities** ☐ ⊤ℐ ⌣
Location 2m NE of city centre off A658
Hotel ★★★ 79% HL Midland Hotel, Forster Square, BRADFORD
☎ 01274 735735 90 en suite

Clayton Thornton View Rd, Clayton BD14 6JX

☎ 01274 880047

Parkland course, difficult in windy conditions.
9 holes, 6300yds, Par 72, SSS 72. Club membership 250.
Visitors Mon-Fri & BHs. Dress code. **Societies** booking required. **Green Fees** not confirmed. ⚐ **Facilities** ⑪ ⑩ ⒧ ☐ ⊤ℐ ⌣ **Conf** Corporate Hospitality Days **Location** 2.5m SW of city centre on A647
Hotel ★★★ 70% HL Novotel Bradford, 6 Roydsdale Way, BRADFORD
☎ 01274 683683 119 en suite

East Bierley South View Rd, East Bierley BD4 6PP

☎ 01274 681023 🖹 01274 683666

e-mail: rjwelch@talktalk.net

Hilly moorland course with narrow fairways. Two Par 3 holes over 200yds.
9 holes, 4700yds, Par 64, SSS 63, Course record 59.
Club membership 300.
Visitors Tue, Thu & Fri except BHs. Handicap certificate. Dress code.
Societies Booking welcome. **Green Fees** Phone. ⚐ **Prof** J. Whittam
Facilities ☐ ⊤ℐ ⌣ 🖻 **Location** 4m SE of city centre off A650
Hotel ★★★ 70% HL Novotel Bradford, 6 Roydsdale Way, BRADFORD
☎ 01274 683683 119 en suite

Headley Headley Ln, Thornton BD13 3LX

☎ 01274 833481 🖹 01274 833481

e-mail: danny.britton@headleygolfclub.co.uk

web: www.headleygolfclub.co.uk

Hilly moorland course, short but very testing, windy, fine views.
9 holes, 4864yds, Par 65, SSS 65, Course record 57.
Club membership 256.
Visitors Mon-Sun & BHs. Booking required Sat & Sun. Dress code.
Societies Welcome. **Green Fees** Phone. ⚐ **Facilities** ⑪ ⑩ ⒧ ☐ ⊤ℐ ⌣
Conf Corporate Hospitality Days **Location** 4m W of city centre off B6145 at Thornton
Hotel ★★★ 79% HL Midland Hotel, Forster Square, BRADFORD
☎ 01274 735735 90 en suite

Queensbury Brighouse Rd, Queensbury BD13 1QF

☎ 01274 882155 & 816864 🖹 01274 882155

web: www.queensburygc.co.uk

Undulating woodland and parkland.
9 holes, 5024yds, Par 66, SSS 65, Course record 59.
Club membership 350.
Visitors Mon-Fri & BHs. Booking required Sat & Sun. Dress code. **Societies** Booking required. **Green Fees** Phone. ⚐ **Prof** Nathan Stead **Course Designer** Jonathan Gaunt **Facilities** ⑪ ⑩ ⒧ ☐ ⊤ℐ ⌣ 🖻 ⚐ 🖻 🏌 **Conf** Corporate Hospitality Days **Location** 4m from Bradford on A647
Hotel ★★★ 79% HL Midland Hotel, Forster Square, BRADFORD
☎ 01274 735735 90 en suite

South Bradford Pearson Rd, Odsal BD6 1BH

☎ 01274 673346 (pro shop) & 679195 🖹 01274 690643

Hilly course with good greens, trees and ditches. Interesting short 2nd hole (Par 3) 200yds, well-bunkered and played from an elevated tee.
9 holes, 6068yds, Par 70, SSS 68, Course record 65.
Club membership 300.
Visitors Mon-Fri except BHs. Booking required. Dress code. **Societies** Booking required. **Green Fees** Phone. **Prof** Paul Cooke **Facilities** ⑪ ⑩
by prior arrangement ⒧ ☐ ⊤ℐ ⌣ 🖻 ⚐ **Location** 2m S of city centre off A638
Hotel ★★★ 70% HL Novotel Bradford, 6 Roydsdale Way, BRADFORD
☎ 01274 683683 119 en suite

West Bowling Newall Hall, Rooley Ln BD5 8LB
☎ 01274 393207 (office) & 728036 (pro) 📄 01274 393207
18 holes, 5769yds, Par 69, SSS 67, Course record 65.
Location Junct M606
Telephone for further details
Hotel ★★★ 70% HL Cedar Court Hotel, Mayo Av, Off Rooley Ln,
BRADFORD ☎ 01274 406606 131 en suite

West Bradford Chellow Grange Rd, Haworth Rd
BD9 6NP
☎ 01274 542767 📄 01274 482079
e-mail: secretary@westbradfordgolfclub.co.uk
web: www.westbradfordgolfclub.co.uk
Parkland course providing a good test for golfers of all abilities with its
undulating terrain, tree-lined fairways and demanding Par 3 holes.
18 holes, 5738yds, Par 69, SSS 68, Course record 63.
Club membership 440.
Visitors Mon-Fri, Sun & BHs. Booking required. Dress code.
Societies Booking required. **Green Fees** £30 per day. **Prof** Warren Kemp
Facilities ⑪🍴🍸☕🍴⚐⚑🏌 **Leisure** snooker room. **Conf** facs
Corporate Hospitality Days **Location** 3.5 m W of city centre off B6144
Hotel ★★★★ 78% HL Marriott Hollins Hall Hotel & Country Club, Hollins
Hill, Baildon, SHIPLEY ☎ 0870 400 7227 122 en suite

BRIGHOUSE MAP 07 SE12

Willow Valley Golf Highmoor Ln, Clifton HD6 4JB
☎ 01274 878624
e-mail: sales@wvgc.co.uk
web: www.wvgc.co.uk
A championship length 18-hole course offering a unique golfing
experience, featuring island greens, shaped fairways and bunkers, and
multiple teeing areas. The nine-hole course offers an exciting challenge
to less experienced golfers and the 18 hole course, Pine Valley, is
suitable for golfers of all abilities.

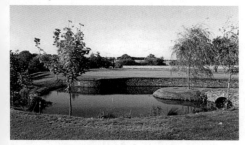

Willow Valley: 18 holes, 7030yds, Par 72, SSS 74,
Course record 69.
Pine Valley: 18 holes, 5032yds, Par 67, SSS 64.
Fountain Ridge: 9 holes, 2039yds, Par 62, SSS 60.
Club membership 350.
Visitors Mon-Sun & BHs. Dress code. **Societies** Booking required. **Green**
Fees Willow Valley: £25 per round, Pine Valley: £12.50 per round, Fountain
Ridge: £7.50 per round (£35/£14.50/£9 Sat, Sun & BHs). **Prof** Julian Haworth
Course Designer Jonathan Gaunt **Facilities** ⑪🍴 by prior arrangement
🍸☕🍴⚐⚑⚑🏌 **Leisure** 3 hole floodlit academy course.
Conf Corporate Hospitality Days **Location** M62 junct 25, A644 towards
Brighouse, right at rdbt onto A643, course 2m on right
Hotel ★★★ 71% HL Healds Hall Hotel, Leeds Rd, Liversedge, DEWSBURY
☎ 01924 409112 24 en suite

CLECKHEATON MAP 08 SE12

Cleckheaton & District Bradford Rd BD19 6BU
☎ 01274 851266 📄 01274 871382
e-mail: info@cleckheatongolf.co.uk
web: www.cleckheatongolfclub.co.uk
Parkland with gentle hills and easy walking. Feature holes: 5th, 16th
and 17th.
18 holes, 5706yds, Par 70, SSS 68, Course record 61.
Club membership 550.
Visitors Mon-Sun except Bhs. Handicap certificate. Dress code. **Societies**
Booking required **Green Fees** May-Sep: £35 per day, £30 per round. Nov-
Apr: £25 per day. **Prof** Mike Ingham **Course Designer** Dr A MacKenzie
Facilities ⑪🍴🍸☕🍴⚐⚑🏌 **Conf** facs **Location** M62
junct 26, towards Oakenshaw, 100yds on left, signed Low Moor
Hotel ★★★ 77% HL Gomersal Park Hotel, Moor Ln, GOMERSAL
☎ 01274 869386 100 en suite

DEWSBURY MAP 08 SE22

Hanging Heaton White Cross Rd WF12 7DT
☎ 01924 461606 📄 01924 430100
e-mail: derek.atkinson@hhgc.org
web: www.h.h.gc.org.uk
Arable land, easy walking, fine views. Testing 4th hole (Par 3).
9 holes, 5836yds, Par 69, SSS 68. Club membership 500.
Visitors Mon-Fri except BHs. Booking required. **Societies** Booking required.
Green Fees £17 per round. 🌐 **Prof** Gareth Moore **Facilities** ⑪ by prior
arrangement 🍴 by prior arrangement 🍸 by prior arrangement ☕🍴⚐
🍴 **Conf** facs Corporate Hospitality Days **Location** 0.75m NE off A653
Hotel ★★★ 71% HL Healds Hall Hotel, Leeds Rd, Liversedge, DEWSBURY
☎ 01924 409112 24 en suite

ELLAND MAP 07 SE12

Elland Hammerstone, Leach Ln HX5 0TA
☎ 01422 372505 & 374886 (pro)
9 holes, 5498yds, Par 66, SSS 67, Course record 65.
Location M62 junct 24, signs to Blackley
Telephone for further details
Hotel ★★★★ 68% HL Cedar Court Hotel, Ainley Top, HUDDERSFIELD
☎ 01422 375431 114 en suite

FENAY BRIDGE MAP 08 SE11

Woodsome Hall HD8 0LQ
☎ 01484 602739 📄 01484 608260
e-mail: thesecretary@woodsome.co.uk
web: www.woodsome.co.uk
A parkland course with good views and a historic clubhouse.

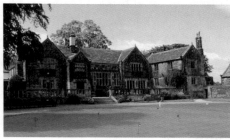

18 holes, 6096yds, Par 70, SSS 69, Course record 67.
Club membership 800.
Visitors Mon-Sun & BHs. Booking required Tue, Sat & Sun. Handicap certificate. Dress code. **Societies** Booking required. **Green Fees** not confirmed. **Prof** M Higginbotton **Facilities** ⊕ ⓘ◎ ↆ ◻️ ℃ 🈁 ♨ 📖 ⚶
Location 1.5m SW off A629
Hotel ★★★ 74% HL Bagden Hall, Wakefield Rd, Scissett, HUDDERSFIELD ☎ 01484 865330 16 en suite

GARFORTH MAP 08 SE43

Garforth Long Ln LS25 2DS
☎ 0113 286 3308 📠 0113 286 3308
e-mail: garforthgcltd@lineone.net
web: www.garforthgolfclub.co.uk
Gently undulating parkland with fine views and easy walking.
18 holes, 6304yds, Par 70, SSS 70, Course record 64.
Club membership 600.
Visitors Mon-Fri & Sun except BHs. Booking required Sun. Dress code. **Societies** Booking required. **Green Fees** £42 per day, £36 per round. ◉
Prof Ken Findlater **Course Designer** Dr Alister Mackenzie **Facilities** ⊕ ⓘ◎
ↆ ◻️ ℃ 🈁 ⛽ ♨ 📖 ⚶ **Conf** Corporate Hospitality Days **Location** 6m E
of Leeds, next to A1/M1 link road
Hotel ★★★ 79% HL Best Western Milford Hotel, A1 Great North Rd, Peckfield, LEEDS ☎ 01977 681800 46 en suite

GUISELEY MAP 08 SE14

Bradford (Hawksworth) Hawksworth Ln LS20 8NP
☎ 01943 875570 📠 01943 875570
e-mail: trevor.eagle@tiscali.co.uk
web: www.bradfordgolfclub.co.uk
Set in undulating countryside, the course is a moorland links laid out on the southern slope of a wooded ridge about 650ft above sea level. The spacious greens with their subtle borrows, together with some tough and uncompromising Par 4s make this a challenging course. The testing Par 4 10th and the Par 3 14th require accurate shots to well-protected greens.
Hawksworth: 18 holes, 6303yds, Par 71, SSS 71, Course record 65. Club membership 650.
Visitors Mon-Fri, Sun & BHs. Booking required. Handicap certificate. Dress code. **Societies** Booking required **Green Fees** £36 per day (£45 Sun & BHs). **Prof** Andrew Hall **Course Designer** W H Fowler **Facilities** ⊕ ⓘ◎
ↆ ◻️ ℃ 🈁 ♨ ⚶ **Conf** facs Corporate Hospitality Days **Location** SW of town centre off A6038
Hotel ★★★★ 78% HL Marriott Hollins Hall Hotel & Country Club, Hollins Hill, Baildon, SHIPLEY ☎ 0870 400 7227 122 en suite

HALIFAX MAP 07 SE02

Halifax Union Ln, Ogden HX2 8XR
☎ 01422 244171
e-mail: halifax.golfclub@virgin.net
web: www.halifaxgolfclub.co.uk
Moorland course crossed by streams, natural hazards and offering fine views of wildlife and the surroundings. Testing 172-yd 17th (Par 3).
18 holes, 6037yds, Par 70, SSS 69, Course record 65.
Club membership 700.
Visitors Mon-Fri. Booking required Thu & Fri. Handicap certificate. Dress code. **Societies** Booking required **Green Fees** £30 per day, £25 per round. **Prof** Michael Allison **Course Designer** A Herd/J Braid **Facilities** ⊕ ⓘ◎ ↆ

◻️ 🈁 ☂ ⚶ ⚶ **Conf** facs Corporate Hospitality Days **Location** 4m from Halifax on A629 Halifax-Keighley road
Hotel ★★★ 83% HL Holdsworth House Hotel, Holdsworth, HALIFAX ☎ 01422 240024 40 en suite

Lightcliffe Knowle Top Rd, Lightcliffe HX3 8SW
☎ 01422 202459 & 204081
A parkland course where positioning of the drive is as important as length. Signature hole is a dog-leg with the second shot over a deep ravine.
9 holes, 5388mtrs, Par 68, SSS 68. Club membership 460.
Visitors Mon, Tue, Thu-Sun & BHs. Booking required Tue. Handicap certificate. Dress code. **Societies** Booking required **Green Fees** £18 per 18 holes (£22 Sun). ◉ **Prof** Robert Tickle **Facilities** ⊕ ↆ ◻️ 🈁 ♨
⚶ **Location** 3.5m E of Halifax on A58
Hotel ★★★ 83% HL Holdsworth House Hotel, Holdsworth, HALIFAX ☎ 01422 240024 40 en suite

West End Paddock Ln, Highroad Well HX2 0NT
☎ 01422 341878 📠 01422 341878
e-mail: westendgc@btinternet.com
web: www.westendgc.co.uk
Semi-moorland course. Tree lined. Two ponds.
18 holes, 5951yds, Par 69, SSS 69, Course record 62.
Club membership 650.
Visitors Mon-Fri, Sun & BHs. Booking required. Dress code. **Societies** Booking required. **Green Fees** £30 per round. ◉ **Prof** David Rishworth **Facilities** ⊕ ⓘ◎ ↆ ◻️ 🈁 ♨ ⚶ ⚶ **Conf** Corporate Hospitality Days
Location W of town centre off A646
Hotel ★★★ 83% HL Holdsworth House Hotel, Holdsworth, HALIFAX ☎ 01422 240024 40 en suite

HEBDEN BRIDGE MAP 07 SD92

Hebden Bridge Great Mount, Wadsworth HX7 8PH
☎ 01422 842896 & 842732
e-mail: hbgc@btconnect.com
web: www.hebdenbridgegolfclub.co.uk
Moorland course, approximately 1000 feet above sea level, with splendid views. Laid out on hillside, making use of the natural contours of the land. Although relatively short, the combination of the terrain and the prevailing weather conditions (generally windy) ensure that you have to place your shots carefully in order to record a good score. Conservation of the natural landscape has been of paramount importance.
9 holes, 5242yds, Par 68, SSS 67, Course record 61.
Club membership 300.
Visitors Mon-Fr except BHs. Dress code. **Societies** Booking required.
Green Fees £12 per 18 holes. ◉ **Facilities** ⊕ ⓘ◎ ↆ ◻️ 🈁 ♨ 📖
Location 1.5m E off A6033
Hotel ★★ 69% HL Old White Lion Hotel, Main St, HAWORTH ☎ 01535 642313 15 en suite

HOLYWELL GREEN MAP 07 SE01

Halifax Bradley Hall HX4 9AN
☎ 01422 374108
18 holes, 6138yds, Par 70, SSS 70, Course record 65.
Location S on A6112
Telephone for further details
Hotel ★★★ 74% HL Best Western Pennine Manor Hotel, Nettleton Hill Rd, Scapegoat Hill, HUDDERSFIELD ☎ 01484 642368 30 en suite

HUDDERSFIELD MAP 07 SE11

Bagden Hall Hotel & Golf Course Wakefield Rd,
Scissett HD8 9LE
☎ 01484 865330 ▤ 01484 861001
e-mail: info@bagdenhallhotel.co.uk
web: www.bagdenhallhotel.co.uk.
Well maintained tree-lined course set in idyllic surroundings and
offering a challenging test of golf for all levels of handicap. Lake
guarded greens require pin-point accuracy.
9 holes, 3002yds, Par 56, SSS 55, Course record 60.
Visitors Mon-Sun & BHs. Dress code. **Societies** welcome. **Green Fees** not
confirmed. **Course Designer** F O'Donnell/R Braithwaite **Facilities** ⑪ ◎
⬟ ▱ ▦ ⬛ ◌ **Conf** facs Corporate Hospitality Days **Location** A636
Wakefield-Denby Dale
Hotel ★★★ 74% HL Bagden Hall, Wakefield Rd, Scissett, HUDDERSFIELD
☎ 01484 865330 16 en suite

Bradley Park Off Bradley Rd HD2 1PZ
☎ 01484 223772 ▤ 01484 451613
e-mail: parnellreilly@pgabroadband.com
web: www.bradleyparkgolf.co.uk
Parkland course, challenging with good mix of long and short holes.
Also 14-bay floodlit driving range and a nine-hole Par 3 course, ideal
for beginners. Superb views.
18 holes, 6284yds, Par 70, SSS 70, Course record 65.
Club membership 300.
Visitors Mon-Sun & BHs. **Societies** Booking required. **Green Fees** £16
(£18 Sat & Sun). **Prof** Parnell E Reilly **Course Designer** Cotton/Pennick/
Lowire & Ptnrs **Facilities** ⑪ ◎ ⬟ ▱ ▦ ⬛ ◌ ⬧ **Leisure** 9
hole Par 3 course. **Conf** facs Corporate Hospitality Days **Location** M62
junct 25, 2.5m
Hotel ★★★★ 68% HL Cedar Court Hotel, Ainley Top, HUDDERSFIELD
☎ 01422 375431 114 en suite

Crosland Heath Felk Stile Rd, Crosland Heath HD4 7AF
☎ 01484 653216 ▤ 01484 461079
e-mail: golf@croslandheath.co.uk
web: www.croslandheath.co.uk
Moorland course with fine views over valley.
18 holes, 6087yds, Par 71, SSS 69. Club membership 650.
Visitors Mon, Tue, Thu & Sun except BHs. Booking required. Handicap
certificate. Dress code. **Societies** Booking required. **Green Fees** £35.50
per day (£40.50 Sun). **Prof** John Eyre **Course Designer** Dr. McKenzie
Facilities ⑪ ◎ ⬟ ▱ ▦ ⬛ ◌ **Conf** facs Corporate Hospitality Days
Location SW off A62
Hotel ★★★ 74% HL Best Western Pennine Manor Hotel, Nettleton Hill Rd,
Scapegoat Hill, HUDDERSFIELD ☎ 01484 642368 30 en suite

Huddersfield Fixby Hall, Lightridge Rd, Fixby HD2 2EP
☎ 01484 426203 ▤ 01484 424623
e-mail: secretary@huddersfield-golf.co.uk
web: www.huddersfield-golf.co.uk
A testing heathland course of championship standard laid out in 1891.
18 holes, 6466yds, Par 71, SSS 71, Course record 63.
Club membership 760.
Visitors Mon-Sun & BHs. Booking required. Handicap certificate. Dress
code. **Societies** Booking required. **Green Fees** £55 per day, £45 per round
(£65/£55 Sat, Sun & BHs). **Prof** Paul Carman **Facilities** ⑪ ◎ ⬟ ▱ ▦ ⬛
⬛ ◌ ⬧ **Conf** facs Corporate Hospitality Days **Location** 2m N off A641
Hotel ★★★★ 68% HL Cedar Court Hotel, Ainley Top, HUDDERSFIELD
☎ 01422 375431 114 en suite

Longley Park Maple St, Off Somerset Rd HD5 9AX
☎ 01484 422304 ▤ 01484 515280
e-mail: longleyparkgolfclub@12freeukisp.co.uk
Lowland course, surrounded by mature woodland.
9 holes, 5212yds, Par 66, SSS 66, Course record 61.
Club membership 440.
Visitors Mon, Tue, Fri, Sun & BHs. Booking required Sun & BHs. Dress code.
Societies Booking required. **Green Fees** Phone. ◉ **Prof** Nick Leeming
Facilities ⑪ ◎ ⬟ facs Corporate Hospitality Days
Location 0.5m SE of town centre off A629
Hotel ★★★★ 68% HL Cedar Court Hotel, Ainley Top, HUDDERSFIELD
☎ 01422 375431 114 en suite

ILKLEY MAP 07 SE14

Ben Rhydding High Wood, Ben Rhydding LS29 8SB
☎ 01943 608759
e-mail: secretary@benrhyddinggc.freeserve.co.uk
Moorland and parkland with splendid views over the Wharfe valley. A
compact but testing course.
9 holes, 4611yds, Par 65, SSS 63, Course record 64.
Club membership 250.
Visitors Mon, Tue, Thu, Fri & BHs. Wed am only & Sat & Sun pm only.
Handicap certificate. Dress code. **Societies** Booking required **Green Fees**
£15 per per day (£20 Sat, Sun & BHs). ◉ **Course Designer** William
Dell **Facilities** ▱ ⬛ **Conf** Corporate Hospitality Days **Location** SE of
town centre. Off Wheatley Ln onto Wheatley Grove, left onto High Wood,
clubhouse on left
Hotel ★★★ 82% HL Best Western Rombalds Hotel & Restaurant, 11 West
View, Wells Rd, ILKLEY ☎ 01943 603201 15 en suite

Ilkley Nesfield Rd, Myddleton LS29 0BE
☎ 01943 600214 ▤ 01943 816130
e-mail: honsec@ilkleygolfclub.co.uk
web: www.ikleygolfclub.co.uk
A beautiful parkland course in Wharfedale. The Wharfe is a hazard
on the first seven holes - in fact, the 3rd is laid out entirely on an
island in the river.
18 holes, 5953yds, Par 69, SSS 70, Course record 64.
Club membership 450.
Visitors Mon-Sun & BHs. Booking required. Handicap certificate. Dress
code. **Societies** Booking required. **Green Fees** £45 (£55 Sat & Sun).
Prof John L Hammond **Course Designer** Mackenzie **Facilities** ⑪ ◎ ⬟
▱ ▦ ⬛ ◌ ⬧ **Leisure** fishing. **Conf** facs Corporate Hospitality Days
Location W side of town centre off A65
Hotel ★★★ 82% HL Best Western Rombalds Hotel & Restaurant, 11
West View, Wells Rd, ILKLEY ☎ 01943 603201 15 en suite

KEIGHLEY MAP 07 SE04

Branshaw Branshaw Moor, Oakworth BD22 7ES
☎ 01535 643235 (sec) ▤ 01535 648011
e-mail: branshaw@golfclub.fslife.co.uk
18 holes, 5823yds, Par 69, SSS 68, Course record 64.
Course Designer James Braid **Location** 2m SW on B6149, signed
Oakworth
Telephone for further details
Hotel ★★ 70% HL Dalesgate Hotel, 406 Skipton Rd, Utley, KEIGHLEY
☎ 01535 664930 20 en suite

Keighley Howden Park, Utley BD20 6DH
☎ 01535 604778 📠 01535 604778
e-mail: manager@keighleygolfclub.com
web: www.keighleygolfclub.com
Parkland course is good quality and has great views down the Aire valley. The 17th hole has been described as 'one of the most difficult and dangerous holes in Yorkshire golf'. The club celebrated its centenary in 2004.
18 holes, 6141yds, Par 69, SSS 70, Course record 64.
Club membership 650.
Visitors Mon-Sun & BHs. Booking required. Handicap certificate. Dress code. **Societies** Booking required. **Green Fees** £43 per day, £35 per round (£47/£39 Sat, Sun & BHs). **Prof** Andrew Rhodes **Course Designer** Henry Smith **Facilities** ⑪ ⑩ ⅃ ♨ ⅃ ♨ ♨ ♨ ♨ **Leisure** Snooker table.
Conf facs Corporate Hospitality Days **Location** 1m NW of town centre off B6265, turn N at Roebuck pub
Hotel ★★ 70% HL Dalesgate Hotel, 406 Skipton Rd, Utley, KEIGHLEY
☎ 01535 664930 20 en suite

LEEDS   MAP 08 SE33

Brandon Hollywell Ln, Shadwell LS17 8EZ
☎ 0113 273 7471
An 18-hole links type course enjoying varying degrees of rough, water and sand hazards.
18 holes, 4000yds, Par 63.
Visitors Mon-Sun & BHs. Booking required. Dress code. **Societies** Booking required. **Green Fees** £9 per round (£10 Sat, Sun & BHs). ⊛ **Prof** Carl Robinson **Course Designer** William Binner **Facilities** ⑪ ⅃ ♨ ♨ ♨ ♨ **Location** Off A58 into Shadwell, onto Main St, right at Red Lion pub
Hotel ★★★ 79% HL Haley's Hotel & Restaurant, Shire Oak Rd, Headingley, LEEDS ☎ 0113 278 4446 22 en suite 6 annexe en suite

Cookridge Hall Golf & Country Club Cookridge Ln LS16 7NL
☎ 0113 2300641 📠 0113 203 0198
e-mail: info@cookridgehall.co.uk
web: www.cookridgehall.co.uk
American-style course designed by Karl Litten. Expect plenty of water hazards, tees for all standards. Large bunkers and fairways between mounds and young trees.
18 holes, 6788yds, Par 72, SSS 72, Course record 69.
Club membership 570.
Visitors Mon-Sun & BHs. Booking required Sat, Sun & BHs. Dress code. **Societies** Booking required **Green Fees** £25 per round (£30 Sat, Sun & BHs). **Prof** Mark Pinkett **Course Designer** Karl Liiten **Facilities** ⑪ ⑩ ⅃ ⅃ ♨ ♨ ♨ ♨ ♨ **Leisure** heated indoor swimming pool, sauna, solarium, gymnasium, chipping and practice bunker. **Conf** Corporate Hospitality Days **Location** 6m NW of Leeds, off A660
Hotel ★★★ 79% HL Haley's Hotel & Restaurant, Shire Oak Rd, Headingley, LEEDS ☎ 0113 278 4446 22 en suite 6 annexe en suite

De Vere Oulton Hall Rothwell Ln, Oulton LS26 8HN
☎ 0113 282 3152 📠 0113 282 6290
27-hole championship-length course. Major refurbishment underway to include a luxury clubhouse and state of the art golf academy.
Hall Course: 9 holes, 3300yds, Par 36, SSS 36.
Park Course: 18 holes, 6428yds, Par 71, SSS 71.
Club membership 200.
Visitors Mon-Sun & BHs. Booking required. Handicap certificate. Dress code. **Societies** booking required **Green Fees** not confirmed. **Prof** Keith Pickard **Course Designer** Dave Thomas **Facilities** ⑪ ⑩ ⅃ ♨ ⅃ ♨ ♨ ♨ ♨ ♨ **Leisure** heated indoor swimming pool, sauna, solarium, gymnasium. **Conf** Corporate Hospitality Days **Location** M62 junct 30
Hotel ★★★★ 81% HL De Vere Oulton Hall, Rothwell Ln, Oulton, LEEDS ☎ 0113 282 1000 152 en suite

Gotts Park Armley Ridge Rd LS12 2QX
☎ 0113 231 1896 & 256 2994
e-mail: maurice.gl@sagainternet.co.uk
18 holes, 4960yds, Par 65, SSS 64, Course record 63.
Location 3m W of city centre off A647
Telephone for further details
Hotel ★★★★ 78% HL Queens Hotel, City Square, LEEDS ☎ 0113 243 1323 217 en suite

Headingley Back Church Ln, Adel LS16 8DW
☎ 0113 267 9573 📠 0113 281 7334
e-mail: manager@headingleygolfclub.co.uk
web: www.headingleygolfclub.co.uk
An undulating course with a wealth of natural features offering fine views from higher ground. Its most striking hazard is the famous ravine at the 18th. Leeds's oldest course, founded in 1892.
18 holes, 6608yds, Par 71, SSS 72. Club membership 700.
Visitors Mon-Sun & BHs. Booking required except BHs. Handicap certificate. Dress code. **Societies** booking required. **Green Fees** not confirmed. **Prof** Neil M Harvey **Course Designer** Dr Mackenzie **Facilities** ⑪ ⑩ ⅃ ♨ ⅃ ♨ ♨ ♨ **Conf** Corporate Hospitality Days **Location** 5.5m N of city centre. A660 to Skipton, right at lights junct Farrar Ln and Church Ln, follow Eccup signs
Hotel BUD Premier Travel Inn Leeds/Bradford Airport, Victoria Av, Yeadon, LEEDS ☎ 08701 977153 40 en suite

Horsforth Layton Rise, Layton Rd, Horsforth LS18 5EX
☎ 0113 258 6819 📠 0113 258 9336
e-mail: secretary@horsforthgolfclubltd.co.uk
web: www.horsforthgolfclubltd.co.uk
Moorland and parkland course combining devilish short holes with some more substantial challenges. Extensive views across Leeds and on a clear day York Minster can be seen from the 14th tee.
18 holes, 6243yds, Par 71, SSS 70, Course record 65.
Club membership 750.
Visitors Mon, Tue, Thu, Fri, Sun & BHs. Booking required. Dress code. **Societies** Booking required. **Green Fees** £36 per round (£40 Sun & BHs). ⊛ **Prof** Dean Stokes/Simon Booth **Course Designer** Alister MacKenzie **Facilities** ⑪ ⑩ ⅃ ♨ ⅃ ♨ ♨ ♨ **Conf** facs Corporate Hospitality Days **Location** 6.5m NW of city centre off A65
Hotel BUD Travelodge Leeds Bradford Airport, White House Ln, LEEDS ☎ 0113 250 3996 48 en suite

Leeds Elmete Ln LS8 2LJ
☎ 0113 265 8775 📄 0113 232 3369
e-mail: secretary@leedsgolfclub.co.uk
web: www.leedsgolfclub.co.uk
Parkland with pleasant views.
18 holes, 6097yds, Par 69, SSS 69, Course record 63.
Club membership 600.
Visitors Mon-Sun except BHs. Booking required. Dress code. **Societies**
Booking required. **Green Fees** £32 per round (£36 Sat & Sun). ● **Prof**
Simon Longster **Course Designer** Alister McKenzie **Facilities** ⑪ ⑩ 🎱 ☞
🏌 ⚒ 🍴 🏌 **Location** 5m NE of city centre on A6120, off A58
Hotel ★★★ 79% HL Haley's Hotel & Restaurant, Shire Oak Rd, Headingley,
LEEDS ☎ 0113 278 4446 22 en suite 6 annexe en suite

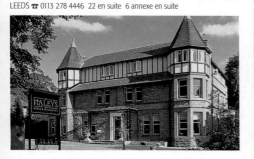

Leeds Golf Centre, Wike Ridge Wike Ridge Ln,
Shadwell LS17 9JW
☎ 0113 288 6000 📄 0113 288 6185
e-mail: info@leedsgolfcentre.com
web: www.leedsgolfcentre.com/aa

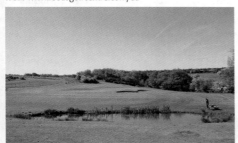

Wike Ridge Course: 18 holes, 6482yds, Par 72, SSS 71.
Oaks: 12 holes, 1610yds, Par 36.
Course Designer Donald Steel **Location** 5m N, A58, course on N side of
Shadwell
Telephone for further details
Hotel ★★★ 79% HL Haley's Hotel & Restaurant, Shire Oak Rd, Headingley,
LEEDS ☎ 0113 278 4446 22 en suite 6 annexe en suite

Middleton Park Municipal Middleton Park, Middleton
LS10 3TN
☎ 0113 270 0449 📄 0113 270 0449
e-mail: lynn@ratcliffel.fsnet.co.uk
18 holes, 5263yds, Par 68, SSS 66, Course record 63.
Location 3m S off A653
Telephone for further details
Hotel ★★★★ 78% HL Queens Hotel, City Square, LEEDS
☎ 0113 243 1323 217 en suite

Moor Allerton Coal Rd, Wike LS17 9NH
☎ 0113 266 1154 📄 0113 237 1124
e-mail: info@magc.co.uk
web: www.magc.co.uk
Lakes Course: 18 holes, 6470yds, Par 71, SSS 72.
Blackmoor Course: 18 holes, 6673yds, Par 71, SSS 73.
High Course: 18 holes, 6841yds, Par 72, SSS 74.
Course Designer Robert Trent Jones **Location** 5.5m N of city centre
on A61
Telephone for further details
Hotel ★★★ 72% HL The Merrion Hotel, Merrion Centre, LEEDS
☎ 0113 243 9191 109 en suite

Moortown Harrogate Rd, Alwoodley LS17 7DB
☎ 0113 268 6521 📄 0113 268 0986
e-mail: secretary@moortown-gc.co.uk ·
web: www.moortown-gc.co.uk
Championship course, tough but fair. Springy moorland turf, natural
hazards of heather, gorse and streams, cunningly placed bunkers
and immaculate greens. No winter tees or greens. Original home of
Ryder Cup in 1929.
18 holes, 6757yds, Par 72, SSS 73, Course record 64.
Club membership 585.
Visitors Mon-Sun & BHs. Booking required. Dress code. **Societies**
booking required. **Green Fees** not confirmed. ● **Prof** Martin Heggie
Course Designer Alistair Mackenzie **Facilities** ⑪ ⑩ 🎱 ☞ 🏌 🏌 🍴
🏌 🍴 🏌 🏌 **Conf** facs Corporate Hospitality Days **Location** 6m N of
city centre on A61
Hotel ★★★ 72% HL The Merrion Hotel, Merrion Centre, LEEDS
☎ 0113 243 9191 109 en suite

Roundhay Park Ln LS8 2EJ
☎ 0113 266 2695 & 266 4225
Attractive municipal parkland course, natural hazards, easy walking.
9 holes, 5223yds, Par 70, SSS 65, Course record 61.
Club membership 240.
Visitors Mon-Sun & BHs. Booking required. Dress code. **Societies** Booking
required. **Green Fees** Phone. ● **Prof** James Pape **Facilities** 🎱 ☞ 🍴 🏌
🍴 🏌 🏌 **Location** 4m NE of city centre off A58
Hotel ★★★ 79% HL Haley's Hotel & Restaurant, Shire Oak Rd, Headingley,
LEEDS ☎ 0113 278 4446 22 en suite 6 annexe en suite

Sand Moor Alwoodley Ln LS17 7DJ
☎ 0113 268 5180 📄 0113 266 1105
e-mail: ian.kerr@sandmoorgolf.co.uk
web: www.sandmoorgolf.co.uk
A beautiful, inland course situated next to Eccup reservoir on the
north side of Leeds. It has been described as the finest example
of golfing paradise being created out of a barren moor. With
magnificent views of the surrounding countryside, the course has
sandy soil and drains exceptionally well.
18 holes, 6446yds, Par 71, SSS 71, Course record 63.
Club membership 600.
Visitors Mon-Fri, Sun & BHs. Booking required. Handicap certificate.
Dress code. **Societies** Booking required. **Green Fees** £55 per day, £45
per round (£55 per round Sun). **Prof** Frank Houlgate **Course Designer**
Dr A Mackenzie **Facilities** ⑪ ⑩ 🎱 ☞ 🏌 🏌 🍴 🏌 🏌 **Conf**
Corporate Hospitality Days **Location** 5m N of city centre off A61
Hotel ★★★★ 71% HL Cedar Court Hotel, Denby Dale Rd, WAKEFIELD
☎ 01924 276310 150 en suite

South Leeds Gipsy Ln, Beeston LS11 5TU
☎ 0113 272 3757
e-mail: pro.slgc@talktalk.net
web: www.southleedsgolfclub.co.uk
Hard-walking parkland, windy but good views. The small undulating greens are a very good test of putting.

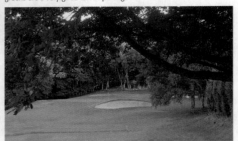

18 holes, 5865yds, Par 69, SSS 68, Course record 63.
Club membership 400.
Visitors Mon-Sun & BHs. **Societies** Booking required. **Green Fees** £26 per day, £21 per round (£28 per round weekends). ● **Prof** Nick Sheard **Course Designer** Dr Alister Mackenzie **Facilities** ⑪ ⑩ ⓛ ☒ ☂ ☒ & **Conf** Corporate Hospitality Days **Location** 3m S of city centre off A653
Hotel ★★★★ 78% HL Queens Hotel, City Square, LEEDS
☎ 0113 243 1323 217 en suite

Temple Newsam Temple-Newsam Rd LS15 0LN
☎ 0113 264 7362
web: www.templenewsamgolfcourse.co.uk
Two parkland courses. Testing long 13th (563yds) on second course.
Lord Irwin: 18 holes, 6460yds, Par 68, SSS 71,
Course record 66.
Lady Dorothy: 18 holes, 6299yds, Par 70, SSS 70,
Course record 67. Club membership 520.
Visitors Mon-Sun & BHs. Booking required Sat, Sun & BHs. **Societies** Booking required **Green Fees** £10 per round (£13 Sat, Sun & BHs).
Prof Adrian Newboult **Facilities** ⑪ ⑩ by prior arrangement ☒ ☒ ☒ ☒ ☂ & **Conf** facs Corporate Hospitality Days **Location** 3.5m E of city centre off A63
Hotel ★★★ 79% HL Haley's Hotel & Restaurant, Shire Oak Rd, Headingley, LEEDS ☎ 0113 278 4446 22 en suite 6 annexe en suite

MARSDEN   MAP 07 SE01

Marsden Mount Rd, Hemplow HD7 6NN
☎ 01484 844253
e-mail: secretary@marsdengolf.co.uk
web: www.marsdengolf.co.uk
Moorland course with good views, natural hazards, windy.
9 holes, 5702yds, Par 68, SSS 68, Course record 64.
Club membership 280.
Visitors Mon, Wed-Fri, Sun & BHs. Booking required. Handicap certificate. Dress code. **Societies** Booking required. **Green Fees** £15 per round (£20 Sun & BHs). ● **Prof** J Crompton **Course Designer** Dr McKenzie **Facilities** ⑪ ⑩ ⓛ ☒ ☒ ☂ **Leisure** tennis courts. **Conf** facs **Location** S side off A62
Hotel ★★ 74% HL Old Bridge Hotel, HOLMFIRTH ☎ 01484 681212 20 en suite

MELTHAM   MAP 07 SE01

Meltham Thick Hollins Hall HD9 4DQ
☎ 01484 850227 (office) & 851521 (pro) 📄 01484 850227
e-mail: melthamgolf@supanet.com
web: www.meltham-golf.co.uk
Parkland with good views. Testing 548yd 13th hole (Par 5).
18 holes, 6139yds, Par 71, SSS 70, Course record 63.
Club membership 756.
Visitors Mon-Sun & BHs. Booking required. **Societies** Booking required **Green Fees** £33 per day, £28 per round (£38/£33 Sat, Sun & BHs). ● **Prof** Paul Davies **Course Designer** Alex Herd **Facilities** ⑪ ⑩ ⓛ ☒ ☒ & ☂ ☂ & **Conf** Corporate Hospitality Days **Location** 0.5m E of Meltham on B6107
Hotel ★★ 80% HL Hey Green Country House Hotel, Waters Rd, MARSDEN ☎ 01484 848000 12 en suite

MIRFIELD   MAP 08 SE21

Dewsbury District Sands Ln WF14 8HJ
☎ 01924 492399 & 496030 📄 01924 492399
e-mail: dewsbury.golf@btconnect.com
web: www.dewsburygolf.co.uk
Moorland or parkland terrain with panoramic views. Ponds in middle of 3rd fairway, left of 5th green and 17th green. A challenging test of golf.
18 holes, 6360yds, Par 71, SSS 71, Course record 64.
Club membership 700.
Visitors Mon-Fri. Sat, Sun & BHs pm only. Booking required. Dress code. **Societies** Booking required. **Green Fees** £28 per day, £22 per round (£17.50 Sat & Sun). **Prof** Nigel P Hirst **Course Designer** Old Tom Morris/Peter Alliss **Facilities** ⑪ ⑩ by prior arrangement ☒ ☒ ☒ ☒ ☂ ☂ & **Leisure** snooker tables. **Conf** facs Corporate Hospitality Days **Location** M62 junct 25, 6m off A644
Hotel ★★★ 71% HL Healds Hall Hotel, Leeds Rd, Liversedge, DEWSBURY ☎ 01924 409112 24 en suite

MORLEY   MAP 08 SE22

Howley Hall Scotchman Ln LS27 0NX
☎ 01924 350100 📄 01924 350104
e-mail: office@howleyhall.co.uk
web: www.howleyhall.co.uk
Easy walking parkland with superb views of the Pennines and the Calder valley.
18 holes, 6092yds, Par 71, SSS 69, Course record 64.
Club membership 700.
Visitors Mon-Fri, Sun & BHs. Dress code. **Societies** Booking required. **Green Fees** £36 per day, £30 per round (£40 Sun & BHs). ● **Prof** Gary Watkinson **Course Designer** MacKenzie **Facilities** ⑪ ⑩ by prior arrangement ☒ ☒ ☒ ☒ ☂ ☂ & **Conf** facs Corporate Hospitality Days **Location** 1.5m S on B6123
Hotel ★★ 72% HL Alder House Hotel, Towngate Rd, Healey Ln, BATLEY ☎ 01924 444777 20 en suite

OSSETT   MAP 08 SE22

Low Laithes Parkmill Ln, Flushdyke WF5 9AP
☎ 01924 274667 & 266067 📄 01924 266266
web: www.lowlaithesgolfclub.co.uk
Testing parkland course.

Continued

18 holes, 6463yds, Par 72, SSS 71, Course record 65.
Club membership 600.
Visitors Mon-Sun & BHs. Booking required Sat, Sun & BHs. Handicap certificate. Dress code. **Societies** Booking required. **Green Fees** £25 per day, £22 per round (£36 Sat, Sun & BHs). ● **Prof** Paul Browning
Course Designer Dr Mackenzie **Facilities** ⓣ ⦿ 🍴 ⬛ ⌷ ⛵ ⚐ ⼂ 🛒 🛍 ✆
Conf Corporate Hospitality Days **Location** M1 junct 40, 0.5m on Dewsbury road, signed
Hotel ★★★ 73% HL Heath Cottage Hotel & Restaurant, Wakefield Rd, DEWSBURY ☎ 01924 465399 22 en suite 6 annexe en suite

OTLEY — MAP 08 SE24

Otley Off West Busk Ln LS21 3NG
☎ 01943 465329 📄 01943 850387
e-mail: office@otley-golfclub.co.uk
web: www.otley-golfclub.co.uk
An expansive course with magnificent views across Wharfedale. It is well wooded with streams crossing the fairway. The 4th is a fine hole which generally needs two woods to reach the plateau green. The 17th is a good short hole. A test of golf as opposed to stamina.
18 holes, 6211yds, Par 70, SSS 70, Course record 62.
Club membership 700.
Visitors Mon, Wed-Fri, Sun & BHs. Booking required. Handicap certificate. Dress code. **Societies** Booking required. **Green Fees** £40 per day, £34 per 18/27 holes (£47/£40 Sun & BHs). **Prof** Steven Tomkinson
Facilities ⓣ ⦿ 🍴 ⬛ ⌷ ⛵ ⼂ 🛒 🛍 ✆ ⟋ **Leisure** practice bunker.
Conf facs Corporate Hospitality Days **Location** 1m W of Otley off A6038
Hotel BUD Premier Travel Inn Leeds/Bradford Airport, Victoria Av, Yeadon, LEEDS ☎ 08701 977153 40 en suite

OUTLANE — MAP 07 SE01

Outlane Slack Ln, Off New Hey Rd HD3 3FQ
☎ 01422 374762 📄 01422 311789
e-mail: secretary@outlanegolfclub.ltd.uk
web: www.outlanegolfclub.ltd.uk
An 18-hole moorland course with undulating fairways. Four Par 3 holes with an 8th hole of 249yds and a 15th regarded as the hardest Par 3 in Yorkshire. The three Par 5s may be reachable on a good day in two strokes but in adverse conditions will take more than three. Smaller than average greens on some holes, which makes for accurate approach shots.
18 holes, 6015yds, Par 71, SSS 69, Course record 67.
Club membership 600.
Visitors Mon-Fri, Sun except BHs. Booking required. Dress code. **Societies** Booking required. **Green Fees** £22 per day (£32 Sun & BHs). ● **Prof** David Chapman **Facilities** ⓣ ⦿ 🍴 ⬛ ⌷ ⛵ ⼂ 🛒 🛍 ✆ **Location** M62 junct 23, A640 New Hey Rd through Outlane
Hotel ★★★ 70% HL The Old Golf House Hotel, New Hey Rd, Outlane, HUDDERSFIELD ☎ 0870 609 6128 52 en suite

PONTEFRACT — MAP 08 SE42

Mid Yorkshire Havercroft Ln, Darrington WF8 3BP
☎ 01977 704522 📄 01977 600823
e-mail: admin@midyorkshiregolfclub.com
web: www.midyorkshiregolfclub.com
An 18-hole championship-standard course opened in 1993, and widely considered to be one of the finest new courses in Yorkshire.

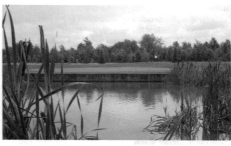

Mid Yorkshire

18 holes, 6308yds, Par 70, SSS 70, Course record 68.
Club membership 500.
Visitors Mon-Sun & BHs. Dress code. **Societies** Booking required **Green Fees** £21 per round (£31 Sat & Sun). **Prof** Michael Hessay **Course Designer** Steve Marnoch **Facilities** ⓣ ⦿ 🍴 ⬛ ⌷ ⛵ ⼂ 🛒 🛍 ✆ ✆ 🏌
Conf facs Corporate Hospitality Days **Location** On A1 0.5m S junct A1/M62
Hotel ★★★ 79% HL Wentbridge House Hotel, Wentbridge, PONTEFRACT ☎ 01977 620444 14 en suite 4 annexe en suite

Pontefract & District Park Ln WF8 4QS
☎ 01977 792241 📄 01977 792241
e-mail: manager@pdgc.co.uk
web: www.pdgc.co.uk
Undulating parkland course, some elevated tees.
18 holes, 6227yds, Par 72, SSS 70, Course record 64.
Club membership 800.
Visitors Mon, Tue, Thu-Sun except BHs. Booking required Sat & Sun. Handicap certificate. Dress code. **Societies** Booking required.
Green Fees £30 per day, £25 per round.(£32 Sat, Sun). ● **Prof** Nick Newman **Course Designer** A McKenzie **Facilities** ⓣ ⦿ 🍴 ⬛ ⌷ ⛵ ⼂ 🛒 ✆
Conf Corporate Hospitality Days **Location** W of Pontefract. A639 onto B6134, club 1m on right
Hotel ★★★ 79% HL Wentbridge House Hotel, Wentbridge, PONTEFRACT ☎ 01977 620444 14 en suite 4 annexe en suite

PUDSEY — MAP 08 SE23

Calverley Golf Club Woodhall Ln LS28 5QY
☎ 0113 256 9244 📄 0113 256 4362
e-mail: golf@cgc1.freeserve.co.uk
Gently undulating parkland. The small greens require accurate approach shots.

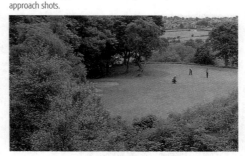

18 holes, 5590yds, Par 68, SSS 67, Course record 62.
9 holes, 3000yds, Par 36. Club membership 553.

Continued

Visitors Mon-Fri. Sat, Sun & BHs pm onluy. Booking required. Handicap certificate. Dress code. **Societies** Booking required. **Green Fees** £14 per round (£17 Sat & Sun). **Prof** Neil Wendel-Jones **Facilities** ⓤ ⑩ ﹗ ⅃ ▱ ㏒ 🕍 ⅃ 🏌 🍴 🏌 **Conf** Corporate Hospitality Days **Location** Signed Calverley from A647
Hotel BUD Travelodge Bradford, 1 Mid Point, Dick Ln, PUDSEY
☎ 08700 850 950 48 en suite

Fulneck LS28 8NT
☎ 0113 256 5191
9 holes, 5456yds, Par 66, SSS 67, Course record 65.
Location Pudsey, between Leeds
Telephone for further details
Hotel ★★★ 70% HL Novotel Bradford, 6 Roydsdale Way, BRADFORD
☎ 01274 683683 119 en suite

Woodhall Hills Calverley LS28 5UN
☎ 0113 255 4594 📄 0113 255 4594
e-mail: whhgc@tiscali.co.uk
Meadowland course, recently redeveloped with an improved layout and open ditches around the course. A challenging opening hole, a good variety of Par 3s and testing holes at the 6th and 11th.
18 holes, 6184yds, Par 71, SSS 70, Course record 64. Club membership 550.
Visitors Mon-Fri, Sun & BHs. Booking required. Dress code. **Societies** Booking required. **Green Fees** £26 per round (£30 Sat & Sun, £15 Twilight). 🏌 **Prof** Warren Lockett **Facilities** ⓤ ⑩ ﹗ ⅃ ▱ 🕍 ⅃ 🏌 🍴 🏌 **Conf** facs Corporate Hospitality Days **Location** 1m NW off A647
Hotel BUD Travelodge Bradford, 1 Mid Point, Dick Ln, PUDSEY
☎ 08700 850 950 48 en suite

RIDDLESDEN   MAP 07 SE04

Riddlesden Howden Rough BD20 5QN
☎ 01535 602148
Undulating moorland course with prevailing west winds and beautiful views. Nine Par 3 holes and spectacular 6th and 15th holes played over old quarry sites.
18 holes, 4295yds, Par 63, SSS 61, Course record 59. Club membership 300.
Visitors Mon-Sun & BHs. **Societies** Booking required. **Green Fees** £16 per day (£21 Sat & Sun). 🏌 **Facilities** ⓤ ⑩ ﹗ ⅃ ▱ 🕍 ⅃ **Conf** Corporate Hospitality Days **Location** 1m NW
Hotel ★★ 70% HL Dalesgate Hotel, 406 Skipton Rd, Utley, KEIGHLEY
☎ 01535 664930 20 en suite

SCARCROFT   MAP 08 SE34

Scarcroft Syke Ln LS14 3BQ
☎ 0113 289 2311 📄 0113 289 3835
e-mail: secretary@scarcroftgolfclub.com
web: www.scarcroftgolfclub.com
Undulating parkland course with prevailing west wind and easy walking.
18 holes, 6456yds, Par 71, SSS 69. Club membership 650.
Visitors Mon-Sun & BHs. Booking required. Handicap certificate. Dress code. **Societies** Booking required. **Green Fees** Phone. **Prof** David Hughes **Course Designer** Charles Mackenzie **Facilities** ⓤ ⑩ ﹗ ⅃ ▱ 🕍 ⅃ 🏌🍴 🏌 **Conf** facs **Location** 0.5m N of village off A58
Hotel ★★★ 72% HL The Merrion Hotel, Merrion Centre, LEEDS
☎ 0113 243 9191 109 en suite

SHIPLEY   MAP 07 SE13

Marriott Hollins Hall Hotel & Country Club Hollins Hill, Otley Rd BD17 7QW
☎ 01274 534212 📄 01274 534220
e-mail: mhrs.lbags.golf@marriotthotels.com
web: www.marriotthollinshall.com
Set in 200 acres of natural heathland amongst the beautiful Yorkshire moors and dales. The 6671 yard course offers multiple teeing areas which challenge any standard of golfer and is majestic, challenging and classically designed in the spirit of the game.

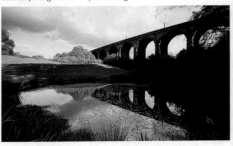

18 holes, 6671yds, Par 71, SSS 71, Course record 65. Club membership 350.
Visitors Mon-Sun & BHs. Dress code. **Societies** Booking required **Green Fees** £55 per day, £40 per round (£75/£50 Fri-Sun & BHs). **Prof** Brian Rumney **Course Designer** Ross McMurray **Facilities** ⓤ ⑩ ﹗ ⅃ ▱ ㏒ 🕍 ⅃ 🏌🍴 🏌 **Leisure** heated indoor swimming pool, sauna, solarium, gymnasium. **Conf** facs Corporate Hospitality Days **Location** 3m N on the A6038
Hotel ★★★★ 78% HL Marriott Hollins Hall Hotel & Country Club, Hollins Hill, Baildon, SHIPLEY ☎ 0870 400 7227 122 en suite

Northcliffe High Bank Ln BD18 4LJ
☎ 01274 596731 📄 01274 584148
e-mail: northcliffegc@hotmail.com
web: www.northcliffegolfclubshipley.co.uk
Parkland with magnificent views of moors. Testing 1st hole, dog-leg left over a ravine. The 18th hole is one of the most picturesque and difficult Par 3s in the country, with a green 100feet below the tee and protected by bunkers, water and trees.
18 holes, 6104yds, Par 71, SSS 70, Course record 64. Club membership 700.
Visitors Mon-Fri, Sun & BHs. Booking required. Dress code. **Societies** Booking required. **Green Fees** £30 per day, £25 per round (£30 per round Sat, Sun & BHs). 🏌 **Prof** M Hillas **Course Designer** James Braid **Facilities** ⓤ ⑩ ⅃ ▱ ㏒ 🕍 ⅃ 🏌🍴 🏌 **Conf** Corporate Hospitality Days **Location** 1.25m SW of Shipley, off A650
Hotel ★★★★ 78% HL Marriott Hollins Hall Hotel & Country Club, Hollins Hill, Baildon, SHIPLEY ☎ 0870 400 7227 122 en suite

---

SILSDEN   MAP 07 SE04

Silsden Brunthwaite Ln, Brunthwaite BD20 0ND
☎ 01535 652998 📄 01535 654273
e-mail: info@silsdengolfclub.co.uk
web: www.silsdengolfclub.co.uk
18 holes, 5062yds, Par 67, SSS 64, Course record 62.
Location E of town off Howden Rd onto Hawber Ln
Telephone for further details
Hotel ★★ 70% HL Dalesgate Hotel, 406 Skipton Rd, Utley, KEIGHLEY
☎ 01535 664930 20 en suite

SOWERBY · MAP 07 SE02

Ryburn The Shaw, Norland HX6 3QP
☎ 01422 831355
Moorland course, easy walking. Panoramic views of the Ryburn and Calder valleys.
9 holes, 5127yds, Par 66, SSS 65, Course record 64.
Club membership 300.
Visitors Mon-Fri. Handicap certificate. Dress code. **Societies** Booking required. **Green Fees** £20 per round. ☻ **Facilities** ⊕ ⦾ ⓛ ☐ ⌾ 🏌 🎗
Conf Corporate Hospitality Days **Location** 1m S of Sowerby Bridge off A58
Hotel ★★★ 63% HL Imperial Crown Hotel, 42/46 Horton St, HALIFAX
☎ 0870 609 6114 41 en suite 15 annexe en suite

TODMORDEN · MAP 07 SD92

Todmorden Rive Rocks, Cross Stone Rd OL14 8RD
☎ 01706 812986 ▤ 01706 812986
A tough but fair moorland course with spectacular scenery.
9 holes, 5874yds, Par 68, SSS 68, Course record 67.
Club membership 240.
Visitors Mon, Tue, Wed Fri & BHs. Restricted Thu & Sat. Dress code.
Societies booking required. **Green Fees** not confirmed. ☻ **Facilities** ⊕ ⓛ ☐ ⌾ 🏌 **Conf** Corporate Hospitality Days **Location** NE off A646
Hotel ★★★ 83% HL Holdsworth House Hotel, Holdsworth, HALIFAX
☎ 01422 240024 40 en suite

WAKEFIELD · MAP 08 SE32

City of Wakefield Horbury Rd WF2 8QS
☎ 01924 360282
18 holes, 6319yds, Par 72, SSS 70, Course record 64.
Course Designer J S F Morrison **Location** 1.5m W of city centre on A642
Telephone for further details
Hotel ★★★ 81% HL Best Western Waterton Park Hotel, Walton Hall, The Balk, Walton, WAKEFIELD ☎ 01924 257911 & 249800 ▤ 01924 259686 25 en suite 43 annexe en suite

Lofthouse Hill Leeds Rd WF3 3LR
☎ 01924 823703 ▤ 01924 823703
e-mail: lofthousehillgolfclub@fsmail.net
web: www.lofthousehillgolfclub.co.uk
New parkland course.
18 holes, 5988yds, Par 70, SSS 69.
Visitors Mon-Sun & BHs. Booking required. Handicap certificate. Dress code. **Societies** Booking required. **Green Fees** £12 per 18 holes.
Prof Simon Hotham/Derek Johnson **Facilities** ⊕ ⦾ ⓛ ☐ ⌾ 🏌 🏨 🎗
Conf facs Corporate Hospitality Days **Location** 2m from Wakefield off A61
Hotel ★★★ 81% HL Best Western Waterton Park Hotel, Walton Hall, The Balk, Walton, WAKEFIELD ☎ 01924 257911 & 249800 ▤ 01924 259686 25 en suite 43 annexe en suite

Normanton Hatfield Hall, Aberford Rd WF3 4JP
☎ 01924 377943 ▤ 01924 200777
web: normantongolf.co.uk
18 holes, 6205yds, Par 72, SSS 71.
Location M62 junct 30, A642 towards Wakefield, 2m on right
Telephone for further details
Hotel ★★★ 74% HL Best Western Stoneleigh Hotel, Doncaster Rd, WAKEFIELD ☎ 01924 369461 28 en suite

Painthorpe House Painthorpe Ln, Painthorpe, Crigglestone WF4 3HE
☎ 01924 254737 & 255083 ▤ 01924 252022
Undulating meadowland course, easy walking.
9 holes, 4544yds, Par 62, SSS 62, Course record 63.
Club membership 100.
Visitors Mon-Sat & BHs. Sun after 1.30pm **Societies** booking required.
Green Fees not confirmed. ☻ **Facilities** 🏌 **Leisure** bowling green.
Location 2m S off A636
Hotel ★★★★ 71% HL Cedar Court Hotel, Denby Dale Rd, WAKEFIELD
☎ 01924 276310 150 en suite

Wakefield Woodthorpe Ln, Sandal WF2 6JH
☎ 01924 258778 (sec) ▤ 01924 242752
Well-sheltered meadowland and parkland with easy walking and good views.
18 holes, 6653yds, Par 72, SSS 72, Course record 67.
Club membership 540.
Visitors Mon-Sun & BHs. Booking required. Handicap certificate. Dress code. **Societies** Booking required. **Green Fees** £37 per day, £32 per round (£40 Sun & Sat). ☻ **Prof** Ian M Wright **Course Designer** A McKenzie/S Herd **Facilities** ⊕ ⦾ ⓛ ☐ ⌾ 🏌 🏨 🎗 **Conf** Corporate Hospitality Days
Location 3m S of Wakefield, off A61
Hotel Ⓤ Hotel St Pierre, Barnsley Rd, Newmillerdam, WAKEFIELD
☎ 01924 255596 54 en suite

WETHERBY · MAP 08 SE44

Wetherby Linton Ln LS22 4JF
☎ 01937 580089 ▤ 01937 581915
e-mail: info@wetherbygolfclub.co.uk
web: www.wetherbygolfclub.co.uk
A medium length parkland course renowned for its lush fairways. Particularly memorable holes are the 7th, a Par 4 which follows the sweeping bend of the River Wharfe, and the 14th (the quarry hole), an intimidating Par 3.
18 holes, 6213yds, Par 71, SSS 70, Course record 63.
Club membership 950.
Visitors Mon-Fri, Sun except BHs. Booking required. Handicap certificate. Dress code. **Societies** booking required. **Green Fees** not confirmed. ☻
Prof Mark Daubney **Facilities** ⊕ ⦾ ⓛ ☐ ⌾ 🏌 🏨 🎗 **Conf** facs Corporate Hospitality Days **Location** 1m W off A661
Hotel ★★★★ CHH Wood Hall Hotel, Trip Ln, Linton, WETHERBY
☎ 01937 587271 14 en suite 30 annexe en suite

WIKE · MAP 08 SE34

The Village Golf Course Backstone Gill Ln LS17 9JU
☎ 0113 273 7471 & 07759012364
A 12-hole pay and play course in an elevated position enjoying long panoramic views. The holes are Par 3, 4 and 5s and include water hazards and shaped large greens.
12 holes, 5780yds, Par 75, SSS 68, Course record 66.
Visitors Mon-Sun & BHs. Booking required. Dress code. **Societies** Booking required. **Green Fees** £10 per 18 holes, £8 per 12 holes (£12/£9 Sat & Sun). ☻ **Prof** Deborah Snowden **Course Designer** William Binner **Facilities** ⊕ ☐ 🎗 **Leisure** fishing. **Conf** facs Corporate Hospitality Days **Location** Signed, 1m off A61, 2m off A58
Hotel ★★★ 72% HL Jurys Inn Leeds, Kendell St, Brewery Place, Brewery Wharf, LEEDS ☎ 0113 283 8800 248 en suite

WOOLLEY
MAP 08 SE31

Woolley Park New Rd WF4 2JS
☎ 01226 380144 📠 01226 390295
web: www.woolleyparkgolfclub.co.uk
A demanding course set in a mature wooded parkland. With many water features in play and undulating greens, the course offers a challenge to all golfers.
18 holes, 6636yds, Par 71, SSS 72.
Visitors Mon-Sun & BHs. Booking required. Dress code. **Societies** Booking required. **Green Fees** £19 per 18 holes (£26 Sat & Sun). **Prof** Jon Baldwin **Course Designer** M Shattock **Facilities** ⊕ ⅃ ➘ ♀ ♪ ⊞ ⌦ ✔
Conf Corporate Hospitality Days **Location** M1 junct 38, off A61 between Wakefield & Barnsley
Hotel ★★★★ 71% HL Cedar Court Hotel, Denby Dale Rd, WAKEFIELD
☎ 01924 276310 150 en suite

CHANNEL ISLANDS
ALDERNEY

ALDERNEY
MAP 16

Alderney Route des Carrieres GY9 3YD
☎ 01481 822835
9 holes, 5006yds, Par 64, SSS 65, Course record 65.
Location 1m E of St Annes
Telephone for further details

GUERNSEY

L'ANCRESSE VALE
MAP 16

Royal Guernsey GY3 5BY
☎ 01481 246523 📠 01481 243960
e-mail: bob.rggc@cwgsy.net
web: www.royalguernseygolfclub.com
Not quite as old as its neighbour Royal Jersey, Royal Guernsey is a sporting course which was redesigned after World War II by Mackenzie Ross, who has many fine courses to his credit. It is a pleasant links, well-maintained, and administered by the States of Guernsey. The 8th hole, a good Par 4, requires an accurate second shot to the green set among the gorse and thick rough. The 18th, with lively views, needs a strong shot to reach the green well down below. The course is windy, with hard walking.
18 holes, 6215yds, Par 70, SSS 70, Course record 64.
Club membership 934.
Visitors Mon-Wed, Fri & BHs. Thu & Sat am only. Booking required. Handicap certificate. Dress code. **Green Fees** £45 per day. **Prof** Norman Wood **Course Designer** Mackenzie Ross **Facilities** ⊕ ⏀ ⅃ ➘ ♀ ♪ ➘ **Location** 3m N of St Peter Port
Hotel ★★★★ 77% HL St Pierre Park Hotel, Rohais, ST PETER PORT
☎ 01481 728282 131 en suite

CASTEL
MAP 16

La Grande Mare Golf & Country Club Vazon Bay GY5 7LL
☎ 01481 253544 📠 01481 255197
e-mail: golf@lagrandemare.com
web: www.lgm.guernsey.net
This hotel and golf complex is set in over 120 acres of grounds. The Hawtree designed parkland course opened in 1994 and was originally designed around 14 holes with four double greens. Water hazards on 15 holes.
18 holes, 4755yards, Par 64, SSS 64, Course record 65.
Club membership 800.
Visitors Mon-Sun & BHs. Dress code. **Societies** Booking required.
Green Fees £34 per 18 holes (£38 Sat & Sun). **Prof** Matt Groves **Course Designer** Hawtree **Facilities** ⊕ ⏀ ⅃ ➘ ♀ ♪ ➘ ⌦ ◇ ✔ **Leisure** hard tennis courts, outdoor and indoor heated swimming pools, fishing, sauna, gymnasium, sports massage. **Conf** facs Corporate Hospitality Days **Hotel** ★★★ 72% HL Hotel Hougue du Pommier, Hougue du Pommier Rd, CATEL ☎ 01481 256531 37 en suite 6 annexe en suite

ST PETER PORT
MAP 16

St Pierre Park Golf Club Rohais GY1 1FD
☎ 01481 728282 📠 01481 712041
e-mail: stppark@itl.net
web: www.stpierrepark.co.uk
Par 3 parkland course with delightful setting, with lakes, streams and many tricky holes.
9 holes, 2610yds, Par 54, SSS 50, Course record 52.
Club membership 200.
Visitors Mon-Sun & BHs. Dress code. **Societies** welcome. **Green Fees** not confirmed. **Prof** Roy Corbet **Course Designer** Jacklin **Facilities** ⊕ ⏀ ⅃ ➘ ♀ ♪ ➘ ⌦ ◇ ✔ **Leisure** hard tennis courts, heated indoor swimming pool, sauna, solarium, gymnasium. **Conf** facs **Location** 1m W off Rohais Rd
Hotel ★★★★ 77% HL St Pierre Park Hotel, Rohais, ST PETER PORT
☎ 01481 728282 131 en suite

JERSEY

GROUVILLE
MAP 16

Royal Jersey Le Chemin au Greves JE3 9BD
☎ 01534 854416 📠 01534 854684
e-mail: thesecretary@royaljersey.com
web: www.royaljersey.com
18 holes, 6100yds, Par 70, SSS 70, Course record 63.
Location 4m E of St Helier off coast road
Telephone for further details
Hotel ★★★ 74% HL Old Court House Hotel, GOREY ☎ 01534 854444 58 en suite

LA MOYE   MAP 16

La Moye La Route Orange JE3 8GQ
☎ 01534 743401 📄 01534 747289
e-mail: secretary@lamoyegolfclub.co.uk
web: www.lamoyegolfclub.co.uk
Seaside championship links course (venue for the Jersey Seniors Open) situated in an exposed position on the south western corner of the island overlooking St Ouen's Bay. Offers spectacular views, two start points, full course all year - no temporary greens.
18 holes, 6664yds, Par 72, SSS 73, Course record 65.
Club membership 1300.
Visitors Mon-Sun & BHs. Booking required. Handicap certificate. Dress code. **Societies** Booking required. **Green Fees** £55 per 18 holes (£60 Sat, Sun & BHs). **Prof** Mike Deeley **Course Designer** James Braid
Facilities ⑪ 🍴 ⌂ ♨ ⚐ ☂ 🛒 🏌 **Location** W of village off A13
Hotel ★★★★ HL The Atlantic Hotel, Le Mont de la Pulente, ST BRELADE ☎ 01534 744101 50 en suite

ST CLEMENT   MAP 16

St Clement Jersey Recreation Grounds JE2 6PN
☎ 01534 721938 📄 01534 721012
Very tight moorland course. Impossible to play to scratch. Suitable for middle to high handicaps.
9 holes, 2244yds, Par 30, SSS 31, Course record 29.
Club membership 500.
Visitors Mon, Wed-Fri & BHs. **Green Fees** £22 per day, £12 per 9 holes.
Prof Lee Elstone **Facilities** ⑪ 🍴 ⌂ ♨ ⚐ ☂ 🛒 🏌 **Leisure** hard tennis courts, squash, bowls. **Location** E of St Helier on A5
Hotel ★★★★ HL Longueville Manor Hotel, ST SAVIOUR ☎ 01534 725501 29 en suite 1 annexe en suite

ST OUEN   MAP 16

Les Mielles Golf & Country Club JE3 7FQ
☎ 01534 482787 📄 01534 485414
e-mail: enquiry@lesmielles.co.je
web: www.lesmielles.com
Challenging championship course with bent grass greens, dwarf rye fairways and picturesque ponds situated in the Island's largest conservation area within St Ouen's Bay.

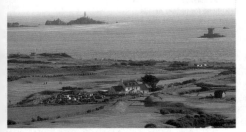

18 holes, 5261yds, Par 70, SSS 68, Course record 65.
Club membership 1500.
Visitors contact club for details. **Societies** booking required. **Green Fees** not confirmed. **Prof** W Osmand/L Cummins/A Jones **Course Designer** J Le Brun/R Whitehead **Facilities** ⑪ 🍴 ⌂ ♨ ⚐ ☂ 🛒 🏌 **Leisure**

Laser clay pigeon shooting, 'Breakers' realistic golf course. **Conf** facs Corporate Hospitality Days **Location** Centre of St Ouen's Bay
Hotel ★★★★ 80% HL L'Horizon Hotel and Spa, St Brelade's Bay, ST BRELADE ☎ 01534 743101 106 en suite

ISLE OF MAN

CASTLETOWN   MAP 06 SC26

Castletown Golf Links Fort Island, Derbyhaven IM9 1UA
☎ 01624 822220 📄 01624 829661
e-mail: 1sttee@manx.net
web: www.golfiom.com
Set on the Langness peninsula, this superb championship course is surrounded on three sides by the sea, and holds many surprises from its Championship tees.

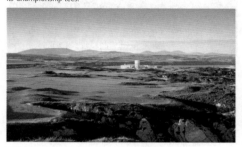

18 holes, 6707yds, Par 72, SSS 72, Course record 64.
Club membership 500.
Visitors Mon-Sun & BHs. Booking required. Handicap certificate. Dress code. **Societies** welcome. **Green Fees** not confirmed. **Prof** Michael Brookes **Course Designer** McKenzie Ross/Old Tom Morris **Facilities** ⑪ 🍴 ⌂ ♨ ⚐ ☂ 🛒 ◇ 🏌 **Leisure** heated indoor swimming pool, sauna, snooker. **Conf** Corporate Hospitality Days
Hotel ★★ 69% HL Falcon's Nest, The Promenade, PORT ERIN ☎ 01624 834077 35 en suite

DOUGLAS   MAP 06 SC37

Douglas Pulrose Park IM2 1AE
☎ 01624 675952 📄 01624 616865
e-mail: mug@hotmail.co.uk
Hilly, parkland and moorland course under the control of Douglas Corporation.
18 holes, 5937yds, Par 69, SSS 69, Course record 62.
Club membership 330.
Visitors Mon-Sun & BHs. Booking required Tue, Wed, Sat & Sun. **Societies** Booking required. **Green Fees** £11 per day (£16 Sat & Sun). ⊛ **Prof** Mike Vipond **Course Designer** Dr A Mackenzie **Facilities** ⑪ ⌂ ♨ ⚐ ☂ 🛒 🏌 **Conf** Corporate Hospitality Days **Location** 1m from Douglas on Castletown road on Pulrose Estate
Hotel ★★★ 75% HL The Empress Hotel, Central Promenade, DOUGLAS ☎ 01624 661155 102 en suite

England

Mount Murray Hotel & Country Club Mount Murray, Santon IM4 2HT

☎ 01624 661111 📠 01624 611116

e-mail: hotel@mountmurray.com

web: www.mountmurray.com

A challenging course with many natural features, lakes, streams etc. Five Par 5s, six Par 3s and the rest Par 4. Fine views over the whole island.

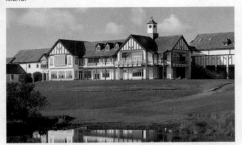

18 holes, 6356yds, Par 71, SSS 71, Course record 66.
Club membership 378.
Visitors Mon-Sun & BHs. Booking required Sat, Sun & BHs. Dress code. **Societies** Booking required. **Green Fees** £25 per round (£30 Sat & Sun). **Prof** Andrew Dyson **Course Designer** Bingley Sports Research **Facilities** ⑪🍴🏪 🖵 🏋 🚾 🏌️ ☕ ✓ 🛥 ✓ 🏌️ **Leisure** heated indoor swimming pool, squash, sauna, solarium, gymnasium. **Conf** facs Corporate Hospitality Days **Location** 5m from Douglas towards airport
Hotel ★★★★ 74% HL Mount Murray Hotel & Country Club, Santon, DOUGLAS ☎ 01624 661111 90 en suite

ONCHAN
MAP 06 SC47

King Edward Bay Golf & Country Club Howstrake, Groudle Rd IM3 2JR

☎ 01624 672709 & 620430

e-mail: mail@kebgc.com

web: kebgc.com

18 holes, 5492yds, Par 67, SSS 65, Course record 58.
Course Designer Tom Morris **Location** E of town off A11
Telephone for further details
Hotel ★★★★ 77% HL Sefton Hotel, Harris Promenade, DOUGLAS ☎ 01624 645500 96 en suite

PEEL
MAP 06 SC28

Peel Rheast Ln IM5 1BG

☎ 01624 842227 & 843456 📠 01624 843456

e-mail: peelgc@.manx.net

web: www.peelgolfclub.com

Moorland course, with natural hazards and easy walking. Good views. The drop down to the 12th and climb back up to the 13th interrupt an otherwise fairly level course. The long, dog-legged 11th hole is an outstanding Par 4, where the gorse must be carried to get a good second shot to the green. Most notable of the short holes are the 10th and 17th where an errant tee shot finds bunker, gorse or thick rough.

18 holes, 5850yds, Par 69, SSS 69, Course record 64.
Club membership 856.
Visitors Mon-Sun & BHs. Booking required. Handicap certificate. Dress code. **Societies** Booking required. **Green Fees** £22 per round (£30 Sat

& Sun). **Prof** Paul O'Reilly **Course Designer** James Braide **Facilities** ⑪ 🖵 🏪🍴🏋 🚾 🏌️ ✓ **Leisure** snooker. **Conf** Corporate Hospitality Days
Location SE of town centre on A1
Hotel ★★★ 75% HL The Empress Hotel, Central Promenade, DOUGLAS ☎ 01624 661155 102 en suite

PORT ERIN
MAP 06 SC16

Rowany Rowany Dr IM9 6LN

☎ 01624 834108 or 834072 📠 01624 834072

e-mail: rowany@iommail.net

web: www.rowanygolfclub.com

Undulating seaside course with testing later holes, which cut through gorse and rough. However, those familiar with this course maintain that the 7th and 12th holes are the most challenging.

18 holes, 5840yds, Par 70, SSS 69, Course record 62.
Club membership 500.
Visitors Mon-Sun & BHs. Booking required. **Societies** Booking required. **Green Fees** Phone. ✆ **Course Designer** G Lowe **Facilities** ⑪ 🍴 by prior arrangement 🏪 🖵🍴🏋 🚾 🏌️ ✓ 🛥 ✓ **Conf** Corporate Hospitality Days **Location** N of village off A32

PORT ST MARY
MAP 06 SC26

Port St Mary Kallow Point Rd

☎ 01624 834932

Slightly hilly course with beautiful scenic views over Port St Mary and the Irish Sea.

9 holes, 5702yds, Par 68, SSS 68, Course record 62.
Club membership 324.
Visitors contact club for details. **Societies** welcome. **Green Fees** not confirmed. **Course Designer** George Duncan **Facilities** 🏋 🚾 🛥 ✓ **Leisure** hard tennis courts, Croquet lawn. **Conf** Corporate Hospitality Days **Location** Signed entering Port St Mary, one-way system, 2nd left to end , 1st right

RAMSEY
MAP 06 SC49

Ramsey Brookfield IM8 2AH

☎ 01624 812244 📠 01624 815833

e-mail: ramseygolfclub@manx.net

web: www.ramseygolfclub.com

18 holes, 5960yds, Par 70, SSS 69, Course record 63.
Course Designer James Braid **Location** SW of town centre
Telephone for further details
Hotel ★★★ 75% HL The Empress Hotel, Central Promenade, DOUGLAS ☎ 01624 661155 102 en suite

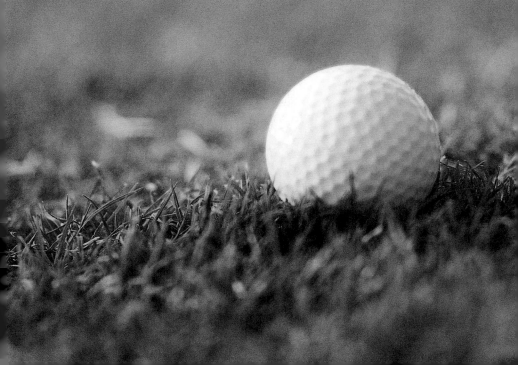

Scotland

CITY OF ABERDEEN

ABERDEEN MAP 15 NJ90

Auchmill Bonnyview Rd, West Heatheryfold AB16 7FQ
☎ 01224 714577 📠 01224 648693
18 holes, 5123metres, Par 70, SSS 67, Course record 67.
Course Designer Neil Coles/Brian Hugget **Location** Outskirts Aberdeen,
A96 Aberdeen-Inverness
Telephone for further details
Hotel ★★★ 77% HL The Craighaar Hotel, Waterton Rd, Bucksburn,
ABERDEEN ☎ 01224 712275 55 en suite

Balnagask St Fitticks Rd AB11 3QT
☎ 01224 876407 📠 01224 648693
18 holes, 5986yds, Par 70, SSS 69.
Location 2m E of city centre
Telephone for further details
Hotel ★★★ 74% HL Maryculter House Hotel, South Deeside Rd,
Maryculter, ABERDEEN ☎ 01224 732124 40 en suite

Craibstone Golf Centre Craibstone Estate, Bucksburn
AB21 9YA
☎ 01224 716777 & 711012 📠 01224 711298
e-mail: craibstonegolf@sac.co.uk
web: www.sac.ac.uk/craibstone/
18 holes, 5757yards, Par 69, SSS 69, Course record 66.
Location NW of city off A96 Aberdeen-Inverness road. A96 through
Bucksburn. Before next rdbt left signed Forrit Brae. At top of road club
signed
Telephone for further details
Hotel ★★★★ 77% HL Aberdeen Marriott Hotel, Overton Circle, Dyce,
ABERDEEN ☎ 01224 770011 155 en suite

Deeside Golf Rd, Bieldside AB15 9DL
☎ 01224 869457 📠 01224 861800
e-mail: admin@deesidegolfclub.com
web: www.deesidegolfclub.com
An interesting riverside course with several tree-lined fairways. A
stream comes into play at nine of the 18 holes on the main course.
In recent years major reconstruction work has taken place to provide
a testing course in which only five of the original holes are virtually
unchanged. These include the 15th (the old 6th) which bears the
name of James Braid who advised the club during previous course
alterations. Various water features are incorporated into the course
including pools at the 4th, 10th and 17th.
Haughton: 18 holes, 6286yds, Par 70, SSS 71,
Course record 65.
Blairs: 9 holes, 5042yds, Par 68, SSS 64.
Club membership 1000.
Visitors Mon-Sun & BHs. Booking required. Handicap certificate. Dress
code. **Societies** Booking required. **Green Fees** Phone. **Prof** Frank J Coutts
Course Designer Archie Simpson **Facilities** ⊕ ⦿ ⓮ ⌼ ☚ ⚑ ⚘ ⚑
Conf Corporate Hospitality Days **Location** 3m W of city centre off A93
Hotel ★★★★ 77% HL Mercure Ardoe House, South Deeside Rd, Blairs,
ABERDEEN ☎ 0870 194 2104 109 en suite

Hazelhead Hazlehead Av AB15 8BD
☎ 01224 321830 📠 01224 810452
e-mail: golf@aberdeencity.gov.uk
web: www.aberdeencity.gov.uk
Three picturesque courses and a pitch and putt course which provide a
true test of golfing skills with gorse and woodlands being a hazard for
any wayward shots.
No 1 Course: 18 holes, 6224yds, Par 70, SSS 70.
No 2 Course: 18 holes, 5764yds, Par 67, SSS 67.
Visitors Mon-Sun & BHs. Dress code. **Societies** booking required. **Green
Fees** not confirmed. ⊛ **Prof** C Nelson **Facilities** ⚑ **Leisure** 9 hole pitch &
putt course. **Location** 4m W of city centre off A944
Hotel ★★★★ 77% HL Mercure Ardoe House, South Deeside Rd, Blairs,
ABERDEEN ☎ 0870 194 2104 109 en suite

Kings Links Golf Rd AB24 1RZ
☎ 01224 632269 📠 01224 648693
18 holes, 6384yds, Par 72, SSS 71.
Location 0.75m NE of city centre
Telephone for further details

Murcar Links Bridge of Don AB23 8BD
☎ 01224 704354 📠 01224 704354
e-mail: golf@murcarlinks.com
web: www.murcarlinks.com
Seaside links course with a prevailing south-west wind. Its main
attraction is the challenge of playing round and between gorse, heather
and sand dunes. The additional hazards of burns and out of bounds
give any golfer a testing round of golf.

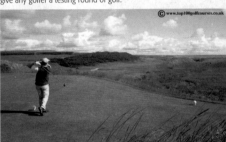

Murcar Links: 18 holes, 6500yds, Par 71, SSS 72,
Course record 64.
Strabathie: 9 holes, 2680yds, Par 35, SSS 35.
Club membership 650.
Visitors Mon, Thur, Fri & BHs. Tue, Sat & Sun; pm only. Wed; am only.
Handicap certificate. Dress code. **Societies** Booking required. **Green Fees**
£90 per day, £65 per round (£85 per round Sat & Sun). Strabathie: £28
per day, £14 per round (£44/£22 Sat & Sun). **Prof** Gary Forbes **Course
Designer** A Simpson/J Braid/G Webster **Facilities** ⊕ ⦿ ⓮ ⌼ ⚑ ⚘ ☚
⚑ ⚘ ⚑ **Location** 5m NE of city centre off A90
Hotel ★★★ 77% HL The Craighaar Hotel, Waterton Rd, Bucksburn,
ABERDEEN ☎ 01224 712275 55 en suite

Royal Aberdeen Links Rd, Balgownie, Bridge of Don
AB23 8AT
☎ 01224 702571 📠 01224 826591
e-mail: admin@royalaberdeengolf.com
web: www.royalaberdeengolf.com
Championship links course with undulating dunes. Windy, easy
walking. *Continued*

Scotland

Balgownie Course: 18 holes, 6504yds, Par 71, SSS 71, Course record 63.
Silverburn Course: 18 holes, 4066yds, Par 60, SSS 60.
Club membership 500.
Visitors Mon-Sun & BHs. Booking required. Handicap certificate. Dress code. **Societies** Booking required. **Green Fees** £150 per day, £100 per round (£120 per round Sun & Sat). **Prof** Ronnie MacAskill **Course Designer** Baird & Simpson **Facilities** ⑪ ⓑ ⌸ ⓜ ⌼ ⚘ ⌸ ❦ ⚘ **Location** 2.5m N of city centre off A92

Westhill Westhill Heights, Westhill AB32 6RY
☎ 01224 740159 🗐 01224 749124
e-mail: westhillgolf@btconnect.com
web: www.westhillgolfclub.co.uk
A challenging parkland course.
18 holes, 5921yds, Par 69, SSS 69, Course record 65.
Club membership 808.
Visitors Mon-Sun & BHs. Booking required. Dress code. **Societies** Booking required. **Green Fees** £25 per day, £20 per round (£30/£25 Sat & Sun).
Prof George Bruce **Course Designer** Charles Lawrie **Facilities** ⑪ ⑩ ⓑ ⌸ ⓜ ⌼ ⚘ ❦ ⚘ **Leisure** Snooker table. **Conf** facs Corporate Hospitality Days **Location** 7m NW of city centre off A944

PETERCULTER   MAP 15 NJ80

Peterculter Oldtown, Burnside Rd AB14 0LN
☎ 01224 734994(shop) & 735245(office)
🗐 01224 735580
e-mail: info@petercultergolfclub.co.uk
web: www.petercultergolfclub.co.uk
Surrounded by wonderful scenery and bordered by the River Dee, a variety of birds, deer and foxes may be seen on the course, which also has superb views up the Dee Valley.
18 holes, 6219yds, Par 71, SSS 70, Course record 64.
Club membership 1035.
Visitors Mon-Fri & BHs. Booking Required. Dress code. **Societies** Booking required. **Green Fees** £32 per day, £25 per round (£38/£30 Sat & Sun). **Prof** Dean Vannet **Course Designer** Greens of Scotland **Facilities** ⑪ ⑩ ⓑ ⌸ ⓜ ⌼ ⚘ ❦ ⚘ **Location** On A93

ABERDEENSHIRE

ABOYNE   MAP 15 NO59

Aboyne Formaston Park AB34 5HP
☎ 013398 86328 🗐 013398 87592
e-mail: aboynegolfclub@btconnect.com
web: www.aboynegolfclub.co.uk
Beautiful parkland with outstanding views. Two lochs on course.
18 holes, 6009yds, Par 68, SSS 69, Course record 62.
Club membership 970.
Visitors Mon-Sun & BHs. Booking required. Handicap certificate. Dress code. **Societies** Welcome. **Green Fees** £32 per day, £25 per round (£38/£28 Sat & Sun). **Prof** Stephen Moir **Facilities** ⑪ ⑩ ⓑ ⌸ ⓜ ⌼ ⚘ **Conf** Corporate Hospitality Days **Location** E side of village, N of A93
Hotel ★★★ 79% HL Loch Kinord Hotel, Ballater Rd, Dinnet, BALLATER ☎ 013398 85229 20 en suite

---

ALFORD   MAP 15 NJ51

Alford Montgarrie Rd AB33 8AE
☎ 019755 62178 🗐 019755 64910
e-mail: info@alford-golf-club.co.uk
web: www.alford-golf-club.co.uk
Flat parkland in scenic countryside. The course is challenging, testing golfers of all skills and abilities. Divided into sections by a road, a narrow-gauge railway and a burn.
18 holes, 5483yds, Par 69, SSS 65, Course record 64.
Club membership 800.
Visitors Mon-Sun & BHs. Booking required Sat. Dress code. **Societies** Booking required. **Green Fees** £25 per day / £20 per round (£30/£25 Sat & Sun). **Facilities** ⑪ ⑩ ⓑ ⌸ ⓜ ⌼ ⚘ ❦ ⚘ **Conf** Corporate Hospitality Days **Location** In village centre on A944
Hotel ★★ 65% HL Gordon Arms Hotel, The Square, HUNTLY ☎ 01466 792288 13 en suite

---

AUCHENBLAE   MAP 15 NO77

Auchenblae AB30 1WQ
☎ 01561 320002
e-mail: parks@auchenblae.org.uk
web: www.auchenblae.org.uk/golf
Short but demanding course set in spectacular scenery and renowned for its excellent greens. A mixture of short and long holes, small and large greens add to the challenge and enjoyment of the course.
9 holes, 2217yds, Par 32, SSS 61, Course record 61.
Club membership 500.
Visitors Mon-Sun & BHs. **Societies** Booking required. **Green Fees** £12 per day (£15 Sat & Sun). ⊜ **Course Designer** Robin Hiseman **Facilities** ⌸ ⌼ ⚘ **Leisure** hard tennis courts. **Location** 10m S of Stonehaven off A90

BALLATER   MAP 15 NO39

Ballater Victoria Rd AB35 5QX
☎ 013397 55567
e-mail: sec@ballatergolfclub.co.uk
web: www.ballatergolfclub.co.uk
Heather covered course with testing long holes and beautiful scenery.
18 holes, 5638yds, Par 67, SSS 67, Course record 62.
Club membership 750.
Visitors Mon-Sun & BHs. Dress code. **Societies** Booking required. **Green Fees** £24 per round (£28 Sat & Sun). **Prof** Bill Yule **Facilities** ⑪ ⑩ ⓑ ⌸ ⓜ ⌼ ⚘ ❦ ⚘ **Leisure** hard tennis courts, fishing, snooker. **Conf** Corporate Hospitality Days **Location** W side of town
Hotel ★★★ 79% HL Loch Kinord Hotel, Ballater Rd, Dinnet, BALLATER ☎ 013398 85229 20 en suite

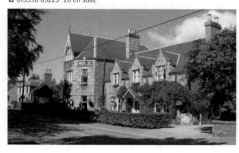

Scotland

Scotland

BALMEDIE   MAP 15 NJ91

East Aberdeenshire Golf Centre Millden AB23 8YY
☎ 01358 742111 🖹 01358 742123
e-mail: info@eagolf.com
web: www.eagolf.com
Designed as two loops of nine holes each, starting and finishing outside the clubhouse. Skilful use of 130 acres of rolling Buchan farmland has resulted in a challenging course of 6276yds in length. Even in the short history of the course, the Par 3 holes have gained the reputation of being equal to any in the north of Scotland.
18 holes, 6276yrds, Par 71, SSS 71, Course record 69.
Club membership 400.
Visitors Mon-Sun & BHs. **Societies** Welcome. **Green Fees** £24 (£30 Sat, Sun & BHs). **Prof** Ian Bratton **Course Designer** Ian Cresswell **Facilities** ⊕ ⎯ ⊾ ⌷ ⎯ ⌷ ⌷ ⌷ ⌷ **Conf** facs Corporate Hospitality Days **Hotel** [U] HL The Udny Arms Hotel, Main St, NEWBURGH ☎ 01358 789444 25 en suite

BANCHORY   MAP 15 NO69

Banchory Kinneskie Rd AB31 5TA
☎ 01330 822365 🖹 01330 822491
e-mail: info@banchorygolfclub.co.uk
web: www.banchorygolfclub.co.uk
Sheltered parkland beside the River Dee, with easy walking and woodland scenery. Testing 12th and 13th holes.
18 holes, 5801yds, Par 69, SSS 68, Course record 63.
Club membership 975.
Visitors Mon, Wed-Fri & BHs. Limited play Sat & Sun. Booking required. Dress code. **Societies** Booking required. **Green Fees** £35 per day, £26 per round (£45/£35 Sat & Sun). **Prof** David Naylor **Facilities** ⊕ ⎯ ⊾ ⌷ ⎯ ⌷ ⌷ ⌷ ⌷ **Conf** facs **Location** A93, 300yds from W end of High St **Hotel** ★★★ 81% CHH Banchory Lodge Hotel, BANCHORY ☎ 01330 822625 22 en suite

Inchmarlo Golf Club Inchmarlo AB31 4BQ
☎ 01330 826422 🖹 01330 826425
e-mail: info@inchmarlo.com
web: www.inchmarlogolf.com
The Laird's (18-hole course) is laid out on the gentle parkland slopes of the Inchmarlo Estate in the Dee Valley and the designer has take advantage of the natural contours of the land and its many mature trees. The nine-hole Queen's course is a tricky and testing course with ponds, meandering burns and dry stone dykes combining with the more traditional bunkers to test the skill of even the most accomplished player.

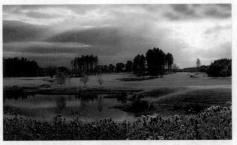

Laird's Course: 18 holes, 6218yards, Par 71, SSS 71, Course record 65.

Queen's Course: 9 holes, 2150yds, Par 32, SSS 31.
Club membership 900.
Visitors Mon-Fri, Sun & BHs. Sat after 3pm. Booking required. Dress code. **Societies** Booking required. **Green Fees** Laird's Course £32 per round (£37 Sat & Sun), Queens Course £16 per 18 holes, £11 per 9 holes (£18 / £12 Sun & Sat). **Prof** Patrick Lovie **Course Designer** Graeme Webster **Facilities** ⊕ ⎯ ⎯ ⌷ ⌷ ⌷ ⌷ ⌷ ⌷ ⌷ ⌷ **Conf** facs Corporate Hospitality Days **Location** 0.5m from A93 Aberdeen-Braemar road

BANFF   MAP 15 NJ66

Duff House Royal The Barnyards AB45 3SX
☎ 01261 812062 🖹 01261 812224
e-mail: duff_house_royal@btinternet.com
web: www.theduffhouseroyalgolfclub.co.uk
Well-manicured flat parkland, bounded by woodlands and the River Deveron. Well bunkered and renowned for its large, two-tier greens. The river is a hazard for those who wander off the tee at the 7th, 16th and 17th holes.
18 holes, 6161yds, Par 68, SSS 70, Course record 62.
Club membership 1000.
Visitors Mon-Sun. Booking required. Handicap certificate. Dress code. **Societies** booking required. **Green Fees** not confirmed. **Prof** Gary Holland **Course Designer** Dr McKenzie **Facilities** ⊕ ⊕ ⎯ ⌷ ⌷ ⌷ ⎯ ⌷ ⌷ **Conf** Corporate Hospitality Days **Location** 0.5m S on A98 **Hotel** ★★★ 77% HL Banff Springs Hotel, Golden Knowes Rd, BANFF ☎ 01261 812881 31 en suite

BRAEMAR   MAP 15 NO19

Braemar Cluniebank Rd AB35 5XX
☎ 013397 41618 🖹 013397 41400
e-mail: info@braemargolfclub.co.uk
web: www.braemargolfclub.co.uk
Flat course, set amid beautiful countryside on Royal Deeside, with River Clunie running through several holes. The 2nd hole is one of the most testing in the area.
18 holes, 5000yds, Par 65, SSS 64, Course record 59.
Club membership 450.
Visitors Mon-Sun & BHs. Booking required. **Societies** Booking required. **Green Fees** £25 per day, £20 per round (£30/£25 Sat & Sun). **Course Designer** Joe Anderson **Facilities** ⊕ ⊕ ⎯ ⌷ ⌷ ⌷ ⎯ ⌷ ⌷ **Location** 0.5m S

CRUDEN BAY   MAP 15 NK03

Cruden Bay Aulton Rd AB42 0NN
☎ 01779 812285 🖹 01779 812945
e-mail: cbaygc@aol.com
web: www.crudenbaygolfclub.co.uk
A typical links course which epitomises the old fashioned style of rugged links golf. The drives require accuracy with bunkers and protecting greens, blind holes and undulating greens. The 10th provides a panoramic view of half the back nine down at beach level, and to the east can be seen the outline of the spectacular ruin of Slains Castle featured in Bram Stoker's Dracula. The figure eight design of the course is quite unusual.
Main Course: 18 holes, 6395yds, Par 70, SSS 72, Course record 65.
St Olaf Course: 9 holes, 5106yds, Par 64, SSS 65.
Club membership 1100.

Continued

Scotland

Visitors Mon-Sun & BHs. Booking required. Handicap certificate. Dress code. **Societies** Booking required. **Green Fees** £60 per round/£80 per day (£70 per round Sat & Sun). **Prof** Robbie Stewart **Course Designer** Thomas Simpson **Facilities** ⓣ ⓞ ⓛ ⓓ ⓔ ⓕ ⓖ ⓗ ⓘ ⓙ **Conf** Corporate Hospitality Days **Location** SW side of village on A975

Hotel ★★ 69% HL Red House Hotel, Aulton Rd, CRUDEN BAY ☎ 01779 812215 6 rms (5 en suite)

ELLON   MAP 15 NJ93

McDonald Hospital Rd AB41 9AW
☎ 01358 720576 📄 01358 720001
e-mail: mcdonald.golf@virgin.net
web: www.ellongolfclub.co.uk
Tight, parkland course with streams.
18 holes, 5986yds, Par 70, SSS 70, Course record 62.
Club membership 710.
Visitors Mon-Sun & BHs. Booking required Sat-Sun & BHs. Dress code.
Societies Booking required. **Green Fees** £30 per day, £24 per round (£35/£30 Sat & Sun). **Prof** Ronnie Urquhart **Facilities** ⓣ ⓞ ⓛ ⓓ ⓔ ⓕ ⓗ ⓘ **Conf** Corporate Hospitality Days **Location** 0.25m N on A948
Hotel Ⓤ HL The Udny Arms Hotel, Main St, NEWBURGH ☎ 01358 789444 25 en suite

FRASERBURGH   MAP 15 NJ96

Fraserburgh Philorth Links AB43 8TL
☎ 01346 516616 📄 01346 516616
e-mail: secretary@fraserburghgolfclub.org
web: www.fraserburghgolfclub.org
Testing seaside course, natural links. An extremely scenic course, surrounded and protected by substantial sand dunes. Fraserburgh is the seventh oldest golf club in the world.
Corbie: 18 holes, 6308yds, Par 70, SSS 71,
Course record 63.
Rosehill: 9 holes, 2416yds, Par 66, SSS 63.
Club membership 650.
Visitors Mon-Sun & BHs. **Societies** Welcome. **Green Fees** Corbie £40 per day, £35 per round (£45/ £35 Sat & Sun). Rosehill £12 per day/9 holes. ⓔ
Course Designer James Braid **Facilities** ⓣ ⓞ ⓛ ⓓ ⓔ ⓕ ⓗ ⓘ **Leisure** Various open competitions throughout the year. **Conf** Corporate Hospitality Days **Location** 1m SE on B9033

HUNTLY   MAP 15 NJ53

Huntly Cooper Park AB54 4SH
☎ 01466 792643 📄 01466 794574
e-mail: huntlygc1@tiscali.co.uk
web: www.huntlygc.com
Parkland between the rivers Deveron and Bogie.
18 holes, 5399yds, Par 67, SSS 66. Club membership 700.
Visitors Mon-Sun & BHs. Booking required Sat, Sun & BHs. **Societies** Booking required. **Green Fees** £24 per day, £18 per round (£28/£22 Sat & Sun). **Facilities** ⓣ ⓞ ⓛ ⓓ ⓕ ⓗ ⓘ ⓔ ⓕ **Location** N side of Huntly, turn off A96 at bypass rdbt
Hotel ★★ 65% HL Gordon Arms Hotel, The Square, HUNTLY ☎ 01466 792288   13 en suite

INSCH   MAP 15 NJ62

Insch Golf Ter AB52 6JY
☎ 01464 820363 📄 01464 820363
e-mail: administrator@inschgolfclub.co.uk
web: www.inschgolfclub.co.uk
A challenging 18-hole course, a mixture of flat undulating parkland, with trees, stream and pond. The most challenging hole of the course is the 9th, a testing Par 5 of 534yds requiring long and accurate play. This follows the Par 3 8th, a hole which demands a well-positioned tee shot played over a large water hazard to a long narrow green. Although a relatively short course, the natural woodland, water hazards and large contoured greens require accurate play.
18 holes, 5350yds, Par 69, SSS 67. Club membership 400.
Visitors Mon-Sun & BHs. **Societies** Booking Required. **Green Fees** £16 per day (£22 Sat & Sun) reductions during winter. **Course Designer** Greens of Scotland **Facilities** ⓣ by prior arrangement ⓞ by prior arrangement ⓛ ⓓ ⓕ ⓗ ⓘ ⓔ ⓕ **Conf** Corporate Hospitality Days **Location** A96

INVERALLOCHY   MAP 15 NK06

Inverallochy Whitelink AB43 8XY
☎ 01346 582000
Seaside links course with natural hazards, tricky Par 3s and easy walking.
18 holes, 5351yds, Par 67, SSS 66, Course record 57.
Club membership 600.
Visitors Mon-Sun & BHs. Booking required. Dress code **Societies** Booking required. **Green Fees** £25 per day, £17 per round (Sat & Sun £30/£20).
ⓔ **Facilities** ⓣ ⓞ ⓛ ⓓ ⓕ ⓗ ⓘ ⓔ ⓕ **Leisure** Bowling green. **Location** E side of village off B9107

INVERURIE   MAP 15 NJ72

Inverurie Davah Wood AB51 5JB
☎ 01467 624080 📄 01467 672869
e-mail: administrator@inveruriegc.co.uk
web: www.inveruriegc.co.uk
Parkland course, part of which is through a wood.
18 holes, 5711yds, Par 69, SSS 68, Course record 63.
Club membership 750.
Visitors Mon-Sun & BHs. Booking required. Dress code. **Societies** Welcome. **Green Fees** £24 per day; £20 per round (£30/£24 Sat & Sun). ⓔ
Prof John Logue **Facilities** ⓣ ⓞ ⓛ ⓓ ⓕ ⓗ ⓘ ⓔ ⓕ **Location** Off Blackhall rdbt off A96 bypass

KEMNAY   MAP 15 NJ71

Kemnay Monymusk Rd AB51 5RA
☎ 01467 642225 (shop) 📄 01467 643746
e-mail: administrator@kemnaygolfclub.co.uk
web: www.kemnaygolfclub.co.uk
Parkland with stunning views, incorporating tree-lined and open fairways, and a stream crossing four holes. The course is not physically demanding but a challenge is presented to every level of golfer due to the diverse characteristics of each hole.
18 holes, 6362yds, Par 71, SSS 71, Course record 66.
Club membership 800.
Visitors Mon-Sun & BHs. Booking required. **Societies** Welcome.
Green Fees £26 per day; £20 per round (£30/£24 Sat & Sun).
Prof Ronnie McDonald **Course Designer** Greens of Scotland
Facilities ⓣ ⓞ ⓛ ⓓ ⓕ ⓗ ⓘ ⓔ ⓕ ⓖ **Conf** Corporate Hospitality Days **Location** W side of village on B993

KINTORE
MAP 15 NJ71

Kintore Balbithan AB51 0UR
☎ 01467 632631 🖥 01467 632995
e-mail: kintoregolfclub@lineone.net
web: www.kintoregolfclub.net
The course covers a large area of ground, from the Don Basin near the clubhouse, to mature woodland at the far perimeter. The 1st is one of the toughest opening holes in the North East, and the 7th requires an accurate drive followed by a second shot over a burn which runs diagonally across the front of the green. The 11th is the longest hole on the course, made longer by the fact that it slopes upwards all the way to the green. The final holes are short, relatively hilly and quite tricky but offer spectacular views to the Bennachie and Grampian hills.
18 holes, 6019yds, Par 70, SSS 69, Course record 62. Club membership 700.
Visitors Mon-Fri, Sun & BHs. Dress code **Societies** Booking required.
Green Fees Phone. **Facilities** ⑪ ⑩ ᕦ ☷ ⑪ ᗱ ᖆ ᵺ
Conf Corporate Hospitality Days **Location** 1m from village centre on B977

MACDUFF
MAP 15 NJ76

Royal Tarlair Buchan St AB44 1TA
☎ 01261 832897 🖥 01261 833455
e-mail: info@royaltarlair.co.uk
web: www.royaltarlair.co.uk
Seaside clifftop course. Testing 13th, Clivet (Par 3).
18 holes, 5866yds, Par 71, SSS 68, Course record 62. Club membership 350.
Visitors Mon-Sun & BHs. Booking required Sat & Sun. **Societies** Booking required. **Green Fees** £25 per day, £20 per round (£30/£25 Sat & Sun). ☻
Facilities ⑪ ⑩ ᕦ ☷ ⑪ ᗱ ᖆ ᵺ **Conf** Corporate Hospitality Days
Location 0.75m E off A98
Hotel ★★★ 77% HL Banff Springs Hotel, Golden Knowes Rd, BANFF
☎ 01261 812881 31 en suite

MINTLAW
MAP 15 NJ94

Longside West End, Longside AB42 4XJ
☎ 01779 821558 🖥 01779 821564
e-mail: info@longsidegolf.wanadoo.co.uk
Flat parkland course with a river winding through, providing a challenging course which requires accurate play.
18 holes, 5225yds, Par 66, SSS 66, Course record 64. Club membership 700.
Visitors Mon-Sat & BHs, Sun after 10:30am. Booking required.
Societies Booking required. **Green Fees** £18 per day, £13 per round (£24/£19 Sun). ☻ **Facilities** ⑪ ⑩ ᕦ ☷ ⑪ ᗱ ᵺ **Location** 4m W of Peterhead on New Pitsligo road
Hotel ★★★ 73% HL Palace Hotel, Prince St, PETERHEAD ☎ 01779 474821
64 en suite

NEWBURGH
MAP 15 NJ92

Newburgh on Ythan Beach Rd AB41 6BE
☎ 01358 789058 & 789084
e-mail: secretary@newburghgolfclub.co.uk
web: www.newburghgolfclub.co.uk
This seaside course was founded in 1888 and is adjacent to a bird sanctuary. The course was extended in 1996 and the nine new holes, the outward half, are characterised by undulations and hills, with elevated tees and greens requiring a range of shot making. The original inward nine demands accurate golf from tee to green. Testing 550yd dog-leg (Par 5).
18 holes, 6373yds, Par 72, SSS 71, Course record 68. Club membership 800.
Visitors Mon-Sun. Booking required. **Societies** Booking required.
Green Fees £40 per day, £30 per round (£50/£35 Sat & Sun). **Prof** Ian Bratton **Facilities** ⑪ ⑩ ᕦ ☷ ⑪ ᗱ ᖆ ᵺ **Leisure** hard tennis courts. **Conf** facs Corporate Hospitality Days **Location** 10m N of Aberdeen on A975
Hotel 🄷 HL The Udny Arms Hotel, Main St, NEWBURGH ☎ 01358 789444 25 en suite

NEWMACHAR
MAP 15 NJ81

Newmachar Swailend AB21 7UU
☎ 01651 863002 🖥 01651 863055
e-mail: info@newmachargolfclub.co.uk
web: www.newmachargolfclub.co.uk
Hawkshill is a championship-standard parkland course designed by Dave Thomas. Several lakes affect five of the holes and there are well-developed birch and Scots pine trees. Swailend is a parkland course, also designed by Dave Thomas and opened in 1997. It provides a test all of its own with some well-positioned bunkering and testing greens.
Hawkshill Course: 18 holes, 6700yds, Par 72, SSS 74, Course record 67.
Swailend Course: 18 holes, 6388yds, Par 72, SSS 71, Course record 67. Club membership 900.
Visitors Mon-Sun & BHs. Booking required Sat-Sun & BHs. Handicap certificate. Dress code. **Societies** Booking required. **Green Fees** Phone.
Prof Andrew Cooper **Course Designer** Dave Thomas/Peter Allis
Facilities ⑪ ⑩ ᕦ ☷ ⑪ ᗱ ᖆ ᵺ **Conf** Corporate Hospitality Days **Location** 2m N of Dyce, off A947

OLDMELDRUM
MAP 15 NJ82

Old Meldrum Kirk Brae AB51 0DJ
☎ 01651 872648 🖥 01651 873555
e-mail: admin@oldmeldrumgolf.co.uk
web: www.oldmeldrumgolf.co.uk
Parkland with tree-lined fairways and superb views. Challenging 196yd, Par 3 11th over two ponds to a green surrounded by bunkers.
18 holes, 5988yds, Par 70, SSS 69, Course record 66. Club membership 850.
Visitors Contact club for details. **Societies** Booking required. **Green Fees** £24 per round (£30 Sat & Sun). **Prof** Hamish Love **Facilities** ⑪ ⑩ ᕦ ☷ ⑪ ᗱ ᖆ ᵺ **Location** E side of village off A947

PETERHEAD
MAP 15 NK14

Peterhead Craigewan Links, Riverside Dr AB42 1LT
☎ 01779 472149 & 480725 🖥 01779 480725
e-mail: phdgc@freenetname.co.uk
web: www.peterheadgolfclub.co.uk
Old Course: 18 holes, 6173yds, Par 70, SSS 71, Course record 64. New Course: 9 holes, 2228yds, Par 31.
Course Designer W Park/ L Auchterconie/J Braid **Location** N side of town centre off A90
Telephone for further details

PORTLETHEN

MAP 15 NO99

Portlethen Badentoy Rd AB12 4YA
☎ 01224 782575 & 781090 📄 01224 783383
e-mail: info@portlethengc.fsnet.co.uk
Set in pleasant parkland, this new course features mature trees and a stream which affects a number of holes.
18 holes, 6707yds, Par 72, SSS 72, Course record 63.
Club membership 1200.
Visitors Mon-Fri, Sun & BHs. Booking Required. Handicap certificate. Dress code. **Societies** Booking required. **Green Fees** £33 per day; £22 per round (£40/£32 Sat, Sun & BHs). **Prof** Muriel Thomson **Course Designer** Cameron Sinclair **Facilities** ⑪ ⚘⃝ ⚘ ▱ ⚘⃠ ⚘ ⚘ ⚘ **Conf** facs **Location** Off A90 S of Aberdeen

STONEHAVEN

MAP 15 NO88

Stonehaven Cowie AB39 3RH
☎ 01569 762124 📄 01569 765973
e-mail: stonehaven.golfclub@virgin.net
web: www.stonehavengolfclub.com
Challenging meadowland course overlooking sea with three gullies and splendid views.
18 holes, 5103yds, Par 66, SSS 65, Course record 61.
Club membership 850.
Visitors Mon-Sun & BHs. Booking required. Dress code. **Societies** Welcome. **Green Fees** £25 per day, £18 per round (£28/£20 Sat & Sun). **Course Designer** C Simpson **Facilities** ⑪ ⚘ ▱ ⚘⃠ ⚘ ⚘ ⚘ **Leisure** snooker. **Location** 1m N off A92

TARLAND

MAP 15 NJ40

Tarland Aberdeen Rd AB34 4TB
☎ 013398 81000 📄 013398 81000
e-mail: rw.joseph@btinternet.com
web: www.tarlandgolfclub.co.uk
Difficult upland course, but easy walking. Some spectacular holes, mainly 4th (Par 4) and 5th (Par 3) and fine scenery. A challenge to golfers of all abilities.
9 holes, 5888yds, Par 67, SSS 68, Course record 65.
Club membership 325.
Visitors Phone **Societies** Booking required. **Green Fees** £18 per day (£24 Sun & Sat). ⚘ **Course Designer** Tom Morris **Facilities** ⚘ ▱ ⚘⃠ ⚘ ⚘ **Conf** Corporate Hospitality Days **Location** E side of village off B9119 **Hotel** ★★★ 79% HL Loch Kinord Hotel, Ballater Rd, Dinnet, BALLATER ☎ 013398 85229 20 en suite

TORPHINS

MAP 15 NJ60

Torphins Bog Rd AB31 4JU
☎ 013398 82115
e-mail: stuartmacgregor5@btinternet.com
Heathland and parkland course built on a hill with views of the Cairngorms.
9 holes, 4800yds, Par 64, SSS 64, Course record 59.
Club membership 310.
Visitors Mon-Sun & BHs. **Societies** Booking required. **Green Fees** £14 per day (£15 Sun & Sat). £7 per 9 holes. ⚘ **Facilities** ⚘ ⚘ **Location** 0.25m W of village off A980

TURRIFF

MAP 15 NJ75

Turriff Rosehall AB53 4HD
☎ 01888 562982 📄 01888 568050
e-mail: grace@turriffgolf.sol.co.uk
web: www.turriffgolfclub.com
An inland course with tight fairways, well-paced greens and well-sighted bunkers to test all golfers. The Par 5 12th hole sets a challenge for the longest driver while the short Par 3 4th, with its green protected by bunkers is a challenge in its own right.

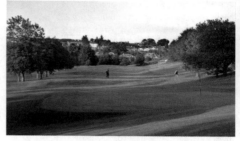

18 holes, 5664yds, Par 68, SSS 68. Club membership 650.
Visitors Mon-Sun & BHs. Booking required Fri-Sun & BHs. Handicap certificate. Dress code. **Societies** Booking required. **Green Fees** £26 per day, £22 per round (£32/£26 Sun, Sat & BHs). ⚘ **Facilities** ⑪ ⚘⃝ ⚘ ▱ ⚘⃠ ⚘ ⚘ ⚘ **Conf** Corporate Hospitality Days **Location** 1m W off B9024 **Hotel** ★★★ 77% HL Banff Springs Hotel, Golden Knowes Rd, BANFF ☎ 01261 812881 31 en suite

ANGUS

ARBROATH

MAP 12 NO64

Arbroath Elliot DD11 2PE
☎ 01241 875837 📄 01241 875837
e-mail: arbroathgolf@btinternet.com
A typical links layout, predominately flat, with the prevailing south westerly wind facing for the first seven holes, making a big difference to how certain holes play. When the wind is in a northerly direction the back nine holes are very tough. The greens are well protected by deep riveted pot bunkers. Fast tricky greens make for difficult putting.
18 holes, 6185yds, Par 70, SSS 69, Course record 64.
Club membership 550.
Visitors Mon-Sun & BHs. Booking required Sat, Sun & BHs. Dress code. **Societies** Booking required. **Green Fees** £30 per day, £25 per round (£35/£30 Sat & Sun). **Prof** Lindsay Ewart **Course Designer** Braid **Facilities** ⑪ ⚘⃝ ⚘ ▱ ⚘⃠ ⚘ ⚘ ⚘ ⚘ **Location** 1m SW on A92

Letham Grange Golf Ltd Colliston DD11 4RL
☎ 01241 890373 📄 01241 890725
e-mail: lethamgrangegolf@yahoo.co.uk
Often referred to as the 'Augusta of Scotland', the Old Course provides championship standards in spectacular surroundings with attractive lochs and burns. The Glens Course is less arduous and shorter using many natural features of the estate.
Old Course: 18 holes, 6632yds, Par 73, SSS 73, Course record 67.
Glens Course: 18 holes, 5528yds, Par 68, SSS 68, Course record 60. Club membership 600.

Continued

Scotland

Visitors Mon-Sun & BHs. Booking required. Dress code. **Societies** Booking required. **Green Fees** Old Course: £45 (£50 Sat & Sun). Glens Course: £25 (£30 Sat & Sun). **Course Designer** G K Smith/Donald Steel **Facilities** ⑪ ⑩ 🝙 ⌨ ⁂ ⚘ ☎️ ♦ ✎ 🝙 ✎ **Conf** facs Corporate Hospitality Days **Location** 4m N on A933

BARRY MAP 12 NO53

Panmure Burnside Rd DD7 7RT
☎ 01241 855120 📠 01241 859737
e-mail: secretary@panmuregolfclub.co.uk
web: www.panmuregolfclub.co.uk
A nerve-testing, adventurous course which opens quietly and builds its challenge amongst the sandhills further out. The course is used for Open championship final qualifying rounds.
18 holes, 6317yds, Par 70, SSS 71, Course record 62.
Club membership 700.
Visitors Mon, Wed-Fri, Sun & BHs. Dress code. **Societies** Booking required. **Green Fees** £85 per day; £65 per round. **Prof** Neil Mackintosh **Course Designer** James Braid **Facilities** ⑪ ⑩ 🝙 ⌨ ⁂ 🝙 ⚘ ✎ 🝙 ✎ 🝙 **Conf** Corporate Hospitality Days **Location** S side of village off A930
Hotel BUD Premier Travel Inn Dundee East, 115-117 Lawers Dr, Panmurefield Village, BROUGHTY FERRY ☎ 0870 9906324 60 en suite

BRECHIN MAP 15 NO56

Brechin Trinity DD9 7PD
☎ 01356 622383 & 625270 📠 01356 625270
e-mail: brechingolfclub@tiscali.co.uk
web: www.brechingolfclub.co.uk
Rolling parkland with easy walking and good views of the Grampian mountains. Set among many tree-lined fairways with excellent greens and lush green fairways. A wide variation of holes with dog legs, long Par 3s, tricky Par 4s and reachable in two Par 5s, where the longer hitters can take a more challenging tee shot.
18 holes, 6092yds, Par 72, SSS 70, Course record 66.
Club membership 850.
Visitors Mon-Sun & BHs. Booking required. **Societies** Booking required. **Green Fees** £35 per day, £28 per round (£40/£30 Sat & Sun). **Prof** Stephen Rennie **Course Designer** James Braid (partly) **Facilities** ⑪ ⑩ 🝙 ⌨ ⁂ 🝙 ⚘ ✎ 🝙 ✎ **Leisure** squash. **Conf** Corporate Hospitality Days **Location** 1m N on B966
Hotel ★★★ 66% HL Glenesk Hotel, High St, EDZELL ☎ 01356 648319 24 en suite

CARNOUSTIE MAP 12 NO53

Carnoustie Golf Links see page 315

EDZELL MAP 15 NO66

Edzell High St DD9 7TF
☎ 01356 647283 (Secretary) 📠 01356 648094
e-mail: secretary@edzellgolfclub.net
web: www.edzellgolfclub.net
This delightful, gentle, flat course is situated in the foothills of the Highlands and provides good golf as well as conveying a feeling of peace and quiet to everyone who plays here. The village of Edzell is one of the most picturesque in Scotland.
18 holes, 6367yds, Par 71, SSS 71, Course record 62.
West Water: 9 holes, 2057yds, Par 32, SSS 31.
Club membership 855.
Visitors Mon-Sun & BHs. Booking required. Handicap certificate. Dress code. **Societies** Booking required. **Green Fees** £45 per day; £33 per round (£56/£40 Sat & Sun). West Water: £15 per 16 holes, £12 per 9 holes. **Prof** A J Webster **Course Designer** Bob Simpson **Facilities** ⑪ ⑩ 🝙 ⌨ ⁂ 🝙 ⚘ ✎ ✎ 🝙 **Location** On B966, S end of Edzell
Hotel ★★★ 66% HL Glenesk Hotel, High St, EDZELL ☎ 01356 648319 24 en suite

FORFAR MAP 15 NO45

Forfar Cunninghill, Arbroath Rd DD8 2RL
☎ 01307 463773 📠 01307 468495
e-mail: forfargolfclub@uku.co.uk
web: forfargolfclub.com
18 holes, 6066yds, Par 69, SSS 70, Course record 61.
Course Designer James Braid **Location** 1.5m E of Forfar on A932
Telephone for further details
Hotel ★★★ CHH Castleton House Hotel, Castleton of Eassie, GLAMIS ☎ 01307 840340 6 en suite

KIRRIEMUIR MAP 15 NO35

Kirriemuir Shielhill Rd, Northmuir DD8 4LN
☎ 01575 573317 📠 01575 574608
e-mail: kirriemuirgolfclub@fsmail.net
Parkland and heathland course set at the foot of the Angus glens, with good view.
18 holes, 5553yds, Par 68, SSS 67, Course record 62.
Club membership 750.
Visitors Mon-Sun & BHs. Booking required. Dress code.
Societies booking required. **Green Fees** not confirmed. **Prof** Karyn Dallas **Course Designer** James Braid **Facilities** ⑪ ⑩ 🝙 ⌨ ⁂ 🝙 ⚘ ✎ **Location** 1m N off B955
Hotel ★★★ CHH Castleton House Hotel, Castleton of Eassie, GLAMIS ☎ 01307 840340 6 en suite

CHAMPIONSHIP COURSE

ANGUS — CARNOUSTIE

CARNOUSTIE GOLF LINKS

Map 12 NO53

20 Links Pde DD7 7JE
☎ **01241 853789 bookings**
🖷 **01241 852720**
e-mail: golf@carnoustiegolflinks.co.uk
web: www.carnoustiegolflinks.co.uk
Championship: 18 holes, 6941yds, Par 72, SSS 75, Course record 64.
Burnside: 18 holes, 6028yds, Par 68, SSS 70.
Buddon Links: 18 holes, 5420yds, Par 66, SSS 67.
Visitors Mon-Sun & BHs. Booking required. Dress code. **Societies** Booking required.
Green Fees Championship course £115, Burnside £33, Buddon £28. Play all 3 courses £135.
Prof Colin Sinclair **Course Designer** James Braid
Facilities 🕐 🍴 🛢 🖥 🍽 🏌 🛍 ⛳ ◇ ⚒ 🏌
Leisure heated indoor pool, sauna, solarium, gym. **Conf** Corporate Hospitality Days
Location SW of town centre off A930

This Championship Course has been voted the top course in Britain by many golfing greats and described as Scotland's ultimate golfing challenge. The course developed from origins in the 1560s; James Braid added new bunkers, greens and tees in the 1920s. The Open Championship first came to the course in 1931 and Carnoustie hosted the Scottish Open in 1995 and 1996, and was the venue for the 1999 Open Championship and will stage the Championship in 2007. The Burnside Course is enclosed on three sides by the Championship Course and has been used for Open Championship qualifying rounds. The Buddon Course has been extensively remodelled, making it ideal for mid to high handicappers.

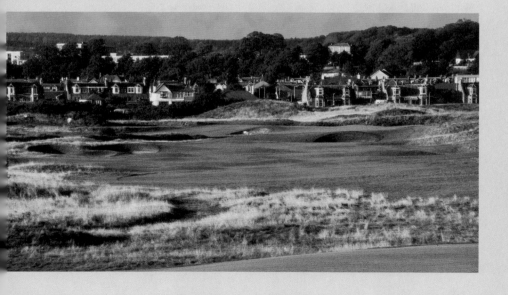

<table>
<tr><td>

MONIFIETH

MAP 12 NO43

Monifieth Princes St DD5 4AW
☎ 01382 532767 (Medal) & 532967 (Ashludie)
🖹 01382 535816
The chief of the two courses at Monifieth is the Medal Course. It has been one of the qualifying venues for the Open Championship on more than one occasion. A seaside links, but divided from the sand dunes by a railway which provides the principal hazard for the first few holes. The 10th hole is outstanding, the 17th is excellent and there is a delightful finishing hole. The other course here is the Ashludie, and both are played over by a number of clubs who share the links.

</td></tr>
</table>

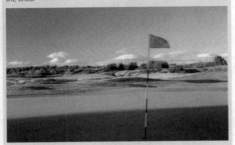

Medal Course: 18 holes, 6655yds, Par 71, SSS 72, Course record 63.
Ashludie Course: 18 holes, 5123yds, Par 68, SSS 66.
Club membership 1750.
Visitors Mon-Sun & BHs. Booking required. Handicap certificate. Dress code. **Societies** booking required. **Green Fees** not confirmed. **Prof** Ian McLeod **Facilities** ⊕ ⊠ ⤢ ⧉ ▯ ⊠ ⚐ ⚑ ⚙ ⌀ **Location** NE side of town on A930
Hotel BUD Premier Travel Inn Dundee East, 115-117 Lawers Dr, Panmurefield Village, BROUGHTY FERRY ☎ 0870 9906324   60 en suite

---

MONTROSE

MAP 15 NO75

Montrose Golf Links Traill Dr DD10 8SW
☎ 01674 672932 🖹 01674 671800
e-mail: secretary@montroselinks.co.uk
web: www.montroselinks.co.uk
The links at Montrose like many others in Scotland are on commonland and are shared by three clubs. The Medal Course at Montrose - the fifth oldest in the world - is typical of Scottish links, with narrow, undulating fairways and problems from the first hole to the last. The Broomfield course is flatter and easier.

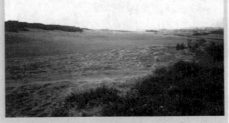

Medal Course: 18 holes, 6544yds, Par 71, SSS 72, Course record 63.

Broomfield Course: 18 holes, 4830yds, Par 66, SSS 63.
Club membership 1300.
Visitors Mon-Sun & BHs. Booking required Sat & Sun. Handicap certificate. Dress code. Must contact in advance. **Societies** Booking required. **Green Fees** Medal: £57 per day; £45 per round (£65/£50 Sat & Sun). Broomfield: £18 per round (£20 weekends). **Prof** Jason J Boyd **Course Designer** W Park/Tom Morris **Facilities** ⊕ ⊠ ⤢ ⧉ ▯ ⚐ ⚑ ⚙ **Location** NE side of town off A92

See advert on opposite page

ARGYLL & BUTE

CARDROSS

MAP 10 NS37

Cardross Main Rd G82 5LB
☎ 01389 841754 🖹 01389 842162
e-mail: golf@cardross.com
web: www.cardross.com
Undulating, testing parkland course with good views.
18 holes, 6469yds, Par 71, SSS 72, Course record 64.
Club membership 800.
Visitors Mon-Fri except BHs. Booking required. Handicap certificate. Dress code. **Societies** Booking required. **Green Fees** £50 per day., £35 per round. **Prof** Robert Farrell **Course Designer** James Braid **Facilities** ⊕ ⊠ by prior arrangement ⤢ ▯ ⧉ ⚐ ⧉ ⚙ ⌀ **Conf** Corporate Hospitality Days **Location** In village centre on A814
Hotel ★★★★★ 81% HL De Vere Cameron House, BALLOCH ☎ 01389 755565   96 en suite

---

CARRADALE

MAP 10 NR83

Carradale The Arch PA28 6QT
☎ 01583 431321
Pleasant seaside course built on a promontory overlooking the Isle of Arran. Natural terrain and small greens are the most difficult natural hazards. Described as the most sporting nine-hole course in Scotland. Testing 7th hole (240yds), Par 3.
9 holes, 2358yds, Par 65, SSS 64, Course record 62.
Club membership 246.
Visitors Mon-Sun & BHs. **Societies** booking required. **Green Fees** not confirmed. ⊛ **Facilities** ⤢ ⚐ ⌀ **Location** S side of village, on B842

DALMALLY

MAP 10 NN12

Dalmally Old Saw Mill PA33 1AE
☎ 01866 822708
e-mail: golfclub@lock-awe.com
A nine-hole flat parkland course bounded by the River Orchy and surrounded by mountains. Many water hazards and bunkers.
9 holes, 2257yds, Par 64, SSS 63, Course record 64.
Club membership 130.
Visitors Mon-Fri & BHs. **Societies** welcome. **Green Fees** not confirmed. ⊛ **Course Designer** MacFarlane Barrow Co **Facilities** ⤢ ⚐ ⌀ **Location** On A85, 1.5m W of Dalmally
Hotel ★★★ 81% HL Loch Fyne Hotel & Leisure Club, INVERARAY ☎ 0870 950 6270   74 en suite

Scotland

DUNOON
MAP 10 NS17

Cowal Ardenslate Rd PA23 8LT
☎ 01369 705673 📠 01369 705673
e-mail: secretary@cowalgolfclub.com
web: www.cowalgolfclub.com

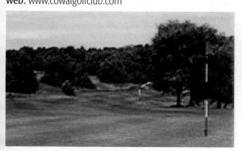

18 holes, 6063yds, Par 70, SSS 70, Course record 63.
Course Designer James Braid **Location** 1m N
Telephone for further details
Hotel ★★ 69% HL Selborne Hotel, Clyde St, West Bay, DUNOON
☎ 01369 702761 98 en suite

ERISKA
MAP 10 NM94

Isle of Eriska PA37 1SD
☎ 01631 720371 📠 01631 720531
e-mail: gc@eriska-hotel.co.uk
web: www.eriska-hotel.co.uk
This remote and most beautiful six-hole course, set around the owners'
hotel, is gradually being upgraded to a testing nine-hole challenge,
complete with stunning views. The signature 5th hole provides a 140yd
carry to a green on a hill surrounded by rocks and bunkers.
6 holes, 1588yds, Par 22. Club membership 40.
Visitors Mon-Sun & BHs. **Green Fees** £10 per day. **Course Designer** H
Swan **Facilities** ⊕ ⊡ ⊞⊓ ⊿ ⊶◇⊘ ⅀ **Leisure** hard tennis courts, heated
indoor swimming pool, sauna, gymnasium. **Location** A828 Connel-Fort
William, signed 4m N of Benderloch
Hotel ★★★★★ CHH Isle of Eriska, Eriska, Ledaig, BY OBAN
☎ 01631 720371 17 en suite

GIGHA ISLAND
MAP 10 NR64

Isle of Gigha PA41 7AA
☎ 01583 505242 📠 01583 505244
e-mail: golf@gigha.net
web: www.gigha.org
A nine-hole course with scenic views of the Sound of Gigha and
Kintyre. Ideal for the keen or occasional golfer.
9 holes, 5042yds, Par 66, SSS 65. Club membership 40.
Visitors Mon-Sun & BHs. **Societies** Booking Required **Green Fees** £10
per day. ⊛ **Course Designer** Members **Facilities** ⊿ ⊶ **Location** Near
ferry landing

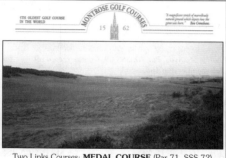

Two Links Courses: **MEDAL COURSE** (Par 71, SSS 72)
BROOMFIELD COURSE (Par 66, SSS 63)
MEDAL COURSE RANKED FIFTH OLDEST IN THE WORLD
OPEN CHAMPIONSHIP FINAL QUALIFYING COURSE –
1999 and 2007
Individual Round and Day Tickets Available on Both Courses
All Visitors and Parties Welcome – Group Discounts available
SPECIAL PACKAGES AVAILABLE INCLUDING
CATERING AND IN CONJUNCTION WITH LOCAL
HOTELS

Enquiries to: **Mrs M Stewart, Secretary,**
Montrose Golf Links Ltd, Traill Drive,
Montrose, Angus, DD10 8SW.
Tel:- (01674) 672932
Fax: (01674) 671800
E-mail: secretary@montroselinks.co.uk
Website: www.montroselinks.co.uk

HELENSBURGH
MAP 10 NS28

Helensburgh 25 East Abercromby St G84 9HZ
☎ 01436 674173 📠 01436 671170
e-mail: thesecretary@helensburghgolfclub.co.uk
web: www.helensburghgolfclub.co.uk
Testing moorland course with superb views of Loch Lomond and River
Clyde.
18 holes, 6104yds, Par 69, SSS 70, Course record 62.
Club membership 875.
Visitors Mon-Fri & BHs. Booking required. Handicap certificate. Dress code.
Societies Booking required. **Green Fees** £40 per day, £30 per round.
Prof Fraser Hall **Course Designer** Old Tom Morris **Facilities** ⊕ ⊺⊙⊺ ⅃ ⊡
⊺⊓ ⊿ ⊜ ⊶ ⊘ ⊞ ⊘ **Conf** Corporate Hospitality Days **Location** NE side
of town off B832
Hotel ★★★★★ 81% HL De Vere Cameron House, BALLOCH
☎ 01389 755565 96 en suite

INNELLAN
MAP 10 NS17

Innellan Knockamillie Rd PA23 7SG
☎ 01369 830242 & 702573
Situated above the village of Innellan, this undulating hilltop, parkland
course has extensive views of the Firth of Clyde.
9 holes, 4683yds, Par 64, SSS 64, Course record 63.
Club membership 199.
Visitors Mon-Sat & BHs. **Societies** Booking Required. **Green Fees** £13
per day. £10 per round. (£15 at Sat & Sun). ⊛ **Facilities** ⊵ ⊡ ⊺⊓ ⊶
Location 4m S of Dunoon
Hotel ★★ 79% HL Royal Marine Hotel, Hunters Quay, DUNOON
☎ 01369 705810 31 en suite 10 annexe en suite

INVERARAY — MAP 10 NN00

Inveraray North Cromalt PA32 8XT
☎ 01499 302116
Testing parkland course with beautiful views overlooking Loch Fyne.
9 holes, 5628yds, Par 70, SSS 69, Course record 69.
Club membership 160.
Visitors Mon-Sun & BHs. Booking required Sun. **Societies** Booking required. **Green Fees** £15 per day. ● **Facilities** ⚒ ⚐ **Location** 1m S of Inveraray
Hotel ★★★ 81% HL Loch Fyne Hotel & Leisure Club, INVERARAY
☎ 0870 950 6270 74 en suite

LOCHGILPHEAD — MAP 10 NR88

Lochgilphead Blarbuie Rd PA31 8LE
☎ 01546 602340 510383
9 holes, 2242yds, Par 64, SSS 63, Course record 58.
Course Designer Dr I McCamond **Location** Next to hospital, signed from village
Telephone for further details

MACHRIHANISH — MAP 10 NR62

Machrihanish PA28 6PT
☎ 01586 810213 📠 01586 810221
e-mail: secretary@machgolf.com
web: www.machgolf.com
Magnificent natural links of championship status. The 1st hole is the famous drive across the Atlantic. Sandy soil allows for play all year round. Large greens, easy walking, windy. Fishing.
18 holes, 6225yds, Par 70, SSS 71, Course record 63.
The Pans Course: 9 holes, 2376yds, Par 34, SSS 69.
Club membership 1400.
Visitors Mon-Sun & BHs. Booking Required Sat & Sun
Societies Booking required. **Green Fees** Mon-Fri & Sun £60 per day, £40 per round. (Sat £75£50). The Pans course £12 per day. **Prof** Ken Campbell **Course Designer** Tom Morris **Facilities** ⚒ ⛳ ▥ ⬜ ⛳⬛ ⚒ ⬛ ⚐ ⬛ ⚐ **Location** 5m W of Campbeltown on B843

OBAN — MAP 10 NM83

Glencruitten Glencruitten Rd PA34 4PU
☎ 01631 564604
e-mail: obangolf@btinternet.com
web: www.obangolf.com
There is plenty of space and considerable variety of hole on this downland course - popular with holidaymakers. In a beautiful, isolated situation, the course is hilly and testing, particularly the 1st and 12th (Par 4s) and 10th and 17th (Par 3s).
18 holes, 4452yds, Par 61, SSS 63, Course record 55.
Club membership 500.
Visitors Mon-Sun & BHs. Booking required Sat. Dress code.
Societies Welcome. **Green Fees** Mon-Fri £25 per day. (£30 Sat & Sun). **Course Designer** James Braid **Facilities** ⚒ ⛳ ▥ ⬜ ⛳⬛ ⚒ ⬛ ⚐ ⬛
Location NE side of town centre off A816
Hotel ★★★ 80% HL Manor House Hotel, Gallanach Rd, OBAN
☎ 01631 562087 11 en suite

SOUTHEND — MAP 10 NR60

Dunaverty PA28 6RW
☎ 01586 830677 📠 01586 830677
e-mail: dunavertygc@aol.com
web: www.dunavertygolfclub.com
Undulating, seaside course with spectacular views of Ireland and the Ayrshire coast.
18 holes, 4799yds, Par 66, SSS 63, Course record 58.
Club membership 400.
Visitors Mon-Sun & BHs. Dress code **Societies** Booking Required. **Green Fees** £28 per day, £20 per round (£24/£32 Sat & Sun). ● **Facilities** ⚐ ⛳ ▥ ⬜ ⚒ ⬛ ⚐ **Leisure** fishing. **Location** 10m S of Campbeltown on B842

TARBERT — MAP 10 NR86

Tarbert PA29 6XX
☎ 01546 606896
Hilly parkland with views over West Loch Tarbert.
9 holes, 4460yds, Par 66, SSS 63, Course record 62.
Club membership 90.
Visitors Mon-Sun & BHs. **Societies** Booking required. **Green Fees** £20 per day, £10 per round. ● **Location** N1m W on B8024

TIGHNABRUAICH — MAP 10 NR97

Kyles of Bute PA212AB
☎ 01700 811603
Moorland course which is hilly and exposed. Fine mountain and sea views. Heather, whin and burns provide heavy penalties for inaccuracy. Wild life abounds.
9 holes, 4778yds, Par 66, SSS 64, Course record 62.
Club membership 150.
Visitors Mon-Sat & BHs, Sun after 1:30pm. **Societies** Booking required. **Green Fees** £10 per day. ● **Facilities** ⚒ ⚐ ⚐ **Location** 1.25m S off B8000
Hotel ★★★ 85% SHL An Lochan, Shore Rd, TIGHNABRUAICH
☎ 01700 811239 11 en suite

CLACKMANNANSHIRE

ALLOA — MAP 11 NS89

Alloa Schawpark, Sauchie FK10 3AX
☎ 01259 724476 📠 01259 724476
e-mail: davieherd@btinternet.com
web: alloagolfpage.co.uk
Set in 150 acres of rolling parkland beneath the Ochil Hills, this course will challenge the best golfers while offering great enjoyment to the average player. The challenging finishing holes, 15th to 18th, consist of two long Par 3s split by two long and demanding Par 4s which will test any golfer's ability. Privacy provided by mature tree-lined fairways.
18 holes, 6229yds, Par 69, SSS 71, Course record 63.
Club membership 910.
Visitors Mon-Fri, Sun & BHs. Booking required. Dress code. **Societies** Booking required. **Green Fees** £38 per day, £28 per round (£34 Sun). **Prof** David Herd **Course Designer** James Braid **Facilities** ⚒ ⛳ ▥ ⬜ ⛳⬛ ⚒ ⬛ ⚐ **Conf** Corporate Hospitality Days **Location** 1.5m NE on A908

Braehead Cambus FK10 2NT
☎ 01259 725766 📠 01259 214070
e-mail: braehead.gc@btinternet.com
web: www.braeheadgolfclub.co.uk
Attractive parkland at the foot of the Ochil Hills, having spectacular views.
18 holes, 6053yds, Par 70, SSS 69, Course record 63.
Club membership 800.
Visitors Mon-Sun & BHs. Handicap certificate. Dress code. **Societies** Booking required. **Green Fees** £32 per day, £24 per round (£40/£32 weekends). **Prof** Jamie Stevenson **Course Designer** Robert Tait **Facilities** ⛳ 🍴 🛒 🏌 🅿 🏊 🏨 🥢 ✏ 🚗 ✏ **Conf** Corporate Hospitality Days
Location 1m W on A907

ALVA   MAP 11 NS89

Alva Beauclerc St FK12 5LD
☎ 01259 760431
e-mail: alva@alvagolfclub.wanadoo.com
web: www.alvagolfclub.com
9 holes, 2423yds, Par 66, SSS 64, Course record 63.
Location 7m from Stirling, A91 Stirling-St Andrews
Telephone for further details
Hotel ★★★ 75% HL Best Western Royal Hotel, Henderson St, BRIDGE OF ALLAN ☎ 01786 832284 32 en suite

---

DOLLAR   MAP 11 NS99

Dollar Brewlands House FK14 7EA
☎ 01259 742400 📠 01259 743497
e-mail: info@dollargolfclub.com
web: www.dollargolfclub.com
Compact hillside course with magnificent views along the Ochil Hills.
18 holes, 5242yds, Par 69, SSS 66, Course record 60.
Club membership 450.
Visitors Mon-Sun & BHs. Booking required. Dress code. **Societies** booking required. **Green Fees** not confirmed. ⛳ **Course Designer** Ben Sayers **Facilities** ⛳ 🍴 🛒 🏌 🏊 🥢 ✏ **Leisure** snooker table. **Conf** Corporate Hospitality Days **Location** 0.5m N off A91
Hotel ★★★ 75% HL Best Western Royal Hotel, Henderson St, BRIDGE OF ALLAN ☎ 01786 832284 32 en suite

---

MUCKHART   MAP 11 NO00

Muckhart FK14 7JH
☎ 01259 781423 & 781493 📠 01259 781544
e-mail: enquiries@muckhartgolf.com
web: www.muckhartgolf.com
Scenic heathland and downland course comprising 27 holes in three combinations of nine, all of which start and finish close to the clubhouse. Each of the nine holes requires a different approach, demanding tactical awareness and a skilful touch with all the clubs in the bag. There are superb views from the course's many vantage points, including the aptly named 5th 'Top of the World'.
Cowden: 9 holes, 3251yds, Par 36.
Naemoor Course: 9 holes, 3234yds, Par 35.
Arndean: 9 holes, 2835yds, Par 35. Club membership 750.
Visitors Mon-Sun & BHs. Booking required. Dress code **Societies** Booking Required. **Green Fees** Phone. **Prof** Keith Salmoni **Facilities** ⛳ 🍴 🛒 🏌 🏊 🥢 🚗 ✏ **Location** S of village between A91 & A911
Hotel ★★ 75% SHL Castle Campbell Hotel, 11 Bridge St, DOLLAR ☎ 01259 742519 9 en suite

---

TILLICOULTRY   MAP 11 NS99

Tillicoultry Alva Rd FK13 6BL
☎ 01259 750124 📠 01259 750124
e-mail: miket@tillygc.freeserve.co.uk
Parkland at foot of the Ochil Hills. Some hard walking but fine views.
9 holes, 5004metres, Par 68, SSS 67, Course record 64.
Club membership 400.
Visitors Mon-Sun & BHs. Booking required Sat & Sun. Dress code.
Societies Booking required. **Green Fees** £12 per 18 holes (£18 Sat, Sun & BHs). ⛳ **Facilities** ⛳ 🛒 🏌 🥢 🏊 **Conf** Corporate Hospitality Days
Location A91, 9m E of Stirling
Hotel ★★★ 75% HL Best Western Royal Hotel, Henderson St, BRIDGE OF ALLAN ☎ 01786 832284 32 en suite

---

DUMFRIES & GALLOWAY

CASTLE DOUGLAS   MAP 11 NX76

Castle Douglas Abercromby Rd DG7 1BA
☎ 01556 502801 & 502509 📠 01556 502509
e-mail: cdgolfclub@aol.com
2006 saw the layout of a new testing parkland course, featuring the region's longest Par 5, the 603yd 6th hole.
9 holes, 6254yds, Par 70, SSS 70, Course record 61.
Club membership 320.
Visitors may play Mon-Sun & BHs. **Societies** Booking required. **Green Fees** not confirmed. ⛳ **Facilities** ⛳ 🍴 🛒 🏌 🥢 🏊 **Leisure** pool table.
Conf Corporate Hospitality Days **Location** 0.5m from town centre on A713 Abercrombie road
Hotel ★★ 68% HL Imperial Hotel, 35 King St, CASTLE DOUGLAS ☎ 01556 502086 12 en suite

---

COLVEND   MAP 11 NX85

Colvend Sandyhills DG5 4PY
☎ 01556 630398 📠 01556 630495
e-mail: thesecretary@colvendgolfclub.co.uk
web: www.colvendgolfclub.co.uk
Picturesque and challenging course on the Solway coast. Superb views.
18 holes, 5250yds, Par 68, SSS 67, Course record 64.
Club membership 490.
Visitors Mon-Sun & BHs. **Societies** Welcome. **Green Fees** £30 per day, £25 per round. **Course Designer** Allis & Thomas **Facilities** ⛳ 🍴 🛒 🏌 🥢 🚗 🥢 ✏ **Location** 6m SE from Dalbeattie on A710
Hotel ★★★ 85% HL Balcary Bay Hotel, AUCHENCAIRN ☎ 01556 640217 & 640311 📠 01556 640272 20 en suite

---

CUMMERTREES   MAP 11 NY16

Powfoot DG12 5QE
☎ 01461 204100 📠 01461204111
e-mail: info@powfootgolfclub.com
web: www.powfootgolfclub.com
This British Championship course is on the Solway Firth, playing at this delightfully compact semi-links seaside course is a scenic treat. Lovely holes include the 2nd, the 8th and the 11th. The 9th includes a Second World War bomb crater.
18 holes, 6255yds, Par 69, SSS 69, Course record 63.
Club membership 660.

Continued

Scotland

Visitors Mon-Fri, Sun & BHs. Booking required. Handicap certificate. Dress code. **Societies** Booking required. **Green Fees** £46 per day, £35 per round (£57/£41 Sat & Sun). **Course Designer** J Braid **Facilities** ⑪ ⑩ ⓦ ⌷ ⑂ ⚘ 🛆 🏌 ✦ **Location** 0.5m off B724
Hotel ★★★ 73% HL Best Western Hetland Hall Hotel, CARRUTHERSTOWN ☎ 01387 840201 14 en suite 15 annexe en suite

DALBEATTIE   MAP 11 NX86

Dalbeattie 19 Maxwell Park DG5 4LR
☎ 01556 610666 📄 01556 612247
e-mail: ocm@associates-ltd.fsnet.co.uk
web: dalbeattiegc.co.uk
This nine-hole course provides an excellent challenge for golfers of all abilities. There are a few gentle slopes to negotiate but compensated by fine views along the Urr Valley. The 363yd 4th hole is a memorable Par 4, with views across to the Lake District.
9 holes, 5710yds, Par 68, SSS 68. Club membership 250.
Visitors Mon-Sun & BHs. Dress code. **Societies** booking required. **Green Fees** not confirmed. ⚘ **Course Designer** Bryan C Moor **Facilities** 🍴 🛆 ✦ 🚶 **Location** Signed off B794. Access by Maxwell Park
Hotel ★★ 68% HL Imperial Hotel, 35 King St, CASTLE DOUGLAS ☎ 01556 502086 12 en suite

DUMFRIES   MAP 11 NX97

Dumfries & County Nunfield, Edinburgh Rd DG1 1JX
☎ 01387 253585 📄 01387 253585
e-mail: dumfriesc@aol.com
web: thecounty.org.uk
Parkland alongside the River Nith, with views of the Queensberry Hills. Greens built to USPGA specifications. Nature trails link the fairways.

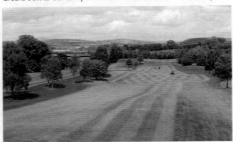

Nunfield: 18 holes, 5918yds, Par 69, SSS 69, Course record 61. Club membership 800.
Visitors Mon-Fri, Sun & BHs. Booking required. Dress code. **Societies** Booking required **Green Fees** £40 per day, £35 per 27 holes, £30 per round (£45/£40/£35 Sun & BHs). **Prof** Stuart Syme **Course Designer** William Fernie **Facilities** ⑪ ⑩ ⓦ ⌷ ⑂ 🛆 ⚘ ✦ 🚶 **Conf** Corporate Hospitality Days **Location** 1m NE of Dumfries on A701
Hotel ★★★ 75% HL Cairndale Hotel & Leisure Club, English St, DUMFRIES ☎ 01387 254111 91 en suite

Dumfries & Galloway 2 Laurieston Av DG2 7NY
☎ 01387 263848 📄 01387 263848
e-mail: info@dandggolfclub.co.uk
web: www.dandggolfclub.co.uk
Attractive parkland course, a good test of golf but not physically demanding.

18 holes, 6309yds, Par 70, SSS 71. Club membership 800.
Visitors Mon-Fri. Booking required. Handicap certificate. Dress code. **Societies** Booking required. **Green Fees** £38 per day, £30 per round (£45/£35 Sat & Sun). ⚘ **Prof** Joe Fergusson **Course Designer** W Fernie **Facilities** ⑪ ⑩ ⓦ ⌷ ⑂ 🛆 ⚘ ✦ 🚶 ✦ **Location** W of town centre on A780
Hotel ★★★ 79% HL Best Western Station Hotel, 49 Lovers Walk, DUMFRIES ☎ 01387 254316 32 en suite

Pines Golf Centre Lockerbie Rd DG1 3PF
☎ 01387 247444 📄 01387 249600
e-mail: admin@pinesgolf.com
web: www.pinesgolf.com
A mixture of parkland and woodland with numerous water features and dog-legs. Excellent greens.
18 holes, 5604yds, Par 68, SSS 68, Course record 66. Club membership 280.
Visitors Mon-Sun & BHs. **Societies** booking required. **Green Fees** not confirmed. ⚘ **Prof** Brian Gemmell/Bruce Gray **Course Designer** Duncan Gray **Facilities** ⑪ ⑩ ⓦ ⌷ ⑂ 🛆 ⚘ ✦ 🚶 ✦ **Conf** Corporate Hospitality Days **Location** Just off A701 Lockerbie Road, beside A75 Dumfries bypass
Hotel ★★★ 75% HL Cairndale Hotel & Leisure Club, English St, DUMFRIES ☎ 01387 254111 91 en suite

GATEHOUSE OF FLEET   MAP 11 NX55

Gatehouse Laurieston Rd DG7 2BE
☎ 01644 450260 📄 01644 450260
e-mail: gatehousegolf@sagainternet.co.uk
Set against a background of rolling hills with scenic views of Fleet Bay and the Solway Firth.
9 holes, 2521yds, Par 66, SSS 66, Course record 62. Club membership 300.
Visitors Mon-Sun & BHs. Booking required Sun. Dress code. **Societies** Booking required. **Green Fees** £15 per round. ⚘ **Course Designer** Tom Fernie **Facilities** 🛆 **Location** 0.25m N of town
Hotel ★★★★ 79% HL Cally Palace Hotel, GATEHOUSE OF FLEET ☎ 01557 814341 55 en suite

GLENLUCE   MAP 10 NX15

Wigtownshire County Mains of Park DG8 0NN
☎ 01581 300420 📄 01581 300420
e-mail: enquiries@wigtownshirecountygolfclub.com
web: www.wigtownshirecountygolfclub.com
Seaside links course on the shores of Luce Bay, easy walking but affected by winds. The 12th hole, a dog-leg with out of bounds to the right, is named after the course's designer, Gordon Cunningham.
18 holes, 5977yds, Par 70, SSS 69, Course record 63. Club membership 450.
Visitors Mon-Sun & BHs. Dress code. **Societies** Booking required. **Green Fees** £32 per day, £25 per round (£34/£27 Sat & Sun). **Course Designer** W Gordon Cunningham **Facilities** ⑪ ⑩ ⓦ ⌷ ⑂ 🛆 ⚘ ✦ 🚶 ✦ **Conf** Corporate Hospitality Days **Location** 1.5m W off A75, 200yds off A75 on shores of Luce Bay
Hotel ★★★★ 76% HL North West Castle Hotel, STRANRAER ☎ 01776 704413 70 en suite 2 annexe en suite

GRETNA
MAP 11 NY36

Gretna Kirtle View DG16 5HD
☎ 01461 338464 📄 01461 337362
9 holes, 3214yds, Par 72, SSS 71, Course record 71.
Course Designer N Williams **Location** 0.5m W of Gretna on B721, signed
Telephone for further details
Hotel ★★★ 74% HL Garden House Hotel, Sarkfoot Rd, GRETNA
☎ 01461 337621 38 en suite

KIRKCUDBRIGHT
MAP 11 NX65

Brighouse Bay Brighouse Bay, Borgue DG6 4TS
☎ 01557 870409 📄 01557 870409
e-mail: leisureclub@brighouse-bay.co.uk
web: www.gillespie-leisure.co.uk
18 holes, 6366yds, Par 73, SSS 73.
Course Designer D Gray **Location** 3m S of Borgue off B727
Telephone for further details
Hotel ★★ 67% HL Arden House Hotel, Tongland Rd, KIRKCUDBRIGHT
☎ 01557 330544 9 rms (8 en suite)

Kirkcudbright Stirling Crescent DG6 4EZ
☎ 01557 330314 📄 01557 330314
e-mail: david@kirkcudbrightgolf.co.uk
web: kirkcudbrightgolf.co.uk
Hilly parkland with good views over the harbour town of Kirkcudbright
and the Dee estuary.
18 holes, 5739yds, Par 69, SSS 69, Course record 63.
Club membership 500.
Visitors Mon-Sun & BHs. Booking required. Handicap certificate. Dress
code. **Societies** booking required. **Green Fees** not confirmed. ☺ **Course
Designer** E. Shamash **Facilities** ⓘ ⌾ ⓘ ⓛ ☐ ⓘ ⚒ ⚑ ⚔ ⛳ ⚑ **Location**
NE side of town off A711
Hotel ★★ 67% HL Arden House Hotel, Tongland Rd, KIRKCUDBRIGHT
☎ 01557 330544 9 rms (8 en suite)

LANGHOLM
MAP 11 NY38

Langholm Whiteside DG13 0JR
☎ 07724 875151
e-mail: golf@langholmgolfclub.co.uk
web: www.langholmgolfclub.co.uk
Hillside course with fine views, easy to medium walking.
9 holes, 6180yds, Par 70, SSS 69, Course record 65.
Club membership 200.
Visitors contact club for details. Dress code. **Societies** booking required.
Green Fees not confirmed. ☺ **Facilities** ⓘ by prior arrangement ⌾
by prior arrangement ⓛ by prior arrangement ⓘ ⚒ **Location** E side of
village off A7

LOCHMABEN
MAP 11 NY08

Lochmaben Castlehillgate DG11 1NT
☎ 01387 810552
e-mail: lgc@naims.co.uk
web: www.lochmabengolf.co.uk
Attractive parkland surrounding Kirk Loch. Excellent views from this
well-maintained course.
18 holes, 5890yds, Par 70, SSS 69, Course record 60.
Club membership 850.

Visitors Mon- Sun & BHs. Booking required. Handicap certificate. Dress
code. **Societies** welcome. **Green Fees** not confirmed. ☺ **Course
Designer** James Braid **Facilities** ⓘ ⌾ ⓘ ⓛ ☐ ⓘ ⚒ ⚑ ⚔ **Leisure** fishing.
Conf Corporate Hospitality Days **Location** 4m from Lockerbie on A74. S
side of village off A709
Hotel ★★★ 79% HL The Dryfesdale Country House Hotel, Dryfebridge,
LOCKERBIE ☎ 01576 202427 16 en suite

LOCKERBIE
MAP 11 NY18

Lockerbie Corrie Rd DG11 2ND
☎ 01576 203363 📄 01576 203363
e-mail: enquiries@lockerbiegolf.com
web: www.lockerbiegolf.com
Parkland course with fine views and featuring the only pond hole in
Dumfriesshire. Pond comes into play at 3 holes.
18 holes, 5614yds, Par 68, SSS 67, Course record 64.
Club membership 620.
Visitors Mon-Sun & BHs. Dress code. **Societies** Booking required. **Green
Fees** £26 per 18 holes (£28 weekends). ☺ **Course Designer** James Braid
Facilities ⓘ ⓛ ☐ ⓘ ⚒ ⚑ ⚔ ⛳ ⚑ **Conf** Corporate Hospitality Days
Location E side of town centre off B7068
Hotel ★★★ 79% HL The Dryfesdale Country House Hotel, Dryfebridge,
LOCKERBIE ☎ 01576 202427 16 en suite

MOFFAT
MAP 11 NT00

Moffat Coatshill DG10 9SB
☎ 01683 220020
e-mail: bookings@moffatgolfclub.co.uk
web: www.moffatgolfclub.co.uk
Scenic moorland course overlooking the town, with panoramic views
of southern uplands.
18 holes, 5259yds, Par 69, SSS 67, Course record 60.
Club membership 350.
Visitors Mon-Sun & BHs. Dress code. **Societies** Booking required. **Green
Fees** £28 per day, £22 per round (£36/£30 weekends and bank holidays).
Course Designer Ben Sayers **Facilities** ⓘ ⌾ ⓘ ⓛ ☐ ⓘ ⚒ ⚑ ⚔ ⛳ ⚔
Leisure snooker. **Conf** Corporate Hospitality Days **Location** From A74(M)
junct 15, take A701 to Moffat, course signposted on left after 30mph limit
sign
Hotel ★★★ 71% HL Best Western Moffat House Hotel, High St, MOFFAT
☎ 01683 220039 20 en suite

MONREITH
MAP 10 NX34

St Medan DG8 8NJ
☎ 01988 700358
Scotland's most southerly course. This links nestles in Monreith Bay
with panoramic views across to the Isle of Man. The testing nine-hole
course is a challenge to both high and low handicaps.
9 holes, 4520yds, Par 64, SSS 64, Course record 60.
Club membership 300.
Visitors Mon-Sun & BHs. Booking required Wed pm, Fri & Sun.
Societies Booking welcome. **Green Fees** £24 per day, £15 per 18 holes,
£10 per 9 holes. ☺ **Course Designer** James Braid **Facilities** ⓛ ☐ ⓘ ⚒
⚑ ⚔ **Location** 3m S of Port William off A747

NEW GALLOWAY — MAP 11 NX67

New Galloway High St DG7 3RN
☎ 01644 420737 & 450685 📠 01644 450685
web: www.nggc.com
Set on the edge of the Galloway Hills and overlooking Loch Ken, the course has excellent tees, no bunkers and first class greens. The course rises through the first two fairways to a plateau with all round views that many think unsurpassed.
9 holes, 5006yds, Par 68, SSS 67, Course record 64.
Club membership 250.
Visitors Mon-Sun & BHs. Booking required. **Societies** Booking required.
Green Fees £18 per day. 🅿 **Course Designer** James Braid **Facilities** ⌷
🍴 ⚌ ⚑ ☎ ♂ **Conf** Corporate Hospitality Days **Location** S side of town on A762
Hotel ★★ 68% HL Imperial Hotel, 35 King St, CASTLE DOUGLAS
☎ 01556 502086 12 en suite

NEWTON STEWART — MAP 10 NX46

Newton Stewart Kirroughtree Av, Minnigaff DG8 6PF
☎ 01671 402172 📠 01671 402172
e-mail: newtonstewartgc@btconnect.com
web: www.newtonstewartgolfclub.com
A parkland course in a picturesque setting. A good test for all standards of golfer with a variety of shots required. Many mature trees on the course and the five short holes have interesting features.
18 holes, 5903yds, Par 69, SSS 70, Course record 66.
Club membership 380.
Visitors Mon-Sun & BHs. Dress code. **Societies** Booking required.
Green Fees £27 per round (£31 Sat & Sat). 🅿 **Facilities** ⌷🍴 ⚌ ⌷🍴
⚌ ⚑ ☎ ♂ **Location** 0.5m N of town centre off A75
Hotel ★★★ HL Kirroughtree House, Minnigaff, NEWTON STEWART
☎ 01671 402141 17 en suite

PORTPATRICK — MAP 10 NX05

Lagganmore Hotel DG9 9AB
☎ 01776 810499
e-mail: lagganmoregolf@aol.com
web: www.lagganmoregolf.co.uk
Parkland and heath course with many water features. The signature hole is the 7th, considered the best in the county.
18 holes, 5698yds, Par 69, SSS 68, Course record 66.
Club membership 50.
Visitors Mon-Sun & BHs. Booking required Sat. **Societies** booking required.
Green Fees not confirmed. **Course Designer** Stephen Hornby
Facilities ⌷🍴 ⚌ ⌷🍴 ⚑ ♂ ☎ ♂ ♪ **Conf** facs Corporate
Hospitality Days **Location** on A77
Hotel ★★★ 80% HL Fernhill Hotel, Heugh Rd, PORTPATRICK
☎ 01776 810220 27 en suite 9 annexe en suite

Portpatrick Golf Course Rd DG9 8TB
☎ 01776 810273 📠 01776 810811
e-mail: enquiries@portpatrickgolfclub.com
web: www.portpatrickgolfclub.com
Seaside links-type course, set on cliffs overlooking the Irish Sea, with magnificent views.
Dunskey Course: 18 holes, 5913yds, Par 70, SSS 69, Course record 63.
Dinvin Course: 9 holes, 1504yds, Par 27, SSS 27, Course record 23. Club membership 750.

Visitors Mon-Sun & BHs. Booking required. Handicap certificate. Dress code. **Societies** Booking required. **Green Fees** £42.50 per day, £32 per round (£48.50/£37.50 Sat & Sun). **Prof** Haldane Lee
Course Designer Charles Hunter **Facilities** ⌷🍴 ⚌ ⌷🍴 ⚌ ☎ ♂ ♪
♂ **Location** Entering village fork right at war memorial, signed 300yds
Hotel ★★★ 80% HL Fernhill Hotel, Heugh Rd, PORTPATRICK
☎ 01776 810220 27 en suite 9 annexe en suite

SANQUHAR — MAP 11 NS70

Sanquhar Euchan Golf Course, Blackaddie Rd DG4 6JZ
☎ 01659 50577
e-mail: tich@rossirence.fsnet.co.uk
Easy walking parkland, fine views. A good test for all standards of golfer.
9 holes, 5594yds, Par 70, SSS 68, Course record 66.
Club membership 200.
Visitors Mon-Sun & BHs. Dress code. **Societies** Welcome.
Green Fees £10 per day (£12 weekends). 🅿 **Course Designer** Willie Fernie **Facilities** ⌷ by prior arrangement 🍴 by prior arrangement ⚌ by prior arrangement ⌷ by prior arrangement ⚌ **Leisure** snooker, pool.
Conf Corporate Hospitality Days **Location** 0.5m SW off A76

SOUTHERNESS — MAP 11 NX95

Solway Links KIrkbean DG2 8BE
☎ 01387 880323 & 880623 📠 01387 880555
e-mail: info@solwaygolf.co.uk
web: www.solwaygolf.co.uk
Solway Links is an 18 hole pay and play links golf course in a stunning coastal location near Southerness holiday village and beaches. The golf course overlooks the Solway Firth with spectacular views of the surrounding countryside and across the sea to the Lake District. Built on an ancient raised beach with excellent, well drained, undulating fairways.
18 holes, 5005yds, Par 67.
Visitors Mon-Sun & BHs. **Societies** Booking required. **Green Fees** £16 per day/round, £11 per 9 holes. 🅿 **Course Designer** Gordon Gray **Facilities**
⌷ ⚑ ♂ ☎ ♂ **Leisure** clay pigeon shooting. **Location** On A710 Dumfries to Dalbeattie road.
Hotel ★★ 85% CHH Cavens, KIRKBEAN ☎ 01387 880234 6 en suite

Southerness DG2 8AZ
☎ 01387 880677 📠 01387 880644
e-mail: admin@southernessgc.sol.co.uk
web: www.southernessgolfclub.com
Natural links, championship course with panoramic views. Heather and bracken abound.
18 holes, 6105yds, Par 69, SSS 70, Course record 64.
Club membership 830.
Visitors Mon-Sun & BHs. Booking required. Handicap certificate. Dress code. **Societies** Booking required. **Green Fees** £60 per day; £45 per round (£70/£55 weekends). **Course Designer** McKenzie Ross **Facilities** ⌷ 🍴
⌷🍴 ⚌ ♂ **Location** 3.5m S of Kirkbean off A710
Hotel ★★ 85% CHH Cavens, KIRKBEAN ☎ 01387 880234 6 en suite

STRANRAER

MAP 10 NX06

Stranraer Creachmore DG9 0LF
☎ 01776 870245 📋 01776 870445
e-mail: stranraergolf@btclick.com
web: www.stranraergolfclub.net
Parkland with beautiful views over Loch Ryan to Ailsa Craig, Arran and beyond. Several notable holes including the 3rd, where a winding burn is crossed three times to a green set between a large bunker and a steep bank sloping down to the burn; the scenic 5th with spectacular views; the 11th requiring a demanding tee shot with trees and out of bounds to the left, then a steep rise to a very fast green. The 15th is a difficult Par 3 where accuracy is paramount with ground sloping away either side of the green.
18 holes, 6308yds, Par 70, SSS 72, Course record 66.
Club membership 700.
Visitors may play Mon-Sun & BHs. Dress code **Societies** welcome.
Green Fees £28 per 18 holes (£33 weekends). **Course Designer** James Braid **Facilities** ⑪ ⑩ ▦ ⬜ ⬛ ⬜ ⬜ ⬜ ⬜ **Location** 2.5m NW on A718 from Stranraer
Hotel ★★★★ 76% HL North West Castle Hotel, STRANRAER
☎ 01776 704413 70 en suite 2 annexe en suite

THORNHILL

MAP 11 NX89

Thornhill Blacknest DG3 5DW
☎ 01848 331779 & 330546
e-mail: info@thornhillgolfclub.co.uk
web: www.thornhillgolfclub.co.uk
Moorland and parkland with fine views of the southern uplands.
18 holes, 6085yds, Par 71, SSS 70, Course record 67.
Club membership 560.
Visitors Mon-Sun & BHs. Booking required. Dress code. **Societies** Booking required. **Green Fees** £40 per day, £30 per round (£45/£35 Sat & Sun).
⬤ **Course Designer** Willie Fernie **Facilities** ⑪ ⑩ ▦ ⬜ ⬛ ⬜ ⬜ ⬜
Location 1m E of town off A76

WIGTOWN

MAP 10 NX45

Wigtown & Bladnoch Lightlands Ter DG8 9DY
☎ 01988 403354
Slightly hilly parkland with fine views over Wigtown Bay to the Galloway Hills.
9 holes, 5462yds, Par 68, SSS 67, Course record 62.
Club membership 150.
Visitors Mon-Sun & BHs. Booking required Sat-Sun. **Societies** booking required. **Green Fees** not confirmed. ⬤ **Course Designer** W Muir
Facilities ⬜ ⬛ ⬜ ⬜ **Location** SW on A714
Hotel ★★★ HL Kirroughtree House, Minnigaff, NEWTON STEWART
☎ 01671 402141 17 en suite

CITY OF DUNDEE

DUNDEE

MAP 11 NO43

Ballumbie Castle 2 Old Quarry Rd DD4 0SY
☎ 01382 730026 (club) & 770028 (pro) 📋 01382 730008
e-mail: ballumbie2000@yahoo.com
web: www.ballumbiecastlegolfclub.com
Parkland/heathland course built in 2000. No two holes go in the same direction and every golf club is required. Water comes into play on 4 holes.
18 holes, 6127yds, Par 69, SSS 70, Course record 65.
Club membership 550.
Visitors Mon-Sun & BHs. Booking required. Dress code. **Societies** booking required. **Green Fees** not confirmed. **Prof** Lee Sutherland **Facilities** ⑪ ⑩ ▦ ⬜ ⬛ ⬜ ⬜ ⬜ ⬜ **Conf** Corporate Hospitality Days **Location** NE outskirts of town, signed off A90
Hotel BUD Premier Travel Inn Dundee East, 115-117 Lawers Dr, Panmurefield Village, BROUGHTY FERRY ☎ 0870 9906324 60 en suite

Caird Park Mains Loan DD4 9BX
☎ 01382 438871 📋 01382 433211
e-mail: la.bookings@dundeecity.gov.uk
web: www.dundeecity.gov.uk/golf
A pay and play course situated in extensive parkland in the heart of Carnoustie countryside. A reasonably easy start belies the difficulty of the middle section (holes 7-13) and the back nine cross the Gelly Burn four times.
18 holes, 6280yds, Par 72, SSS 69, Course record 65.
Club membership 1800.
Visitors Mon-Sun & BHs. Booking required Sat-Sun. Dress code.
Societies booking required. **Green Fees** not confirmed. ⬤ **Prof** J Black
Facilities ⬜ ⬛ ⬜ ⬜ ⬜ ⬜ **Leisure** sports stadium.
Location Off A90 Kingsway onto Forfar Rd, left onto Claverhouse Rd, 1st left into Caird Park
Hotel ★★★★ 81% HL Apex City Quay Hotel & Spa, 1 West Victoria Dock Rd, DUNDEE ☎ 01382 202404 & 0845 365 0000 📋 01382 201401 153 en suite

Camperdown Camperdown Park, Coupar Angus Rd DD2 4TF
☎ 01382 431820 📋 01382 433486
web: www.dundeecity.gov.uk/~golf
18 holes, 6548yds, Par 71, SSS 72.
Location A90 Kingsway onto A923 CouPar Angus Rd into Camperdown Park
Telephone for further details

Downfield Turnberry Av DD2 3QP
☎ 01382 825595 📋 01382 813111
e-mail: downfieldgc@aol.com
web: www.downfieldgolf.co.uk
A 2007 Open Qualifying venue. A course with championship credentials providing an enjoyable test for all golfers.
18 holes, 6803yds, Par 73, SSS 73, Course record 65.
Club membership 750.
Visitors Mon-Fri, Sun & BHs. Booking required. Dress code. **Societies** Booking required. **Green Fees** £59 per day, £49 per round. **Prof** Kenny Hutton **Course Designer** James Braid **Facilities** ⑪ ⑩ ▦ ⬜ ⬛ ⬜ ⬜ ⬜ ⬜ ⬜ ⬜ **Leisure** snooker room. **Conf** Corporate Hospitality Days **Location** N of city centre, signed at junct A90

Scotland

Scotland

EAST AYRSHIRE

GALSTON
MAP 11 NS53

Loudoun Edinburgh Rd KA4 8PA
☎ 01563 821993 📠 01563 820011
e-mail: secy@loudoungowfclub.co.uk
web: www.loudoungowfclub.co.uk
Pleasant, fairly flat parkland with many mature trees, in the Irvine valley. Excellent test of golf skills without being too strenuous.
18 holes, 6005yds, Par 68, SSS 69, Course record 60.
Club membership 850.
Visitors Mon-Fri. Booking required. Dress code **Societies** Booking required. **Green Fees** £35 per day, £25 per 18 holes. **Facilities** ⑪ ⑩ ⑤ 💺 🚻 ⚞
🏌 🍴 ♂ **Conf** Corporate Hospitality Days **Location** NE side of town on A71
Hotel ★★★ 79% HL Best Western Strathaven Hotel, Hamilton Rd, STRATHAVEN ☎ 01357 521778 22 en suite

KILMARNOCK
MAP 10 NS43

Annanhill Irvine Rd KA1 2RT
☎ 01563 521644 & 521512 (Starter)
Municipal, tree-lined parkland course.
18 holes, 6269yds, Par 71, SSS 70, Course record 66.
Club membership 274.
Visitors Mon-Sun & BHs. Booking required. Dress code. **Societies** Booking required. **Green Fees** Phone. 🎁 **Course Designer** Jack McLean
Facilities 💺 🚻 **Location** 1m N on B7081
Hotel BUD Premier Travel Inn Kilmarnock, Annadale, KILMARNOCK
☎ 08701 977148 40 en suite

Caprington Ayr Rd KA1 4UW
☎ 01563 523702 & 521915 (Gen Enq)
18 holes, 5810yds, Par 68, SSS 68.
Location 1.5m S on B7038
Telephone for further details
Hotel BUD Travelodge Kilmarnock, Kilmarnock By Pass, KILMARNOCK
☎ 08700 850 950 40 en suite

MAUCHLINE
MAP 11 NS42

Ballochmyle Catrine Rd KA5 6LE
☎ 01290 550469 📠 01290 553657
e-mail: secretary@ballochmylegolf.wanadoo.co.uk
Parkland course.
18 holes, 5972yds, Par 70, SSS 69, Course record 64.
Club membership 730.
Visitors Mon-Fri & Sun except BHs. Dress code. **Societies** Booking required. **Green Fees** £32.50 36 holes, £22.50 18 holes (£37.50/£27.50).
Facilities ⑪ ⑩ ⑤ 💺 🚻 ⚞ 🏌 🍴 ♂ **Leisure** snooker. **Location** 1m SE on B705
Hotel BUD Travelodge Kilmarnock, Kilmarnock By Pass, KILMARNOCK
☎ 08700 850 950 40 en suite

NEW CUMNOCK
MAP 11 NS61

New Cumnock Lochhill, Cumnock Rd KA18 4PN
☎ 01290 338848
9 holes, 5176yds, Par 68, SSS 68, Course record 63.
Course Designer Willie Fernie **Location** 0.75m N on A76
Telephone for further details

PATNA
MAP 10 NS41

Doon Valley Hillside Park KA6 7JT
☎ 01292 531607
Established parkland course located on an undulating hillside.
9 holes, 5886yds, Par 70, SSS 70, Course record 56.
Club membership 100.
Visitors Mon-Sun & BHs. Booking required. Dress code. **Societies** Booking required. **Green Fees** £14 per 18 holes. 🎁 **Facilities** 🚻 ⚞ **Leisure** fishing, fitness and games hall nearby. **Location** 10m S of Ayr on the A713
Hotel ★★ HL Ladyburn, MAYBOLE ☎ 01655 740585 5 en suite

EAST DUNBARTONSHIRE

BALMORE
MAP 11 NS57

Balmore Golf Course Rd G64 4AW
☎ 01360 620284 📠 01360 622742
e-mail: balmoregolf@btconnect.com
web: www.balmoregolfclub.co.uk
Parkland with fine views. Greens to USGA standards.
18 holes, 5530yds, Par 66, SSS 67, Course record 61.
Club membership 700.
Visitors Mon-Fri except BHs. Handicap certificate. Dress code. **Societies** Booking required. **Green Fees** £40 per day; £30 per round. **Prof** Paul Morrison **Course Designer** Harry Vardon **Facilities** ⑪ ⑩ ⑤ 💺 🚻 ⚞ 🏌 🍴 ♂ **Location** N off A807
Hotel BUD Premier Travel Inn Glasgow (Bearsden), Milngavie Rd, BEARSDEN ☎ 0870 9906532 61 en suite

BEARSDEN
MAP 11 NS57

Bearsden Thorn Rd G61 4BP
☎ 0141 586 5300
e-mail: secretary@bearsdengolfclub.com
web: www.bearsdengolfclub.com
Parkland course with 16 greens and 11 teeing grounds. Easy walking and views of city and the Campsie Hills.
9 holes, 6014yds, Par 68, SSS 69, Course record 64.
Club membership 560.
Visitors Mon-Sun. Booking required. Handicap certificate. Dress code. **Societies** booking required. **Green Fees** not confirmed. 🎁 **Facilities** ⑪ ⑩ 💺 🚻 ⚞ **Location** 1m W off A809
Hotel BUD Premier Travel Inn Glasgow (Bearsden), Milngavie Rd, BEARSDEN ☎ 0870 9906532 61 en suite

Douglas Park Hillfoot G61 2TJ
☎ 0141 942 2220 (Clubhouse) 📠 0141 942 0985
e-mail: secretary@douglasparkgolfclub.co.uk
web: www.douglasparkgolfclub.co.uk
Undulating parkland course with a variety of holes.
18 holes, 5962yds, Par 69, SSS 69, Course record 64.
Club membership 960.

Continued

Visitors Mon-Sun & BHs. Booking required. Dress Code. **Societies** Booking
required. **Green Fees** £35 per day; £25 per round (£30 Sat, Sun & BHs). ☻
Prof David Scott **Course Designer** Willie Fernie **Facilities** ⊕ ⫶◐⫶ ⓛ ⊡ 🕱
⟰ 🖃 ⬥ ⚋ **Location** E side of town on A81
Hotel BUD Premier Travel Inn Glasgow (Bearsden), Milngavie Rd,
BEARSDEN ☎ 0870 9906532 61 en suite

Glasgow Killermont G61 2TW
☎ 0141 942 2011 🖹 0141 942 0770
e-mail: secretary@glasgow-golf.com
web: www.glasgowgolfclub.com
One of the finest parkland courses in Scotland.
Killermont: 18 holes, 5977yds, Par 70, SSS 69,
Course record 64. Club membership 800.
Visitors Mon-Fri. Booking required. Handicap certificate. Dress code.
Societies Booking required. **Green Fees** £70 per day, £55 per round.
Prof J Steven **Course Designer** Tom Morris Snr **Facilities** ⊕ ⫶◐⫶ ⓛ ⊡
🕱 ⟰ 🖃🗭 ⬥ ⚋ **Conf** Corporate Hospitality Days **Location** SE side
off A81

Windyhill Baljaffray Rd G61 4QQ
☎ 0141 942 2349 🖹 0141 942 5874
e-mail: secretary@windyhill.co.uk
web: www.windyhillgolfclub.co.uk
Interesting parkland and moorland course with panoramic views of
Glasgow and beyond; testing 12th hole.
18 holes, 6254yds, Par 71, SSS 70, Course record 64.
Club membership 800.
Visitors Mon-Fri. Booking required. Handicap certificate. Dress code.
Societies Booking required. **Green Fees** £25 per round/£35 per day.
Prof Chris Duffy **Course Designer** James Braid **Facilities** ⊕ ⫶◐⫶ ⓛ ⊡🕱
⟰ 🖃🗭 ⬥ **Location** 2m NW off B8050, 1.5m from Bearsden cross, just
off Drymen road
Hotel BUD Premier Travel Inn Glasgow (Bearsden), Milngavie Rd,
BEARSDEN ☎ 0870 9906532 61 en suite

BISHOPBRIGGS   MAP 11 NS67
Bishopbriggs Brackenbrae Rd G64 2DX
☎ 0141 772 1810 & 772 8938 🖹 762 2532
e-mail: secretarybgc@yahoo.co.uk
web: www.bishopbriggsgolfclub.com
18 holes, 6041yds, Par 69, SSS 69, Course record 63.
Course Designer James Braid **Location** 0.5m NW off A803
Telephone for further details
Hotel ★★★★ 76% HL Glasgow Marriott Hotel, 500 Argyle St, Anderston,
GLASGOW ☎ 0870 400 7230 300 en suite

Cawder Cadder Rd G64 3QD
☎ 0141 761 1281 🖹 0141 761 1285
e-mail: secretary@cawdergolfclub.org.uk
web: www.cawdergolfclub.org.uk
Cawder Course: 18 holes, 6295yds, Par 70, SSS 71,
Course record 63.
Keir Course: 18 holes, 5877yds, Par 68, SSS 68.
Course Designer James Braid **Location** 5 m NE off A803
Telephone for further details
Hotel ★★★★ 76% HL Glasgow Marriott Hotel, 500 Argyle St, Anderston,
GLASGOW ☎ 0870 400 7230 300 en suite

Littlehill Auchinairn Rd G64 1UT
☎ 0141 772 1916
Municipal parkland course.
18 holes, 6240yds, Par 70, SSS 70.
Visitors Mon-Sun & BHs. Booking required. **Societies** Booking required
Green Fees £10 per round. ☻ **Facilities** ⊡ ⚋ **Location** 3m NE of
Glasgow city centre on A803
Hotel ★★★★ 76% HL Glasgow Marriott Hotel, 500 Argyle St, Anderston,
GLASGOW ☎ 0870 400 7230 300 en suite

KIRKINTILLOCH   MAP 11 NS67
Hayston Campsie Rd G66 1RN
☎ 0141 776 1244 🖹 0141 776 9030
e-mail: secretary@haystongolf.com
web: www.haystongolf.com
An undulating, tree-lined course with a sandy subsoil.
18 holes, 6042yds, Par 70, SSS 70, Course record 60.
Club membership 800.
Societies booking required. **Green Fees** not confirmed. ☻ **Prof** Steven
Barnett **Course Designer** James Braid **Facilities** ⊕ ⫶◐⫶ ⓛ ⊡🕱 ⟰ 🖃 ⬥
Location 1m NW off A803
Hotel ★★★★ 74% HL The Westerwood Hotel, 1 St Andrews Dr,
Westerwood, CUMBERNAULD ☎ 01236 457171 100 en suite

Kirkintilloch Todhill, Campsie Rd G66 1RN
☎ 0141 776 1256 & 775 2387 🖹 0141 775 2424
e-mail: secretary@kirkintillochgolfclub.co.uk
web: www.kirkintillochgolfclub.co.uk
Rolling parkland in the foothills of the Campsie Fells. The course was
extended some years ago giving testing but enjoyable holes over the
whole 18.
18 holes, 5860yds, Par 70, SSS 69, Course record 64.
Club membership 650.
Visitors Mon-Fri & BHs. Booking required. Dress code. **Societies** Booking
required. **Green Fees** £30 per 36 holes, £20 per 18 holes. ☻ **Prof** Jamie
Good **Course Designer** James Braid **Facilities** ⊕ ⫶◐⫶ ⓛ ⊡🕱 ⟰ 🖃
Conf facs Corporate Hospitality Days **Location** 1m NW off A803
Hotel ★★★★ 74% HL The Westerwood Hotel, 1 St Andrews Dr,
Westerwood, CUMBERNAULD ☎ 01236 457171 100 en suite

LENNOXTOWN   MAP 11 NS67
Campsie Crow Rd G66 7HX
☎ 01360 310244 🖹 01360 310244
e-mail: campsiegolfclub@aol.com
web: www.campsiegolfclub.org.uk
Scenic hillside course.
18 holes, 5507yds, Par 70, SSS 68, Course record 69.
Club membership 620.
Visitors Mon-Sun & BHs. Booking required Sat & Sun. **Societies** Booking
required **Green Fees** £15 per round (£20 Sat & Sun). ☻ **Prof** Mark
Brennan **Course Designer** W Auchterlonie **Facilities** ⊕ ⫶◐⫶ ⓛ ⊡🕱 ⚋
🖃 **Conf** Corporate Hospitality Days **Location** 0.5m N on B822
Hotel ★★★★ 74% HL The Westerwood Hotel, 1 St Andrews Dr,
Westerwood, CUMBERNAULD ☎ 01236 457171 100 en suite

Scotland

Scotland

LENZIE
MAP 11 NS67

Lenzie 19 Crosshill Rd G66 5DA
☎ 0141 776 1535 & 812 3018 📠 0141 777 7748
& 0141 812 3018
e-mail: scottdavidson@lenziegolfclub.demon.co.uk
web: www.lenziegolfclub.co.uk
18 holes, 5984yds, Par 69, SSS 69, Course record 64.
Location N of Glasgow, M80 exit Kirkintilloch
Telephone for further details
Hotel ★★★★ 74% HL The Westerwood Hotel, 1 St Andrews Dr,
Westerwood, CUMBERNAULD ☎ 01236 457171 100 en suite

MILNGAVIE
MAP 11 NS57

Clober Craigton Rd G62 7HP
☎ 0141 956 1685 📠 0141 955 1416
e-mail: clobergolfclub@btopenworld.com
web: www.clober.co.uk
Short parkland course that requires skill in chipping with eight Par 3s.
Testing 5th hole, Par 3 with out of bounds left and right and a burn in
front of the tee.
18 holes, 4824yds, Par 66, SSS 65, Course record 61.
Club membership 600.
Visitors Mon-Fri. Booking required. Handicap certificate. Dress code.
Societies Booking required. **Green Fees** £15 per round. **Prof** J McFadyen
Course Designer George Lyle **Facilities** ⊕ ⁺◎ ⁅ ⏛ ⏛ ⊟ ⼈ ⼀ ⼀
Location NW side of town
Hotel BUD Premier Travel Inn Glasgow (Milngavie), 103 Main St,
MILNGAVIE ☎ 08701 977112 60 en suite

Esporta, Dougalston Strathblane Rd G62 8HJ
☎ 0141 955 2404 📠 0141 955 2406
e-mail: hilda.everett@esporta.com
A course of tremendous character set in 300 acres of beautiful
woodland dotted with drumlins, lakes and criss-crossed by streams
and ditches. The course makes excellent use of the natural features to
create mature, tree-lined fairways. The course has been upgraded to
improve drainage and introduce three new holes as well as clearing
shrubbery to widen some others.
18 holes, 6120yds, Par 70, SSS 71, Course record 65.
Club membership 800.
Visitors Mon-Fri, Sat-Sun after 1pm. Booking required. Handicap certificate.
Dress code. **Societies** Booking required. **Green Fees** Phone. **Prof** Craig
Everett **Course Designer** Commander Harris **Facilities** ⊕ ⁺◎ ⁅ ⏛ ⏛ ⼈
⊟ ⼀ ⼀ ⼀ **Leisure** hard tennis courts, heated indoor swimming pool,
sauna, solarium, gymnasium. **Conf** Corporate Hospitality Days **Location**
NE side of town on A81
Hotel BUD Premier Travel Inn Glasgow (Milngavie), 103 Main St,
MILNGAVIE ☎ 08701 977112 60 en suite

Hilton Park Auldmarroch Estate, Stockiemuir Rd
G62 7HB
☎ 0141 956 4657 📠 0141 956 1215
e-mail: info@hiltonparkgolfclub.fsnet.co.uk
web: www.hiltonpark.co.uk
Moorland courses set amid magnificent scenery.
Hilton Course: 18 holes, 6054yds, Par 70, SSS 70,
Course record 65.
Allander Course: 18 holes, 5487yards, Par 69, SSS 67,
Course record 65. Club membership 1300.
Visitors Mon-Sun & BHs. Booking required. Dress code. **Societies** Booking
required. **Green Fees** £35 per day, £28 per round (£35 Sat & Sun). **Prof**

Gordon Simpson **Course Designer** James Braid **Facilities** ⊕ ◎ ⁅ ⏛
⼁ ⼈ ⊟ ⼀ ⼀ ⼀ **Conf** Corporate Hospitality Days **Location** 3m NW of
Milngavie, on A809
Hotel BUD Premier Travel Inn Glasgow (Milngavie), 103 Main St,
MILNGAVIE ☎ 08701 977112 60 en suite

EAST LOTHIAN

ABERLADY
MAP 12 NT47

Kilspindie EH32 0QD
☎ 01875 870358 📠 01875 870358
e-mail: kilspindie@btconnect.com
web: www.golfeastlothian.com
Traditional Scottish seaside links, short but good challenge of golf
and well-bunkered. Situated on the shores of the River Forth with
panoramic views.
Kilspindie: 18 holes, 5502yds, Par 69, SSS 66,
Course record 59. Club membership 800.
Visitors Mon-Sun & BHs. Booking required. Dress code. **Societies** Booking
required. **Green Fees** £52.50 per day, £34 per round (£62.50/£43
weekends). **Prof** Graham J Sked **Course Designer** Park & Ross with
additions by Braid **Facilities** ⊕ ◎ ⁅ ⊟ ⼁ ⼈ ⊟ ⼀ ⼀ ⼀ ⼀
Conf Corporate Hospitality Days **Location** N side of village off A198.
Private access at E end of Aberlady
Hotel ★★★ HL Greywalls Hotel, Muirfield, GULLANE ☎ 01620 842144
17 en suite 6 annexe en suite

Luffness New EH32 0QA
☎ 01620 843336 📠 01620 842933
e-mail: secretary@luffnessnew.com
Links course, national final qualifying course for the Open
Championship.
18 holes, 6122yds, Par 69, SSS 70, Course record 63.
Club membership 750.
Visitors Mon-Fri. Booking required. Handicap certificate. Dress code.
Societies Booking required. **Green Fees** £95 per day, £70 per round.
Course Designer Tom Morris **Facilities** ⊕ ◎ ⊟ ⼁ ⼈ ⼀
Location 1m E Aberlady on A198
Hotel ★★★ HL Greywalls Hotel, Muirfield, GULLANE ☎ 01620 842144
17 en suite 6 annexe en suite

DUNBAR
MAP 12 NT67

Dunbar East Links EH42 1LL
☎ 01368 862317 📠 01368 865202
e-mail: secretary@dunbargolfclub.sol.co.uk
web: www.dunbar-golfclub.co.uk
Another of Scotland's old links. It is said that it was some Dunbar
members who first took the game of golf to the north of England. A
natural links course on a narrow strip of land, following the contours
of the sea shore. There is a wall bordering one side and the shore
on the other side making this quite a challenging course for all levels
of player. The wind, if blowing from the sea, is a problem. Qualifying
course for the Open Championship.
18 holes, 6406yds, Par 71, SSS 71, Course record 62.
Club membership 1000.
Visitors Mon-Wed, Fri-Sun & BHs. Booking required. Dress code.
Societies Booking required. **Green Fees** £65 per day, £50 per round
(£85/£60 Sat & Sun). Discounts after 3pm. **Prof** Jacky Montgomery
Course Designer Tom Morris **Facilities** ⊕ ◎ ⁅ ⊟ ⼁ ⼈ ⊟ ⼀ ⼀
⼀ **Conf** Corporate Hospitality Days **Location** 0.5m E off A1087
Hotel ★★★★ 80% HL Macdonald Marine Hotel, Cromwell Rd, NORTH
BERWICK ☎ 0870 400 8129 83 en suite

CHAMPIONSHIP COURSE

EAST LOTHIAN — GULLANE

MUIRFIELD

(HONOURABLE COMPANY OF EDINBURGH GOLFERS)

Map 12 NT48

Muirfield EH31 2EG
☎ 01620 842123 📠 01620 842977
e-mail: hceg@muirfield.org.uk
web: www.muirfield.org.uk
Muirfield Course: 18 holes, 6673yds, Par 70,
SSS 73, Course record 63.
Club membership 700.
Visitors Tue & Thu. Booking required. Handicap
certificate. Dress code. **Societies** Booking
required. **Green Fees** £180 per 36 holes, £145
per 18 holes. **Course Designer** Harry Colt
Facilities ⑪ by prior arrangement 🖵 🕎 🛆
🍴 ✂ **Location** NE of village, off A198 next to
Greywalls Hotel

The course at Muirfield was designed by Old Tom Morris in 1891 and is generally considered to be one of the top ten courses in the world. The club itself has an excellent pedigree: it was founded in 1744, making it just 10 years older than the Royal and Ancient but not as old as Royal Blackheath. Muirfield is the only course to have hosted the Open (15 times, the most recent in 2002), the Amateur, the Mid Amateur, the Ryder Cup, the Walker Cup and the Curtis Cup. It is consistently ranked as one of the world's best golf courses.

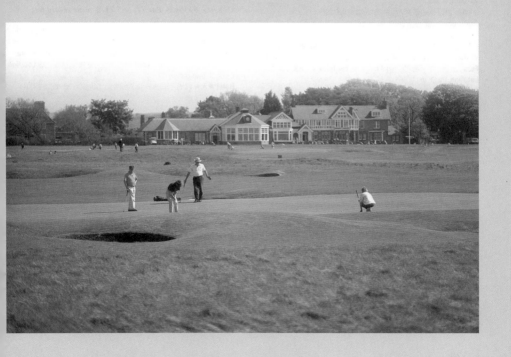

Winterfield North Rd EH42 1AU

☎ 01368 863562
e-mail: kevinphillips@tiscali.co.uk
Seaside course with superb views.
18 holes, 5155yds, Par 65, SSS 64, Course record 61.
Club membership 350.
Visitors Mon-Sun & BHs. Booking required Sat-Sun. Dress code. **Societies** booking required. **Green Fees** not confirmed. **Prof** Kevin Phillips **Facilities** ⊕ ⚲ ⓘ ⚲ ☐ ☷ ☓ ⚸ ⛳ ⚐ ⚑ **Location** W side of town off A1087
Hotel ★★★★ 80% HL Macdonald Marine Hotel, Cromwell Rd, NORTH BERWICK ☎ 0870 400 8129 83 en suite

---

GIFFORD   MAP 12 NT56

Castle Park Castlemains EH41 4PL

☎ 01620 810733 ▤ 01620 810691
e-mail: castleparkgolf@hotmail.com
web: www.castleparkgolfclub.co.uk
Naturally undulating parkland course in beautiful setting with much wild life. Wide rolling fairways on the first nine with tantalising water and dyke hazards. The mature back nine is shorter but full of hidden surprises requiring good golfing strategy as you pass Yester Castle.
18 holes, 6126yds, Par 72, SSS 70, Course record 71.
Club membership 430.
Visitors Mon-Sun & BHs. Dress code. **Societies** Welcome. **Green Fees** £22 per 18 holes, £11 per 9 holes (£30/£15 Sat & Sun). **Prof** Derek Small **Course Designer** Archie Baird **Facilities** ⊕ ⓘ ⚲ ☐ ⚲ ☓ ⛳ ⚸ ⚐ **Conf** Corporate Hospitality Days **Location** off B6355, 2m S of Gifford
Guesthouse ★★★★★ GA Kippielaw Farmhouse, EAST LINTON ☎ 01620 860368 2 rms (1 en suite)

Gifford Edinburgh Rd EH41 4JE

☎ 01620 810267
e-mail: thesecretary@giffordgolfclub.fsnet.co.uk
web: www.giffordgolfclub.com
Parkland with easy walking.
9 holes, 6057yds, Par 71, SSS 69. Club membership 600.
Visitors Mon-Sun & BHs. Dress code **Societies** Booking required **Green Fees** £20 per 18 holes, £14 per 9 holes. ⊛ **Facilities** ⚲ ☐ ⚲ ☓ ⚸ ⚐ **Location** 1m SW off B6355
Guesthouse ★★★★★ GA Kippielaw Farmhouse, EAST LINTON ☎ 01620 860368 2 rms (1 en suite)

GULLANE   MAP 12 NT48

Gullane West Links Rd EH31 2BB

☎ 01620 842255 ▤ 01620 842327
e-mail: bookings@gullanegolfclub.com
web: www.gullanegolfclub.com
Gullane is a delightful village and one of Scotland's great golf centres. The game has been played on the 3 links courses for over 300 years and was formed in 1882. The first tee of the Championship No. 1 course (a Final Qualifier when The Open is played at Muirfield) is literally in the village and the three courses stretch out along the coast line. All have magnificent views over the Firth of the Fourth, standing on the highest point at the 7th Tee is reported as one of the "finest views in golf".
Course No 1: 18 holes, 6466yds, Par 71, SSS 72, Course record 65.
Course No 2: 18 holes, 6244yds, Par 71, SSS 71, Course record 64.

Course No 3: 18 holes, 5252yds, Par 68, SSS 66.
Club membership 1200.
Visitors Mon-Sun & BHs. Booking required. Dress code. Handicap certificate required for Course 1 **Societies** Welcome. **Green Fees** Course 1: £85 per round (£100 Sat & Sun). Course 2: £40 per round (£45 Sat & Sun). Course 3: £25 per round (£30 Sat & Sun). **Prof** Alasdair Good **Course Designer** Various **Facilities** ⊕ ⓘ ⚲ ☐ ⚲ ☓ ⚸ ⛳ ⚐ ⚑ **Leisure** golf museum. **Conf** facs Corporate Hospitality Days **Location** W end of village on A198
Hotel ★★★ HL Greywalls Hotel, Muirfield, GULLANE ☎ 01620 842144 17 en suite 6 annexe en suite

Honourable Company of Edinburgh Golfers see page 327

Hotel ★★★ HL Greywalls Hotel, Muirfield, GULLANE ☎ 01620 842144 17 en suite 6 annexe en suite
Hotel ★★★ 77% SHL The Open Arms Hotel, DIRLETON ☎ 01620 850241 Fax 01620 850570 10 en suite
Hotel ★★★★ 80% HL Macdonald Marine Hotel, Cromwell Rd, NORTH BERWICK ☎ 0870 400 8129 Fax 01620 894480 83 en suite
Hotel ★★ 69% HL Nether Abbey Hotel, 20 Dirleton Av, NORTH BERWICK ☎ 01620 892802 Fax 01620 895298 13 en suite

---

HADDINGTON   MAP 12 NT57

Haddington Amisfield Park EH41 4PT

☎ 01620 822727 & 823627 ▤ 01620 826580
e-mail: info@haddingtongolf.co.uk
web: www.haddingtongolf.co.uk
A slightly undulating parkland course within the grounds of a former country estate beside the River Tyne. New ponds and bunkers have been constructed to improve the course even more.
18 holes, 6335yds, Par 71, SSS 71, Course record 64.
Club membership 850.
Visitors Mon-Sun & BHs. Booking required. Dress code. **Societies** Booking required. **Green Fees** £40 per day, £25 per round (£50/£35 Sat & Sun). ⊛ **Prof** John Sandilands **Facilities** ⊕ ⓘ ⚲ ☐ ⚲ ☓ ⚸ ⛳ ⚐ **Leisure** driving net, practice bunker. **Conf** facs Corporate Hospitality Days **Location** E side of town centre
Hotel ★★★ HL Greywalls Hotel, Muirfield, GULLANE ☎ 01620 842144 17 en suite 6 annexe en suite

---

LONGNIDDRY   MAP 12 NT47

Longniddry Links Rd EH32 0NL

☎ 01875 852141 ▤ 01875 853371
e-mail: secretary@longniddrygolfclub.co.uk
web: www.longniddrygolfclub.co.uk
Undulating seaside links and partial woodland course with no Par 5s. One of the numerous courses which stretch east from Edinburgh to Dunbar. The inward half is more open than the wooded outward half, but can be difficult in prevailing west wind.
18 holes, 6260yds, Par 68, SSS 70, Course record 62.
Club membership 1100.
Visitors Mon-Sun & BHs. Booking required. Handicap certificate. Dress code. **Societies** Booking required. **Green Fees** £65 per day, £42 per round (£60 Sat & Sun). **Prof** John Gray **Course Designer** H S Colt **Facilities** ⊕ ⓘ ⚲ ☐ ⚲ ☓ ⚸ ⛳ ⚐ ⚑ **Conf** Corporate Hospitality Days **Location** N side of village off A198
Hotel ★★★ HL Greywalls Hotel, Muirfield, GULLANE ☎ 01620 842144 17 en suite 6 annexe en suite

MUSSELBURGH

MAP 11 NT37

Musselburgh Monktonhall EH21 6SA
☎ 0131 665 2005 📄 0131 665 4435
e-mail: secretary@themusselburghgolfclub.com
web: www.themusselburghgolfclub.com
Testing parkland course with natural hazards including trees and a
burn; easy walking.
18 holes, 6725yds, Par 71, SSS 72, Course record 65.
Club membership 1000.
Visitors Mon-Fri, Sun & BHs. Booking required. Dress Code. **Societies**
Booking required. **Green Fees** £45 per day, £35 per round (£50/£40 Sat &
Sun). **Prof** Fraser Mann **Course Designer** James Braid **Facilities** ⑪ ⑩ ⓛ 🏊
🖵 🍴 🏌 🏠 🔫 ✓ 🍴 ✓ **Conf** Corporate Hospitality Days **Location** 1m
S on B6415
Hotel BUD Premier Travel Inn Edinburgh (Inveresk), Carberry Rd, Inveresk,
Musselburgh, EDINBURGH ☎ 08701 977092   40 en suite

Musselburgh Links, The Old Golf Course 10 Balcarres
Rd EH21 7SD
☎ 0131 665 5438 (Starter) & 665 6981(clubhouse)
📄 0131 665 5438
e-mail: info@musselburgholdlinks.co.uk
web: www.musselburgholdlinks.co.uk
A delightful nine-hole links course weaving in and out of the famous
Musselburgh Race Course. This course is steeped in the history and
tradition of golf. Mary Queen of Scots reputedly played golf at the
old course in 1567, but documentary evidence dates back to 1672.
The 1st hole is a Par 3 and the next three holes play eastward from the
grandstand at the racecourse. The course turns north-west towards the
sea then west for the last four holes. Designed by nature and defined
over the centuries by generations of golfers, the course has many
natural features and hazards.
9 holes, 2874yds, Par 34, SSS 34, Course record 29.
Club membership 300.
Visitors Mon-Sun & BHs. Booking required Sun & BHs. Dress code
Societies Welcome. **Green Fees** £9 per 9 holes, £18 per 18 holes
(£9.50/£19 Sun & Sat). **Facilities** 🏌 ⓡ ✓ **Conf** facs **Location** 1m E of
town off A1
Hotel BUD Premier Travel Inn Edinburgh (Inveresk), Carberry Rd, Inveresk,
Musselburgh, EDINBURGH ☎ 08701 977092   40 en suite

NORTH BERWICK

MAP 12 NT58

Glen East Links, Tantallon Ter EH39 4LE
☎ 01620 892726 📄 01620 895447
e-mail: secretary@glengolfclub.co.uk
web: www.glengolfclub.co.uk
A popular course with a good variety of holes including the
famous 13th, Par 3 Sea Hole. The views of the town, the Firth of Forth
and the Bass Rock are breathtaking.
18 holes, 6243yds, Par 70, SSS 70, Course record 67.
Club membership 650.
Visitors Mon-Sun & BHs. Booking required. Dress code. **Societies** booking
required. **Green Fees** not confirmed. **Course Designer** Ben Sayers/James
Braid **Facilities** ⑪ ⑩ ⓛ 🖵 🍴 🏌 🏠 ⓡ ✓ **Conf** facs Corporate
Hospitality Days **Location** A1 onto A198 to North Berwick. Right at seabird
centre sea-wall road
Hotel ★★ 69% HL Nether Abbey Hotel, 20 Dirleton Av, NORTH BERWICK
☎ 01620 892802   13 en suite

Royal Musselburgh Golf Club
1774   18 holes, par 70, 6237 yards

This Parkland course was designed by James Braid and in
contract to many of East Lothian's courses offers golfers views
of Edinburgh and Arthur's Seat. The golfing challenge comes
on the homeward stretch where a series of par 4s are well
protected by trees. One of the oldest clubs in the world, the
magnificent clubhouse has a superb collection of golfing
memorabilia.

Special feature: the par 3 14th, 'The Gully', penalises short
approach shots with a 30 foot drop just in front of the putting
surface. The club were privileged to host The World Junior
Open in July 2002.

Prestongrange House, Prestonpans, East Lothian, EH32 9RP

Tel / fax: **01875 810 276**

Email: **royalmusselburgh@btinternet.com**

Website: **www.royalmusselburgh.co.uk**

North Berwick Beach Rd EH39 4BB
☎ 01620 892135 📄 01620 893274
e-mail: secretary@northberwickgolfclub.com
web: www.northberwickgolfclub.com
Another of East Lothian's famous courses, the links at North Berwick
is still popular. A classic championship links, it has many hazards
including the beach, streams, bunkers, light rough and low walls.
The great hole on the course is the 15th, the famous Redan.
West Links: 18 holes, 6420yds, Par 71, SSS 72,
Course record 63. Club membership 730.
Visitors Mon-Sun & BHs. Booking required. Handicap certificate.
Dress code. **Societies** booking required. **Green Fees** not confirmed.
Prof D Huish **Facilities** ⑪ ⑩ ⓛ 🖵 🍴 🏌 🏠 ⓡ ✓ **Conf** Corporate
Hospitality Days **Location** W side of town on A198
Hotel ★★★★ 80% HL Macdonald Marine Hotel, Cromwell Rd, NORTH
BERWICK ☎ 0870 400 8129   83 en suite

Whitekirk Whitekirk EH39 5PR
☎ 01620 870300 📄 01620 870330
e-mail: countryclub@whitekirk.com
web: www.whitekirk.com
Scenic coastal course with lush green fairways, gorse covered rocky
banks and stunning views. Natural water hazards and strong sea
breezes make this well-designed course a good test of golf.
18 holes, 6526yds, Par 72, SSS 72, Course record 64.
Club membership 400.

Continued

Scotland

Visitors Mon-Sun & BHs. Booking required Fri-Sun & BHs. Dress code.
Societies Booking required. **Green Fees** £40 per day, £28 per round
(£62/£42 Sun & Sat). **Prof** Paul Wardell **Course Designer** Cameron Sinclair
Facilities ⊕ ⦿ ⤮ ⤴ ♢ ⤵ ♠ ⏏ ✓ ⛴ ✓ ⏩ **Leisure** indoor swimming
pool, sauna, solarium, gymnasium, health spa. **Conf** facs Corporate
Hospitality Days **Location** A198 off A1 to A199, on A198 4m SE of North
Berwick
Hotel ★★ 69% HL Nether Abbey Hotel, 20 Dirleton Av, NORTH BERWICK
☎ 01620 892802 13 en suite

PRESTONPANS · MAP 11 NT37

Royal Musselburgh · Prestongrange House EH32 9RP
☎ 01875 810276 📠 01875 810276
e-mail: royalmusselburgh@btinternet.com
web: www.royalmusselburgh.co.uk

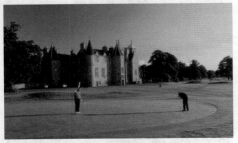

18 holes, 6237yds, Par 70, SSS 70, Course record 64.
Course Designer James Braid **Location** W of town centre on B1361 to
North Berwick
Telephone for further details
Hotel BUD Premier Travel Inn Edinburgh (Inveresk), Carberry Rd, Inveresk,
Musselburgh, EDINBURGH ☎ 08701 977092 40 en suite

See advert on page 329

EAST RENFREWSHIRE

BARRHEAD · MAP 11 NS45

Fereneze · Fereneze Av G78 1HJ
☎ 0141 880 7058 📠 0141 881 7149
e-mail: ferenezegc@lineone.net
web: www.ferenezegolfclub.co.uk
Hilly moorland course, with a good view at the end of a hard climb to
the 3rd, then levels out.
18 holes, 5962yds, Par 71, SSS 69, Course record 65.
Club membership 750.
Visitors Mon-Fri. Booking required. Dress code. **Societies** Booking
required. **Green Fees** £35 per day, £30 per round. ⊛ **Prof** James
Smallwood **Facilities** ⊕ ⦿ ⤮ ⤴ ♢ ⤵ ♠ ✓ **Location** NW side of town
off B774
Hotel ★★ 76% HL Uplawmoor Hotel, Neilston Rd, UPLAWMOOR
☎ 01505 850565 14 en suite

CLARKSTON · MAP 11 NS55

Cathcart Castle · Mearns Rd G76 7YL
☎ 0141 638 9449 📠 0141 638 1201
Tree-lined parkland course, with undulating terrain.
18 holes, 5861yds, Par 69, SSS 69. Club membership 995.

Visitors Mon-Fri & BHs. Booking required. Dress code. **Societies** Booking
required. **Green Fees** £45 per day; £30 per round. ⊛ **Prof** Stephen
Duncan **Facilities** ⊕ ⦿ ⤮ ⤴ ♢ ⤵ ♠ ✓ **Location** 0.75m SW off
A726
Hotel BUD Premier Travel Inn Glasgow East Kilbride West, Eaglesham Rd,
EAST KILBRIDE ☎ 0870 9906542 40 en suite

EAGLESHAM · MAP 11 NS55

Bonnyton · Kirktonmoor Rd G76 0QA
☎ 01355 302781 📠 01355 303151
Dramatic moorland course offering spectacular views of beautiful
countryside as far as snow-capped Ben Lomond. Tree-lined fairways,
plateau greens, natural burns and well-situated bunkers and a unique
variety of holes offer golfers both challenge and reward.
18 holes, 6255yds, Par 72, SSS 71. Club membership 960.
Visitors Mon & Thu. Booking required. Dress code. **Societies** booking
required. **Green Fees** not confirmed. ⊛ **Prof** Kendal McWade **Facilities**
⊕ ⦿ ⤮ ⤴ ♢ ⤵ ♠ ⏏ ✓ **Location** 0.25m SW off B764

NEWTON MEARNS · MAP 11 NS55

East Renfrewshire · Pilmuir G77 6RT
☎ 01355 500256 📠 01355 500323
e-mail: secretary@eastrengolfclub.co.uk
web: www.eastrengolfclub.co.uk
Undulating moorland with loch; prevailing south-west wind. Extensive
views of Glasgow and the southern Highlands.
18 holes, 6107yds, Par 70, SSS 70, Course record 63.
Club membership 900.
Visitors Mon-Fri. Booking required. Handicap certificate. Dress code.
Societies Booking required. **Green Fees** £40 per round/£50 per day.
Prof Stewart Russell **Course Designer** James Braid **Facilities** ⊕ ⦿ ⤮
♢ ⤴ ♠ ⤵ ♠ ✓ **Conf** Corporate Hospitality Days **Location** 3m SW of
Newton Mearns on A77, junct 5
Hotel ★★ 76% HL Uplawmoor Hotel, Neilston Rd, UPLAWMOOR
☎ 01505 850565 14 en suite

Eastwood · Muirshield, Loganswell G77 6RX
☎ 01355 500280 📠 01355 500333
e-mail: eastwoodgolfclub@btconnect.com
web: www.eastwoodgolfclub.co.uk
An undulating moorland course situated in a scenic setting. Originally
built in 1937, the course was redesigned in 2003. The greens are now
of modern design, built to USGA specification.
18 holes, 6071yds, Par 70, SSS 70. Club membership 900.
Visitors Mon-Sun & BHs. Booking required. Dress code. **Societies** Booking
required. **Green Fees** £40 per day; £30 per round. **Prof** Iain J Darroch
Course Designer Graeme J. Webster/Theodore Moone **Facilities** ⊕ ⦿ ⤮
♢ ⤴ ♠ ⤵ ✓ **Location** 2.5m S of Newton Mearns, on A77
Hotel ★★ 76% HL Uplawmoor Hotel, Neilston Rd, UPLAWMOOR
☎ 01505 850565 14 en suite

UPLAWMOOR · MAP 10 NS45

Caldwell · G78 4AU
☎ 01505 850366 (Secretary) & 850616 (Pro)
📠 01505 850604
e-mail: secretary@caldwellgolfclub.co.uk
web: cgc.uplowmoor.net
Parkland course.

Continued

18 holes, 6294yds, Par 71, SSS 71, Course record 62.
Club membership 600.
Visitors Mon-Fri. Booking required. Handicap certificate. Dress code
Societies Booking required. **Green Fees** £25 per round/£35 per day.
Prof Craig Everett **Course Designer** W. Fernie **Facilities** ⑪ ⑩ ⑂ ⌷ ⑂
⚹ ⑁ ⚿ **Conf** Corporate Hospitality Days **Location** 5m SW of Barrhead
on A736 Irvine road
Hotel ★★ 76% HL Uplawmoor Hotel, Neilston Rd, UPLAWMOOR
☎ 01505 850565 14 en suite

CITY OF EDINBURGH

EDINBURGH   MAP 11 NT27

Baberton 50 Baberton Av, Juniper Green EH14 5DU
☎ 0131 453 4911 📠 0131 453 4678
e-mail: manager@baberton.co.uk
web: www.baberton.co.uk
Parkland course offering the golfer a variety of interesting and
challenging holes. The outward half follows the boundary of the course
and presents some demanding Par 3 and 4 holes over the undulating
terrain. The inward half has some longer, equally challenging holes
contained within the course and presents some majestic views of the
Pentland Hills and the Edinburgh skyline.
18 holes, 6129yds, Par 69, SSS 70, Course record 64.
Club membership 900.
Visitors Mon-Fri, Sun & BHs. Booking required. Dress code. **Societies**
Booking required. **Green Fees** £37 per day, £27 per round (£40/£30
Sun). **Prof** Ken Kelly **Course Designer** Willie Park Jnr **Facilities** ⑪ ⑩
⑂ ⌷ ⑂ ⚹ ⑁ ⚿ ⚿ **Leisure** Snooker. **Conf** Corporate Hospitality Days
Location 5m W of city centre off A70
Hotel ★★★★ 76% HL Edinburgh Marriott Hotel, 111 Glasgow Rd,
EDINBURGH ☎ 0131 334 9191 245 en suite

Braid Hills 27 Braid Hills Approach EH10 6JY
☎ 0131 447 6666 📠 0131 651 2299
e-mail: golf@edinburghleisure.co.uk
web: edinburghleisure.co.uk
Municipal heathland course with superb views of Edinburgh and the
Firth of Forth, quite challenging.
Course No 1: 18 holes, 5345yds, Par 70, SSS 66.
Visitors Mon-Sun & BHs. Booking required. **Societies** Booking required.
Green Fees £18 per round (£22 Sat & Sun). **Course Designer** Peter
McEwan & Bob Ferguson **Facilities** ⑪ by prior arrangement ⑩ by prior
arrangement ⑂ by prior arrangement ⌷ ⚹ ⑁ ⚿ **Conf** Corporate
Hospitality Days **Location** 2.5m S of city centre off A702
Hotel ★★★ 80% HL Best Western Braid Hills Hotel, 134 Braid Rd,
EDINBURGH ☎ 0131 447 8888 67 en suite

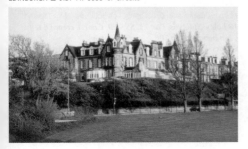

See advert on this page

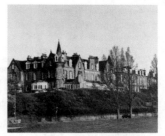

THE BRAID HILLS
HOTEL
134 Braid Road, Edinburgh, EH10 6JD
Magnificently situated only two miles from
the city centre, yet a world away from the
noise and congestion of the centre itself, the
Braid Hills Hotel is your ideal choice when
visiting Edinburgh.
To make your reservation in this

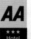 independently-owned hotel
Tel: 0131 447 8888
Fax: 0131 452 8477

AA ★★★ Hotel

Bruntsfield Links Golfing Society 32 Barnton Av
EH4 6JH
☎ 0131 336 1479 📠 0131 336 5538
e-mail: secretary@bruntsfield.sol.co.uk
web: www.sol.co.uk/b/bruntsfieldlinks
Mature parkland course with magnificent views over the Firth of
Forth and to the west. Greens and fairways are generally immaculate.
Challenging for all categories of handicap.
Bruntsfield Links: 18 holes, 6428yds, Par 71, SSS 71,
Course record 63. Club membership 1180.
Visitors Mon-Sun & BHs. Booking required. Handicap certificate. Dress
code. **Societies** Booking required. **Green Fees** £80 per day, £55 per round
(£85/£65 Sat & Sun). **Prof** Brian Mackenzie **Course Designer** Willie Park
Jr, A Mackenzie, Hawtree **Facilities** ⑪ ⑩ ⑂ ⌷ ⑂ ⚹ ⑁ ⚿ ⚿ ⚿
Conf Corporate Hospitality Days **Location** 4m NW of city centre off A90

Carrick Knowe Carrick Knowe, Glendevon Park
EH12 5UZ
☎ 0131 337 1096 📠 0131 651 2299
e-mail: info.carrickknowe@edinburghleisure.co.uk
Flat parkland course. Played over by two clubs, Carrick Knowe and
Carrick Vale.
18 holes, 5697yds, Par 70, SSS 69.
Visitors Mon-Sun & BHs. **Societies** Welcome. **Green Fees** £15 per round
(£18 Sat, Sun & BHs). **Facilities** ⑪ ⑩ ⑂ ⌷ ⚹ ⑁ ⚿ **Location** 3m W of
city centre, S of A8

Craigentinny Fillyside Rd EH7 6RG
☎ 0131 554 7501 📄 0131 651 2299
e-mail: info.craigentinny@edinburghleisure.co.uk
web: www.edinburghleisure.co.uk
An interesting mix of holes on an undulating parkland layout. From some tricky Par 3s to some testing Par 4s, this relatively short course will suit all abilities. The greens are surrounded by some awkward bunkers, requiring a great deal of forethought and an amount of accuracy to make par. The dog-leg 414yd Par 4 10th requires a long tee shot to beyond the trees and an equally long second to the front of the green.
18 holes, 5205yds, Par 67, SSS 65, Course record 62.
Visitors Mon-Sun & BHs. Booking required. **Societies** Booking required.
Green Fees £13 per round (£15 Sat, Sun & BHs). **Prof** Steve Craig
Facilities ♉ ⚲ 🏌 ⛳ ✆ **Location** NE side of city, between Leith & Portobello
Hotel ★★★ 78% HL Best Western Kings Manor, 100 Milton Rd East, EDINBURGH ☎ 0131 669 0444 & 468 8003 📄 0131 669 6650 95 en suite

Craigmillar Park 1 Observatory Rd EH9 3HG
☎ 0131 667 0047 📄 0131 662 8091
e-mail: secretary@craigmillarpark.co.uk
web: www.craigmillarpark.co.uk
18 holes, 5851yds, Par 70, SSS 69, Course record 63.
Course Designer James Braid **Location** 2m S of city centre off A7
Telephone for further details
Hotel ★★★ 80% HL Best Western Braid Hills Hotel, 134 Braid Rd, EDINBURGH ☎ 0131 447 8888 67 en suite

Duddingston Duddingston Rd West EH15 3QD
☎ 0131 661 4301 📄 0131 661 4301
e-mail: duddingstonproshop@hotmail.com
web: www.duddingstongolfclub.com
Easy walking parkland with a burn as a natural hazard. Testing 11th hole.
18 holes, 6525yds, Par 72, SSS 72, Course record 63.
Club membership 700.
Visitors Mon-Fri & BHs, Sat & Sun; pm only. Dresscode **Societies** Booking required. **Green Fees** £48 per day, £38 per round. **Prof** Alastair McLean
Course Designer Willie Park Jnr **Facilities** ⊕ 🍴 🏌 ⚲ 🍺 ⚲ 🏌 🍽 ⛳ ✆ ✆ **Conf** facs Corporate Hospitality Days **Location** 2.5m SE of city centre off A1
Hotel ★★★ 78% HL Best Western Kings Manor, 100 Milton Rd East, EDINBURGH ☎ 0131 669 0444 & 468 8003 📄 0131 669 6650 95 en suite

Kingsknowe 326 Lanark Rd EH14 2JD
☎ 0131 441 1145 (Secretary) 📄 0131 441 2079
e-mail: louis@kingsknowe.com
web: www.kingsknowe.com
Picturesque parkland course set amid gently rolling hills. This course provides a varied and interesting challenge for all levels of golfers.

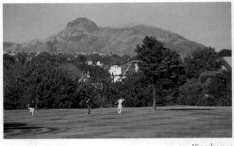

Kingsknowe

18 holes, 5981yds, Par 69, SSS 69, Course record 63.
Club membership 930.
Visitors Mon-Fri & BHs. Booking required. Dress code. **Societies** Booking required. **Green Fees** £32 per day, £25 per round. ● **Prof** Chris Morris
Course Designer A Herd/James Braid **Facilities** ⊕ 🍴 🏌 ⚲ 🍽 ⚲ 🍺 ⛳ ✆ ✆ **Leisure** Indoor teaching/practice facility. **Conf** Corporate Hospitality Days **Location** 4m SW of city centre on A70
Hotel ★★★ 81% HL Best Western Bruntsfield Hotel, 69 Bruntsfield Place, EDINBURGH ☎ 0131 229 1393 71 en suite

Liberton 297 Gilmerton Rd EH16 5UJ
☎ 0131 664 3009 (sec) 📄 0131 666 0853
e-mail: info@libertongc.co.uk
web: www.libertongc.co.uk
Undulating, wooded parkland.
18 holes, 5344yds, Par 67, SSS 66, Course record 62.
Club membership 846.
Visitors Mon-Sun & BHs. Dress code. **Societies** Booking required.
Green Fees £30 per day, £25 per round (£30 Sat & Sun). ● **Prof** Iain Seath **Facilities** ⊕ 🍴 🏌 ⚲ 🍽 ⚲ 🍺 🏌 ⛳ ✆ **Conf** Corporate Hospitality Days **Location** 3m SE of city centre on A7
Hotel ★★★ 83% HL Dalhousie Castle and Aqueous Spa, Bonnyrigg, EDINBURGH ☎ 01875 820153 29 en suite 7 annexe en suite

Lothianburn 106A Biggar Rd, Fairmilehead EH10 7DU
☎ 0131 445 2288 📄 0131 445 5067
e-mail: info@lothianburngc.co.uk
web: www.lothianburngc.co.uk
Situated to the south-west of Edinburgh, on the slopes of the Pentland Hills, the course rises from the clubhouse some 300ft to its highest point at the 13th green. There is only one real climb of note, after playing the 2nd shot to the 9th green. The course is noted for its excellent greens, and challenging holes include the 5th, where one drives for position in order to pitch at almost right angles to a plateau green; and the 14th, longest hole on the course, three-quarters of which is downhill with out of bounds on both sides of the fairway.
18 holes, 5662yds, Par 71, SSS 69, Course record 64.
Club membership 700.
Visitors Mon-Fri & BHs. Booking required. Dress code. **Societies** Booking required. **Green Fees** £20 per round. ● **Prof** Kurt Mungall **Course Designer** J Braid (re-designed 1928) **Facilities** ⊕ 🍴 🏌 ⚲ 🍽 ⚲ 🍺 ⛳ ✆ **Location** 4.5m S of city centre on A702
Hotel ★★★ 80% HL Best Western Braid Hills Hotel, 134 Braid Rd, EDINBURGH ☎ 0131 447 8888 67 en suite

CHAMPIONSHIP COURSE

CITY OF EDINBURGH – EDINBURGH

MARRIOTT DALMAHOY HOTEL

Map 11 NT27

Kirknewton EH27 8EB
☎ 0131 335 1845 📠 0131 335 1433
e-mail: mhrs.golf@marriotthotels.com
web: www.marriott.com/edigs
East Course: 18 holes, 7055yds, Par 73,
SSS 74, Course record 70.
West Course: 18 holes, 5168yds, Par 68,
SSS 66, Course record 60.
Club membership 822.
Visitors Mon-Sun & BHs. Booking required.
Handicap certificate. Dress code.
Societies Booking required. **Green Fees** East
Course: £65 per 18 holes (£80 Sat, Sun & BHs).
West: £40 (£45 Sat, Sun & BHs). Reduced winter
rates. **Prof** Scott Dixon **Course Designer** James
Braid **Facilities** ⑪ ⑩ ⓵ ▭ ☐ ◈ ⏚ ⌂ ☙ ◇ ⌑
⚬ ⚐ **Leisure** hard tennis courts, heated indoor
swimming pool, sauna, solarium, gymnasium,
fitness studio, golf academy, health salon.
Conf facs Corporate Hospitality Days
Location 7m W of city on A71

The Championship East Course has hosted many major events including the Solheim Cup and the Charles Church Seniors PGA Championship of Scotland. The course has long sweeping fairways and generous greens protected by strategic bunkers. Many of the long Par 4 holes offer a serious challenge to any golfer. The signature 18th hole has the green set in front of Dalmahoy's historic hotel with a testing approach over a wide ravine. The shorter West Course offers a different test with tighter fairways requiring more accuracy from the tee. The finishing holes incorporate the Golgar burn meandering through the fairway to create a tough finish to the course.

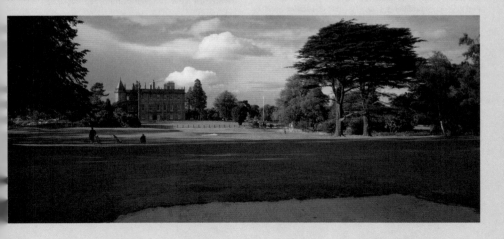

Marriott Dalmahoy Hotel Golf & Country Club see page 333

Hotel ★★★★ 80% HL Marriott Dalmahoy Hotel & Country Club, Kirknewton, EDINBURGH ☎ 0131 333 1845 43 en suite 172 annexe en suite
Hotel ★★★★ 77% HL Macdonald Houstoun House, UPHALL
☎ 0870 1942107 Fax 01506 854220 24 en suite 47 annexe en suite
Hotel ★★★★ 76% HL Edinburgh Marriott Hotel, 111 Glasgow Rd, EDINBURGH ☎ 0131 334 9191 Fax 0131 316 4507 245 en suite

Merchants of Edinburgh 10 Craighill Gardens EH10 5PY
☎ 0131 447 1219 ▤ 0131 446 9833
e-mail: admin@merchantsgolf.com
web: www.merchantsgolf.com
18 holes, 4889yds, Par 65, SSS 64, Course record 59.
Course Designer Ben Sayers **Location** 2m SW of city centre off A702
Telephone for further details
Hotel ★★★ 80% HL Best Western Braid Hills Hotel, 134 Braid Rd, EDINBURGH ☎ 0131 447 8888 67 en suite

Mortonhall 231 Braid Rd EH10 6PB
☎ 0131 447 6974 ▤ 0131 447 8712
e-mail: clubhouse@mortonhallgc.co.uk
web: www.mortonhallgc.co.uk
Moorland and parkland with views over Edinburgh.
18 holes, 6502yds, Par 72, SSS 72, Course record 66.
Club membership 525.
Visitors Mon-Sun & BHs. Booking Required **Societies** Booking required
Green Fees £55 per day, £40 per round. **Prof** Malcolm Leighton **Course Designer** James Braid/F Hawtree **Facilities** ⊕ ▙ ⌹ ⌾ 兀 ㅗ 合 ⚐ 🍴 🏌
Location 3m S of city centre off A702
Hotel ★★★ 80% HL Best Western Braid Hills Hotel, 134 Braid Rd, EDINBURGH ☎ 0131 447 8888 67 en suite

Murrayfield 43 Murrayfield Rd EH12 6EU
☎ 0131 337 3478 ▤ 0131 313 0721
e-mail: marjorie@murrayfieldgolfclub.co.uk
web: www.murrayfieldgolfclub.co.uk
Parkland on the side of Corstorphine Hill, with fine views.
18 holes, 5725yds, Par 70, SSS 69. Club membership 815.
Visitors Mon-Fri. Booking required. Dress code.
Societies Booking required. **Green Fees** £45 per day, £35 per round.
Prof K. Stevenson **Facilities** ⊕ ▙ ⌹ 兀 ㅗ 合 ⚐ 🏌 **Location** 2m W of city centre off A8

Portobello Stanley St EH15 1JJ
☎ 0131 669 4361 & 557 5457(bookings) ▤ 0131 557 5170
9 holes, 2252yds, Par 32, SSS 32.
Location 3m E of city centre off A1
Telephone for further details
Hotel ★★★ 78% HL Best Western Kings Manor, 100 Milton Rd East, EDINBURGH ☎ 0131 669 0444 & 468 8003 ▤ 0131 669 6650 95 en suite

Prestonfield 6 Priestfield Rd North EH16 5HS
☎ 0131 667 9665 ▤ 0131 667 9665
e-mail: generalmanager@prestonfieldgolfclub.co.uk
web: www.prestonfieldgolfclub.co.uk
18 holes, 6212yds, Par 70, SSS 70, Course record 66.
Course Designer James Braid **Location** 1.5m S of city centre off A68
Telephone for further details
Hotel ★★★★★ TH Prestonfield, Priestfield Rd, EDINBURGH
☎ 0131 225 7800 24 en suite

Ravelston 24 Ravelston Dykes Rd EH4 3NZ
☎ 0131 315 2486 ▤ 0131 315 2486
Parkland on the north-east side of Corstorphine Hill, overlooking the Firth of Forth.
9 holes, 5230yds, Par 66, SSS 66, Course record 64.
Club membership 610.
Visitors Mon-Fri. Handicap certificate. Dress code. **Green Fees** not confirmed. ● **Course Designer** James Braid **Facilities** ⌹ ㅗ
Location 3m W of city centre off A90
Hotel ★★★★ 76% HL Edinburgh Marriott Hotel, 111 Glasgow Rd, EDINBURGH ☎ 0131 334 9191 245 en suite

Royal Burgess 181 Whitehouse Rd, Barnton EH4 6BU
☎ 0131 339 2075 ▤ 0131 339 3712
e-mail: secretary@royalburgess.co.uk
web: www.royalburgess.co.uk
No mention of golf clubs would be complete without the Royal Burgess, which was instituted in 1735 and is the oldest golfing society in Scotland. Its course is a pleasant parkland, and one with a great deal of variety. A club which anyone interested in the history of the game should visit.
18 holes, 6111yds, Par 68, SSS 69. Club membership 635.
Visitors Mon-Sun & BHs. Booking required. Handicap certificate. Dress code. **Societies** Booking requried. **Green Fees** £55 per day (£75 Sat & Sun). **Prof** Steven Brian **Course Designer** Tom Morris **Facilities** ⊕ 🍴 ▙ ⌹ 兀 ㅗ 合 ⚐ 🏌 **Conf** Corporate Hospitality Days **Location** 5m W of city centre off A90

Silverknowes Silverknowes, Parkway EH4 5ET
☎ 0131 336 3843
e-mail: golf@edinburghleisure.co.uk
web: www.edinburghleisure.co.uk
Public links course on coast overlooking the Firth of Forth with magnificent views, generous fairways and expansive greens.
The 601yd 18th will be a final test that will make or break your game.
The ball needs to be kept low against the prevailing westerlies.
18 holes, 6070yds, Par 71, SSS 70.
Visitors Mon-Sun & BHs. **Societies** Welcome. **Green Fees** £14 per day, per round (£18/£15 Sat & Sun). **Facilities** ⊕ 🍴 ▙ ⌹ 兀 ㅗ 合 ⚐ 🏌
Conf Corporate Hospitality Days **Location** 4m NW of city centre, easy access from city bypass

Swanston New 111 Swanston Rd, Fairmilehead EH10 7DS
☎ 0131 445 2239 ▤ 0131 445 2239
e-mail: stewart.snedden@swanston.co.uk
web: www.swanstongolf.co.uk
Short yet challenging course situated on the lower slopes of the Pentland Hills with fine views over the city of Edinburgh and the Firth of Forth. The small greens require the golfer's short game to be on form.
18 holes, 5024yds, Par 66, SSS 65, Course record 58.
Club membership 500.
Visitors Mon-Sun & BHs. **Societies** Booking required **Green Fees** Phone.
Course Designer Herbert More **Facilities** ⊕ 🍴 ▙ ⌹ 兀 ㅗ 合 ⚐ 🏌 🍴
Conf Corporate Hospitality Days **Location** 4m S of city centre off B701
Hotel ★★★ 80% HL Best Western Braid Hills Hotel, 134 Braid Rd, EDINBURGH ☎ 0131 447 8888 67 en suite

Torphin Hill Torphin Rd, Colinton EH13 0PG
☎ 0131 441 1100 📠 0131 441 7166
e-mail: torphinhillgc@btconnect.com
web: www.torphinhillgc.co.uk
Beautiful hillside, heathland course, with fine views of Edinburgh and the Forth Estuary. From 600 to 700ft above sea level with 14 holes set on a relatively flat plateau.
18 holes, 5285yds, Par 68, SSS 67, Course record 64.
Club membership 550.
Visitors Mon-Fri & BHs. Dress code. **Societies** booking required.
Green Fees not confirmed. **Prof** Jamie Browne **Facilities** ⊕ 🍴 🏌 ♨ ☂ ▯🍴 ⚒ 🏌 ⚒ **Conf** Corporate Hospitality Days **Location** 5m SW of city centre S of A720
Hotel ★★★ 80% HL Best Western Braid Hills Hotel, 134 Braid Rd, EDINBURGH ☎ 0131 447 8888 67 en suite

Turnhouse 154 Turnhouse Rd EH12 0AD
☎ 0131 339 1014
e-mail: secretary@turnhousegc.com
web: www.turnhousegc.com
Challenging tree-lined course with numerous Par 4s in excess of 400yds. Large sloping greens give a real challenge and the golfer is virtually guaranteed to use all the clubs in the bag.
18 holes, 6171yds, Par 69, SSS 70, Course record 62.
Club membership 800.
Visitors Mon-Fri, Sun & BHs. Booking required Fri, Sun & BHs. Dress code.
Societies Booking required. **Green Fees** £30 per day/round (£38/£25 Sun & Sat). **Prof** John Murray **Course Designer** J Braid **Facilities** ⊕ 🍴 🏌 ☂ ▯🍴 ♨ 🏌 ⚒ 🏌 ⚒ **Conf** facs Corporate Hospitality Days **Location** 6m W of city centre N of A8
Hotel ★★★★ 76% HL Edinburgh Marriott Hotel, 111 Glasgow Rd, EDINBURGH ☎ 0131 334 9191 245 en suite

---

RATHO   **MAP 11 NT17**

Ratho Park EH28 8NX
☎ 0131 335 0068 & 335 0069 📠 0131 333 1752
e-mail: secretary@rathoparkgolfclub.co.uk
web: www.rathoparkgolfclub.co.uk
Easy walking parkland, with a converted mansion as the clubhouse.
18 holes, 5960yds, Par 69, SSS 68, Course record 62.
Club membership 850.
Visitors Mon-Sun & BHs. Booking required. Dress code. **Societies** Booking required. **Green Fees** £45 per day, £32 per round (£45 per round Sun & Sat). **Prof** Alan Pate **Course Designer** James Braid **Facilities** ⊕ 🍴 🏌 ☂ ▯🍴 ♨ **Conf** Corporate Hospitality Days **Location** 0.75m E, N of A71
Hotel ★★★★ 84% HL Norton House Hotel & Restaurant, Ingliston, EDINBURGH ☎ 0131 333 1275 47 en suite

---

SOUTH QUEENSFERRY   **MAP 11 NT17**

Dundas Parks Dundas Estate EH30 9SS
☎ 0131 331 4252
e-mail: cmkwood@btinternet.com
Parkland course situated on the estate of Dundas Castle, with excellent views. For 18 holes, the nine are played twice.
9 holes, 6100yds, Par 70, SSS 69, Course record 62.
Club membership 500.
Visitors Mon-Fri & BHs. Booking required. Dress code. **Societies** Booking required. **Green Fees** £15 per round. ♨ **Facilities** ⊕ by prior arrangement ♨ **Location** 0.5m S on A8000
Hotel BUD Premier Travel Inn (South Queensferry), Builyeon Rd, SOUTH QUEENSFERRY ☎ 08701 977094 46 en suite

---

FALKIRK   **MAP 11 NS88**

Falkirk Carmuirs, 136 Stirling Rd, Camelon FK2 7YP
☎ 01324 611061 (club) 📠 01324 639573 (Sec)
e-mail: falkirkgolfclub@btconnect.com
web: www.falkirkcarmuirsgolfclub.co.uk
Parkland with gorse and streams.
Carmuirs: 18 holes, 6230yds, Par 71, SSS 70, Course record 65. Club membership 800.
Visitors Sun-Fri & BHs. Dress code. **Societies** Booking required. **Green Fees** £35 per day, £25 per round (£50/£40 Sun). **Prof** Stewart Craig **Course Designer** James Braid **Facilities** ⊕ 🍴 🏌 ☂ ▯🍴 ♨ 🏌 ⚒ 🏌 **Conf** Corporate Hospitality Days **Location** 1.5m W on A9
Hotel ★★★★ 75% HL Macdonald Inchyra Grange Hotel, Grange Rd, POLMONT ☎ 01324 711911 101 en suite

---

LARBERT   **MAP 11 NS88**

Falkirk Tryst 86 Burnhead Rd FK5 4BD
☎ 01324 562054 📠 01324 562054
e-mail: falkirktrystgc@tiscali.co.uk
Links-type course, fairly level with trees and broom, well-bunkered. Winds can affect play.
18 holes, 6053yds, Par 70, SSS 69, Course record 62.
Club membership 850.
Visitors Sun-Fri & BHs. Booking required. Dress code. **Societies** booking required. **Green Fees** not confirmed. ♨ **Prof** Steven Dunsmore **Facilities** ⊕ 🏌 ☂ ▯🍴 ♨ 🏌 ⚒ 🏌 ⚒ **Location** On A88
Hotel ★★★★ 75% HL Macdonald Inchyra Grange Hotel, Grange Rd, POLMONT ☎ 01324 711911 101 en suite

Glenbervie Stirling Rd FK5 4SJ
☎ 01324 562605 📠 01324 551054
e-mail: secretary@glenberviegolfclub.com
web: www.glenberviegolfclub.com
Parkland course set amidst mature trees with outstanding views of the Ochil Hills
18 holes, 6438yds, Par 71, SSS 71, Course record 63.
Club membership 700.
Visitors Mon-Fri. Dress code. **Societies** Booking required. **Green Fees** £50 per day, £35 per round. **Prof** David Ross **Course Designer** James Braid **Facilities** ⊕ 🍴 🏌 ☂ ▯🍴 ♨ 🏌 ⚒ **Conf** facs Corporate Hospitality Days **Location** 2m NW on A9
Hotel ★★★★ 75% HL Macdonald Inchyra Grange Hotel, Grange Rd, POLMONT ☎ 01324 711911 101 en suite

---

POLMONT   **MAP 11 NS97**

Grangemouth Polmont Hill FK2 0YE
☎ 01324 503840 📠 01324 503841
e-mail: greg.mcfarlane@falkirk.gov.uk
Windy parkland. Testing holes: 3rd, 4th (Par 4s); 5th (Par 5); 7th (Par 3) 216yds over reservoir (elevated green); 8th, 9th, 18th (Par 4s).
18 holes, 6314yds, Par 71, SSS 71, Course record 65.
Club membership 800.
Visitors Mon-Sun & BHs. Dress code. **Societies** Booking required. **Green Fees** £17 per round (£21 Sat & Sun). ♨ **Prof** Greg McFarlane **Facilities** ⊕ 🍴 🏌 ☂ ▯🍴 ♨ 🏌 ⚒ **Location** M9 junct 4, 0.5m N
Hotel ★★★★ 75% HL Macdonald Inchyra Grange Hotel, Grange Rd, POLMONT ☎ 01324 711911 101 en suite

Scotland

Polmont Manuelrigg, Maddiston FK2 0LS

☎ 01324 711277 🖷 01324 712504
e-mail: polmontgolfclub@btconnect.com
Hilly parkland with small greens protected by bunkers. Views of the
River Forth and the Ochil Hills.
9 holes, 3073yds, Par 72, SSS 69, Course record 66.
Club membership 300.
Visitors Mon-Fri, Sun & BHs. Dress code. **Societies** Welcome. **Green Fees**
£10 per round (weekends £15). 🍴 **Facilities** ⑪ by prior arrangement
🍴 by prior arrangement 🛄 by prior arrangement ⌷ ⚞ ⛳ **Conf** facs
Location A805 from Falkirk, 1st right after fire brigade headquarters
Hotel ★★★★ 75% HL Macdonald Inchyra Grange Hotel, Grange Rd,
POLMONT ☎ 01324 711911 101 en suite

FIFE

ABERDOUR   MAP 11 NT18

Aberdour Seaside Place KY3 0TX

☎ 01383 860080 🖷 01383 860050
e-mail: manager@aberdourgolfclub.co.uk
web: www.aberdourgolfclub.co.uk
Parkland with lovely views over Firth of Forth.

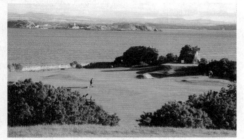

18 holes, 5460yds, Par 67, SSS 66, Course record 59.
Club membership 800.
Visitors Mon-Fri, Sun & BHs. Booking required. Dress code. **Societies**
Booking required. **Green Fees** £35 per day, £25 per round (£40
Sun). **Prof** David Gemmell **Facilities** ⑪ 🍴 🛄 ⌷ ⚞ 🎒 ⛳ ⚞
Location S side of village
Hotel ★★ 69% HL Aberdour Hotel, 38 High St, ABERDOUR
☎ 01383 860325 12 en suite 4 annexe en suite

ANSTRUTHER   MAP 12 NO50

Anstruther Marsfield, Shore Rd KY10 3DZ

☎ 01333 310956 🖷 01333 310956
e-mail: captain@anstruthergolf.co.uk
web: anstruthergolf.co.uk
A tricky links course with some outstanding views of the river Forth.
The nine holes consist of four Par 4s and five Par 3s. The 5th hole is
rated one of the hardest Par 3s anywhere, measuring 235yds from the
medal tees.
9 holes, 2249yds, Par 62, SSS 63, Course record 60.
Club membership 550.
Visitors Mon-Sun. Booking required Sat & Sun. Dress code. **Societies**
Booking required. **Green Fees** £20 per round, £14 for 9 holes. 🍴 **Course**
Designer Tom Morris **Facilities** ⑪ 🍴 🛄 ⌷ ⚞ ⛳ **Location** Turn
right at Craw's Hotel, SW off A917
Hotel ★★ 68% SHL Balcomie Links Hotel, Balcomie Rd, CRAIL
☎ 01333 450237 15 rms (13 en suite)

BURNTISLAND   MAP 11 NT28

Burntisland Golf House Club Dodhead, Kirkcaldy Rd
KY3 9LQ

☎ 01592 874093 (Office) & 872116 (Golf)
🖷 01592 873247
e-mail: infobghc@aol.com
web: www.burntislandgolfhouseclub.co.uk
A lush, testing course offering magnificent views over the Forth estuary.

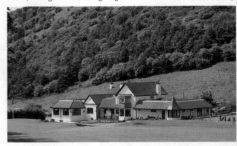

18 holes, 5965yds, Par 70, SSS 70, Course record 62.
Club membership 800.
Visitors Mon-Sun & BHs. Booking required. Dress code. **Societies** Booking
required. **Green Fees** £30 per day; £25 per round (£42/£35 weekends).
Prof Paul Wytrazek **Course Designer** Willie Park Jnr **Facilities** ⑪ 🍴
🛄 ⌷ ⚞ 🛄 ⚞ 🎒 ⚞ ⚞ ⛳ **Conf** facs Corporate Hospitality Days
Location 1m E on B923
Hotel ★★ 79% HL Inchview Hotel, 65-69 Kinghorn Rd, BURNTISLAND
☎ 01592 872239 16 en suite

COLINSBURGH   MAP 12 NO40

Charleton Golf & Country Club Charleton KY9 1HG

☎ 01333 340505 🖷 01333 340583
e-mail: clubhouse@charleton.co.uk
web: www.charleton.co.uk
Parkland with wonderful views over the Firth of Forth.
18 holes, 6443yds, Par 72, SSS 72, Course record 64.
Club membership 400.
Visitors Mon-Sun & BHs. Booking requested. **Societies** Booking required.
Green Fees £44 per day, £27 per round (£54/£32 Sat & Sun). **Prof** George
Finlayson **Course Designer** J Salvesen **Facilities** ⑪ 🍴 🛄 ⌷ ⚞ 🛄 ⚞
⚞ ⛳ **Location** Off B942, NW of Colinsburgh

COWDENBEATH   MAP 11 NT19

Cowdenbeath Seco Place KY4 8PD

☎ 01383 511918
A parkland-based 18 hole golf course.
Dora Course: 18 holes, 6300yds, Par 71, SSS 71,
Course record 64. Club membership 250.
Visitors Mon-Sun & BHs. Booking required. Dress code. **Societies** booking
required. **Green Fees** not confirmed. 🍴 **Facilities** ⑪ 🍴 ⌷ ⚞ 🛄 ⚞ 🎒
Location Off A92 into Cowdenbeath, 2nd right signed
Hotel ★★ 69% HL Aberdour Hotel, 38 High St, ABERDOUR
☎ 01383 860325 12 en suite 4 annexe en suite

CRAIL
MAP 12 NO60

Crail Golfing Society Balcomie Clubhouse, Fifeness KY10 3XN
☎ 01333 450686 & 450960 📠 01333 450416
e-mail: info@crailgolfingsociety.co.uk
web: www.crailgolfingsociety.co.uk
Perched on the edge of the North Sea, the Crail Golfing Society's courses at Balcomie are picturesque and sporting. Crail Golfing Society began its life in 1786 and the course is highly thought of by students of the game both for its testing holes and the standard of its greens. Craighead Links has panoramic seascape and country views. With wide sweeping fairways and USGA specification greens it is a testing but fair challenge.
Balcomie Links: 18 holes, 5922yds, Par 69, SSS 70, Course record 62.
Craighead Links: 18 holes, 6700yds, Par 72, SSS 74, Course record 69. Club membership 1600.
Visitors Mon-Sun & BHs. Booking required. Dress code **Societies** Booking required. **Green Fees** Balcomie £65 per day, (£78 Sat & Sun). Craighead Balcomie £55 per day, £40 per round (£68/£50 Sat & Sun). **Prof** Graeme Lennie **Course Designer** Tom Morris **Facilities** ⑪ ⑩ ⓛ ☐ ☰ ⚑ ☂ ▲ ☎ ⚐ ⚐ ⚑ **Location** 2m NE off A917
Hotel ★★ 68% SHL Balcomie Links Hotel, Balcomie Rd, CRAIL ☎ 01333 450237 15 rms (13 en suite)
Hotel ★★★★ 81% GA The Spindrift, Pittenweem Rd, ANSTRUTHER ☎ 01333 310573 Fax 01333 310573 8 rms (7 en suite)

CUPAR
MAP 11 NO31

Cupar Hilltarvit KY15 5JT
☎ 01334 653549 📠 01334 653549
e-mail: cupargc@fsmail.net
web: www.cupargolfclub.co.uk
Hilly parkland with fine views over north-east Fife. The 5th/14th hole is most difficult - uphill into the prevailing wind. Said to be the oldest nine-hole club in the UK.
9 holes, 5153yds, Par 68, SSS 66, Course record 61. Club membership 400.
Visitors Mon-Sun & BHs. Booking required Sat. **Societies** Booking required. **Green Fees** £20 per day. ⊛ **Course Designer** Allan Robertson **Facilities** ⑪ ⓛ ☐ ⚑ ▲ ⚐ **Location** 0.75m S off A92

Elmwood Stratheden KY15 5RS
☎ 01334 658780 📠 01334 658781
e-mail: clubhouse@elmwood.co.uk
web: www.elmwoodgc.co.uk
A new parkland course set in a rural location, offering fine views of the Lomond Hills to the west and the Tarvit Hills to the east.
18 holes, 5653yds, Par 70, SSS 68. Club membership 750.
Visitors Mon-Sun & BHs. Booking required. Dress code. **Societies** Booking required. **Green Fees** £22 per round (£25 Sat, Sun & BHs). **Prof** Graeme McDowall **Course Designer** John Salveson **Facilities** ⑪ ⑩ ⓛ ☐ ⚑ ▲ ☰ ⚐ ⚐ **Conf** facs Corporate Hospitality Days **Location** M90 junct 8, A91 to St Andrews, 0.5m before Cupar. At Wisemans Dairy right, right at next junct, course 400yds on left

DUNFERMLINE
MAP 11 NT08

Canmore Venturefair Av KY12 0PE
☎ 01383 724969 📠 01383 731649
e-mail: canmoregolfclub@aol.com
web: www.canmoregolf.co.uk
Parkland course with excellent turf, moderate in length but a good test of accuracy demanding a good short game. Ideal for 36-hole play, and suitable for all ages.
18 holes, 5376yds, Par 67, SSS 66, Course record 61. Club membership 650.
Visitors contact club for more details. Dress code. **Societies** booking required. **Green Fees** not confirmed. **Prof** Daryn Cochrane **Course Designer** Ben Sayers & others **Facilities** ⑪ ⑩ ⓛ ☐ ⚑ ▲ ☰ ⚐ ⚐ **Location** 1m N on A823
Hotel ★★★ 79% HL Best Western Keavil House Hotel, Crossford, DUNFERMLINE ☎ 01383 736258 47 en suite

Dunfermline Pitfirrane, Crossford KY12 8QW
☎ 01383 723534 & 729061 📠 01383 723547
e-mail: secretary@dunfermlinegolfclub.com
web: www.dunfermlinegolfclub.com
Gently undulating parkland course with interesting contours. Five Par 5s, five Par 3s. No water hazards. Centre of the course is a disused walled garden, which is a haven for wildlife.
18 holes, 6121yds, Par 72, SSS 70, Course record 65. Club membership 720.
Visitors Sun-Fri & BHs. Booking required. Dress code. **Societies** booking required. **Green Fees** not confirmed. ⊛ **Prof** Chris Nugent **Course Designer** J R Stutt **Facilities** ⑪ ⑩ ⓛ ☐ ⚑ ▲ ☰ ⚐ ⚐ **Location** 2m W of Dunfermline on A994
Hotel ★★★ 79% HL Best Western Keavil House Hotel, Crossford, DUNFERMLINE ☎ 01383 736258 47 en suite

Forrester Park Pitdinnie Rd, Cairneyhill KY12 8RF
☎ 01383 880505 📠 01383 882505
e-mail: forresterpark@aol.com
web: www.forresterparkresort.com
Set in the heart of 350 acres of parkland on what was originally the Keavil Estate. Ponds and streams come into play on 9 holes and all greens have been constructed to USGA specifications.
18 holes, 7000yds, Par 72, SSS 74, Course record 69. Club membership 700.
Visitors Mon-Sun & BHs. Booking required Sat/Sun & BHs. Dress code. **Societies** welcome. **Green Fees** not confirmed. ⊛ **Prof** R Forrester **Facilities** ⑪ ⑩ ⓛ ☐ ⚑ ▲ ☰ ⚐ ⚐ ⚑ **Location** 2.5m W of Dunfermline in village of Cairneyhill
Hotel ★★★ 79% HL Best Western Keavil House Hotel, Crossford, DUNFERMLINE ☎ 01383 736258 47 en suite

Pitreavie Queensferry Rd KY11 8PR
☎ 01383 722591 📠 01383 722592
e-mail: secpdgc@btconnect.com
Picturesque woodland course with panoramic view of the Forth valley. Testing golf.
18 holes, 6086yds, Par 70, SSS 69, Course record 64. Club membership 700.
Visitors contact club for details. Dress code. **Societies** booking required. **Green Fees** not confirmed. ⊛ **Prof** Paul Brookes **Course Designer** Dr Alister McKenzie **Facilities** ⑪ ⑩ ⓛ ☐ ⚑ ▲ ☰ ⚐ **Conf** Corporate Hospitality Days **Location** SE side of town on A823
Hotel ★★★ 70% HL King Malcolm Hotel, Queensferry Rd, DUNFERMLING ☎ 01383 722611 48 en suite

Scotland

ELIE
MAP 12 NO40

Golf House Club KY9 1AS
☎ 01333 330301 🖹 01333 330895
e-mail: secretary@golfhouseclub.org
web: www.golfhouseclub.org
One of Scotland's most delightful holiday courses with panoramic views over the Firth of Forth. Some of the holes out towards the rocky coastline are splendid. This is the course which has produced many good professionals, including James Braid.
18 holes, 6273yds, Par 70, SSS 70, Course record 62.
Club membership 600.
Visitors Mon-Sun & BHs. Booking required. Handicap certificate. Dress code. **Societies** Booking required. **Green Fees** £80 per day, £60 per round (£90/£70 Sat & Sun). **Prof** Ian Muir **Facilities** ⑪ ⑩ ⓛ ▭ ◻ 🍴 △ 🏠 ⛳ ♂ 🌀 **Leisure** hard tennis courts. **Location** W side of village off A917

FALKLAND
MAP 11 NO20

Falkland The Myre KY15 7AA
☎ 01337 857404
A flat, well-kept course with excellent greens and views of East Lomond Hill and Falkland Palace.
9 holes, 4988yds, Par 67, SSS 65, Course record 62.
Visitors Mon-Fri. **Societies** must contact in advance. **Green Fees** Phone. 🐾 **Facilities** ⑪ by prior arrangement ⓛ ▭ 🍴 △ **Location** N side of town on A912
Hotel ★★★★ HL Balbirnie House, Balbirnie Park, MARKINCH
☎ 01592 610066 30 en suite

GLENROTHES
MAP 11 NO20

Glenrothes Golf Course Rd KY6 2LA
☎ 01592 754561 🖹 01592 754561
e-mail: secretary@glenrothesgolf.org.uk
web: www.glenrothesgolf.org.uk
Mature parkland, challenging back nine with burn crossing four fairways. Wide fairways offer opportunities for long hitters and birdy chances for those with good short game.
18 holes, 6444yds, Par 71, SSS 71, Course record 67.
Club membership 750.
Green Fees Phone. 🐾 **Course Designer** J R Stutt **Facilities** ⑪ ⑩ ⓛ ▭ 🍴 △ 🏠 ⛳ ♂ **Location** W side of town off B921
Hotel ★★★★ HL Balbirnie House, Balbirnie Park, MARKINCH
☎ 01592 610066 30 en suite

KINCARDINE
MAP 11 NS98

Tulliallan Alloa Rd FK10 4BB
☎ 01259 730798 🖹 01259 733950
e-mail: tulliallangolf@btconnect.com
web: www.tulliallangolf.co.uk
Pleasant parkland with scenic views of the Ochil Hills and the River Forth. A burn meanders through the course, which combined with maturing trees make this a challenging test of golf. The course is renowned for it's true greens.
18 holes, 5965yds, Par 69, SSS 69, Course record 63.
Club membership 700.
Visitors Mon-Fri, Sun & BHs. Dress code. **Societies** Booking required. **Green Fees** £36 per day, £22 per round (£45 Sun). **Prof** Steven Kelly

Facilities ⑪ ⑩ ⓛ ▭ ◻ 🍴 △ 🏠 ⛳ ♂ **Conf** facs Corporate Hospitality Days **Location** 1m NW on A977
Hotel BUD Premier Travel Inn Falkirk North, Bowtrees Farm, KINCARDINE BRIDGE ☎ 08701 977099 40 en suite

KINGHORN
MAP 11 NT28

Kinghorn Macduff Cres KY3 9RE
☎ 01592 890345 & 890978
Municipal course, 300ft above sea level with views over the Firth of Forth and the North Sea. Undulating and quite testing. Facilities shared by Kinghorn Ladies.
18 holes, 5269yds, Par 65, SSS 67, Course record 62.
Club membership 190.
Visitors Mon-Sun & BHs. Booking required Sat & Sun. **Societies** Booking required. **Green Fees** £19 per round, £30 per day (£24/£42 Sat & Sun). 🐾 **Course Designer** Tom Morris **Facilities** ▭ 🍴 △ **Location** S side of town on A921
Hotel ★★★ 72% HL Dean Park Hotel, Chapel Level, KIRKCALDY
☎ 01592 261635 34 en suite 12 annexe en suite

KIRKCALDY
MAP 11 NT29

Dunnikier Park Dunnikier Way KY1 3LP
☎ 01592 261599 🖹 01592 642541
e-mail: dunnikierparkgolfclub@btinternet.com
Parkland, rolling fairways, not heavily bunkered, views of the Firth of Forth.
18 holes, 6036metres, Par 72, SSS 72, Course record 65.
Club membership 700.
Visitors Mon-Sun & BHs. Booking required. Dress code. **Societies** Booking required. **Green Fees** Phone. 🐾 **Prof** Gregor Whyte **Course Designer** R Stutt **Facilities** ⑪ ⑩ ⓛ ▭ ◻ 🍴 △ 🏠 ⛳ **Conf** facs Corporate Hospitality Days **Location** 2m N on B981, next to Kirkcaldy High School
Hotel ★★★ 72% HL Dean Park Hotel, Chapel Level, KIRKCALDY
☎ 01592 261635 34 en suite 12 annexe en suite

Kirkcaldy Balwearie Rd KY2 5LT
☎ 01592 205240 & 203258 (Pro Shop) 🖹 01592 205240
e-mail: enquiries@kirkcaldygolfclub.co.uk
web: kirkcaldygolfclub.co.uk
A challenging parkland course in countryside, with beautiful views. A burn meanders by five holes. The club celebrated its centenary in 2004.
18 holes, 6086yds, Par 71, SSS 69, Course record 65.
Club membership 892.
Visitors Mon-Sun & BHs. Booking required. Dress code. **Societies** welcome. **Green Fees** not confirmed. **Prof** Anthony Caira **Course Designer** Tom Morris **Facilities** ⑪ ⑩ ⓛ ▭ ◻ 🍴 △ 🏠 ⛳ ♂ 🍽 ♂ **Conf** facs Corporate Hospitality Days **Location** SW side of town off A910
Hotel ★★★ 72% HL Dean Park Hotel, Chapel Level, KIRKCALDY
☎ 01592 261635 34 en suite 12 annexe en suite

LADYBANK
MAP 11 NO30

Ladybank Annsmuir KY15 7RA
☎ 01337 830814 📠 01337 831505
e-mail: info@ladybankgolf.co.uk
web: www.ladybankgolf.co.uk

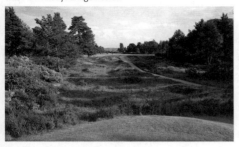

18 holes, 6601yds, Par 71, SSS 72, Course record 63.
Course Designer Tom Morris **Location** N of town off A92
Telephone for further details
Hotel ★★★ 74% HL Fernie Castle, Letham, CUPar ☎ 01337 810381
20 en suite

LESLIE
MAP 11 NO20

Leslie Balsillie Laws KY6 3EZ
☎ 01592 620040
9 holes, 4686yds, Par 63, SSS 64, Course record 63.
Course Designer Tom Morris **Location** N side of town off A911
Telephone for further details

LEUCHARS
MAP 12 NO42

Drumoig Hotel & Golf Course Drumoig KY16 0BE
☎ 01382 541800 (Starter) & 541898 📠 01382 541898
e-mail: drumoig@btconnect.com
web: www.drumoigleisure.com
A developing but challenging young championship course. Set in
a parkland environment, the course is links-like in places. Features
include Whinstone Quarries and views over to St Andrews and
Carnoustie. Water features are demanding, especially on the 9th where
the fairway runs between Drumoig's two tiny lochs.
18 holes, 6835yds, Par 72, SSS 73, Course record 67.
Club membership 350.
Visitors Mon-Sun & BHs. Booking required Sat, Sun & BHs. Dress code
Societies Booking required **Green Fees** £26 per day, £18 per round (£38/£30
Sat & Sun). **Facilities** ⑪ ⑩ ⓑ ♨ 🏌 🏌 🍴 ⛳ **Conf** Corporate
Hospitality Days **Location** On A914 between St Andrews & Dundee
Hotel ★★★★ HL Rufflets Country House & Garden Restaurant,
Strathkinness Low Rd, ST ANDREWS ☎ 01334 472594 19 en suite
5 annexe en suite

St Michaels KY16 0DX
☎ 01334 839365 📠 01334 838789
e-mail: honsec@stmichaelsgolf.co.uk
web: www.stmichaelsgolf.co.uk
Parkland with open views over Fife and Tayside. The undulating course
weaves its way through tree plantations. The short Par 4 17th, parallel
to the railway and over a pond to a stepped green, poses an interesting
challenge.

18 holes, 5802yds, Par 70, SSS 68, Course record 66.
Club membership 500.
Visitors Mon-Sun & BHs. Booking required. Dress code. **Societies** Booking
required. **Green Fees** Phone. **Facilities** ⑪ ⑩ by prior arrangement ⓑ ♨
🏌 🏌 ⚑ ⛳ **Location** NW side of village on A919

LEVEN
MAP 11 NO30

Leven Links The Promenade KY8 4HS
☎ 01333 428859 & 421390 📠 01333 428859
e-mail: secretary@leven-links.com
web: www.leven-links.com
Leven has the classic ingredients which make up a golf links in
Scotland; undulating fairways with hills and hollows, out of bounds
and a burn or stream. Turning into the prevailing west wind at
the 13th leaves the golfer with a lot of work to do before one
of the finest finishing holes in golf. A top class championship links
course used for Open final qualifying stages, it has fine views over
Largo Bay.

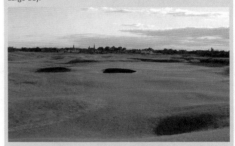

18 holes, 6506yds, Par 71, SSS 72, Course record 63.
Club membership 1000.
Visitors Mon-Fri, Sun & BHs. Booking required Fri & Sun. Dress code.
Societies Welcome. **Green Fees** £60 per day, £45 per round (weekends
£70/£55). **Course Designer** Tom Morris **Facilities** ⑪ ⑩ ⓑ ♨ 🏌 🏌
🍴 ⛳

Scoonie North Links KY8 4SP
☎ 01333 307007 & 423437 (Starter) 📠 01333 307008
e-mail: manager@scooniegolfclub.com
web: www.scooniegolfclub.com
A pleasant inland links course suitable for all ages.
18 holes, 5494mtrs, Par 67, SSS 66, Course record 62.
Club membership 200.
Visitors contact club for details. **Societies** welcome. **Green Fees** not
confirmed. ⓦ **Facilities** ⑪ ⓑ ♨ 🏌 🏌

LOCHGELLY
MAP 11 NT19

Lochgelly Cartmore Rd KY5 9PB
☎ 01592 780174
Easy walking parkland, often windy.
18 holes, 5491yds, Par 68, SSS 67, Course record 62.
Club membership 300.
Visitors Mon-Sun & BHs. Booking required. Handicap certificate. Dress
code. **Societies** Booking required. **Green Fees** Phone. ⓦ **Prof** Martin
Goldie **Course Designer** Ian Marchbanks **Facilities** ⑪ ⑩ ⓑ ♨ 🏌 🏌 ⓐ
🍴 ⛳ **Location** W side of town off A910
Hotel ★★★ 72% HL Dean Park Hotel, Chapel Level, KIRKCALDY
☎ 01592 261635 34 en suite 12 annexe en suite

Scotland

Lochore Meadows Lochore Meadows Country Park, Crosshill, Lochgelly KY5 8BA

☎ 01592 414300 📠 01592 414345
e-mail: info@lochore-meadows.co.uk
web: www.lochore-meadows.co.uk
Lochside course with a stream running through it and woodland nearby. Country park offers many leisure facilities.
9 holes, 3207yds, Par 72, SSS 71. Club membership 240.
Visitors Mon-Sun & BHs. Booking required. Dress code. **Societies** booking required. **Green Fees** not confirmed. ⊕ **Facilities** ⊕ ♡ ⚲
Leisure fishing, outdoor education centre, childrens play park. **Conf** facs
Location 0.5m W off B920
Hotel ★★★★ 75% HL The Green Hotel, 2 The Muirs, KINROSS
☎ 01577 863467 46 en suite

LUNDIN LINKS   MAP 12 NO40

Lundin Golf Rd KY8 6BA

☎ 01333 320202 📠 01333 329743
e-mail: secretary@lundingolfclub.co.uk
web: www.lundingolfclub.co.uk
A complex links course with open burns, an internal out of bounds(the old railway line), and strategic bunkering. Lundin presents a challenge for the thinking golfer where position from the tee rather than distance will yield just rewards on the scorecard. Renowned for its beautiful greens and some of the most demanding short Par 4's in the game of golf.

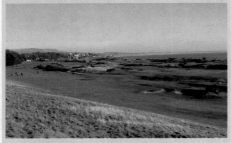

18 holes, 6371yds, Par 71, SSS 71, Course record 63.
Club membership 895.
Visitors Mon-Sun & BHs. Booking required. Dress code. **Societies** Booking required. **Green Fees** £65 per day, £47 per round (£50 Sat & Sun). **Prof** David Webster **Course Designer** James Braid **Facilities** ⊕
🅞 🖢 ♡ ⏳ ⚲ 🖴 ✂ **Location** W side of village off A915

Lundin Ladies Woodielea Rd KY8 6AR

☎ 01333 320832 & 320022
e-mail: llgolfclub@tiscali.co.uk
web: www.lundinladies.co.uk
Short, lowland course with Bronze Age standing stones on the second fairway and coastal views.
9 holes, 2365yds, Par 68, SSS 68, Course record 64.
Club membership 350.
Visitors Mon-Sun. Booking required Wed. **Societies** Booking required.
Green Fees Phone. ⊕ **Course Designer** James Braid **Facilities** ♡ ⚲ ✂
Location W side of village off A915

MARKINCH   MAP 11 NO20

Balbirnie Park Balbirnie Park KY7 6NR

☎ 01592 612095 & 752006 (tee times)
📠 01592 612383/752006
e-mail: craigfdonnelly@aol.com
web: www.balbirniegolf.com
Set in the magnificent Balbirnie Park, a fine example of the best in traditional parkland design, with natural contours the inspiration behind the layout. A course that will suit all standards of golfers.

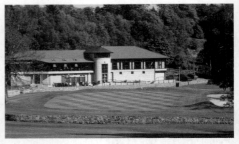

18 holes, 6214yds, Par 71, SSS 71, Course record 66.
Club membership 900.
Visitors Mon-Sun & BHs. Booking required. Dress code. **Societies** Booking required. **Green Fees** £40 per round, £50 per day (£45/£60 Sat & Sun). **Prof** Craig Donnelly **Course Designer** Fraser Middleton **Facilities** ⊕
🅞 🖢 ♡ 🖘 ⏳ ⚲ 🖴 ⚲ ◇ ✂ 🖴 ✂ **Conf** facs Corporate Hospitality Days
Location 2m E of Glenrothes, off A92
Hotel ★★★★ HL Balbirnie House, Balbirnie Park, MARKINCH
☎ 01592 610066 30 en suite

ST ANDREWS   MAP 12 NO51

British Golf Museum

☎ 01334 460046 (situated opposite Royal & Ancient Golf Club)
The museum which tells the history of golf from its origins to the present day, is of interest to golfers and non-golfers alike. Themed galleries and interactive displays explore the history of the major championships and the lives of the famous players, and trace the development of golfing equipment.
Open Mar-Oct, Mon-Sat 9.30am-5.30pm Sun 10am-5pm (Nov-Mar, Mon-Sun 10am-4pm). **Admission** There is a charge. ☎ for details.

CHAMPIONSHIP COURSE

FIFE — ST ANDREWS

ST ANDREWS LINKS

Map 12 NO51

Pilmour House KY16 9SF
☎ 01334 466666 📄 01334 479555
e-mail: linkstrust@standrews.org.uk
web: www.standrews.org.uk
Old Course: 18 holes, 6609yds, Par 72, SSS 72, Course record 62.
New Course: 18 holes, 6604yds, Par 71, SSS 73.
Jubilee Course: 18 holes, 6742yds, Par 72, SSS 73, Course record 63.
Eden Course: 18 holes, 6112yds, Par 70, SSS 70.
Strathtyrum Course: 18 holes, 5094yds, Par 69, SSS 69.
Balgove Course: 9 holes, 1530yds, Par 30, SSS 30.
Visitors Old Course: contact course for booking details. Handicap certificate required. Other courses: 1 month advance booking required New/Jubilee/Eden/Strath. **Societies** booking required. **Green Fees** Old £59-£120 according to season. New £28-£57. Jubilee £28-£57. Eden £17-£34. Strathtyrum £11-£23. Balgove £7-£10.
Prof Steve North **Facilities** ⑪ ⑩ 🏨 🖵 🍴 🏌
🍴 🚄 🔧 🏌 **Conf** Corporate Hospitality Days
Location Off A91

Golf was first played here around 1400 and the Old Course is acknowledged worldwide as the home of golf. The Old Course has played host to the greatest golfers in the world and many of golf's most dramatic moments. The New Course (6604yds) was opened in 1895, having been laid out by Old Tom Morris. The Jubilee was opened in 1897 and is 6805yds long from the medal tees. A shorter version of the Jubilee Course is also available, known as the Bronze Course, measuring 5674yds. There is no handicap limit for the shorter course and it is best for lower and middle handicap golfers. The Starthtyrum has a shorter, less testing layout, best for high handicap golfers. The nine-hole Balgrove Course, upgraded and re-opened in 1993, is best for beginners and children. The facilities and courses at St Andrews make this the largest golf complex in Europe.

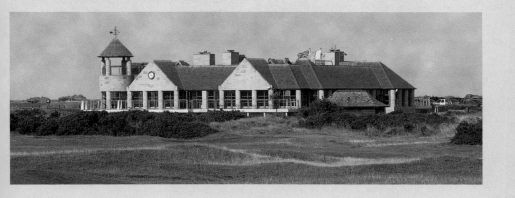

The Duke's Course Craigtoun KY16 8NS
☎ 01334 474371 📄 01334 479456
e-mail: reservations@oldcoursehotel.co.uk
web: www.oldcoursehotel.co.uk
Now owned and managed by the Old Course Hotel, with a spectacular setting above St Andrews. Blending the characteristics of a links course with an inland course, Duke's offers rolling fairways, undulating greens and a testing woodland section, and magnificent views over St Andrews Bay towards Carnoustie. Five separate tees at every hole and buggy paths running throughout the course.

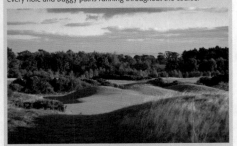

18 holes, 6749yds, Par 71, SSS 73, Course record 67. Club membership 500.
Visitors Mon-Sun & BHs. Booking required. Dress code **Societies** booking required. **Green Fees** not confirmed. **Prof** Ron Walker **Course Designer** Tim Liddy **Facilities** ⊕ ⊘ 🍴 🛒 ♨ 🏊 ⚑ **Leisure** heated indoor swimming pool, sauna, solarium, gymnasium, computer swing analyses. **Conf** facs Corporate Hospitality Days **Location** A91 to St Andrews, turn off for Strathkiness
Hotel ★★★★★ HL The Old Course Hotel, Golf Resort & Spa, ST ANDREWS ☎ 01334 474371 144 en suite

Fairmont St Andrews KY16 8PN
☎ 01334 837000 📄 01334 471115
e-mail: standrews.scotland@fairmont.com
web: www.fairmont.com
The Torrance course is a traditional Scottish layout, which works its way around the hotel before bursting open to reveal a cross section of the remaining 12 holes, which wind down towards the coastal edge. The Devlin is a stunning clifftop course with unique characteristics and requiring a well-devised strategy of play. One of the longest courses in the UK.

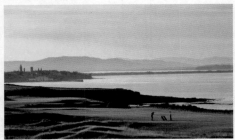

Torrance: 18 holes, 7037yds, Par 72, SSS 74.
Devlin: 18 holes, 7049yds, Par 72, SSS 74.
Visitors Mon-Sun & BHs. Booking required. Dress code. **Societies** Booking required. **Green Fees** £45-£95. **Prof** John Kerr **Course Designer** Sam Torrance/Gene Sarazen **Facilities** ⊕ ⊘ 🍴 🛒 ♨ 🏊 ⚑

Leisure heated indoor swimming pool, sauna, gymnasium. **Conf** facs Corporate Hospitality Days
Hotel ★★★★★ 83% HL Fairmont St Andrews, ST ANDREWS ☎ 01334 837000 209 en suite 8 annexe en suite

St Andrews Links see page 341
Hotel ★★★★★ HL The Old Course Hotel, Golf Resort & Spa, ST ANDREWS ☎ 01334 474371 144 en suite
Hotel ★★★ HL St Andrews Golf Hotel, 40 The Scores, ST ANDREWS ☎ 01334 472611 Fax 01334 472188 22 en suite
Hotel ★★★★ HL Rufflets Country House & Garden Restaurant, Strathkinness Low Rd, ST ANDREWS ☎ 01334 472594 Fax 01334 478703 19 en suite 5 annexe en suite
Hotel ★★★★★ 83% HL Fairmont St Andrews, ST ANDREWS ☎ 01334 837000 Fax 01334 471115 209 en suite 8 annexe en suite
Hotel ★★★★ 72% HL Macdonald Rusacks Hotel, Pilmour Links, ST ANDREWS ☎ 0870 400 8128 Fax 01334 477896 68 en suite
Hotel ★★★ 74% HL Best Western Scores Hotel, 76 The Scores, ST ANDREWS ☎ 01334 472451 Fax 01334 473947 30 en suite

SALINE   MAP 11 NT09
Saline Kinneddar Hill KY12 9LT
☎ 01383 852591 📄 01383 852591
e-mail: salinegolfclub@btconnect.com
web: www.saline-golf-club.co.uk
Hillside parkland course with excellent turf and panoramic view of the Forth Valley.
9 holes, 5384yds, Par 68, SSS 66, Course record 62. Club membership 300.
Visitors Mon-Fri, Sun & BHs. Booking required Sun. Handicap certificate. Dress code. **Societies** Booking required. **Green Fees** £7.50 per 9 holes, £11.50 per 18 holes (£14 Sun). 🍴 **Facilities** ⊕ by prior arrangement 🍴 by prior arrangement 🛒 ♨ 🏊 ⚑ **Location** M90 junct 4,7m W following signs for Dollar
Hotel ★★★ 70% HL King Malcolm Hotel, Queensferry Rd, DUNFERMLING ☎ 01383 722611 48 en suite

TAYPORT   MAP 12 NO42
Scotscraig Golf Rd DD6 9DZ
☎ 01382 552515 📄 01382 553130
e-mail: scotscraig@scotscraiggolfclub.com
web: www.scotscraiggolfclub.com
Combined with heather and rolling fairways, the course is part heathland, part links, with the greens being renowned for being fast and true.
18 holes, 6550yds, Par 71, SSS 72, Course record 62. Club membership 835.
Visitors Mon-Sun & BHs. Booking required. Dress code. **Societies** Booking required. **Green Fees** £65 per day, £47 per round (£80/£60am/ £52pm Sat & Sun). **Prof** Craig Mackie **Course Designer** James Braid **Facilities** ⊕ ⊘ 🍴 🛒 ♨ 🏊 ⚑ **Conf** Corporate Hospitality Days **Location** S side of village off B945
Hotel ★★ 68% HL Sandford Country House Hotel, Newton Hill, Wormit, DUNDEE ☎ 01382 541802 16 en suite

THORNTON
MAP 11 NT29

Thornton Station Rd KY1 4DW
☎ 01592 771111 📠 01592 774955
e-mail: thorntongolf@btconnect.com
web: www.thorntongolfclubfife.co.uk
A relatively flat, lightly tree-lined parkland course, bounded on three sides by a river that comes into play at holes 14 to 16.
18 holes, 6170yds, Par 70, SSS 69, Course record 61.
Club membership 700.
Visitors Mon-Sun & BHs. Booking required. Dress code. **Societies** Booking required. **Green Fees** £35 per day, £25 per round (£50/£35 Fri-Sun). ⊜
Facilities ⊗ ⦶ ⓛ 🝤 ⚒ 🝲 ♣ **Conf** Corporate Hospitality Days
Location 1m E of town off A92
Hotel ★★★★ HL Balbirnie House, Balbirnie Park, MARKINCH
☎ 01592 610066   30 en suite

CITY OF GLASGOW

GLASGOW
MAP 11 NS56

Alexandra Alexandra Park, Alexandra Pde G31 8SE
☎ 0141 556 1294
Hilly parkland with some woodland. Many bunkers and a barrier of trees between 1st and 9th fairway. Work has been in progress to improve the fairways.
9 holes, 2800yds, Par 31, Course record 25.
Club membership 85.
Visitors Mon-Sun & BHs. Booking required Sat, Sun & BHs **Societies** Welcome. **Green Fees** Phone. ⊛ **Course Designer** G McArthur **Facilities** ⚒ **Leisure** bowling green. **Location** 2m E of city centre off M8/A8

Cowglen Barrhead Rd G43 1AU
☎ 0141 632 0556 📠 01505 503000
e-mail: r.jamieson-accountants@rsmail.net
web: www.cowglengolfclub.co.uk
Undulating and challenging parkland course with good views over the Clyde valley to the Campsie Hills. Club and line selection is most important on many holes due to the strategic placing of copses on the course.

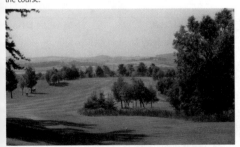

18 holes, 6053yds, Par 70, SSS 69, Course record 64.
Club membership 805.
Visitors Mon-Fri & BHs, Sun after 3pm. Handicap certificate. Dress code
Societies Booking required. **Green Fees** £35 per day, £27.50 per round.
⊛ **Prof** Simon Payne **Course Designer** David Adams/James Braid
Facilities ⊗ ⦶ ⓛ 🝤 ⚒ 🝲 ♣ **Conf** facs Corporate Hospitality
Days **Location** M77 S from Glasgow, Pollok/Barrhead slip road, left at lights club 0.5m right
Hotel BUD Travelodge Glasgow Paisley Road, 251 Paisley Rd, GLASGOW
☎ 08700 850 950   75 en suite

Haggs Castle 70 Dumbreck Rd, Dumbreck G41 4SN
☎ 0141 427 1157 📠 0141 427 1157
e-mail: secretary@haggscastlegolfclub.com
web: www.haggscastlegolfclub.com
Wooded, parkland course where Scottish National Championships and the Glasgow and Scottish Open have been held.
18 holes, 6426yds, Par 72, SSS 71, Course record 63.
Club membership 900.
Visitors Mon-Fri. Booking required. Handicap certificate. Dress code.
Societies Booking required. **Green Fees** £40 per round; £50 per day. **Prof** Campbell Elliott **Course Designer** Dave Thomas (1998)
Facilities ⊗ ⦶ ⓛ 🝤 ⚒ 🝲 ♣ **Conf** Corporate Hospitality Days **Location** M77 junct 1, 2.5m SW of city centre

Kirkhill Greenless Rd, Cambuslang G72 8YN
☎ 0141 641 8499 📠 0141 641 8499
e-mail: carol.downes@btconnect.com
web: www.kirkhillgolfclub.org.uk
Meadowland course designed by James Braid.
18 holes, 6030yds, Par 70, SSS 70, Course record 63.
Club membership 650.
Visitors Mon-Fri. Booking required. Handicap certificate. Dress code.
Societies Booking required. **Green Fees** Phone. **Prof** Duncan Williamson **Course Designer** J Braid **Facilities** ⊗ ⦶ ⓛ 🝤 ⚒ 🝲
Location 5m SE of city centre off A749
Hotel ★★★ 74% HL Bothwell Bridge Hotel, 89 Main St, BOTHWELL
☎ 01698 852246   90 en suite

Knightswood Lincoln Av G13 5QZ
☎ 0141 959 6358
9 holes, 5586yds, Par 68, SSS 67.
Location 4m W of city centre off A82
Telephone for further details
Hotel ★★★ 81% HL Best Western Glasgow Pond Hotel, Great Western Rd, GLASGOW ☎ 0141 334 8161   137 en suite

Lethamhill 1240 Cumbernauld Rd, Millerston G33 1AH
☎ 0141 770 6220 & 0141 770 7135 📠 1041 770 0520
18 holes, 5859yds, Par 70, SSS 69.
Location 3m NE of city centre on A80
Telephone for further details
Hotel ★★★★ 77% HL Millennium Hotel Glasgow, George Square, GLASGOW ☎ 0141 332 6711   117 en suite

Linn Park Simshill Rd G44 5EP
☎ 0141 633 0377
18 holes, 4952yds, Par 65, SSS 65, Course record 61.
Location 4m S of city centre off B766
Telephone for further details

Pollok 90 Barrhead Rd G43 1BG
☎ 0141 632 4351 📠 0141 649 1398
e-mail: secretary@pollokgolf.com
web: www.pollokgolf.com
Parkland with woods and river. Gentle walking until the 18th hole.
18 holes, 6358yds, Par 71, SSS 71, Course record 62.
Club membership 620.
Visitors Contact club for details. **Societies** Booking required.
Green Fees £50 per round. **Course Designer** J Douglas & Alistair McKenzie **Facilities** ⊗ ⓛ 🝤 ⚒ 🝲 ♣ **Conf** facs Corporate Hospitality Days **Location** M77 junct 2, S to A762 Barrhead Rd, 1m E

Williamwood Clarkston Rd G44 3YR
☎ 0141 637 1783 📠 0141 571 0166
e-mail: secretary@williamwoodgc.co.uk
Undulating parkland with mature woods.
18 holes, 5878yds, Par 68, SSS 69, Course record 61.
Club membership 800.
Visitors Mon-Thur. Booking required. Handicap certificate. Dress code.
Societies Booking required. **Green Fees** £40 per day, £30 per round. **Prof**
Stewart Marshall **Course Designer** James Braid **Facilities** ⊕ �🝙 ℔ ℗ ℡
⌖ 🛍 🏌 **Location** 5m S of city centre on B767

HIGHLAND

ALNESS   MAP 14 NH66

Alness Ardross Rd IV17 0QA
☎ 01349 883877
e-mail: info@alness-golfclub.co.uk
web: www.alness-golfclub.co.uk
A testing, parkland course with beautiful views over the Cromarty Firth
and the Black Isle. It is located on the north west edge of the village
of Alness and four holes run parallel to the gorge of the River Averon.
Golfers of all abilities will find the course interesting and challenging.
A particular test of skill is required at the 14th hole where the tee is
located far above the green which lies beside the gorge at a distance
of 406yds.
18 holes, 4886yds, Par 67, SSS 64, Course record 62.
Club membership 350.
Visitors Mon-Sun & BHS. Booking required Sat & Sun. **Societies** Welcome.
Green Fees £23 (£28 weekends). **Prof** Gary Lister **Facilities** ⊕ �🝙 ℔ ℗
℡ ⌖ 🛍 🏌 🍴 ✦ **Leisure** fishing. **Conf** facs Corporate Hospitality Days
Location 0.5m N off A9

ARISAIG   MAP 13 NM68

Traigh Traigh PH39 4NT
☎ 01687 450337 📠 01678 450293
web: www.traighgolf.co.uk
According to at least one newspaper Traigh is 'probably the most
beautifully sited nine-hole golf course in the world'. True or not,
Traigh lies alongside sandy beaches with views to Skye and the Inner
Hebrides. The feature of the course is a line of grassy hills, originally
sand dunes, that rise to some 60ft, and provide a challenge to the
keenest golfer.
9 holes, 2456yds, Par 68, SSS 65, Course record 67.
Club membership 150.
Visitors Mon-Sun & BHs. **Societies** Booking required. **Green Fees** £16
per day. ⊛ **Course Designer** John Salvesen 1994 **Facilities** ℗ 🛍 🍴
Location A830 to Arisaig, signed onto B8008, 2m N of Arisaig

AVIEMORE   MAP 14 NH81

Spey Valley Aviemore Highland Resort PH22 1PJ
☎ 01479 815100 📠 01479 812128
e-mail: golf@ahresort.co.uk
web: www.speyvalleygolf.com
Opened in Spring 2006 with a total length of 7200 yards and featuring
one of the longest Par 5 holes in the country, Creag Eabraich, which
measures 641 yards from the championship tee. Situated beneath the
Cairngorm Mountains with breathtaking views.
18 holes, 7153yds, Par 72. Club membership 300.

Visitors Mon-Sun & BHs. Handicap certificate. Dress code. **Societies**
Booking required. **Green Fees** Phone. **Course Designer** Dave Thomas
Facilities ⊕ �🝙 ℔ ℗ ℡ ⌖ 🛍 🏌 ✦ 🍴 ✦ **Conf** facs Corporate
Hospitality Days **Location** leave A9 signposted Aviemore on B970. Follow
road to village then turn off for Dalfaber and follow signs for golf course.
Guesthouse ★★★★ GH Ravenscraig Guest House, Grampian Rd,
AVIEMORE ☎ 01479 810278 6 en suite 6 annexe en suite

BOAT OF GARTEN   MAP 14 NH91

Boat of Garten PH24 3BQ
☎ 01479 831282 📠 01479 831523
e-mail: office@boatgolf.com
web: www.boatgolf.com
In the heart of the Cairngorm National Park, this prime example
of James Braid's design genius is cut through moorland and birch
forest, maximising the natural landscape. A beautiful and challenging
course set amid stunning scenery.

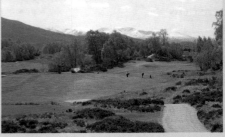

18 holes, 5876yds, Par 70, SSS 69, Course record 67.
Club membership 650.
Visitors Mon-Sun & BHs. Booking required. Handicap certificate. Dress
code. **Societies** Booking required. **Green Fees** £42 per day; £32 per
round (£47/£37 Sat & Sun). **Prof** Ross Harrower **Course Designer** James
Braid **Facilities** ⊕ �🝙 ℔ ℗ ℡ ⌖ 🛍 🏌 ✦ **Leisure** hard tennis
courts. **Conf** Corporate Hospitality Days **Location** E side of village
Hotel ★★★ 85% HL Boat Hotel, BOAT OF GARTEN ☎ 01479 831258
& 831696 📠 01479 831414 22 en suite

BONAR BRIDGE   MAP 14 NH69

Bonar Bridge-Ardgay Migdale Rd IV24 3EJ
☎ 01863 766199
e-mail: bonar-ardgay-golf@tiscali.co.uk
Wooded moorland course with picturesque views of hills and loch.
9 holes, 5162yds, Par 68, SSS 65. Club membership 250.
Visitors Mon-Sun & BHs **Societies** Booking required. **Green Fees** £15
per day. ⊛ **Course Designer** Various **Facilities** ⊕ ℔ ℗ ⌖ 🛍 ✦
Location 0.5m E
Guesthouse ★★★ GH Kyle House, Dornoch Rd, BONAR BRIDGE
☎ 01863 766360 5 rms (3 en suite)

BRORA
MAP 14 NC90

Brora Golf Rd KW9 6QS
☎ 01408 621417 📠 01408 622157
e-mail: secretary@broragolf.co.uk
web: www.broragolf.co.uk
Natural seaside links with little rough and fine views. Some testing holes including the 17th Tarbatness, so called because of the lighthouse which gives the line; the elevated tee is one of the best driving holes in Scotland.
18 holes, 6110yds, Par 69, SSS 70, Course record 61.
Club membership 704.
Visitors Mon-Sun & BHs. **Societies** Booking required. **Green Fees** £45 per day, £35 per round (£50/£40 Sat & Sun). **Prof** Brian Anderson **Course Designer** James Braid **Facilities** ⑪ ⑩ ⒧ ⌑ ⒲ ⤸ ⒧ ⊼ ☎ ⍨ ✔ ⛴ ✔
Location E side of village, signs to Beach Car Park
Hotel ★★★ 78% HL Royal Marine Hotel, Golf Rd, BRORA
☎ 01408 621252   22 en suite

CARRBRIDGE
MAP 14 NH92

Carrbridge Inverness Rd PH23 3AU
☎ 0844 414 1415 📠 0871 288 1014
e-mail: katie@carrbridgegolf.co.uk
web: www.carrbridgegolf.com
Challenging part-parkland, part-moorland course with magnificent views of the Cairngorms.
9 holes, 5402yds, Par 71, SSS 68, Course record 63.
Club membership 450.
Visitors Mon-Sun & BHs. Booking required. **Societies** Booking required.
Green Fees £25 per day, £16 per 9 holes. ☻ **Facilities** ⑪ ⑩ by prior arrangement ⒧ ⌑ ⊼ ☎ ⍨ ✔ **Conf** Corporate Hospitality Days
Location N side of village
Hotel ★★★ 74% SHL Dalrachney Lodge Hotel, CARRBRIDGE
☎ 01479 841252   11 en suite

DORNOCH
MAP 14 NH78

Royal Dornoch Golf Rd IV25 3LW
☎ 01862 810219 ext.185 📠 01862 810792
e-mail: bookings@royaldornoch.com
web: www.royaldornoch.com
The championship course was recently rated among the world's top courses and is a links of rare subtlety. It appears amicable but proves very challenging in play with stiff breezes and tight lies. The 18-hole Struie links course provides, in a gentler style, an enjoyable test of a golfer's accuracy for players of all abilities.

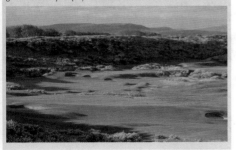

Championship: 18 holes, 6514yds, Par 70, SSS 73.
Struie Course: 18 holes, 6276yds, Par 72, SSS 70.
Club membership 1700.
Visitors Mon-Sun & BHs. Booking required for Championship Course. Handicap certificate. **Societies** Booking required.
Green Fees Championship course: £78 per round (£88 Sat & Sun). Struie course: £45 per day, £35 per round. **Prof** A Skinner
Course Designer Tom Morris **Facilities** ⑪ ⑩ ⒧ ⌑ ⍦ ⊼ ☎ ⍨
✔ ⛴ ✔ **Leisure** hard tennis courts. **Conf** facs Corporate Hospitality
Days **Location** E side of town

See advert on page 347

DURNESS
MAP 14 NC46

Durness Balnakeil IV27 4PG
☎ 01971 511364 📠 01971 511321
e-mail: lucy@durnessgolfclub.org
web: www.durnessgolfclub.org
A nine-hole course set in tremendous scenery overlooking Balnakeil Bay. Part links and part inland with water hazards. Off alternative tees for second nine holes giving surprising variety. Tremendous last hole played over a deep gully to the green over 100yds away.
9 holes, 5555yds, Par 70, SSS 67, Course record 69.
Club membership 150.
Visitors Mon-Sun & BHs. Booking required Sun. **Societies** Booking required. **Green Fees** £15 per day (£10 after 5pm). ☻ **Course Designer** F Keith **Facilities** ⑪ ⌑ ⊼ ⍨ ✔ **Leisure** fishing. **Conf** Corporate Hospitality Days **Location** 1m W of village overlooking Balnakeil Bay

FORT AUGUSTUS
MAP 14 NH30

Fort Augustus Markethill PH32 4DP
☎ 01320 366660 & 366758
web: www.fagc.com
Moorland course, with narrow fairways and good views. Bordered by the tree-lined Caledonian Canal to the north and heather clad hills to the south.
9 holes, 5379yds, Par 67, SSS 67, Course record 67.
Club membership 100.
Visitors Mon-Sun & BHs. **Societies** Welcome. **Green Fees** £20 per day, £15 per round. ☻ **Course Designer** Colt **Facilities** ⍨ ✔ **Location** 1m SW on A82
Hotel Ⓤ Lovat Arms Hotel, Loch Ness Side, FORT AUGUSTUS
☎ 0845 450 1100 & 01456 459250 📠 01320 366697 24 en suite 6 annexe en suite

FORTROSE

MAP 14 NH75

Fortrose & Rosemarkie Ness Rd East IV10 8SE
☎ 01381 620529 🖹 01381 621328
e-mail: secretary@fortrosegolfclub.co.uk
web: www.fortrosegolfclub.co.uk
Links set on a peninsula with the sea on three sides. Easy walking, good views. Designed by James Braid. The club was formed in 1888.

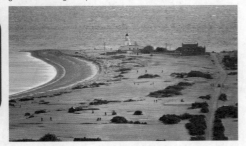

18 holes, 5881yds, Par 71, SSS 69, Course record 63.
Club membership 770.
Visitors Mon-Sun & BHs. Booking required. **Societies** Booking required. **Green Fees** £32 per round/£45 per day (weekends £38/£45).
Course Designer James Braid **Facilities** ⊕ ⏸ ⓛ 坐 ✆ ⼻ ⊟ 占 ゑ ♥ ⼻
Conf Corporate Hospitality Days **Location** A9 N over Kessock Bridge, signs to Munlochy
Hotel ★★★★ 74% HL Inverness Marriott Hotel, Culcabock Rd, INVERNESS ☎ 01463 237166 76 en suite 6 annexe en suite

FORT WILLIAM

MAP 14 NN17

Fort William Torlundy PH33 6SN
☎ 01397 704464
e-mail: fwgolf41@msn.com
web: www.fortwilliamgolf.co.uk
Spectacular moorland location looking onto the north face of Ben Nevis.
18 holes, 6217yds, Par 72, SSS 71, Course record 67.
Club membership 420.
Visitors Mon-Sun & BHs. Booking required. Dress code. **Societies** Booking required. **Green Fees** £20 per round (£22 Sat & Sun). **Course Designer** Hamilton Stutt **Facilities** ⓛ 坐 ✆ ⼻ 坐 ♥ ⼻ **Conf** Corporate Hospitality Days **Location** 3m NE on A82
Hotel ★★★ 79% HL Moorings Hotel, Banavie, FORT WILLIAM ☎ 01397 772797 27 en suite

GAIRLOCH

MAP 14 NG87

Gairloch IV21 2BE
☎ 01445 712407 🖹 01445 712865
e-mail: gairlochgolfclub@hotmail.co.uk
web: www.gairlochgolfclub.co.uk
Fine seaside links course running along Gairloch Sands with good views over the sea to Skye. In windy conditions each hole is affected. Founded in 1898, the course, although short is challenging for all golfers.
9 holes, 4108yds, Par 62, SSS 62, Course record 57.
Club membership 275.
Visitors Mon-Sun & BHs. Booking required. Dress code. **Societies** Booking required. **Green Fees** Phone. **Course Designer** Capt Burgess **Facilities** ⊕ ⓛ 坐 ✆ ⼻ 坐 ⊟ ♥ ⼻ **Conf** Corporate Hospitality Days **Location** 1m S on A832

GOLSPIE

MAP 14 NH89

Golspie Ferry Rd KW10 6ST
☎ 01408 633266 🖹 01408 633393
e-mail: info@golspie-golf-club.co.uk
web: www-golspie-golf-club.co.uk
Founded in 1889 and redesigned in 1926 by James Braid, Golspie's seaside course offers easy walking and natural hazards including beach heather and whins. Spectacular scenery.
18 holes, 5980yds, Par 68, SSS 68, Course record 64.
Club membership 300.
Visitors Mon-Sun & BHs. Booking required. **Societies** Booking required.
Green Fees £40 per day, £30 per round. **Course Designer** James Braid
Facilities ⊕ ⏸ ⓛ 坐 ✆ ⼻ 坐 ⊟ 占 ♥ ⼻ 坐 ⼻ **Location** 0.5m S off A9 at S entry to Golspie
Hotel ★★★ 78% HL Royal Marine Hotel, Golf Rd, BRORA ☎ 01408 621252 22 en suite

GRANTOWN-ON-SPEY

MAP 14 NJ02

Craggan Craggan PH26 3NT
☎ 01479 873283 🖹 01479 872325
e-mail: fhglaing@btopenworld.com
web: www.cragganforleisure.co.uk
A golf course in miniature set in stunning scenery on the edge of the Cairngorms National Park.
18 holes, 2400yds, Par 54, SSS 54, Course record 52.
Club membership 400.
Visitors Mon-Sun & BHs. **Societies** welcome. **Green Fees** not confirmed.
Course Designer Bill Mitchel **Facilities** ⊕ ⓛ 坐 ✆ ⼻ ⊟ 占 ♥ ⼻ **Leisure** fishing, biking. **Location** off A95, 1m S of Grantown-on-Spey
Hotel ★★ 85% SHL Culdearn House, Woodlands Ter, GRANTOWN ON SPEY ☎ 01479 872106 7 en suite

Grantown-on-Spey Golf Course Rd PH26 3HY
☎ 01479 872079 🖹 01479 873725
e-mail: secretary@grantownonspeygolfclub.co.uk
web: www.grantownonspeygolfclub.co.uk
Parkland and woodland course. Part easy walking, remainder hilly. The 7th to 13th holes really sort out the golfers.

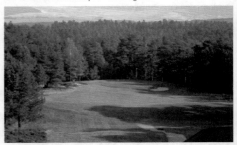

18 holes, 5710yds, Par 70, SSS 68, Course record 60.
Club membership 800.
Visitors Mon-Sun & BHs. Booking required. Dress code. **Societies** Booking required. **Green Fees** Phone. **Course Designer** A Brown/W Park/J Braid
Facilities ⊕ ⏸ by prior arrangement ⓛ 坐 ✆ ⼻ 坐 ⊟ 占 ♥ ⼻ 坐 ⼻
Conf Corporate Hospitality Days **Location** NE side of town centre
Hotel ★★ 85% SHL Culdearn House, Woodlands Ter, GRANTOWN ON SPEY ☎ 01479 872106 7 en suite

Scotland

HELMSDALE
MAP 14 ND01

Helmsdale Golf Rd KW8 6JL
☎ 01431 821063
Sheltered, undulating course following the line of the Helmsdale River.
9 holes, 1860yds, Par 60, SSS 60. Club membership 58.
Visitors Mon-Sun & BHs. **Societies** Booking required. **Green Fees** £15
per 18 holes. **Facilities** ⚲ **Location** NW side of town on A896
Hotel ★★★ 78% HL Royal Marine Hotel, Golf Rd, BRORA
☎ 01408 621252 22 en suite

INVERGORDON
MAP 14 NH76

Invergordon King George St IV18 0BD
☎ 01349 852715 🖹 01349 852715
e-mail: invergordongolf@tiscali.co.uk
web: www.invergordongolf.co.uk
Fairly easy but windy 18-hole parkland course, with woodland, wide
fairways and good views over Cromarty Firth. Very good greens and a
fair challenge, especially if the wind is from the west. Four Par 3s and
one Par 5.
18 holes, 6030yds, Par 69, SSS 69, Course record 63.
Club membership 240.
Visitors Mon-Sun & BHs. Booking required Tue, Thu, Sat-Sun. **Societies**
booking required. **Green Fees** not confirmed. **Course Designer** A Rae
Facilities ⚙ ⚑ ⚐ ⚑ ⚲ ☏ ⚡ **Location** W side of town centre on B817

INVERNESS
MAP 14 NH64

Inverness Culcabock IV2 3XQ
☎ 01463 239882 🖹 01463 240616
e-mail: igc@freeuk.com
web: www.invernessgolfclub.co.uk
Fairly flat parkland. A burn runs through and alongside several of
the holes, and also acts as a lateral water hazard and out of bounds
elsewhere. Considered short by modern day standards, it is an
excellent test of golf rewarding straight drives and accurate iron play to
well-manicured greens.

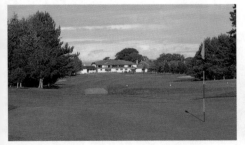

18 holes, 6256yds, Par 69, SSS 70, Course record 64.
Club membership 1182.
Visitors Mon-Sun & BHs. Booking required. Handicap certificate. Dress
code. **Societies** Booking required. **Green Fees** £48 per day, £35 per
round. **Prof** Alistair P Thomson **Course Designer** J Fraser/G Smith
Facilities ⚙ ⚑ ⚐ ⚑ ⚑ ⚲ ☏ ⚡ **Conf** Corporate Hospitality Days
Location 1m E of town centre on Culcabock Rd
Hotel ★★★★ 74% HL Inverness Marriott Hotel, Culcabock Rd,
INVERNESS ☎ 01463 237166 76 en suite 6 annexe en suite

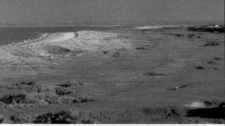

THE ROYAL DORNOCH GOLF CLUB
Golf Road, Dornoch IV25 3LW

Tel Reservations: 01862 810219 Ext 185
Fax: 01862 810792
e-mail: bookings@royaldornoch.com
Web Site: www.royaldornoch.com

Royal Dornoch has two fabulous 18 hole courses that
follow the natural links terrain.

The Championship Course is rated 3rd in the world
outside the USA and the Struie Course is enjoyable
and entertaining for the whole family with the
capacity to test the lower handicap player.

Loch Ness Fairways, Castle Heather IV2 6AA
☎ 01463 713335 🖹 01463 712695
e-mail: info@golflochness.com
web: www.golflochness.com
Course with two 18 hole options and a 9 hole family course with
seven Par 3's and two Par 4's and small undulating greens and deep
bunkers to test short game skills. The New and Old courses combine
several holes giving a great variety from the 550 yard 2nd hole to
the 76 yard hole called Chance which is played over a deep gully.

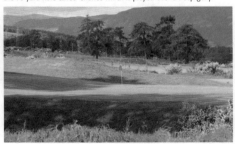

18 holes, 6772yds, Par 73, SSS 72, Course record 67.
New Course: 18 holes, 5907yds, Par 70, SSS 69,
Course record 68.
Wee Course: 9 holes, 1442yds, Par 29.
Club membership 600.

Continued

Scotland

Visitors Mon-Sun & BHs. Booking required. Dress code. **Societies** Booking required. **Green Fees** £40-£50 per day, £25-£35 per round. Wee course £10. **Prof** Martin Piggot **Course Designer** Caddies Golf Course Design **Facilities** ⓣ ⓞ ⓘ 🅱 ⬜ 🏴 👤 ⛳ 🏌 🛒 ⛳ 🚩 **Leisure** indoor bowls, petanque, woodland walks. **Conf** facs Corporate Hospitality Days **Location** SW outskirts of Inverness, along bypass
Hotel ★★★ 66% HL Loch Ness House Hotel, Glenurquhart Rd, INVERNESS ☎ 01463 231248 21 en suite

Torvean Glenurquhart Rd IV3 8JN
☎ 01463 711434 (Starter) & 225651 (Office)
📠 01463 711417
e-mail: info@torveangolfclub.com
web: www.torveangolfclub.co.uk
Public parkland course, easy walking, good views. One of the longest Par 5s in the north at 565yds. Three ponds come into play at the 8th, 15th and 17th holes.
18 holes, 5799yds, Par 69, SSS 68. Club membership 950.
Visitors Mon-Sun & BHs. Booking required. **Societies** Booking required. **Green Fees** £24 per round (£26.50 Sat & Sun). **Course Designer** Hamilton **Facilities** ⓣ ⓞ ⓘ 🅱 ⬜ 🏴 👤 ⛳ 🏌 **Conf** Corporate Hospitality Days **Location** 1.5m SW on A82
Hotel ★★★ 66% HL Loch Ness House Hotel, Glenurquhart Rd, INVERNESS ☎ 01463 231248 21 en suite

KINGUSSIE   MAP 14 NH70

Kingussie Gynack Rd PH21 1LR
☎ 01540 661600 📠 01540 662066
e-mail: sec@kingussie-golf.co.uk
web: www.kingussie-golf.co.uk
Upland course with natural hazards and magnificent views. Stands about 1000ft above sea level at its highest point, and the River Gynack, which runs through the course, comes into play on five holes. Golf has been played here for over 100years and some tight fairways and deceptive Par threes make the course a challenge for all golfers.
18 holes, 5500yds, Par 67, SSS 68, Course record 61.
Club membership 650.
Visitors Mon-Sun & BHs. Booking required. Dress code. **Societies** Booking required. **Green Fees** £32 per day, £24 per round(£34/£32 Sat & Sun). **Course Designer** Vardon **Facilities** ⓣ ⓞ ⓘ 🅱 ⬜ 🏴 👤 ⛳ 🏌 🛒 ⛳ **Location** 0.25m N off A86

LOCHCARRON   MAP 14 NG83

Lochcarron IV54 8YS
☎ 01599 577219
e-mail: mail@lochcarrongolf.co.uk
web: www.lochcarrongolf.co.uk
Seaside links course with some parkland with an interesting 1st hole. A short course but great accuracy is required.
9 holes, 3575yds, Par 60, SSS 60, Course record 58.
Club membership 130.
Visitors Mon-Sun & BHs. **Societies** booking required. **Green Fees** not confirmed. 🅿 **Facilities** ⓣ 🅱 ⬜ 👤 🚩 **Location** 1m E of Lochcarron by A896
Hotel ★★ 76% HL The Plockton Hotel, 41 Harbour St, PLOCKTON ☎ 01599 544274 11 en suite 4 annexe en suite

LYBSTER   MAP 15 ND23

Lybster Main St KW3 6AE
☎ 01593 721486 & 721316
web: www.lybstergolfclub.co.uk
9 holes, 1896yds, Par 62, SSS 61, Course record 57.
Location E side of village
Telephone for further details
Hotel ★★ 75% HL Mackay's Hotel, Union St, WICK ☎ 01955 602323 30 en suite

MUIR OF ORD   MAP 14 NH55

Muir of Ord Great North Rd IV6 7SX
☎ 01463 870825 📠 01463 871867
e-mail: muirgolf@supanet.com-email
web: golfhighland.co.uk
Long-established (1875) heathland course with tight fairways and easy walking. Testing Par 3 13th, Castle Hill.
18 holes, 5596yds, Par 68, SSS 68, Course record 61.
Club membership 750.
Visitors Mon-Fri, Sat pm only, Sun & BHs. Booking required. **Societies** Booking required **Green Fees** £20 per round/£25 per day (weekends £30/£35). **Course Designer** James Braid **Facilities** ⓣ by prior arrangement ⓞ by prior arrangement 🅱 by prior arrangement ⬜ 🏴 👤 ⛳ 🏌 🛒 ⛳ **Conf** Corporate Hospitality Days **Location** S side of village on A862
Hotel ★★★ 74% HL Priory Hotel, The Square, BEAULY ☎ 01463 782309 34 en suite

NAIRN   MAP 14 NH85

Nairn Seabank Rd IV12 4HB
☎ 01667 453208 📠 01667 456328
e-mail: secretary@nairngolfclub.co.uk
web: www.nairngolfclub.co.uk
18 holes, 6430yds, Par 71, SSS 73, Course record 64.
Newton: 9 holes, 3542yds, Par 58, SSS 57.
Course Designer A Simpson/Old Tom Morris/James Braid **Location** 16m E of Inverness on A96
Telephone for further details

Nairn Dunbar Lochloy Rd IV12 5AE
☎ 01667 452741 📠 01667 456897
e-mail: secretary@nairndunbar.com
web: www.nairndunbar.com
18 holes, 6765yds, Par 72, SSS 74, Course record 64.
Location E side of town off A96
Telephone for further details
Hotel ★★ 65% HL Alton Burn Hotel, Alton Burn Rd, NAIRN ☎ 01667 452051 & 453325 📠 01667 456697 23 en suite

NETHY BRIDGE   MAP 14 NJ02

Abernethy PH25 3EB
☎ 01479 821305 📠 01479 821305
e-mail: info@abernethygolfclub.com
web: www.abernethygolfclub.com
Traditional Highland course built on moorland surrounded by pine trees and offering a great variety of shot making for the low handicapped or casual visitor. The 2nd hole, although very short is played across bogland and a B road to a two-tiered green. The small
Continued

Scotland

and fast greens are the most undulating and tricky in the valley. The Abernethy forest lies on the boundary and from many parts of the course there are splendid views of Strathspey.

9 holes, 2526yds, Par 66, SSS 66. Club membership 400.
Visitors Mon-Sun & BHs. Booking Required Sun. **Societies** Welcome.
Green Fees £17 per day (£19 Sun & Sat). ⊛ **Facilities** ⑪ ⑩ ⅼ ⌷ ⅄ 🖾 ↱º ⌀ **Conf** Corporate Hospitality Days **Location** N side of village on B970

NEWTONMORE   MAP 14 NN79

Newtonmore Golf Course Rd PH20 1AT
☎ 01540 673878 🖹 01540 673878
e-mail: secretary@newtonmoregolf.com
web: www.newtonmoregolf.com
Inland course beside the River Spey. Beautiful views and easy walking. Testing 17th hole (Par 3).

18 holes, 6031yds, Par 70, SSS 69, Course record 64.
Club membership 420.
Visitors Mon-Sun & BHs. **Societies** Booking required **Green Fees** Phone.
⊛ **Prof** Robert Henderson **Facilities** ⑪ ⑩ ⅼ ⌷ ⅊ ⅄ 🖾 ↱º ⌀ 🖾 ⌀
Location E side of town off A9
Hotel ★★ 72% SHL The Scot House Hotel, Newtonmore Rd, KINGUSSIE
☎ 01540 661351 9 en suite

REAY   MAP 14 NC96

Reay KW14 7RE
☎ 01847 811288 🖹 01847 894189
e-mail: info@reaygolfclub.co.uk
web: www.reaygolfclub.co.uk
Picturesque seaside links with natural hazards, following the contours of Sandside Bay. Most northerly 18-hole links on the British mainland. The 581yd Par 5 4th hole Sahara requires a solid tee shot and fairway wood to set up an approach to a sheltered green protected by a burn. The 196yd Par 3 7th Pilkington is a beautiful short hole played across Reay burn to a raised green. The two-tiered 18th protected by its greenside bunkers provides a formidable finishing hole. Unique feature in that it opens and closes with a Par 3 and the sea is visible from every hole. An excellent natural seaside links.

18 holes, 5831yds, Par 69, SSS 69, Course record 64.
Club membership 250.
Visitors Mon-Sun & BHs. Contact club for details. **Societies** booking required. **Green Fees** not confirmed. ⊛ **Course Designer** Braid **Facilities** ⑪ by prior arrangement by prior arrangement ⅼ by prior arrangement ⌷ ↱º ⅄ ↱º 🖾 ⌀ **Leisure** see web site. **Conf** Corporate Hospitality Days **Location** 11m W of Thurso on A836

STRATHPEFFER   MAP 14 NH45

Strathpeffer Spa IV14 9AS
☎ 01997 421219 & 421011 🖹 01997 421011
e-mail: mail@strathpeffergolf.co.uk
web: www.strathpeffergolf.co.uk
Beautiful, testing upland course in this historic village. Many natural hazards mean only three sand bunkers on the course and the course's claim to fame is the 1st hole which features the longest drop from tee to green in Scotland. Stunning views.

18 holes, 4956yds, Par 67, SSS 65, Course record 62.
Club membership 400.
Visitors Mon-Sun & BHs. Booking required Sun, Sat & BHs. Handicap certificate. Dress code. **Societies** Booking required. **Green Fees** £30 per day, £20 per round (£35/£25 Sat & Sun). **Course Designer** Willie Park/Tom

---

Morris **Facilities** ⑪ ⅼ ⌷ ↱º ⅄ 🖾 ↱º 🖾 ⌀ **Conf** Corporate Hospitality Days **Location** 0.25m N of village off A834, signed
Hotel ★★★ 74% SHL Achilty Hotel, CONTIN ☎ 01997 421355 9 en suite 2 annexe en suite

---

TAIN   MAP 14 NH78

Tain Chapel Rd IV19 1JE
☎ 01862 892314 🖹 01862 892099
e-mail: info@tain-golfclub.co.uk
web: www.tain-golfclub.co.uk
Links course with river affecting three holes; easy walking, fine views.

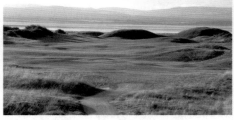

18 holes, 6404yds, Par 70, SSS 71, Course record 68.
Club membership 600.
Visitors Mon-Sun & BHs. **Societies** Booking required. **Green Fees** £55 per day; £40 per round (£60/£45 weekends). **Course Designer** Old Tom Morris **Facilities** ⑪ ⑩ ⅼ ⌷ ↱º ⅄ 🖾 ⌀ 🖾 ⌀ **Leisure** Practice net. **Conf** Corporate Hospitality Days **Location** E side of town centre off B9174

THURSO   MAP 15 ND16

Thurso Newlands of Geise KW14 7XD
☎ 01847 893807
web: europgolf.com
Parkland course, windy, but with fine views of Dunnet Head and the Orkney Islands. Tree-lined fairways but 4th and 16th holes are testing into the prevailing wind. The 13th is a short Par 4 but has a testing drive over a burn with heather on left and punishing rough on right.

18 holes, 5853yds, Par 69, SSS 69, Course record 61.
Club membership 400.
Visitors Mon-Fri, Sun & BHs Satpm only **Societies** Booking required.
Green Fees £20 per day. ⊛ **Course Designer** W S Stewart **Facilities** ⌷ ↱º ⅄ ↱º 🖾 **Conf** Corporate Hospitality Days **Location** 2m SW of Thurso on B874

ULLAPOOL

Ullapool The Clubhouse, North Rd, Morefield IV26 2TH
☎ 01854 613323 🖹 01854 612911
web: www.ullapool-golf.co.uk
Seaside/parkland course with fine views.

9 holes, 5281yds, Par 70, SSS 67, Course record 68.
Club membership 160.
Visitors Mon-Fri & BHs. Dress code. **Societies** Booking required.
Green Fees £18 per day, £15 per 9 holes. ⊛ **Facilities** ⌷ ⅄ 🖾 ↱º ⌀ **Conf** Corporate Hospitality Days **Location** On A835 at N end of village

WICK
MAP 15 ND35

Wick Reiss KW1 4RW
☎ 01955 602726
e-mail: wickgolfclub@hotmail.com
web: www.wickgolfclub.fsnet.co.uk/
Typical seaside links course, fairly flat, easy walking. Nine holes straight out and straight back. Normally breezy.
18 holes, 6123yds, Par 69, SSS 71, Course record 63.
Club membership 352.
Visitors Mon-Sun & BHs. Contact club for details. **Societies** welcome.
Green Fees not confirmed. ◉ **Course Designer** James Braid **Facilities** ⓑ ◻◻◻ ⚒ ⚑ ✦ **Conf** Corporate Hospitality Days **Location** 3.5m N off A9
Hotel ★★ 75% HL Mackay's Hotel, Union St, WICK ☎ 01955 602323 30 en suite

---

INVERCLYDE

GOUROCK
MAP 10 NS27

Gourock Cowal View PA19 1HD
☎ 01475 631001 & 636834 (pro) 📄 01475 638307
e-mail: secretary@gourockgolfclub.com
18 holes, 6408yds, Par 73, SSS 72, Course record 64.
Course Designer J Braid/H Cotton **Location** SW side of town off A770
Telephone for further details
Hotel BUD Premier Travel Inn Greenock, 1-3 James Watt Way, GREENOCK ☎ 08701 977120 40 en suite

GREENOCK
MAP 10 NS27

Greenock Forsyth St PA16 8RE
☎ 01475 720793 📄 01475 791912
Testing moorland course with panoramic views of Clyde Estuary.
18 holes, 5838yds, Par 69, SSS 69. Club membership 700.
Visitors Mon-Sun & BHs. Booking required. Handicap certificate. Dress code. **Societies** Booking required. **Green Fees** Phone. ◉ **Course Designer** James Braid **Facilities** ⓘ ◻ ⓑ ◻◻◻ ⚒ ⚑ ✦ **Location** SW side of town off A770
Hotel BUD Premier Travel Inn Greenock, 1-3 James Watt Way, GREENOCK ☎ 08701 977120 40 en suite

Greenock Whinhill Beith Rd PA16 9LN
☎ 01475 724694 (evenings & weekends only)
Picturesque heathland public course.
18 holes, 5504yds, Par 68, SSS 67, Course record 64.
Club membership 200.
Visitors Mon-Sun & BHs. Booking required Wed, Sat & Sun. Dress code.
Green Fees Phone. ◉ **Course Designer** William Fernie **Facilities** ⓘ ◻ ⓑ ◻◻◻ ⚒ **Location** 1.5m SW off B7054

KILMACOLM
MAP 10 NS36

Kilmacolm Porterfield Rd PA13 4PD
☎ 01505 872139 📄 01505 874007
e-mail: secretary@kilmacolmgolf.com
web: www.kilmacolmgolfclub.com
18 holes, 5961yds, Par 69, SSS 69, Course record 64.
Course Designer Willie Campbell **Location** SE side of town off A761
Telephone for further details
Hotel ★★★ 80% HL Gleddoch House Hotel, LANGBANK ☎ 01475 540711 70 en suite

PORT GLASGOW
MAP 10 NS37

Port Glasgow Devol Rd PA14 5XE
☎ 01475 704181
e-mail: secretary@portglasgowgolfclub.com
web: www.portglasgowgolfclub.com
A moorland course set on a hilltop overlooking the Clyde, with magnificent views to the Cowal hills.
18 holes, 5712yds, Par 68, SSS 68. Club membership 390.
Visitors Mon-Fri, Sun & BHs. Dress code. **Societies** Booking required.
Green Fees £30 per day, £22 per round (£40/£30 Sun). **Facilities** ⓘ ◻ ⓑ ◻◻◻ ⚒ **Location** 1m S
Hotel ★★★ 80% HL Gleddoch House Hotel, LANGBANK ☎ 01475 540711 70 en suite

---

MIDLOTHIAN

BONNYRIGG
MAP 11 NT36

Broomieknowe 36 Golf Course Rd EH19 2HZ
☎ 0131 663 9317 📄 0131 663 2152
e-mail: administrator@broomieknowe.com
web: www.broomieknowe.com
Easy walking mature parkland course laid out by Ben Sayers and extended by James Braid. Elevated site with excellent views.
18 holes, 6150yds, Par 70, SSS 70, Course record 65.
Club membership 900.
Visitors Mon-Sun & BHs. Dress code. **Societies** Booking required.
Green Fees Phone. ◉ **Prof** Mark Patchett **Course Designer** Ben Sayers/Hawtree **Facilities** ⓘ ◻ ⓑ ◻◻◻ ⚒ ⚑ ✦ **Conf** Corporate Hospitality Days **Location** 0.5m NE off B704
Hotel ★★★ 83% HL Dalhousie Castle and Aqueous Spa, Bonnyrigg, EDINBURGH ☎ 01875 820153 29 en suite 7 annexe en suite

DALKEITH
MAP 11 NT36

Newbattle Abbey Rd EH22 3AD
☎ 0131 663 2123 & 0131 663 1819 📄 0131 654 1810
e-mail: mail@newbattlegolfclub.com
web: www.newbattlegolfclub.com
Gently undulating parkland course, dissected by the South Esk river and surrounded by woods.
18 holes, 6025yds, Par 69, SSS 69, Course record 61.
Club membership 700.
Visitors Mon-Fri, Sun pm only. Dress code. **Societies** Booking required.
Green Fees £35 per day, £25 per round. ◉ **Prof** Scott McDonald
Course Designer S Colt **Facilities** ⓘ ◻ ⓑ ◻◻◻ ⚒ ⚑ ✦
Conf Corporate Hospitality Days **Location** SW side of town off A68
Hotel ★★★ 83% HL Dalhousie Castle and Aqueous Spa, Bonnyrigg, EDINBURGH ☎ 01875 820153 29 en suite 7 annexe en suite

GOREBRIDGE
MAP 11 NT36

Vogrie Vogrie Estate Country Park EH23 4NU
☎ 01875 821716 📄 01875 823958
e-mail: ritchie.fraser@midlothian.gov.uk
web: www.midlothian.gov.uk
A 9-hole municipal course located within a country park. The wide fairways are particularly suited to beginners.
9 holes, 2530yds, Par 33.

Continued

Visitors Mon-Fri & BHs. Booking advised Sat/Sun & BHs. **Green Fees** not confirmed. ⊕ **Facilities** ⑪ ⊾ ⊑ ⅄ ✔ **Location** Off B6372
Hotel ★★★ 83% HL Dalhousie Castle and Aqueous Spa, Bonnyrigg, EDINBURGH ☎ 01875 820153 29 en suite 7 annexe en suite

LASSWADE
MAP 11 NT36

Kings Acre EH18 1AU
☎ 0131 663 3456 📄 0131 663 7076
e-mail: info@kings-acregolf.com
web: www.kings-acregolf.com
Parkland course set in countryside location and making excellent use of the natural contours of the land with strategically placed water hazards and over 50 bunkers leading to large undulating greens. The naturally sandy based soil ensures excellent play all year.
18 holes, 6031yds, Par 70, SSS 69. Club membership 300.
Visitors Mon-Sun & BHs. Booking required. Dress code. **Societies** Booking required. **Green Fees** £35 per day, £25 per 18 holes (£34 Sat & Sun).
Prof Alan Murdoch **Course Designer** Graeme Webster **Facilities** ⑪ ⏴❑
⊾ ⊑ ⅋❑ ⅄ ☎❅ ✦ ✔ ✔ ☂ **Conf** facs Corporate Hospitality Days
Location off A720, City of Edinburgh bypass road

PENICUIK
MAP 11 NT25

Glencorse Milton Bridge EH26 0RD
☎ 01968 677189 & 676481 📄 01968 674399
e-mail: glencorsegc@btconnect.com
web: www.glencorsegolfclub.com
Picturesque parkland with a burn affecting 10 holes. Testing 5th hole (237yds) Par 3.
18 holes, 5217yds, Par 64, SSS 66, Course record 60.
Club membership 700.
Visitors Mon-Fri, Sun pm & BHs. Booking required. Dress code. **Societies** booking required. **Green Fees** £32 per day, £25 per round. **Prof** Cliffe Jones **Course Designer** Willie Park **Facilities** ⑪ ⏴❑ ⊾ ⊑ ⅋❑ ⅄ ☎❅
✔ **Location** 9m S of Edinburgh on A701 Peebles Road
Inn ★★★ INN The Original Roslin Inn, 4 Main St, ROSLIN
☎ 0131 440 2384 6 en suite

MORAY

BALLINDALLOCH
MAP 15 NJ13

Ballindalloch Castle Lagmore AB37 9AA
☎ 01807 500305 📄 01807 500226
e-mail: golf@ballindallochcastle.co.uk
web: www.ballindallochcastle.co.uk
Course nestling among mature trees on the banks of the river Avon with fine views of the surrounding hills and woods.
9 holes, 6495yds, Par 72, SSS 71, Course record 64.
Visitors Mon-Sun & BHs. **Societies** Booking required. **Green Fees** £20 per 18 holes, £15 per 9 holes. **Course Designer** Donald Steel **Facilities**
⊾ ⊑ ⅋❑ ⅄ ☎❅ ❅ ✔ ✦ **Conf** Corporate Hospitality Days **Location** off A95 13 NE of Grantown-on-Spey

BUCKIE
MAP 15 NJ46

Buckpool Barhill Rd, Buckpool AB56 1DU
☎ 01542 832236 📄 01542 832236
e-mail: golf@buckpoolgolf.com
web: www.buckpoolgolf.com
Links course with superlative view over Moray Firth, easy walking.
18 holes, 6097yds, Par 70, SSS 69, Course record 63.
Club membership 430.
Visitors Mon-Sun & BHs. **Societies** Booking required. **Green Fees** £25 per day, £20 per round (£30/£25 Sat & Sat). ⊕ **Course Designer** J H Taylor **Facilities** ⑪ ⏴❑ by prior arrangement ⊾ ⊑ ⅋❑ ⅄ ✔ ✔ **Leisure** squash, snooker. **Location** Off A98

Strathlene Buckie Portessie AB56 2DJ
☎ 01542 831798 📄 01542 831798
e-mail: strathgolf@ukonline.co.uk
web: www.strathlenegolfclub.co.uk
Raised seaside links course with magnificent view. A special feature of the course is approach shots to raised greens (holes 4, 5, 6 and 13).
18 holes, 5980yds, Par 69, SSS 69, Course record 64.
Visitors Mon-Sun & BHs. Dress code. **Societies** Booking required.
Green Fees £22 per day; £18 per round (£30/£21 Sat & Sun). ⊕
Course Designer George Smith **Facilities** ⊑ ⅋❑ ⅄ ☎❅ ✦
Conf Corporate Hospitality Days **Location** 2m E of Buckie on A942

CULLEN
MAP 15 NJ56

Cullen The Links AB56 4WB
☎ 01542 840685
e-mail: cullengolfclub@btinternet.com
web: www.cullen-golf-club.co.uk
Interesting links on three levels with rocks and ravines offering some challenging holes. Spectacular scenery.
18 holes, 4610yds, Par 63, SSS 62, Course record 55.
Club membership 400.
Visitors Mon-Sun & BHs. Booking required. **Societies** Booking required.
Green Fees £20 per round. **Course Designer** Tom Morris/Charlie Neaves
Facilities ⑪ ⏴❑ ⊾ ⊑ ⅋❑ ⅄ ☎❅ ✔ **Conf** Corporate Hospitality Days
Location 0.5m W off A98

DUFFTOWN
MAP 15 NJ34

Dufftown Tomintoul Rd AB55 4BS
☎ 01340 820325 📄 01340 820325
e-mail: admin@dufftowngolfclub.com
web: www.dufftowngolfclub.com
A short and undulating inland course with spectacular views. The tee of the highest hole, the 9th, is over 1200ft above sea level.
18 holes, 5308yds, Par 67, SSS 67, Course record 64.
Club membership 350.
Visitors Mon-Sat & BHs. Booking required Sun and Sat. Dress code. **Societies** Welcome. **Green Fees** £20 per day, £15 per round.
Course Designer Members **Facilities** ⑪ by prior arrangement ⏴❑ by prior arrangement ⊾ by prior arrangement ⊑ by prior arrangement ⅋❑
⅄ ☎❅ ✦ **Conf** facs Corporate Hospitality Days **Location** 0.75m SW off B9009
Hotel ★★★ 85% HL Craigellachie Hotel, CRAIGELLACHIE
☎ 01340 881204 26 en suite

ELGIN   MAP 15 NJ26

Elgin Hardhillock, Birnie Rd, New Elgin IV30 8SX
☎ 01343 542338 🖹 01343 542341
e-mail: secretary@elgingolfclub.com
web: www.elgingolfclub.com
Possibly the finest inland course in the north of Scotland, with
undulating greens and compact holes that demand the highest
accuracy. There are 13 Par 4s and one Par 5 hole on its parkland
layout, eight of the Par 4s being over 400yds long.

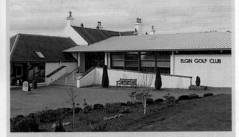

Hardhillock: 18 holes, 6416yds, Par 68, SSS 69,
Course record 63. Club membership 1000.
Visitors Mon-Sun & BHs. Booking required. Handicap certificate.
Dress code. **Societies** booking required. **Green Fees** not confirmed.
Prof Kevin Stables **Course Designer** John Macpherson **Facilities** ⑪ ⦿
🍴 ♨ ⚑ ⚒ ⛳ **Conf** facs **Location** 1m S on A941
Hotel ★★★ 79% HL Mansion House Hotel, The Haugh, ELGIN
☎ 01343 548811   23 en suite

FORRES   MAP 14 NJ05

Forres Muiryshade IV36 2RD
☎ 01309 672250 🖹 01309 672250
e-mail: sandy@forresgolf.demon.co.uk
web: www.forresgolf.demon.co.uk
An all-year parkland course laid on light, well-drained soil in wooded
countryside. Walking is easy despite some hilly holes. A test for the
best golfers.
18 holes, 6240yds, Par 70, SSS 70, Course record 60.
Club membership 1000.
Visitors Mon-Sun & BHs. Dress code. **Societies** Booking required.
Green Fees £30 per round/£40 per day. **Prof** Sandy Aird
Course Designer James Braid/Willie Park **Facilities** ⑪ ⦿ 🍴 ♨ ⚑
♨ ⚑ ⚒ ⛳ **Conf** Corporate Hospitality Days **Location** SE side
of town centre off B9010
Hotel ★★★ 73% HL Ramnee Hotel, Victoria Rd, FORRES
☎ 01309 672410   20 en suite

GARMOUTH   MAP 15 NJ36

Garmouth & Kingston Spey St IV32 7NJ
☎ 01343 870388 🖹 01343 870388
e-mail: garmouthgolfclub@aol.com
Flat seaside course with several parkland holes and tidal waters.
The 8th hole measures only 328yds from the medal tee but the fairway
is bounded by a ditch on either side, the left hand one being out
of bounds for the entire length of the hole. The Par 5 17th Whinny
Side has gorse bordering on both sides of the fairway which can be
intimidating to any level of golfer.
18 holes, 5545yds, Par 69, SSS 67. Club membership 500.
Visitors Mon, Thur & Fri. Booking required. **Societies** Booking required.
Green Fees £25 per day, £20 per round (£28/£25 weekends). **Course**
Designer George Smith **Facilities** ⑪ by prior arrangement ⦿ by prior
arrangement 🍴 ♨ ⚒ **Conf** Corporate Hospitality Days
Location In village on B9015
Hotel ★★★ 79% HL Mansion House Hotel, The Haugh, ELGIN
☎ 01343 548811   23 en suite

HOPEMAN   MAP 15 NJ16

Hopeman Clubhouse IV30 5YA
☎ 01343 830578 🖹 01343 830152
e-mail: hopemangc@aol.com
web: www.hopemangc.co.uk
Links-type course with beautiful views over the Moray Firth. The 12th
hole, called the Priescach, is a short hole with a drop of 100ft from tee
to green. It can require anything from a wedge to a wood depending
on the wind.
18 holes, 5624yds, Par 68, SSS 68. Club membership 700.
Visitors Mon-Sun & BHs. Booking required. **Societies** Booking required.
Green Fees £20 per round (£25 Sat & Sun). **Facilities** ⑪ ⦿ 🍴 ♨ ⚒ ♨
♨ ⚑ ⛳ **Location** E side of village off B9040
Hotel ★★★ 79% HL Mansion House Hotel, The Haugh, ELGIN
☎ 01343 548811   23 en suite

KEITH   MAP 15 NJ45

Keith Fife Park AB55 5DF
☎ 01542 882469 🖹 01542 888176
e-mail: secretary@keithgolfclub.org.uk
web: www.keithgolfclub.org.uk
Parkland course, with natural hazards over first 9 holes. Testing 7th
hole, 232 yds, Par 3.
18 holes, 5767yds, Par 69, SSS 68, Course record 65.
Club membership 500.
Visitors Mon-Sun & BHs. Contact club for details. **Societies** booking
required. **Green Fees** not confirmed. ⦿ **Course Designer** Roy Phimister
Facilities ⑪ ⦿ 🍴 ♨ ⚒ **Location** NW of town centre, A96 onto B9014
right
Hotel ★★★ 85% HL Craigellachie Hotel, CRAIGELLACHIE
☎ 01340 881204   26 en suite

Scotland

LOSSIEMOUTH MAP 15 NJ27

Moray Stotfield Rd IV31 6QS
☎ 01343 812018 📄 01343 815102
e-mail: secretary@moraygolf.co.uk
web: www.moraygolf.co.uk
Two fine Scottish Championship links courses, known as Old and New (Moray), and situated on the Moray Firth where the weather is unusually mild.
Old Course: 18 holes, 6643yds, Par 71, SSS 73,
Course record 65. New Course: 18 holes, 6004yds, Par 69,
SSS 69, Course record 62. Club membership 1550.
Visitors Mon-Sun & BHs. Booking required. Dress code.
Societies Booking required. **Green Fees** Phone. **Prof** Alistair Thomson
Course Designer Tom Morris & Henry Cotton **Facilities** ⊕ ⍟ ☕ ☂
🏌 ⛳ ☂ ⚐ ✦ ✦ **Conf** Corporate Hospitality Days **Location** N side of town
Hotel ★★★ 79% HL Mansion House Hotel, The Haugh, ELGIN
☎ 01343 548811 23 en suite

ROTHES MAP 15 NJ24

Rothes Blackhall AB38 7AN
☎ 01340 831443 (evenings) 📄 01340 831443
e-mail: enquiries@rothesgolfclub.co.uk
web: www.rothesgolfclub.co.uk
A parkland course on an elevated site with fine views over the Spey Valley Lush tree lined fairways and well maintained greens.
9 holes, 4972yds, Par 68, SSS 64. Club membership 260.
Visitors Mon-Sun & BHs. **Societies** Booking required. **Green Fees** £12 (£15 Sat & Sun). ⊗ **Course Designer** John Souter **Facilities** ⊕ ⍟ ☕ ☂
🏌 ⛳ **Conf** Corporate Hospitality Days **Location** on A941 10m S of Elgin
Hotel ★★★ 85% HL Craigellachie Hotel, CRAIGELLACHIE
☎ 01340 881204 26 en suite

SPEY BAY MAP 15 NJ36

Spey Bay IV32 7PJ
☎ 01343 820424 📄 01343 829282
e-mail: info@speybay.com
web: www.speybay.com
18 holes, 6182yds, Par 70, SSS 70, Course record 65.
Course Designer Ben Sayers **Location** 4.5m N of Fochabers on B9104
Telephone for further details
Guesthouse ★★★★★ GH Underwood Country Guest House, The Hill,
MILLOM ☎ 01229 771116 5 en suite

NORTH AYRSHIRE

BEITH MAP 10 NS35

Beith Threepwood Rd KA15 2JR
☎ 01505 503166 & 506814 📄 01505 506814
e-mail: beith_secretary@btconnect.com
web: www.beithgolfclub.co.uk
Hilly course, with panoramic views over seven counties.
18 holes, 5616yds, Par 68, SSS 68. Club membership 487.
Visitors Mon-Sun & BHs. Booking required Sat/Sun & BHs. Handicap certificate. Dress code. **Societies** booking required. **Green Fees** not confirmed. **Course Designer** Members **Facilities** ⊕ ⍟ ☕ ☂ ☂ 🏌 ⛳
Location 1st left on Beith bypass, S on A737
Guesthouse ★★★★ GH Whin Park, 16 Douglas St, LARGS
☎ 01475 673437 4 en suite

GREAT CUMBRAE ISLAND MAP 10 NS15
(MILLPORT)

Millport Golf Rd KA28 OHB
☎ 01475 530305 (Prof) 📄 01475 530306
e-mail: secretary@millportgolfclub.co.uk
web: www.millportgolfclub.co.uk
18 holes, 5828yds, Par 68, SSS 69, Course record 64.
Course Designer James Braid **Location** 4m from ferry slip
Telephone for further details
Hotel ★★ 81% HL Willowbank Hotel, 96 Greenock Rd, LARGS
☎ 01475 672311 & 675435 📄 01475 689027 30 en suite

IRVINE MAP 10 NS34

Glasgow Gailes KA11 5AE
☎ 0141 942 2011 📄 0141 942 0770
e-mail: secretary@glasgow-golf.com
web: www.glasgowgailes-golf.com
A lovely seaside links. The turf of the fairways and all the greens is truly glorious and provides tireless play. Established in 1882, this is a qualifying course for the Open Championship.
Glasgow Gailes: 18 holes, 6535yds, Par 71, SSS 72,
Course record 63. Club membership 1200.
Visitors Mon-Sun & BHs. Booking required. Contact club for details.
Societies booking required. **Green Fees** not confirmed. **Prof** J Steven
Course Designer W Park Jnr **Facilities** ⊕ ⍟ by prior arrangement 🏌
☂ 🏌 ⛳ ☂ ✦ ✦ ✦ **Conf** Corporate Hospitality Days **Location** Off A78 at Newhouse junct, S of Irvine
Hotel ★★★ 75% HL Montgreenan Mansion House Hotel, Montgreenan Estate, KILWINNING ☎ 01294 850005 21 en suite

Irvine Bogside KA12 8SN
☎ 01294 275979 📄 01294 278209
e-mail: secretary@theirvinegolfclub.co.uk
web: www.theirvinegolfclub.co.uk
Testing links course; only two short holes.
18 holes, 6400yds, Par 71, SSS 73, Course record 65.
Club membership 450.
Societies Booking required **Green Fees** Phone. **Prof** Jim McKinnon
Course Designer James Braid **Facilities** ⊕ ⍟ ☕ ☂ ☂ 🏌 ⛳ ✦
Location N side of town off A737
Hotel ★★★ 75% HL Montgreenan Mansion House Hotel, Montgreenan Estate, KILWINNING ☎ 01294 850005 21 en suite

Irvine Ravenspark 13 Kidsneuk Ln KA12 8SR
☎ 01294 271293
e-mail: secretary@irgc.co.uk
web: www.irgc.co.uk
18 holes, 6457yds, Par 71, SSS 71, Course record 65.
Location N side of town on A737
Telephone for further details
Hotel ★★★ 75% HL Montgreenan Mansion House Hotel, Montgreenan Estate, KILWINNING ☎ 01294 850005 21 en suite

Scotland

Western Gailes Gailes by Irvine KA11 5AE
☎ 01294 311649 📄 01294 312312
e-mail: enquiries@westerngailes.com
web: www.westerngailes.com
A magnificent seaside links with glorious turf and wonderful greens.
The view is open across the Firth of Clyde to the neighbouring
islands. It is a well-balanced course crossed by three burns. There
are two Par 5s, the 6th and 14th, and the 11th is a testing 445yd
Par 4 dog-leg.
18 holes, 6639yds, Par 71, SSS 74, Course record 65.
Visitors Mon, Wed, Fri & BHs. Sun pm. Booking required. Dress code.
Societies Booking required. **Green Fees** £110 per 18 holes, £160
per 36 holes (both including lunch). £120 Sun (no lunch). **Facilities** ⓣ
⦿ by prior arrangement 🍴 ⬚ ⛳ ⚍ 🛍 *♂* **Conf** Corporate Hospitality
Days **Location** 2m S off A737
Hotel ★★★ 75% HL Montgreenan Mansion House Hotel, Montgreenan
Estate, KILWINNING ☎ 01294 850005 21 en suite

KILBIRNIE   MAP 10 NS35

Kilbirnie Place Largs Rd KA25 7AT
☎ 01505 684444 & 683398
e-mail: kilbirnie.golfclub@tiscali.co.uk
18 holes, 5543yds, Par 69, SSS 67, Course record 65.
Location 1m W from Kilbirnie Cross on A760
Telephone for further details
Hotel ★★ 81% HL Willowbank Hotel, 96 Greenock Rd, LARGS
☎ 01475 672311 & 675435 📄 01475 689027 30 en suite

LARGS   MAP 10 NS25

Largs Irvine Rd KA30 8EU
☎ 01475 673594 📄 01475 673594
e-mail: secretary@largsgolfclub.co.uk
web: www.largsgolfclub.co.uk
A parkland, tree-lined course with views to the Clyde coast and the
Arran Isles.
18 holes, 6140yds, Par 70, SSS 71, Course record 63.
Club membership 850.
Visitors Mon, Tues, Thurs, Fri & Sun. Booking required Mon, Fri & Sun.
Dress code **Societies** Booking required. **Green Fees** £48 per day, £36 per
round (£48 per round Sun). **Prof** Kenneth Docherty **Course Designer** H
Stutt **Facilities** ⓣ ⦿ ⠐ ⬚ ⛳ ⚍ 🛍 ♀ *♂* **Location** 1m S of town centre
on A78
Hotel ★★ 81% HL Willowbank Hotel, 96 Greenock Rd, LARGS
☎ 01475 672311 & 675435 📄 01475 689027 30 en suite

Routenburn Routenburn Rd KA30 8QA
☎ 01475 673230 & 686475 📄 01475 687240
Heathland course with fine views over the Firth of Clyde.
18 holes, 5675yds, Par 68, SSS 68, Course record 63.
Club membership 300.
Visitors Mon-Fri, Sun & BHs. Booking required. **Societies** Booking required.
Green Fees Phone. **Prof** J Grieg McQueen
Course Designer James Braid **Facilities** ⓣ by prior arrangement ⬚ ⛳
⚍ 🛍 ♀ *♂* *♂* **Conf** Corporate Hospitality Days **Location** 1m N off
A78
Hotel ★★ 81% HL Willowbank Hotel, 96 Greenock Rd, LARGS
☎ 01475 672311 & 675435 📄 01475 689027 30 en suite

SKELMORLIE   MAP 10 NS16

Skelmorlie Beithglass PA17 5ES
☎ 01475 520152
e-mail: sec@skelmorliegolf.co.uk
web: www.skelmorliegolf.co.uk
Parkland and moorland course with magnificent views over the Firth
of Clyde.
18 holes, 5030yds, Par 65, SSS 65, Course record 63.
Club membership 450.
Visitors Mon-Sun & BHs. Booking required Sat. **Societies** Booking
required. **Green Fees** £27 per day, £22 per round (£32/£27 Sun & Sat). ⦾
Course Designer James Braid **Facilities** ⬚ ⛳ ⚍ *♂* **Location** E side of
village off A78
Hotel ★★ 81% HL Willowbank Hotel, 96 Greenock Rd, LARGS
☎ 01475 672311 & 675435 📄 01475 689027 30 en suite

STEVENSTON   MAP 10 NS24

Ardeer Greenhead KA20 4LB
☎ 01294 464542 & 465316 📄 01294 465316
e-mail: peewee_watson@lineone.net
web: www.ardeergolfclub.com
Parkland with natural hazards, including several water features.
18 holes, 6401yds, Par 72, SSS 71, Course record 66.
Club membership 650.
Visitors Mon-Sun & BHs. Booking required. **Societies** Welcome. **Green
Fees** £40 per day; £25 per round (£50/£35 Sun). ⦾ **Course Designer**
Stutt **Facilities** ⓣ ⠐ ⬚ ⛳ ⚍ 🛍 *♂* **Leisure** snooker. **Conf** facs
Corporate Hospitality Days **Location** 0.5m N off A78
Hotel ★★★ 75% HL Montgreenan Mansion House Hotel, Montgreenan
Estate, KILWINNING ☎ 01294 850005 21 en suite

WEST KILBRIDE   MAP 10 NS24

West Kilbride 33-35 Fullerton Dr, Seamill KA23 9HT
☎ 01294 823911 📄 01294 829573
e-mail: golf@westkilbridegolfclub.com
web: www.westkilbridegolfclub.com
Seaside links course on the Firth of Clyde, with fine views of Isle of
Arran from every hole.
18 holes, 5974yds, Par 70, SSS 70, Course record 63.
Club membership 840.
Visitors Mon-Fri. Booking required. **Societies** Booking required.
Green Fees Phone. **Prof** Graham Ross **Course Designer** James Braid
Facilities ⓣ ⦿ ⠐ ⬚ ⛳ ⚍ 🛍 ♀ *♂* **Location** W side of town off A78
Hotel ★★ 81% HL Willowbank Hotel, 96 Greenock Rd, LARGS
☎ 01475 672311 & 675435 📄 01475 689027 30 en suite

NORTH LANARKSHIRE

AIRDRIE   MAP 11 NS76

Airdrie Rochsoles ML6 0PQ
☎ 01236 762195 📄 01236 760584
e-mail: airdriegolfclub@virgin.net
Picturesque parkland course with good views.
18 holes, 6004yds, Par 69, SSS 68, Course record 61.
Club membership 450.
Visitors Mon, Wed-Fri, Sun & BHs. Booking required. Handicap certificate.
Dress code. **Societies** Booking required. **Green Fees** £30 per day; £25 per

Continued

round. ⊛ **Prof** S McLean **Course Designer** J Braid **Facilities** ⑪ ⑩ ⓛ ⌺ ⌶ ⌲ ⌙ ✔ **Location** 1m N on B802
Hotel ★★★★ 74% HL The Westerwood Hotel, 1 St Andrews Dr, Westerwood, CUMBERNAULD ☎ 01236 457171   100 en suite

Easter Moffat Mansion House, Station Rd, Plains ML6 8NP
☎ 01236 842878 📄 01236 842904
e-mail: secretary@emgc.org.uk
A challenging moorland and parkland course which enjoys good views of the Campsie and Ochil hills. Although fairways are generous, accurate placement from the tee is essential on most holes. The signature hole on the course, the 18th is a truly memorable Par 3, played from an elevated tee, to a receptive green in front of the clubhouse.
18 holes, 6221yds, Par 72, SSS 70, Course record 66.
Club membership 500.
Visitors Mon-Fri. Booking required. Dress code. **Societies** booking required. **Green Fees** not confirmed. ⊛ **Prof** Graham King **Facilities** ⑪ ⑩ ⓛ ⌺ ⌶ ⌲ ⌙ ✔ **Location** 2m E of Airdrie on A89
Hotel ★★★★ 74% HL The Westerwood Hotel, 1 St Andrews Dr, Westerwood, CUMBERNAULD ☎ 01236 457171   100 en suite

---

BELLSHILL   MAP 11 NS76

Bellshill Community Rd, Orbiston ML4 2RZ
☎ 01698 745124 📄 01698 292576
e-mail: info@bellshillgolfclub.com
Tree-lined 18 holes situated in the heart of Lanarkshire near Strathclyde Park. First opened for play in 1905 and extended in 1970. The 2nd hole has been redesigned by Mark James and Andrew Mair. The first five holes are extremely demanding but are followed by the gentler birdie alley where shots can be recovered. The signature hole is the 17th, a Par 3 which involves a tricky tee shot from an elevated tee to a small well-bunkered green with out of bounds on the right.
18 holes, 6272yds, Par 70, SSS 69. Club membership 700.
Visitors Mon-Fri, Sun & BHs. Booking required. Dress code. **Societies** Booking required. **Green Fees** Summer £32 per day; £20 per round. Winter reduced rates. **Facilities** ⑪ ⑩ ⓛ ⌺ ⌶ **Location** 1m SE off A721
Hotel BUD Premier Travel Inn Glasgow (Bellshill), Belziehill Farm, New Edinburgh Rd, BELLSHILL ☎ 08701 977106   40 en suite

---

COATBRIDGE   MAP 11 NS76

Drumpellier Drumpellier Av ML5 1RX
☎ 01236 424139 📄 01236 428723
e-mail: administrator@drumpelliergc.freeserve.co.uk
web: www.drumpellier.com
Parkland with rolling fairways and fast greens.

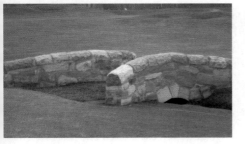

18 holes, 6227yds, Par 71, SSS 70, Course record 62.
Club membership 827.
Visitors Mon-Fri. Booking required. Handicap certificate. Dress code. **Societies** booking required. **Green Fees** not confirmed. **Prof** Jaimie Carver **Course Designer** W Fernie **Facilities** ⑪ ⑩ ⓛ ⌺ ⌶ ⌲ ⌙ ✔ ⊟ ✔ **Conf** facs   Corporate Hospitality Days **Location** 0.75m W off A89
Hotel ★★★ 74% HL Bothwell Bridge Hotel, 89 Main St, BOTHWELL ☎ 01698 852246   90 en suite

---

CUMBERNAULD   MAP 11 NS77

Dullatur 1A Glen Douglas Dr G68 0DW
☎ 01236 723230 📄 01236 727271
e-mail: graeme.campbell@dullaturgolf.com
web: www.dullaturgolf.com
Dullatur Carrickstone is a parkland course, with natural hazards and wind. Dullatur Antonine, designed by Dave Thomas, is a modern course.

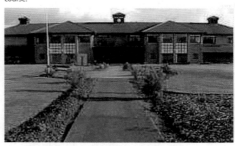

Carrickstone: 18 holes, 6204yds, Par 70, SSS 70, Course record 68.
Antonine: 18 holes, 5875yds, Par 69, SSS 68.
Club membership 700.
Visitors Booking required. **Societies** booking required. **Green Fees** not confirmed. **Prof** Duncan Sinclair **Course Designer** James Braid **Facilities** ⑪ ⑩ ⓛ ⌺ ⌶ ⌲ ⌙ ✔ ⊟ ✔ **Leisure** hard tennis courts, sauna, solarium, gymnasium, bowling green. **Conf**   Corporate Hospitality Days **Location** 1.5m N of A80 at Cumbernauld
Hotel ★★★★ 74% HL The Westerwood Hotel, 1 St Andrews Dr, Westerwood, CUMBERNAULD ☎ 01236 457171   100 en suite

Palacerigg Palacerigg Country Park G67 3HU
☎ 01236 734969 & 721461 📄 01236 721461
e-mail: palacerigg-golfclub@lineone.net
web: www.palacerigggolfclub.co.uk
Well-wooded parkland course set in Palacerigg Country Park, with good views to the Campsie Hills.
18 holes, 6444yds, Par 72, SSS 72, Course record 65.
Club membership 300.
Visitors Mon-Sun & BHs. Booking required Sat, Sun & BHs. Dress code. **Societies** Booking required. **Green Fees** £8 per round/£12 per day (weekend £10 per round). ⊛ **Course Designer** Henry Cotton **Facilities** ⑪ ⑩ ⓛ ⌺ ⌶ ⌲ ⌙ ✔ ⊟ ✔ **Conf**   Corporate Hospitality Days **Location** 2m S of Cumbernauld on Palacerigg road off Lenziemill road B8054
Hotel ★★★★ 74% HL The Westerwood Hotel, 1 St Andrews Dr, Westerwood, CUMBERNAULD ☎ 01236 457171   100 en suite

Scotland

Westerwood Hotel 1 St Andrews Dr, Westerwood
G68 0EW
☎ 01236 725281 ▤ 01236 738478
e-mail: wesgolf@ghotels.com
web: www.ghotels.co.uk
Undulating parkland and woodland course designed by Dave Thomas
and Seve Ballasteros. holes meander through silver birch, firs, heaths
and heather, and the spectacular 15th, The Waterfall, has its green set
against a 40ft rockface. Buggie track. Hotel facilities.
Westerwood: 18 holes, 6557yds, Par 72, SSS 72,
Course record 65. Club membership 400.
Visitors Mon-Sun & BHs. Booking required. Handicap certificate. Dress
code. **Societies** Booking required. **Green Fees** Apr-Oct £35 per round
(£40 Sat & Sun). Nov-Mar £20. **Prof** Vincent Brown **Course Designer**
Seve Ballesteros/Dave Thomas **Facilities** ⑪ ⍵ ⋎ ⟁ ▱ 𝍐 ⋏ 🛆 ⛾⋎ ◇
⋎ 🛒 ⋎ **Leisure** hard tennis courts, heated indoor swimming pool,
sauna, gymnasium, Beauty salon. **Conf** facs Corporate Hospitality Days
Location By A80, 14m from Glasgow
Hotel ★★★★ 74% HL The Westerwood Hotel, 1 St Andrews Dr,
Westerwood, CUMBERNAULD ☎ 01236 457171 100 en suite

GARTCOSH   MAP 11 NS66

Mount Ellen Johnston Rd G69 8EY
☎ 01236 872277 ▤ 01236 872249
18 holes, 5525yds, Par 68, SSS 67, Course record 67.
Location 0.75m N off A752
Telephone for further details
Hotel ★★★★ 77% HL Millennium Hotel Glasgow, George Square,
GLASGOW ☎ 0141 332 6711 117 en suite

KILSYTH   MAP 11 NS77

Kilsyth Lennox Tak Ma Doon Rd G65 0RS
☎ 01236 824115 ▤ 01236 823089
e-mail: mail@klgc.co.uk
web: www.kilsythlennox.com
Hilly moorland course, hard walking.
18 holes, 6612yds, Par 71, SSS 71, Course record 66.
Club membership 667.
Visitors Mon-Fri, Sun & BHs. Booking required Sun & BHs. Dress code.
Societies must contact in advance. **Green Fees** £33 per day; £23 per round
(£38/£28 Sun). **Prof** William Erskine **Facilities** ⑪ ⍵ ⋎ ⟁ ▱ 𝍐 ⋏ 🛆 ⛾ 🛒
Location N side of town off A803
Hotel ★★★★ 74% HL The Westerwood Hotel, 1 St Andrews Dr,
Westerwood, CUMBERNAULD ☎ 01236 457171 100 en suite

MOTHERWELL   MAP 11 NS75

Colville Park New Jerviston House, Jerviston Estate,
Merry St ML1 4UG
☎ 01698 265779 (pro) ▤ 01698 230418
18 holes, 6250yds, Par 71, SSS 70, Course record 63.
Course Designer James Braid **Location** 1.25m NE of Motherwell town
centre on A723
Telephone for further details
Hotel ★★★ 74% HL Bothwell Bridge Hotel, 89 Main St, BOTHWELL
☎ 01698 852246 90 en suite

MUIRHEAD   MAP 11 NS66

Crow Wood Garnkirk House, Cumbernauld Rd G69 9JF
☎ 0141 779 1943 ▤ 0141 779 9148
e-mail: crowwood@golfclub.fsbusiness.co.uk
web: www.golfagent.co.uk
18 holes, 6261yds, Par 71, SSS 71, Course record 62.
Course Designer James Braid **Location** Off A80 to Stirling, between
Stepps
Telephone for further details
Hotel ★★★ 85% HL Malmaison, 278 West George St, GLASGOW
☎ 0141 572 1000 72 en suite

SHOTTS   MAP 11 NS86

Shotts Blairhead ML7 5BJ
☎ 01501 822658 ▤ 01501 822650
web: www.shottsgolfclub.co.uk
Moorland course with fine panoramic views. A good test for all abilities.
18 holes, 6205yds, Par 70, SSS 70, Course record 63.
Club membership 800.
Visitors Mon-Sun & BHs. Booking required **Societies** Booking required.
Green Fees £28 per day, £20 per round (£25 per round Sat & Sun).
Prof John Strachan **Course Designer** James Braid **Facilities** ⑪ ⍵ ⋎ ⟁ ▱
𝍐 ⋏ 🛆 ⛾ 🛒 ⋎ **Location** 2m from M8 off Benhar Road
Hotel ★★★ 77% HL Best Western The Hilcroft Hotel, East Main St,
WHITBURN ☎ 01501 740818 32 en suite

WISHAW   MAP 11 NS75

Wishaw 55 Cleland Rd ML2 7PH
☎ 01698 372869 (club house) & 357480 (admin)
▤ 01698 356930
e-mail: jwdouglas@btconnect.com
web: www.wishawgolfclub.com
Parkland with many tree-lined fairways. Bunkers protect 17 of the 18
greens.
18 holes, 5999yds, Par 69, SSS 69, Course record 62.
Club membership 984.
Visitors Mon-Fri, Sun & BHs. Booking required. Dress code. **Societies**
Booking required. **Green Fees** £35 per day, £25 per round (£39/£29 Sun).
Prof Stuart Adair **Course Designer** James Braid **Facilities** ⑪ ⍵ ⋎ ⟁ ▱ 𝍐
🛆 ⛾ 🛒 ⋎ **Location** NW side of town off A721
Hotel ★★★ 81% HL Best Western Popinjay Hotel & Leisure Club, Lanark
Rd, ROSEBANK ☎ 01555 860441 34 en suite

PERTH & KINROSS

ABERFELDY   MAP 14 NN84

Aberfeldy Taybridge Rd PH15 2BH
☎ 01887 820535 ▤ 01887 820535
e-mail: abergc@tiscali.com.uk
web: www.aberfeldygolf.co.uk
Founded in 1895, this flat, parkland course is situated by the River Tay
near the famous Wade Bridge and Black Watch Monument, and enjoys
some splendid scenery. The new layout will test the keen golfer.
18 holes, 5283yds, Par 68, SSS 66, Course record 67.
Club membership 250.
Visitors Mon-Sun & BHs. Booking required. Dress code. **Societies** Booking
required. **Green Fees** Phone. **Course Designer** Soutars **Facilities** ⑪ ⍵
⋎ ▱ 𝍐 ⋏ 🛆 ⛾ 🛒 ⋎ **Conf** Corporate Hospitality Days **Location** N side
of town centre

ALYTH
MAP 15 NO24

Alyth Pitcrocknie PH11 8HF
☎ 01828 632268 🖹 01828 633491
e-mail: enquiries@alythgolfclub.co.uk
web: www.alythgolfclub.co.uk
Windy, heathland course with easy walking.
18 holes, 6205yds, Par 71, SSS 71, Course record 64.
Club membership 1000.
Visitors Mon-Sun & BHs. Booking required. **Societies** Booking required
Green Fees Phone. **Prof** Tom Melville **Course Designer** James Braid
Facilities ⓣ ⓘ◎ ⒧ ⌷ 🜂 🛪 🕾 🕈 ☞ **Conf** facs **Location** 1m
E on B954
Hotel ★★★ 67% HL Angus Hotel, Wellmeadow, BLAIRGOWRIE
☎ 01250 872455 81 en suite

Strathmore Golf Centre Leroch PH11 8NZ
☎ 01828 633322 🖹 01828 633533
e-mail: enquiries@strathmoregolf.com
web: www.strathmoregolf.com
The Rannaleroch Course is set on rolling parkland and heath with
splendid views over Strathmore.It is generous off the tee but beware
of the udulating, links-style greens. Among the challenging holes is
the 480yd 5th with a 180yd carry over water from a high tee position.
The nine-hole Leitfie Links has been specially designed with beginners,
juniors and older golfers in mind.

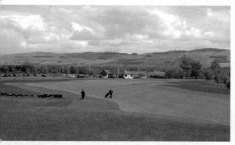

Rannaleroch Course: 18 holes, 6454yds, Par 72, SSS 72,
Course record 65.
Leitfie Links: 9 holes, 1719yds, Par 29, SSS 29.
Club membership 450.
Visitors Mon-Sun & BHs. Dress code. **Societies** Booking required.
Green Fees £26 per round. Leitfie £10 per round (£32/£12 Sat & Sun).
Prof Margot Smith **Course Designer** John Salvesen **Facilities** ⓣ ⓘ◎ ⒧ ⌷
🜂 🛪 🕾 🕈 ☞ **Conf** Corporate Hospitality Days **Location** 2m SE of
Alyth, B954 at Meigle onto A926, signed from Blairgowrie
Hotel ★★★ 67% HL Angus Hotel, Wellmeadow, BLAIRGOWRIE
☎ 01250 872455 81 en suite

AUCHTERARDER
MAP 11 NN91

Auchterarder Orchil Rd PH3 1LS
☎ 01764 662804 (Sec) 🖹 01764 664423(Sec)
e-mail: secretary@auchterardergolf.co.uk
web: www.auchterardergolf.co.uk
Flat parkland course, part woodland with pine, larch and silver birch. It
may be short but tricky with cunning dog-legs and guarded greens that
require accuracy rather than sheer power. The 14th Punchbowl hole is
perhaps the trickiest. A blind tee shot needs to be hit accurately over

the left edge of the cross bunker to a long and narrow green - miss
and you face a difficult downhill chip shot from deep rough.
18 holes, 5775yds, Par 69, SSS 68, Course record 61.
Club membership 820.
Visitors Mon-Sun & BHs. Booking required. Handicap certificate. Dress
code. **Societies** Booking required. **Green Fees** £25 per round/£35 per day
(weekends £30/£45). ⓦ **Prof** Gavin Baxter **Course Designer** Ben Sayers
Facilities ⓣ ⓘ◎ ⒧ ⌷ 🜂 🛪 🕾 🕈 **Conf** Corporate Hospitality Days
Location 0.75m SW on A824
Hotel ★★★★★ HL The Gleneagles Hotel, AUCHTERARDER
☎ 01764 662231 266 en suite

Gleneagles Hotel see page 359

Hotel ★★★★★ HL The Gleneagles Hotel, AUCHTERARDER
☎ 01764 662231 266 en suite
Hotel ★★ 85% HL Cairn Lodge, Orchil Rd, AUCHTERARDER
☎ 01764 662634 Fax 01764 662866 10 en suite
Hotel ★★★ 78% HL Best Western Huntingtower Hotel, Crieff Rd, PERTH
☎ 01738 583771 Fax 01738 583777 31 en suite 3 annexe en suite

BLAIR ATHOLL
MAP 14 NN86

Blair Atholl Invertilt Rd PH18 5TG
☎ 01796 481407 🖹 01796 481292
Easy walking parkland with a river alongside three holes.
9 holes, 5816yds, Par 70, SSS 68, Course record 65.
Club membership 368.
Visitors Mon-Sun & BHs. Booking required Sun, Sat & BHs. Dress code.
Societies Booking required. **Green Fees** £21 per day (£23 Sat & Sun).
ⓦ **Course Designer** Tom Morriss **Facilities** ⓣ ⒧ ⌷ 🛪 🜂 🕈 🕾
Location 0.5m S off B8079
Hotel ★★ 76% HL Atholl Arms Hotel, Old North Rd, BLAIR ATHOLL
☎ 01796 481205 30 en suite

BLAIRGOWRIE
MAP 15 NO14

Blairgowrie Golf Course Rd, Rosemount PH10 6LG
☎ 01250 872622 🖹 01250 875451
e-mail: office@theblairgowriegolfclub.co.uk
web: www.theblairgowriegolfclub.co.uk
Two 18-hole championship heathland/woodland courses, also a
nine-hole course.

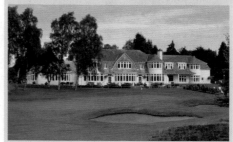

Rosemount Course: 18 holes, 6590yds, Par 72, SSS 72,
Course record 64.
Lansdowne Course: 18 holes, 6834yds, Par 72, SSS 73,
Course record 66.
Wee Course: 9 holes, 2352yds, Par 32.
Club membership 1724.

Continued

Scotland

Visitors Mon-Sun & BHs. Booking required. Handicap certificate. Dress code. **Societies** Booking required. **Green Fees** Phone. **Prof** Charles Dernie **Course Designer** J Braid/P Allis/D Thomas/Old Tom Morris **Facilities** ⑪ ⑩ ⓘ ﹗ ⊾ ⌷ ⍥ ⌴ ☂ ☏ ♥ ▩ ✔ **Conf** Corporate Hospitality Days **Location** Off A93 Rosemount
Hotel ★★★ 67% HL Angus Hotel, Wellmeadow, BLAIRGOWRIE
☎ 01250 872455 81 en suite

COMRIE   MAP 11 NN72

Comrie Laggan Braes PH6 2LR
☎ 01764 670055
e-mail: enquiries@comriegolf.co.uk
web: www.comriegolf.co.uk
9 holes, 6040yds, Par 70, SSS 70, Course record 62.
Course Designer Col. Williamson **Location** E side of village off A85
Telephone for further details
Hotel ★★★ 82% HL The Four Seasons Hotel, Loch Earn, ST FILLANS
☎ 01764 685333 12 en suite 6 annexe en suite

CRIEFF   MAP 11 NN82

Crieff Ferntower, Perth Rd PH7 3LR
☎ 01764 652909 ▤ 01764 655096
e-mail: bookings@crieffgolf.co.uk
web: www.crieffgolf.co.uk
Set in dramatic countryside, Crieff Golf Club was established in 1891. The Ferntower championship course has magnificent views over the Strathearn valley and offers all golfers an enjoyable round. The short nine-hole Dornoch course, which incorporates some of the James Braid designed holes from the original 18 holes, provides an interesting challenge for juniors, beginners and others short of time.

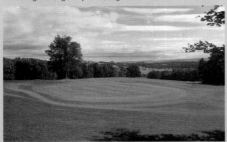

Ferntower Course: 18 holes, 6502yds, Par 71, SSS 72, Course record 63.
Dornock Course: 9 holes, 2372yds, Par 32, SSS 63.
Club membership 720.
Visitors Mon-Sun & BHs. Booking required. Handicap certificate.
Societies Booking required. **Green Fees** Ferntower: May & Oct £30, Jun-Sep £33 per round (£36/£40 Sat & Sun). Dornock £12 for 9 holes, £16 for 18 holes. **Prof** David Murchie **Course Designer** James Braid **Facilities** ⌷ ﹗ ⊾ ☂ ☏ ♥ ▩ ✔ **Conf** Corporate Hospitality Days **Location** 0.5m NE on A85
Hotel ★★★ 80% HL Royal Hotel, Melville Square, COMRIE
☎ 01764 679200 11 en suite

DUNKELD   MAP 11 NO04

Dunkeld & Birnam Fungarth PH8 0ES
☎ 01350 727524 ▤ 01350 728660
e-mail: secretary-dunkeld@tiscali.co.uk
web: dunkeldandbirnamgolfclub.co.uk
Interesting and challenging course with spectacular views of the surrounding countryside. The original nine-hole heathland course is now augmented by an additional nine holes of parkland character close to the Loch of the Lowes.
18 holes, 5511yds, Par 70, SSS 67, Course record 63.
Club membership 600.
Visitors Mon-Sun & BHs. Booking required. Dress code. **Societies** Booking required. **Green Fees** Phone. **Course Designer** D A Tod **Facilities** ⑪ ⑩ ⓘ ﹗ ⊾ ⌷ ﹗ ⊾ ☂ ☏ ♥ ✔ **Conf** Corporate Hospitality Days **Location** 1m N of village on A923
Hotel ★★★★ HL Kinnaird, Kinnaird Estate, DUNKELD ☎ 01796 482440 9 en suite

---

DUNNING   MAP 11 NO01

Dunning Rollo Park, Station Rd PH2 0QX
☎ 01764 684747
A pleasant parkland course with some testing holes, complicated by the burn which is a feature of four of the nine holes.
9 holes, 4836yds, Par 66, SSS 63, Course record 62.
Club membership 480.
Visitors Mon-Fri. Sat & Sun pm only. Booking required. Dress code.
Societies Booking required. **Green Fees** £18 per 18 holes. ❀ **Prof** Stuart Barker **Facilities** ⊾ by prior arrangement ⌷ ⊾ ♥ ✔ **Location** 4m N of Auchterarder, 1.5m off A9 on B9146
Hotel ★★★ 74% HL Lovat Hotel, 90 Glasgow Rd, PERTH ☎ 01738 636555 30 en suite

Whitemoss Whitemoss Rd PH2 0QX
☎ 01738 730300 ▤ 01738 730490
e-mail: info@whitemossgolf.com
web: www.whitemossgolf.com

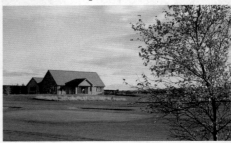

18 holes, 5595yds, Par 68, SSS 68, Course record 63.
Course Designer Whitemoss Leisure **Location** Off A9 at Whitemoss Rd junct, 3m N of Gleneagles
Telephone for further details
Hotel ★★ 85% HL Cairn Lodge, Orchil Rd, AUCHTERARDER
☎ 01764 662634 10 en suite

CHAMPIONSHIP COURSE

PERTH AND KINROSS — AUCHTERARDER

GLENEAGLES HOTEL

Map 11 NN91

PH3 1NF
☎ 01764 662231 📠 01764 662134
e-mail: resort.sales@gleneagles.com
web: www.gleneagles.com
King's Course: 18 holes, 6471yds, Par 70,
SSS 73, Course record 60.
Queen's Course: 18 holes, 5965yds, Par 68,
SSS 70, Course record 62.
PGA Centenary Course: 18 holes, 6787yds,
Par 73, SSS 74, Course record 63.
Visitors Booking required. **Societies** Booking
required. **Green Fees** May-Sept £115 up
to 3pm, £75 after 3pm, £40 after 5pm. Reduced
rates rest of the year. **Prof** Russell Smith
Course Designer James Braid/Jack Nicklaus
Facilities ⑨ 🍴 🛍 ☞ 🍴 ⚲ 🛍 ⛳ ◇ ⚑ 🚗
⚑ ☞ **Leisure** hard and grass tennis courts,
outdoor and indoor heated pools, fishing, sauna,
gym, golf academy, horse riding, shooting,
falconry, off road driving. **Conf** Corporate
Hospitality Days **Location** 2m SW of A823

The PGA Centenary Course, created by
Jack Nicklaus, and launched in May 1993,
has an American-Scottish layout with many
water hazards, elevated tees and raised
contoured greens. It is the selected venue
for the Ryder Cup 2014. It has a five-tier
tee structure making it both the longest
and shortest playable course, as well as
the most accommodating to all standards
of golfer. The King's Course, with its
abundance of heather, gorse, raised greens
and plateau tees, is set within the valley of
Strathearn with the Grampian mountains
spectacularly in view to the north. The
shorter Queen's Course, with fairways lined
with Scots pines and water hazards, is set
in a softer landscape and is considered
an easier test of golf. You can improve
your game at the golf academy where the
philosophy is that golf should be fun and
fun in golf comes from playing better.
A corporate golf package is available.

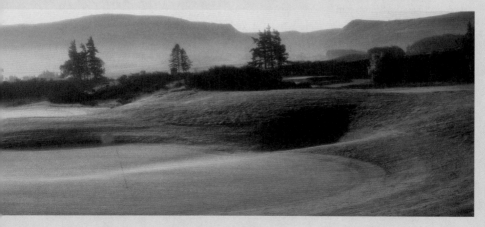

Scotland

GLENSHEE (SPITTAL OF)   MAP 15 NO17

Dalmunzie Dalmunzie Estate PH10 7QE
☎ 01250 885226
e-mail: enquiries@dalmunziecottages.com
web: www.dalmunziecottages.com
Well-maintained Highland course. Testing short course with small but good greens. One of the highest courses in Britain at 1200ft.
9 holes, 2099yds, Par 30, SSS 30. Club membership 91.
Visitors Mon-Sun & BHs. **Societies** Booking required. **Green Fees** £14 per day. ☻ **Course Designer** Alistair Campbell **Facilities** ⑪ ⑩ ⅃ ▱ ⛾ ▤ ⛾ ◇ **Leisure** hard tennis courts, fishing, mountain bikes. **Conf** facs Corporate Hospitality Days **Location** 2m NW of Spittal of Glenshee
Hotel ★★★ 81% CHH Dalmunzie House Hotel, SPITTAL OF GLENSHEE
☎ 01250 885224   17 en suite

KENMORE   MAP 14 NN74

Kenmore PH15 2HN
☎ 01887 830226 🖷 01887 830775
e-mail: info@taymouth.co.uk
web: www.taymouth.co.uk
Testing course in mildly undulating natural terrain. Beautiful views in tranquil setting by Loch Tay. The Par 5 4th is 560yds and only one of the Par 4s, the 2nd, is under 400yds - hitting from the tee out of a mound of trees down a snaking banking fairway which encourages the ball to stay on the fairway. The slightly elevated green is surrounded by banks to help hold the ball on the green. The fairways are generous and the rough turn, which tends to encourage an unhindered round.
9 holes, 6052yds, Par 70, SSS 69, Course record 67.
Club membership 200.
Visitors Mon-Sun & BHs. Booking required Sat, Sun & BHs. **Societies** Welcome. **Green Fees** £30 per day, £20 per 18 holes, £15 per 9 holes (£35/£25/£17 Sat & Sun). **Course Designer** Robin Menzies **Facilities** ⑪ ⑩ ⅃ ▱ ▤ ⅃ ▱ ☘ ◇ ☘ ☘ **Leisure** fishing. **Conf** Corporate Hospitality Days **Location** On A827, beside Kenmore Bridge
Hotel ★★★ 74% HL Kenmore Hotel, The Square, KENMORE
☎ 01887 830205   27 en suite   13 annexe en suite

KINROSS   MAP 11 NO10

Kinross The Green Hotel, 2 The Muirs KY13 8AS
☎ 01577 863407 🖷 01577 863180
e-mail: bookings@golfkinross.com
web: www.golfkinross.com

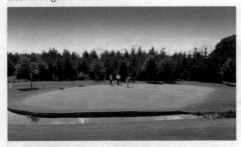

Two interesting and picturesque parkland courses, with easy walking. Many of the fairways are bounded by trees and plantations. A number of holes have views over Loch Leven to the hills beyond. The more challenging of the two is the Montgomery which has recently been enhanced by the addition of a pond in front of the 11th green and 19 extra bunkers. The Bruce is slightly shorter but still provides a stern test of golf with notable features being the 6th Pond Hole and the run of four Par 5's in six holes on the front nine.

Bruce: 18 holes, 6231yds, Par 73, SSS 71.
Montgomery: 18 holes, 6452yds, Par 71, SSS 72.
Club membership 600.
Visitors Mon-Sun & BHs. Dress code. **Societies** Booking required. **Green Fees** The Bruce £35 per day, £25 per round (£45/£35 Sat & Sun). The Montgomery £45 per day, £30 per round (£40/£55 Sat & Sun). **Prof** Stuart Geraghty **Course Designer** Sir David Montgomery **Facilities** ⑪ ⑩ ⅃ ▱ ▱ ⅄ ▤ ⛾ ◇ ☘ ⛾ ◇ **Leisure** hard tennis courts, heated indoor swimming pool, squash, fishing, sauna, solarium, gymnasium, 4 sheet curling rink, croquet. **Conf** facs Corporate Hospitality Days **Location** NE side of town on B996
Hotel ★★★★ 75% HL The Green Hotel, 2 The Muirs, KINROSS
☎ 01577 863467   46 en suite

MILNATHORT   MAP 11 NO10

Milnathort South St KY13 9XA
☎ 01577 864069
e-mail: milnathort.gc@btconnect.com
Undulating inland course with lush fairways and excellent greens for most of the year. Strategically placed copses require accurate tee shots. Different tees and greens for some holes will make for more interesting play.
9 holes, 5969yds, Par 71, SSS 69, Course record 62.
Club membership 575.
Visitors Mon-Fri & Sun. Booking required. Dress code. **Societies** Booking required. **Green Fees** Weekdays £22 per day, £15 per round (weekends £25/£17). ☻ **Facilities** ⑪ ⑩ ⅃ ▱ ▱ ⅄ ▱ ☘ **Conf** Corporate Hospitality Days **Location** S side of town on A922
Hotel ★★★★ 75% HL The Green Hotel, 2 The Muirs, KINROSS
☎ 01577 863467   46 en suite

MUTHILL   MAP 11 NN81

Muthill Peat Rd PH5 2DA
☎ 01764 681523 🖷 01764 681557
e-mail: muthillgolfclub@lineone.net
web: muthillgolfclub.co.uk
A nine-hole course that, although short, requires accurate shot making to match the SSS. The three Par 3s are all challenging holes with the 9th, a 205yd shot to a small well-bunkered green making a fitting end to nine holes characterised by great views and springy well-maintained fairways.
9 holes, 4700yds, Par 66, SSS 63, Course record 62.
Club membership 285.
Visitors Mon-Sun & BHs. Booking required. Dress code. **Societies** booking required. **Green Fees** not confirmed. ☻ **Course Designer** Members **Facilities** ⑪ ▱ ⅄ ▱ ☘ **Location** W side of village off A822
Hotel ★★ 85% HL Cairn Lodge, Orchil Rd, AUCHTERARDER
☎ 01764 662634   10 en suite

PERTH
MAP 11 NO12

Craigie Hill Cherrybank PH2 0NE
☎ 01738 622644 (pro) 🖹 01738 620829
e-mail: golf@craigiehill.com
web: www.craigiehill.scottishgolf.com
Slightly hilly, heathland course. Panoramic views of Perth and the surrounding hills.
18 holes, 5386yds, Par 66, SSS 67, Course record 60.
Club membership 600.
Visitors Mon-Fri, Sun & BHs. Booking required. Dress code.
Societies booking required. **Green Fees** not confirmed. ⊛ **Prof** Kris Esson
Course Designer Fernie/Anderson **Facilities** ⊕ ⏦ ⓛ ⌴ ⛴ ⚑ ⬆ ⚙ ⚷
Conf facs Corporate Hospitality Days **Location** 1m SW of city centre off A952
Hotel ★★★ 72% HL Best Western Queens Hotel, Leonard St, PERTH ☎ 01738 442222 50 en suite

King James VI Moncreiffe Island PH2 8NR
☎ 01738 445132 (Secretary) & 632460 (Pro)
🖹 01738 445132
e-mail: kingjamesvi@fsmail.net
web: www.kingjamesvi.com
Parkland course on island in the River Tay. Easy walking.
18 holes, 6038yds, Par 70, SSS 69, Course record 62.
Club membership 650.
Visitors Mon-Sun & BHs. Booking required. Dress code. **Societies** Booking required. **Green Fees** £32 per day, £24 per round (£34/£26 Sat & Sun).
Prof Andrew Crerar **Course Designer** Tom Morris **Facilities** ⊕ ⏦ ⓛ ⌴
⛴ ⬆ ⚑ ⚷ ⚙ ⚷ **Location** SE side of city centre
Hotel ★★★ 72% HL Best Western Queens Hotel, Leonard St, PERTH ☎ 01738 442222 50 en suite

Murrayshall Country House Hotel Murrayshall, Scone PH2 7PH
☎ 01738 552784 & 551171 🖹 01738 552595
e-mail: info@murrayshall.com
web: www.murrayshall.com
Murrayshall Course: *18 holes, 6441yds, Par 73, SSS 72.*
Lyndoch Course: *18 holes, 5800yds, Par 69.*
Course Designer Hamilton Stutt **Location** E side of village off A94
Telephone for further details
Hotel ★★★ 85% HL Murrayshall Country House Hotel & Golf Course, New Scone, PERTH ☎ 01738 551171 27 en suite 14 annexe en suite

North Inch North Inch, off Hay St PH1 5PH
☎ 01738 636481
e-mail: es@pkc.gov.uk
18 holes, 5442yds, Par 68, SSS 66, Course record 62.
Course Designer Tom Morris **Location** N of City
Telephone for further details
Hotel ★★★ 72% HL Best Western Queens Hotel, Leonard St, PERTH ☎ 01738 442222 50 en suite

PITLOCHRY
MAP 14 NN95

Pitlochry Golf Course Rd PH16 5QY
☎ 01796 472792 🖹 01796 473947
e-mail: pro@pitlochrygolf.co.uk
web: www.pitlochrygolf.co.uk
A varied and interesting heathland course with fine views and posing many problems. Its SSS permits few errors in its achievement.
18 holes, 5670yds, Par 69, SSS 69, Course record 60.
Club membership 400.
Societies Booking required. **Green Fees** £37 per day, £27 per round (£45/£35 weekends). **Prof** Mark Pirie **Course Designer** Willy Fernie
Facilities ⊕ ⏦ ⓛ ⌴ ⛴ ⬆ ⚑ ⚷ ⚙ **Location** Off A924 onto Larchwood Rd
Hotel ★★ 76% HL Moulin Hotel, 11-13 Kirkmichael Rd, Moulin, PITLOCHRY ☎ 01796 472196 15 en suite

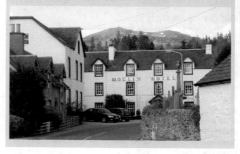

ST FILLANS
MAP 11 NN62

St Fillans South Loch Earn Rd PH6 2NJ
☎ 01764 685312 🖹 01764 685312
web: www.stfillans-golf.com
Fairly flat, beautiful parkland course. Beside the river Earn and set amongst the Perthshire hills. Wonderfully rich in flora, animal and bird life. Easy to play but hard to score.
9 holes, 6054yds, Par 69, SSS 69, Course record 73.
Club membership 400.
Visitors Mon-Sun & BHs. Booking advised. Dress code. **Societies** welcome.
Green Fees not confirmed. ⊛ **Course Designer** W Auchterlonie
Facilities ⊕ ⏦ ⓛ ⌴ ⛴ ⬆ ⚑ ⚷ ⚙ ⚷ **Location** E side of village off A85
Hotel ★★★ 82% HL The Four Seasons Hotel, Loch Earn, ST FILLANS ☎ 01764 685333 12 en suite 6 annexe en suite

STRATHTAY
MAP 14 NN95

Strathtay Lyon Cottage PH9 0PG
☎ 01887 840373 🖹 01887 840777
e-mail: aivr@aol.com
Very attractive Highland course in a charming location. Steep in places but with fine views of surrounding hills and the Tay valley.
9 holes, 4082yds, Par 63, SSS 62, Course record 61.
Club membership 212.
Visitors Mon-sun & BHs. Contact club for details. **Societies** welcome.
Green Fees not confirmed. ⊛ **Facilities** ⬆ ⚷ **Location** E of village centre off A827

Scotland

RENFREWSHIRE

BISHOPTON
MAP 10 NS47

Erskine PA7 5PH
☎ 01505 862108 📠 01505 862302
e-mail: peter@erskinegc.wanadoo.co.uk
Parkland on the south bank of the River Clyde, with views of the hills beyond.
18 holes, 6372yds, Par 71, SSS 71. Club membership 800.
Visitors Mon-Fri & BHs. Dress code. **Societies** booking required. **Green Fees** not confirmed. **Prof** Peter Thomson **Facilities** ⊕ ⏺ ⓘ ⓛ ⓒ ⚑ ⓘ ⚐ ⚒ ⓕ ⚐ **Location** 0.75 NE off B815

BRIDGE OF WEIR
MAP 10 NS36

Old Course Ranfurly Ranfurly Place PA11 3DE
☎ 01505 613612 📠 01505 613214
e-mail: secretary@oldranfurly.com
web: www.oldranfurly.com
A Par 70 course that is both fun and challenging to play. From the higher, moorland part of the course the River Clyde comes into view and makes a spectacular backdrop, with Ben Lomond and the Campsie Fells in the distance.
18 holes, 6061yds, Par 70, SSS 70, Course record 63. Club membership 819.
Visitors Mon-Fri. Booking required. Handicap certificate. Dress code. **Societies** booking required. **Green Fees** not confirmed. **Prof** Grant Miller **Course Designer** W Park **Facilities** ⊕ ⏺ ⓘ ⓛ ⓒ ⓕ ⚐ **Conf** Corporate Hospitality Days **Location** 6m S of Glasgow Airport

Ranfurly Castle The Clubhouse, Golf Rd PA11 3HN
☎ 01505 612609 📠 01505 610406
e-mail: secretary@ranfurlycastlegolfclub.co.uk
web: www.ranfurlycastlegolfclub.co.uk
A picturesque, highly challenging 240-acre moorland course.
18 holes, 6261yds, Par 70, SSS 71, Course record 65. Club membership 825.
Visitors Mon,Tue, Thur-Sun. Booking required Sat & Sun. Handicap certificate. Dress code. **Societies** Booking required. **Green Fees** £30 per round; £40 per day. **Prof** Tom Eckford **Course Designer** A Kirkcaldy/W Auchterlomie **Facilities** ⊕ ⏺ ⓘ ⓛ ⓒ ⓕ ⚐ ⓛ ⚐ ⓕ **Location** 5m NW of Johnstone
Hotel BUD Premier Travel Inn Glasgow (Paisley), Phoenix Retail Park, PAISLEY ☎ 08701 977113 40 en suite

JOHNSTONE
MAP 10 NS46

Cochrane Castle Scott Av, Craigston PA5 0HF
☎ 01505 328465 📠 01505 325338
web: www.cochranecastle.scottishgolf.com
Fairly hilly parkland, wooded with two small streams running through.
18 holes, 6194yds, Par 71, SSS 71, Course record 63. Club membership 721.
Visitors Mon-Fri. Booking required. Handicap certificate. Dress code. **Societies** Booking required. **Green Fees** £30 per day; £22 per round. 🏢 **Prof** Alan J Logan **Course Designer** J Hunter **Facilities** ⊕ ⏺ ⓘ ⓛ ⓒ ⓕ ⚐ ⓛ ⓕ **Location** 1m from town centre, off Beith Rd

Elderslie 63 Main Rd, Elderslie PA5 9AZ
☎ 01505 323956 📠 01505 340346
e-mail: eldersliegolfclub@btconnect.com
web: www.eldersliegolfclub.net
Undulating parkland with good views.
18 holes, 6175yds, Par 70, SSS 70, Course record 61. Club membership 940.
Visitors Mon-Fri & BHs. Booking required. Dress code. **Societies** Booking required. **Green Fees** £50 per day, £30 per round. **Prof** Richard Bowman **Course Designer** J Braid **Facilities** ⊕ ⏺ ⓘ ⓛ ⓒ ⓕ ⚐ ⓛ ⓕ **Leisure** snooker tables. **Conf** Corporate Hospitality Days **Location** E side of town on A737

LANGBANK
MAP 10 NS37

Gleddoch Golf and Country Club PA14 6YE
☎ 01475 540304 📠 01475 540201
e-mail: golf@gleddochhouse.co.uk
web: www.gleddochhouse.co.uk
18 holes, 6330yds, Par 71, SSS 71, Course record 64.
Course Designer Hamilton Strutt **Location** B789-Old Greenock Road
Telephone for further details
Hotel ★★★ 80% HL Gleddoch House Hotel, LANGBANK ☎ 01475 540711 70 en suite

LOCHWINNOCH
MAP 10 NS35

Lochwinnoch Burnfoot Rd PA12 4AN
☎ 01505 842153 & 01505 843029 📠 01505 843668
18 holes, 6243yds, Par 71, SSS 71, Course record 63.
Location W side of town off A760
Telephone for further details

PAISLEY
MAP 11 NS46

Barshaw Barshaw Park PA1 3TJ
☎ 0141 889 2908
18 holes, 5703yds, Par 68, SSS 67, Course record 63.
Course Designer J R Stutt **Location** 1m E off A737
Telephone for further details
Hotel ★★★ 77% HL Glynhill Hotel & Leisure Club, Paisley Rd, RENFREW ☎ 0141 886 5555 145 en suite

Paisley Braehead Rd PA2 8TZ
☎ 0141 884 3903 & 884 2292 📠 0141 884 3903
e-mail: paisleygolfclub@btconnect.com
web: www.paisleygolfclub.co.uk
Moorland course with good views which suits all handicaps. The course has been designed in two loops of nine holes. holes feature trees and gorse.
18 holes, 6466yds, Par 71, SSS 72, Course record 64. Club membership 810.
Visitors Mon-Fri & Sun. Booking required. Handicap certificate. Dress code. **Societies** Booking required. **Green Fees** £40 per day, £30 per round. **Prof** David Gordon **Course Designer** John Stutt **Facilities** ⊕ ⏺ ⓘ ⓛ ⓒ ⓕ ⚐ ⓛ ⓕ ⚐ ⓕ ⚐ **Conf** facs **Location** Exit M8 junct 27, Renfrew Rd and continue through lights. Left at Causeyside St, right at Jet filling station, left at rdbt, at top of hill
Hotel ★★★ 77% HL Glynhill Hotel & Leisure Club, Paisley Rd, RENFREW ☎ 0141 886 5555 145 en suite

Scotland

Ralston Strathmore Av, Ralston PA1 3DT
☎ 0141 882 1349 📄 0141 883 9837
e-mail: thesecretary@ralstongolf.co.uk
web: www.ralstongolfclub.co.uk
Parkland course.
18 holes, 6071yds, Par 70, SSS 69, Course record 62.
Club membership 750.
Visitors Mon-Fri & BHs. Booking required. Dress code. **Societies** booking
required. **Green Fees** not confirmed. **Prof** Colin Munro **Course Designer**
J Braid **Facilities** ⊕ ⍾ 🏐 ⬜ 🍴 ⚘ 🏌 **Conf** facs Corporate Hospitality
Days **Location** 2m E of Paisley town centre on A761
Hotel BUD Premier Travel Inn Glasgow (Paisley), Phoenix Retail Park,
PAISLEY ☎ 08701 977113 40 en suite

RENFREW   MAP 11 NS46

Renfrew Blythswood Estate, Inchinnan Rd PA4 9EG
☎ 0141 886 6692 📄 0141 886 1808
e-mail: secretary@renfrew.scottishgolf.co.uk
web: www.renfrewgolfclub.com
A tree-lined parkland course.
18 holes, 6818yds, Par 72, SSS 73, Course record 65.
Club membership 800.
Visitors Mon, Tue, Thu & Sun. Dress code. **Societies** Booking required.
Green Fees £40 per day, £30 per round. **Prof** David Grant **Course
Designer** Commander Harris **Facilities** ⊕ ⍾ 🏐 ⬜ 🍴 🏌 🏠 ⚘
Location 0.75m W off A8
Hotel ★★★ 77% HL Glynhill Hotel & Leisure Club, Paisley Rd, RENFREW
☎ 0141 886 5555 145 en suite

SCOTTISH BORDERS

ASHKIRK   MAP 12 NT42

Woll New Woll Estate TD7 4PE
☎ 01750 32711
e-mail: wollgolf@btinternet.com
web: www.wollgolf.co.uk
Flat parkland course with mature trees and a natural burn and ponds.
The course is gentle but testing for all standards of golfer. Set in
outstanding countryside in the Ale valley.
18 holes, 6051yds, Par 70, SSS 69.
Visitors Mon-Sun & BHs. Booking required. Dress code. **Societies** Booking
required. **Green Fees** £32 per day, £26 per round. **Prof** Murray Cleghorn
Course Designer Alec Cleghorn **Facilities** ⊕ ⍾ 🏐 ⬜ 🍴 🏌 🏠 ◇
⚘ ⚘ **Conf** facs Corporate Hospitality Days **Location** Off A7 at village
of Ashkirk

COLDSTREAM   MAP 12 NT83

Hirsel Kelso Rd TD12 4NJ
☎ 01890 882678 & 882233 📄 01890 882233
e-mail: bookings@hirselgc.co.uk
web: www.hirselgc.co.uk
A beautifully situated parkland course set in the Hirsel Estate, with
panoramic views of the Cheviot Hills. Each hole offers a different
challenge especially the 7th, a 170yd Par 3 demanding accuracy of
flight and length from the tee to ensure achieving a par.
18 holes, 6024yds, Par 70, SSS 70, Course record 65.
Club membership 680.

Visitors Mon-Sun & BHs. Booking required. Dress code. **Societies** Booking
required. **Green Fees** £32 per day (£38 Sat & Sun). **Facilities** ⊕ ⍾ 🏐 ⬜
🍴 🏌 ⚘ ⚘ ⚘ **Conf** Corporate Hospitality Days **Location** On A697 at
W end of Coldstream
Guest Accommodation ★★★★ RR Wheatsheaf at Swinton, SWINTON
☎ 01890 860257 10 en suite

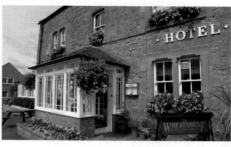

DUNS   MAP 12 NT75

Duns Hardens Rd TD11 3NR
☎ 01361 882194 📄 01361 883599
e-mail: secretary@dunsgolfclub.com
web: www.dunsgolfclub.com
Interesting upland course, with natural hazards of water and hilly
slopes. Views south to the Cheviot Hills. A burn comes into play at
seven of the holes.
18 holes, 6298yds, Par 71, SSS 70, Course record 67.
Club membership 426.
Visitors Mon-Sun & BHs. Booking required Sat, Sun & BHs. Dress code.
Societies Booking details. **Green Fees** £32 per day, £25 per round
(£38/£30 Sat, Sun & BHs). ⊚ **Course Designer** A H Scott **Facilities** ⊕ ⍾
🏐 ⬜ 🍴 🏌 🏠 ⚘ 🍴 ⚘ **Conf** Corporate Hospitality Days **Location** 1m
W off A6105
Hotel ★★★ 72% HL Marshall Meadows Country House Hotel, BERWICK-
UPON-TWEED ☎ 01289 331133 19 en suite

EYEMOUTH   MAP 12 NT96

Eyemouth Gunsgreen Hill TD14 5SF
☎ 01890 750551 (clubhouse) & 750004 (Pro shop)
e-mail: eyemouth@gxn.co.uk
web: www.eyegolfclub.co.uk
A superb course set on the coast, containing interesting and
challenging holes, in particular the intimidating 6th hole, a formidable
Par 3 across a vast gully with the waves crashing below and leaving
little room for error. The clubhouse overlooks the picturesque fishing
village of Eyemouth and provides panoramic views over the course
and the North Sea.
18 holes, 6520yds, Par 72, SSS 72, Course record 66.
Club membership 400.
Visitors Mon-Sun & BHs. Dress code. **Societies** Booking required. **Green
Fees** £30 per day, £25 per round (£35/£30 Sat & Sun). **Prof** Michael Hackett
Course Designer J R Bain **Facilities** ⊕ 🏐 ⬜ 🍴 🏌 🏠 ⚘ 🍴 ⚘ **Conf**
Corporate Hospitality Days **Location** E side of town, 8m N of Berwick
and 2m off A1
Hotel ★★★ 72% HL Marshall Meadows Country House Hotel, BERWICK-
UPON-TWEED ☎ 01289 331133 19 en suite

GALASHIELS MAP 12 NT43

Galashiels Ladhope Recreation Ground TD1 2NJ
☎ 01896 753724
e-mail: secretary@galashiels-golfclub.co.uk
web: www.galashiels-golfclub.co.uk
Hillside course, superb views from the top; 10th hole very steep.
18 holes, 5185yds, Par 67, SSS 66, Course record 61.
Club membership 86.
Visitors Mon-Sun & BHs. Booking required Sat & Sun. **Societies** Booking
required. **Green Fees** £12 per 9 holes, £20 per 18 holes (£15/£25 Sat &
Sun). ☻ **Course Designer** James Braid **Facilities** ⊕ by prior arrangement
🍴 by prior arrangement ♨ by prior arrangement ⊑ by prior arrangement
🏌 ⚒ ✆ **Location** N side of town centre off A7
Hotel ★★★ 73% HL Kingsknowes Hotel, Selkirk Rd, GALASHIELS
☎ 01896 758375 12 en suite

Torwoodlee Edinburgh Rd TD1 2NE
☎ 01896 752260 📄 01896 752306
e-mail: thesecretary@torwoodleegolfclub.org.uk
web: www.torwoodleegolfclub.org.uk
A picturesque course flanked by the River Gala and set among a mix of
mature woodland and rolling parkland.
18 holes, 6021yds, Par 69, SSS 70, Course record 63.
Club membership 550.
Visitors Mon-Sun & BHs. Booking required **Societies** Booking required.
Green Fees £40 per day, £30 per round. **Course Designer** Willie Park
Facilities ⊕ 🍴 🍺 ⊑ 🏌 ♨ ⚒ ✆ **Location** 1.75m NW of Galashiels
off A7
Hotel ★★★ 73% HL Kingsknowes Hotel, Selkirk Rd, GALASHIELS
☎ 01896 758375 12 en suite

HAWICK MAP 12 NT51

Hawick Vertish Hill TD9 0NY
☎ 01450 372293
e-mail: thesecretary@hawickgolfclub.fsnet.co.uk
web: www.hawickgolfclub.com
Hill course with good views.
18 holes, 5933yds, Par 68, SSS 69, Course record 61.
Club membership 600.
Visitors Mon-Sun & BHs. Booking required. Handicap certificate. Dress
code. **Societies** Booking required. **Green Fees** £30 per day. ☻ **Facilities**
⊕ 🍴 🍺 ⊑ 🏌 ♨ ⚒ ✆ ⚒ ✆ **Conf** Corporate Hospitality Days
Location SW side of town

INNERLEITHEN MAP 11 NT33

Innerleithen Leithen Water, Leithen Rd EH44 6NL
☎ 01896 830951
Moorland course, with easy walking. Burns and rivers are natural
hazards. Testing 5th hole (100yds) Par 3.
9 holes, 6066yds, Par 70, SSS 69, Course record 65.
Club membership 280.
Visitors contact club for details. **Societies** welcome. **Green Fees** not
confirmed. ☻ **Course Designer** Willie Park **Facilities** 🍺 ⊑ 🏌 ♨
Conf Corporate Hospitality Days **Location** 1.5m N on B709
Hotel ★★★★ 75% HL Peebles Hotel Hydro, PEEBLES ☎ 01721 720602
128 en suite

JEDBURGH MAP 12 NT62

Jedburgh Dunion Rd TD8 6TA
☎ 01835 863587
web: www.tweeddalepress.co.uk/jedburghgolfclub.htlm
9 holes, 5760yds, Par 68, SSS 67, Course record 62.
Course Designer William Park **Location** 1m W on B6358
Telephone for further details
Hotel ★★★ 81% HL Jedforest Hotel, Camptown, JEDBURGH
☎ 01835 840222 8 en suite 4 annexe en suite

KELSO MAP 12 NT73

Kelso Racecourse Rd TD5 7SL
☎ 01573 223009 📄 01573 228490
18 holes, 6046yds, Par 70, SSS 69, Course record 64.
Course Designer James Braid **Location** N side of town centre off B6461
Telephone for further details
Hotel ★★★ 73% HL Cross Keys Hotel, 36-37 The Square, KELSO
☎ 01573 223303 27 en suite

Roxburghe Heiton TD5 8JZ
☎ 01573 450331 📄 01573 450611
e-mail: hotel@roxburghe.net
web: www.roxburghe.net
An exceptional parkland layout designed by Dave Thomas and
opened in 1997. Surrounded by natural woodland on the banks
of the River Teviot. Owned by the Duke of Roxburghe, this course
has numerous bunkers, wide rolling and sloping fairways and
strategically placed water features. The signature hole is the 14th.

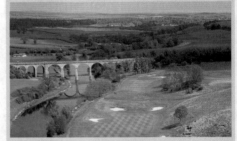

18 holes, 6925yds, Par 72, SSS 74, Course record 66.
Club membership 300.
Visitors Mon-Sun & BHs. Booking required. Handicap certificate.
Dress code. **Societies** booking required. **Green Fees** not confirmed.
Prof Craig Montgomerie **Course Designer** Dave Thomas
Facilities ⊕ 🍴 🍺 ⊑ 🏌 ♨ ⚒ 🏇 ♦ ⚒ ✆ 🏹 **Leisure** fishing, Clay
pigeon shooting, falconry, archery, mountain bikes. **Conf** facs Corporate
Hospitality Days **Location** 2m W of Kelso on A698
Hotel ★★★ 83% HL The Roxburghe Hotel & Golf Course, Heiton,
KELSO ☎ 01573 450331 16 en suite 6 annexe en suite

LAUDER

MAP 12 NT54

Lauder Galashiels Rd TD2 6RS
☎ 01578 722240 📠 01578 722526
e-mail: secretary@laudergolfclub.org.uk
web: www.laudergolfclub.org.uk
Inland course and practice area on gently sloping hill with stunning views of the Lauderdale district. The signature holes are The Wood, a dog-leg Par 4 played round the corner of a wood which is itself out of bounds, and The Quarry, a 150yd Par 3 played over several old quarry holes into a bowl shaped green.
9 holes, 6050yds, Par 72, SSS 69, Course record 66. Club membership 260.
Visitors Mon-Sun & BHs. Booking required Sun. Dress code. **Societies** Booking required. **Green Fees** £15 per day. ● **Prof** Craig Lumsden **Course Designer** Willie Park Jnr **Facilities** 🍴 🖓 🏌 **Conf** Corporate Hospitality Days **Location** Off A68, 0.5m from Lauder
Hotel ★★ 68% HL Lauderdale Hotel, 1 Edinburgh Rd, LAUDER ☎ 01578 722231   10 en suite

MELROSE

MAP 12 NT53

Melrose Dingleton TD6 9HS
☎ 01896 822855
Undulating tree-lined fairways with spendid views. Many bunkers.
9 holes, 5562yds, Par 70, SSS 68, Course record 61. Club membership 380.
Visitors Mon-Fri & BHs. Booking required Tue & Sat-Sun. Dress code. **Societies** welcome. **Green Fees** not confirmed. ● **Course Designer** James Braid **Facilities** 🖓 🏌 **Location** S side of town centre on B6359
Hotel ★★★ 75% HL Burt's Hotel, Market Square, MELROSE ☎ 01896 822285   20 en suite

MINTO

MAP 12 NT52

Minto TD9 8SH
☎ 01450 870220 📠 01450 870126
e-mail: pat@mintogolfclub.freeserve.co.uk
web: mintogolf.co.uk
Pleasant, undulating parkland, featuring mature trees and panoramic views of the border country. Short but quite testing course.
18 holes, 5542yds, Par 69, SSS 67, Course record 63. Club membership 500.
Visitors Mon-Sun & BHs. Booking required. Handicap certificate. Dress code. **Societies** Booking required. **Green Fees** £35 per day, £30 per round (£45/£40 Sat, Sun & BHs). **Course Designer** Thomas Telford **Facilities** ⑪ 🍴 🍺 🖓 🏌 🏌 🍴 🍴 **Conf** Corporate Hospitality Days **Location** 5m NE from Hawick off B6405
Hotel ★★★ 77% HL Dryburgh Abbey Hotel, ST BOSWELLS ☎ 01835 822261   38 en suite

NEWCASTLETON

MAP 12 NY48

Newcastleton Holm Hill TD9 0QD
☎ 01387 375608
Hilly course with scenic views over the Liddesdale valley and Newcastleton.
9 holes, 5491yds, Par 69, SSS 70, Course record 67. Club membership 100.
Visitors Mon-Sun & BHs. Booking required Sat-Sun. Handicap certificate. Dress code. **Societies** Booking required. **Green Fees** £10 per day. ●

Course Designer J Shade **Facilities** 🏌 🍴 **Leisure** fishing. **Location** W side of village
Hotel ★★★ 74% HL Garden House Hotel, Sarkfoot Rd, GRETNA ☎ 01461 337621   38 en suite

PEEBLES

MAP 11 NT24

Macdonald Cardrona Hotel, Golf & Country Club
Cardrona EH45 6LZ
☎ 01896 833600 📠 01896 831166
e-mail: golf.cardrona@macdonald-hotels.co.uk
web: www.macdonaldhotels.co.uk
Opened for play in 2001 and already a settled and inspiring test. The terrain is a mixture of parkland, heathland and woodland with an additional 20,000 trees planted. The USPGA specification greens are mostly raised and mildly contoured with no two being the same shape.
18 holes, 6856yds, Par 72, SSS 74, Course record 64. Club membership 200.
Visitors Mon-Sun & BHs. Booking required. Dress code. **Societies** booking required. **Green Fees** not confirmed. **Prof** Ross Harrower **Course Designer** Dave Thomas **Facilities** ⑪ 🍴 🍺 🖓 🍴 🏌 🍺 🍴 ◇ 🍴 🍴 **Leisure** heated indoor swimming pool, fishing, sauna, solarium, gymnasium. **Conf** facs   Corporate Hospitality Days **Location** off A72, 3m S of Peebles
Hotel ★★★★ 77% HL Macdonald Cardrona Hotel Golf & Country Club, Cardrona Mains, PEEBLES ☎ 0870 1942114   99 en suite

Peebles Kirkland St EH45 8EU
☎ 01721 720197
e-mail: secretary@peeblesgolfclub.co.uk
web: peeblesgolfclub.co.uk
This parkland course is one of the most picturesque courses in Scotland, shadowed by the rolling border hills and Tweed valley and set high above the town. The tough opening holes are balanced by a more generous stretch through to the 14th hole but from here the closing five prove a challenging test.
18 holes, 6160yds, Par 70, SSS 70, Course record 63. Club membership 750.
Visitors Sun-Fri, Sun & BHs. Booking required Sun & BHs. Dress code. **Societies** Booking required. **Green Fees** £50 per day, £38 per round. **Prof** Craig Imlah **Course Designer** H S Colt **Facilities** ⑪ 🍴 🍺 🖓 🍴 🏌 🍺 🍴 🍴 **Conf** Corporate Hospitality Days **Location** W side of town centre off A72
Hotel ★★★★ 75% HL Peebles Hotel Hydro, PEEBLES ☎ 01721 720602   128 en suite

ST BOSWELLS

MAP 12 NT53

St Boswells Braeheads TD6 0DE
☎ 01835 823527
web: www.stboswellsgolfclub.co.uk
Attractive, easy walking parkland by the River Tweed.
9 holes, 5274yds, Par 68, SSS 66. Club membership 350.
Visitors Mon-Sun & BHs. **Societies** welcome. **Green Fees** £24 per day, £20 per 18 holes, £12 per 9 holes. ● **Course Designer** W Park **Facilities** 🏌 **Location** 500yds off A68 east end of village
Hotel ★★★ 77% HL Dryburgh Abbey Hotel, ST BOSWELLS ☎ 01835 822261   38 en suite

Scotland *(side tab)*

SELKIRK   MAP 12 NT42

Selkirk Selkirk Hill TD7 4NW
☎ 01750 20621 & 20857 (pm)
e-mail: secretary@selkirkgolfclub.co.uk
Pleasant moorland course with gorse and heather, set around Selkirk Hill. A testing course for all golfers. Unrivalled views.
9 holes, 5620yds, Par 68, SSS 68, Course record 61.
Club membership 300.
Visitors Mon-Fri & BHs. Handicap certificate. Dress code. **Societies** Booking required. **Green Fees** £22 per 18 holes, £11 per 9 holes. ◉ **Facilities** ▜⏴
⚲ **Location** 1m S on A7
Hotel ★★★ 75% HL Burt's Hotel, Market Square, MELROSE
☎ 01896 822285 20 en suite

WEST LINTON   MAP 11 NT15

Rutherford Castle Golf Club EH46 7AS
☎ 01968 661 233 🖹 01968 661 233
e-mail: rcgc@btconnect.com
Undulating parkland set beneath the Pentland Hills. The many challenging holes are a good test for the better player while offering great enjoyment to the average player.
18 holes, 6525yds, Par 72, SSS 71. Club membership 120.
Visitors Mon-Sun & BHs. Booking required Sat & Sun **Green Fees** Phone. ◉ **Course Designer** Bryan Moore **Facilities** ▙ ⌂⏴ & ✓ **Location** On A702 towards Carlisle
Hotel ★★★★ 75% HL Peebles Hotel Hydro, PEEBLES ☎ 01721 720602 128 en suite

West Linton EH46 7HN
☎ 01968 660970 🖹 01968 660622
e-mail: secretarywlgc@btinternet.com
web: www.wlgc.co.uk
Moorland course with beautiful views of Pentland Hills. This well-maintained course offers a fine challenge to all golfers with ample fairways and interesting layouts. The wildlife and natural scenery give added enjoyment.
18 holes, 6161yds, Par 69, SSS 70, Course record 63.
Club membership 1000.
Visitors Mon-Sun & BHs. Booking required. Dress code. **Societies** Booking required. **Green Fees** £40 per day, £30 per round (£40 per round Sat & Sun). ◉ **Prof** Ian Wright **Course Designer** Millar/Braid/Fraser
Facilities ⏴⏴▙ ⌂⏴⚲ & ✓ & ✓ **Conf** Corporate Hospitality Days
Location NW side of village off A702
Hotel ★★★★ 75% HL Peebles Hotel Hydro, PEEBLES ☎ 01721 720602 128 en suite

SOUTH AYRSHIRE

AYR   MAP 10 NS32

Belleisle Belleisle Park KA7 4DU
☎ 01292 441258 🖹 01292 442632
e-mail: belleisle.golf@south-ayrshire.gov.uk
web: www.golfsouthayrshire.com
Parkland course with beautiful sea views. First-class conditions.
Belleisle Course: 18 holes, 6431yds, Par 71, SSS 72, Course record 63.
Seafield Course: 18 holes, 5498yds, Par 68, SSS 67.

Visitors Mon-Sun & BHs. Booking required. Dress code. **Societies** booking required. **Green Fees** not confirmed. **Prof** David Gemmell **Course Designer** James Braid **Facilities** ⏴⏴▙ ⌂⏴⚲ & ✓ ◊ ✓ **Conf** facs
Location 2m S of Ayr on A719
Hotel ★★★ 79% HL Savoy Park Hotel, 16 Racecourse Rd, AYR
☎ 01292 266112 15 en suite

Dalmilling Westwood Av KA8 0QY
☎ 01292 263893 🖹 01292 610543
web: www.golfsouthayrshire.com/dalmilling.html
Meadowland course, with easy walking. Tributaries of the River Ayr add interest to early holes.
18 holes, 5724yds, Par 69, SSS 68, Course record 61.
Club membership 260.
Visitors Mon-Sun & BHs. Booking required. Dress code. **Societies** Booking required. **Green Fees** £20 per day, £14 per round (£27/£17.50 Sat & Sun). **Prof** Philip Cheyney **Facilities** ⏴⏴▙ ⌂⏴⚲ & ✓ **Location** 1.5m E of town centre off A77
Hotel ★★★★ 80% HL Fairfield House Hotel, 12 Fairfield Rd, AYR
☎ 01292 267461 40 en suite 4 annexe en suite

BARASSIE   MAP 10 NS33

Kilmarnock (Barassie) 29 Hillhouse Rd KA10 6SY
☎ 01292 313920 🖹 01292 318300
e-mail: secretary@kbgc.co.uk
web: www.kbgc.co.uk
The club has a 27-hole layout. Magnificent seaside links, relatively flat with much heather and small, undulating greens.
18 holes, 6817yds, Par 72, SSS 74, Course record 63.
9 hole course: 9 holes, 2888yds, Par 34.
Club membership 600.
Visitors Mon, Tue, Thu & Fri. Booking required. Dress code. **Societies** Booking required. **Green Fees** £65 for up to 36 holes.
Prof Gregor Howie **Course Designer** Theodore Moone **Facilities** ⏴⏴ ⏴⏴▙ ⌂⏴⚲ & ✓ **Location** E side of village on B746, 2m N of Troon
Hotel ★★★★ 75% HL Paramount Marine Hotel, Crosbie Rd, TROON
☎ 01292 314444 89 en suite

GIRVAN   MAP 10 NX19

Brunston Castle Golf Course Rd, Dailly KA26 9GD
☎ 01465 811471 🖹 01465 811545
e-mail: golf@brunstoncastle.co.uk
web: www.brunstoncastle.co.uk
Burns: 18 holes, 6662yds, Par 72, SSS 72, Course record 63.
Course Designer Donald Steel **Location** 5m E of Girvan
Telephone for further details
Hotel ★★★ 81% HL Malin Court, TURNBERRY ☎ 01655 331457
18 en suite

Girvan Golf Course Rd KA26 9HW
☎ 01465 714346 🖹 01465 714272
18 holes, 5098yds, Par 64, SSS 65, Course record 61.
Course Designer D Kinnell/J Braid **Location** N side of town off A77
Telephone for further details
Hotel ★★★ 81% HL Malin Court, TURNBERRY ☎ 01655 331457
18 en suite

CHAMPIONSHIP COURSE

ROYAL TROON

Map 10 NS33

Craigend Rd KA10 6EP

☎ 01292 311555 📄 01292 318204

e-mail: bookings@royaltroon.com

web: www.royaltroon.com

Old Course: 18 holes, 6641yds, Par 71, SSS 73, Course record 64.

Portland: 18 holes, 6289yds, Par 71, SSS 71, Course record 65.

Craigend: 9 holes.

Club membership 800.

Visitors Mon-Tue & Thu. Booking required. Handicap certificate. Dress code.

Societies Booking required. **Green Fees** £220 per day including coffee/lunch, 1 round over Old & 1 round over Portland **Prof** R B Anderson **Course Designer** C Hunter/G Strath/W Fernie **Facilities** ⑪ ⑩ 🍴 🍺 ☕ 🍽 ⚒ 🍴 ⚐ ⚒ ⛳ **Location** S of town on B749. 5m from Prestwick airport

Troon was founded in 1878 with just five holes on linksland. In its first decade it grew from five holes to six, then 12, and finally 18 holes. It became Royal Troon in 1978 on its 100th anniversary. Royal Troon's reputation is based on its combination of rough and sandy hills, bunkers, and a severity of finish that has diminished the championship hopes of many. The most successful players have relied on an equal blend of finesse and power. The British Open Championship has been played at Troon eight times - in 1923, 1950, 1962, 1973, 1982, 1989, 1997, and lastly in 2004 when it hosted the 133rd tournament. It has the shortest hole of courses hosting the Open. Ten new bunkers and four new tees were added after the 1997 competition. It is recommended that you apply to the course in advance for full visitor information.

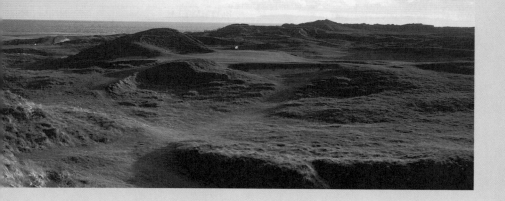

Scotland

MAYBOLE
MAP 10 NS20

Maybole Municipal Memorial Park KA19 7DX
☎ 01655 889770
9 holes, 2635yds, Par 33, SSS 65, Course record 64.
Location Off A77 S of town
Telephone for further details
Hotel ★★ HL Ladyburn, MAYBOLE ☎ 01655 740585 5 en suite

PRESTWICK
MAP 10 NS32

Prestwick 2 Links Rd KA9 1QG
☎ 01292 477404 🗎 01292 477255
e-mail: bookings@prestwickgc.co.uk
web: www.prestwickgc.co.uk
Seaside links with natural hazards, tight fairways and difficult fast
undulating greens.
18 holes, 6544yds, Par 71, SSS 73, Course record 67.
Club membership 575.
Visitors Mon-Fri, Sun & BHs. Booking required. Handicap certificate.
Dress code. **Societies** Booking required. **Green Fees** £110 per
round, £165 per day (Sun £140 per round). **Prof** D A Fleming
Course Designer Tom Morris **Facilities** ⑪ ⅂⅃ ⊑ ⅋⅃ ⅂ 🏻 ⅌
Conf Corporate Hospitality Days **Location** In town centre off A79
Hotel ★★★ 75% HL Parkstone Hotel, Esplanade, PRESTWICK
☎ 01292 477286 30 en suite

Prestwick St Cuthbert East Rd KA9 2SX
☎ 01292 477101 🗎 01292 671730
e-mail: secretary@stcuthbert.co.uk
web: www.stcuthbert.co.uk
Parkland with easy walking and natural hazards. Sometimes windy.
Tree-lined fairways and well bunkered.
18 holes, 6470yds, Par 71, SSS 71, Course record 64.
Club membership 880.
Visitors Mon, Tue, Thur & Fri. Dress code. **Societies** Booking required.
Green Fees £45 per day, £30 per round. **Course Designer** Stutt &
Co **Facilities** ⑪ ⅃⅁⅃ ⊑ ⅀⅃ ⅂ ⅌ **Conf** Corporate Hospitality Days
Location 0.5m E of town centre off A77
Hotel ★★★ 75% HL Parkstone Hotel, Esplanade, PRESTWICK
☎ 01292 477286 30 en suite

Prestwick St Nicholas Grangemuir Rd KA9 1SN
☎ 01292 477608 🗎 01292 473900
e-mail: secretary@prestwickstnicholas.com
web: www.prestwickstnicholas.com
Classic seaside links course with views across the Firth of Clyde to the
Isle of Arran to the west and Ailsa Craig to the south.
18 holes, 5952yds, Par 69, SSS 69, Course record 63.
Club membership 750.
Visitors Mon-Fri, Sun & BHs. Dress code. **Societies** Booking required.
Green Fees £65 per day, £55 per round (£60 per round Sun).
Course Designer Charles Hunter **Facilities** ⑪ ⅃◯⅃ ⅂⅃ ⊑ ⅀⅃ ⅂ 🏻 ⅌
Location S side of town off A79
Hotel ★★★ 75% HL Parkstone Hotel, Esplanade, PRESTWICK
☎ 01292 477286 30 en suite

TROON
MAP 10 NS33

Royal Troon see page 367

Hotel ★★★★ 75% HL Paramount Marine Hotel, Crosbie Rd, TROON
☎ 01292 314444 89 en suite
Hotel ★★★★ CHH Lochgreen House Hotel, Monktonhill Rd, Southwood,
TROON ☎ 01292 313343 Fax 01292 318661 31 en suite 7 annexe en suite
Hotel ★★★ 86% HL Piersland House Hotel, Craigend Rd, TROON
☎ 01292 314747 Fax 01292 315613 15 en suite 15 annexe en suite

Troon Municipal Harling Dr KA10 6NE
☎ 01292 312464 🗎 01292 312578
e-mail: troongolf@south-ayrshire.gov.uk
web: www.golfsouthayrshire.com
Three links courses, two of championship standard.
Lochgreen Course: 18 holes, 6820yds, Par 74, SSS 73.
Darley Course: 18 holes, 6360yds, Par 71, SSS 63.
Fullarton Course: 18 holes, 4870yds, Par 66, SSS 64.
Visitors Mon-Sun & BHs. Booking required. Dress code. **Societies** booking
required. **Green Fees** not confirmed. **Prof** Gordon McKinlay **Facilities** ⑪
⅃◯⅃ ⅂⅃ ⊑ ⅀⅃ ⅂ 🏻 ⅌ **Location** 100yds from railway station
Hotel ★★★★ 75% HL Paramount Marine Hotel, Crosbie Rd, TROON
☎ 01292 314444 89 en suite

TURNBERRY
MAP 10 NS20

Westin Turnberry Resort see page 369

Hotel ★★★★★ HL The Westin Turnberry Resort, TURNBERRY
☎ 01655 331000 130 en suite 89 annexe en suite
Hotel ★★★ 81% HL Malin Court, TURNBERRY ☎ 01655 331457
Fax 01655 331072 18 en suite
Hotel ★★ HL Ladyburn, MAYBOLE ☎ 01655 740585 Fax 01655 740580
5 en suite

SOUTH LANARKSHIRE

BIGGAR
MAP 11 NT03

Biggar The Park, Broughton Rd ML12 6AH
☎ 01899 220618(club) & 220319(course)
18 holes, 5600yds, Par 68, SSS 67, Course record 61.
Course Designer W Park Jnr **Location** S side of town
Telephone for further details
Hotel ★★★ 80% CHH Shieldhill Castle, Quothquan, BIGGAR
☎ 01899 220035 16 en suite

BOTHWELL
MAP 11 NS75

Bothwell Castle Uddingston Rpad G71 8TD
☎ 01698 801971 & 801972 🗎 01698 801971
Flattish tree-lined parkland course in a residential area.
18 holes, 6220yds, Par 70, SSS 70, Course record 62.
Club membership 1000.
Visitors Mon-Fri. Booking required. Dress code. **Societies** welcome.
Green Fees not confirmed. **Prof** Alan McCloskey **Facilities** ⊑ ⅀⅃ 🏻 ⅌
⅌ **Conf** Corporate Hospitality Days **Location** NW of village off B7071
Hotel ★★★ 74% HL Bothwell Bridge Hotel, 89 Main St, BOTHWELL
☎ 01698 852246 90 en suite

CHAMPIONSHIP COURSE

SOUTH AYRSHIRE — TURNBERRY

WESTIN TURNBERRY RESORT

Map 10 NS20

KA26 9LT
☎ 01655 331000 📄 01655 331069
e-mail: turnberry@westin.com
web: www.westin.com/turnberry
Ailsa Course: 18 holes, 6440yds, Par 69, SSS 72, Course record 63.
Kintyre Course: 18 holes, 6376yds, Par 71, SSS 72, Course record 63.
Arran Course: 9 holes, 1996, Par 31, SSS 31.
Visitors Mon-Sun & BHs. Booking required. Dress code. **Societies** booking required.
Green Fees Phone. **Prof** Paul Burley
Course Designer Mackenzie Ross/Donald Steel **Facilities** 🕦 🍴 🍺 🖥 🕯 🏊 🛍 🎿 ◇ 🚗 ✂ 🦮 **Leisure** hard tennis courts, heated indoor swimming pool, fishing, sauna, solarium, gymnasium, Colin Montgomerie Links Golf Academy. **Conf** Corporate Hospitality Days
Location 15m SW of Ayr on A77

For thousands of players of all nationalities, Turnberry is one of the finest of all golf destinations, where some of the most remarkable moments in Open history have taken place. The legendary Ailsa Course is complemented by the new highly acclaimed Kintyre Course, while the nine-hole Arran Course, created by Donald Steel and Colin Montgomerie, has similar challenges such as undulating greens, tight tee shots, pot bunkers and thick Scottish rough. With the famous hotel on the left and the magnificent Ailsa Craig away to the right, there are few vistas in world golf to match the 1st tee here. To help you prepare for your game the Colin Montgomerie Links Golf Academy, alongside the luxurious and extensive clubhouse, was opened in April 2000; it features 12 driving bays, four short-game bays, two dedicated teaching rooms and a group teaching room.

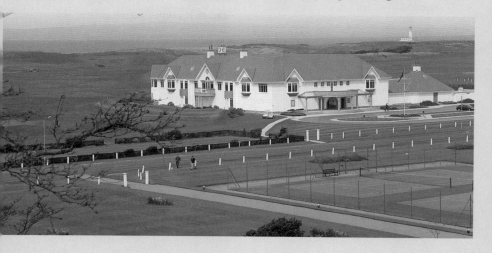

BURNSIDE · MAP 11 NS65

Blairbeth Fernbrae Av, Fernhill G73 4SF
☎ 0141 634 3355 & 634 3325
e-mail: bgc1910@yahoo.co.uk
Parkland with some small elevated greens and views over Glasgow and the Clyde valley.
18 holes, 5537yds, Par 70, SSS 68, Course record 63.
Club membership 480.
Visitors Mon-Sun & BHs. Booking required Sat, Sun & BHs. Dress code.
Societies Booking required. **Green Fees** £25 per day, £18 per round.
Facilities ⊕ ⦿1 ☷ ⌂ ⬚ 🖈 ⌇ ♨ **Conf** Corporate Hospitality Days
Location 2m S of Rutherglen off Burnside Rd

Cathkin Braes Cathkin Rd G73 4SE
☎ 0141 634 6605
e-mail: secretary@cathkinbraesgolfclub.co.uk
web: www.cathkinbraesgolfclub.co.uk
Moorland course, 600ft above sea level but relatively flat with a prevailing westerly wind and views over Glasgow. A small loch hazard at 5th hole. Very strong finishing holes.
18 holes, 6200yds, Par 71, SSS 71, Course record 62.
Club membership 920.
Visitors Mon-Fri. Booking required. Dress code. **Societies** Booking required. **Green Fees** £45 per day, £35 per round. ♨ **Prof** Stephen Bree
Course Designer James Braid **Facilities** ⊕ ⦿1 ☷ ⌂ 🖈1 ⬚ 🖈♨ ⌇ ♨ ⌇
Conf Corporate Hospitality Days **Location** 1m S on B759

CARLUKE · MAP 11 NS85

Carluke Mauldslie Rd, Hallcraig ML8 5HG
☎ 01555 770574 & 771070
e-mail: carlukegolfsecy@tiscali.co.uk
web: www.carlukegolfclub.com/
Parkland course with views over the Clyde Valley. Testing 11th hole, Par 3.
18 holes, 5919yds, Par 70, SSS 69, Course record 63.
Club membership 750.
Visitors Mon-Fri. Dress code. **Societies** Booking required **Green Fees** £35 per day, £25 per round. ♨ **Prof** Craig Ronald **Facilities** ⊕ ⦿1 ☷ ⌂ 🖈1
⬚ 🖃 ⌇ **Location** 1m W off A73
Hotel ★★★ 81% HL Best Western Popinjay Hotel & Leisure Club, Lanark Rd, ROSEBANK ☎ 01555 860441 34 en suite

CARNWATH · MAP 11 NS94

Carnwath 1 Main St ML11 8JX
☎ 01555 840251 🖨 01555 841070
e-mail: carnwathgc@hotmail.co.uk
web: www.carnwathgc.co.uk
Picturesque parkland, slightly hilly, panoramic views. The small greens call for accuracy.
18 holes, 5222yds, Par 66, SSS 66, Course record 63.
Club membership 586.
Visitors Sun-Fri & BHs. Booking required Mon, Wed, Fri, Sun & BHs.
Dress code. **Societies** Welcome. **Green Fees** £30 per day, £20 per round
(£36/£26 Sun). ♨ **Facilities** ⊕ ⦿1 ☷ ⌂ 🖈1 ⬚ ⌇ **Location** W side of village on A70
Hotel ★★★ 75% CHH Cartland Bridge Hotel, Glasgow Rd, LANARK
☎ 01555 664426 20 rms (18 en suite)

EAST KILBRIDE · MAP 11 NS65

East Kilbride Chapelside Rd, Nerston G74 4PF
☎ 01355 247728
18 holes, 6419yds, Par 71, SSS 71, Course record 64.
Location 0.5m N off A749
Telephone for further details

Torrance House Calderglen Country Park, Strathaven Rd
G75 0QZ
☎ 01355 248638 🖨 01355 570916
18 holes, 6476yds, Par 72, SSS 69, Course record 71.
Course Designer Hawtree & Son **Location** 1.5m SE of East Kilbride on
A726
Telephone for further details

HAMILTON · MAP 11 NS75

Hamilton Carlisle Rd, Ferniegair ML3 7UE
☎ 01698 282872 🖨 01698 204650
e-mail: secretary@hamiltongolfclub.co.uk
Beautiful parkland.
18 holes, 6498yds, Par 70, SSS 70, Course record 62.
Visitors Mon-Sun & BHs. Booking required. **Societies** Welcome.
Green Fees Phone. **Prof** Derek Wright **Course Designer** James Braid
Facilities ⬚ 🖈 ⌂ ⌇ ♨ **Location** 1.5m SE on A72
Hotel BUD Premier Travel Inn Glasgow (Hamilton), Hamilton Motorway
Service Area, HAMILTON ☎ 08701 977124 36 en suite

Strathclyde Park Mote Hill ML3 6BY
☎ 01698 429350
Municipal wooded parkland course with views of the Strathclyde Park sailing loch. Surrounded by a nature reserve and Hamilton racecourse.
9 holes, 3113yds, Par 36, SSS 70, Course record 68.
Club membership 120.
Visitors Mon-Sun & BHs. Booking required. Dress code. **Societies** Booking required. **Green Fees** £3.55 per 9 holes. ♨ **Prof** William Walker **Facilities**
⬚ ⌂ ⌇ ♨ 🖈 **Location** N side of town off B7071
Hotel BUD Premier Travel Inn Glasgow (Hamilton), Hamilton Motorway
Service Area, HAMILTON ☎ 08701 977124 36 en suite

LANARK · MAP 11 NS84

Lanark The Moor, Whitelees Rd ML11 7RX
☎ 01555 663219 & 661456 🖨 01555 663219
e-mail: lanarkgolfclub@supanet.com
web: www.lanarkgolfclub.co.uk
Lanark is renowned for its smooth fast greens, natural moorland fairways and beautiful scenery. The course is built on a substrate of glacial sands, providing a unique feeling of tackling a links course at 600ft above sea level. The Par of 70 can be a real test when the prevailing wind blows.
Old Course: 18 holes, 6306yds, Par 70, SSS 71,
Course record 63.
Wee Course: 9 holes, 1489yds, Par 28.
Club membership 880.
Visitors Mon-Fri. Booking required. Dress code. **Societies** Booking required. **Green Fees** £50 per day, £40 per round. Wee Course £8 per day. **Prof** Alan White **Course Designer** Tom Morris **Facilities** ⊕ ⦿1 ☷
⬚ 🖈1 ⬚ ⌇ ♨ ⌇ **Conf** Corporate Hospitality Days **Location** E side of town centre off A73
Hotel ★★★ 75% CHH Cartland Bridge Hotel, Glasgow Rd, LANARK
☎ 01555 664426 20 rms (18 en suite)

LARKHALL
MAP 11 NS75

Larkhall Burnhead Rd ML9 3AA
☎ 01698 889597 & 881113 (bookings)
Small, inland parkland course.
9 holes, 6234yds, Par 70, SSS 70, Course record 69.
Club membership 130.
Visitors Mon-Fri, Sun & BHs. Booking required. Societies Welcome. **Green Fees** Phone. ● **Facilities** ☐ ☜🗓 ⚲ ✔ **Location** E side of town on B7019
Hotel ★★★ 81% HL Best Western Popinjay Hotel & Leisure Club, Lanark Rd, ROSEBANK ☎ 01555 860441 34 en suite

LEADHILLS
MAP 11 NS81

Leadhills 51 Main St ML12 6XP
☎ 01659 74456
e-mail: harry@glenfranka.fsnet.co.uk
A testing, hilly course. At 1500ft above sea level it is the highest golf course in Scotland.
9 holes, 4354yds, Par 66, SSS 64. Club membership 80.
Visitors Mon-Sun & BHs. Booking required. **Societies** Welcome.
Green Fees £10 per day. ● **Facilities** by prior arrangement by prior arrangement by prior arrangement by prior arrangement **Location** E side of village off B797

LESMAHAGOW
MAP 11 NS83

Holland Bush Acretophead ML11 0JS
☎ 01555 893484 & 893646 📄 01555 893984
e-mail: mail@hollandbushgolfclub.co.uk
web: www.hollandbushgolfclub.co.uk
18 holes, 6246yds, Par 71, SSS 70, Course record 63.
Course Designer J Lawson/K Pate **Location** 3m S of Lesmahagow on Coalburn Rd
Telephone for further details
Hotel ★★★ 79% HL Best Western Strathaven Hotel, Hamilton Rd, STRATHAVEN ☎ 01357 521778 22 en suite

RIGSIDE
MAP 11 NS83

Douglas Water Ayr Rd ML11 9NP
☎ 01555 880361 📄 01555 880361
A 9-hole course with good variety and some hills and spectacular views. An interesting course with a challenging longest hole of 564 yards but, overall, not too testing for average golfers.
9 holes, 5890yds, Par 72, SSS 69, Course record 63.
Club membership 150.
Visitors Mon-Sun & BHs. Booking required Sat. Dress code.
Societies Welcome. **Green Fees** £10 per day (£12 Sat & Sun). ●
Facilities ☐ ⚲ **Location** On A70
Hotel ★★★ 75% CHH Cartland Bridge Hotel, Glasgow Rd, LANARK ☎ 01555 664426 20 rms (18 en suite)

STRATHAVEN
MAP 11 NS74

Strathaven Glasgow Rd ML10 6NL
☎ 01357 520421 📄 01357 520539
e-mail: info@strathavengc.com
web: www.strathavengc.com
Gently undulating, tree-lined, championship parkland course with views over the town and the Avon valley.

18 holes, 6250yds, Par 71, SSS 71, Course record 65.
Club membership 1050.
Visitors Mon-Fri. Booking required. Handicap certificate. Dress code.
Societies Booking required. **Green Fees** £41 per day, £31 per round. **Prof** Stuart Kerr **Course Designer** Willie Fernie/J Stutt **Facilities** ⑪ ⑨ 🝙 ☐ ☜🗓 ⚲ 🖴 ✔ 🝙 ✔ **Conf** facs **Location** NE side of town on A726
Hotel ★★★ 79% HL Best Western Strathaven Hotel, Hamilton Rd, STRATHAVEN ☎ 01357 521778 22 en suite

UDDINGSTON
MAP 11 NS66

Calderbraes 57 Roundknowe Rd G71 7TS
☎ 01698 813425
Parkland with good views of Clyde valley. Testing 4th hole (Par 4), hard uphill.
9 holes, 5046yds, Par 66, SSS 67, Course record 65.
Club membership 230.
Visitors Mon-Fri & BHs. Dress code. **Societies** booking required. **Green Fees** not confirmed. ● **Facilities** ⑪ ⑨ 🝙 ☐ ☜🗓 ⚲ **Location** 1.5m NW off A74
Hotel ★★★ 74% HL Bothwell Bridge Hotel, 89 Main St, BOTHWELL ☎ 01698 852246 90 en suite

STIRLING

ABERFOYLE
MAP 11 NN50

Aberfoyle Braeval FK8 3UY
☎ 01877 382493
Scenic heathland course with mountain views.
18 holes, 5210yds, Par 66, SSS 66, Course record 64.
Club membership 485.
Visitors Mon-Sun & BHs. Booking required Sat-Sun. Handicap certificate.
Societies Booking required. **Green Fees** £18 per round, £24 per day (£24/30 weekends). ● **Facilities** ⑪ ⑨ 🝙 ☐ ☜🗓 ⚲ 🝙 ✔ **Conf** Corporate Hospitality Days **Location** 1m E on A81
Hotel ★★★★ 75% HL Macdonald Forest Hills Hotel & Resort, Kinlochard, ABERFOYLE ☎ 0870 1942105 54 en suite

BANNOCKBURN
MAP 11 NS89

Brucefields Family Golfing Centre Pirnhall Rd FK7 8EH
☎ 01786 818184 📄 01786 817770
e-mail: christine.frost@brucefields.co.uk
Gently rolling parkland with fine views. Most holes can be played without too much difficulty with the exception of the 2nd which is a long and tricky Par 4 and the 6th, a Par 3 which requires exact club selection and a straight shot.
Main Course: 9 holes, 2513yds, Par 68, SSS 68,
Course record 66. Club membership 300.
Visitors Mon-Sun & BHs. Dress code. **Societies** Booking required.
Green Fees £18 per 18 holes, £11 per 9 holes (£20/£12 Sat & Sun).
Prof Gregor Monks **Course Designer** Souters Sportsturf **Facilities** ⑪ ⑨ 🝙 ☐ ☜🗓 ⚲ 🖴 🝚 🖴 ✔ 🝛 **Leisure** golf academy, Par 3 9 hole course. **Conf** facs Corporate Hospitality Days **Location** M80/M9 junct 9, A91, 1st left signed

Scotland

BRIDGE OF ALLAN — MAP 11 NS79

Bridge of Allan Sunnylaw FK9 4LY
☎ 01786 832332
e-mail: secretary@bofagc.com
web: www.bofagc.co.uk
Very hilly parkland with good views of Stirling Castle and beyond to the Trossachs. Testing Par 3 1st hole, 221yds uphill, with a 6ft wall 25yds before green.
9 holes, 4932yds, Par 66, SSS 66, Course record 59.
Club membership 400.
Visitors Mon-Sun. Booking required Sun & Sat Dress code. **Societies** Booking required. **Green Fees** Phone. ◉ **Course Designer** Tom Morris **Facilities** 🍴 ⬚ ⛏ ⛳ **Location** 0.5m N off A9
Hotel ★★★ 75% HL Best Western Royal Hotel, Henderson St, BRIDGE OF ALLAN ☎ 01786 832284 32 en suite

CALLANDER — MAP 11 NN60

Callander Aveland Rd FK17 8EN
☎ 01877 330090 & 330975 📄 01877 330062
e-mail: callandergc@nextcall.net
web: www.callandergolfclub.co.uk
Challenging parkland course with tight fairways and a number of interesting holes. Designed by Tom Morris Snr and overlooked by the Trossachs.
18 holes, 5151yds, Par 66, SSS 65, Course record 61.
Club membership 600.
Visitors Mon-Sun & BHs. Dress code. **Societies** booking required. **Green Fees** not confirmed. **Prof** Allan Martin **Course Designer** Morris/Fernie **Facilities** ⊕ ⋒ 🍴 ⬚ ⛏ 🛍 ⛳ 🍴 **Conf** Corporate Hospitality Days **Location** E side of town off A84
Hotel ★★★ 83% HL Roman Camp Country House Hotel, CALLANDER ☎ 01877 330003 14 en suite

DRYMEN — MAP 11 NS48

Buchanan Castle G63 0HY
☎ 01360 660307 📄 01360 660993
e-mail: info@buchanancastlegolfclub.co.uk
web: www.buchanancastlegolfclub.com
Easy walking parkland with and good views. A quiet and relaxed place to play golf, with views of the old castle. Owned by the Duke of Montrose.
18 holes, 6059yds, Par 70, SSS 69. Club membership 830.
Visitors Mon-Sun & BHs. Booking required. Dress code. **Societies** Booking required. **Green Fees** £48 per day, £38 per round. **Prof** Keith Baxter **Course Designer** James Braid **Facilities** ⊕ ⋒ 🍴 ⬚ ⛏ 🛍 ⛳ **Conf** facs Corporate Hospitality Days **Location** 1m W
Hotel ★★★ 79% HL Best Western Winnock Hotel, The Square, DRYMEN ☎ 01360 660245 48 en suite

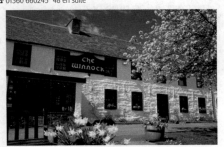

Strathendrick G63 0AA
☎ 01360 660695
e-mail: melvinquyn@hotmail.com
Hillside course with breathtaking views of the Campsie and Luss Hills and Ben Lomond. Mainly natural hazards with few bunkers. Greens are comparatively small but in immaculate condition.
9 holes, 4982yards, Par 66, SSS 64, Course record 60.
Club membership 470.
Visitors Mon-Fri & BHs. **Societies** Booking required. **Green Fees** £18 per 18 holes, £12 per 9 holes. ◉ **Facilities** ⛏ ⛳ **Leisure** hard tennis courts, driving net. **Location** 0.5m S of Drymen via access lane E of A811
Hotel ★★★★ 81% HL De Vere Cameron House, BALLOCH ☎ 01389 755565 96 en suite

DUNBLANE — MAP 11 NN70

Dunblane New Golf Club Perth Rd FK15 0LJ
☎ 01786 821521 📄 01786 825066
e-mail: secretary@dngc.co.uk
web: www.dngc.co.uk
Well-maintained parkland course. Testing Par 3 holes.
18 holes, 5930yds, Par 69, SSS 69. Club membership 1000.
Visitors Mon-Fri, Sun & BHs. Booking required. Handicap certificate. Dress code. **Societies** Booking required. **Green Fees** £40 per day, £30 per round. **Prof** Bob Jamieson **Course Designer** James Braid **Facilities** ⊕ 🍴 ⬚ ⛏ 🛍 ⛳ **Conf** facs Corporate Hospitality Days **Location** Off fourways rdbt in town centre
Hotel CHH Cromlix House Hotel, Kinbuck, DUNBLANE ☎ 01786 822125 14 en suite

KILLIN — MAP 11 NN53

Killin FK21 8TX
☎ 01567 820312 & 07795 483107 📄 01567 820312
e-mail: info@killingolfclub.co.uk
web: www.killingolfclub.co.uk
Parkland course at the west end of Loch Tay with outstanding views. Challenging nine-hole course with 14 different tees.

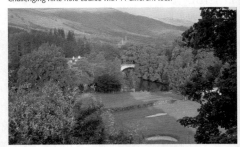

9 holes, 2600yds, Par 66, SSS 65, Course record 61.
Club membership 250.
Visitors contact club for details. Dress code. **Societies** booking required. **Green Fees** not confirmed. **Course Designer** John Duncan/J Braid **Facilities** ⊕ 🍴 ⬚ ⛏ 🛍 ⛳ **Conf** Corporate Hospitality Days **Location** 0.5m N of village centre on A827

STIRLING
MAP 11 NS79

Stirling Queens Rd FK8 3AA
☎ 01786 464098 🖷 01786 460090
e-mail: enquiries@stirlinggolfclub.tv
web: www.stirlinggolfclub.com
Undulating parkland with magnificent views of Stirling Castle and the Grampian Mountains. Testing 15th, Cotton's Fancy, 384yds (Par 4).
18 holes, 6438yds, Par 72, SSS 71, Course record 64.
Club membership 1100.
Visitors Mon-Fri, Sun & BHs. Booking required. **Societies** Booking required. **Green Fees** £45 per day, £30 per round. **Prof** Ian Collins
Course Designer Henry Cotton **Facilities** ⊕ ⦿ ⓛ ⦿ ᔑ 杤 ⚘ 📇 ⚐ ✦ ✦
✦ **Conf** Corporate Hospitality Days **Location** W side of town on B8051

WEST DUNBARTONSHIRE

BALLOCH
MAP 10 NS48

De Vere Cameron House Hotel Loch Lomond
G83 8QZ
☎ 01389 755565
e-mail: stewart.smith@cameronhouse.co.uk
New 18 hole course. The Carrick on Loch Lomond opened 2007.

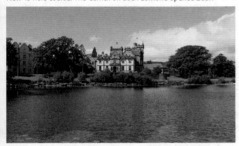

Carrick on Loch Lomond: 18 holes, 7200yds, Par 71.
Wee Demon: 9 holes, 3200yds, Par 32.
Club membership 250.
Visitors Mon-Sun & BHs. Booking required. Handicap certificate (Carrick course). **Societies** booking required. **Green Fees** not confirmed.
Prof Stewart Smith **Facilities** ⊕ ⦿ ⓛ ⦿ 杤 ⚘ 📇 ⚐ ♦ ✦ ✦
Leisure hard tennis courts, heated indoor swimming pool, squash, fishing, sauna, solarium, gymnasium. **Conf** facs Corporate Hospitality Days
Location M8 (W) junct 30 for Erskine Bridge, then A82 for Crainlarich. Course adjacent 1m past Balloch roundabout
Hotel ★★★★★ 81% HL De Vere Cameron House, BALLOCH
☎ 01389 755565 96 en suite

BONHILL
MAP 10 NS37

Vale of Leven North Field Rd G83 9ET
☎ 01389 752351 🖷 0870 749 8950
e-mail: rbarclay@volgc.org
web: www.volgc.org
Moorland course, tricky with many natural hazards - gorse, burns, trees. Overlooks Loch Lomond.
18 holes, 5277yds, Par 67, SSS 67, Course record 63 or ,
SSS 2. Club membership 750.
Visitors Mon-Fri, Sun & BHs. Booking required Fri, Sun & BHs. Dress code.
Societies Booking required. **Green Fees** £30 per day, £20 per round
(£37.50/£25 Sun). **Prof** Barry Campbell **Facilities** ⊕ ⦿ ⓛ ⦿ 杤 ⚘ 📇 ⚐
✦ **Conf** facs Corporate Hospitality Days **Location** E side of town off A813
Hotel ★★★★★ 81% HL De Vere Cameron House, BALLOCH
☎ 01389 755565 96 en suite

CLYDEBANK
MAP 11 NS56

Clydebank & District Glasgow Rd, Hardgate G81 5QY
☎ 01389 383831 & 383833 🖷 01389 383831
e-mail: clydebankanddgc@yahoo.com
An undulating parkland course established in 1905, overlooking Clydebank.
18 holes, 5823yds, Par 68, SSS 69, Course record 64.
Club membership 889.
Visitors Mon-Fri. Booking required. Dress code. **Societies** Booking required. **Green Fees** Phone. ⊛ **Prof** A Waugh **Course Designer** Members **Facilities** ⊕ ⦿ ⓛ ⦿ 杤 ⚘ 📇 ✦ **Conf** facs Corporate Hospitality Days **Location** 2m E of Erskine Bridge
Hotel BUD Premier Travel Inn Glasgow (Bearsden), Milngavie Rd, BEARSDEN ☎ 0870 9906532 61 en suite

Clydebank Municipal Overtoun Rd, Dalmuir G81 3RE
☎ 0141 952 6372
Dalmuir Municipal Golf Course: 18 holes, 5349yds, Par 67, SSS 66, Course record 63.
Location 2m NW of town centre
Telephone for further details
Hotel ★★★★ 78% HL Beardmore Hotel, Beardmore St, CLYDEBANK
☎ 0141 951 6000 166 en suite

DUMBARTON
MAP 10 NS37

Dumbarton Broadmeadow G82 2BQ
☎ 01389 732830 & 765995
e-mail: captain@dumbartongolfclub.co.uk
web: www.dumbartongolfclub.co.uk
Flat parkland.
18 holes, 6017yds, Par 71, SSS 69, Course record 64.
Club membership 800.
Visitors Mon-Fri. Dress code. **Societies** Booking required. **Green Fees** £32 per day, £22 per round. ⊛ **Prof** David Muir. **Facilities** ⊕ ⦿ ⓛ ⦿ 杤 ⚘ 📇 ✦ **Conf** Corporate Hospitality Days **Location** 0.25m N off A814
Guesthouse ★★★★★ GA Kirkton House, Darleith Rd, CARDROSS
☎ 01389 841951 6 en suite

Scotland

WEST LOTHIAN

BATHGATE
MAP 11 NS96

Bathgate Edinburgh Rd EH48 1BA
☎ 01506 630553 & 652232/630505 📄 01506 636775
e-mail: bathgate.golfclub@lineone.net
web: www.bathgategolfclub.visps.com
Moorland course. Easy walking. Testing 11th hole, Par 3.
18 holes, 6328yds, Par 71, SSS 71, Course record 58.
Club membership 900.
Visitors Mon-Sat. Booking required. Dress code. **Societies** Booking
required. **Green Fees** £25 per day, £20 per round (£35/£25 Sat). 🍽
Prof Sandy Strachan **Course Designer** W Park **Facilities** ⑪ ⌾ ⓣ ⌂ 🍴 ⌨ ☂ ⚐ ☂ 🏌 **Conf** Corporate Hospitality Days **Location** E side
of town off A89
Hotel ★★★ 77% HL Best Western The Hilcroft Hotel, East Main St,
WHITBURN ☎ 01501 740818 32 en suite

BROXBURN
MAP 11 NT07

Niddry Castle Castle Rd, Winchburgh EH52 6RQ
☎ 01506 891097 📄 01506 891097
e-mail: info@niddrycastlegc.co.uk
web: www.niddrycastlegc.co.uk
An 18-hole parkland course, requiring accurate golf to score well.
18 holes, 5914yds, Par 70, SSS 69, Course record 63.
Club membership 600.
Visitors Mon-Wed & Fri. Booking required. Dress code. **Societies** Booking
required. **Green Fees** Phone. 🍽 **Course Designer** A Scott **Facilities** ⑪
⌾ ⓣ ⌂ 🍴 ⌨ ☂ ⚐ 🏌 **Conf** Corporate Hospitality Days **Location** 9m W
of Edinburgh on B9080
Hotel ★★★★ 77% HL Macdonald Houstoun House, UPHALL
☎ 0870 1942107 24 en suite 47 annexe en suite

FAULDHOUSE
MAP 11 NS96

Greenburn 6 Greenburn Rd EH47 9HJ
☎ 01501 770292 📄 01501 772615
e-mail: administrator@greenburngolfclub.freeserve.co.uk
web: www.greenburngolfclub.co.uk
A testing course, with a mixture of parkland and moorland. Water
features on 14 of the 18 holes, with a burn crossing most of the holes
on the back 9.
18 holes, 6067yds, Par 71, SSS 70, Course record 63.
Club membership 750.
Visitors Mon-Sun & BHs. Booking required. Dress code. **Societies** Booking
required. **Green Fees** £29 per day, £22 per round (weekends £35/£28).
🍽 **Prof** Scott Catlin **Facilities** ⑪ ⌾ ⓣ ⌂ 🍴 ☂ 🏌 **Location** 3m SW
of Whitburn
Hotel ★★★ 77% HL Best Western The Hilcroft Hotel, East Main St,
WHITBURN ☎ 01501 740818 32 en suite

LINLITHGOW
MAP 11 NS97

Linlithgow Braehead EH49 6QF
☎ 01506 844356 (Pro) & 842585 (sec) 📄 01506 842764
e-mail: info@linlithgowgolf.co.uk
web: www.linlithgowgolf.co.uk
A short but testing undulating parkland course with panoramic views
of the Forth valley.
18 holes, 5800yds, Par 70, SSS 68, Course record 64.
Club membership 450.
Visitors Mon, Tue, Thu, Fri am, Sun & BHs. Booking required. Dress code.
Societies Booking required. **Green Fees** £35 per day, £25 per round
(£40/£30 Sun). 🍽 **Prof** Steven Rosie **Course Designer** R Simpson of
Carnoustie **Facilities** ⑪ ⌾ ⓣ ⌂ 🍴 ☂ ⚐ 🏌 ☂ **Conf** Corporate
Hospitality Days **Location** 1m S off A706
Hotel ★★★★ 75% HL Macdonald Inchyra Grange Hotel, Grange Rd,
POLMONT ☎ 01324 711911 101 en suite

West Lothian Airngath Hill EH49 7RH
☎ 01506 825060 📄 01506 826462
web: www.thewestlothiangolfclub.co.uk
18 holes, 6249yds, Par 71, SSS 70.
Course Designer Fraser Middleton **Location** 1m N off A706
Telephone for further details
Hotel ★★★★ 75% HL Macdonald Inchyra Grange Hotel, Grange Rd,
POLMONT ☎ 01324 711911 101 en suite

LIVINGSTON
MAP 11 NT06

Deer Park Golf & Country Club Golf Course Rd
EH54 8AB
☎ 01506 446699 📄 01506 435608
e-mail: deerpark@muir-group.co.uk
web: www.deer-park.co.uk
18 holes, 6690yds, Par 72, SSS 72, Course record 65.
Course Designer Alliss/Thomas **Location** M8 junct 3, to N side of town
Telephone for further details
Hotel BUD Premier Travel Inn Livingston (Nr Edinburgh), Deer Park Av,
Knightsridge, LIVINGSTON ☎ 08701 977161 83 en suite

Pumpherston Drumshoreland Rd, Pumpherston
EH53 0LH
☎ 01506 433336 & 433337 (pro) 📄 01506 438250
e-mail: sheena.corner@tiscali.co.uk
web: www.pumpherstongolfclub.co.uk
Undulating, well-bunkered parkland course with very testing 2nd
and 15th holes. The course has water features at five holes and has
won several environmental awards. Panoramic views of Edinburgh and
the Pentland Hills.
18 holes, 6006yds, Par 70, SSS 72. Club membership 800.
Visitors Mon-Sun & BHs. Dress code. **Societies** Booking required.
Green Fees Phone. **Prof** Richard Fyvie **Course Designer** G Webster
Facilities ⑪ ⌾ by prior arrangement ⓣ ⌂ 🍴 ☂ 🏌 **Leisure** Pool
table. **Conf** Corporate Hospitality Days **Location** 1m E of Livingston off
B8046
Hotel BUD Premier Travel Inn Livingston (Nr Edinburgh), Deer Park Av,
Knightsridge, LIVINGSTON ☎ 08701 977161 83 en suite

UPHALL
MAP 11 NT07

Uphall EH52 6JT
☎ 01506 856404 📠 01506 855358
e-mail: uphallgolfclub@btconnect.com
web: www.uphallgolfclub.com
A compact and challenging parkland course with easy walking.
18 holes, 5588yds, Par 69, SSS 67, Course record 61.
Club membership 650.
Visitors Mon-Sun & BHs. Booking required. Handicap certificate. Dress code. **Societies** Booking required. **Green Fees** Phone. 🅟 **Prof** Gordon Law **Facilities** ⑪ 🍴 ⓦ ⏚ ⚐ 🏌 ⚒ 👜 ✆ **Location** W side of village on A899
Hotel ★★★★ 77% HL Macdonald Houstoun House, UPHALL
☎ 0870 1942107 24 en suite 47 annexe en suite

WEST CALDER
MAP 11 NT06

Harburn EH55 8RS
☎ 01506 871131 & 871256 📠 01506 870286
e-mail: info@harburngolfclub.co.uk
web: www.harburngolfclub.co.uk
Parkland with a variety of beech, oak and pine trees. The 11th and 12th holes were extended in 2004. Fine views of the Pentlands

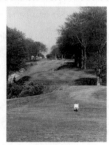

18 holes, 6125yds, Par 71, SSS 70, Course record 64.
Club membership 870.
Visitors Mon-Sun & BHs. Booking required. Dress code. **Societies** Booking required. **Green Fees** £30 per day, £25 per round (Fri £35/£30, Sat-Sun £40/£35). 🅟 **Prof** Stephen Mills **Facilities** ⑪ 🍴 ⏚ ⓦ 🏌 ⚐ 👜 ⚒ ✆ **Conf** facs Corporate Hospitality Days **Location** 2m S of West Calder on B7008
Hotel ★★★ 77% HL Best Western The Hilcroft Hotel, East Main St, WHITBURN ☎ 01501 740818 32 en suite

---

WHITBURN
MAP 11 NS96

Polkemmet Country Park EH47 0AD
☎ 01501 743905 📠 01506 846256
e-mail: mail@beecraigs.com
web: www.beecraigs.com
Public parkland course surrounded by mature woodland and rhododendron bushes and bisected by a river. Interesting and demanding last hole.
9 holes, 2946mtrs, Par 37.
Visitors Mon-Sun & BHs. **Societies** booking required. **Green Fees** not confirmed. **Facilities** ⑪ ⏚ ⓦ ⚐ ✆ 🏊 **Leisure** bowling green.
Location 2m W of Whitburn on B7066
Hotel ★★★ 77% HL Best Western The Hilcroft Hotel, East Main St, WHITBURN ☎ 01501 740818 32 en suite

---

ARRAN, ISLE OF

BLACKWATERFOOT
MAP 10 NR92

Shiskine Shore Rd KA27 8HA
☎ 01770 860226 📠 01770 860205
e-mail: info@shiskinegolf.com
web: www.shiskinegolf.com
Unique 12-hole links course with gorgeous outlook to the Mull of Kintyre. The course is crossed by two burns and includes the longest Par 5 on the island at 509yds. There are several blind holes at which various signals indicate when the green is clear and it is safe to play.
12 holes, 2990yds, Par 42, SSS 42, Course record 38.
Club membership 751.
Visitors Mon-Sun & BHs. Booking required. Handicap certificate. **Societies** Booking required. **Green Fees** £30 per day, £18 per round (£35/£22 Sat & Sun). **Prof** Douglas Bell **Course Designer** Fernie of Troon **Facilities** ⑪ 🍴 by prior arrangement ⏚ ⓦ 🏌 ⚐ 👜 🏳 ⚒ ✆ **Leisure** hard tennis courts, bowling green, golf practice nets. **Conf** Corporate Hospitality Days **Location** W side of village off A841
Hotel ★★★ HL Kilmichael Country House Hotel, Glen Cloy, BRODICK
☎ 01770 302219 4 en suite 3 annexe en suite

BRODICK
MAP 10 NS03

Brodick KA27 8DL
☎ 01770 302349 📠 01770 302349
e-mail: info@brodickgolfclub.org
web: www.brodickgolfclub.org
18 holes, 4747yds, Par 65, SSS 64, Course record 60.
Location N side of village, 0.5m N of Brodick Ferry Terminal
Telephone for further details
Hotel ★★★★ 79% HL Auchrannie House Hotel, BRODICK
☎ 01770 302234 28 en suite

LAMLASH
MAP 10 NS03

Lamlash KA27 8JU
☎ 01770 600296 📠 01770 600296
e-mail: lamlashgolfclub@connectfree.co.uk
web: www.lamlashgolfclub.co.uk
Undulating heathland course with magnificent views of the mountains and sea.
18 holes, 4510yds, Par 64, SSS 64, Course record 58.
Club membership 480.
Visitors Mon-Sun & BHs. Booking required. **Societies** Welcome.
Green Fees Phone. **Course Designer** Auchterlonie **Facilities** ⑪ 🍴 ⏚ ⓦ 🏳 🏌 👜 ✆ 🏊 ✆ **Location** 0.75m N of Lamlash on A841
Hotel ★★★★ 79% HL Auchrannie House Hotel, BRODICK
☎ 01770 302234 28 en suite

375

LOCHRANZA
MAP 10 NR95

Lochranza KA27 8HL
☎ 01770 830273
e-mail: office@lochgolf.demon.co.uk
web: www.lochranzagolf.com
This course is mainly on the level, set amid spectacular scenery where the fairways are grazed by wild red deer, while overhead buzzards and golden eagles may be seen. There are water hazards including the river which is lined by mature trees. The final three holes, nicknamed the Bermuda Triangle, provide an absorbing finish right to the 18th hole - a 530yd dogleg through trees and over the river. The large greens, six single and six double, are played off 18 tees.
18 holes, 5033mtrs, Par 70, SSS 67, Course record 72.
Visitors Mon-Sun & BHs. **Societies** Welcome. **Green Fees** £18 per 18 holes;£12 per 9 holes;£24 per day. ⊕ **Course Designer** re laid 1991 I Robertson **Facilities** ⊕ ⚑ ⚐ ⚒ 🍴 ⚐ 𝄞 **Location** In Lochranza village
Hotel ★★★ HL Kilmichael Country House Hotel, Glen Cloy, BRODICK
☎ 01770 302219 4 en suite 3 annexe en suite

MACHRIE
MAP 10 NR83

Machrie Bay KA27 8DZ
☎ 01770 840259 ▤ 01770 840266
e-mail: office@dougarie.com
web: www.dougarie.com
Fairly flat seaside course. Designed at the start of the 20th century by William Fernie.
9 holes, 4556yds, Par 66, SSS 63, Course record 63.
Club membership 350.
Visitors Mon-Sun & BHs. **Societies** Booking required. **Green Fees** £15 per day. ⊕ **Course Designer** W Fernie **Facilities** ⊕ ⚐ ⚒ ⚐ 𝄞 **Leisure** hard tennis courts. **Location** 9m W of Brodick via String Rd
Hotel ★★★ HL Kilmichael Country House Hotel, Glen Cloy, BRODICK
☎ 01770 302219 4 en suite 3 annexe en suite

SANNOX
MAP 10 NS04

Corrie KA27 8JD
☎ 01770 810223 & 810606
A heathland course on the coast with beautiful mountain scenery. An upward climb to 6th hole then a descent from the 7th. All these holes are subject to strong winds in bad weather.
9 holes, 1948yds, Par 62, SSS 61, Course record 56.
Club membership 300.
Visitors Mon-Fri, Sun & BHs. **Societies** booking required. **Green Fees** not confirmed. ⊕ **Facilities** ⊕ 🍴 ⚐ ⚒ **Location** 6m N of A841
Hotel ★★★★ 79% HL Auchrannie House Hotel, BRODICK
☎ 01770 302234 28 en suite

WHITING BAY
MAP 10 NS02

Whiting Bay KA27 8QT
☎ 01770 700487
Heathland course.
18 holes, 4405yds, Par 63, SSS 63, Course record 59.
Club membership 350.
Visitors Mon-Fri & BHs. Booking required Sat, Sun & BHs. **Societies** welcome. **Green Fees** not confirmed. **Facilities** ⚑ ⚐ ⚒ 🍴 ⚐ 𝄞 🍴 𝄞
Location NW side of village off A841
Hotel ★★★ HL Kilmichael Country House Hotel, Glen Cloy, BRODICK
☎ 01770 302219 4 en suite 3 annexe en suite

BUTE, ISLE OF

KINGARTH
MAP 10 NS05

Bute St Ninians, 32 Marine Place, Ardbeg, Rothesay
PA20 0LF
☎ 01700 502158
e-mail: info@butegolfclub.com
web: www.butegolfclub.com
Flat seaside course with good fenced greens and fine views over the Sound of Bute to Isle of Arran. Challenging Par 3 along sea.
9 holes, 2361mtrs, Par 68, SSS 64, Course record 61.
Club membership 250.
Visitors Mon-Fri, Sun & BHs. Sat after 11.30am. **Societies** Booking required. **Green Fees** £10 per day. ⊕ **Facilities** ⚒ **Location** 6m from Rothesay pier on A845
Hotel ★★★ 85% SHL An Lochan, Shore Rd, TIGHNABRUAICH
☎ 01700 811239 11 en suite

PORT BANNATYNE
MAP 10 NS06

Port Bannatyne Bannatyne Mains Rd PA20 0PH
☎ 01700 505142
e-mail: scrumbick@aol.com
web: www.geocities.com/~golftraveler/
Seaside hill course with panoramic views. Almost unique in having 13 holes, with the first five being played again before a separate 18th. Difficult 4th (Par 3).
13 holes, 5085yds, Par 68, SSS 65, Course record 61.
Club membership 170.
Visitors Mon-Sun. Booking Required Sat & Sun. **Societies** Welcome.
Green Fees £13 per day, £10 per round. (£18/£13 Sat & Sun). ⊕ **Course Designer** Peter Morrison **Facilities** ⊕ ⚑ ⚐ 🍴 ⚒ **Location** W side of village off A886
Hotel ★★★ 85% SHL An Lochan, Shore Rd, TIGHNABRUAICH
☎ 01700 811239 11 en suite

ROTHESAY

MAP 10 NS06

Rothesay Canada Hill PA20 9HN
☎ 01700 503554 📄 01700 503554
e-mail: thepro@rothesaygolfclub.com
web: www.rothesaygolfclub.com
18 holes, 5419yds, Par 69, SSS 66, Course record 62.
Course Designer James Braid & Ben Sayers **Location** 500yds SE from main ferry terminal
Telephone for further details
Hotel ★★★ 85% SHL An Lochan, Shore Rd, TIGHNABRUAICH
☎ 01700 811239   11 en suite

COLONSAY, ISLE OF

SCALASAIG

MAP 10 NR39

Colonsay Machrins Farm PA61 7YR
☎ 01951 200290 📄 01951 200290
Traditional links course on natural machair (hard wearing short grass), challenging, primitive.
18 holes, 4775yds, Par 72, SSS 72. Club membership 200.
Visitors Mon-Sun & BHs. Handicap certificate. **Societies** Booking required.
Green Fees not confirmed. ⊛ **Facilities** ⚏ ⚏ **Location** 2m W on A870

ISLAY, ISLE OF

PORT ELLEN

MAP 10 NR34

Machrie Hotel Machrie PA42 7AN
☎ 01496 302310 📄 01496 302404
e-mail: machrie@machrie.com
web: www.machrie.com
Championship links course opened in 1891, where golf's first £100 Open Championship was played in 1901. Fine turf and many blind holes. Par 4.
18 holes, 6226yds, Par 71, SSS 71, Course record 66.
Club membership 340.
Visitors Mon-Sun & BHs. Dress code **Societies** Booking required.
Green Fees £65 per day, £47 per round. **Course Designer** W Campbell **Facilities** ⚏ ⚏ ⚏ ⚏ ⚏ ⚏ ⚏ ⚏ ⚏ ⚏ ⚏ **Leisure** fishing, snooker, table tennis. **Conf** facs   Corporate Hospitality Days **Location** 4m N off A846
Guest Accommodation ★★★★★ RR The Harbour Inn and Restaurant, BOWMORE ☎ 01496 810330   7 en suite

LEWIS, ISLE OF

STORNOWAY

MAP 13 NB43

Stornoway Lady Lever Park HS2 0XP
☎ 01851 702240
e-mail: admin@stornowaygolfclub.co.uk
web: www.stornowaygolfclub.co.uk
A short but tricky undulating parkland course set in the grounds of Lewis Castle with fine views over the Minch to the mainland. The terrain is peat based and there has been substantial investment in drainage works.
18 holes, 5252yds, Par 68, SSS 67, Course record 61.
Club membership 500.

Visitors Mon-Sat & BHs. Booking required Sat. **Societies** Booking required.
Green Fees £20 per day. ⊛ **Course Designer** J & R Stutt **Facilities** ⚏ by prior arrangement ⚏ ⚏ ⚏ ⚏ ⚏ ⚏ ⚏ **Conf** facs **Location** 0.5m from town centre off A857

MULL, ISLE OF

CRAIGNURE

MAP 10 NM73

Craignure Scallastle PA65 6BA
☎ 01680 300402 📄 01680 300402
e-mail: mullair@btinternet.com
9 holes, 5357yds, Par 69, SSS 66, Course record 72.
Location 1.5m N of Craignure A849
Telephone for further details
Hotel ★★★ 71% HL Isle of Mull Hotel, CRAIGNURE ☎ 0870 950 6267 85 en suite

TOBERMORY

MAP 13 NM55

Tobermory PA75 6PG
☎ 01688 302743 📄 0870 052 3091
e-mail: enquiries@tobermorygolfclub.com
web: www.tobermorygolfclub.com
A beautifully maintained hilltop course with superb views over the Sound of Mull. Testing 7th hole (Par 3). Often described as the best nine-hole course in Scotland.
9 holes, 4912yds, Par 64, SSS 64, Course record 65.
Club membership 150.
Visitors Mon-Sun & BHs. **Societies** Booking required. **Green Fees** £18 per day. ⊛ **Course Designer** David Adams
Facilities ⚏ ⚏ ⚏ ⚏ ⚏ ⚏ ⚏ **Location** 0.5m N off A848

ORKNEY

KIRKWALL

MAP 16 HY41

Orkney Grainbank KW15 1RB
☎ 01856 872457
e-mail: les@orkneygolfclub.co.uk
web: www.orkneygolfclub.co.uk
Open parkland course with few hazards and superb views over Kirkwall and Islands. Very exposed to the elements which can make play tough.
18 holes, 5411yds, Par 70, SSS 67, Course record 63.
Club membership 350.
Visitors Mon-Sun & BHs. Booking required Sat-Sun. **Societies** booking required. **Green Fees** not confirmed. ⊛ **Facilities** ⚏ ⚏ ⚏ ⚏ ⚏ ⚏
Conf   Corporate Hospitality Days **Location** 0.5m W off A965

Scotland

STROMNESS   MAP 16 HY20

Stromness Ness KW16 3DW
☎ 01856 850772
e-mail: sgc@stromnessgc.co.uk
web: www.stromnessgc.co.uk
Testing parkland and seaside course with easy walking. Magnificent views of Scapa Flow.
18 holes, 4762yds, Par 65, SSS 64, Course record 61.
Club membership 350.
Visitors Mon-Sun & BHs. Contact club for details. **Societies** welcome. **Green Fees** not confirmed. ⊕ **Facilities** ⌨ ⊮ ⚘ ⚐ ⚒ **Leisure** hard tennis courts, Bowling. **Location** S side of town centre off A965

SHETLAND

LERWICK   MAP 16 HU44

Shetland Dale Golf Course Gott ZE2 9SB
☎ 01595 840369 🖷 01595 840369
e-mail: shetlandgolfclub@btopenworld.com
web: www.shetlandgolfclub.co.uk
Challenging moorland course, hard walking. A burn runs the full length of the course and provides a natural hazard. Testing holes include the 4th (Par 4), 7th (par4),14th (Par 3)and 15th (Par 4). Every hole provides a new and varied challenge with no two holes similar in layout or appearance.
Dale Course: 18 holes, 5562yds, Par 68, SSS 68,
Course record 68. Club membership 430.
Visitors Mon, Wed-Fri & BHs. Restricted play Tue, Sat & Sun. Booking required Tue, Wed, Sat & Sun. Dress code **Societies** Booking required. **Green Fees** £20 per day. ⊕ **Course Designer** Fraser Middleton **Facilities** ⚏ ⌨ ⊮ ⚘ ⚐ ⚒ **Conf** facs Corporate Hospitality Days **Location** 4m N on A970
Hotel ★★★ 73% HL Lerwick Hotel, 15 South Rd, LERWICK
☎ 01595 692166 34 en suite

WHALSAY, ISLAND OF   MAP 16 HU56

Whalsay Skaw Taing ZE2 9AA
☎ 01806 566450 566705
The most northerly golf course in Britain, with a large part of it running round the coastline, offering spectacular holes in an exposed but highly scenic setting. There are no cut fairways as yet; these are defined by marker posts, with preferred lies in operation all year round.
18 holes, 6140yds, Par 71, SSS 69, Course record 69.
Club membership 205.
Visitors Mon-Sun & BHs. **Societies** booking required. **Green Fees** not confirmed. ⊕ **Facilities** ⑪ by prior arrangement ⌨ ⊮ ⚘ **Location** Whalsay Island

SKYE, ISLE OF

SCONSER   MAP 13 NG53

Isle of Skye IV48 8TD
☎ 01478 650414
e-mail: info@isleofskyegolfclub.co.uk
web: www.isleofskyegolfclub.co.uk
Seaside course with spectacular views; nine holes with 18 tees, different settings on the back nine. Suitable for golfers of all abilities.
18 holes, 4677yds, Par 66, SSS 64, Course record 62.
Club membership 200.
Visitors Mon-Sun & BHs. **Societies** Booking required. **Green Fees** £27 per day, £21 per round, 9 holes £14. **Facilities** ⑪ ⚏ ⌨ ⚘ ⚑ ⚐ ⚒ **Conf** Corporate Hospitality Days **Location** On A87 between Broadford **Hotel** ★★ 75% HL Rosedale Hotel, Beaumont Crescent, PORTREE
☎ 01478 613131 18 en suite

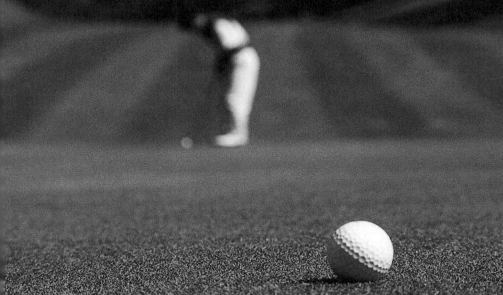

Wales

ANGLESEY, ISLE OF

AMLWCH
MAP 06 SH49

Bull Bay LL68 9RY
☎ 01407 830960 ▤ 01407 832612
e-mail: secretary@bullbaygolf.freeserve.co.uk
web: ww.bullbaygc.co.uk
Wales's northernmost course, Bull Bay is a pleasant coastal, heathland course with natural rock, gorse and wind hazards. Views from several tees across the Irish Sea to the Isle of Man, and across Anglesey to Snowdonia.
18 holes, 6217yds, Par 70, SSS 70, Course record 60.
Club membership 700.
Visitors Mon-Sun & BHs. Booking required. Handicap certificate. Dress code. **Societies** welcome. **Green Fees** not confirmed. ● **Prof** John Burns **Course Designer** W H Fowler **Facilities** ⌕ 🏌 🍴 ✔ 🏀 ✔
Conf Corporate Hospitality Days **Location** 1m W of Amlwch on A5025
Hotel ★★ 76% HL Lastra Farm Hotel, Penrhyd, AMLWCH ☎ 01407 830906
5 en suite 3 annexe en suite

BEAUMARIS
MAP 06 SH67

Baron Hill LL58 8YW
☎ 01248 810231 ▤ 01248 810231
e-mail: golf@baronhill.co.uk
web: www.baronhill.co.uk
Undulating course with natural hazards of rock and gorse. Testing 3rd and 4th holes (Par 4s). Hole 5/14 plays into the prevailing wind with an elevated tee across two streams. The hole is between two gorse covered mounds.
9 holes, 5572yds, Par 68, SSS 68, Course record 65.
Club membership 350.
Visitors Mon, Wed, Fri, Sat & BHs, Tue & Thu am only. Booking required. Dress code. **Societies** Booking required. **Green Fees** £15 per day.
● **Course Designer** R Dawson **Facilities** ⌕ 🏌 🍴 ✔ 🏀 ✔ ✔
Conf Corporate Hospitality Days **Location** A545 from Menai Bridge to Beaumaris, course signed on approach to town
Hotel ★★ 83% HL Ye Olde Bulls Head Inn, Castle St, BEAUMARIS
☎ 01248 810329 12 en suite 1 annexe en suite

Henllys Henllys Hall LL58 8HU
☎ 01248 811717 ▤ 01248 811511
e-mail: hg@hpb.co.uk
web: www.henllysgolfclub.co.uk
The Menai Straits and the Snowdonia mountains form a magnificent backdrop to the course. Full use has been made of the mature parkland trees and natural water hazards to provide a really testing and enjoyable game of golf.
18 holes, 6062yards, Par 71, SSS 69, Course record 65.
Club membership 300.
Visitors Mon-Sun & BHs. Booking required. **Societies** Booking required.
Green Fees £24 (£30 Sat & Sun). **Prof** Peter Maton & David Gadsby
Course Designer Roger Jones **Facilities** ⌕ 🏌 🍴 ✔ 🏀 ✔ ✔
Location A545 through Beaumaris, 0.25m Henllys Hall signed on left
Hotel ★★ 83% HL Ye Olde Bulls Head Inn, Castle St, BEAUMARIS
☎ 01248 810329 12 en suite 1 annexe en suite

HOLYHEAD
MAP 06 SH28

Holyhead Lon Garreg Fawr, Trearddur Bay LL65 2YL
☎ 01407 763279 ▤ 01407 763279
web: www.holyheadgolfclub.co.uk
Treeless, undulating seaside course which provides a varied and testing game, particularly in a south wind. The fairways are bordered by gorse, heather and rugged outcrops of rock. Accuracy from most tees is paramount as there are 43 fairway and greenside bunkers and lakes. Designed by James Braid.

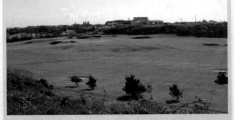

18 holes, 6058yds, Par 70, SSS 70, Course record 64.
Club membership 1350.
Visitors Mon-Sun & BHs. Booking required. Handicap certificate. Dress code. **Societies** Booking required **Green Fees** £35 per day (£40 Sat & Sun). ● **Prof** Stephen Elliot **Course Designer** James Braid **Facilities** ⌕ 🏌 🍴 ✔ ⌕ 🏀 ✔ ✔ **Conf** facs Corporate Hospitality Days **Location** A55 to rdbt at Holyhead, left onto B4545 to Trearddur Bay 1m
Hotel ★★★ 79% HL Trearddur Bay Hotel, TREARDDUR BAY
☎ 01407 860301 34 en suite 6 annexe en suite

RHOSNEIGR
MAP 06 SH37

Anglesey Station Rd LL64 5QX
☎ 01407 811127 & 811202 ▤ 01407 811127
e-mail: info@theangleseygolfclub.com
web: www.theangleseygolfclub.co.uk
18 holes, 6330yds, Par 70, SSS 71, Course record 64.
Course Designer H Hilton **Location** NE side of village on A4080
Telephone for further details
Hotel ★★★ 79% HL Trearddur Bay Hotel, TREARDDUR BAY
☎ 01407 860301 34 en suite 6 annexe en suite

BLAENAU GWENT

NANTYGLO
MAP 03 SO11

West Monmouthshire Golf Rd, Winchestown NP23 4QT
☎ 01495 310233
e-mail: care@westmongolfclub.co.uk
web: www.westmongolfclub.co.uk
Established in 1906, this mountain and heathland course was officially designated by the Guinness Book of Records in 1994 as being the highest above sea level, with the 14th tee at a height of 1513ft. The course has plenty of picturesque views, hard walking and natural hazards. Testing 3rd hole, Par 5, and 7th hole, Par 4.
18 holes, 6300yds, Par 71, SSS 69, Course record 65.
Club membership 350.

Continued

Visitors Mon-Sun & BHs. Booking required. Dress code. **Societies** Booking required. **Green Fees** £15 per day (£18 weekends). ⊕ **Course Designer** Ben Sayers **Facilities** ⑪ ⑩ ⬥ ⬜ ⅋⬜ ⬥ ⬤ ⭤ **Conf** facs Corporate Hospitality Days **Location** 0.25m W off A467
Hotel ★★ 79% HL Llanwenarth Hotel & Riverside Restaurant, Brecon Rd, ABERGAVENNY ☎ 01873 810550 17 en suite

---

TREDEGAR
MAP 03 SO10

Tredegar and Rhymney Cwmtysswg, Rhymney NP2 3BQ
☎ 01685 840743 (club)
e-mail: tandrgc@googlemail.com
web: www.tandrgc.co.uk
Mountain course with lovely views. The course has now been developed into an 18-hole course with easy walking.
18 holes, 6250yds, Par 67, SSS 67, Course record 68.
Club membership 194.
Visitors Mon-Sun & BHs. Booking required. Handicap certificate. Dress code. **Societies** Booking required. **Green Fees** £15 per day. ⊕
Facilities ⑪ ⑩ ⬥ ⬜ ⅋⬜ ⬥ ⭤ ⬤ **Conf** Corporate Hospitality Days **Location** 1.75m SW on B4256
Hotel ★★★ 72% HL Bessemer Hotel, Hermon Close, Dowlais, MERTHYR TYDFIL ☎ 01685 350780 17 en suite

---

BRIDGEND

BRIDGEND
MAP 03 SS97

Coed-Y-Mwstwr The Clubhouse, Bryn Rd, Coychurch CF35 6AF
☎ 01656 864934 🖺 01656 864934
e-mail: secretary@coed-y-mwstwr.co.uk
web: www.coed-y-mwstwr.co.uk
Previously 12 holes but extended to 18 holes during 2005. The new holes are now fully bedded in. The 2nd hole, a 212 yard Par 3 to a well guarded green is a real tester. The fairways are lush and new tees for 2007 will enhance the courses playability. Generous fairways allow the golfer to open their shoulders but the surrounding woodland is a trap for the wayward drive.
18 holes, 5703yds, Par 69, SSS 68, Course record 69.
Club membership 300.
Visitors Mon-Fri, & BHs. Sun pm only. Booking required BHs. Handicap certificate. Dress code. **Societies** Booking required. **Green Fees** £22 per 18 holes (£26.50 Sun & BHs). **Course Designer** Chapman/Warren **Facilities** ⑪ ⬥ ⬜ ⅋⬜ ⬥ ⬤ ⭤ **Conf** facs Corporate Hospitality Days **Location** M4 junct 35, A473 into Coychurch, course 1m N
Hotel ★★★★ 74% CHH Coed-y-Mwstwr Hotel, Coychurch, BRIDGEND ☎ 01656 860621 28 en suite

---

Southerndown Ogmore By Sea CF32 0QP
☎ 01656 880476 🖺 01656 880317
e-mail: southerndowngolf@btconnect.com
web: www.southerndowngolfclub.co.uk
Downland-links championship course with rolling fairways and fast greens. Golfers who successfully negotiate the four Par 3s still face a testing finish with three of the last four holes played into the prevailing wind. The Par 3 5th is played across a valley and the 18th, with its split-level fairway, is a demanding finishing hole. Superb views.
18 holes, 6449yds, Par 70, SSS 72, Course record 63.
Club membership 710.

Visitors Mon-Sun & BHs. Booking required. Handicap certificate. Dress code. **Societies** Booking required. **Green Fees** £50 per 18 holes £65 per day (£70 Sat & Sun). **Prof** D G McMonagle **Course Designer** W Park/W Fernie & others **Facilities** ⑪ ⑩ ⬥ ⬜ ⅋⬜ ⬥ ⬤ ⭤ ⬥ ⬤ ⭤ **Conf** Corporate Hospitality Days **Location** 3m SW of Bridgend on B4524
Hotel ★★★ 73% HL Best Western Heronston Hotel, Ewenny Rd, BRIDGEND ☎ 01656 668811 & 666084 🖺 01656 767391 69 en suite 6 annexe en suite

---

MAESTEG
MAP 03 SS89

Maesteg Mount Pleasant, Neath Rd CF34 9PR
☎ 01656 734106 🖺 01656 731822
e-mail: ijm@fsmail.net
web: www.maesteg-golf.co.uk
Reasonably flat hill-top course with scenic views.
18 holes, 5929yds, Par 70, SSS 69, Course record 69.
Club membership 789.
Visitors Mon-Fri & BHs. Booking required. Handicap certificate. Dress code. **Societies** Booking required. **Green Fees** Phone. **Course Designer** James Braid **Facilities** ⑪ ⑩ by prior arrangement ⬥ ⬜ ⅋⬜ ⬥ ⬤ **Conf** facs Corporate Hospitality Days **Location** 0.5m W off B4282
Hotel ★★★ 72% HL Best Western Aberavon Beach Hotel, PORT TALBOT ☎ 01639 884949 52 en suite

---

PENCOED
MAP 03 SS98

St Mary's Hotel Golf & Country Club St Mary Hill CF35 5EA
☎ 01656 868900 🖺 01656 863400
A parkland course with many American-style features. The Par 3 10th, called Alcatraz, has a well-deserved reputation.
St Mary's Course: 18 holes, 5291yds, Par 68, SSS 66, Course record 65.
Kingfisher: 12 holes, 3125yds, Par 35.
Club membership 600.
Visitors Mon-Sun & BHs. Booking required. Dress code. **Societies** Booking required **Green Fees** £22 per round, Kingfisher £7.50 (£27/£8.50 Sun & Mon). **Prof** Leighton Janes **Course Designer** Peter Johnson **Facilities** ⑪ ⑩ ⬥ ⬜ ⅋⬜ ⬥ ⬤ ⬥ ⬤ ⭤ **Leisure** tennis courts. **Location** M4 junct 35, 5m
Hotel ★★★ 71% HL St Mary's Hotel & Country Club, St Marys Golf Club, PENCOED ☎ 01656 861100 24 en suite

---

PORTHCAWL
MAP 03 SS87

Royal Porthcawl Rest Bay CF36 3UW
☎ 01656 782251 🖺 01656 771687
e-mail: royalporthcawl@btconnect.com
web: www.royalporthcawl.com
One of the great links courses, Royal Porthcawl is unique in that the sea is in full view from every single hole. The course enjoys a substantial reputation with heather, broom, gorse and a challenging wind demanding a player's full skill and attention.
18 holes, 6440yds, Par 72, SSS 73. Club membership 800.
Visitors Tue, Thu & Fri. Booking required. Handicap certificate. Dress code. **Societies** booking required. **Green Fees** not confirmed. **Prof** Peter Evans **Course Designer** Ramsey Hunter **Facilities** ⑪ ⑩ ⬥ ⬜ ⅋⬜ ⬥ ⬤ ⭤ ⬥ **Location** M4 junct 37, proceed to Rest Bay
Hotel ★★★ 68% HL Seabank Hotel, The Promenade, PORTHCAWL ☎ 01656 782261 67 en suite

PYLE   MAP 03 SS88

Pyle & Kenfig Waun-Y-Mer CF33 4PU
☎ 01656 783093 📠 01656 772822
e-mail: secretary@pandkgolfclub.co.uk
web: www.pandkgolfclub.co.uk
Links and downland course, with dunes. Easy walking.
18 holes, 6776yds, Par 71, SSS 73, Course record 61.
Club membership 950.
Visitors Mon-Fri, Sun in summer & BHs. Booking required. Handicap
certificate. Dress code. **Societies** booking required. **Green Fees** not
confirmed. **Prof** Robert Evans **Course Designer** Colt **Facilities** ⑪ ⑩ ⅃
⌁ ⑩ ⌁ ⌁ ⌁ ⌁ **Location** M4 junct 37, S side of Pyle off A4229
Hotel ★★★ 68% HL Seabank Hotel, The Promenade, PORTHCAWL
☎ 01656 782261 67 en suite

CAERPHILLY

BARGOED   MAP 03 ST19

Bargoed Heolddu CF81 9GF
☎ 01443 836179 📠 01143 830608
Mountain parkland course, a challenging Par 70 with panoramic views.
Easy walking.
18 holes, 6049yds, Par 70, SSS 70, Course record 64.
Club membership 600.
Visitors Mon-Fri & BHs. Handicap certificate. Dress code. **Societies** Booking
required. **Green Fees** £17.50 per round. **Prof** Craig Easton **Facilities**
⑪ ⑩ ⅃ ⌁ ⑩ ⌁ ⌁ ⌁ **Conf** facs Corporate Hospitality Days
Location NW side of town
Hotel ★★★ 70% HL Maes Manor Hotel, BLACKWOOD ☎ 01495 220011
13 en suite 14 annexe en suite

BLACKWOOD   MAP 03 ST19

Blackwood Cwmgelli NP12 1BR
☎ 01495 222121 (Office) & 223152 (Club)
Heathland course with sand bunkers. Undulating, with hard walking.
Testing 2nd hole Par 4. Good views.
9 holes, 5332yds, Par 67, Course record 62.
Club membership 310.
Visitors Mon-Sun & BHs. Dress code. **Societies** Booking required.
Green Fees £15 per round. ⊛ **Facilities** ⑪ ⅃ ⌁ ⑩ ⌁ **Location** 0.25m
N of Blackwood, off A4048
Hotel ★★★ 70% HL Maes Manor Hotel, BLACKWOOD ☎ 01495 220011
13 en suite 14 annexe en suite

CAERPHILLY   MAP 03 ST18

Caerphilly Pencapel, Mountain Rd CF83 1HJ
☎ 029 2088 3481 & 2086 3441 📠 029 2086 3441
18 holes, 5732yds, Par 71, SSS 69.
Location 0.5m S on A469
Telephone for further details
Hotel ★★★ 72% HL Manor Parc Country Hotel & Restaurant, Thornhill Rd,
Thornhill, CARDIFF ☎ 029 2069 3723 21 en suite

Mountain Lakes & Castell Heights Blaengwynlais
CF83 1NG
☎ 029 2086 1128 & 2088 6666 📠 029 2086 3243
e-mail: sales@golfclub.co.uk
web: www.golfclub.co.uk
The nine-hole Castell Heights course within the Mountain Lakes
complex was established in 1982 on a 45-acre site. In 1988 a
further 18-hole course, Mountain Lakes was designed by Bob Sandow
to take advantage of 160 acres of mountain heathland, combining both
mountain-top golf and parkland. Most holes are tree-lined and there
are 20 lakes as hazards. Host to major PGA tournaments.
Mountain Lakes Course: 18 holes, 6046mtrs, Par 74,
SSS 73, Course record 69.
Castell Heights Course: 9 holes, 2751mtrs, Par 35, SSS 32,
Course record 32. Club membership 500.
Visitors contact club for details. **Societies** welcome. **Prof** Sion Bebb
Course Designer Bob Sandow **Facilities** ⌁ ⌁ ⌁ ⌁ ⌁ ⌁
Conf facs Corporate Hospitality Days **Location** M4 junct 32, near Black
Cock Inn, Caerphilly Mountain
Hotel ★★★ 72% HL Manor Parc Country Hotel & Restaurant, Thornhill Rd,
Thornhill, CARDIFF ☎ 029 2069 3723 21 en suite

MAESYCWMMER   MAP 03 ST19

Bryn Meadows Golf & Country Hotel Mr G Mayo
CF82 7FN
☎ 01495 225590 & 224103 📠 01495 228272
e-mail: information@brynmeadows.co.uk
Heavily wooded parkland with panoramic views of the Brecon
Beacons.
18 holes, 6132yds, Par 72, SSS 69, Course record 68.
Club membership 540.
Visitors Mon-Sat & BHs. Booking required. **Societies** Booking required.
Green Fees Phone. **Prof** Bruce Hunter **Course Designer** Mayo/Jeffries
Facilities ⑪ ⑩ ⅃ ⌁ ⑩ ⌁ ⌁ ⌁ ⌁ ⌁ ⌁ **Leisure** heated indoor
swimming pool, sauna, solarium, gymnasium. **Conf** facs Corporate
Hospitality Days **Location** On A4048 Blackwood-Ystrad Mynach road
Hotel ★★★ 70% HL Maes Manor Hotel, BLACKWOOD ☎ 01495 220011
13 en suite 14 annexe en suite

NELSON   MAP 03 ST19

Whitehall The Pavilion CF46 6ST
☎ 01443 740245
e-mail: m.wilde001@tiscali.co.uk
web: www.whitehallgolfclub1922.co.uk
Hilltop course. Testing 4th hole (225yds) Par 3, and 6th hole (402yds)
Par 4. Pleasant views.
9 holes, 5666yds, Par 69, SSS 68, Course record 63.
Club membership 300.
Visitors Mon-Sat & BHs. Booking required Fri, Sat & BHs. Handicap
certificate. Dress code. **Societies** Booking required. **Green Fees** £10
per 18 holes. ⊛ **Facilities** ⑪ ⑩ ⅃ ⌁ ⑩ ⌁ **Leisure** snooker.
Conf facs Corporate Hospitality Days **Location** 1m SW of Nelson off A4054
Hotel ★★★ 73% HL Llechwen Hall Hotel, Llanfabon, PONTYPRIDD
☎ 01443 742050 & 743020 📠 01443 742189 12 en suite 8 annexe en suite

Wales

OAKDALE
MAP 03 ST19

Oakdale Llwynon Ln NP12 0NF
☎ 01495 220044 220440
9 holes, 1344yds, Par 28, Course record 27.
Course Designer Ian Goodenough **Location** Off B4251 at Oakdale
Telephone for further details
Hotel ★★★ 70% HL Maes Manor Hotel, BLACKWOOD ☎ 01495 220011
13 en suite 14 annexe en suite

CARDIFF

CARDIFF
MAP 03 ST17

Cardiff Sherborne Av, Cyncoed CF23 6SJ
☎ 029 2075 3320 🖹 029 2068 0011
e-mail: cardiff.golfclub@virgin.net
web: www.cardiffgc.co.uk
Parkland where trees form natural hazards. Interesting variety of holes, mostly bunkered. A stream flows through course and comes into play on nine separate holes.
18 holes, 6116yds, Par 70, SSS 70, Course record 66.
Club membership 900.
Visitors Mon, Wed-Fri, Sun & BHs. Tue pm only. Booking required. Handicap certificate. Dress code. **Societies** Booking required. **Green Fees** Phone. **Prof** Terry Hanson **Facilities** ⚙ 🍴 ⬛ 🏌 ⬛ 🏹 ⛳ 🏌 **Leisure** snooker. **Conf** facs Corporate Hospitality Days **Location** 3m N of city centre
Hotel BUD Hotel Ibis Cardiff Gate, Malthouse Av, Cardiff Gate Business Park, Pontprennau, CARDIFF ☎ 029 2073 3222 78 en suite

Cottrell Park Cottrell Park, St Nicholas CF5 6SJ
☎ 01446 781781 🖹 01446 781187
e-mail: admin@golfwithus.com
web: www.golfwithus.com
Two well-designed courses situated in historic parkland with spectacular views, across the Brecon Beacons to the Mendips over the Bristol Channel. An enjoyable yet testing game of golf for players of all abilities.

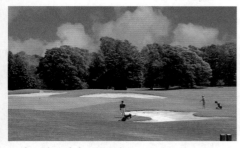

Mackintosh: 18 holes, 6052yds, Par 72, SSS 69, Course record 66.
Gwinnett: 18 holes, 5777yds, Par 71, SSS 68.
Club membership 1465.
Visitors Mon-Sun & BHs. Booking required. Dress code. **Societies** Booking required. **Green Fees** £30 per 18 holes (£40 Fri-Sun). **Prof** Steve Birch **Course Designer** MRM Sandow **Facilities** ⚙ 🍴 ⬛ 🏌 ⬛ 🏹 ⬛ 🏌 ⛳ 🏌 **Conf** facs Corporate Hospitality Days **Location** 6.5m W of Cardiff off A48, NW of St Nicholas
Hotel ★★★★ 70% HL Copthorne Hotel Cardiff - Caerdydd, Copthorne Way, Culverhouse Cross, CARDIFF ☎ 029 2059 9100 135 en suite

---

Llanishen Cwm Lisvane CF14 9UD
☎ 029 2075 5078 🖹 029 2076 5253
e-mail: secretary.llanishen@virgin.net
Picturesque sloping course overlooking England & the Bristol Channel.
18 holes, 5338yds, Par 68, SSS 67, Course record 63.
Club membership 900.
Visitors Tue, Thu, Fri & Sun. Booking required. Handicap certificate. Dress code. **Societies** Booking required. **Green Fees** Phone. ⊛ **Prof** Adrian Jones **Facilities** ⚙ 🍴 ⬛ 🏌 ⬛ 🏹 ⛳ 🏌 **Conf** Corporate Hospitality Days **Location** 5m N of city off A469
Hotel ★★★ 71% HL Quality Hotel & Suites Cardiff, Merthyr Rd, Tongwynlais, CARDIFF ☎ 029 2052 9988 95 en suite

Peterstone Lakes Peterstone, Wentloog CF3 2TN
☎ 01633 680009 🖹 01633 680563
e-mail: peterstone_lakes@yahoo.com
web: www.peterstonelakes.com
Parkland course with abundant water features and several long drives (15th, 601yds).
18 holes, 6555yds, Par 72. Club membership 600.
Visitors contact club for details. Dress code. **Societies** welcome. **Green Fees** not confirmed. **Prof** Paul Glyn **Course Designer** Bob Sandow **Facilities** ⚙ 🍴 ⬛ 🏌 ⬛ 🏹 ⛳ 🏌 ⛳ 🏌 **Conf** facs **Location** 3m from Castleton off A48
Hotel ★★★ 72% HL Best Western St Mellons Hotel & Country Club, Castleton, CARDIFF ☎ 01633 680355 21 en suite 20 annexe en suite

Radyr The Clubhouse, Drysgol Rd, Radyr CF15 8BS
☎ 029 2084 2408 🖹 029 2084 3914
e-mail: manager@radyrgolf.co.uk
web: www.radyrgolf.co.uk
Parkland course that celebrated its centenary in 2002. Good views. Venue for many county and national championships.
18 holes, 6078yds, Par 69, SSS 70, Course record 62.
Club membership 935.
Visitors Mon-Fri. Booking required. Handicap certificate. Dress code. **Societies** Booking required. **Green Fees** £40 per day. **Prof** Simon Swales **Course Designer** Colt **Facilities** ⚙ 🍴 ⬛ 🏌 ⬛ 🏹 ⬛ 🏌 ⛳ 🏌 ⛳ 🏌 **Leisure** Table tennis. **Conf** facs Corporate Hospitality Days **Location** M4 junct 32, 4.5m NW of city off A4119
Hotel ★★★ 72% HL Manor Parc Country Hotel & Restaurant, Thornhill Rd, Thornhill, CARDIFF ☎ 029 2069 3723 21 en suite

St Mellons St Mellons CF3 2XS
☎ 01633 680408 🖹 01633 681219
e-mail: stmellons@golf2003.fsnet.co.uk
web: www.stmellonsgolfclub.co.uk
Opened in 1936, St Mellons is a parkland course on the eastern edge of Cardiff. The course is laid out in the shape of a clover leaf and provides one of the best tests of golf in south Wales. The course comprises three Par 5s, five Par 3s and 10 Par 4s. The Par 3s will make or break your card but the two finishing Par 4 holes are absolutely superb.
18 holes, 6275yds, Par 70, SSS 70, Course record 63.
Club membership 700.
Visitors Mon, Tue & Thu. Fri am only. Booking required. Handicap certificate. Dress code. **Societies** Booking required. **Green Fees** £32 per round, £40 per day. **Prof** Barry Thomas **Course Designer** Colt & Morrison **Facilities** ⚙ 🍴 ⬛ 🏌 ⬛ 🏹 ⛳ 🏌 **Conf** Corporate Hospitality Days **Location** M4 junct 30, 2m E off A48
Hotel ★★★ 72% HL Best Western St Mellons Hotel & Country Club, Castleton, CARDIFF ☎ 01633 680355 21 en suite 20 annexe en suite

Wales

Whitchurch Pantmawr Rd, Whitchurch CF14 7TD

☎ 029 2062 0985 🖷 029 2052 9860

e-mail: secretary@whitchurchcardiffgolfclub.com

This undulating parkland course is an urban oasis and offers panoramic views of the city. It is an easy walk and always in good condition with excellent drainage and smooth, quick greens.

18 holes, 6258yds, Par 71, SSS 71, Course record 62.
Club membership 750.

Visitors Mon-Sun & BHs. Booking required. Handicap certificate. Dress code. **Societies** Booking required. **Green Fees** £40 per day (£45 per round Sat & Sun). **Prof** Rhys Davies **Course Designer** F Johns **Facilities** ⛳ 🍴 🛍 ⬛ 🖥 🔌 🏌 🛒 ✓ **Conf** Corporate Hospitality Days **Location** M4 junct 32, 0.5m S on A470

Hotel ★★★ 72% HL Manor Parc Country Hotel & Restaurant, Thornhill Rd, Thornhill, CARDIFF ☎ 029 2069 3723 21 en suite

---

CREIGIAU (CREIYIAU) MAP 03 ST08

Creigiau Llantwit Rd CF15 9NN

☎ 029 2089 0263 🖷 029 2089 0706

e-mail: manager@creigiaugolf.co.uk

web: www.creigiaugolf.co.uk

Downland course, with small greens and many interesting water hazards.

18 holes, 6063yds, Par 71, SSS 70, Course record 64.
Club membership 800.

Visitors Mon-Sun & BHs. Booking required. Handicap certificate. Dress code. **Societies** Booking required. **Green Fees** £35 per day. **Prof** Iain Luntz **Facilities** ⛳ 🍴 🛍 ⬛ 🖥 🏌 🛒 ✓ **Location** 6m NW of Cardiff on A4119

Hotel ★★★★ 71% CHH Miskin Manor Country Hotel, Pendoylan Rd, MISKIN ☎ 01443 224204 34 en suite 9 annexe en suite

---

CARMARTHENSHIRE

AMMANFORD MAP 03 SN61

Glynhir Glynhir Rd, Llandybie SA18 2TF

☎ 01269 851365 🖷 01269 851365

e-mail: glynhir.golfclub@virgin.net

web: www.glynhirgolfclub.co.uk

Parkland with good views. Last holes close to Upper Loughor River and the 14th is a 394yd dog-leg.

18 holes, 5917yds, Par 69, SSS 70, Course record 66.
Club membership 700.

Visitors Mon-Sun & BHs. Booking required. Handicap certificate. Dress code. **Societies** Booking required. **Green Fees** Winter £12, Summer £18 (£15/£25 Sat & Sun). **Prof** Duncan Prior **Course Designer** F Hawtree **Facilities** ⛳ 🍴 🛍 ⬛ 🖥 🔌 🏌 🛒 🍷 ◇ ✓ 🏁 **Conf** facs Corporate Hospitality Days **Location** 2m N of Ammanford

---

BURRY PORT MAP 02 SN40

Ashburnham Cliffe Ter SA16 0HN

☎ 01554 832269 & 833846

e-mail: golf@ashburnhamgolfclub.co.uk

web: www.ashburnhamgolfclub.co.uk

This course has a lot of variety. In the main it is of the seaside type although the holes in front of the clubhouse are of an inland character. The front nine are played in a westerly direction into the prevailing wind, which can vary from a mild breeze to a near

gale, the 1st and 9th being particularly tough. The second nine, usually wind assisted, opens with a long Par 5 and has a testing last few holes finishing with an elevated treacherous green at the 18th.

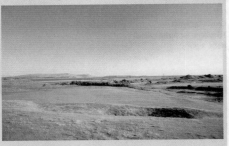

18 holes, 6916yds, Par 72, SSS 74, Course record 66.
Club membership 650.

Visitors Mon-Sun & BHs. Booking required Sun, Sat & BHs. Handicap certificate. Dress code **Societies** Booking required. **Green Fees** £60 per day, £50 per round (£75/£65 Sat, Sun & BHs). **Prof** Martin Stimson **Course Designer** J H Taylor **Facilities** ⛳ by prior arrangement 🍴 by prior arrangement 🛍 ⬛ 🖥 🏌 🛒 🍷 ✓ **Conf** facs Corporate Hospitality Days **Location** W of town centre on A484

Hotel ★★ 72% HL Ashburnham Hotel, Ashburnham Rd, Pembrey, LLANELLI ☎ 01554 834343 & 834455 🖷 01554 834483 13 en suite

See advert on opposite page

CARMARTHEN MAP 02 SN42

Carmarthen Blaenycoed Rd SA33 6EH

☎ 01267 281588 🖷 01267 281493

e-mail: carmarthengolfc@aol.com

web: www.carmarthengolfclub.com

A well maintained Heathland course with tricky greens. Magnificent clubhouse and scenery.

18 holes, 6245yds, Par 71, SSS 71, Course record 66.
Club membership 600.

Visitors Mon-Sun & BHs. Booking required. Dress code. **Societies** booking required. **Green Fees** not confirmed. ◉ **Prof** Jon Hartley **Course Designer** J H Taylor **Facilities** ⛳ 🍴 🛍 ⬛ 🖥 🔌 🏌 ✓ 🛒 ✓ **Conf** facs Corporate Hospitality Days **Location** 4m N of town

Hotel ★★ 71% HL Falcon Hotel, Lammas St, CARMARTHEN ☎ 01267 234959 & 237152 🖷 01267 221277 16 en suite

Derllys Court Llysonnen Rd, Bancyfelin SA33 5DT

☎ 01267 211575 🖷 01267 211575

e-mail: derllys@hotmail.com

web: www.derllyscourtgolfclub.com

The back and front halves provide an interesting contrast. The greens on the front 9 are extremely undulating as opposed to the relatively flat greens of the back 9. Water hazards and bunkers come into play providing an interesting challenge. Fine views.

18 holes, 5847yds, Par 70, SSS 68, Course record 69.
Club membership 220.

Visitors Mon-Sun & BHs. Booking required Sat & Sun. Dress code. **Societies** Booking required. **Green Fees** Phone. **Prof** Robert Ryder **Course Designer** Peter Johnson/Stuart Finney **Facilities** ⛳ 🍴 🛍 ⬛ 🖥 🏌 🛒 ◇ 🛒 ✓ **Conf** Corporate Hospitality Days **Location** Off A40 between Carmarthen and St Clears

Hotel ★★ 71% HL Falcon Hotel, Lammas St, CARMARTHEN ☎ 01267 234959 & 237152 🖷 01267 221277 16 en suite

GARNANT   MAP 03 SN61

Garnant Park Dinefwr Rd SA18 1NP
☎ 01269 823365
web: www.parcgarnantgolf.co.uk
Superb setting in the Brecon Beacons, designed to high standards for all abilities of golfer.
18 holes, 6670yds, Par 72, SSS 72, Course record 69.
Club membership 400.
Visitors Mon-Sun & BHs. Booking required Sat/Sun. Dress code. **Societies** Booking required. **Green Fees** £15 (£20 weekends and bank holidays). **Prof** Gethin Collins **Course Designer** Roger Jones **Facilities** ⑪ ⑩ ⚑ ⛳ ╘ ╬ ╩ ⚐ ♪ ☀ ✦ **Leisure** Par 3 course. **Conf** facs Corporate Hospitality Days **Location** M4 junct48, off A474 in village of Garnant, signed

KIDWELLY   MAP 02 SN40

Glyn Abbey Trimsaran SA17 4LB
☎ 01554 810278 📠 01554 810889
e-mail: course-enquiries@glynabbey.co.uk
web: www.glynabbey.co.uk
Beautiful parkland course with spectacular views of the Gwendraeth valley, set in 200 acres with mature wooded backdrops. USGA greens and tees.
18 holes, 6173yds, Par 70, SSS 70, Course record 68.
Club membership 420.
Visitors Mon-Sun & BHs. Dress code. **Societies** Booking required. **Green Fees** £18 per round (£25 Sat, Sun & BHs). **Course Designer** Hawtree **Facilities** ⑪ ⑩ ⚑ ⛳ ╘ ╬ ╩ ⚐ ♪ ☀ ✦ **Leisure** solarium, gymnasium, 9 hole Par 3 course. **Conf** facs Corporate Hospitality Days **Location** E of Kidwelly on B4317 between Trimsaran & Carway
Hotel ★★ 72% HL Ashburnham Hotel, Ashburnham Rd, Pembrey, LLANELLI ☎ 01554 834343 & 834455 📠 01554 834483 13 en suite

LLANELLI   MAP 03 SS59

Machynys Peninsula Golf & Country Club Nicklaus Av, Machynys SA15 2DG
☎ 01554 744888 📠 01554 744680
e-mail: info@machynys.com
web: www.machynys.com
A picturesque course with stunning views over Carmarthen Bay and the Gower Peninsula and including 25 acres of salt and fresh water lakes. The most challenging and interesting holes are the 4th, 5th, 16th and 18th. The 16th is a Par 4 played across a lake and the view of the bay from the green is spectacular.
18 holes, 7051yds, Par 72, SSS 75. Club membership 400.
Visitors Mon-Sun & BHs. Booking required. Handicap certificate. Dress code. **Societies** Booking required. **Green Fees** Summer: £50 per round Winter: £30 (£55/£35 Sat & Sun). **Prof** Reed, Peters, Lewis & Minty **Course Designer** Gary Nicklaus **Facilities** ⑪ ⑩ ⚑ ⛳ ╘ ╬ ╩ ☀ ✦ **Leisure** sauna, gymnasium, health spa. **Conf** facs Corporate Hospitality Days **Location** M4 junct 47/48, follow directions for Llanelli. Take B4034 to Machynys, golf club on left
Hotel ★★ 67% HL Hotel Miramar, 158 Station Rd, LLANELLI ☎ 01554 754726 12 en suite

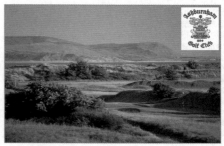

Ashburnham Golf Club
Cliffe Terrace, Burry Port, SA16 0HN

Ashburnham is regarded as one of the best links courses in Britain. The Course is basically the layout designed by J. H. Taylor in 1910; a straight out and straight back course. The front nine are played in a westerly direction into the prevailing wind, which can vary in strength from a mild breeze to a formidable near gale. In recent years it has been the venue for both the Men's and Ladies Home Internationals; British Youths, British Ladies and British Senior Ladies Championships; Welsh Golfing Union Championships and also Welsh PGA events.

ProShop: tel 01554 833846 **Office:** tel 01554 832269
Catering: tel 01554 832466
Website: www.ashburnhamgolfclub.co.uk
Email: golf@ashburnhamgolfclub.co.uk

RHOS   MAP 02 SN44

Saron Saron, Penwern SA44 5EL
☎ 01559 370705
e-mail: c9mbl@sarongolf.freeserve.co.uk
web: www.saron-golf.com
Set in 50 acres of mature parkland with large trees and magnificent Teifi valley views. Numerous water hazards and bunkers.
9 holes, 2400yds, Par 32, Course record 34.
Visitors Mon-Sun & BHs. **Societies** Booking required. **Green Fees** £12 per 18 holes, £9 per 9 holes. ⊛ **Course Designer** Adas **Facilities** ⚑ ♦ ✦ **Location** Off A484 at Saron, between Carmarthen and Newcastle Emlyn

CEREDIGION

ABERYSTWYTH   MAP 06 SN58

Aberystwyth Brynymor Rd SY23 2HY
☎ 01970 615104 📠 01970 626622
e-mail: aberystwythgolf@talk21.com
web: www.aberystwythgolfclub.com
Undulating meadowland course. Testing holes: 16th (The Loop), Par 3; 17th, Par 4; 18th, Par 3. Good views over Cardigan Bay.
18 holes, 5801yds, Par 70, SSS 69. Club membership 400.
Visitors Mon-Sun & BHs. Booking required. Dress code. **Societies** booking required. **Green Fees** not confirmed. ⊛ **Prof** Jim McLeod **Course Designer** Harry Vardon **Facilities** ⑪ ⑩ ⚑ ⛳ ╘ ╬ ╩ ☀ ✦ **Conf** facs **Location** N side of town
Hotel ★★★ 74% HL Belle Vue Royal Hotel, Marine Ter, ABERYSTWYTH ☎ 01970 617558 37 rms (34 en suite)

Wales

BORTH
MAP 06 SN69

Borth & Ynyslas SY24 5JS
☎ 01970 871202 🖹 01970 871202
e-mail: secretary@borthgolf.co.uk
web: www.borthgolf.co.uk
Traditional championship links course with superb scenery. Provides a true test of golf for all standards of player.
18 holes, 6116yds, Par 70, SSS 70, Course record 61.
Club membership 550.
Visitors Mon-Sun & BHs. Handicap certificate. Dress code.
Societies booking required. **Green Fees** not confirmed. **Prof** J G Lewis
Course Designer Harry Colt **Facilities** ⑨ ⑩ by prior arrangement 🚾 ⏣
🎲 ⚘ 🎯 🐾 🖋 **Conf** Corporate Hospitality Days **Location** 0.5m N on B4353
Hotel ★★★ CHH Ynyshir Hall, EGLWYSFACH ☎ 01654 781209 & 781268 🖹 01654 781366 7 en suite 2 annexe en suite

CARDIGAN
MAP 02 SN14

Cardigan Gwbert-on-Sea SA43 1PR
☎ 01239 621775 & 612035 🖹 01239 621775
e-mail: golf@cardigan.fsnet.co.uk
web: www.cardigangolf.co.uk
A links course, very dry in winter, with wide fairways, light rough and gorse. Every hole overlooks the sea.
18 holes, 6687yds, Par 72, SSS 73, Course record 68.
Club membership 600.
Visitors Mon-Sun & BHs. Booking required. Dress code. **Societies** booking required. **Green Fees** not confirmed. **Prof** Colin Parsons **Course Designer** Grant/Hawtree **Facilities** ⑨ ⑩ 🚾 ⏣ 🎲 🐾 ⚘ 🎯 🖋 🐾 🖋
Leisure squash, squash courts. **Location** 3m N off A487
Hotel ★★★ 77% HL The Cliff Hotel, GWBERT-ON-SEA ☎ 01239 613241 70 en suite

GWBERT ON SEA
MAP 02 SN15

Cliff Hotel SA43 1PP
☎ 01239 613241 🖹 01239 615391
e-mail: reservations@cliffhotel.com
This is a short course with two Par 4s and the remainder are challenging Par 3s. Particularly interesting holes are played across the sea on to a small island.

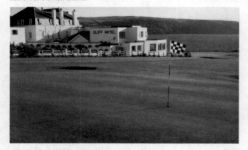

9 holes, 1545yds, Par 29.
Visitors Mon-Sun & BHs. **Societies** Booking required. **Green Fees** from £7.
Facilities ⑨ ⑩ 🚾 ⏣ 🎲 🎯 ✧ 🐾 🖋 **Leisure** heated outdoor swimming pool, fishing, sauna, solarium, gymnasium. **Conf** facs Corporate Hospitality Days **Location** 3m N 0f Cardigan off B4548
Hotel ★★★ 77% HL The Cliff Hotel, GWBERT-ON-SEA ☎ 01239 613241 70 en suite

LLANRHYSTUD
MAP 06 SN56

Penrhos Golf & Country Club SY23 5AY
☎ 01974 202999 🖹 01974 202100
e-mail: info@penrhosgolf.co.uk
web: www.penrhosgolf.co.uk
Beautifully scenic course incorporating lakes and spectacular coastal and inland views.
Championship: 18 holes, 6641yds, Par 72, SSS 73, Course record 70.
Academy: 9 holes, 1827yds, Par 31. Club membership 300.
Visitors Mon-Sun & BHs. Booking required. Dress code. **Societies** Booking required. **Green Fees** Main £25 Academy £5 (£35/£5 Sat & Sun). **Prof** Paul Diamond **Course Designer** Jim Walters **Facilities** ⑨ ⑩ 🚾 ⏣ 🎲 🐾 🎯 ✧ 🐾 🖋 🖋 **Leisure** hard tennis courts, heated indoor swimming pool, sauna, solarium, gymnasium, bowling green. **Conf** facs Corporate Hospitality Days **Location** A487 onto B4337 in Llanrhystud, course 0.25m on left
Hotel ★★★ 82% CHH Conrah Hotel, Ffosrhydygaled, Chancery, ABERYSTWYTH ☎ 01970 617941 11 en suite 6 annexe en suite

CONWY

ABERGELE
MAP 06 SH97

Abergele Tan-y-Gopa Rd LL22 8DS
☎ 01745 824034 🖹 01745 824772
e-mail: secretary@abergelegolfclub.co.uk
web: abergelegolfclub.co.uk
A beautiful parkland course with views of the Irish Sea and Gwyrch Castle. There are splendid finishing holes: a testing Par 5 16th; a 185yd 17th to an elevated green; and a superb Par 5 18th with out of bounds just behind the green.
18 holes, 6520yds, Par 72, SSS 71, Course record 66.
Club membership 1250.
Visitors Sun-Fri & BHs. Booking required. Handicap certificate. Dress code.
Societies booking required. **Green Fees** not confirmed. **Prof** Iain R Runcie
Course Designer Hawtree **Facilities** ⑨ ⑩ 🚾 ⏣ 🎲 🐾 ⚘ 🖋 🐾 🖋
Conf facs **Location** 0.5m W off A547
Hotel ★★★ 71% HL Kinmel Manor Hotel, St George's Rd, ABERGELE ☎ 01745 832014 51 en suite

BETWS-Y-COED
MAP 06 SH75

Betws-y-Coed LL24 0AL
☎ 01690 710556
e-mail: info@golf-betws-y-coed.co.uk
web: www.golf-betws-y-coed.co.uk
Attractive flat meadowland course set between two rivers in Snowdonia National Park, known as the Jewel of the Nines.
9 holes, 4998yds, Par 64, SSS 64, Course record 63.
Club membership 300.
Visitors Mon-Sun. Booking required Tue-Wed & Sat-Sun. Handicap certificate. Dress code. **Societies** booking required. **Green Fees** not confirmed. ⊕ **Facilities** ⑨ ⑩ 🚾 ⏣ 🎲 🎯 ⚘ 🖋 **Location** NE side of village off A5
Hotel ★★★ 83% HL The Royal Oak Hotel, Holyhead Rd, BETWS-Y-COED ☎ 01690 710219 27 en suite

COLWYN BAY　　　MAP 06 SH87

Old Colwyn Woodland Av, Old Colwyn LL29 9NL
☎ 01492 515581
web: www.oldcolwyngolfclub.co.uk
9 holes, 5243yds, Par 68, SSS 66, Course record 62.
Course Designer James Braid **Location** E of town centre on B5383
Telephone for further details
Hotel ★★★ 68% HL Hopeside Hotel, 63-67 Princes Dr, West End,
COLWYN BAY ☎ 01492 533244　16 en suite

CONWY　　　MAP 06 SH77

Conwy (Caernarvonshire) Beacons Way, Morfa
LL32 8ER
☎ 01492 592423 📄 01492 593363
e-mail: secretary@conwygolfclub.co.uk
web: www.conwygolfclub.co.uk
Founded in 1890, Conwy has hosted national and international
championships since 1898. Set among sand hills, possessing true
links greens and a profusion of gorse on the latter holes, especially
the 16th, 17th and 18th. This course provides the visitor with real
golfing enjoyment in stunning scenery.
18 holes, 6100yds, Par 72, SSS 72.
Club membership 1050.
Visitors Mon-Sun & BHs. Booking required. Handicap certificate. Dress
code. **Societies** Booking required. **Green Fees** £43 per day, £38 per
round (£48/£42 Sat, Sun & BHs). **Prof** Peter Lees **Facilities** ⑪ ⎟◎⎥ ⭙ ⬓
⑪⎥ ⏏ 🛍 ⛱ ⛳ 🛒 ⛳ **Leisure** snooker tables. **Location** 1m W of town
centre on A55
Hotel ★★★ 78% HL Castle Hotel Conwy, High St, CONWY
☎ 01492 582800　28 en suite

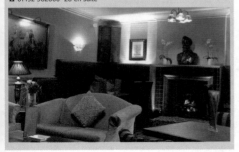

LLANDUDNO　　　MAP 06 SH78

Llandudno (Maesdu) Hospital Rd LL30 1HU
☎ 01492 876450 📄 01492 876450
e-mail: secretary@maesdugolfclub.co.uk
web: www.maesdugolfclub.co.uk
Part links, part parkland, this championship course starts and finishes
on one side of the main road, the remaining holes, more seaside
in nature, being played on the other side. The holes are pleasantly
undulating and present a pretty picture when the gorse is in bloom.
Often windy, this varied and testing course is not for beginners.
18 holes, 6545yds, Par 72, SSS 72, Course record 62.
Club membership 1120.
Visitors Mon-Sun & BHs. Dress code. **Societies** Booking required.
Green Fees £35 per day, £25 per round (£40/£30 Sat & Sun).

Prof Simon Boulden **Facilities** ⑪ ⎟◎⎥ ⭙ ⬓ ⑪⎥ ⏏ 🛍 ⛱ ⛳ 🛒 ⛳
Leisure snooker. **Location** S of town centre on A546
Hotel ★★★ 81% HL Imperial Hotel, The Promenade, LLANDUDNO
☎ 01492 877466　100 en suite

North Wales 72 Bryniau Rd, West Shore LL30 2DZ
☎ 01492 875325 📄 01492 873355
e-mail: golf@nwgc.freeserve.co.uk
web: www.northwalesgolfclub.co.uk
Challenging seaside links with superb views of Anglesey and
Snowdonia. It possesses hillocky fairways, awkward stances and the
occasional blind shot. Heather and gorse lurk beyond the fairways
and several of the greens are defended by deep bunkers. The first
outstanding hole is the 5th, a Par 5 that dog-legs into the wind along
a rollercoasting, bottleneck fairway. Best Par 4s include the 8th,
played through a narrow valley menaced by a railway line and the
beach and the 11th, which runs uphill into the wind and where the
beach again threatens. The finest Par 3 is the 16th, with a bunker to
the left of a partially hidden, bowl-shape green.
18 holes, 6287yds, Par 71, SSS 71, Course record 66.
Club membership 670.
Visitors Mon-Sun & BHs. Booking required. Dress code.
Societies booking required. **Green Fees** not confirmed. **Prof** Richard
Bradbury **Course Designer** Tancred Cummins **Facilities** ⑪ ⎟◎⎥ ⭙ ⬓ ⑪⎥
⛱ 🛍 ⛳ 🛒 ⛳ **Leisure** snooker. **Location** W side of town on A546
Hotel ★★ HL St Tudno Hotel and Restaurant, The Promenade,
LLANDUDNO ☎ 01492 874411　18 en suite

Rhos-on-Sea Penryhn Bay LL30 3PU
☎ 01492 548115 (Prof) & 549641 (clubhouse)
📄 01492 549100
18 holes, 6064yds, Par 69, SSS 69, Course record 68.
Course Designer J J Simpson **Location** 0.5m W of Llandudno off A55
Telephone for further details
Hotel ★★★ 68% HL Hopeside Hotel, 63-67 Princes Dr, West End,
COLWYN BAY ☎ 01492 533244　16 en suite

LLANFAIRFECHAN　　　MAP 06 SH67

Llanfairfechan Llannerch Rd LL33 0ES
☎ 01248 680144 & 680524
Hillside course with panoramic views of coast. All holes Par but 7
over 200 yds.
9 holes, 3119yds, Par 54, SSS 57, Course record 53.
Club membership 191.
Visitors Mon-Sun & BHs. Booking required Sat-Sun & BHs. Handicap
certificate. Dress code. **Societies** booking required. **Green Fees**
not confirmed. ⊕ **Facilities** ⭙ **Conf** Corporate Hospitality Days
Location W side of town on A55

PENMAENMAWR　　　MAP 06 SH77

Penmaenmawr Conway Old Rd LL34 6RD
☎ 01492 623330 📄 01492 622105
e-mail: clubhouse@pengolfclub.co.uk
web: www.pengolf.co.uk
Hilly course with magnificent views across the bay to Llandudno and
Anglesey. Drystone wall hazards.
9 holes, 5350yds, Par 67, SSS 66, Course record 62.
Club membership 600.

Continued

Wales

Wales

Visitors Mon-Sun & BHs. Booking required Sat & BHs. Handicap certificate. Dress code. **Societies** Booking required. **Green Fees** £15 per round (£20 Sat, Sun & BHs). ⚘ **Facilities** ⑪ ⚏ ⚑ ⑨ ⚐ ⚒ ✦ **Conf** Corporate Hospitality Days **Location** 1.5m NE off A55
Hotel ★★★ 78% HL Castle Hotel Conwy, High St, CONWY
☎ 01492 582800 28 en suite

DENBIGHSHIRE

BODELWYDDAN   MAP 06 SJ07

Kimnel Park LL18 5SR
☎ 01745 833548 ▤ 01745 833544
Kimnel Park Golf Course: 9 holes, 3100, Par 58, SSS 58.
Telephone for further details
Hotel ★★★ 79% HL Oriel House Hotel, Upper Denbigh Rd, ST ASAPH
☎ 01745 582716 39 en suite

DENBIGH   MAP 06 SJ06

Bryn Morfydd Hotel Llanrhaedr LL16 4NP
☎ 01745 589090 ▤ 01745 589093
e-mail: reception@brynmorfyddhotelgolf.co.uk
web: www.brynmorfyddhotelgolf.co.uk
In a beautiful setting in the Vale of Clwyd, the original nine-hole Duchess Course was designed by Peter Alliss in 1982. In 1992, the 18-hole Dukes Course was completed: a parkland course designed to encourage finesse in play.
Dukes Course: 18 holes, 5650yds, Par 70, SSS 67, Course record 74.
Duchess Course: 9 holes, 2098yds, Par 27.
Club membership 200.
Visitors Mon-Sun & BHs. Dress code. **Societies** Welcome. **Green Fees** Dukes £15 (£20 Sat & Sun). Duchess £5 per 18 holes. **Prof** Richard Hughes **Course Designer** Peter Allis **Facilities** ⑪ ⑨⚏ ⚑ ⑨ ⚐ ⚒ ⚘✦ ✦ **Conf** facs Corporate Hospitality Days **Location** On A525 between Denbigh and Ruthin
Hotel ★★★ 75% HL Ruthin Castle, RUTHIN ☎ 01824 702664 58 en suite

Denbigh Henllan Rd LL16 5AA
☎ 01745 814159 & 816669 ▤ 01745 814888
e-mail: denbighgolfclub@aol.com
web: www.denbighgolfclub.co.uk
Parkland course, giving a testing and varied game. Good views.
18 holes, 5712yds, Par 69, SSS 68, Course record 64.
Club membership 725.
Visitors Mon-Sun & BHs. Booking required. Dress code. **Societies** Booking required. **Green Fees** £30 per day , £24 per round (£35/£30 Sat & Sun). ⚘ **Prof** Mike Jones **Course Designer** John Stockton **Facilities** ⑪ ⑨⚏ ⚑ ⑨ ⚐ ⚒ ⚘✦ ✦ **Conf** Corporate Hospitality Days **Location** 1.5m NW on B5382
Hotel ★★★ 79% HL Oriel House Hotel, Upper Denbigh Rd, ST ASAPH
☎ 01745 582716 39 en suite

LLANGOLLEN   MAP 07 SJ24

Vale of Llangollen Holyhead Rd LL20 7PR
☎ 01978 860906
Parkland in superb scenery by the River Dee.
18 holes, 6705yds, Par 72, SSS 73, Course record 66.
Club membership 800.

Visitors contact club for details. Handicap certificate. Dress code. **Societies** booking required. **Green Fees** not confirmed. **Prof** David Vaughan **Facilities** ⑪ ⚏ ⚑ ⑨ ⚐ ⚒ ✦ ⚘ ✦ **Location** 1.5m E on A5

PRESTATYN   MAP 06 SJ08

Prestatyn Marine Rd East LL19 7HS
☎ 01745 854320 ▤ 01745 854320
e-mail: prestatyngcmanager@freenet.co.uk
web: www.prestatyngolfclub.co.uk
Set besides rolling sand dunes and only a few hundred yards from the sea, this course enjoys a temperate climate and its seaside location ensures that golfers can play on superb greens all year round. Some holes of note are the Par 5 3rd with out of bounds on the left dog-leg followed by the Ridge, a Par 4 of 468yds normally played with the prevailing wind. The pretty 9th is surrounded by a moat where birdies and double bogies are common followed by the challenging Par 4 450yd 10th.
18 holes, 6568yds, Par 72, SSS 72, Course record 65.
Club membership 673.
Visitors Mon, Wed-Fri & Sun. Tue pm only. Handicap certificate. Dress code. **Societies** Booking required. **Green Fees** £25 per round (£30 Sun). **Prof** David Ames **Course Designer** S Collins **Facilities** ⑪ ⑨⚏ ⚑ ⑨ ⚐ ⚒ ⚘ ✦ ✦ **Leisure** snooker. **Conf** facs Corporate Hospitality Days **Location** 0.5m N off A548
Guesthouse ★★★★ ⚐ RR Barratt's at Ty'N Rhyl, Ty'N Rhyl, 167 Vale Rd, RHYL ☎ 01745 344138 & 0773 095 4994 ▤ 01745 344138 3 en suite

St Melyd The Paddock, Meliden Rd LL19 8NB
☎ 01745 854405 ▤ 01745 856908
e-mail: info@stmelydgolf.co.uk
web: www.stmelydgolf.co.uk
9 holes, 5829yds, Par 68, SSS 68, Course record 65.
Location 0.5m S on A547
Telephone for further details
Hotel ★★★ 79% HL Oriel House Hotel, Upper Denbigh Rd, ST ASAPH
☎ 01745 582716 39 en suite

RHUDDLAN   MAP 06 SJ07

Rhuddlan Meliden Rd LL18 6LB
☎ 01745 590217 (Sec) & 590898(Pro) ▤ 01745 590472
e-mail: secretary@rhuddlangolfclub.co.uk
web: www.rhuddlangolfclub.co.uk
Attractive, gently undulating parkland with good views. Well bunkered with trees and water hazards. The 476yd 8th and 431yd 11th require both length and accuracy.
18 holes, 6471yds, Par 71, SSS 71, Course record 66.
Club membership 1133.
Visitors Mon, Wed-Sat. Handicap certificate. Dress code. **Societies** Booking required. **Green Fees** £35 per day, £30 per round (£35 per round Sat). **Prof** Andrew Carr **Course Designer** Hawtree & Son **Facilities** ⑪ ⑨⚏ ⚑ ⑨ ⚐ ⚒ ⚘ ✦ **Conf** Corporate Hospitality Days **Location** E side of town on A547
Hotel ★★★ 71% HL Kinmel Manor Hotel, St George's Rd, ABERGELE
☎ 01745 832014 51 en suite

RHYL
MAP 06 SJ08

Rhyl Coast Rd LL18 3RE
☎ 01745 353171 📠 01745 360007
e-mail: rhylgolfclub@i12.com
web: www.rhylgolfclub.com
Flat links course with challenging holes.
9 holes, 6220yds, Par 71, SSS 70, Course record 64.
Club membership 500.
Visitors Mon-Sun & BHs. Booking required Thu, Sat & BHs. Handicap
certificate. Dress code. **Societies** Booking required. **Green Fees** £15 per
round (£20 Sat & Sun). **Prof** John Stubbs **Course Designer** James Braid
Facilities ⊛ ⚑ ♨ by prior arrangement ⚑ ⊒ ♨ ⚑ ⚑ ✦ **Conf**
Corporate Hospitality Days **Location** 1m E on A548
Guesthouse ★★★★ 🏨 RR Barratt's at Ty'N Rhyl, Ty'N Rhyl, 167 Vale Rd,
RHYL ☎ 01745 344138 & 0773 095 4994 📠 01745 344138 3 en suite

RUTHIN
MAP 06 SJ15

Ruthin-Pwllglas Pwllglas LL15 2PE
☎ 01824 702296 & 702383
Parkland course established in 1905 with panoramic views of the Vale
of Clwyd. Three testing Par 3 holes.
10 holes, 5362yds, Par 66, SSS 66, Course record 62.
Club membership 380.
Visitors Mon-Sun & BHs. **Societies** Booking required. **Green Fees** £16 per
day (£22 Sat, Sun & BHs). ⊛ **Prof** M Jones **Course Designer** Dai Rees
Facilities ⊛ ⚑ ⚑ ⊒ ♨ ⚑ ✦ ⚑ ✦ **Conf** Corporate Hospitality Days
Location 2.5m S off A494
Hotel ★★★ 75% HL Ruthin Castle, RUTHIN ☎ 01824 702664 58 en suite

ST ASAPH
MAP 06 SJ07

Llannerch Park North Wales Golf Range, Llannerch Park
LL17 0BD
☎ 01745 730805
e-mail: steve@parkgolf.co.uk
web: www.parkgolf.co.uk
Mainly flat parkland with one dog-leg hole. Fine views towards the
Clwydian Range.
9 holes, 1587yds, Par 30, Course record 27.
Visitors Mon-Sun & BHs. **Societies** Welcome. **Green Fees** £5 per 9 holes.
⊛ **Prof** Andrew Barnett **Course Designer** B Williams **Facilities** ⊒ 🍴 ♨
🎣 **Leisure** fishing. **Location** 200yds S off A525
Hotel ★★ 74% SHL Plas Elwy Hotel & Restaurant, The Roe, ST ASAPH
☎ 01745 582263 & 582089 📠 01745 583864 7 en suite 6 annexe en suite

FLINTSHIRE

BRYNFORD
MAP 07 SJ17

Holywell Brynford CH8 8LQ
☎ 01352 713937 & 710040 📠 01352 713937
e-mail: holywell_golf_club@lineone.net
web: www.hoywellgc.co.uk
Links type course on well-drained mountain turf, with bracken and
gorse flanking undulating fairways. 720ft above sea level.
18 holes, 6100yds, Par 70, SSS 70, Course record 67.
Club membership 505.
Visitors Mon-Fri, Sun & BHs. Booking required. Dress code. **Societies**
Booking required. **Green Fees** £20 per round (£25 Sun & BHs). ⊛

Prof Matt Parsley **Facilities** ⊛ ⚑ 🍴 ⚑ ⊒ ♨ ⚑ ⚑ ⚑ ✦ **Location** 1.25m
SW off B5121
Hotel ★★ 72% HL Stamford Gate Hotel, Halkyn Rd, HOLYWELL
☎ 01352 712942 12 en suite

FLINT
MAP 07 SJ27

Flint Cornist Park CH6 5HJ
☎ 01352 735645
e-mail: paulm@jearrinsurance.co.uk
web: flintgolfclub.netsales.co.uk
Parkland incorporating woods and streams. Excellent views of Dee
estuary and the Welsh hills.
9 holes, 6084yds, Par 70, SSS 69, Course record 65.
Club membership 200.
Visitors Mon-Fri & BHs. Dress code. **Societies** Booking required. **Green
Fees** £12 per day, £10 per 18 holes, £5 per 9 holes. ⊛ **Course Designer** H
G Griffith **Facilities** ⊛ ⚑ ⚑ ⊒ ♨ ⚑ **Location** 1m W of Flint, signs for
Cornist Hall Golf Club
Hotel ★★★ 73% HL Mountain Park Hotel, Northop Rd, Flint Mountain,
FLINT ☎ 01352 736000 & 730972 📠 01352 736010 21 annexe en suite

HAWARDEN
MAP 07 SJ36

Hawarden Groomsdale Ln CH5 3EH
☎ 01244 531447 & 520809 📠 01244 536901
e-mail: secretary@hawardengolfclub.co.uk
Parkland course with comfortable walking and good views.
18 holes, 5842yds, Par 69, SSS 69. Club membership 750.
Visitors Sun-Fri & BHs. Booking required. Handicap certificate. Dress code.
Societies booking required. **Green Fees** not confirmed. ⊛ **Prof** Alex
Rowland **Facilities** ⊛ ⚑ ⚑ ⊒ ♨ ⚑ ⚑ **Location** W side of town off
B5125
Hotel Ⓤ The Gateway To Wales Hotel, Welsh Rd, Sealand, Deeside,
CHESTER ☎ 01244 830332 40 en suite

MOLD
MAP 07 SJ26

Old Padeswood Station Ln, Padeswood CH7 4JL
☎ 01244 547401 & 547701 📠 01244 545082
e-mail: oldpad@par72.fsbusiness.co.uk
web: www.oldpadeswoodgolfclub.co.uk
Situated in the beautiful Alyn valley, part bounded by the River Alyn,
this challenging course suits all categories of golfers. Nine holes are flat
and nine are gently undulating. The signature hole is the 18th, a Par 3
that needs a carry to the green as a valley waits below.
18 holes, 6685yds, Par 72, SSS 72, Course record 66.
Club membership 600.
Visitors Mon-Sun & BHs. Booking required. Dress code. **Societies** Booking
required. **Green Fees** £25 per round (£30 Sat, Sun & BHs). ⊛ **Prof** Tony
Davies **Course Designer** Jeffries **Facilities** ⊛ ⚑ ⚑ ⊒ ♨ ⚑ ⚑ ⚑ ✦ ⚑
✦ **Conf** facs Corporate Hospitality Days **Location** 3m SE off A5118
Hotel ★★★ 73% HL Beaufort Park Hotel, Alltami Rd, New Brighton, MOLD
☎ 01352 758646 106 en suite

Wales

Padeswood & Buckley The Caia, Station Ln, Padeswood
CH7 4JD
☎ 01244 550537 📄 01244 541600
e-mail: admin@padeswoodgolf.plus.com
Bounded by the banks of the River Alyn, gently undulating parkland
with natural hazards and good views of the Welsh hills.
18 holes, 6042yds, Par 70, SSS 69. Club membership 800.
Visitors Mon-Fri. Dress code. **Societies** Booking required. **Green Fees**
£25 per round weekdays. **Prof** David Ashton **Course Designer** Williams
Partnership **Facilities** ⑪ ⑩ ⒧ ⏳ ⑲ ⑳ ⏛ ⑨ ✔ ℰ ⑨ **Leisure** snooker
tables. **Conf** Corporate Hospitality Days **Location** 3m SE off A5118
Hotel ★★★ 73% HL Beaufort Park Hotel, Alltami Rd, New Brighton, MOLD
☎ 01352 758646 106 en suite

NORTHOP   MAP 07 SJ26

Northop Golf & Country Club CH7 6WA
☎ 01352 840440 📄 01352 840445
18 holes, 6750yds, Par 72, SSS 73, Course record 64.
Course Designer John Jacobs **Location** 150yds from Connahs Quay
turning on A55
Telephone for further details
Hotel ★★★★ 76% HL De Vere St David's Park, St Davids Park, EWLOE
☎ 01244 520800 147 en suite

PANTYMWYN   MAP 07 SJ16

Mold Cilcain Rd CH7 5EH
☎ 01352 741513 📄 01352 741517
e-mail: info@moldgolfclub.co.uk
web: www.moldgolfclub.co.uk
Meadowland course with some hard walking and natural hazards.
Fine views.
18 holes, 5603yds, Par 68, SSS 67, Course record 63.
Club membership 700.
Visitors Mon-Sun & BHs. Booking required. Dress code. **Societies** Booking
required. **Green Fees** winter: £15 per day (£25 Sat, Sun & BHs) £22 per
round. summer: £27.50 per day (£33 Sat, Sun & BHs) £25 per round.
Prof Mark Jordan **Course Designer** Hawtree **Facilities** ⑪ ⑩ ⒧ ⌨ 𝍌 ⑳
⏛ 🞉 ⑨ ✔ 🞈 ℰ **Conf** facs Corporate Hospitality Days **Location** E side
of village
Hotel ★★★ 73% HL Beaufort Park Hotel, Alltami Rd, New Brighton, MOLD
☎ 01352 758646 106 en suite

WHITFORD   MAP 06 SJ17

Pennant Park CH8 9AE
☎ 01745 563000
e-mail: enquiries@pennant-park.co.uk
web: www.pennant-park.co.uk
Parkland course set in rolling countryside with fine quality greens and
spectacular views.
18 holes, 6059yds, Par 70, SSS 70, Course record 69.
Club membership 220.
Visitors Mon-Sun & BHs. Booking required Sat, Sun & BHs. Dress code.
Societies Booking required. **Green Fees** £20 per round (£25 Sat & Sun).
Course Designer Roger Jones **Facilities** ⑪ ⑩ ⒧ ⏳ 𝍌 ⑳ ⏛ 🞉 ⑨ ✔ 🞈
Conf Corporate Hospitality Days **Location** from Chester take A55 towards
Holyhead. Exit at junct 32 to Holywell, follow signs for Pennant Park
Hotel ★★ 72% HL Stamford Gate Hotel, Halkyn Rd, HOLYWELL
☎ 01352 712942 12 en suite

GWYNEDD

ABERDYFI   MAP 06 SN69

Aberdovey see page 391

ABERSOCH   MAP 06 SH32

Abersoch LL53 7EY
☎ 01758 712622(shop) 712636(office) 📄 01758 712777
e-mail: admin@abersochgolf.co.uk
web: www.abersochgolf.co.uk

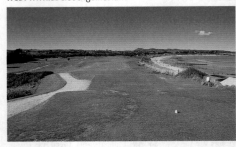

18 holes, 5819yds, Par 69, SSS 68, Course record 66.
Course Designer Harry Vardon **Location** S side of village
Telephone for further details
Hotel ★★ 79% HL Neigwl Hotel, Lon Sarn Bach, ABERSOCH
☎ 01758 712363 9 en suite

See advert on page 393

BALA   MAP 06 SH93

Bala Penlan LL23 7YD
☎ 01678 520359 & 521361 📄 01678 521361
e-mail: balagolfclub@one-tel.com
Upland course with natural hazards. All holes except first and last
affected by wind. First hole is a most challenging Par 3. Irrigated greens
and spectacular views of surrounding countryside.
10 holes, 4962yds, Par 66, SSS 64, Course record 64.
Club membership 235.
Visitors Mon-Sun & BHs. Booking required Sat-Sun & BHs.
Societies Booking required. **Green Fees** £20 (£30 Sat, Sun & BHs).
🖲 **Prof** A R Davies **Course Designer** Syd Collins **Facilities** ⒧ by prior
arrangement 𝍌 ⑳ ⏛ ⏳ 🞉 ⑨ ✔ **Location** 0.5m SW off A494
Hotel ★★ 69% SHL Plas Coch Hotel, High St, BALA ☎ 01678 520309
10 en suite

BANGOR   MAP 06 SH57

St Deiniol Penbryn LL57 1PX
☎ 01248 353098 📄 01248 370792
e-mail: secretary@stdeiniol.fsbusiness.co.uk
web: st-deiniol.co.uk
Elevated parkland course with panoramic views of Snowdonia, the
Menai Strait and Anglesey. Designed by James Braid in 1906 this
course is a test test of accuracy and course management. The 3rd
has a narrow driving area and a shot to an elevated green. The 4th,
one of six Par 3s, provides a choice of pitching the green or utilising

Continued

ABERDOVEY

Map 06 SN69

LL35 0RT
☎ **01654 767493** 🖨 **01654 767027**
e-mail: info@aberdoveygolf.co.uk
web: www.aberdoveygolf.co.uk
18 holes, 6454yds, Par 71, SSS 72,
Course record 66.
Club membership 1000.
Visitors Mon-Sun & BHs. Booking required.
Handicap certificate. Dress code.
Societies Booking required. **Green Fees** £50
per day, £40 per round (£60/£45 Sat & Sun).
Prof John Davies **Course Designer** J Braid
Facilities ⑪ ⑩ ⓲ ⌑ 🖵 🎱 ⚖ 🏠 ◇ 🪒 🚗 🪒
Leisure snooker. **Conf** facs **Location** 0.5m W
on A493

Golf was first played at Aberdovey in 1886, with the club founded six years later. The links has since developed into one of the finest championship courses in Wales. The club has hosted many prestigious events over the years, and is popular with golfing societies and clubs who regularly return here. Golfers can enjoy spectacular views and easy walking alongside the dunes of this characteristic seaside links. Fine holes include the 3rd, 11th and a good short hole at the 12th. The late Bernard Darwin, a former president and captain at the club, was a golf correspondent for the Times. Many of his writings feature the course, which he referred to as 'the course that my soul loves best of all the courses in the world.' Darwin was a major contributor to its success, and he would easily recognise the course today.

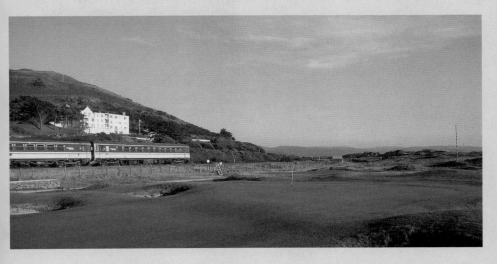

the contours, making it one of the most difficult holes on the course. The 13th, a dog-leg Par 4, is the last hole of the course's own Amen Corner with its out of bounds to the right and left. Centenary in 2006.
18 holes, 5421yds, Par 68, SSS 67, Course record 61.
Club membership 300.
Visitors Mon-Sun & BHs. Booking required. Dress code **Societies** booking required. **Green Fees** not confirmed. **Course Designer** James Braid **Facilities** ⊕ ⑩ ⧠ ☐ ⑪ ⚐ ⚑ 🏌 **Location** A55 junct 11, E of town centre off A5122

CAERNARFON   MAP 06 SH46

Caernarfon Llanfaglan LL54 5RP
☎ 01286 678359 📄 01286 673783
e-mail: pro@caernarfongolfclub.co.uk
web: www.caernarfongolfclub.co.uk
Parkland with gentle gradients. Immaculately kept course with excellent greens and tree-lined fairways.
18 holes, 5941yds, Par 69, SSS 68, Course record 63.
Club membership 660.
Visitors Mon-Sun & BHs. Booking required. Handicap certificate. Dress code. **Societies** Booking required. **Green Fees** £35 per day, £30 per round (£35 per round Sun & Sat). **Prof** Aled Owen **Facilities** ⊕ ⑩ ⧠ ☐ ⑪ ⚐ ⚑ 🏌 **Conf** Corporate Hospitality Days **Location** 1.75m SW
Hotel ★★★ 77% HL Celtic Royal Hotel, Bangor St, CAERNARFON
☎ 01286 674477 110 en suite

CRICCIETH   MAP 06 SH43

Criccieth Ednyfed Hill LL52 0PH
☎ 01766 522154
e-mail: aaguide@criccieethgolfclub.co.uk
web: www.criccieethgolfclub.co.uk
Hilly course on high ground, with generous fairways and natural hazards. The 16th tee has panoramic views in all directions.
18 holes, 5787yds, Par 69, SSS 68. Club membership 200.
Visitors Mon-Sun & BHs. **Societies** Booking required. **Green Fees** £25 per day May-Sep (£15 all other times). ⊕ **Facilities** ⊕ ⑩ ⧠ ☐ ⑪ ⚐ ⚑ **Location** 1m NE
Hotel ★★★ 83% CHH Bron Eifion Country House Hotel, CRICCIETH
☎ 01766 522385 19 en suite

DOLGELLAU   MAP 06 SH71

Dolgellau Hengwrt Estate, Pencefn Rd LL40 2ES
☎ 01341 422603 📄 01341 422603
e-mail: richard@dolgellaugolfclub.com
web: www.dolgellaugolfclub.com
Undulating parkland course set on former hunting grounds of the last Welsh prince, with ancient oak and holly trees. Good views of mountains and the Mawddach estuary.
9 holes, 4671yds, Par 66, SSS 63, Course record 62.
Club membership 300.
Visitors Mon-Sun & BHs. Booking required Sat, Sun & BHs. Dress code. **Societies** Booking required. **Green Fees** £18 per day (£22.50 Sat, Sun & BHs). **Prof** Richard Stockdale **Course Designer** Jack Jones **Facilities** ⊕ ⑩ ⧠ ☐ ⑪ ⚐ 🏌 ⚑ **Conf** facs **Location** 0.5m N, near Town Bridge

---

FFESTINIOG   MAP 06 SH93

Ffestiniog Y Cefn LL41 4LS
☎ 01766 762637
e-mail: info@ffestinioggolf.org
web: www.ffestiniog.org
Moorland course set in Snowdonia National Park.
9 holes, 4570yds, Par 68, SSS 66. Club membership 150.
Visitors Mon-Sat. Booking required Sun & BHs. Dress code. **Societies** Booking required. **Green Fees** £10 per day. ⊕ **Facilities** ⧠ **Location** 1m E of Ffestiniog on B4391
Hotel ★★★ 78% HL Maes y Neuadd Country House Hotel, TALSARNAU
☎ 01766 780200 15 en suite

HARLECH   MAP 06 SH53

Royal St Davids LL46 2UB
☎ 01766 780361 📄 01766 781110
e-mail: secretary@royalstdavids.co.uk
web: www.royalstdavids.co.uk
Championship links with easy walking. Natural hazards demand strength and accuracy. Under the gaze of Harlech Castle, with a magnificent backdrop of the Snowdonia mountains.

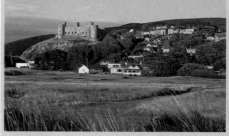

18 holes, 6263yds, Par 69, SSS 71, Course record 61.
Club membership 900.
Visitors Mon-Sun & BHs. Booking required. Handicap certificate. Dress code. **Societies** Booking required. **Green Fees** £55 per day, £45 per round, £28 after 3pm (£65/£55/£34 Sat & Sun). **Prof** John Barnett **Course Designer** Harold Finch-Hatton **Facilities** ⊕ ⑩ ⧠ ☐ ⑪ ⚐ 🏌 ⚑ **Conf** facs Corporate Hospitality Days **Location** W side of town on A496
Hotel ★★ 68% SHL Ty Mawr Hotel, LLANBEDR ☎ 01341 241440 10 en suite

---

MORFA NEFYN   MAP 06 SH24

Nefyn & District LL53 6DA
☎ 01758 720966 📄 01758 720476
e-mail: nefyngolf@tesco.net
web: nefyn-golf-club.com
A 27-hole course played as two separate 18s, Nefyn is a cliff-top links where you never lose sight of the sea. A well-maintained course which will be a very tough test for the serious golfer, but still user friendly for the casual visitor. Every hole has a different challenge and the old 13th fairway is some 30yds across from sea to sea. The

Continued

course has the bonus of a pub on the beach roughly halfway round for those whose golf may need some bolstering.
Old Course: 18 holes, 6201yds, Par 71, SSS 71, Course record 67. New Course: 18 holes, 6317yds, Par 71, SSS 71, Course record 66. Club membership 800.
Societies booking required. **Prof** John Froom **Course Designer** James Braid **Facilities** ⓦ ⓘⓞ 🍴 ⛽ 🏌 ⚐ 🅿 🏪 ⛳ 🏆 **Conf** facs
Location 0.75m NW
Hotel ★★★ 78% CHH Porth Tocyn Hotel, Bwlch Tocyn, ABERSOCH
☎ 01758 713303   17 en suite

PORTHMADOG   MAP 06 SH53

Porthmadog Morfa Bychan LL49 9UU
☎ 01766 514124 📠 01766 514124
e-mail: secretary@porthmadog-golf-club.co.uk
web: www.porthmadog-golf-club-co.uk
Seaside links, very interesting but with easy walking and good views.
18 holes, 6322yds, Par 71, SSS 71. Club membership 1000.
Visitors Mon-Sun & BHs. Booking required. Handicap certificate. Dress code. **Societies** Booking required. **Green Fees** £37 per day, £30 per round (£42/£35 Sun, Sat & BHs). **Prof** Peter L Bright **Course Designer** James Braid **Facilities** ⛽ 🏪 🏌 🏆 **Leisure** snooker. **Conf** Corporate Hospitality Days **Location** 1.5m SW of Porthmadog
Hotel ★★★ 83% CHH Bron Eifion Country House Hotel, CRICCIETH
☎ 01766 522385   19 en suite

PWLLHELI   MAP 06 SH33

Pwllheli Golf Rd LL53 5PS
☎ 01758 701644 📠 01758 701644
e-mail: admin@pwllheligolfclub.co.uk
web: www.pwllheligolfclub.co.uk
Easy walking on flat seaside course, 9 holes links, 9 holes parkland. Outstanding views of Snowdon, Cader Idris and Cardigan Bay.

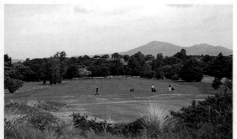

18 holes, 6091yds, Par 69, SSS 70, Course record 66. Club membership 880.
Visitors Mon-Sun & BHs. Dress code. **Societies** Booking required.
Green Fees £34 per day (£39 Sat, Sun & BHs). **Prof** Stuart Pilkington **Course Designer** Tom Morris **Facilities** ⓦ ⓘⓞ 🍴 ⛽ 🏌 🏪 ⚐ 🏪 ⛳ **Conf** Corporate Hospitality Days **Location** 0.5m SW off A497
Hotel ★★★ 78% CHH Porth Tocyn Hotel, Bwlch Tocyn, ABERSOCH
☎ 01758 713303   17 en suite

See advert on this page

Pwllheli Golf Club

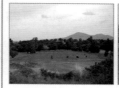
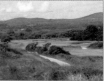

Situated on the south coast of the Lleyn Peninsula Pwllheli Golf Club has unrivalled views of Snowdonia over Cardigan Bay. Established in 1900 this mature course designed by Tom Morris and James Braid has often been described as a unique golf course with 9 holes of gentle parkland and 9 holes a true test of links golf. In 1998, in a survey for Golf Monthly magazine by a group of independent golf panellists, amongst them Walker Cup Captain Peter McEvoy, Pwllheli was listed as only one of seven Welsh golf clubs to appear on the "Top 200 Courses to Play in Britain" – a fact that the Club is proud of, and a standard that has been maintained to the present day.

Pwllheli Golf Club, Golf Road, Pwllheli, Gwynedd LL53 5PS

Tel: 01758 701644 (office)
01758 701644 (professional)
Email: admin@pwllheligolfclub.co.uk
Website: www.pwllheligolfclub.co.uk

— Clwb Golf Abersoch —

Located at Abersoch on the Llyn Peninsula in Gwynedd, Wales, UK – Clwb Golff Abersoch / Abersoch Golf Club offers-18 holes of links and parkland golf.

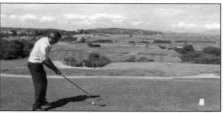

Designed by Harry Varden in 1907, the original 9 hole links course opened in 1908. Today we offer a full 18 holes of links and parkland golf. The sandy soil and the unique microclimate ensures golf for 365-days a year.

We pride ourselves in the condition of the course and the warm welcome extended to members and visitors alike.

Please browse the website for all the latest information, green fees and facilities offered, then visit the local www.abersoch.co.uk website for further details about the resort's surrounding area.

Clwb Golf Abersoch	Tel: Admin 01758 712636
Abersoch	Email: admin@abersochgolf.co.uk
Pwllheli	Web: www.abersochgolf.co.uk
Gwynedd	Pro: Tel: 01758 712622
LL53 7NN	Email: pro@abersochgolf.co.uk

MERTHYR TYDFIL

MERTHYR TYDFIL — MAP 03 SO00

Merthyr Tydfil Cilsanws Mountain, Cefn Coed CF48 2NT
☎ 01685 723308
Mountain-top course in the Brecon Beacons National Park with beautiful views of the surrounding area. The course plays longer than its card length and requires accuracy off the tee.
18 holes, 5625yds, Par 69, SSS 68, Course record 65.
Club membership 160.
Visitors Mon-Sat & BHs. Booking required. Dress code. **Societies** Booking required. **Green Fees** £10 per day (£15 Sat, Sun & BHs). ● **Course Designer** V Price/R Mathias **Facilities** ⑪ by prior arrangement ⊙ by prior arrangement ⬩ by prior arrangement ⬩ by prior arrangement ⬩ ⬩
Location Off A470 at Cefn Coed

Morlais Castle Pant, Dowlais CF48 2UY
☎ 01685 722822 📄 01685 388555
e-mail: morlaiscastlegolfclub@uk2.net
web: www.morlaiscastle-golfclub.com
Beautiful moorland course with excellent views of the Brecon Beacons and surrounding countryside. The interesting layout makes for a testing game.
18 holes, 6320yds, Par 71, SSS 71, Course record 64.
Club membership 600.
Visitors Mon-Fri, Sun & BHs. Booking required. Handicap certificate. Dress code. **Societies** Booking required. **Green Fees** Phone. ● **Prof** H Jarrett **Course Designer** James Braid **Facilities** ⑪ ⊙ ⬩ ⬩ ⬩ ⬩ ⬩ ⬩ ⬩ ⬩ **Conf** facs Corporate Hospitality Days **Location** 2.5m N off A465. Follow signs for Mountain Railway. Course entrance opposite railway car park

MONMOUTHSHIRE

ABERGAVENNY — MAP 03 SO21

Monmouthshire Gypsy Ln, LLanfoist NP7 9HE
☎ 01873 852606 📄 01873 850470
e-mail: monmouthshiregc@btconnect.com
web: www.themonmouthshiregolfclub.com
This parkland course is very picturesque, with the beautifully wooded River Usk running alongside. There are a number of Par 3 holes and a testing Par 4 at the 15th.
18 holes, 5806yds, Par 70, SSS 69, Course record 65.
Club membership 600.
Visitors Mon-Sun. Booking required Mon & Thu-Sun. Handicap certificate. Dress code. **Societies** Booking required. **Green Fees** Phone. **Prof** B Edwards **Course Designer** James Braid **Facilities** ⑪ ⊙ by prior arrangement ⬩ ⊙ ⬩ ⬩ ⬩ **Location** 2m S off B4269
Hotel ★★ 79% HL Llanwenarth Hotel & Riverside Restaurant, Brecon Rd, ABERGAVENNY ☎ 01873 810550 17 en suite

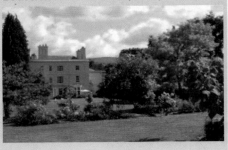
Hotel ★★★★★ 86% GA Glangrwyney Court, CRICKHOWELL
☎ 01873 811288 Fax 01873 810317 5 rms (4 en suite)

Wernddu Golf Centre Old Ross Rd NP7 8NG
☎ 01873 856223 📄 01873 852177
e-mail: info@wernddu-golf-club.co.uk
web: www.wernddu-golf-club.co.uk
A parkland course with magnificent views, wind hazards on several holes in certain conditions, and water hazards on four holes. This gently undulating course has a long front nine and a shorter back nine, while the final hole, a Par 3, is an outstanding finish.
18 holes, 5572yds, Par 69, SSS 67, Course record 63.
Club membership 550.
Visitors Mon-Sun & BHs. Booking required. Dress code. **Societies** Booking required. **Green Fees** £18 per round. **Prof** Tina Tetley **Course Designer** G Watkins **Facilities** ⑪ ⬩ ⊙ ⬩ ⬩ ⬩ ⬩ ⬩ ⬩ ⬩ **Leisure** fishing, 9 hole pitch & putt course. **Location** 1.5m NE on B4521
Hotel ★★★ 77% CHH Llansantffraed Court Hotel, Llanvihangel Gobion, ABERGAVENNY ☎ 01873 840678 21 en suite

BETTWS NEWYDD — MAP 03 SO30

Alice Springs Kemeys Commander NP15 1JY
☎ 01873 880708 📄 01873 881381
e-mail: alice_springs@btconnect.com
web: www.alicespringsgolfclub.co.uk
Two 18-hole undulating parkland courses set back to back with magnificent views of the Usk Valley. The Monow course has testing 7th and 15th holes.

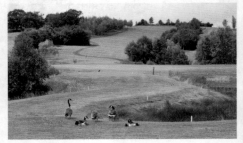

Monow Course: 18 holes, 5544yds, Par 69, SSS 69.
Usk Course: 18 holes, 5934yds, Par 70, SSS 70.
Club membership 450.
Visitors Mon-Sun & BHs. Booking required Tue, Fri-Sun & BHs. Dress code. **Societies** Booking required. **Green Fees** not confirmed. **Prof** Stuart Steel **Course Designer** Keith R Morgan **Facilities** ⑪ ⊙ ⬩ ⊙ ⬩ ⬩ ⬩ ⬩ ⬩ ⬩ **Conf** facs Corporate Hospitality Days **Location** N of Usk on B4598
Hotel ★★★ 64% HL Three Salmons Hotel, Bridge St, USK ☎ 01291 672133 10 en suite 14 annexe en suite

Wales

CHAMPIONSHIP COURSE

MONMOUTHSHIRE — CHEPSTOW

MARRIOTT ST PIERRE HOTEL

Map 03 ST59

St Pierre Park NP16 6YA
☎ **01291 625261** 🖷 **01291 627977**
e-mail: mhrs.cwlgs.golf@marriotthotels.co.uk
web: www.marriottstpierre.co.uk
Old Course: 18 holes, 6733yds, Par 71, SSS 72,
Course record 64.
Mathern Course: 18 holes, 5732yds, Par 68,
SSS 67.
Club membership 800.
Visitors Mon-Sun & BHs. Booking required.
Dress code. **Societies** Booking required.
Green Fees Old from £68, Mathern from £37.
Winter: Old Course from £32, Mathern from £25.
Prof Craig Dun **Course Designer** Henry Cotton
Facilities ⑪ 🍽 ⅃ 🖵 🎱 ♨ 🏌 ⛳ 🚃 ⛴ ⚒
Leisure hard tennis courts, heated indoor pool,
fishing, sauna, solarium, gymnasium, halfway
house on Old Course, health & beauty suite,
chipping green. **Conf** facs Corporate Hospitality
Days **Location** M48 junct 2, A466 towards
Chepstow, at 2nd rdbt take exit for Caerwent.
Hotel after 2m

Set in 400 acres of beautiful parkland,
Marriott St Pierre offers two 18-hole
courses. The Old Course is one of the
finest in the country and has played host
to over 14 European Tour events. The
Par 3 18th hole is famous for its tee shot
over the lake to an elevated green. The
Mathern has its own challenges and is
highly enjoyable for golfers of all abilities.
The hotel has teaching professionals as
well as hire of clubs and equipment.

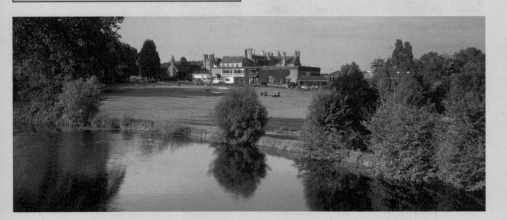

CAERWENT — MAP 03 ST49

Dewstow NP26 5AH
☎ 01291 430444 📠 01291 425816
e-mail: info@dewstow.com
web: www.dewstow.co.uk
Valley Course: 18 holes, 6110yds, Par 72, SSS 70,
Course record 64.
Park Course: 18 holes, 6226yds, Par 69, SSS 69,
Course record 67
Location 0.5m S of Caerwent
Telephone for further details
Hotel BUD Travelodge Magor Newport, Magor Service Area, MAGOR
☎ 08700 850 950 43 en suite

CHEPSTOW — MAP 03 ST59

Marriott St Pierre Hotel Country Club see page 395
Hotel ★★★★ 75% HL Marriott St Pierre Hotel & Country Club, St Pierre Park, CHEPSTOW ☎ 01291 625261 148 en suite
Hotel ★★ 68% HL Castle View Hotel, 16 Bridge St, CHEPSTOW
☎ 01291 620349 Fax 01291 627397 9 en suite 4 annexe en suite

MONMOUTH — MAP 03 SO51

Monmouth Leasbrook Ln NP25 3SN
☎ 01600 712212 (clubhouse) 📠 01600 772399
e-mail: sec.mongc@barbox.net
web: ww.monmouthgolfclub.co.uk
Parkland on high undulating land with beautiful views. The 8th hole, Cresta Run, is renowned as one of Britain's most extraordinary golf holes.

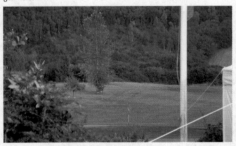

18 holes, 5698yds, Par 69, SSS 69, Course record 67.
Club membership 500.
Visitors Mon-Sun & BHs. Booking required. Handicap certificate. Dress code. **Societies** Booking required. **Green Fees** £28 per day, £20 per round (£30/£24 Sat, Sun & BHs). **Prof** Mike Waldron **Course Designer** George Walden **Facilities** ⊕ ⓘ 🍴 ⚑ ⚑ 🏌 🏌 🏌 🏌 🏌 **Conf** Corporate Hospitality Days **Location** Turn into Leasbrook Lane, 150 yds past Dixon rdbt on Monmouth to Ross on Wye dual carriageway. Club 0.5m up lane on right

Rolls of Monmouth The Hendre NP25 5HG
☎ 01600 715353 📠 01600 713115
e-mail: sandra@therollsgolfclub.co.uk
web: www.therollsgolfclub.co.uk
A hilly and challenging parkland course encompassing several lakes and ponds and surrounded by woodland. Set within a beautiful private estate complete with listed mansion and panoramic views towards the Black Mountains. The short 4th has a lake beyond the green and both the 17th and 18th holes are magnificent holes with which to end your round.
18 holes, 6733yds, Par 72, SSS 73, Course record 69.
Club membership 160.
Visitors Mon-Sun & BHs. Booking required. Dress code.
Societies Booking required. **Green Fees** £40 per day (£44 Sat & Sun).
Facilities ⊕ ⓘ 🍴 ⚑ ⚑ 🏌 🏌 🏌 🏌 **Location** 4m W on B4233

RAGLAN — MAP 03 SO40

Raglan Parc Parc Lodge, Station Rd NP5 2ER
☎ 01291 690077
18 holes, 6604yds, Par 72, SSS 73, Course record 67.
Location Off junct A449
Telephone for further details
Hotel ★★★ 77% CHH Llansantffraed Court Hotel, Llanvihangel Gobion, ABERGAVENNY ☎ 01873 840678 21 en suite

NEATH PORT TALBOT

GLYNNEATH — MAP 03 SN80

Glynneath Pen-y-graig, Pontneathvaughan SA11 5UH
☎ 01639 720452 & 720872 📠 01639 720452
e-mail: enquiries@glynneathgolfclub.co.uk
web: www.glynneathgolfclub.co.uk
Attractive hillside golf overlooking the Vale of Neath in the foothills of the Brecon Beacons National Park. Reasonably level parkland and wooded course.
18 holes, 6211yds, Par 71, SSS 70, Course record 69.
Club membership 603.
Visitors Mon-Sun & BHs. Booking required Sat/Sun. Dress code. **Societies** booking required. **Green Fees** not confirmed. ⊕ **Prof** Shane McMenamin **Course Designer** Cotton/Pennick/Lawrie/williams **Facilities** ⊕ ⓘ 🍴 ⚑ ⚑ 🏌 🏌 🏌 🏌 **Leisure** Snooker. **Conf** facs Corporate Hospitality Days **Location** 2m NE of Glynneath on B4242 then take Pontneath Vaughan Rd **Hotel** ★★★ 70% HL Castle Hotel, The Parade, NEATH ☎ 01639 641119 29 en suite

MARGAM — MAP 03 SS78

Lakeside Water St SA13 2PA
☎ 01639 899959
web: www.lakesidegolf.co.uk
A parkland course with bunkers and natural hazards. Eight Par 4's and ten Par 3's.
18 holes, 4550yds, Par 63, SSS 63, Course record 65.
Club membership 250.
Visitors Mon-Sun & BHs. Dress code. **Societies** Booking required. **Green Fees** £15 per round. **Prof** Mathew Wootton **Course Designer** Matthew Wootton **Facilities** ⊕ ⓘ 🍴 ⚑ ⚑ 🏌 🏌 🏌 🏌 **Conf** Corporate Hospitality Days **Location** M4 junct 38, off B4283
Hotel ★★★ 72% HL Best Western Aberavon Beach Hotel, PORT TALBOT ☎ 01639 884949 52 en suite

NEATH   MAP 03 SS79

Earlswood Jersey Marine SA10 6JP
☎ 01792 321578
Earlswood is a hillside course offering spectacular scenic views over Swansea Bay. The terrain is gently undulating downs with natural hazards and is designed to appeal to both the new and the experienced golfer.
18 holes, 5084yds, Par 68, SSS 68.
Visitors Mon-Sun & BHs. **Societies** Booking required. **Green Fees** £10 per round. ● **Prof** Mike Day **Course Designer** Gorvett Estates **Facilities** ⓑ ▯⚲🍴▯🏌 **Location** 4m E of Swansea, off A483
Hotel ★★★ 70% HL Castle Hotel, The Parade, NEATH ☎ 01639 641119 29 en suite

Neath Cadoxton SA10 8AH
☎ 01639 643615 (clubhouse) & 632759 📠 01639 632759
e-mail: neathgolf@btconnect.com
web: www.neathgolfclub.com
Mountain course, with spectacular views of the Brecon Beacons to the north and the Bristol Channel to the south.

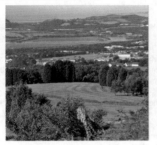

18 holes, 6490yds, Par 72, SSS 72, Course record 66.
Club membership 700.
Visitors Mon-Sun. Booking required. Handicap certificate. Dress code.
Societies booking required. **Green Fees** not confirmed. ● **Prof** R Bennett **Course Designer** James Braid **Facilities** ⓑ▯🍴▯🏌 **Leisure** snooker. **Conf** Corporate Hospitality Days **Location** 2m NE off A4230
Hotel ★★★ 70% HL Castle Hotel, The Parade, NEATH ☎ 01639 641119 29 en suite

Swansea Bay Jersey Marine SA10 6JP
☎ 01792 812198 & 814153
Fairly level seaside links with part dunes.
18 holes, 6605yds, Par 72, SSS 71, Course record 69.
Club membership 500.
Visitors Mon-Sun & BHs. Handicap certificate. Dress code. **Societies** Booking required. **Green Fees** £18 per round (£25 Sat, Sun & BHs). ● **Prof** Mike Day **Facilities** ⓑ🍴▯🏌 **Conf** Corporate Hospitality Days **Location** M4 junct 42, onto A483, 1st right onto B4290 towards Jersey Marine, 1st right to clubhouse

Hotel ★★★ 72% HL Best Western Aberavon Beach Hotel, PORT TALBOT ☎ 01639 884949 52 en suite

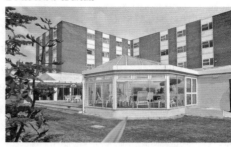

PONTARDAWE   MAP 03 SN70

Pontardawe Cefn Llan SA8 4SH
☎ 01792 863118 📠 01792 830041
e-mail: pontardawe@btopenworld.com
web: pontardawegc.co.uk
Meadowland course situated on plateau 600ft above sea level with good views of the Bristol Channel and the Brecon Beacons.
18 holes, 6101yds, Par 70, SSS 70, Course record 64.
Club membership 500.
Visitors Mon-Fri, Sun & BHs. Booking required except Mon. Handicap certificate. Dress code. **Societies** Booking required. **Green Fees** £20 per day. ● **Prof** Gary Hopkins **Facilities** ⓑ🍴▯🏌 **Leisure** snooker & pool rooms. **Conf** Corporate Hospitality Days **Location** M4 junct 45, off A4067 N of town centre
Hotel ★★★ 70% HL Castle Hotel, The Parade, NEATH ☎ 01639 641119 29 en suite

PORT TALBOT   MAP 03 SS78

British Steel Port Talbot Sports & Social Club, Margam SA13 2NF
☎ 01639 791938
e-mail: tony.edwards@ntlworld.com
9 holes, 4726yds, Par 62, SSS 63, Course record 60.
Location M4 junct 40
Telephone for further details
Hotel ★★★ 72% HL Best Western Aberavon Beach Hotel, PORT TALBOT ☎ 01639 884949 52 en suite

Wales

YSTRADGYNLAIS   **MAP 03 SN71**

Palleg Lower Cwmtwrch SA9 2QQ
☎ 01639 842193 📇 01639 845661
e-mail: gc.gcgs@btinternet.com
web: www.palleg-golf.co.uk
Meadowland course with fine views. An attractive ravine runs through the back nine holes.
18 holes, 5902yds, Par 72, SSS 72. Club membership 300.
Visitors Mon-Sun & BHs. Booking required Sat, Sun & BHs. Dress code.
Societies Booking required. **Green Fees** £20 per day, £12 per round.
Prof Baden Jones **Facilities** ⊕ ⑩ ⚏ ♬ ♉ ⚐ ⚑ 🏌 🍴 ⚬ **Leisure** practice nets. **Conf** facs Corporate Hospitality Days **Location** M4 junct 45, N on A4067 towards Brecon. At 6th roundabout (Powys sign) turn left to Cwmtwrch for 500 yds. Turn right at mini roundabout, up hill into Palleg Rd. Course 1m on left
Hotel ★★★ 70% HL Castle Hotel, The Parade, NEATH ☎ 01639 641119 29 en suite

NEWPORT

CAERLEON   **MAP 03 ST39**

Caerleon NP6 1AY
☎ 01633 420342 📇 01633 420342
9 holes, 2900yds, Par 34, SSS 34, Course record 29.
Course Designer Steel **Location** M4 junct 24, B4236 to Caerleon, 1st left after Priory Hotel, follow road to bottom
Telephone for further details
Hotel ★★★★★ 85% HL The Celtic Manor Resort, Coldra Woods, NEWPORT ☎ 01633 413000 400 en suite

LLANWERN   **MAP 03 ST38**

Llanwern Tennyson Av NP18 2DY
☎ 01633 412029 (sec) & 413233 (pro) 📇 01633 412029
e-mail: llanwerngolfclub@btconnect.com
web: www.llanwerngolfclub.co.uk
Established in 1928, a mature, parkland course in a picturesque village setting.
18 holes, 6177yds, Par 70, SSS 70, Course record 66. Club membership 650.
Visitors Mon-Sat. Handicap certificate. Dress code. **Societies** Booking required. **Green Fees** £35 per day, £25 per round (£40/£30 Sat & Sun). **Prof** Stephen Price **Facilities** ⊕ ⑩ ⚏ ♬ ♉ 🏌 🍴 **Conf** Corporate Hospitality Days **Location** 0.5m S off A455, signed
Hotel ★★★★★ 85% HL The Celtic Manor Resort, Coldra Woods, NEWPORT ☎ 01633 413000 400 en suite

NEWPORT   **MAP 03 ST38**

Celtic Manor Resort see page 399

Hotel ★★★★★ 85% HL The Celtic Manor Resort, Coldra Woods, NEWPORT ☎ 01633 413000 400 en suite
Hotel ★★★ 68% HL Newport Lodge Hotel, Bryn Bevan, Brynglas Rd, NEWPORT ☎ 01633 821818 Fax 01633 856360 27 en suite
Hotel ★★★ 68% HL The Kings Hotel, High St, NEWPORT
☎ 01633 842020 Fax 01633 244667 61 en suite

Newport Great Oak, Rogerstone NP10 9FX
☎ 01633 892643 📇 01633 896676
e-mail: newportgolfclub.gwent@euphony.net
web: newportgolfclub.org.uk
Undulating parkland on an inland plateau 300ft above sea level, with views over the surrounding wooded countryside. There are no blind holes, but plenty of natural hazards and bunkers.
18 holes, 6460yds, Par 72, SSS 71, Course record 63. Club membership 800.
Visitors Mon-Sun except BHs. Booking required. Dress code.
Societies Booking required. **Green Fees** £35 per day; £30 per round (£40 weekends & bank holidays). ⊛ **Prof** Paul Mayo
Course Designer W Fernie **Facilities** ⊕ ⑩ ⚏ ♬ ♉ ⚐ 🏌 🍴 ⚬ **Conf** Corporate Hospitality Days **Location** M4 junct 27, 1m NW on B4591
Hotel ★★★★★ 85% HL The Celtic Manor Resort, Coldra Woods, NEWPORT ☎ 01633 413000 400 en suite

Parc Church Ln, Coedkernew NP10 8TU
☎ 01633 680933 📇 01633 681011
e-mail: enquiries@parcgolf.co.uk
web: www.parcgolf.co.uk
A challenging but enjoyable 18-hole course with water hazards and accompanying wildlife. The 38-bay driving range is floodlit until 10pm.
18 holes, 5619yds, Par 70, SSS 68, Course record 66. Club membership 400.
Visitors Mon-Sun & BHs. Booking required. Dress code. **Societies** Booking required. **Green Fees** Weekdays £15 (£20 Sun, Sat & BHs). **Prof** R Dinsdale/J Wills/N Humphries **Course Designer** B Thomas/T F Hicks **Facilities** ⊕ ⑩ ⚏ ♬ ♉ ⚐ 🏌 🍴 ⚬ 🚩 **Leisure** 9 hole astra turf short course. **Conf** facs Corporate Hospitality Days **Location** 3m SW of Newport, off A48
Hotel ★★★ 68% HL The Kings Hotel, High St, NEWPORT
☎ 01633 842020 61 en suite

Tredegar Park Parc-y-Brain Rd, Rogerstone NP10 9TG
☎ 01633 894433 📇 01633 897152
e-mail: secretary@tredegarparkgolfclub.co.uk
web: www.tredegarparkgolfclub.co.uk
A course completed in 1999 with two balanced halves, mostly in view from the clubhouse. A rolling, open course with fine scenic views.
18 holes, 6545yds, Par 72, SSS 72. Club membership 822.
Visitors Mon-Sun & BHs. Booking required. Handicap certificate. Dress code. **Societies** Booking required. **Green Fees** Phone. **Prof** Lee Pagett **Course Designer** R Sandow **Facilities** ⊕ ⑩ ⚏ ♬ ♉ ⚐ 🏌 🍴 ⚬ **Conf** facs **Location** M4 junct 27, B4591 N, club signed
Hotel ★★★ 68% HL The Kings Hotel, High St, NEWPORT
☎ 01633 842020 61 en suite

Wales

CHAMPIONSHIP COURSE

CELTIC MANOR RESORT

Map 03 ST38

Coldra Woods NP18 1HQ
☎ 01633 413000 📠 01633 410269
e-mail: golf@celtic-manor.com
web: www.celtic-manor.com
Roman Road: 18 holes, 6030yds, Par 70, SSS 72, Course record 63.
Coldra Woods: 18 holes, 3539yds, Par 59, SSS 61.
Wentwood Hills: 18 holes, 6211yds, Par 71, SSS 75, Course record 61.
Club membership 580.
Visitors Mon-Sun & BHs. Booking required. Dress code. **Societies** booking required.
Green Fees Apr-Oct: Wentworth Hills £60, Roman Road £60, Coldra Woods £25.
Prof Kevin Carpenter **Course Designer** Robert Trent Jones **Facilities** ⑨ ⑩ ┗ ◻ ⑨ ⛳ 🏠 ⛳ ◇ ◢ 🛒 ◢ ⚑ **Leisure** hard tennis courts, heated indoor pool, fishing, sauna, solarium, gym, Health spa, Golf Academy with 18 hole course, Shooting school. **Conf** facs Corporate Hospitality Days **Location** M4 junct 24, B4237 towards Newport, 300yds right

This relatively new resort has quickly become a world-renowned venue for golf, set in 1400 acres of beautiful, unspoiled parkland at the southern gateway to Wales. Boasting three championship courses, Celtic Manor offers a challenge for all levels of play, complemented by a golf school and one of the largest clubhouses in Europe, as well as extensive leisure facilities. In 2010, The Celtic Manor Resort will host the 38th Ryder Cup on the world's first ever course to be specifically designed for this prestigious tournament. The new course opened in spring 2007, featuring nine holes from the original Wentwood Hills course and nine spectacular new holes in the valley of the River Usk.

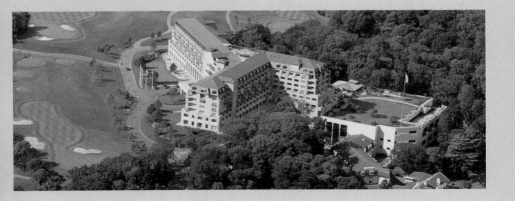

PEMBROKESHIRE

HAVERFORDWEST
MAP 02 SM91

Haverfordwest Arnolds Down SA61 2XQ
☎ 01437 764523 & 768409 🖹 01437 764143
e-mail: haverfordwestgc@btconnect.com
web: www.haverfordwestgolfclub.co.uk
Fairly flat parkland course, a good challenge for golfers of all handicaps.
Set in attractive surroundings with fine views over the Preseli Hills.
18 holes, 5966yds, Par 70, SSS 69, Course record 63.
Club membership 770.
Visitors Mon-Sun & BHs. Booking required. Dress code. **Societies** Booking
required **Green Fees** Phone. **Prof** Alex Pile **Facilities** ⊕ ⊠ ↳ ♿ ⛿ 🖥 ⚘
🖨 ☂ 🛒 ♿ **Conf** facs Corporate Hospitality Days **Location** 1m E on A40
Hotel ★★ 67% HL Hotel Mariners, Mariners Square, HAVERFORDWEST
☎ 01437 763353 28 en suite

LETTERSTON
MAP 02 SM92

Priskilly Forest Castlemorris SA62 5EH
☎ 01348 840276 🖹 01348 840276
e-mail: jevans@priskilly-forest.co.uk
web: www.priskilly-forest.co.uk
Challenging parkland course with panoramic views and a stunning 18th
hole. Immaculate greens and fairways surrounded by rhododendrons,
established shrubs and trees. Testing lies.
9 holes, 5874yds, Par 70, SSS 68, Course record 73.
Club membership 180.
Visitors Mon-Sun & BHs. Booking required Thu. Dress code. **Societies**
Welcome. **Green Fees** £24 per day, £20 per 18 holes, £14 per 9 holes. **Prof**
S Parsons **Course Designer** J Walters **Facilities** ⊕ ⊠ ↳ ♿ ⛿ 🖥 🖨 ☂
◇ ♿ 🛒 **Leisure** fishing. **Conf** facs Corporate Hospitality Days **Location**
Off B4331 between Letterston
Hotel ★★ 76% CHH Wolfscastle Country Hotel, WOLF'S CASTLE
☎ 01437 741688 & 741225 🖹 01437 741383 20 en suite 1 annexe en suite

MILFORD HAVEN
MAP 02 SM90

Milford Haven Woodbine House, Hubberston SA73 3RX
☎ 01646 697762 🖹 01646 697870
e-mail: cerithmhgc@aol.com
web: www.mhgc.co.uk
Parkland course with excellent greens and views of the Milford Haven
waterway.
18 holes, 6030yds, Par 71, SSS 70, Course record 64.
Club membership 550.
Visitors Mon-Sun & BHs. Booking required. Dress code. **Societies** Booking
required. **Green Fees** Phone. **Facilities** ⊕ ⊠ ↳ ♿ ⛿ 🖥 ☂ 🖨 ☂ 🛒 ♿
Location 1.5m W of Milford Haven
Hotel ★★★ 64% HL Cleddau Bridge Hotel, Essex Rd, PEMBROKE DOCK
☎ 01646 685961 24 en suite

NEWPORT (PEMBROKESHIRE)
MAP 02 SN03

Newport (Pemb) Newport Links Golf Club SA42 0NR
☎ 01239 820244 🖹 01239 820085
e-mail: newportgc@lineone.net
web: www.newportlinks.co.uk
Seaside links course situated in a National Park, with easy walking and
good view of the Preselli Hills and Newport Bay.
9 holes, 6002yds, Par 70, SSS 69, Course record 64.
Club membership 510.
Visitors Mon-Sun & BHs. Dress code. **Societies** Booking required **Green
Fees** £22 per round (£25 Sat & Sun). **Prof** Alun Evans **Course Designer**
James Baird **Facilities** ⊕ ⊠ ↳ ♿ ⛿ 🖥 ☂ ◇ ♿ 🛒 ♿ **Conf** facs
Corporate Hospitality Days **Location** 1.25m N
Hotel ★★ 71% HL Trewern Arms, NEVERN ☎ 01239 820395 10 en suite

PEMBROKE DOCK
MAP 02 SM90

South Pembrokeshire Military Rd SA72 6SE
☎ 01646 621453 & 682442 🖹 01646 621453
web: www.southpembsgolf.co.uk
A hillside course on an elevated site overlooking the Cleddau and
Haven waterway.
18 holes, 6100yds, Par 71, SSS 70, Course record 65.
Club membership 350.
Visitors Mon-Sun & BHs. Booking required. Dress code. **Societies** Booking
required **Green Fees** Phone. **Course Designer** Committee **Facilities** ⊕
⊠ ↳ ♿ ⛿ 🖥 ☂ 🛒 ♿ **Conf** facs Corporate Hospitality Days **Location** SW
of town centre off B4322

TENBY
MAP 02 SN10

Tenby The Burrows SA70 7NP
☎ 01834 844447 & 842978 🖹 01834 842978
e-mail: tenbygolfclub@uku.co.uk
web: www.tenbygolf.co.uk
The oldest club in Wales, this fine seaside links, with sea views and
natural hazards, provides good golf all the year round.
18 holes, 6224yds, Par 69, SSS 71, Course record 65.
Club membership 700.
Visitors Mon-Sun & BHs. Booking required. Handicap certificate. Dress
code. **Societies** Booking required. **Green Fees** Phone ● **Prof** Mark
Hawkey **Course Designer** James Braid **Facilities** ⊕ ⊠ ↳ ♿ ⛿ 🖥 ☂ 🖨
🛒 🛒 ♿ **Conf** Corporate Hospitality Days **Location** Near railway
station
Hotel ★★★ 77% HL Atlantic Hotel, The Esplanade, TENBY
☎ 01834 842881 42 en suite

Trefloyne Golf, Bar & Restaurant Trefloyne Park,
Penally SA70 7RG
☎ 01834 842165 🖹 01834 844288
e-mail: enquiries@trefloyne
web: www.trefloyne.com
Idyllic parkland course with backdrop of mature mixed woodlands and
distant views of Tenby, Carmarthen Bay and Caldey Island. Opened
in 1996, natural features and hazards such as the Old Quarry make for
exciting and challenging golf.
18 holes, 6635yds, Par 71, SSS 73. Club membership 400.

Continued

Visitors Mon-Sun & BHs. Booking required Sat, Sun & BHs. Dress code.
Societies booking required. **Green Fees** not confirmed. **Prof** Steven
Laidler **Course Designer** F H Gillman **Facilities** ⑪ ⑩ ⓘ ▣ ☐ ⌁ ⌂
⌐ ⌂ ⌂ ⌂ **Leisure** lessons by PGA Professional. **Conf** facs Corporate
Hospitality Days **Location** In Trefloyne Park, just W of Tenby
Hotel ★★★ 72% HL Fourcroft Hotel, North Beach, TENBY
☎ 01834 842886 40 en suite

POWYS

BRECON   MAP 03 SO02

Brecon Newton Park LD3 8PA
☎ 01874 622004
Easy walking parkland. Natural hazards include two rivers on the
boundary. Good river and mountain scenery.
9 holes, 5476yds, Par 68, SSS 66, Course record 63.
Club membership 360.
Visitors Mon-Sun & BHs. Contact club for details. Handicap certificate. Dress
code. **Societies** booking required. **Green Fees** not confirmed. ◎ **Course**
Designer James Braid **Facilities** ⑪ ⑩ ⓘ ▣ ☐ ⌁ ⌂ ⌂ **Conf**
Corporate Hospitality Days **Location** 0.75m W of town centre on A40
Hotel ★★ 68% HL The Castle of Brecon Hotel, Castle Square, BRECON
☎ 01874 624611 30 en suite 12 annexe en suite

Cradoc Penoyre Park, Cradoc LD3 9LP
☎ 01874 623658 ▤ 01874 611711
e-mail: secretary@cradoc.co.uk
web: www.cradoc.co.uk
Parkland with wooded areas, ponds and spectacular views over the
Brecon Beacons. Challenging golf.

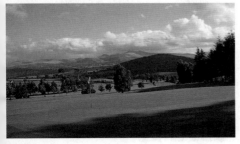

18 holes, 6188yds, Par 71, SSS 71, Course record 65.
Club membership 700.
Visitors Mon-Sun & BHs. Booking advised. Handicap certificate. Dress code.
Prof Richard Davies **Course Designer** C K Cotton **Facilities** ⑪ ⑩ ⓘ ▣ ☐
⌁ ⌂ ☐ ⌐ ⌂ ⌂ ⌂ **Location** 2m N of Brecon off B4520
Hotel ★★ 68% HL The Castle of Brecon Hotel, Castle Square, BRECON
☎ 01874 624611 30 en suite 12 annexe en suite

BUILTH WELLS   MAP 03 SO05

Builth Wells Golf Links Rd LD2 3NF
☎ 01982 553296 ▤ 01982 551064
e-mail: info@builthwellsgolf.co.uk
web: www.builthwellsgolf.co.uk
Well-guarded greens and a stream running through the centre of the
course add interest to this 18-hole undulating parkland course. The
clubhouse is a converted 16th-century Welsh longhouse.
18 holes, 5424yds, Par 66, SSS 67, Course record 62.
Club membership 380.
Visitors Mon-Sun & BHs. Booking required. Handicap certificate. Dress
code. **Societies** Booking required. **Green Fees** £30 per day, £22 per round
(£32/£25 Sat, Sun & BHs). **Prof** Simon Edwards **Facilities** ⑪ ⑩ ⓘ ▣ ☐ ⌁ ⌂
⌐ ⌂ ☐ ⌂ ⌂ **Conf** Corporate Hospitality Days **Location** N of A483
Hotel ★★★ 75% HL Caer Beris Manor Hotel, BUILTH WELLS
☎ 01982 552601 23 en suite

KNIGHTON   MAP 07 SO27

Knighton Ffrydd Wood LD7 1DL
☎ 01547 528046 (Sec)
Upland course with some hard walking. Fine views over the England
border.
9 holes, 5362yds, Par 68, SSS 66, Course record 65.
Club membership 150.
Visitors Mon-Sat & BHs. Booking required Sat & BHs. Dress code.
Societies Booking required. **Green Fees** £10 per day (£15 Sat & BHs). ◎
Course Designer Harry Vardon **Facilities** ⑪ by prior arrangement ▣ by
prior arrangement ☐ ⌂ ⌁ **Location** 0.5m S off B4355
Hotel ★★ 85% HL Milebrook House Hotel, Milebrook, KNIGHTON
☎ 01547 528632 10 en suite

LLANDRINDOD WELLS   MAP 03 SO06

Llandrindod Wells The Clubhouse LD1 5NY
☎ 01597 823873 (sec) ▤ 01597 823873
e-mail: secretary@lwgc.co.uk
web: www.lwgc.co.uk
An upland links course, designed by Harry Vardon, with easy walking
and panoramic views.
18 holes, 5759yds, Par 69, SSS 69, Course record 65.
Club membership 465.
Visitors Mon-Sun & BHs. Booking required Fri-Sun & BHs. Dress code.
Societies Booking required. **Green Fees** £32 per day, £24 per round
(£36/£30 Sat, Sun & BHs). ◎ **Prof** Philip Davies **Course Designer**
H Vardon **Facilities** ⑪ ⑩ ⓘ ▣ ☐ ⌁ ⌂ ⌂ ⌐ ⌂ ☐ ⌂ **Conf** facs
Corporate Hospitality Days **Location** 1m SE off A483
Hotel ★★★ 80% HL The Metropole, Temple St, LLANDRINDOD WELLS
☎ 01597 823700 120 en suite

Wales

LLANGATTOCK
MAP 03 SO21

Old Rectory NP8 1PH
☎ 01873 810373 📄 018373 810373
e-mail: stu@rectoryhotel.co.uk
web: www.rectoryhotel.co.uk
Sheltered course with easy walking.
9 holes, 2200yds, Par 54, SSS 59, Course record 53.
Club membership 80.
Visitors Mon-Sat & BHs. Dress code. **Societies** Booking required **Green Fees** £10 per day. **Facilities** ⑪ ⑥ ᐟ ᐟ ☋ ᐟ ᐟ ⛄ **Leisure** fishing. **Conf** facs **Location** SW of village
Hotel ★★★ 80% HL Gliffaes Country House Hotel, CRICKHOWELL
☎ 01874 730371 19 en suite 4 annexe en suite

LLANIDLOES
MAP 06 SN98

St Idloes Penrallt SY18 6LG
☎ 01686 412559
Hill-course, slightly undulating but walking is easy. Good views, partly lined with trees. Sand and grass bunkers.
9 holes, 5540yds, Par 66, SSS 66, Course record 61.
Club membership 339.
Visitors Mon-Sun & BHs. Dress code. **Societies** Welcome. **Green Fees** £20 day, £15 per 18 holes, £10 per 9 holes. ⊕ **Facilities** ⑪ by prior arrangement ⑥ by prior arrangement ᐟ ☋ ᐟ ᐟ **Conf** facs
Location 1m N off B4569
Inn ★★★ INN Mount Inn, China St, LLANIDLOES ☎ 01686 412247
3 en suite 6 annexe en suite

MACHYNLLETH
MAP 06 SH70

Machynlleth SY20 8UH
☎ 01654 702000 📄 01654 702928
Lowland course with mostly natural hazards.
9 holes, 5726yds, Par 68, SSS 68, Course record 65.
Club membership 200.
Visitors Mon-Sun & BHs. Dress code. **Societies** booking required. **Green Fees** not confirmed. ⊕ **Course Designer** James Braid **Facilities** ⑪ ⑥ ᐟ ☋ ᐟ ᐟ ᐟ **Location** 0.5m E off A489
Hotel ★★★ 70% HL Wynnstay Hotel, Maengwyn St, MACHYNLLETH
☎ 01654 702941 23 en suite

NEWTOWN
MAP 06 SO19

St Giles Pool Rd SY16 3AJ
☎ 01686 625844 📄 01686 625844
e-mail: stgilesgolf@tiscali.co.uk
Inland country course with easy walking. Testing 2nd hole, Par 3, and 4th hole, Par 4. River Severn skirts four holes.
9 holes, 6012yds, Par 70, SSS 70, Course record 67.
Club membership 350.
Visitors Contact club for details. Dress code. **Societies** booking required. **Green Fees** not confirmed. ⊕ **Prof** D P Owen **Facilities** ⑪ by prior arrangement ⑥ by prior arrangement ⑥ by prior arrangement ☋ by prior arrangement ᐟ ᐟ **Location** 0.5m NE on A483
Hotel ★★★ 70% HL Wynnstay Hotel, Maengwyn St, MACHYNLLETH
☎ 01654 702941 23 en suite

WELSHPOOL
MAP 07 SJ20

Welshpool Golfa Hill SY21 9AQ
☎ 01938 850249 📄 01938 850249
e-mail: welshpool.golfclub@virgin.net
web: www.welshpoolgolfclub.co.uk
Undulating, hilly, heathland course with bracing air. Testing holes are 2nd (Par 5), 14th (Par 3), 17th (Par 3) and a memorable 18th.
18 holes, 5716yds, Par 71, SSS 68, Course record 68.
Club membership 400.
Visitors Mon-Sun & BHs. Booking required. **Societies** Booking required. **Green Fees** £15.50 per day (£25.50 Sat & Sun, £15.50 winter months). ⊕ **Prof** Bob Barlow **Course Designer** James Braid **Facilities** ⑪ ⑥ ᐟ ☋ ᐟ ᐟ ☋ ᐟ ᐟ ᐟ **Conf** Corporate Hospitality Days **Location** 3m W off A458
Hotel ★★★ 73% HL Royal Oak Hotel, The Cross, WELSHPOOL
☎ 01938 552217 25 en suite

RHONDDA CYNON TAFF

ABERDARE
MAP 03 SO00

Aberdare Abernant CF44 0RY
☎ 01685 872797 📄 01685 872797
e-mail: sec-age@tiscali.co.uk
Mountain course with parkland features overlooking the Brecon Beacons. Tree-lined with many mature oaks.
18 holes, 5875yds, Par 69, SSS 69, Course record 64.
Club membership 550.
Visitors Mon-Sun & BHs. Contact club for details. Handicap certificate. Dress code. **Societies** booking required. **Green Fees** not confirmed. ⊕ **Prof** A Palmer **Facilities** ⑪ ⑥ ᐟ ☋ ᐟ ᐟ ☋ ᐟ ᐟ ᐟ **Leisure** 3 practice nets.
Conf facs Corporate Hospitality Days **Location** 1m NE of town centre. Past hospital, 400yds on right

MOUNTAIN ASH
MAP 03 ST09

Mountain Ash Cefnpennar CF45 4DT
☎ 01443 479459 📄 01443 479628
e-mail: geoff@magc.fsnet.co.uk
web: www.mountainash.co.uk
18 holes, 5553yds, Par 69, SSS 67, Course record 60.
Location 1m NW off A4059
Telephone for further details

PENRHYS
MAP 03 ST09

Rhondda Golf Club House CF43 3PW
☎ 01443 441384 📄 01443 441384
e-mail: rhondda@btinternet.com
Mountain course with good views.
18 holes, 6205yds, Par 70, SSS 71, Course record 67.
Club membership 600.
Visitors Mon-Fri. Booking required. Handicap certificate. Dress code.
Societies booking required. **Green Fees** not confirmed. ⊕ **Facilities** ⑪ by prior arrangement ⑥ by prior arrangement ᐟ ☋ ᐟ ᐟ ☋ ᐟ ᐟ ᐟ
Conf facs **Location** 0.5m W off B4512

Wales

PONTYPRIDD
MAP 03 ST08

Pontypridd Ty Gwyn Rd CF37 4DJ
☎ 01443 409904 🖹 01443 491622
Well-wooded mountain course with springy turf. Good views of the Rhondda Valley and coast.
18 holes, 5721yds, Par 69, SSS 68, Course record 65. Club membership 850.
Visitors Mon-Sun & BHs. Handicap certificate. Dress code. **Societies** Booking required **Green Fees** £20 per 18 holes. ☻ **Prof** Wade Walters **Facilities** ⑪ 🍴 🍻 💪 🖵 🍴 🛄 ⚐ 🛄 ⚐ **Location** E of town centre off A470

TALBOT GREEN
MAP 03 ST08

Llantrisant & Pontyclun Off Ely Valley Rd CF72 8AL
☎ 01443 228169 🖹 01443 224601
e-mail: lpgc@barbox.net
Scenic, undulating parkland.
18 holes, 5328yds, Par 68, SSS 66. Club membership 600.
Visitors Mon-Fri. Booking required. Handicap certificate. **Societies** telephone in advance **Green Fees** not confirmed. **Prof** Steve Hurley & Matt Vanstone **Facilities** ⑪ 🍴 🍻 💪 🖵 🍴 🛄 ⚐ **Conf** Corporate Hospitality Days **Location** M4 junct 34, A4119 to Llantrisant, over 1st rdbt, left at 2nd lights to Talbot Green, right at minirdbt, club 50yds on left
Hotel ★★★★ 71% CHH Miskin Manor Country Hotel, Pendoylan Rd, MISKIN ☎ 01443 224204 34 en suite 9 annexe en suite

SWANSEA

CLYDACH
MAP 03 SN60

Inco SA6 5QR
☎ 01792 842929
e-mail: secretaryinco.golf@amserve.com
Flat meadowland course bordered by meandering River Tawe and the Swansea valley. Recently completed an ambitious development programme.
18 holes, 6064yds, Par 70, SSS 69, Course record 68. Club membership 450.
Visitors Mon-Sun & BHs. Dress code. **Societies** Booking required. **Green Fees** £18 per round (£23 Sat & Sun). ☻ **Facilities** ⑪ 🍴 🍻 💪 🖵 🍴 🛄 **Leisure** outdoor bowling green. **Conf** Corporate Hospitality Days **Location** M4 junct 45, 1.5m NE on A4067
Hotel BUD Premier Travel Inn Swansea North, Upper Fforest Way, Morriston, SWANSEA ☎ 08701 977246 40 en suite

PONTLLIW
MAP 02 SS69

Allt-y-Graban Allt-y-Grabam Rd SA4 1DT
☎ 01792 885757
9 holes, 2210yds, Par 66, SSS 66, Course record 63.
Course Designer F G Thomas **Location** M4 junct 47, A48 towards Pontardulais, left after Glamorgan Arms
Telephone for further details
Hotel BUD Travelodge Swansea (M4), Penllergaer, SWANSEA ☎ 08700 850 950 50 en suite

SOUTHGATE
MAP 02 SS58

Pennard 2 Southgate Rd SA3 2BT
☎ 01792 233131 & 233451 🖹 01792 234797
e-mail: sec@pennardgolfclub.com
web: www.pennardgolfclub.com
Undulating, cliff-top seaside links with good coastal views. At first sight it can be intimidating with steep hills that make club selection important - there are a few blind shots to contend with. The difficulties are not insurmountable unless the wind begins to blow in calm weather. Greens are slick and firm all year.
18 holes, 6265yds, Par 71, SSS 72, Course record 69. Club membership 1020.
Visitors Mon & Wed-Sun. Contact club for details. Handicap certificate. Dress code. **Societies** booking required. **Green Fees** not confirmed. **Prof** M V Bennett **Course Designer** James Braid **Facilities** ⑪ 🍴 🍻 💪 🖵 🍴 🛄 ⚐ 🛄 ⚐ 🛄 **Location** 8m W of Swansea by A4067 and B4436
Hotel ★★★ CHH Fairyhill, REYNOLDSTON ☎ 01792 390139 8 en suite

SWANSEA
MAP 03 SS69

Clyne 120 Owls Lodge Ln, The Mayals, Blackpyl SA3 5DP
☎ 01792 401989 🖹 01792 401078
e-mail: clynegolfclub@supanet.com
web: www.clynegolfclub.com
Challenging moorland course with excellent greens and scenic views of Swansea Bay and the Gower. Many natural hazards with a large number of bunkers and gorse and bracken in profusion.
18 holes, 6334yds, Par 70, SSS 72, Course record 64. Club membership 900.
Visitors Mon-Sun & BHs. Booking required. Handicap certificate. Dress code. **Societies** Booking required. **Green Fees** £30 per round (£40 Sat, Sun & BHs), Winter £20 including bar meal. ☻ **Prof** Jonathan Clewett **Course Designer** H S Colt & Harries **Facilities** ⑪ 🍴 🍻 💪 🖵 🍴 🛄 ⚐ 🛄 ⚐ **Leisure** chipping green,driving nets,indoor practice net. **Location** 3.5m SW on B4436

Langland Bay Langland Bay SA3 4QR
☎ 01792 361721 🖹 01792 361082
e-mail: info@langlandbaygolfclub.com
web: www.langlandbaygolfclub.com
Parkland situated on cliff tops and land between Caswell and Langland Bay. The Par 4 6th is an uphill dog-leg open to the wind, and the Par 3 16th (151yds) is aptly named Death or Glory.
18 holes, 5857yds, Par 70, SSS 70, Course record 63 or 18 holes, 5717yds. Club membership 850.
Visitors Mon, Wed-Sun & BHs. Booking required. Handicap certificate. Dress code. **Societies** Booking required. **Green Fees** £40 per round (£50 Sat, Sun & BHs). ☻ **Prof** Mark Evans **Facilities** ⑪ 🍴 🍻 💪 🖵 🍴 🛄 ⚐ 🛄 ⚐ **Location** 6m SW off B4593

Morriston 160 Clasemont Rd SA6 6AJ
☎ 01792 796528 🖹 01792 796528
e-mail: morristongolf@btconnect.com
18 holes, 5891yds, Par 68, SSS 68, Course record 61.
Location M4 junct 46, 1m E on A48
Telephone for further details
Hotel BUD Premier Travel Inn Swansea North, Upper Fforest Way, Morriston, SWANSEA ☎ 08701 977246 40 en suite

Wales

THREE CROSSES
MAP 02 SS59

Gower Cefn Goleu SA4 3HS
☎ 01792 872480 (Off) 🖷 01792 875535
e-mail: info@gowergolf.co.uk
web: www.gowergolf.co.uk
Set in attractive rolling countryside, this Donald Steel designed course provides good strategic hazards, including trees, water and bunkers. Outstanding views and a challenging game of golf.
18 holes, 6441yds, Par 71, SSS 72, Course record 66.
Club membership 400.
Visitors Mon-Sun & BHs. Booking required. Handicap certificate. Dress code. **Societies** Booking required. **Green Fees** £24 per round (£30 Sun & Sat), £15 winter rate. **Prof** Alan Williamson **Course Designer** Donald Steel **Facilities** ⑪ � ⅃ ▱ ⚐ ⚲ ☒ ➿ ◇ ✔ 👜 ✔ **Conf** facs Corporate Hospitality Days **Location** Off A4118 Swansea to Gower, signed from Three Crosses
Hotel ★★ 68% HL Beaumont Hotel, 72-73 Walter Rd, SWANSEA
☎ 01792 643956 16 en suite

UPPER KILLAY
MAP 02 SS59

Fairwood Park Blackhills Ln SA2 7JN
☎ 01792 297849 🖷 01792 297849
e-mail: info@fairwoodpark.com
web: www.fairwoodpark.com
Parkland championship course on the beautiful Gower peninsula, being both the flattest and the longest course in Swansea. Surrounded by vast areas of woodland on all sides, each fairway is well defined with lakes and bunkers to test the nerve of any golfer.
18 holes, 6650yds, Par 73, SSS 73, Course record 68.
Club membership 500.
Visitors Mon-Sun & BHs. Dress code. **Societies** Booking required.
Green Fees £22 per round, (£27 Fri-Sun). **Prof** Gary Hughes
Course Designer Hawtree **Facilities** ⑪ 101 ⅃ ▱ ⚐ ⚲ ☒ ➿ ◇ ✔ 👜
✔ **Conf** Corporate Hospitality Days **Location** 1.5m S off A4118

TORFAEN

CWMBRAN
MAP 03 ST29

Green Meadow Golf & Country Club Treherbert Rd, Croesyceiliog NP44 2BZ
☎ 01633 869321 & 862626 🖷 01633 868430
e-mail: info@greenmeadowgolf.com
web: www.greenmeadowgolf.com
Undulating parkland with panoramic views. Tree-lined fairways, water hazards and pot bunkers. The greens are excellent and are playable all year round.

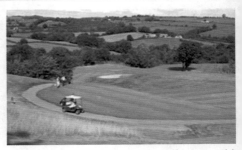
Green Meadow Golf & Country Club

18 holes, 6029yds, Par 70, SSS 70, Course record 64.
Club membership 400.
Visitors Mon-Fri & BHs. Booking required Fri-Sun. Dress code. **Societies** Booking required. **Green Fees** £22 per round (£19 Mon, £27 Sat, Sun & BHs). **Prof** Dave Woodman **Course Designer** Peter Richardson **Facilities** ⑪ 101 ⅃ ▱ ⚐ ⚲ ☒ ◇ 👜 101 **Leisure** hard tennis courts, sauna, gymnasium. **Conf** facs Corporate Hospitality Days **Location** NE of town off A4042
Hotel ★★★★ 70% HL Best Western Parkway Hotel, Cwmbran Dr, CWMBRAN ☎ 01633 871199 70 en suite

See advert on opposite page

Pontnewydd Maesgwyn Farm, Upper Cwmbran NP44 1AB
☎ 01633 482170 🖷 01633 838598
e-mail: ct.phillips@virgin.net
Mountainside course with hard walking. Good views across the Severn estuary.
11 holes, 5278yds, Par 68, SSS 67, Course record 61.
Club membership 502.
Visitors Mon, Tue, Thu, Fri, Sun & BHs. Booking required Mon & BHs. Handicap certificate. Dress code. **Societies** Booking required **Green Fees** £15 per round. ⊜ **Facilities** ⑪ 101 ⅃ ▱ ⚐ ☒ **Location** N of town centre
Hotel ★★★★ 70% HL Best Western Parkway Hotel, Cwmbran Dr, CWMBRAN ☎ 01633 871199 70 en suite

PONTYPOOL
MAP 03 SO20

Pontypool Lasgarn Ln, Trevethin NP4 8TR
☎ 01495 763655 🖷 01495 755564
e-mail: pontypoolgolf@btconnect.com
web: pontypoolgolf.co.uk
Undulating mountain course with magnificent views of the Bristol Channel.
18 holes, 5963yds, Par 69, SSS 69, Course record 64.
Club membership 638.
Visitors Mon-Fri. booking required. Handicap certificate. Dress code. **Societies** welcome. **Green Fees** not confirmed. ⊜ **Prof** Neil Matthews **Facilities** ⑪ 101 ⅃ ▱ ⚐ ☒ ☒ 👜 ✔ **Leisure** indoor teaching academy with video analysis. **Conf** Corporate Hospitality Days **Location** 1.5m N off A4043

Woodlake Park Golf & Country Club Glascoed
NP4 0TE
☎ 01291 673933 🖥 01291 673811
e-mail: golf@woodlake.co.uk
web: www.woodlake.co.uk
Undulating parkland with magnificent views over the Llandegfedd Reservoir. Superb greens constructed to USGA specification. holes 4, 7 and 16 are Par 3s, which are particularly challenging. holes 6 and 17 are long Par 4s, which can be wind affected.
18 holes, 6278yds, Par 71, SSS 72, Course record 67. Club membership 500.
Visitors Mon-Sun & BHs. Booking required. Handicap certificate. Dress code. **Societies** Booking required. **Green Fees** £35 per day, £25 per round (£42/£32 Fri-Sun & BHs). **Prof** Leon Lancey **Facilities** ⓘ �𝄞 ⚑ ⌨ 🍴 ⚲ 🏌 🐟 🏹 🏌 **Leisure** fishing. **Conf** Corporate Hospitality Days **Location** Overlooking Llandegfedd Reservoir

VALE OF GLAMORGAN

BARRY   MAP 03 ST16

Brynhill Port Rd CF62 8PN
☎ 01446 720277 🖥 01446 740422
e-mail: postbox@brynhillgolfclub.co.uk
web: www.brynhillgolfclub.co.uk
Meadowland course with some hard walking. Prevailing west wind.
18 holes, 6516yds, Par 72, SSS 71. Club membership 750.
Visitors Mon-Sat & BHs. Handicap certificate. Dress code. **Societies** booking required. **Green Fees** not confirmed. 🚶 **Prof** Duncan Prior
Facilities ⚲ 🏌 ⚑ 🏌 🏌 **Location** 1.25m N on B4050
Hotel ★★★ 74% HL Best Western Mount Sorrel Hotel, Porthkerry Rd, BARRY ☎ 01446 740069 42 en suite

RAF St Athan Clive Rd, St Athan CF62 4JD
☎ 01446 751043 🖥 01446 751862
e-mail: rafstathan@golfclub.fsbusiness.co.uk
Parkland affected by strong winds straight from the sea. Further interest is added by this being a very tight course with lots of trees. Beware of low-flying RAF jets.
9 holes, 6480yds, Par 72, SSS 72. Club membership 450.
Visitors Mon-Fri. Handicap certificate. Dress code. **Societies** Booking requested. **Green Fees** £15 per day. 🚶 **Course Designer** the members
Facilities ⓘ 🏌 🏌 ⚑ 🍴 ⚲ **Location** Between Barry & Llantwit Major
Hotel ★★★ 79% CHH Egerton Grey Country House Hotel, Porthkerry, BARRY ☎ 01446 711666 10 en suite

St Andrews Major Coldbrook Rd East, Cadoxton
CF63 1BL
☎ 01446 722227 🖥 01446 748953
A scenic 18-hole parkland course, suitable for all standards of golfer. The greens are designed to US specifications. The course provides excellent challenges to all levels of golfers without being physically exerting.
18 holes, 5300yds, Par 69, SSS 70. Club membership 400.
Visitors Mon-Sun & BHs. Dress code. **Societies** Booking required. **Green Fees** £18 per round (£20 Sat & Sun). **Prof** Iestyn Taylor **Course Designer** Richard Hurd **Facilities** ⓘ 🍴 🏌 ⚑ 🏌 🏌 🏌 🏌 **Conf** facs Corporate Hospitality Days **Location** 1.5m NE of Barry off A4231
Hotel ★★★ 79% CHH Egerton Grey Country House Hotel, Porthkerry, BARRY ☎ 01446 711666 10 en suite

Green Meadow Golf & Country Club
Treherbert Road, Croesyceiliog, Cwmbran, Gwent, NP44 2BZ

Beautiful 18-hole, par 70, Parkland Course measuring 6,200 yds; a good test of golf for all categories of player.

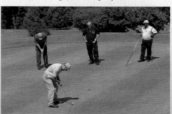

• **Conferences facilities with full catering provision, seven days a week.** • **Excellent changing facilities**
• **Fitness Suite with saunas** • **26-Bay Driving Range**
• **Buggy and Trolly Hire.**

Pro Shop: 01633 862626
Clubhouse: 01633 869321
Email: info@greenmeadowgolf.com
Web: www.greenmeadowgolf.com

** JUST 10mins FROM J26 M4, on A4042.**

DINAS POWYS   MAP 03 ST17

Dinas Powis High Walls Av CF64 4AJ
☎ 029 2051 2727 🖥 029 2051 2727
Parkland/downland course with views over the Bristol Channel and the seaside resort of Barry.
18 holes, 5532yds, Par 68, SSS 67, Course record 64. Club membership 550.
Visitors Mon-Sun & BHs. Booking required Sat, Sun & BHs. Handicap certificate. Dress code. **Societies** Booking required **Green Fees** £20 per round summer, £15 winter (£30/£20 Sat & Sun). 🚶 **Prof** Gareth Bennett
Facilities ⓘ 🍴 🏌 ⚑ 🏌 ⚲ 🏌 🏌 🏌 **Location** NW side of village
Hotel ★★★ 74% HL Best Western Mount Sorrel Hotel, Porthkerry Rd, BARRY ☎ 01446 740069 42 en suite

---

HENSOL   MAP 03 ST07

Vale Hotel Golf & Spa Resort Hensol Park CF72 8JY
☎ 01443 665899 🖥 01443 222220
e-mail: smetson@vale-hotel.com
web: www.vale-hotel.com
Two championship courses set in 200 acres of glorious countryside, with views over Hensol Lake and castle. The Wales National with greens constructed to USGA standard will prove a stern test for even the very best players. The aptly named Lake course has water coming into play on 12 holes. The signature hole, the 12th, has an island green reached via a stone bridge. The club is also home to the Welsh PGA.

Continued

Lake: 18 holes, 6426yds, Par 72, SSS 71.
Wales National: 18 holes, 7414yds, Par 73, SSS 73,
Course record 64. Club membership 1100.
Visitors Mon-Sun & BHs. Booking required. Handicap certificate. Dress code. **Societies** Booking required **Green Fees** Phone. **Prof** Llewellyn, Coombs, Williams **Course Designer** Peter Johnson & Terry Jones **Facilities** ⊕ ⦵ 🝖 ⌷ ⟆ ⟤ ⌑ ⍾⚲ ◇ ✦ 🝖 ✦ **Leisure** hard tennis courts, heated indoor swimming pool, squash, fishing, sauna, solarium, gymnasium, short game area, video analysis. **Conf** facs Corporate Hospitality Days **Location** M4 junct 34, signed
Hotel ★★★★ 79% HL Vale Hotel Golf & Spa Resort, Hensol Park, HENSOL ☎ 01443 667800 29 en suite 114 annexe en suite

PENARTH   MAP 03 ST17

Glamorganshire Lavernock Rd CF64 5UP
☎ 029 2070 1185 🖹 029 2070 1185
e-mail: glamgolf@btconnect.com
web: www.glamorganshiregolfclub.co.uk
Parkland overlooking the Bristol Channel.
18 holes, 6184yds, Par 70, SSS 70, Course record 64.
Club membership 1000.
Visitors Mon, Wed-Fri & Sun. Booking required. Handicap certificate. Dress code. **Societies** Booking required. **Green Fees** not confirmed. **Prof** Andrew Kerr-Smith **Course Designer** James Braid **Facilities** ⊕ ⦵ 🝖 ⌷ 🝖 ⟤ ⟆ ⍾⚲ ◇ ⚲ ◇ **Location** S of town centre on B4267
Hotel ★★★ 74% HL Best Western Mount Sorrel Hotel, Porthkerry Rd, BARRY ☎ 01446 740069 42 en suite

WREXHAM

CHIRK   MAP 07 SJ23

Chirk Golf Club LL14 5AD
☎ 01691 774407 🖹 01691 773878
e-mail: chirkjackbarker@btinternet.com
web: www.jackbarker.com
Overlooked by the National Trust's Chirk Castle, a championship-standard 18-hole course with a 664yd Par 5 at the 9th - one of the longest in Europe. Also a nine-hole course, driving range and golf academy.
18 holes, 7045yds, Par 72, SSS 73, Course record 69.
Club membership 300.
Visitors Mon-Sun & BHs. Booking required. Dress code. **Societies** Booking required. **Green Fees** £14 per round (£16 Fri, £18 Sat & Sun). **Prof** M Maddison **Facilities** ⊕ ⦵ 🝖 ⌷ 🝖 ⟤ ⟆ ⍾⚲ ◇ ⚲ ◇ **Leisure** 9 hole Par 3 course. **Conf** facs **Location** 1m NW of Chirk, near Chirk Castle

EYTON   MAP 07 SJ34

Plassey Oaks Golf Complex LL13 0SP
☎ 01978 780020 🖹 01978 781397
e-mail: ljones@plasseygolf.com
web: www.plasseygolf.com
Picturesque nine-hole course in undulating parkland.
9 holes, 5002yds, Par 68, SSS 66, Course record 62.
Club membership 222.
Visitors Mon-Sun & BHs. Booking required Sat, Sun & BHs. Dress code. **Societies** Booking required **Green Fees** £12 per 18 holes, £10 per 9 holes. **Course Designer** Welsh Golf Union **Facilities** ⊕ ⦵ 🝖 ⌷ ⟆ ⟤ ⍾⚲ ⚲ ◇ ✦ **Leisure** hard and grass tennis courts, fishing. **Conf** Corporate Hospitality Days **Location** 4m S of Wrexham off B5426, signed
Hotel ★★★ 75% HL Best Western Cross Lanes Hotel & Restaurant, Cross Lanes, Bangor Rd, Marchwiel, WREXHAM ☎ 01978 780555 16 en suite

WREXHAM   MAP 07 SJ35

Clays Bryn Estyn Rd, Llan-y-Pwll LL13 9UB
☎ 01978 661406 🖹 01978 661406
e-mail: claysgolf@claysgolf.co.uk
web: www.claysgolf.co.uk
Gently undulating parkland course in countryside with views of the Welsh mountains. Noted for its difficult Par 3s.
18 holes, 6010yds, Par 69, SSS 69, Course record 62.
Club membership 420.
Visitors Mon-Sun & BHs **Societies** Welcome. **Green Fees** £19 per round (£25 Sat & Sun). **Prof** David Larvin **Course Designer** R D Jones **Facilities** ⊕ ⦵ 🝖 ⌷ ⟆ 🝖 ⟤ ⍾⚲ ⚲ ◇ ✦ ⚲ ◇ ✦ **Conf** facs Corporate Hospitality Days **Location** Off A534

Wrexham Holt Rd LL13 9SB
☎ 01978 364268 🖹 01978 362168
e-mail: info@wrexhamgolfclub.co.uk
web: www.wrexhamgolfclub.co.uk
Inland, sandy course with easy walking. Testing dog-leg 7th hole (Par 4), and short 14th hole (Par 3) with full carry to green.
18 holes, 6233yds, Par 70, SSS 70, Course record 64.
Club membership 680.
Visitors Mon-Sun except BHs. Booking required. Handicap certificate. Dress code. **Societies** Booking required. **Green Fees** Phone. ☻ **Prof** Paul Williams **Course Designer** James Braid **Facilities** ⊕ ⦵ 🝖 ⌷ ⟆ 🝖 ⟤ ⍾⚲ ⚲ ◇ **Conf** facs Corporate Hospitality Days **Location** 2m NE on A534

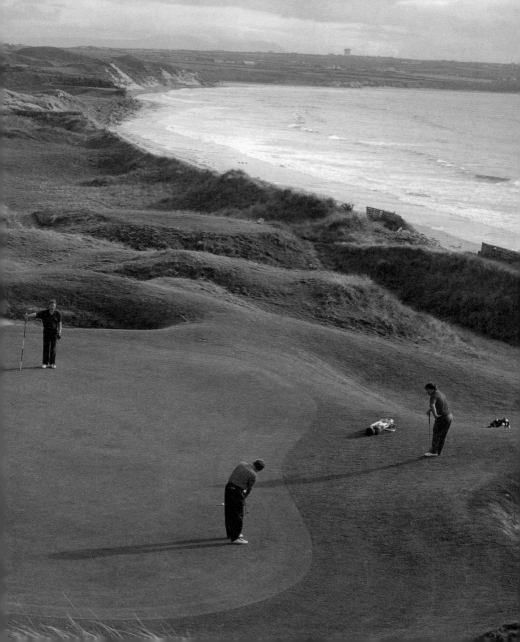

Ireland

NORTHERN IRELAND

CO ANTRIM

ANTRIM MAP 01 D5

Massereene 51 Lough Rd BT41 4DQ
☎ 028 9442 8096 📠 028 9448 7661
e-mail: info@massereene.com
web: www.massereene.com
The first nine holes are parkland, while the second, adjacent to the shore of Lough Neagh, have more of a links character with sandy ground.
18 holes, 6602yds, Par 72, SSS 72, Course record 63. Club membership 1050.
Visitors Mon-Sun & BHs. Booking required. Dress code. **Societies** Booking required. **Green Fees** £22 per round (£30 Sun & Sat). **Prof** Jim Smyth **Course Designer** F Hawtree/H Swan **Facilities** **Conf** facs Corporate Hospitality Days **Location** 1m SW of town
Hotel ★★★★ 69% HL Galgorm Manor, BALLYMENA ☎ 028 2588 1001 24 en suite

BALLYCASTLE MAP 01 D6

Ballycastle Cushendall Rd BT54 6QP
☎ 028 2076 2536 📠 028 2076 9909
e-mail: info@ballycastlegolfclub.com
web: www.ballycastlegolfclub.com
An unusual mixture of terrain beside the sea, lying at the foot of one of the nine glens of Antrim, with magnificent views from all parts. The first five holes are parkland with natural hazards; the middle holes are links type and the rest on adjacent upland. Accurate iron play is essential for good scoring while the undulating greens will test putting skills.
18 holes, 5927mtrs, Par 71, SSS 70, Course record 64. Club membership 825.
Visitors Mon-Sun & BHs. Booking required Sat, Sun & BHs. Dress code. **Societies** Booking required. **Green Fees** £25 per round (£35 Sat, Sun & BHs). **Prof** Ian McLaughlin **Facilities** **Conf** facs Corporate Hospitality Days **Location** Between Portrush & Cushendall (A2)
Hotel ★★★ 74% HL Bayview Hotel, 2 Bayhead Rd, PORTBALLINTRAE ☎ 028 2073 4100 25 en suite

BALLYCLARE MAP 01 D5

Ballyclare 23 Springdale Rd BT39 9JW
☎ 028 9332 2696 📠 028 9332 2696
e-mail: ballyclaregolfclub@supanet
web: www.ballyclaregolfclub.com
18 holes, 5745mtrs, Par 71, SSS 71, Course record 66.
Course Designer T McCauley **Location** 1.5m N of Ballyclare
Telephone for further details
Hotel ★★★★ 69% HL Galgorm Manor, BALLYMENA ☎ 028 2588 1001 24 en suite

Greenacres 153 Ballyrobert Rd BT39 9RT
☎ 028 9335 4111 📠 028 9335 4166
Designed and built into the rolling countryside, and with the addition of lakes at five of the holes, provides a challenge for both the seasoned golfer and the higher-handicapped player.
18 holes, 6031yds, Par 71, SSS 69. Club membership 520.
Visitors Mon-Fri, Sun & BHs. Dress code **Societies** Booking required. **Green Fees** not confirmed. **Facilities** **Conf** facs Corporate Hospitality Days **Location** 12m from Belfast city centre
Hotel ★★★ 72% HL Headfort Arms Hotel, Headfort Place, KELLS ☎ 0818 222800 & 046 9240063 📠 046 9240587 45 en suite

BALLYGALLY MAP 01 D5

Cairndhu 192 Coast Rd BT40 2QG
☎ 028 2858 3954 📠 028 2858 3324
e-mail: cairndhugc@btconnect.com
Built on a hilly headland, this course is both testing and scenic, with wonderful coastal views. The Par 3 second hole can require anything from a 9 to a 3 iron depending on the wind, while the 3rd has a carry of 165 metres over a headland to the fairway. The 10th, 11th and 12th holes constitute Cairndhu's Amen Corner, feared and respected by any standard of golfer.
18 holes, 5611mtrs, Par 70, SSS 69, Course record 64. Club membership 905.
Visitors Mon-Fri , Sun & BHs. Booking required Thu, Fri, Sun & BHs. Handicap certificate. Dress code. **Societies** Booking required **Green Fees** £20 per round (£25 Sun). **Prof** Stephen Hood **Course Designer** Mr Morrison **Facilities** **Conf** facs **Location** 4m N of Larne on coast road
Guesthouse ★★★★ GH Manor Guest House, 23 Older Fleet Rd, Harbour Highway, LARNE ☎ 028 2827 3305 8 en suite

BALLYMENA MAP 01 D5

Ballymena 128 Raceview Rd BT42 4HY
☎ 028 2586 1487 📠 028 2586 1487
18 holes, 5299mtrs, Par 68, SSS 67, Course record 62.
Location 2m E on A42
Telephone for further details
Hotel ★★★★ 69% HL Galgorm Manor, BALLYMENA ☎ 028 2588 1001 24 en suite

Galgorm Castle Golf & Country Club Galgorm Rd BT42 1HL
☎ 028 2564 6161 📠 028 2565 1151
e-mail: golf@galgormcastle.co.uk
web: www.galgormcastle.com
An 18-hole USGA championship course set in 220 acres of mature parkland in the grounds of one of Ireland's most historic castles. The course is bordered by two rivers which come into play and includes five lakes. A course of outstanding beauty offering a challenge to both the novice and low handicapped golfer.

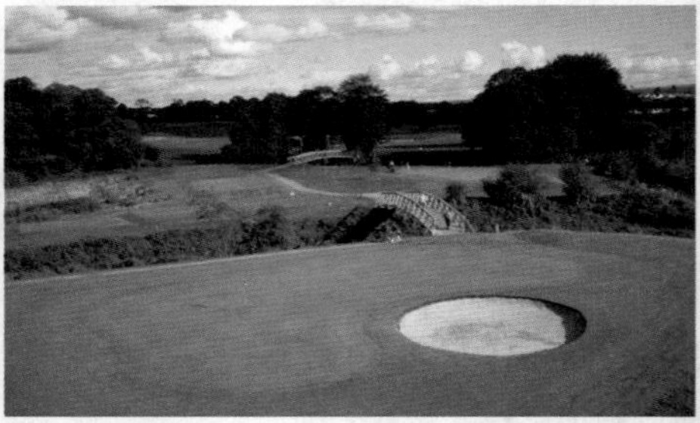

18 holes, 6736yds, Par 72, SSS 72, Course record 67. Club membership 600.

Continued

CHAMPIONSHIP COURSE

CO ANTRIM — PORTRUSH

ROYAL PORTRUSH

Map 01 C6

Dunluce Rd BT56 8JQ
☎ 028 7082 2311 📠 028 7082 3139
e-mail: info@royalportrushgolfclub.com
web: www.royalportrushgolfclub.com
Dunluce: 18 holes, 6641yds, Par 72, SSS 73.
Valley: 18 holes, 6054yds, Par 70, SSS 72.
Club membership 1300.
Visitors Mon-Sun & BHs. Handicap certificate.
Dress code. **Societies** Booking required.
Green Fees Dunluce: £105 per round,
£120 weekends. Valley: £35 per round, £40
weekends. **Prof** Gary McNeill
Course Designer Harry Colt **Facilities** ⑪ ⑩
⮕ ▯ ▤ ⊼ ☕ ⚑ ✀ ⚐ **Location** 0.8km from
Portrush on Bushmills road

This course, designed by Harry S Colt, is considered to be among the best six in the UK. Founded in 1888, it was the venue of the first professional golf event in Ireland, held in 1895, when Sandy Herd beat Harry Vardon in the final. Royal Portrush is spectacular and breathtaking, one of the tightest driving courses known to golfers. On a clear day there's a fine view of Islay and the Paps of Jura from the 3rd tee, and the Giant's Causeway from the 5th. While the greens have to be 'read' from the start, there are fairways up and down valleys, and holes called Calamity Corner and Purgatory (for good reason). The 2nd hole, Giant's Grave, is 509yds, but the 17th is even longer.

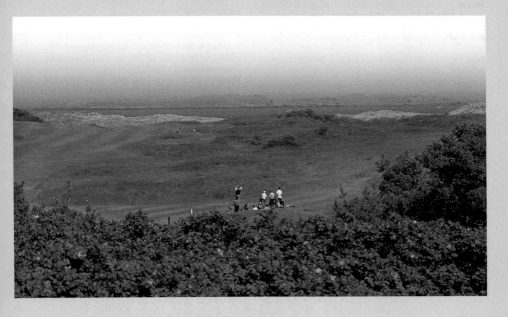

Visitors Mon–Sun & BHs. Booking required. Dress code. **Societies** Booking required. **Green Fees** £32 per round (£40 Sat & Sun). **Prof** Phil Collins **Course Designer** Simon Gidman **Facilities** ⑪ ⑩ 🄻 ♨ ☷ 🕇 🍴 ✆ 🖻 ✆ 🕇 **Leisure** fishing, PGA staffed Academy. **Conf** facs Corporate Hospitality Days **Location** 1m S of Ballymena on A42
Hotel ★★★★ 69% HL Galgorm Manor, BALLYMENA ☎ 028 2588 1001 24 en suite

---

BALLYMONEY   MAP 01 D6

Gracehill 141 Ballinlea Rd, Stranocum BT53 8PX
☎ 028 2075 1209 📄 028 2075 1074
e-mail: info@gracehillgolfclub.co.uk
web: www.gracehillgolfclub.co.uk
Challenging parkland course with some holes played over water and many mature trees coming into play.
18 holes, 6553yds, Par 72, SSS 73, Course record 69.
Club membership 400.
Visitors Mon–Sun & BHs. Booking required. Dress code. **Societies** Booking required. **Green Fees** £25 per round (£30 Sat & Sun). **Course Designer** Frank Ainsworth **Facilities** ⑪ ⑩ 🄻 ♨ 🕇 🍴 ☷ ✆ ✆ 🕇 **Conf** Corporate Hospitality Days **Location** M2 N from Belfast, onto A26 N to Ballymoney, signs for Coleraine. At Ballymoney bypass onto B147/A2 to Sranocum/Ballintoy
Hotel ★★ 76% HL Brown Trout Golf & Country Inn, 209 Agivey Rd, AGHADOWEY ☎ 028 7086 8209 15 en suite

---

CARRICKFERGUS   MAP 01 D5

Carrickfergus 35 North Rd BT38 8LP
☎ 028 9336 3713 📄 028 9336 3023
e-mail: carrickfergusgc@btconnect.com
Parkland course, fairly level but nevertheless demanding, with a notorious water hazard at the 1st. Well-maintained, with an interesting in-course riverway and fine views across Belfast Lough.
18 holes, 5768yds, Par 68, SSS 68. Club membership 850.
Visitors Mon–Fri, Sun & BHs. Booking required. Handicap certificate. Dress code. **Societies** Booking required. **Green Fees** £19 per day, £12 per round (£25/£15 Sat, Sun & BHs). **Prof** Gary Mercer **Facilities** ⑪ ⑩ 🄻 ☷ 🕇 🍴 ♨ 🖻 ✆ **Conf** facs Corporate Hospitality Days **Location** 9m NE of Belfast on A2
Hotel ★★ 68% HL Dobbins Inn Hotel, 6-8 High St, CARRICKFERGUS ☎ 028 9335 1905 15 en suite

Greenisland 156 Upper Rd, Greenisland BT38 8RW
☎ 028 9086 2236
A parkland course nestling at the foot of Knockagh Hill, with scenic views over Belfast Lough.
9 holes, 6045yds, Par 71, SSS 69. Club membership 660.
Visitors Mon–Sun & BHs. **Societies** Welcome. **Green Fees** £12 (£18 Sat & Sun). ◉ **Facilities** ⑪ ⑩ 🄻 ☷ 🕇 🍴 ♨ **Location** N of Belfast, close to Carrickfergus
Hotel ★★ 68% HL Dobbins Inn Hotel, 6-8 High St, CARRICKFERGUS ☎ 028 9335 1905 15 en suite

---

CUSHENDALL   MAP 01 D6

Cushendall 21 Shore Rd BT44 0NG
☎ 028 2177 1318
e-mail: cushendallgc@btconnect.com
Scenic course with spectacular views over the Sea of Moyle and Red Bay to the Mull of Kintyre. The River Dall winds through the course, coming into play in seven of the nine holes. This demands a premium on accuracy rather than length. The signature hole is the Par 3 2nd, requiring a tee shot across the river to a plateau green with a steep slope in front and out of bounds behind.
9 holes, 4386mtrs, Par 66, SSS 63, Course record 59.
Club membership 824.
Visitors Mon–Wed, Fri & BHs. Booking required Thu. Dress code. **Societies** Booking required. **Green Fees** £13 per day (£18 BHs). ◉ **Course Designer** D Delargy **Facilities** 🄻 ☷ 🕇 🍴 ♨ ✆ **Location** In Cushendall beside beach on Antrim coast road
Guesthouse (AA Appointed) The Villa Farm House, 185 Torr Rd, CUSHENDUN ☎ 028 2176 1252 3 en suite

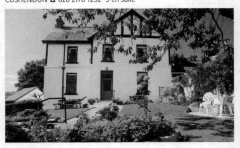

LARNE   MAP 01 D5

Larne 54 Ferris Bay Rd, Islandmagee BT40 3RT
☎ 028 9338 2228 📄 028 9338 2088
e-mail: info@larnegolfclub.co.uk
web: www.larnegolfclub.co.uk
An exposed part links, part heathland course offering a good test, particularly on the last three holes along the sea shore.
9 holes, 6686yds, Par 70, SSS 70, Course record 64.
Club membership 430.
Visitors Contact club for details. **Societies** welcome. **Green Fees** not confirmed. ◉ **Course Designer** G L Bailie **Facilities** ⑪ ⑩ 🄻 ☷ 🕇 🍴 ♨ **Location** 6m N of Whitehead on Browns Bay road

---

LISBURN   MAP 01 D5

Aberdelghy Bell's Ln, Lambeg BT27 4QH
☎ 028 9266 2738 📄 028 926 03432
e-mail: info@mmsportsgolf.com
web: www.mmsportsgolf.com
18 holes, 4139mtrs, Par 66, SSS 62, Course record 64.
Course Designer Alec Blair **Location** 1.5m N of Lisburn off A1
Telephone for further details
Hotel ★★★ 75% HL Malone Lodge Hotel, 60 Eglantine Av, BELFAST ☎ 028 9038 8000 51 en suite

Lisburn 68 Eglantine Rd BT27 5RQ
☎ 028 9267 7216 📠 028 9260 3608
e-mail: lisburngolfclub@aol.com
web: www.lisburngolfclub.com
18 holes, 6647yds, Par 72, SSS 72, Course record 67.
Course Designer Hawtree **Location** 2m from town on A1
Telephone for further details
Hotel ★★★ 75% HL Malone Lodge Hotel, 60 Eglantine Av, BELFAST
☎ 028 9038 8000 51 en suite

MAZE   **MAP 01 D5**

Down Royal Park Dunygarton Rd BT27 5RT
☎ 028 9262 1339 📠 028 9262 1339
18 holes, 6824yds, Par 72, SSS 72, Course record 69.
Valley Course: 9 holes, 2019, Par 33.
Location Inside Down Royal Race Course
Telephone for further details
Hotel ★★★ 75% HL Malone Lodge Hotel, 60 Eglantine Av, BELFAST
☎ 028 9038 8000 51 en suite

PORTBALLINTRAE   **MAP 01 C6**

Bushfoot 50 Bushfoot Rd, Portballintrae BT57 8RR
☎ 028 2073 1317 📠 028 2073 1852
e-mail: bushfootgolfclub@btconnect.com
A seaside links course with superb views in an area of outstanding beauty. A challenging Par 3 7th is ringed by bunkers with out of bounds beyond, while the 3rd has a blind approach. Also a putting green and pitch and putt course.
9 holes, 6075yds, Par 70, SSS 68, Course record 68.
Club membership 850.
Visitors Mon, Wed-Fri, Sun & BHs. Booking required. **Societies** Booking required. **Green Fees** £16 per round (£20 Sat, Sun & BHs). **Facilities** ⊕ ◎ ⬙ ♨ ♫ ⚐ ⚲ **Location** Off Ballaghmore road
Hotel ★★★ 74% HL Bayview Hotel, 2 Bayhead Rd, PORTBALLINTRAE
☎ 028 2073 4100 25 en suite

PORTRUSH   **MAP 01 C6**

Royal Portrush see page 409
Hotel ★★★ 74% HL Bayview Hotel, 2 Bayhead Rd, PORTBALLINTRAE
☎ 028 2073 4100 25 en suite

WHITEHEAD   **MAP 01 D5**

Bentra Slaughterford Rd BT38 9TG
☎ 028 9337 8996

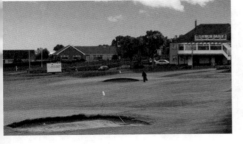

9 holes, 5952yds, Par 37, SSS 35.
Location 6m from Carrickfergus
Telephone for further details
Hotel ★★ 68% HL Dobbins Inn Hotel, 6-8 High St, CARRICKFERGUS
☎ 028 9335 1905 15 en suite

Whitehead McCrae's Brae BT38 9NZ
☎ 028 9337 0820 & 9337 0822 📠 028 9337 0825
e-mail: robin@whiteheadgc.fsnet.co.uk
web: www.whiteheadgolfclub.com
Undulating parkland course with magnificent sea views.
18 holes, 5952yds, Par 70, SSS 69, Course record 65.
Club membership 962.
Visitors Mon, Sat, Sun & BHs. Booking required Thu & Sun. Dress code.
Societies Booking required. **Green Fees** £18 per round (£22 Sun & BHs).
Prof Colin Farr **Course Designer** A B Armstrong **Facilities** ⊕ ◎ ⬙ ⬚ ♫ ♨ ⚐ ⚲ **Conf** Corporate Hospitality Days **Location** 1m from town
Hotel ★★ 68% HL Dobbins Inn Hotel, 6-8 High St, CARRICKFERGUS
☎ 028 9335 1905 15 en suite

CO ARMAGH

ARMAGH   **MAP 01 C5**

County Armagh The Demesne, Newry Rd BT60 1EN
☎ 028 3752 5861 & 3752 8768 📠 028 3752 5861
e-mail: june@golfarmagh.co.uk
web: www.golfarmagh.co.uk
Mature parkland course with excellent views of Armagh city and its surroundings.
18 holes, 6212yds, Par 70, SSS 69, Course record 63.
Club membership 1300.
Visitors Mon, Tue, Thu, Sat, Sun & BHs. Handicap certificate. Dress code. **Societies** Booking required. **Green Fees** not confirmed. **Prof** Alan Rankin **Facilities** ⊕ ◎ ⬙ ⬚ ♫ ♨ ⚐ ⚲ ⚑ **Leisure** snooker. **Conf** Corporate Hospitality Days **Location** On Newry Rd
Hotel ★★ 68% HL The Cohannon Inn & Autolodge, 212 Ballynakilly Rd, DUNGANNON ☎ 028 8772 4488 42 en suite

---

CULLYHANNA   **MAP 01 C5**

Ashfield 44 Cregganduff Rd BT35 0JJ
☎ 028 3086 8611
18 holes, 5840yds, Par 69.
Course Designer Frank Ainsworth
Telephone for further details
Hotel ★★ 69% HL Enniskeen House Hotel, 98 Bryansford Rd, NEWCASTLE
☎ 028 4372 2392 12 en suite

LURGAN   **MAP 01 D5**

Craigavon Golf & Ski Centre Turmoyra Ln, Silverwood BT66 6NG
☎ 028 3832 6606 📠 028 3834 7272
e-mail: michael.stanford@craigavon.gov.uk
web: www.craigavon.gov.uk
Parkland course with a lake and stream providing water hazards.
Silverwood: 18 holes, 6496yds, Par 72, SSS 72.
Club membership 400.

Continued

Visitors Mon-Sun & BHs. Booking required. Dress code. **Societies** Booking required **Green Fees** £16.50 per round (£18.50 Sat, Sun & BHs). **Prof** Michael Stanford **Facilities** ⑪ ☷ ᇰ ʳ⁺ ✔ ♔ **Leisure** Ski slope. **Conf** facs **Location** 2m N at Silverwood off M1

Lurgan The Demesne BT67 9BN
☎ 028 3832 2087 🖹 028 3831 6166
e-mail: lurgangolfclub@btconnect.com
web: www.lurgangolfclub.co.uk
Testing parkland course bordering Lurgan Park Lake with a need for accurate shots. Drains well in wet weather and suits a long straight hitter.
18 holes, 6257yds, Par 70, SSS 70, Course record 66.
Club membership 903.
Visitors Mon-Tue, Thu-Fri, Sun & BHs. Booking required. Dress code.
Societies Booking required. **Green Fees** not confirmed. ⊛ **Prof** Des Paul
Course Designer A Pennink **Facilities** ⑪ ⑨ ᇰ ☷ ᇰ ᐠ ᇰ ✔ **Conf** facs Corporate Hospitality Days **Location** 0.5m from town centre near Lurgan Park

PORTADOWN — MAP 01 D5

Portadown 192 Gilford Rd BT63 5LF
☎ 028 3835 5356 🖹 028 3839 1394
e-mail: portadown.gc@btconnect.com
web: www.portadowngolfclub.co.uk
Well-wooded parkland on the banks of the River Bann, which is one of the water hazards.
18 holes, 6130yds, Par 70, SSS 69, Course record 65.
Club membership 800.
Visitors Mon-Sun & BHs. Booking required. Dress code. **Societies** Booking required. **Green Fees** not confirmed. ⊛ **Prof** Paul Stevenson **Facilities** ⑪
⑨ ᇰ ☷ ᐠ ᇰ ᐠ ✔ **Leisure** squash. **Conf** facs Corporate Hospitality Days **Location** SE via A59
Hotel ★★ 68% HL The Cohannon Inn & Autolodge, 212 Ballynakilly Rd, DUNGANNON ☎ 028 8772 4488 42 en suite

TANDRAGEE — MAP 01 D5

Tandragee Markethill Rd BT62 2ER
☎ 028 3884 1272 🖹 028 3884 0664
e-mail: office@tandragee.co.uk
web: www.tandragee.co.uk
Pleasant parkland course, the signature hole is the demanding Par 3 16th known as 'The Quarry Hole'; the real strength of Tandragee is in the short holes. Pleasant views with the Mourne mountains in the distance.
18 holes, 5747mtrs, Par 71, SSS 70, Course record 65.
Club membership 1018.
Visitors Mon-Fri, Sun & BHs. Booking required. Dress code. **Societies** Booking required. **Green Fees** £16 per round (£21 Sat & Sun). ⊛ **Prof** Dympna Keenan **Course Designer** John Stone **Facilities** ⑪ ⑨ ᇰ ☷ ᐠ ᐠ ᇰ ᐠ ✔ **Leisure** snooker. **Conf** facs Corporate Hospitality Days **Location** On B3 from Tandragee towards Markethill

BELFAST — MAP 01 D5
See also The Royal Belfast, Holywood, Co Down.

Balmoral 518 Lisburn Rd BT9 6GX
☎ 028 9038 1514 🖹 028 9066 6759
e-mail: enquiries@balmoralgolf.com
web: www.balmoralgolf.com
18 holes, 6276yds, Par 69, SSS 70, Course record 64.
Location 2m S next to Kings Hall
Telephone for further details
Hotel ★★★ 75% HL Malone Lodge Hotel, 60 Eglantine Av, BELFAST
☎ 028 9038 8000 51 en suite

Cliftonville 44 Westland Rd BT14 6NH
☎ 028 9074 4158 & 9022 8585
web: www.cliftonvillegolfclub.com
9 holes, 6242yds, Par 70, SSS 70, Course record 65.
Location Between Cavehill Rd & Cliftonville Circus
Telephone for further details
Hotel ★★★ 71% HL Jurys Inn Belfast, Fisherwick Place, Great Victoria St, BELFAST ☎ 028 9053 3500 190 en suite

Dunmurry 91 Dunmurry Ln, Dunmurry BT17 9JS
☎ 028 9061 0834 🖹 028 9060 2540
e-mail: dunmurrygc@hotmail.com
web: www.dunmurrygolfclub.co.uk
Maturing very nicely, this tricky parkland course has several memorable holes which call for skilful shots.
18 holes, 6156yds, Par 70, SSS 69, Course record 65.
Club membership 1100.
Visitors Mon-Fri, Sun & BHs. Booking required Fri, Sun & BHs. Dress code.
Societies Booking required **Green Fees** £27 per round (£37 Sat, Sun & BHs). ⊛ **Prof** John Dolan **Facilities** ⑪ ⑨ ᇰ ☷ ᐠ ᇰ ᐠ ✔
Hotel ★★★ 75% HL Malone Lodge Hotel, 60 Eglantine Av, BELFAST
☎ 028 9038 8000 51 en suite

Fortwilliam Downview Ave BT15 4EZ
☎ 028 9037 0770 (Office) & 9077 0980 (Pro)
🖹 028 9078 1891
e-mail: admin@fortwilliam.co.uk
web: www.fortwilliam.co.uk
Parkland course in most attractive surroundings. The course is bisected by a lane.
18 holes, 5514mtrs, Par 70, SSS 68, Course record 65.
Club membership 1000.
Visitors Mon-Fri, Sun & BHs. Booking required. Handicap certificate. Dress code. **Societies** Booking required. **Green Fees** £22 per round (£29 Sun).
Prof Peter Hanna **Facilities** ⑪ ⑨ ᇰ ☷ ᐠ ᐠ ᇰ ᐠ ✔ ☋ ✔ ♔ **Conf** facs Corporate Hospitality Days **Location** Off Antrim road
Hotel ★★★ 71% HL Jurys Inn Belfast, Fisherwick Place, Great Victoria St, BELFAST ☎ 028 9053 3500 190 en suite

Malone 240 Upper Malone Rd, Dunmurry BT17 9LB
☎ 028 9061 2758 (Office) & 9061 4917 (Pro)
📠 028 9043 1394
e-mail: manager@malonegolfclub.co.uk
web: www.malonegolfclub.co.uk
Two parkland courses, extremely attractive with a large lake, mature trees and flowering shrubs and bordered by the River Lagan. Very well maintained and offering a challenging round.

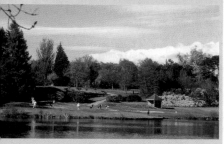

Main Course: 18 holes, 6706yds, Par 71, SSS 72, Course record 65.
Edenderry: 9 holes, 6320yds, Par 72, SSS 70.
Club membership 1450.
Visitors Mon, Thu-Fri, Sun & BHs. Wed am only. Booking required. Dress code. **Societies** Booking required. **Green Fees** Main Course: £65 per day, Edenderry: £20 per day (£75/£25 Sat & Sun). **Prof** Michael McGee **Course Designer** C K Cotton **Facilities** ⑪🍴🍺🏌🍹🛒🏊🏺⛳🏌 **Leisure** fishing, Outdoor bowling green. **Conf** Corporate Hospitality Days **Location** 4.5m S opposite Lady Dixon Park
Hotel ★★★ 75% HL Malone Lodge Hotel, 60 Eglantine Av, BELFAST ☎ 028 9038 8000 51 en suite

Mount Ober Golf & Country Club 24 Ballymaconaghy Rd BT8 6SB
☎ 028 9040 1811 & 9079 5666 📠 028 9070 5862
web: www.mountober.com
Inland parkland course which is a great test of golf for all handicaps.
18 holes, 5022yds, Par 67, SSS 66, Course record 67.
Club membership 400.
Visitors Mon-Fri, Sun & BHs. Contact club for details. Dress code. **Societies** Booking required. **Green Fees** £16.50 per round (£18.50 Sun & BHs). **Prof** Wesley Ramsay **Facilities** ⑪🍴🍺🏌🍹🛒🏺⛳🏌 **Leisure** American billiards & snooker. **Conf** facs Corporate Hospitality Days **Location** Off Saintfield Rd
Hotel ★★★ 75% HL The Crescent Townhouse, 13 Lower Crescent, BELFAST ☎ 028 9032 3349 17 en suite

Ormeau 50 Park Rd BT7 2FX
☎ 028 9064 0700 📠 028 9064 6250
e-mail: ormeau.golfclub@virgin.net
Nine hole parkland course which provides a challenge for low and high handicap golfers, good shots being rewarded and those that play offline receiving due punishment. The long Par 4 5th hole has intimidating out of bounds on the right and a narrow sloping green, well protected by trees and bunkers. Two long Par 3 holes each demand an accurate drive and when playing the 3rd and 12th holes, visitors are advised to look for the Fairy Tree which graces the middle of the fairway. Club folklore states that if a golfer hits this tree he should apologise to the fairies or his game will suffer!

9 holes, 2688yds, Par 68, SSS 66. Club membership 520.
Visitors Mon, Wed-Fri, Sun & BHs. Booking required Fri, Sun & BHs. Dress code. **Societies** Booking required. **Green Fees** not confirmed. 🏌 **Prof** Mr Stephen Rourke **Facilities** ⑪🍴🍺🏌🍹🛒🏊🏺⛳🏌 **Location** S of city centre between Ravenhill & Ormeau roads
Hotel ★★★ 75% HL The Crescent Townhouse, 13 Lower Crescent, BELFAST ☎ 028 9032 3349 17 en suite

Shandon Park 73 Shandon Park BT5 6NY
☎ 028 90805030
e-mail: shandonpark@btconnect.com
Fairly level parkland offering a pleasant challenge.
18 holes, 6261yds, Par 70, SSS 70. Club membership 1100.
Visitors Mon-Fri & BHs. Booking required. Dress code. **Societies** Booking required. **Green Fees** £27.50 per round (£35 Sat & Sun). **Prof** Barry Wilson **Facilities** ⑪🍴🍺🏌🍹🛒🏊🏺⛳🍴🏌 **Conf** facs Corporate Hospitality Days **Location** Off Knock road
Hotel ★★★ 75% HL The Crescent Townhouse, 13 Lower Crescent, BELFAST ☎ 028 9032 3349 17 en suite

DUNDONALD   MAP 01 D5

Knock Summerfield BT16 2QX
☎ 028 9048 3251 📠 028 9048 7277
18 holes, 6435yds, Par 70, SSS 71, Course record 66.
Course Designer Colt, Allison & McKenzie **Location** 5m E of Belfast
Telephone for further details
Hotel ★★★ 87% HL The Old Inn, 15 Main St, CRAWFORDSBURN ☎ 028 9185 3255 29 en suite 1 annexe en suite

NEWTOWNBREDA   MAP 01 D5

The Belvoir Park 73 Church Rd BT8 7AN
☎ 028 9049 1693 📠 028 9064 6113
web: www.belvoirparkgolfclub.com
This undulating parkland course is not strenuous to walk, but is certainly a test of your golf, with tree-lined fairways and a particularly challenging finish at the final four holes.
18 holes, 6516yds, Par 71, SSS 71, Course record 65.
Club membership 1000.
Visitors Mon, Tue & Thu. Booking required. Dress code. **Societies** Booking required. **Green Fees** £45 (£55 Sat, Sun & BHs). **Prof** Michael McGivern **Course Designer** H. S. Holt **Facilities** ⑪🍴🍺🏌🍹🛒🏊🏺 🏌🍴⛳ **Location** 2m from city centre off Saintfield-Newcastle road
Hotel ★★★★ 74% HL Clandeboye Lodge Hotel, 10 Estate Rd, Clandeboye, BANGOR ☎ 028 9185 2500 43 en suite

CO DOWN

ARDGLASS   MAP 01 D5

Ardglass Castle Place BT30 7TP
☎ 028 4484 1219 📠 028 4484 1841
e-mail: info@ardglassgolfclub.com
web: www.ardglassgolfclub.com
A scenic clifftop seaside course with championship standard greens. The first five holes, with the Irish Sea and cliffs tight to the left, should be treated with respect as anything resembling a hook will meet with disaster. The 2nd hole is a daunting Par 3. The tee shot must carry a cliff and canyon - meanwhile the superb views of the Mountains of Mourne should not be missed.

Continued

Ireland

18 holes, 6268yds, Par 70, SSS 69, Course record 65.
Club membership 900.
Visitors Mon-Sun & BHs. Booking required **Societies** Booking
required **Green Fees** £37 per round (£51 Sat & Sun). **Prof** Philip Farrell
Course Designer David Jones **Facilities** ⑨ ⑩ ⓵ ⓵ ⓵ ⓵ ⓵ ⓵ ⓵
Conf facs **Location** 7m from Downpatrick on the B1
Hotel ★★ 69% HL Enniskeen House Hotel, 98 Bryansford Rd, NEWCASTLE
☎ 028 4372 2392 12 en suite

BALLYNAHINCH MAP 01 D5

Spa 20 Grove Rd BT24 8PN
☎ 028 9756 2365 📄 028 9756 4158
e-mail: spagolfclub@btconnect.com
web: www.spagolfclub.net
Parkland course with tree-lined fairways and scenic views of the
Mourne Mountains. A long and demanding course and feature holes
include the Par 3 2nd and 405yd Par 4 11th.

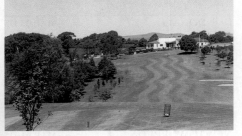

18 holes, 6003mtrs, Par 72, SSS 72, Course record 65.
Club membership 888.
Visitors Mon-Fri, Sun & BHs. Booking required Sun. Dress code.
Societies Booking required. **Green Fees** £20 per round (£25 Sun & BHs).
Course Designer F Ainsworth **Facilities** ⑨ ⑩ ⓵ ⓵ ⓵ ⓵ ⓵ ⓵ ⓵
Leisure gymnasium, outdoor bowls. **Conf** facs Corporate Hospitality Days
Location 1m S
Hotel ★★ 69% HL Enniskeen House Hotel, 98 Bryansford Rd, NEWCASTLE
☎ 028 4372 2392 12 en suite

BANBRIDGE MAP 01 D5

Banbridge 116 Huntly Rd BT32 3UR
☎ 028 4066 2211 📄 028 4066 9400
e-mail: banbridgegolf@btconnect.com
web: www.banbridge-golf.freeserve.co.uk
A mature parkland course with excellent views of the Mourne
mountains. The holes are not long, but are tricky. Signature holes are
the 6th with its menacing pond and the Par 3 10th where playing for a
safe 4 is usually the best option.
18 holes, 5003mtrs, Par 69, SSS 67, Course record 61.
Club membership 800.
Visitors Mon-Fri, Sun & BHs. Dress code. **Societies** Welcome. **Green Fees**
£17 (£22 Sun). ⑨ **Prof** Jason Greenaway **Course Designer** F Ainsworth
Facilities ⑨ ⑩ ⓵ ⓵ ⓵ ⓵ ⓵ ⓵ ⓵ **Location** 0.5m along Huntly Rd

BANGOR MAP 01 D5

Bangor Broadway BT20 4RH
☎ 028 9127 0922 📄 028 9145 3394
e-mail: bangorgolfclubni@btinternet.com
web: www.bangorgolfclubni.co.uk
Undulating parkland course in the town. It is well maintained and
pleasant and offers a challenging round, particularly at the 5th. Scenic
views to Scotland on a clear day.
18 holes, 6410yds, Par 71, SSS 71, Course record 62.
Club membership 1122.
Visitors Mon, Wed-Fri & Sun & BHs. Booking required. Dress code.
Societies Booking required. **Green Fees** Phone. ⑨ **Prof** Michael Bannon
Course Designer James Braid **Facilities** ⑨ ⑩ ⓵ ⓵ ⓵ ⓵ ⓵ ⓵ ⓵
Conf Corporate Hospitality Days **Location** 1m from town centre, 300yds
off Donaghadee Rd
Hotel ★★★ 68% HL Royal Hotel, Seafront, BANGOR ☎ 028 9127 1866
50 en suite

Blackwood Golf Centre 150 Crawfordsburn Rd,
Clandeboye BT19 1GB
☎ 028 9185 2706 📄 028 9185 3785
web: www.blackwoodgolfcentre.com
The golf centre is a pay and play development with a computerised
booking system for the 18-hole championship-standard Hamilton
Course. The course is built on mature woodland with man-made lakes
that come into play on five holes. The Temple course is an 18-hole
Par 3 course with holes ranging from the 75yd 1st to the 185yd 10th,
which has a lake on the right of the green. Banked by gorse with
streams crossing throughout, this Par 3 course is no pushover.
Hamilton Course: 18 holes, 6392yds, Par 71, SSS 70,
Course record 62.
Temple Course: 18 holes, 2492yds, Par 54.
Visitors Mon-Sun & BHs. Booking required Sat, Sun & BHs. Dress code.
Societies Booking required. **Green Fees** Phone. **Prof** Debbie Hanna
Course Designer Simon Gidman **Facilities** ⑨ ⑩ ⓵ ⓵ ⓵ ⓵ ⓵ ⓵ ⓵
Location 2m from Bangor off A2 to Belfast
Hotel ★★★★ 74% HL Clandeboye Lodge Hotel, 10 Estate Rd,
Clandeboye, BANGOR ☎ 028 9185 2500 43 en suite

Carnalea Station Rd BT19 1EZ
☎ 028 9127 0368 📄 028 9127 3989
A scenic course on the shores of Belfast Lough.
18 holes, 5647yds, Par 69, SSS 67, Course record 63.
Club membership 1354.
Visitors Mon-Fri, Sun except BHs. Dress code. **Societies** booking required.
Green Fees not confirmed. ⑨ **Prof** Tom Loughran **Facilities** ⑨ ⑩ ⓵ ⓵
⓵ ⓵ ⓵ ⓵ ⓵ **Location** 2m W next to railway station
Hotel ★★★ 87% HL The Old Inn, 15 Main St, CRAWFORDSBURN
☎ 028 9185 3255 29 en suite 1 annexe en suite

Clandeboye Tower Rd, Conlig, Newtownards BT23 3PN
☎ 028 9127 1767 📄 028 9147 3711
e-mail: cgc-ni@btconnect.com
web: www.cgc-ni.com
Dufferin Course: 18 holes, 6559yds, Par 71, SSS 71.
Ava Course: 18 holes, 5755yds, Par 70, SSS 68.
Course Designer Von Limburger/Allis/Thomas **Location** 2m S on A1
between Bangor & Newtownards
Telephone for further details
Hotel ★★★ 68% HL Royal Hotel, Seafront, BANGOR ☎ 028 9127 1866
50 en suite

Ireland

CHAMPIONSHIP COURSE

CO DOWN — NEWCASTLE

ROYAL COUNTY DOWN

Map 01 D5

36 Golf Links Rd BT33 0AN
☎ **028 43723314** 📄 **028 43726281**
e-mail: **golf@royalcountydown.org**
web: **www.royalcountydown.org**
Championship Course: 18 holes, 7181yds,
Par 71, SSS 74, Course record 66.
Annesley: 18 holes, 4681yds, Par 66, SSS 63.
Club membership 450.
Visitors Mon, Tue, Thu, Fri, Sun & BHs. Booking
required. Dress code. **Societies** Booking
required. **Green Fees** Championship Course:
£135 weekdays, £120 afternoon (£150 Sun).
Prof Kevan Whitson **Course Designer** Tom
Morris **Facilities** ⑨ by prior arrangement 🍴 ☕
🎽 ⚲ 📦 ⛳ ⚔ **Location** N of town centre off
A24

The Championship Course is consistently rated among the world's top ten courses. Laid out beneath the imperious Mourne Mountains, the course has a magnificent setting as it stretches out along the shores of Dundrum Bay. As well as being one of the most-beautiful courses, it is also one of the most challenging, with great swathes of heather and gorse lining fairways that tumble beneath vast sand hills, and wild tussock-faced bunkers defending small, subtly contoured greens. The Annesley Links offers a less formidable yet extremely characterful game, played against the same incomparable backdrop. Recently substantially revised under the direction of Donald Steel, the course begins quite benignly before charging headlong into the dunes. Several charming and one or two teasing holes have been carved out amid the gorse, heather and bracken.

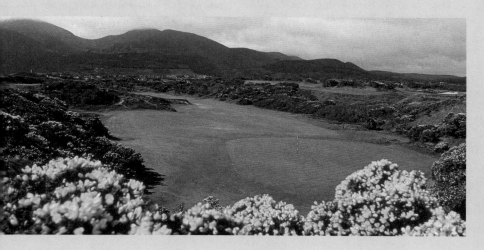

Helen's Bay Golf Rd, Helen's Bay BT19 1TL
☎ 028 9185 2815 & 9185 2601 📠 028 9185 2660
e-mail: mail@helensbaygc.com
web: www.helensbaygc.com
A parkland course on the shores of Belfast Lough with panoramic
views along the Antrim coast. The 4th hole Par 3 is particularly
challenging as the green is screened by high trees.
9 holes, 5644yds, Par 68, SSS 67, Course record 67.
Club membership 750.
Visitors Mon, Wed-Fri, Sun & BHs. Booking required. Dress code.
Societies Booking required. **Green Fees** £19 per 18 holes (£22 Fri-Sun &
BHs). ⊕ **Facilities** ⑪ ⫶⦿⟊ ⊾ ⌴ ⟊ ⌳ ⟊ ✿ ⟊ **Conf** facs **Location** A2
from Belfast
Hotel ★★★ 87% HL The Old Inn, 15 Main St, CRAWFORDSBURN
☎ 028 9185 3255 29 en suite 1 annexe en suite

CARRYDUFF   MAP 01 D5

Rockmount 28 Drumalig Rd, Carryduff BT8 8EQ
☎ 028 9081 2279 📠 020 9081 5851
e-mail: rockmountgc@btconnect.com
web: www.rockmountgolfclub.co.uk
A cleverly designed course incorporating natural features with water
coming into play as streams with a lake at the 11th and 14th.
18 holes, 6373yds, Par 71, SSS 71, Course record 68.
Club membership 750.
Visitors Mon, Tue, Thu, Fri, Sun & BHs. Wed am only. Dress code. **Societies**
Booking required **Green Fees** £24 per round (£28 Sun). **Course Designer**
Robert Patterson **Facilities** ⑪ ⫶⦿⟊ ⊾ ⌴ ⟊ ⊾ ✿ ⟊ ✿ **Conf** facs
Corporate Hospitality Days **Location** 10m S of Belfast

CLOUGHEY   MAP 01 D5

Kirkistown Castle 142 Main Rd, Cloughey BT22 1JA
☎ 028 4277 1233 📠 028 4277 1699
e-mail: kirkistown@supanet.com
web: www.linksgolfkirkistown.com
A seaside part-links, designed by James Braid, popular with visiting
golfers because of its quiet location. The course is exceptionally dry
and remains open when others in the area have to close. The short
but treacherous Par 4 15th hole was known as Braid's Hole. The 2nd
and 10th holes are long Par 4s with elevated greens, which are a
feature of the course. The 10th is particularly distinctive with a long
drive and a slight dog-leg to a raised green with a gorse covered motte
waiting for the wayward approach shot. It has the reputation of being
one of the hardest Par 4s in Ireland.
18 holes, 6167yds, Par 69, SSS 70, Course record 65.
Club membership 1012.
Visitors Mon-Sun & BHs. Booking required Sat, Sun & BHs. Handicap
certificate. Dress code. **Societies** Booking required **Green Fees** £25 per
day (£30 Sat & Sun). ⊕ **Prof** Andrew Ferguson **Course Designer** James
Braid **Facilities** ⑪ ⫶⦿⟊ ⊾ ⌴ ⟊ ⊾ ✿ ⟊ ✿ **Leisure** snooker room. **Conf**
Corporate Hospitality Days **Location** 16m from Newtownards on A2
Hotel ★★★ 87% HL The Old Inn, 15 Main St, CRAWFORDSBURN
☎ 028 9185 3255 29 en suite 1 annexe en suite

COMBER   MAP 01 D5

Mahee Island 14 Mahee Island, Comber BT23 6EP
☎ 028 9754 1234
e-mail: mahee_gents@hotmail.com
An undulating parkland course, almost surrounded by water, with
magnificent views of Strangford Lough and its islands, with Scrabo
Tower in the background. Undulating fairways and tricky greens make
this a good test of golf.
9 holes, 5822yds, Par 71, SSS 70, Course record 66.
Club membership 600.
Visitors Mon-Fri, Sun & BHs. Dress code **Societies** Booking required.
Green Fees £13 per 18 holes, £9 per 9 holes (£18/£12 Sat, Sun & BHs).
⊕ **Course Designer** Mr Robinson **Facilities** ⑪ by prior arrangement ⫶⦿⟊
by prior arrangement ⌴ by prior arrangement ⊾ ⊾ ✿ ⟊ ✿ **Location** Off
Comber-Killyleagh road 0.5m from Comber
Hotel ★★★★ 74% HL Clandeboye Lodge Hotel, 10 Estate Rd,
Clandeboye, BANGOR ☎ 028 9185 2500 43 en suite

DONAGHADEE   MAP 01 D5

Donaghadee Warren Rd BT21 0PQ
☎ 028 9188 3624 📠 028 9188 8891
e-mail: deegolf@freenet.co.uk
Undulating seaside course, part links, part parkland, requiring a certain
amount of concentration. Splendid views.
18 holes, 5616mtrs, Par 71, SSS 69, Course record 64.
Club membership 1200.
Visitors Mon, Wed-Fri, Sun & BHs. Dress code. **Societies** Booking required
Green Fees £23 (£26 Sun). ⊕ **Prof** Gordon Drew **Facilities** ⑪ ⫶⦿⟊ ⊾ ⌴
⊾ ⊾ ✿ ⟊ ⊾ ✿ ⟊ ✿ **Conf** facs Corporate Hospitality Days **Location** 5m
S of Bangor on Coast Rd
Hotel ★★★ 87% HL The Old Inn, 15 Main St, CRAWFORDSBURN
☎ 028 9185 3255 29 en suite 1 annexe en suite

DOWNPATRICK   MAP 01 D5

Bright Castle 14 Coniamstown Rd, Bright BT30 8LU
☎ 028 4484 1319
18 holes, 7300yds, Par 74, SSS 74, Course record 69.
Course Designer Mr Ennis Snr **Location** 5m S
Telephone for further details
Hotel ★★ 69% HL Enniskeen House Hotel, 98 Bryansford Rd, NEWCASTLE
☎ 028 4372 2392 12 en suite

Downpatrick 43 Saul Rd BT30 6PA
☎ 028 4461 5947 📠 028 4461 7502
e-mail: info@downpatrickgolfclub.org.com
web: www.downpatrickgolfclub.org.com
18 holes, 6100yds, Par 70, SSS 69, Course record 66.
Course Designer Hawtree & Son **Location** 1.5m from town centre
Telephone for further details
Hotel ★★ 69% HL Enniskeen House Hotel, 98 Bryansford Rd, NEWCASTLE
☎ 028 4372 2392 12 en suite

Ireland

HOLYWOOD MAP 01 D5

Holywood Nuns Walk, Demesne Rd BT18 9LE
☎ 028 904 23135 📠 028 9042 5040
e-mail: mail@holywoodgolfclub.co.uk
web: www.holywoodgolfclub.co.uk
18 holes, 5480mtrs, Par 69, SSS 68, Course record 64.
Location Off Bangor dual carriageway, behind Holywood
Telephone for further details
Hotel ★★★ 87% HL The Old Inn, 15 Main St, CRAWFORDSBURN
☎ 028 9185 3255 29 en suite 1 annexe en suite

The Royal Belfast Station Rd, Craigavad BT18 0BP
☎ 028 9042 8165 📠 028 9042 1404
e-mail: royalbelfastgc@btclick.com
web: www.royalbelfast.com
18 holes, 6185yds, Par 70, SSS 69.
Course Designer H C Colt **Location** 2m E on A2
Telephone for further details
Hotel ★★★ 87% HL The Old Inn, 15 Main St, CRAWFORDSBURN
☎ 028 9185 3255 29 en suite 1 annexe en suite

KILKEEL MAP 01 D5

Kilkeel Mourne Park BT34 4LB
☎ 028 4176 5095 📠 028 4176 5579
e-mail: kilkeelgolfclub@gmail.com
Picturesquely situated at the foot of the Mourne Mountains. Seven holes have tree-lined fairways with the remainder in open parkland. The 13th hole is testing and a well-positioned tee shot is essential.
18 holes, 6579yds, Par 72, SSS 72, Course record 67.
Club membership 750.
Visitors Mon-Fri, Sun & BHs. Booking required Sun & BHs. Dress code.
Societies Booking required. **Green Fees** £23 per round (£28 Sun & BHs).
Course Designer Babington/Hackett **Facilities** ⑪ ⑭ ⓛ ⌂ ⏂ ⏁ ⏂ ⌕
⌕ **Conf** facs Corporate Hospitality Days **Location** 3m from Kilkeel on Newry road
Hotel ★★ 69% HL Enniskeen House Hotel, 98 Bryansford Rd, NEWCASTLE
☎ 028 4372 2392 12 en suite

KILLYLEAGH MAP 01 D5

Ringdufferin Golf Course 31 Ringdufferin Rd, Toye BT30 9PH
☎ 028 4482 8812 📠 028 4482 8812
9 holes, 4652mtrs, Par 68, SSS 66.
Course Designer Frank Ainsworth **Location** 2m N of Killyleagh
Telephone for further details

MAGHERALIN MAP 01 D5

Edenmore Golf & Country Club Edenmore House, 70 Drumnabreeze Rd BT67 0RH
☎ 028 9261 9241 📠 028 9261 3310
e-mail: info@edenmore.com
web: www.edenmore.com
Set in mature parkland with gently rolling slopes. The front nine holes provide an interesting contrast to the back nine with more open play involved. Many new paths and features have been added. The 13th hole, Edenmore, is the most memorable hole with a small lake protecting a contoured green.
18 holes, 6278yds, Par 71, SSS 69, Course record 70.
Club membership 600.
Visitors Mon-Sun & BHs. Booking required Sat & Sun. Dress code.
Societies Booking required. **Green Fees** £18 (£24 Sat, Sun & BHs).
Prof Andrew Manson **Course Designer** F Ainsworth **Facilities** ⑪ ⑭
ⓛ ⌂ ⏂ ⏁ ⏂ ⌕ ⌕ ⌕ **Leisure** sauna, gymnasium. **Conf** facs
Corporate Hospitality Days **Location** M1 Moira exit, through Moira towards Lurgan. Turn off in Magheralin signed
Hotel ★★★ 87% HL The Old Inn, 15 Main St, CRAWFORDSBURN
☎ 028 9185 3255 29 en suite 1 annexe en suite

NEWCASTLE MAP 01 D5

Royal County Down see page 415
Hotel ★★ 69% HL Enniskeen House Hotel, 98 Bryansford Rd, NEWCASTLE
☎ 028 4372 2392 12 en suite

NEWTOWNARDS MAP 01 D5

Scrabo 233 Scrabo Rd BT23 4SL
☎ 028 9181 2355 📠 028 9182 2919
e-mail: admin.scrabogc@btconnect.com
web: www.scrabo-golf-club.org
18 holes, 5722mtrs, Par 71, SSS 71, Course record 65.
Location Outskirts of Newtownards on Ards peninsula, signs for Scrabo Country Park
Telephone for further details
Hotel ★★★★ 74% HL Clandeboye Lodge Hotel, 10 Estate Rd, Clandeboye, BANGOR ☎ 028 9185 2500 43 en suite

WARRENPOINT MAP 01 D5

Warrenpoint Lower Dromore Rd BT34 3LN
☎ 028 4175 3695 📠 028 4175 2918
e-mail: office@warrenpointgolf.com
web: www.warrenpointgolf.com
Parkland course with marvellous views and a need for accurate shots.
18 holes, 6108yds, Par 71, SSS 70, Course record 61.
Club membership 1460.
Visitors Mon, Thu, Fri, Sun & BHs. Booking required. Handicap certificate.
Dress code. **Societies** Booking required. **Green Fees** £28 per round (£32 Sat, Sun & BHs). **Prof** Nigel Shaw **Course Designer** Tom Craddock/Pat Ruddy **Facilities** ⑪ ⑭ ⓛ ⌂ ⏂ ⏁ ⏂ ⌕ **Leisure** 9 hole Par 3 academy course. **Conf** facs Corporate Hospitality Days **Location** 1m W
Hotel ★★ 69% HL Enniskeen House Hotel, 98 Bryansford Rd, NEWCASTLE
☎ 028 4372 2392 12 en suite

CO FERMANAGH

ENNISKILLEN MAP 01 C5

Ashwoods Golf Centre Sligo Rd BT74 7JY
☎ 028 6632 5321 & 6632 2908 📠 028 6632 9411
14 holes, 1930yds, Par 42.
Course Designer P Loughran **Location** 1.5m W of Enniskillen on Sligo road
Telephone for further details
Hotel ★★★★ 80% HL Killyhevlin Hotel, ENNISKILLEN ☎ 028 6632 3481 70 en suite

Ireland

Castle Hume Castle Hume, Belleek Rd BT93 7ED
☎ 028 6632 7077 📄 028 6632 7076
e-mail: info@castlehumegolf.com
web: www.castlehumegolf.com
Castle Hume is a particularly scenic and challenging course. Set in undulating parkland with large rolling greens, rivers, lakes and water hazards all in play on a championship standard course.
18 holes, 5770mtrs, Par 72, SSS 70, Course record 69.
Club membership 350.
Visitors Mon-Sun & BHs. Booking required Wed, Sat & Sun. Dress code. **Societies** booking required. **Green Fees** not confirmed. **Prof** Shaun Donnelly **Course Designer** B Browne **Facilities** ⑪ ⚬ 🍴 🛍 🖅 ♨ 🏌 🛎 🏈 ✎ 🐴 ⛳ 🏌 **Leisure** fishing. **Conf** facs Corporate Hospitality Days **Location** 4m from Enniskillen on A46 Belleek-Donegal road
Hotel ★★★★ 80% HL Killyhevlin Hotel, ENNISKILLEN ☎ 028 6632 3481 70 en suite

Enniskillen Castlecoole BT74 6HZ
☎ 028 6632 5250 📄 028 6632 5250
e-mail: enniskillengolfclub@mail.com
web: www.enniskillengolfclub.com
Tree lined parkland course offering panoramic views of Enniskillen town and the surrounding lakeland area. Situated beside the National Trust's Castlecoole Estate.
18 holes, 6230yds, Par 71, SSS 69, Course record 67.
Club membership 550.
Visitors Mon-Sun & BHs. Booking required Tue, Sat & Sun. Handicap certificate. Dress code. **Societies** Booking required. **Green Fees** £18 per day (£22 Sat & Sun). **Facilities** ⑪ by prior arrangement 🍴 by prior arrangement 🛍 by prior arrangement ♨ 🖅 🛎 🏈 ✎ 🐴 **Conf** facs Corporate Hospitality Days **Location** 1m E of town centre
Hotel ★★★★ 80% HL Killyhevlin Hotel, ENNISKILLEN ☎ 028 6632 3481 70 en suite

CO LONDONDERRY

AGHADOWEY
MAP 01 C6

Brown Trout Golf & Country Inn 209 Agivey Rd BT51 4AD
☎ 028 7086 8209 📄 028 7086 8878
e-mail: bill@browntroutinn.com
web: www.browntroutinn.com
A challenging course with two Par 5s. During the course of the nine holes, players have to negotiate water seven times and all the fairways are lined with densely packed fir trees.
9 holes, 5510yds, Par 70, SSS 68, Course record 64.
Club membership 100.
Visitors Mon-Sun & BHs. Booking required Sat/Sun. **Societies** booking required. **Green Fees** not confirmed. **Prof** Ken Revie **Course Designer** Bill O'Hara Snr **Facilities** ⑪ ⚬ 🍴 🛍 ♨ 🖅 🛎 🏈 ◇ ✎ **Leisure** fishing, gymnasium. **Location** Junct A54 , 7m S of Coleraine
Hotel ★★ 76% HL Brown Trout Golf & Country Inn, 209 Agivey Rd, AGHADOWEY ☎ 028 7086 8209 15 en suite

CASTLEDAWSON
MAP 01 C5

Moyola Park 15 Curran Rd BT45 8DG
☎ 028 7946 8468 & 7946 8830 (Prof) 📄 028 7946 8626
e-mail: moyolapark@btconnect.com
web: www.moyolapark.com
18 holes, 6519yds, Par 71, SSS 71, Course record 67.
Course Designer Don Patterson **Location** Club signed
Telephone for further details
Hotel ★★★★ 69% HL Galgorm Manor, BALLYMENA ☎ 028 2588 1001 24 en suite

CASTLEROCK
MAP 01 C6

Castlerock 65 Circular Rd BT51 4TJ
☎ 028 7084 8314 📄 028 7084 9440
e-mail: info@castlerockgc.co.uk
web: www.castlerockgc.co.uk
A most exhilarating course with three superb Par 4s, four testing short holes and five Par 5s. After an uphill start, the hazards are many, including the river and a railway, and both judgement and accuracy are called for. The signature hole is the 4th, Leg of Mutton. A challenge in calm weather, any trouble from the elements will test your golf to the limits.
Mussenden Course: 18 holes, 6499yds, Par 73, SSS 71, Course record 64.
Bann Course: 9 holes, 2938yds, Par 34, SSS 33, Course record 60. Club membership 1250.
Visitors Mon-Sun & BHs. Booking required. Dress code.
Societies Booking required. **Green Fees** £60 per day (£75 Sat, Sun & BHs). **Prof** Ian Blair **Course Designer** Ben Sayers **Facilities** ⑪ ⚬ 🛍 🖅 🏈 ♨ 🛎 🏈 ✎ 🐴 ✎ **Location** 6m from Coleraine on A2

KILREA
MAP 01 C5

Kilrea 47a Lisnagrot Rd BT51 5TB
☎ 028 2954 0044
Inland course, winner of an environmental award.
9 holes, 5578yds, Par 68, SSS 68, Course record 66.
Club membership 300.
Visitors Mon-Sun & BHs. Booking required Tue, Wed & Sat. Dress code. **Societies** booking required. **Green Fees** not confirmed. 🐴 **Facilities** ⑪ ⚬ 🛍 ♨ 🖅 🛎 🏈 🐴
Hotel ★★ 76% HL Brown Trout Golf & Country Inn, 209 Agivey Rd, AGHADOWEY ☎ 028 7086 8209 15 en suite

LIMAVADY
MAP 01 C6

Benone 53 Benone Ave BT49 0LQ
☎ 028 7775 0555 📄 028 7775 0919
Beside a beach, a delightful mix of parkland quite testing for the short game. Nestling at the foot of the Binevenagh mountains with picturesque views.
9 holes, 1459yds, Par 27. Club membership 100.
Visitors Mon-Sun & BHs. Booking required, **Societies** booking required. **Green Fees** not confirmed. **Facilities** 🏈 🏌 **Leisure** hard tennis courts, heated outdoor swimming pool. **Location** Between Coleraine & Limavady on A2
Hotel ★★★ 70% HL Gorteen House Hotel, Deerpark, Roemill Rd, LIMAVADY ☎ 028 7772 2333 26 en suite

Ireland

adisson SAS Roe Park Resort Roe Park BT49 9LB
☎ 028 7772 2222 🖷 028 7772 2313
-mail: sales@radissonroepark.com
eb: www.radissonroepark.com
  parkland course opened in 1992 on an historic Georgian estate. The
  urse surrounds the original buildings and a driving range has been
  eated in the old walled garden. Final holes 15-18 are particularly
  emorable with water, trees and out-of-bounds to provide a testing
  ish.
3 holes, 6283yds, Par 70, SSS 70, Course record 67.
lub membership 600.
sitors Mon-Sun & BHs. Booking required. Dress code. **Societies** Booking
quired. **Green Fees** £25 per round (£30 Sat, Sun & BH). **Prof** Shaun
evenney **Course Designer** Frank Ainsworth **Facilities** ⑪ ⑥ ᛒ ♟ ☡ ⊏┒ ⍱
  ⌐ ◇ ⦿ 🝙 ⦿ ┏ **Leisure** heated indoor swimming pool, fishing, sauna,
larium, gymnasium, indoor golf academy. **Conf** facs Corporate Hospitality
ys **Location** Just outside Limavady on A2 Ballykelly-Londonderry road
tel ★★★★ 74% HL Radisson SAS Roe Park Resort, LIMAVADY
  028 7772 2222 118 en suite

ONDONDERRY   MAP 01 C5

ity of Derry 49 Victoria Rd BT47 2PU
☎ 028 7134 6369 🖷 028 7131 0008
mail: cityofderry@aol.com
eb: cityderrygolfclub.com
  rhen Course: 18 holes, 6406yds, Par 71, SSS 71,
  urse record 68.
  unhugh Course: 9 holes, 2354yds, Par 66, SSS 66.
cation 2m S
lephone for further details
tel ★★★ 75% HL Beech Hill Country House Hotel, 32 Ardmore Rd,
NDONDERRY ☎ 028 7134 9279 17 en suite 10 annexe en suite

•yle International Golf Centre 12 Alder Rd BT48 8DB
  028 7135 2222 🖷 028 7135 3967
mail: mail@foylegolf.club24.co.uk
eb: www.foylegolfcentre.co.uk
  yle International has a championship course, a nine-hole Par 3
  urse and a driving range. It is a fine test of golf with water coming
  o play on the 3rd, 10th and 11th holes. The 6th green overlooks the
  elia Earhart centre.
  rhart: 18 holes, 6643yds, Par 71, SSS 71,
  urse record 70.
  oodlands: 9 holes, 1349yds, Par 27.
ub membership 320.
sitors Mon-Sun & BHs. Dress code. **Societies** Welcome. **Green Fees** £16
9 Sat & Sun). **Prof** Derek Morrison, Sean Young **Course Designer** Frank
 sworth **Facilities** ⑪ ⑥ ᛒ ♟ ☡ ⊏┒ ⍱ 🝙 ⌐ ◇ ┏ **Leisure** 9 hole Par 3
  urse. **Conf** facs Corporate Hospitality Days **Location** 1.5m from Foyle
  dge towards Moville

PORTSTEWART   MAP 01 C6

Portstewart 117 Strand Rd BT55 7PG
☎ 028 7083 2015 & 7083 3839 🖷 028 7083 4097
e-mail: bill@portstewartgc.co.uk
web: www.portstewartgc.co.uk
Three links courses with spectacular views, offering a testing round
on the Strand course in particular with every shot in the bag
required.
Strand Course: 18 holes, 6784yds, Par 72, SSS 72,
Course record 67.
Old Course: 18 holes, 4733yds, Par 64, SSS 62.
Riverside: 9 holes, 2622yds, Par 32.
Club membership 1666.
Visitors Mon-Sun & BHs. Booking required. Handicap certificate. Dress
code. **Societies** booking required **Green Fees** not confirmed. **Prof** Alan
Hunter **Course Designer** Des Giffin **Facilities** ⑪ ⑥ ᛒ ♟ ☡ ⊏┒ ⍱ 🝙 ⌐
◇ 🝙 ┏ **Conf** facs

CO TYRONE

COOKSTOWN   MAP 01 C5

Killymoon 200 Killymoon Rd BT80 8TW
☎ 028 8676 3762 & 8676 2254 🖷 028 8676 3762
e-mail: killymoongolf@btconnect.com
web: www.killymoongolfclub.com
Parkland course on elevated, well-drained land. The signature hole is
the aptly named 10th hole - the Giant's Grave. Accuracy is paramount
here and a daunting tee shot into a narrow-necked fairway will
challenge even the most seasoned golfer. The enclosing influence of
the trees continues the whole way to the green.
18 holes, 6202yds, Par 70, SSS 70, Course record 64.
Club membership 830.
Visitors Mon-Wed, Fri, Sun & BHs. Booking required Sun. Dress code.
Societies Booking required. **Green Fees** Tue-Fri £22 per round (£15 Mon,
£28 Sat-Sun). **Prof** Gary Chambers **Course Designer** John Nash **Facilities**
⑪ ⑥ ᛒ ♟ ☡ ⊏┒ ⍱ 🝙 ⌐ ◇ **Leisure** snooker. **Conf** facs Corporate
Hospitality Days **Location** S of Cookstown
Hotel ★★ 68% HL The Cohannon Inn & Autolodge, 212 Ballynakilly Rd,
DUNGANNON ☎ 028 8772 4488 42 en suite

DUNGANNON   MAP 01 C5

Dungannon 34 Springfield Ln BT70 1QX
☎ 028 8772 2098 🖷 028 8772 7338
e-mail: info@dungannongolfclub.com
web: www.dungannongolfclub.com
Parkland course with five Par 3s and tree-lined fairways.
18 holes, 6046yds, Par 72, SSS 69, Course record 62.
Club membership 1100.
Visitors Mon-Fri, Sun & BHs. Booking required Sun & BHs. Handicap
certificate. Dress code. **Societies** Welcome. **Green Fees** £18 per round
(£22 Sat & Sun). ⊛ **Prof** Vivian Teague **Course Designer** Sam Bacon
Facilities ⍱ 🝙 ⌐ ◇ 🝙 ⌐ **Location** 0.5m outside town on Donaghmore
road
Hotel ★★ 68% HL The Cohannon Inn & Autolodge, 212 Ballynakilly Rd,
DUNGANNON ☎ 028 8772 4488 42 en suite

Ireland

FINTONA MAP 01 C5

Fintona Ecclesville Demesne, 1 Kiln St BT78 2BJ
☎ 028 8284 1480 & 8284 0777 (office) 📄 028 8284 1480
9 holes, 5765mtrs, Par 72, SSS 70.
Location 8m S of Omagh
Telephone for further details
Hotel ★★★ 68% HL Mahons Hotel, Mill St, IRVINESTOWN
☎ 028 6862 1656 & 6862 1657 📄 028 6862 8344 24 en suite

NEWTOWNSTEWART MAP 01 C5

Newtownstewart 38 Golf Course Rd BT78 4HU
☎ 028 8166 1466 📄 028 8166 2506
e-mail: newtown.stewart@lineone.net
web: www.globalgolf/newtownstewart.com
Parkland course bisected by a stream. Deer and pheasant are present on the course.
18 holes, 5818yds, Par 70, SSS 69, Course record 65.
Club membership 550.
Visitors Mon-Sun & BHs. Booking required Wed, Sat, Sun & BHs. Dress code. **Societies** booking required. **Green Fees** not confirmed. 🅱
Course Designer Frank Pennick **Facilities** ⚑ ♿ 🍴 🏌 🏖 🍺 ⛳ 🏌 🛒 ⛳
Leisure snooker. **Conf** facs Corporate Hospitality Days **Location** 2m SW on B84

OMAGH MAP 01 C5

Omagh 83a Dublin Rd BT78 1HQ
☎ 028 8224 3160 📄 028 8224 3160
Undulating parkland course beside the River Drumnagh, with the river coming into play on 4 of the holes.
18 holes, 5683mtrs, Par 71, SSS 70. Club membership 850.
Visitors Mon-Sun & BHs. Booking required Fri-Sun. Dress code.
Societies Booking required **Green Fees** £15 per round (£20 Sat, Sun & BHs). 🅱 **Course Designer** Dun Patterson **Facilities** 🅿 by prior arrangement 🍴 by prior arrangement 🏖 by prior arrangement ♿ 🍴 🏌
Conf Corporate Hospitality Days **Location** S outskirts of town

STRABANE MAP 01 C5

Strabane Ballycolman Rd BT82 9HY
☎ 028 7138 2271 & 7138 2007 📄 028 7188 6514
e-mail: strabanegc@btconnect.com
18 holes, 5537mtrs, Par 69, SSS 69, Course record 62.
Course Designer Eddie Hackett/P Jones **Location** 1m from Strabane on Dublin road
Telephone for further details

BORRIS MAP 01 C3

Borris Deerpark
☎ 059 9773310 📄 059 9773750
e-mail: borrisgolfclub@eircom.net
9 holes, 5680mtrs, Par 70, SSS 69, Course record 66.
Telephone for further details
Hotel ★★★★ CHH Mount Juliet Conrad Hotel, THOMASTOWN
☎ 056 7773000 32 en suite 27 annexe en suite

CARLOW MAP 01 C3

Carlow Deerpark
☎ 059 9131695 📄 059 9140065
e-mail: carlowgolfclub@eircom.net
web: www.carlowgolfclub.com
Created in 1922 to a design by Cecil Barcroft, this testing and enjoyable course is set in a wild deer park, with beautiful dry terrain and a varied character. With sandy subsoil, the course is playable all year round. There are water hazards at the 2nd, 10th and 11th and only two Par 5s, both offering genuine birdie opportunities.
18 holes, 6025mtrs, Par 70, SSS 71, Course record 63.
Oakpark: 9 holes, 5650mtrs, Par 70, SSS 69,
Course record 67. Club membership 1200.
Visitors Mon-Sun & BHs. Handicap certificate. Dress code.
Societies Booking required. **Green Fees** €50 per round (€60 Sat).
Oakpark: €20 per 9/18 holes. **Prof** Andrew Gilbert **Course Designer** Cecil Barcroft/Tom Simpson **Facilities** ⊕ 🍴 ⚑ ♿ 🍴 🏌 🏖 🍺 🛒 ⛳
Location 3km N of Carlow on N9
Hotel ★★★ 75% HL Seven Oaks Hotel, Athy Rd, CARLOW
☎ 059 9131308 89 en suite

TULLOW MAP 01 C3

Mount Wolseley Hotel, Spa, Golf & Country Club
☎ 059 9180161 📄 059 9152123
e-mail: golfmountwolseley@hilton.com
web: www.hilton.co.uk/mountwolseley
A magnificent setting, a few hundred yards from the banks of the River Slaney with its mature trees and lakes set against the backdrop of the East Carlow and Wicklow mountains. With wide landing areas the only concession for demanding approach shots to almost every green. There is water in play on 11 holes, with the 11th an all-water carry off the tee of 207yds. The 18th is a fine finishing hole - a fairway lined with mature oak trees, then a second shot uphill across a water hazard to a green.
18 holes, 6558metres, Par 72, SSS 74, Course record 68.
Club membership 300.
Visitors Mon-Sun & BHs. Booking required. Dress code. **Societies** Booking required. **Green Fees** €60 (€90 Sat, Sun & BHs). Winter €40/€60.
Course Designer Christy O'Connor Jnr **Facilities** ⊕ 🍴 ⚑ ♿ 🍴 🏌 🏖 ⛳ 🛒 ⛳ 🍺 ⛳ **Leisure** hard tennis courts, heated indoor swimming pool, sauna, solarium, gymnasium, spa. **Conf** facs Corporate Hospitality Days
Location 1.6km from Tullow centre
Hotel ★★★ 75% HL Seven Oaks Hotel, Athy Rd, CARLOW ☎ 059 9131308 89 en suite

CO CAVAN

BALLYCONNELL
MAP 01 C4

Slieve Russell Hotel Golf & Country Club
☎ 049 9525090 ▤ 049 9526640
e-mail: slieve-russell@quinn-hotels.com
web: www.quinnhotels.com
An 18-hole course opened in 1992 and rapidly establishing itself as one of the finest parkland courses in the country. Forming part of a 300 acre estate, including 50 acres of lakes, the course has been sensitively wrapped around the surrounding landscape. On the main course, the 2nd plays across water while the 16th has water surrounding the green. The course finishes with a 519yd, Par 5 18th.
18 holes, 6048mtrs, Par 72, SSS 72, Course record 65. Club membership 400.
Visitors Mon-Sun & BHs. Booking required. Dress code.
Societies Booking required **Green Fees** €72 per round (€90 Sat).
Prof Liam McCool/ Tristan Mullally **Course Designer** Paddy Merrigan **Facilities** ⑪ ⑩ ⅃ ⅃ ⅂ ⚑ ⅃ ⚑ ☇ ✦ ⚑ ✦ **Leisure** hard tennis courts, heated indoor swimming pool, sauna, solarium, gymnasium.
Conf facs Corporate Hospitality Days **Location** 4km E of Ballyconnell
Hotel ★★★★ 76% HL Slieve Russell Hotel Golf and Country Club, BALLYCONNELL ☎ 049 9526444 219 en suite

BELTURBET
MAP 01 C4

Belturbet Erne Hill
☎ 049 9522287 & 9524044
9 holes, 5011metres, Par 68, SSS 65, Course record 64.
Course Designer Eddie Hackett **Location** 0.8km N of town off N3
Telephone for further details
Hotel ★★★★ 76% HL Slieve Russell Hotel Golf and Country Club, BALLYCONNELL ☎ 049 9526444 219 en suite

BLACKLION
MAP 01 C5

Blacklion Toam
☎ 072 53024 & 53418 ▤ 072 53418
9 holes, 5614mtrs, Par 72, SSS 69.
Course Designer Eddie Hackett
Telephone for further details
Hotel ★★★ 76% HL Sligo Park Hotel, Pearse Rd, SLIGO ☎ 071 9190400 137 en suite

CAVAN
MAP 01 C4

County Cavan Drumelis
☎ 049 4331541 & 049 4371313 ▤ 049 31541
e-mail: info@cavangolf.ie
web: www.cavangolf.ie
Parkland course with number of mature trees, some over 100 years old. The closing six holes are an exacting challenge for both the handicap and professional golfer alike.
18 holes, 5634mtrs, Par 70, SSS 69, Course record 64. Club membership 830.
Visitors Mon-Sun & BHs. **Societies** Booking required. **Green Fees** €30 per round (€35 Sat & Sun). **Prof** Bill Noble **Course Designer** Eddie Hackett, Arthur Spring **Facilities** ⅃ ⅂ ⚑ ⅃ ⅃ ⚑ ☇ ✦ ⚑ **Location** On road towards Killeshandra
Hotel ★★★ 70% HL Kilmore Hotel, Dublin Rd, CAVAN ☎ 049 4332288 39 en suite

VIRGINIA
MAP 01 C4

Virginia
☎ 049 47235 & 48066
9 holes, 4139mtrs, Par 64, SSS 62, Course record 57.
Location By Lough Ramor
Telephone for further details
Hotel ★★ 67% HL The Park Manor House Hotel, Virginia Park, VIRGINIA ☎ 049 8546100 26 en suite

CO CLARE

BODYKE
MAP 01 B3

East Clare
☎ 061 921322 ▤ 061 921717
e-mail: eastclaregolfclub@eircon.net
web: www.eastclare.com
18 holes, 5415metres, Par 71, SSS 71.
Course Designer Dr Arthur Spring
Telephone for further details
Hotel ★★★ 70% HL Temple Gate Hotel, The Square, ENNIS ☎ 065 6823300 70 en suite

ENNIS
MAP 01 B3

Ennis Drumbiggle
☎ 065 6824074 & 6865415 ▤ 065 6841848
e-mail: info@ennisgolfclub.com
web: www.ennisgolfclub.com
On rolling hills, this immaculately manicured course presents an excellent challenge to both casual visitors and aspiring scratch golfers, with tree-lined fairways and well-protected greens.
18 holes, 5706mtrs, Par 70, SSS 70, Course record 65. Club membership 1370.
Visitors Mon-Sat & BHs. Booking required. Handicap certificate. Dress code. **Societies** Booking required. **Green Fees** €35 per round (€40 Sat & Sun). **Facilities** ⑪ ⑩ by prior arrangement ⅃ ⅂ ⚑ ⅃ ⅃ ⚑ ☇ ✦ ⚑
Conf Corporate Hospitality Days **Location** Signed near town
Hotel ★★★ 70% HL Temple Gate Hotel, The Square, ENNIS ☎ 065 6823300 70 en suite

Woodstock Golf and Country Club Shanaway Rd
☎ 065 6829463 & 6842406 ▤ 065 6820304
e-mail: woodstock.ennis@eircon.net
web: www.woodstockgolfclub.com
This parkland course is set in 63 hectares and includes four holes where water is a major hazard. The course is playable all year and the sand-based greens offer a consistent surface for putting.
18 holes, 5864mtrs, Par 71, SSS 71. Club membership 350.
Visitors Mon-Sun and BHs. Booking required Sat, Sun & BHs. Handicap certificate. Dress code. **Societies** Booking required. **Green Fees** €42; 9 holes €20 (€45/€25 Sun, Sat & BHs). **Course Designer** Arthur Spring **Facilities** ⑪ ⑩ ⅃ ⅂ ⚑ ⅃ ⅃ ⚑ ☇ ✦ ⚑ ✦ **Leisure** heated indoor swimming pool, sauna, gymnasium. **Location** Off N85
Hotel ★★★ 70% HL Temple Gate Hotel, The Square, ENNIS ☎ 065 6823300 70 en suite

Ireland

KILKEE — MAP 01 B3

Kilkee East End
☎ 065 9056048 📠 065 9656977
e-mail: kilkeegolfclub@eircom.net
web: www.kilkeegolfclub.ie
Well-established course on the cliffs of Kilkee Bay. Mature championship course with a great variety of challenges - seaside holes, clifftop holes and holes that feature well-positioned water hazards. The spectacular 3rd hole hugs the cliff top. The ever present Atlantic breeze provides golfers with a real test.
18 holes, 5555mtrs, Par 70, SSS 69, Course record 68.
Club membership 770.
Visitors Mon-Sun & BHs. Booking required Sat, Sun & BHs. Dress code.
Societies Booking required. **Green Fees** €30 per round (€35 Sat & Sun).
Course Designer Eddie Hackett **Facilities** ⑪ ⦾ ⬚ ⬚ ▢ ⬚ ⬚ ⬚ ⬚ ⬚ ⬚
Hotel ★★ 64% HL Halpin's Townhouse Hotel, Erin St, KILKEE
☎ 065 9056032 12 en suite

KILRUSH — MAP 01 B3

Kilrush Parknamoney
☎ 065 9051138 📠 065 9052633
e-mail: info@kilrushgolfclub.com
web: www.kilrushgolfclub.com
18 holes, 5474metres, Par 70, SSS 70, Course record 68.
Course Designer Arthur Spring **Location** 0.8km from Kilrush towards Ennis
Telephone for further details
Hotel ★★ 64% HL Halpin's Townhouse Hotel, Erin St, KILKEE
☎ 065 9056032 12 en suite

LAHINCH — MAP 01 B3

Lahinch
☎ 065 708 1592 📠 065 708 1592
e-mail: info@lahinchgolf.com
web: www.lahinchgolf.com
Old Course: 18 holes, 6123metres, Par 72, SSS 73.
Castle Course: 18 holes, 5115metres, Par 70, SSS 70.
Course Designer Alister MacKenzie **Location** 3km W of Ennisstymon on N67
Telephone for further details

MILLTOWN MALBAY — MAP 01 B3

Spanish Point
☎ 065 7084198 📠 065 7084263
e-mail: dkfitzgerald@tinet.ie
web: spanish-point.com
9 holes, 4600mtrs, Par 64, SSS 63, Course record 59.
Location 3km SW of Miltown Malbay on N67
Telephone for further details
Hotel ★★ 64% HL Halpin's Townhouse Hotel, Erin St, KILKEE
☎ 065 9056032 12 en suite

NEWMARKET-ON-FERGUS — MAP 01 B3

Dromoland Castle Golf & Country Club
☎ 061 368444 & 368144 📠 061 363355/368498
e-mail: golf@dromoland.ie
web: www.dromoland.ie
Set in 200 acres of parkland, the course is enhanced by numerous trees and a lake. Three holes are played around the lake which is in front of the castle.

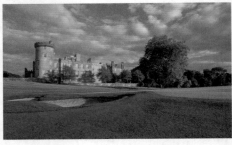

18 holes, 6240mtrs, Par 72, SSS 72, Course record 65.
Club membership 500.
Visitors Mon-Sun & BHs. Booking required. Dress code. **Societies** Booking required **Green Fees** €110 per round (€60 early/twilight). **Prof** David Foley **Course Designer** Ron Kirby & J. B. Carr **Facilities** ⑪ ⦾ ⬚ ▢ ⬚ ⬚ ⬚ ⬚ ⬚ ⬚ ⬚ **Leisure** hard tennis courts, heated indoor swimming pool, fishing, sauna, solarium, gymnasium. **Conf** facs Corporate Hospitality Days **Location** 3km N on Limerick-Galway road
Hotel ★★★★★ HL Dromoland Castle Hotel, NEWMARKET-ON-FERGUS
☎ 061 368144 100 en suite

See advert on opposite page

CO CORK

BANDON — MAP 01 B2

Bandon Castlebernard
☎ 023 41111 📠 023 44690
e-mail: enquiries@bandongolfclub.com
web: www.bandongolfclub.com
Lovely parkland in pleasant countryside. Hazards of water, sand and trees. The course has been extended around the picturesque ruin of Castle Barnard.
18 holes, 5854mtrs, Par 71, SSS 71. Club membership 900.
Visitors Mon, Tue, Thu-Sat & BHs. Dress code. **Societies** Booking required **Green Fees** €45 per round (€55 Sat & BHs). **Prof** Paddy O'Boyle **Facilities** ⑪ ⦾ ⬚ ▢ ⬚ ⬚ ⬚ ⬚ **Leisure** hard tennis courts, caddies available. **Location** 2.5km W
Hotel ★★★ 66% HL Innishannon House Hotel, INNISHANNON
☎ 021 4775121 12 en suite

Ireland

BANTRY
MAP 01 B2

Bantry Bay Donemark
☎ 027 50579 📠 027 53790
e-mail: info@bantrygolf.com
web: www.bantrygolf.com
Designed by Christy O'Connor Jnr and extended in 1997 to 18 holes, this challenging and rewarding course is idyllically set at the head of Bantry Bay. Testing holes include the Par 5 of 487 metres and the little Par 3 of 127 metres where accuracy is all-important.
18 holes, 6117mtrs, Par 71, SSS 72, Course record 71.
Club membership 600.
Visitors Mon-Sun & BHs. Booking required Sat & BHs. **Societies** Booking required. **Green Fees** €45 per round (€50 Sat & Sun). **Course Designer** Christy O'Connor Jnr/Eddie Hackett **Facilities** ⑪ ⑩ ♨ ⬚ ☜ ⚒ ⌁ ⊜ ♈ ⚐ ⚑ ⚒ **Conf** facs Corporate Hospitality Days **Location** 3km N of town on N71
Hotel ★★★ 66% HL Westlodge Hotel, BANTRY ☎ 027 50360 90 en suite

BLACKROCK
MAP 01 B2

Mahon Clover Hill
☎ 021 4294280
18 holes, 4862metres, Par 70, SSS 67, Course record 64.
Course Designer Eddie Hackett
Telephone for further details
Hotel ★★★★ 78% HL Rochestown Park Hotel, Rochestown Rd, Douglas, CORK ☎ 021 4890800 160 en suite

BLARNEY
MAP 01 B2

Muskerry Carrigrohane
☎ 021 4385297 📠 021 4516860
e-mail: muskgc@eircom.net
web: www.muskerrygolfclub.ie
An adventurous game is guaranteed at this course, with its wooded hillsides and the meandering Shournagh River coming into play at a number of holes. The 15th is a notable hole - not long, but very deep - and after that all you need to do to get back to the clubhouse is stay out of the water.
18 holes, 5520mtrs, Par 71, SSS 70.
Club membership 851.
Visitors Mon & Tue, Wed am only & Thu, Sat & Sun pm only. Booking required. Handicap certificate. Dress code. **Societies** Booking required.
Green Fees €40 per round (€50 Sat & Sun). **Prof** W M Lehane
Course Designer Dr A McKenzie **Facilities** ⑪ ♨ ⬚ ⚒ ⌁ ⊜ ♈ ⚒ ⚐ **Location** 4km W of Blarney
Hotel ★★★ 70% HL Blarney Castle Hotel, The Village Green, BLARNEY ☎ 021 4385116 13 en suite

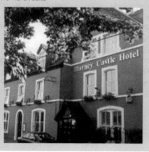

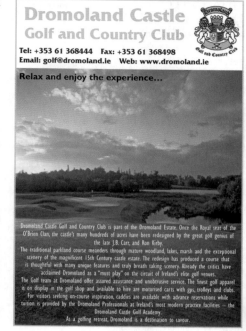

Dromoland Castle
Golf and Country Club
Tel: +353 61 368444   Fax: +353 61 368498
Email: golf@dromoland.ie   Web: www.dromoland.ie

Relax and enjoy the experience...

Dromoland Castle Golf and Country Club is part of the Dromoland Estate. Once the Royal seat of the O'Brien Clan, the castle's many hundreds of acres have been redesigned by the great golf genius of the late J.B. Carr, and Ron Kirby.
The traditional parkland course meanders through mature woodland, lakes, marsh and the exceptional scenery of the magnificent 15th Century castle estate. The redesign has produced a course that is thoughtful with many unique features and truly breath taking scenery. Already the critics have acclaimed Dromoland as a "must play" on the circuit of Ireland's elite golf venues.
The Golf team at Dromoland offer assured assistance and unobtrusive service. The finest golf apparel is on display in the golf shop and available to hire are motorised carts with gps, trolleys and clubs. For visitors seeking on-course inspiration, caddies are available with advance reservations while tuition is provided by the Dromoland Professionals at Ireland's most modern practice facilities – the Dromoland Castle Golf Academy.
As a golfing retreat, Dromoland is a destination to savour.

CARRIGALINE
MAP 01 B2

Fernhill Hotel & Golf Club
☎ 021 4372226 📠 021 4371011
e-mail: fernhill@iol.ie
web: www.fernhillgolfhotel.com
18 holes, 5000mtrs, Par 69, SSS 68.
Course Designer M L Bowes **Location** 3km from Ringaskiddy
Telephone for further details
Hotel ★★★★ 78% HL Rochestown Park Hotel, Rochestown Rd, Douglas, CORK ☎ 021 4890800 160 en suite

CASTLETOWNBERE
(CASTLETOWN BEARHAVEN)
MAP 01 A2

Berehaven Millcove
☎ 027 70700 📠 027 71957
e-mail: info@berehavengolf.com
web: www.berehavengolf.com
Scenic seaside links founded in 1902. Moderately difficult with four holes over water. Testing nine-hole course with different tee positions for the back nine. Water is a dominant feature and comes into play at every hole.
9 holes, 2624mtrs, Par 68, SSS 67, Course record 63.
Club membership 175.
Visitors Mon-Sun & BHs. **Societies** Booking required. **Green Fees** €20 per day (€25 Sat, Sun & BHs). **Course Designer** Royal Navy **Facilities** ⑪ ⑩ ♨ ⬚ ⚒ ⌁ ⊜ ♈ ⚒ **Leisure** hard tennis courts, sauna. **Conf** facs Corporate Hospitality Days **Location** 3km E from Castletownbere on R572
Hotel ★★★ HL Sea View House Hotel, BALLYLICKEY ☎ 027 50073 & 50462 📠 027 51555 25 en suite

Ireland

CHARLEVILLE MAP 01 B2

Charleville

☎ 063 81257 & 81515 📄 063 81274
e-mail: info@charlevillegolf.com
web: www.charlevillegolf.com

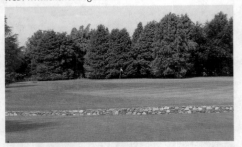

West Course: 18 holes, 5680metres, Par 71, SSS 69,
Course record 65.
East Course: 9 holes, 6128metres, Par 72, SSS 72.
Course Designer Eddie Connaughton **Location** 3km W of town centre
Telephone for further details
Hotel ★★★ CHH Longueville House Hotel, MALLOW ☎ 022 47156
& 47306 📄 022 47459 20 en suite

CLONAKILTY MAP 01 B2

Dunmore Dunmore, Muckross

☎ 023 33352
9 holes, 4082metres, Par 64, SSS 61, Course record 57.
Course Designer E Hackett **Location** 5.5km S of Clonakilty
Telephone for further details
Hotel ★★★★ 81% HL Inchydoney Island Lodge & Spa, CLONAKILTY
☎ 023 33143 67 en suite

CORK MAP 01 B2

Cork Little Island

☎ 021 4353451 📄 021 4353410
e-mail: corkgolfclub@eircom.net
web: www.corkgolfclub.ie
This championship-standard course is kept in superb condition
and is playable all year round. Memorable and distinctive features
include holes at the water's edge and in a disused quarry. The 4th
hole is considered to be among the most attractive and testing holes
in Irish golf.

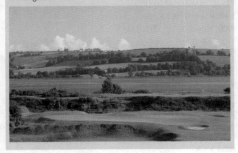

18 holes, 5910mtrs, Par 72, SSS 72, Course record 67.
Club membership 750.
Visitors Mon-Wed, Fri-Sun & BHs. Booking required. Handicap certificate.
Dress code. **Societies** Booking required. **Green Fees** €85 (€95 Sat &
Sun). **Prof** Peter Hickey **Course Designer** Alister Mackenzie **Facilities**
⊕ ⌾ 🍴 🏌 ☂ 🎱 🏌 ⛳ ☕ ⚑ **Conf** Corporate Hospitality Days
Location 8km E of Cork on N25

See advert on opposite page

Fota Island Resort Fota Island

☎ 021 4883700 📄 021 4883713
e-mail: info@fotaisland.ie
web: www.fotaisland.ie
Set in the heart of a 780-acre island in Cork Harbour with an
outstanding landscape. The course is routed among mature woodlands
with occasional views of the harbour. The traditional design features
pot bunkers and undulating putting surfaces.

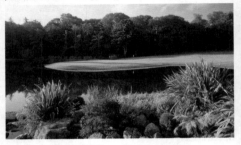

Deerpark: 18 holes, 6334mtrs, Par 71, SSS 73,
Course record 63.
Belvelly: 18 holes, 6511mtrs, Par 72.
Barryscourt: 18 holes, 6732mtrs, Par 73.
Club membership 600.
Visitors Mon-Sun & BHs. Booking required. Dress code.
Societies Welcome. **Green Fees** €75-€120 per round. **Prof** Kevin Morris
Course Designer Jeff Howes **Facilities** ⊕ ⌾ 🍴 🏌 ☂ 🎱 🏌 ⚑ ⚑ ◇ ⛳
🏌 ⛳ ⚑ **Leisure** heated indoor swimming pool, sauna, gymnasium, golf
academy, spa treatments. **Conf** facs Corporate Hospitality Days
Location E of Cork. N25 exit for Cobh, 500 metres on right
Hotel ★★★ 79% HL Midleton Park Hotel & Spa, MIDLETON
☎ 021 4631767 40 en suite

See advert on opposite page

The Ted McCarthy Municipal Golf Course Blackrock

☎ 021 4292543 📄 021 4292604
e-mail: mahon-golf@leisureworldcork.com
Municipal course which stretches alongside the river estuary, with
some holes across water.
18 holes, 5033mtrs, Par 70, SSS 66, Course record 65.
Club membership 400.
Visitors Mon-Sun & BHs. Booking required. **Societies** booking required.
Green Fees not confirmed. ⊕ **Course Designer** E Hackett **Facilities** ☂
🏌 ⚑ 🎱 ⛳ **Location** 3km from city centre
Hotel ★★★★ 77% HL Silver Springs Moran Hotel, Tivoli, CORK
☎ 021 4507533 109 en suite

DONERAILE MAP 01 B2

Doneraile
☎ 022 24137 & 24379
9 holes, 5055metres, Par 68, SSS 67, Course record 61.
Location N of town centre
Telephone for further details
Hotel ★★★ 68% HL Springfort Hall Country House Hotel, MALLOW
☎ 022 21278 49 en suite

DOUGLAS MAP 01 B2

Douglas
☎ 021 4895297 📠 021 4895297
e-mail: admin@douglasgolfclub.ie
web: www.douglasgolfclub.ie
Well-maintained, very flat parkland course with panoramic views from
the clubhouse.
18 holes, 5607mtrs, Par 72, SSS 69. Club membership 900.
Visitors Mon, Thu-Sun except BHs. Booking required. Handicap certificate.
Dress code. **Societies** booking required. **Green Fees** not confirmed.
Prof Gary Nicholson **Course Designer** Peter McEvoy **Facilities** ⚒ 🏠 ⛳
🏌 🏴 **Location** 6km E of Cork
Hotel ★★★★ 78% HL Rochestown Park Hotel, Rochestown Rd, Douglas,
CORK ☎ 021 4890800 160 en suite

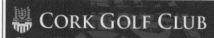
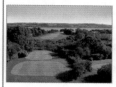
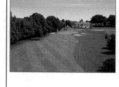
Ireland

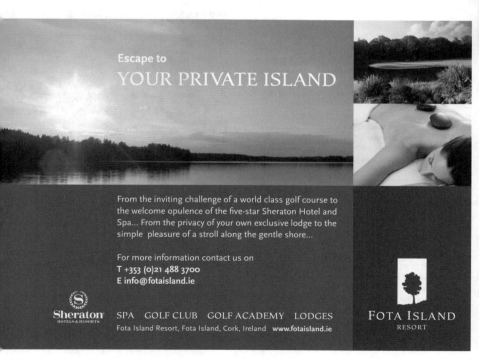

FERMOY
MAP 01 B2

Fermoy Corrin Cross
☎ 025 32694 (office) & 31472 (shop) 📄 025 33072
e-mail: fermoygolfclub@eircom.net
web: www.fermoygolfclub.ie
A mature 18-hole heathland course facing the slopes of Corrin Hill and set in a profusion of natural heather and gorse and bisected by a road. The course commands panoramic views over the plains of East Cork. *18 holes, 5596mtrs, Par 70, SSS 69, Course record 66. Club membership 820.*
Visitors Mon-Fri. Booking required. Dress code. **Societies** Booking required. **Green Fees** €20 per round. **Prof** Brian Moriarty **Course Designer** John Harris **Facilities** ⑪ ⑩ 🍴 🔒 ⬜ 🍴 🛎 🏌 **Location** S of town off N8, signed
Hotel ★★★ CHH Longueville House Hotel, MALLOW ☎ 022 47156 & 47306 📄 022 47459 20 en suite

GLENGARRIFF
MAP 01 B2

Glengarriff
☎ 027 63150 📄 027 63575
Course is surrounded by one of the remaining ancient oak forests of Ireland. The course is set amid mountain scenery of breathtaking beauty, overlooking world renowned Garnish Island and Bantry Bay. *9 holes, 2042metres, Par 66, SSS 62. Club membership 300.*
Visitors Mon-Sun. Booking required Sat-Sun & BHs. Dress code. **Societies** welcome. **Green Fees** not confirmed. ⊚ **Facilities** 🔒 🏌 **Location** On N71
Hotel ★★★ 66% HL Westlodge Hotel, BANTRY ☎ 027 50360 90 en suite

KANTURK
MAP 01 B2

Kanturk Fairyhill
☎ 029 50534 📄 029 20951
Scenic parkland course set in the heart of the Duhallow region with superb mountain views. It provides a good test of skill for golfers of all standards, with tight fairways requiring accurate driving and precise approach shots to small and tricky greens. *18 holes, 5721mtrs, Par 71, SSS 69, Course record 68. Club membership 600.*
Visitors Mon-Sun & BHs. Booking required Fri-Sun & BHs. Dress code. **Societies** Booking required **Green Fees** €25 per round (€30 Sat, Sun & BHs). ⊚ **Course Designer** Richard Barry **Facilities** ⑪ by prior arrangement ⑩ by prior arrangement 🔒 ⬜ 🍴 🛎 🏌 🏌 **Conf** Corporate Hospitality Days **Location** 1.6km SW of Kanturk

KINSALE
MAP 01 B2

Kinsale Farrangalway
☎ 021 4774722 📄 021 4773114
e-mail: office@kinsalegolf.com
web: www.kinsalegolf.com
Set in farmland surrounded by rolling countryside. A stiff yet fair challenge to be enjoyed by all standards of golfers. *Farrangalway: 18 holes, 6043metres, Par 71, SSS 71, Course record 70.*
Ringenane: 9 holes, 4856metres, Par 70, SSS 68. Club membership 800.
Visitors Mon-Sun & BHs. Booking required Sat-Sun & BHs. Dress code. **Societies** booking required. **Green Fees** not confirmed. **Prof** Ger Broderick **Course Designer** Jack Kenneally **Facilities** ⑪ ⑩ 🍴 🔒 ⬜ 🍴 🛎 🏌 🛎 🏌 **Location** Farrangalway N off R607. Ringenane N off R600
Hotel ★★★ 75% HL Trident Hotel, Worlds End, KINSALE ☎ 021 4779300 75 en suite

Old Head
☎ 021 4778444 📄 021 4778022
e-mail: info@oldheadgolf.ie
web: www.oldheadgolflinks.com
Spectacular location on a promontory jutting out into the Atlantic. As well as bringing the sea and cliffs into play, you have to contend with strong prevailing winds - a fine test for serious golfers.

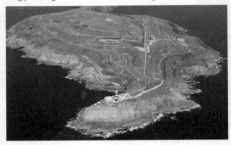

18 holes, 6675meters, Par 72, SSS 73. Club membership 350.
Visitors Mon-Sun & BHs. Booking required. Handicap certificate. Dress code. **Societies** booking required. **Green Fees** not confirmed. **Prof** Danny Brassil **Course Designer** R Kirby/J Carr/P Merrigan/E Hackett **Facilities** ⑪ ⑩ 🍴 🔒 ⬜ 🍴 🛎 🏌 🛎 🏌 **Conf** Corporate Hospitality Days **Location** On R600 towards Cork, signed
Hotel ★★★ 70% HL Blue Haven, 3 Pearse St, KINSALE ☎ 021 4772209 17 en suite

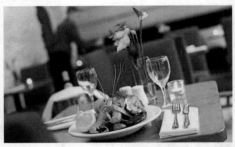

LITTLE ISLAND
MAP 01 B2

Harbour Point Clash Rd
☎ 021 4353094 📄 021 4354408
e-mail: hpoint@iol.ie
18 holes, 5883metres, Par 72, SSS 71, Course record 71.
Course Designer Patrick Merrigan **Location** 8km E of Cork on Rosslare road
Telephone for further details
Hotel ★★★★ 77% HL Silver Springs Moran Hotel, Tivoli, CORK ☎ 021 4507533 109 en suite

MACROOM   MAP 01 B2

Macroom Lackaduve
☎ 026 41072 & 42615 📠 026 41391
e-mail: mcroomgc@iol.ie
18 holes, 5574mtrs, Par 72, SSS 70, Course record 67.
Course Designer Jack Kenneally/Eddie Hackett **Location** Through castle
entrance in town square
Telephone for further details
Hotel ★★★ 78% HL Castle Hotel, Main St, MACROOM ☎ 026 41074
60 en suite

MALLOW   MAP 01 B2

Mallow Ballyellis
☎ 022 21145 📠 022 42501
e-mail: mallowgolfclubmanager@eircom.net
web: www.mallowgolfclub.net
Mallow Golf Club was established in the late 19th century. A well-wooded parkland course overlooking the Blackwater Valley, Mallow is straightforward, but no less a challenge for it. The front nine is by far the longer, but the back nine is demanding in its call for accuracy and the Par 3 18th provides a tough finish.

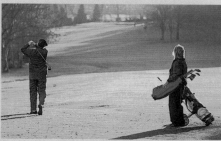

18 holes, 5769mtrs, Par 72, SSS 71, Course record 66.
Club membership 1100.
Visitors Mon-Sun & BHs. Booking required Tue, Wed, Fri-Sun & BHs.
Dress code. **Societies** Booking required **Green Fees** €45 per round
(€50 Sat, Sun & BHs). **Prof** Sean Conway **Course Designer** D W
Wishart **Facilities** ⓘ ⦿ ⓛ ⬛ ⬛ ⬚ ⬛ ⚘ ✪ ✪ ✪ **Leisure** hard tennis
courts, squash. **Location** 1.6km E of Mallow
Hotel ★★★ CHH Longueville House Hotel, MALLOW ☎ 022 47156
& 47306 📠 022 47459 20 en suite

MIDLETON   MAP 01 C2

East Cork Gortacrue
☎ 021 4631687 & 4631273 📠 021 4613695
e-mail: eastcorkgolfclub@eircom.net
web: eastcorkgolfclub.com
A well-wooded course calling for accuracy of shots.
18 holes, 5152mtrs, Par 69, SSS 66, Course record 64.
Club membership 820.
Visitors Mon-Sun & BHs. Booking required Sat. **Societies** Booking
requested **Green Fees** €30 per round (€35 Sat & Sun). **Prof** Don
MacFarlane **Course Designer** E Hackett **Facilities** ⓘ ⦿ ⓛ ⬛ ⬛ ⬚ ⬛
⚘ ✪ **Location** 3km N of Midleton on A626
Hotel ★★★ 79% HL Midleton Park Hotel & Spa, MIDLETON
☎ 021 4631767 40 en suite

Water Rock Water Rock
☎ 021 4613499
e-mail: waterrock@eircom.net
web: www.waterrockgolfcourse.com
18 holes, 6223yds, Par 70.
Course Designer Patrick Merrilas **Location** Next to N25 on outskirts of
Midleton
Telephone for further details
Hotel ★★★ 79% HL Midleton Park Hotel & Spa, MIDLETON
☎ 021 4631767 40 en suite

MITCHELSTOWN   MAP 01 B2

Mitchelstown Limerick Rd
☎ 025 24072 & 087 2650110
e-mail: info@mitchelstown-golf.com
web: www.mitchelstown-golf.com
18 holes, 5493mtrs, Par 71, SSS 70.
Course Designer David Jones **Location** 1km from Mitchelstown
Telephone for further details
Hotel ★★★ CHH Longueville House Hotel, MALLOW ☎ 022 47156
& 47306 📠 022 47459 20 en suite

MONKSTOWN   MAP 01 B2

Monkstown Parkgariffe, Monkstown
☎ 021 4841376
e-mail: office@monkstowngolfclub.com
web: www.monkstowngolfclub.com
Undulating parkland with five tough finishing holes.

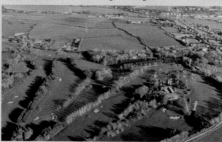

18 holes, 5441mtrs, Par 70, SSS 68, Course record 66.
Club membership 960.
Visitors Mon & Thu-Sun. Booking required Fri-Sun. Handicap certificate.
Dress code. **Societies** Welcome. **Green Fees** €43 per day (€50 Sat &
Sun). **Prof** Batt Murphy **Course Designer** Peter O'Hare & Tom Carey
Facilities ⓘ ⦿ ⓛ ⬛ ⬚ ⬛ ⚘ ✪ ✪ ✪ **Conf** Corporate
Hospitality Days **Location** 0.8km SE of Monkstown
Hotel ★★★★ 73% HL Carrigaline Court Hotel, CARRIGALINE
☎ 021 4852100 91 en suite

OVENS
MAP 01 B2

Lee Valley Golf & Country Club Clashanure
☎ 021 7331721 🖹 021 7331695
e-mail: leevalleygolfclub@eircom.net
web: www.leevalleygcc.ie
18 holes, 5883metres, Par 72, SSS 70, Course record 62.
Course Designer Christy O'Connor **Location** Off N22
Telephone for further details
Hotel ★★★ 78% HL Castle Hotel, Main St, MACROOM ☎ 026 41074
60 en suite

SKIBBEREEN
MAP 01 B2

Skibbereen & West Carbery Licknavar
☎ 028 21227 🖹 028 22994
e-mail: bookings@skibbgolf.com
web: www.skibbgolf.com
Slightly hilly course in scenic location.
18 holes, 5490mtrs, Par 71, SSS 69, Course record 66.
Club membership 700.
Visitors Mon-Sun & BHs. Booking required. **Societies** Booking required
Green Fees €33 per round, Oct-Apr €30. **Course Designer** Jack
Kenneally Ⓦ ⦿ ⓘ ⌨ ♄ ♦ ◊ **Conf** Corporate
Hospitality Days **Location** 1.6km SW on R595
Hotel ★★★ 70% HL Baltimore Harbour Hotel & Leisure Cntr, BALTIMORE
☎ 028 20361 64 en suite

YOUGHAL
MAP 01 C2

Youghal Knockaverry
☎ 024 92787 & 92861 🖹 024 92641
e-mail: youghalgolfclub@eircom.ie
web: www.youghalgolfclub.ie
For many years the host of various Golfing Union championships,
Youghal offers a good test of golf and is well maintained for
year-round play. The Parkland course has recently been extended
with the addition of two new holes. There are panoramic views of
Youghal Bay and the Blackwater estuary.
18 holes, 6175mtrs, Par 72, SSS 72, Course record 68.
Club membership 1050.
Visitors Mon, Tue, Thu-Sun & BHs. Booking required. Handicap
certificate. Dress code. **Societies** Booking required. **Green Fees** €30 per
round (€40 Sat & Sun). **Prof** Liam Burns **Course Designer** Jeff Howes
Golf Design **Facilities** Ⓦ ⦿ ⓘ ⌨ ♄ ♦ ◊ **Conf** Corporate
Hospitality Days **Location** Off N25

CO DONEGAL
(DÚN NA NGALL)

BALLYBOFEY
MAP 01 C5

Ballybofey & Stranorlar Stranorlar
☎ 074 9131093 🖹 074 9130158
18 holes, 5366mtrs, Par 68, SSS 68, Course record 64.
Course Designer P C Carr **Location** 0.4km E of Stranorlar
Telephone for further details

BALLYLIFFIN
MAP 01 C6

Ballyliffin Clonmany
☎ 074 9376119 🖹 074 9376672
e-mail: info@ballyliffingolfclub.com
web: www.ballyliffingolfclub.com
The Old course is a links course with rolling fairways, surrounded by
rolling hills and bounded on one side by the ocean and has received a
facelift from Nick Faldo. The 18-hole Glashedy course offers a modern
championship test.
Old Links: 18 holes, 6039metres, Par 71, SSS 72,
Course record 65.
Glashedy Links: 18 holes, 7135yds, Par 72, SSS 74,
Course record 68. Club membership 1400.
Visitors Mon-Sun & BHs. Booking required. Handicap certificate. Dress
code. **Societies** booking required. **Green Fees** not confirmed. **Prof** John P
Dolan **Course Designer** Nick Faldo/Tom Craddock/Pat Ruddy **Facilities** Ⓦ
⦿ ⓘ ⌨ ♄ ♦ ◊ **Conf** facs Corporate Hospitality Days
Location Off R238

BUNCRANA
MAP 01 C6

Buncrana Railway Rd, Ballymacarry
☎ 074 9362279 074 9320749
e-mail: buncranagc@eircom.net
A nine-hole course with a very challenging Par 3 3rd hole with all
carry out of bounds on either side. Situated on the banks of The White
Strand, overlooking the beautiful Lough Swilly. The 9 hole course offers
a challenge to golfers of all ability.
9 holes, 1969mtrs, Par 62, SSS 60, Course record 59.
Club membership 200.
Visitors Mon-Sun & BHs. Booking required Sat & Sun. **Societies** Booking
required. **Green Fees** €13 per round. ⦿ **Prof** Jim Doherty **Facilities** ⌨
♄ ◊ **Conf** facs

North West Lisfannon, Fahan, Buncrana
☎ 074 9361715 🖹 074 9363284
e-mail: secretary@northwestgolfclub.com
web: www.northwestgolfclub.com
A traditional links course on gently rolling sandy terrain with some
long Par 4s. Good judgement is required on the approaches and the
course offers a satisfying test coupled with undemanding walking.
18 holes, 5457mtrs, Par 70, SSS 70, Course record 64.
Club membership 580.
Visitors Mon-Sun & BHs. Booking required. **Societies** Booking required.
Green Fees €30 per round (€35 Sat & Sun). **Prof** Seamus McBriarty
Course Designer Thompson Davy **Facilities** Ⓦ ⦿ ⓘ ⌨ ♄ ♦
◊ **Location** 1.6km S of Buncrana on R238

BUNDORAN
MAP 01 B5

Bundoran
☎ 071 9841302 📄 071 9842014
e-mail: bundorangolfclub@eircom.net
web: www.bundorangolfclub.com
This popular course, acknowledged as one of the best in the country, runs along the high cliffs above Bundoran beach and has a difficult Par of 70. Designed by Harry Vardon, it offers a challenging game of golf in beautiful surroundings and has been the venue for a number of Irish golf championships.
18 holes, 5688metres, Par 70, SSS 70, Course record 67. Club membership 770.
Visitors Mon-Sun & BHs. Booking required. Handicap certificate. Dress code. **Societies** welcome. **Green Fees** not confirmed. ⊕ **Prof** David T Robinson **Course Designer** Harry Vardon **Facilities** ⚐ 🕳 ♍ 🏌 **Conf** Corporate Hospitality Days **Location** Off Main St onto Sligo-Derry road
Hotel ★★★ 85% HL Sandhouse Hotel, ROSSNOWLAGH
☎ 071 9851777 55 en suite

CRUIT ISLAND (AN CHRUIT)
MAP 01 B5

Cruit Island Kincasslagh
☎ 074 9543296 📄 074 9548028
9 holes, 4833mtrs, Par 68, SSS 66, Course record 62.
Course Designer Michael Doherty **Location** 8km N of Dungloe
Telephone for further details
Hotel ★★★ 72% HL Arnold's Hotel, DUNFANAGHY ☎ 074 9136208
50 en suite

DUNFANAGHY
MAP 01 C6

Dunfanaghy Kill
☎ 074 9136335 📄 074 9136684
e-mail: dunfanaghygolf@eircom.net
web: ww.dunfanaghygolfclub.com
Overlooking Sheephaven Bay, the course has a flat central area with three difficult streams to negotiate. At the Port-na-Blagh end there are five marvellous holes, including one across the beach, while at the Horn Head end, the last five holes are a test for any golfer.
18 holes, 5247mtrs, Par 68, SSS 66, Course record 63. Club membership 335.
Visitors Mon-Sun & BHs. Booking required Wed, Fri-Sun & BHs. Dress code. **Societies** Booking required. **Green Fees** €30 per round (€40 Sat & Sun).
Course Designer Harry Vardon **Facilities** ⚐ 🕳 ♍ 🏌 **Conf** facs **Location** 30m W of Letterkenny on N56
Hotel ★★★ 72% HL Arnold's Hotel, DUNFANAGHY ☎ 074 9136208
50 en suite

GREENCASTLE
MAP 01 C6

Greencastle Geencastle
☎ 074 9381013 📄 074 9381015
e-mail: info@greencastlegolfclub.net
web: ww.greencastlegolfclub.com
A links course along the shores of Lough Foyle, surrounded by rocky headlands and sandy beaches.
18 holes, 5334mtrs, Par 70, SSS 68, Course record 65. Club membership 750.
Visitors Mon-Sat. Booking required. Dress code. **Societies** Booking required **Green Fees** €25 per day, €20 per round (€40/€30 Sat, Sun & BHs). **Course Designer** E Hackett **Facilities** ⚐ 🕳 ♍ 🏌

GWEEDORE (GAOTH DOBHAIR)
MAP 01 B6

Gweedore Derrybeg
☎ 075 31140
With breath taking scenery, this 9-hole links course provides plenty of challenge with two subtle Par 3s and the Par 5 5th/14th at 556yards into the prevailing west wind is a monster.
9 holes, 5699mtrs, Par 71, SSS 68. Club membership 175.
Visitors Mon, Tue & Thu-Sat. Booking required. Handicap certificate.
Societies Booking required. **Green Fees** €20 per 18 holes. ⊕ **Facilities** ⚐ 🕳 ♍ 🏌 **Location** 37m NW of Letterkenny on N56
Hotel ★★★ 65% HL Ostan Na Rosann, Mill Rd, DUNGLOE
☎ 074 9522444 48 en suite

LETTERKENNY
MAP 01 C5

Letterkenny Barnhill
☎ 074 9121150 📄 074 9121175
e-mail: letterkennygolfclub@eircom.net
The fairways are wide and generous, but the rough, when you find it, is short, tough and mean. The flat and untiring terrain on the shores of Lough Swilly provides good holiday golf. The first 11 holes have been redesigned to incorporate 7 new lakes and 5 new greens and bunkers on all holes. The next 7 holes have also been redesigned with bunkers and fairway mounding and 2 new greens
18 holes, 5705mtrs, Par 72, SSS 71, Course record 65. Club membership 700.
Visitors Mon-Sun & BHs. Booking required Sat, Sun & BHs. Dress code. **Societies** Booking required **Green Fees** Phone. **Prof** Seamus Duffy **Course Designer** Eddie Hacket **Facilities** ⊕ 🍴 ⚐ 🕳 ♍ 🏌 **Conf** facs Corporate Hospitality Days **Location** 3km NE of town on R245

MOVILLE
MAP 01 C6

Redcastle Redcastle
☎ 074 9385555 📄 074 9385444
e-mail: info@carltonredcastlehotel.com
web: www.carltonredcastlehotel.com
A testing course with lush greens and mature woodland, enjoying a picturesque setting on the shores of Loch Foyle. The lush greens and mature woodland
9 holes, 2846mtrs, Par 35. Club membership 200.
Visitors Mon-Fri. **Societies** Booking required **Green Fees** €20. **Prof** James Gallagher **Facilities** ⊕ 🍴 ⚐ 🕳 ♍ 🏌 **Leisure** heated indoor swimming pool, gymnasium. **Conf** facs Corporate Hospitality Days **Location** 6km SW on R238
Hotel ★★ 65% HL Malin Hotel, Malin Town, INISHOWEN ☎ 074 9370606
18 en suite

NARIN (NARAN)
MAP 01 B5

Narin & Portnoo
☎ 074 9545107 📄 074 9545994
e-mail: narinportnoo@eircom.net
web: www.narinportnoogolfclub.ie
18 holes, 5322mtrs, Par 69, SSS 68, Course record 63.
Course Designer Leo Wallace/Hugh McNeill **Location** Off R261
Telephone for further details
Hotel ★★★ 65% HL Ostan Na Rosann, Mill Rd, DUNGLOE
☎ 074 9522444 48 en suite

Ireland

PORTSALON — MAP 01 C6

Portsalon
☎ 074 9159459 📠 074 9159919
e-mail: portsalongolfclub@eircom.net
web: www.portsalongolfclub.ie
Another course blessed by nature. The golden beaches of
Ballymastocker Bay lie at one end, while the beauty of Lough Swilly
and the Inishowen Peninsula beyond is a distracting but pleasant
feature to the west. Situated on the Fanad Peninsula, this lovely links
course provides untiring holiday golf at its best.
18 holes, 6185mtrs, Par 72, SSS 72, Course record 71.
Club membership 500.
Visitors Mon-Sun & BHs. Booking required. Handicap certificate. Dress
code. **Societies** Booking required. **Green Fees** €40 per round (€50 Sat,
Sun & BHs). **Prof** Seamus Clinton **Course Designer** Pat Ruddy **Facilities**
⑪ ⑩ ⅃ ⫐ ⊑ ⅊ ⚏ ⚑ ✔ **Conf** Corporate Hospitality Days **Location** Off
R246
Hotel ★★★ 79% HL Fort Royal Hotel, Fort Royal, RATHMULLAN
☎ 074 9158100 11 en suite 4 annexe en suite

RATHMULLAN — MAP 01 C6

Otway Saltpans
☎ 074 918319
e-mail: otway_golf_club@iolfree.ie
One of the oldest courses in Ireland, created in 1861 by British military
personnel as a recreational facility.
9 holes, 3872mtrs, Par 64, SSS 60, Course record 60.
Club membership 112.
Visitors Mon-Sun & BHs. Booking required. Dress code. **Societies** Booking
required. **Green Fees** €15 per day (€20 Sat & Sun). ⊛ **Facilities** ⅊ ⫐
Conf Corporate Hospitality Days **Location** In Rathmullan, turn left at Mace
convenience store, head for Knockalla coast Rd. 2m signed
Hotel ★★★ 79% HL Fort Royal Hotel, Fort Royal, RATHMULLAN
☎ 074 9158100 11 en suite 4 annexe en suite

ROSEPENNA (MACHAIR LOISCTHE) — MAP 01 C6

Rosapenna Downings
☎ 074 9155301 📠 074 9155128
e-mail: rosapenna@tinet.ie
web: www.rosapenna.ie
Dramatic links course offering a challenging round. Originally designed
by Tom Morris and later modified by James Braid and Harry Vardon, it
includes features such as bunkers in mid-fairway. The best part of the
links runs in the low valley along the ocean.
Old Tom Morris: 18 holes, 5734mtrs, Par 70, SSS 71.
Sandy Hills Links: 18 holes, 5812metres, Par 71.
Club membership 400.
Visitors Mon-Sun & BHs. **Societies** Booking required **Green Fees** Old Tom
Morris: €45 per round (€50 Sat, Sun & BHs); Sandy Hills Links: €60 per
round. **Prof** Brian Patterson **Course Designer** Old Tom Morris **Facilities**
⑪ ⑩ ⅃ ⫐ ⊑ ⅊ ⚏ ⚑ ✔ ⚘ ✔ **Leisure** hard tennis courts, heated
indoor swimming pool. **Conf** facs **Location** NE of village off R248
Hotel ★★★ 72% HL Arnold's Hotel, DUNFANAGHY ☎ 074 9136208
30 en suite

CO DUBLIN

BALBRIGGAN — MAP 01 D4

Balbriggan Blackhall
☎ 01 8412229 📠 01 8413927
e-mail: balbriggangolfclub@eircom.net
web: www.balbriggangolfclub.com
A parkland course with great variations and good views of the Mourne
and Cooley mountains.
18 holes, 5922mtrs, Par 71, SSS 71. Club membership 750.
Visitors Mon-Sat & BHs. Booking required Mon-Sat. Dress code.
Societies Booking required. **Green Fees** Phone. **Prof** Nigel Howley
Course Designer Paramoir **Facilities** ⑪ ⑩ ⅃ ⫐ ⊑ ⅊ ⚏ ⚘ ✔
Location 1km S of Balbriggan on N1
Hotel ★★★ 70% HL Boyne Valley Hotel & Country Club, Stameen, Dublin
Rd, DROGHEDA ☎ 041 983 7737 73 en suite

BALLYBOUGHAL — MAP 01 D4

Hollywood Lakes
☎ 01 8433406 📠 01 8433002
e-mail: hollywoodlakesgc@eircom.net
web: www.hollywoodlakesgolfclub.com

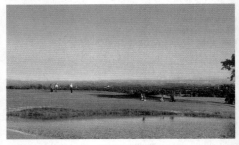

18 holes, 6246mtrs, Par 72, SSS 72, Course record 67.
Course Designer Mel Flanagan **Location** N of village on R108
Telephone for further details

BRITTAS — MAP 01 D4

Slade Valley Lynch Park
☎ 01 4582183 & 4582739 📠 01 4582784
e-mail: sladevalleygc@eircom.net
web: www.sladevalleygolfclub.ie
This is a course for a relaxing game, being fairly easy and in pleasant
surroundings.
18 holes, 5388mtrs, Par 69, SSS 68, Course record 65.
Club membership 954.
Visitors Mon-Fri. Booking required. Dress code. **Societies** Booking
required. **Green Fees** €30 per round (€35 Fri, €40 Sat & Sun). **Prof** John
Dignam **Course Designer** W Sullivan & D O Brien **Facilities** ⑪ ⑩ ⅃ ⫐ ⊑
⅊ ⚏ ⚑ ⚘ ✔ **Location** Off N81

ASTLEKNOCK MAP 01 D4

lm Green

☎ 01 8200797 📠 01 8226668
e-mail: elmgreen@golfdublin.com
web: www.golfdublin.com

ocated a short distance from Dublin, beside Phoenix Park, with a
ne layout, tricky greens and year round playability.
*8 holes, 5300mtrs, Par 71, SSS 66, Course record 65.
Club membership 650.*
Visitors Mon-Sat & BHs. Booking required. **Societies** Booking required.
Green Fees €20 per round (€36 Sat, Sun & BHs). **Prof** Arnold
O'Connor/Paul McGavan **Course Designer** Eddie Hackett **Facilities** ⑪
🍴 🗦 🖳 🖴 ⛳ ✦ 🛒 ✦ ✦ **Leisure** pitch and putt course. **Conf** facs
orporate Hospitality Days **Location** Off N3
otel ★★★ 74% HL Finnstown Country House Hotel, Newcastle Rd,
ucan, DUBLIN ☎ 01 6010700 25 en suite 28 annexe en suite

uttrellstown Castle Dublin15

☎ 01 8089988 📠 01 8089989
mail: golf@luttrellstown.ie
eb: www.luttrellstown.ie

t in the grounds of the magnificent 560-acre Luttrellstown Castle
tate, this championship course has been re-designed to enhance the
olfing experience. The new layout respects and retains the integrity
the mature and ancient parkland. The course is renowned for the
ality of its greens and facilities.
*8 holes, 6378metres, Par 72, SSS 73, Course record 66.
lub membership 400.*

Visitors Mon-Sun & BHs. Booking required. Dress code. **Societies** booking
required. **Prof** Edward Doyle **Course Designer** Donald Steele & Tom
Mackenzie **Facilities** ⑪ 🍴 🗦 🖳 ⛳ 🖴 ⛳ ✦ 🛒 ✦ 🛒 ✦ **Leisure** fishing,
clay shooting. **Conf** facs Corporate Hospitality Days **Location** W of town
off R121
Hotel ★★★ 74% HL Finnstown Country House Hotel, Newcastle Rd,
Lucan, DUBLIN ☎ 01 6010700 25 en suite 28 annexe en suite

CLOGHRAN MAP 01 D4

Forrest Little

☎ 01 8401183 & 8401763 📠 01 8908499
e-mail: margaret@forrestlittle.ie
web: www.forrestlittle.ie

A well-manicured and mature parkland with many water features, large
sand based greens and undulating fairways, playable all year.
*18 holes, 5902mtrs, Par 71, SSS 72, Course record 68.
Club membership 1000.*
Visitors Mon-Fri. Dress code. **Societies** Booking required. **Green Fees**
€50 per 18 holes. **Prof** Tony Judd **Course Designer** Mr Hawtree snr
Facilities ⑪ 🍴 🗦 🖳 🖴 ⛳ 🖴 ⛳ ✦ 🛒 ✦ **Location** N of Dublin Airport
off R132

Deer Park Hotel, Golf and Spa

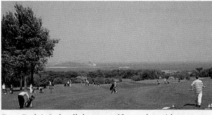
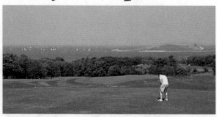

Deer Park is Ireland's largest golf complex with a vast array of golf courses that offer great golf for everyone, including
the guests of Deer Park hotel. It is set in 450 acres of tranquil parkland overlooking the sea and near the picturesque
village of Howth.

The selection of golf is varied. The main course, the Deerpark 18 hole course is in a wonderful parkland setting.
Alongside this are two excellent 9-hole courses, the Grace O'Malley and the St. Fintans nine hole courses, that can
also be played as a second 18-hole course. Deer Park also boasts a full-length 12 holes, Par 3 short course. All of this is
crowned by a championship 18-hole Pitch & Putt course and a large putting green.

Close to Dublin city, with all the amenities of Howth village, Deer Park Hotel offers the best location in Ireland for your
golf vacation.

Deer Park Hotel & Golf Courses Howth, Co. Dublin
Telephone: 00 353 1 832 2624 or 00353 1 832 3489   **Fax:** 00 353 1 839 2405
General Managers: David & Antoinette Tighe
Email: sales@deerpark.iol.ie   **Website:** www.deerpark-hotel.ie

DONABATE
MAP 01 D4

Balcarrick Corballis
☎ 01 8436957 📄 01 8436228
e-mail: balcarr@iol.ie
web: www.balcarrickgolfclub.com
Splendid 18-hole semi-links course with many challenging holes,
located close to the sea. A strong prevailing wind often plays a big part
on every hole and many of the Par 3s are fronted by water.
18 holes, 6273mtrs, Par 73, SSS 71. Club membership 750.
Visitors Mon-Sun & BHs. Booking required Thu, Sat, Sun & BHs. Handicap
certificate. Dress code. **Societies** Booking required **Green Fees** Phone.
Prof Stephen Rayfus **Course Designer** Barry Langan **Facilities** ⓐ ⓘⓒⓛ ⓛ
ⓓⓣ ⓛ ⓐ **Location** Off R126
Hotel ★★★ 72% HL Deer Park Hotel, Golf & Spa, HOWTH ☎ 01 8322624
80 en suite

See advert on page 431

Donabate Balcarrick
☎ 01 8436346 📄 01 8434488
e-mail: info@donabategolfclub.com
web: www.donabategolfclub.com
All greens are USGA standard and water comes into play on
eight holes. Sand-based course playable all year.
27 holes, 6068mtrs, Par 72, SSS 73, Course record 66.
Club membership 1200.
Visitors Mon-Sun & BHs. Booking required Wed, Sat & Sun. Dress code.
Societies Booking required **Green Fees** €40 (€50 Sat & Sun), winter
€35/€40. **Prof** Hugh Jackson **Course Designer** Pat Suttle **Facilities** ⓐ
ⓘⓒⓛ ⓛ ⓓⓣ ⓛ ⓐ ⓕ ⓐ **Conf** Corporate Hospitality Days **Location**
E of town off R126
Hotel ★★★ 72% HL Deer Park Hotel, Golf & Spa, HOWTH ☎ 01 8322624
80 en suite

Island Corballis
☎ 01 8436205 📄 01 8436860
e-mail: info@theislandgolfclub.com
web: www.theislandgolfclub.com

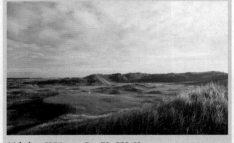

18 holes, 6206mtrs, Par 71, SSS 63.
Course Designer Martin Hawtree **Location** Off R126
Telephone for further details
Hotel ★★★ 72% HL Deer Park Hotel, Golf & Spa, HOWTH
☎ 01 8322624 80 en suite

Turvey Golf Club & Hotel Turvey Av
☎ 01 8435169 📄 01 8435179
e-mail: turveygc@eircom.net
web: www.turveygolfclub.com
A mature parkland course with oak trees over 220 years old. A test of
golf for all levels of golfer.
18 holes, 6068mtrs, Par 71, SSS 72, Course record 64.
Club membership 500.
Visitors Mon-Sun & BHs. Booking required. Dress code. **Societies** Booking
required. **Green Fees** €40 per 18 holes, €20 per 9 holes (€45/€25 Sat &
Sun). **Course Designer** P McGurk **Facilities** ⓐ ⓘⓒⓛ ⓛ ⓓⓣ ⓛ ◇ ⓕ ⓛ
ⓕ ⓕ **Conf** facs Corporate Hospitality Days **Location** M1, 1st junct N after
Dublin airport, 1m on N1 Turvey signed on right
Hotel ★★★ 72% HL Deer Park Hotel, Golf & Spa, HOWTH ☎ 01 8322624
80 en suite

DUBLIN
MAP 01 D4

The Carrickmines Carrickmines
☎ 01 2955972
Meadowland and partly hilly gorseland course.
9 holes, 5554mtrs, Par 71, SSS 69. Club membership 600.
Visitors Mon-Sun & BHs. Booking required. Dress code.Booking required
Green Fees Phone. ⓢ **Facilities** ⓓⓣ ⓛ ⓕ **Location** 11km SE of city
centre off N11

Castle Woodside Dr, Rathfarnham
☎ 01 4904207 📄 01 4920264
e-mail: office@castlegc.ie
web: www.castlegc.ie
A tight, tree-lined parkland course which is very highly regarded by all
who play there.
18 holes, 5732mtrs, Par 70, SSS 71, Course record 66.
Club membership 1350.
Visitors Mon-Fri. Booking required. Handicap certificate. Dress code.
Societies Booking required. **Green Fees** €85 per round. **Prof** David
Kinsella **Course Designer** Harry Colt **Facilities** ⓐ ⓘⓒⓛ ⓛ ⓓⓣ ⓛ ⓐ ⓕ
Location Off Dodder Park Rd

Clontarf Donnycarney House, Malahide Rd
☎ 01 8331892 & 8331520 📄 01 8331933
e-mail: info.cgc@indigo.ie
web: clontarfgolfclub.ie

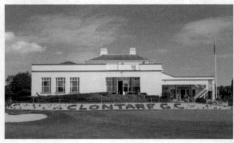

The nearest golf course to Dublin city, with a historic building as a
clubhouse, Clontarf is a parkland type course bordered on one side
by a railway line. Although a relatively short course, its narrow fairways
and punitive rough call for accuracy off the tee and will test players'
golfing skill. There are several challenging holes including the 12th,
which involves playing over a pond and a quarry. *Continued*

18 holes, 5317metres, Par 69, SSS 68, Course record 64.
Club membership 1150.
Visitors Mon-Sun & BHs. Booking required. Dress code. **Societies** booking required. **Green Fees** not confirmed. ⊛ **Prof** Mark Callan **Course Designer** Harry Colt **Facilities** ⓣ ⓞ ⓛ ⓛ ⓓ ⓣ ⓛ ⓔ ☂ ✔ **Leisure** bowling green, snooker room, golf teaching by pro. **Conf** facs Corporate Hospitality Days **Location** 4km NE of city centre via Fairview

Corrstown Corrstown, Kilsallaghan
☎ 01 8640533 & 8640534 📄 01 8640537
e-mail: info@corrstowngolfclub.com
web: www.corrstowngolfclub.com
The 18-hole course has a small river meandering through, coming into play at several holes culminating in a challenging island green finish. Orchard course has mature trees and rolling pastureland offering golfers a relaxing enjoyable game.
River Course: 18 holes, 6077mtrs, Par 72, SSS 71,
Course record 69.
Orchard Course: 9 holes, 2792metres, Par 35, SSS 69.
Club membership 1050.
Visitors Mon-Fri. Booking required. Dress code. **Societies** Booking required. **Green Fees** €50 per round. Orchard course €25 (€60/€30 at & Sun). **Prof** Pat Gittens **Course Designer** Eddie Connaughton **Facilities** ⓣ ⓞ ⓛ ⓓ ⓣ ⓛ ⓔ ✔ ☂ ✔ **Location** 10km N of city centre via St Margarets

Edmondstown Edmondstown Rd, Edmondstown
☎ 01 4931082 & 4932461 📄 01 4933152
e-mail: info@edmondstowngolfclub.ie
web: www.edmondstowngolfclub.ie
A popular and testing parkland course situated at the foot of the Dublin Mountains in the suburbs of the city. Now completely renovated and redesigned. All greens are now sand based to the highest standard. An attractive stream flows in front of the 4th and 6th greens calling for an accurate approach shot. The Par 3 17th will test the best golfers and the 5th and 12th require thoughtful club selection to the green.

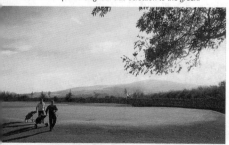

18 holes, 6011mtrs, Par 71, SSS 73, Course record 66.
Club membership 750.
Visitors Mon, Thu-Sat & BHs. Booking required Sat & BHs. Dress code. **Societies** Booking Required **Green Fees** €55 per round (€65 Sat). **Prof** Gareth McShea **Course Designer** McEvoy/Cooke **Facilities** ⓣ ⓞ ⓛ ⓓ ⓛ ⓔ ☂ ✔ ☂ ✔ **Conf** facs Corporate Hospitality Days **Location** M50 Junct 12
Hotel ★★★ 74% HL Jurys Montrose Hotel, Stillorgan Rd, DUBLIN ☎ 01 2693311 178 en suite

Elm Park Golf & Sports Club Nutley House, Nutley Ln, Donnybrook
☎ 01 2693438 📄 01 2694505
e-mail: office@elmparkgolfclub.ie
web: elmparkgolfclub.ie
Interesting parkland course requiring a degree of accuracy, particularly as half of the holes involve crossing the stream.
18 holes, 5380mtrs, Par 69, SSS 69, Course record 64.
Club membership 1900.
Visitors Mon-Sun & BHs. Booking required. **Societies** Booking required **Green Fees** Phone. **Prof** Seamus Green **Course Designer** Paytrick Merrigan **Facilities** ⓣ ⓞ ⓛ ⓓ ⓣ ⓛ ⓔ ☂ ✔ ☂ ✔ **Leisure** hard and grass tennis courts. **Location** 5km SE of city centre off N11

Hollystown Hollystown
☎ 01 8207444 📄 01 8207447
e-mail: info@hollystown.com
web: www.hollystown.com
Red/Yellow: 18 holes, 5829yds, Par 70, SSS 69.
Yellow/Blue: 18 holes, 6216yds, Par 71, SSS 69.
Blue/Red: 18 holes, 6201yds, Par 71, SSS 69.
Course Designer Eddie Hackett **Location** 8m off N3 Dublin-Cavan road at Mulhuddart or off the N2 Dublin-Ashbourne road at Ward
Telephone for further details
Hotel BUD Travelodge Dublin Castleknock, Auburn Av Roundabout, Navan Rd, ☎ 08700 850 950 100 en suite

Howth Carrickbrack Rd, Sutton
☎ 01 8323055 📄 01 8321793
e-mail: secretary@howthgolfclub.ie
web: www.howthgolfclub.ie
A hilly heathland course with scenic views of Dublin Bay. A good challenge to the novice or expert golfer.
18 holes, 5618mtrs, Par 72, SSS 69.
Club membership 1200.
Visitors Mon, Tue & Thu-Sun. Booking required Wed, Sat & Sun. Handicap certificate. Dress code. **Societies** Booking required **Green Fees** €50 per day. **Prof** John McGuirk **Course Designer** James Braid **Facilities** ⓣ by prior arrangement ⓞ by prior arrangement ⓛ ⓓ ⓣ ⓛ ⓔ ☂ ✔ ☂ ✔ **Conf** facs Corporate Hospitality Days **Location** 14.5km NE of city

Milltown Lower Churchtown Rd
☎ 01 4976090 📄 01 4976008
e-mail: info@milltowngolfclub.ie
web: www.milltowngolfclub.ie.
Level parkland three miles from Dublin City Centre.
18 holes, 5638mtrs, Par 71, SSS 70, Course record 64.
Club membership 1400.
Visitors Mon, Thu & Fri. Booking required. Handicap certificate. Dress code. **Societies** Booking required. **Green Fees** €85 per 18 holes. **Prof** John Harnett **Course Designer** Freddie Davis **Facilities** ⓣ ⓞ ⓛ ⓓ ⓣ ⓛ ⓔ ☂ ✔ ✔

Newlands Clondalkin
☎ 01 4593157 & 4593498 📄 01 4593498
e-mail: info@newlandsgolfclub.com
web: www.newlandsgolfclub.com
Mature trees model and soften the landscape of this parkland course once the home of the Lord Chief Justice of ireland.
18 holes, 5982mtrs, Par 71, SSS 70.
Club membership 1000.

Continued

Ireland

Visitors Mon, Thu & Fri. Booking required. Dress code. **Societies** Booking required **Green Fees** €55 per round. **Prof** Karl O'Donnell **Course Designer** James Braid **Facilities** ⓦ ⓘ ⓛ ⌂ ⍩ ⚑ ⍨ ⚓ ⚴ ⛳ ✦ ⚇
Hotel ★★★ 74% HL Lynch Green Isle Hotel, Naas Rd, Newlands Cross, Naas Rd, DUBLIN 22 ☎ 01 4593406 240 en suite

Rathfarnham Newtown
☎ 01 4931201 & 4931561 📠 01 4931561
e-mail: rgc@oceanfree.net
Parkland course designed by John Jacobs in 1962.
14 holes, 5815mtrs, Par 71, SSS 70, Course record 69.
Club membership 685.
Visitors Mon, Wed-Fri. Booking required. Dress code. **Societies** Booking required **Green Fees** €40 (€40 per 18 holes. ⊛ **Prof** Brian O'Hara **Course Designer** John Jacobs **Facilities** ⓦ ⓛ ⌂ ⍩ ⚑ ⚓ ⚴ ✦ **Location** 5km S of city centre off N81

Royal Dublin North Bull Island Reserve, Dollymount
☎ 01 8336346 📠 01 8336504
e-mail: info@theroyaldublingolfclub.com
web: www.theroyaldublingolfclub.com
A popular course with visitors, for its design subtleties, the condition of the links and the friendly atmosphere. Founded in 1885, the club moved to its present site in 1889 and received its Royal designation in 1891. A notable former club professional was Christy O'Connor, who was appointed in 1959 and immediately made his name. Along with its many notable holes, Royal Dublin has a fine and testing finish. The 18th is a sharp dog-leg Par 4, with out of bounds along the right-hand side. The decision to try the long carry over the 'garden' is one many visitors have regretted.
18 holes, 6297mtrs, Par 72, SSS 74, Course record 63.
Club membership 1250.
Visitors Mon, Tue, Thu and Fri. Booking required. Handicap certificate. Dress code. **Societies** Booking required. **Green Fees** €150 per round. **Prof** Leonard Owens **Course Designer** H S Colt **Facilities** ⓦ ⓘ ⓛ ⌂ ⍩ ⚑ ⚓ ⚴ ⛳ ⚇ **Conf** facs Corporate Hospitality Days
Location 5.5km NE of city centre
Hotel ✉ Longfield's Hotel, Fitzwilliam St Lower, DUBLIN 2 ☎ 01 6761367 26 en suite

St Margaret's Golf & Country Club St Margaret's
☎ 01 8640400 📠 01 8640408
e-mail: reservations@stmargaretsgolf.com
web: www.stmargaretsgolf.com
A championship standard course which measures nearly 7,000 yards off the back tees, but flexible teeing offers a fairer challenge to the middle and high handicap golfer. The modern design makes wide use of water hazards and mounding. The Par 5 8th hole is set to become notorious - featuring lakes to the left and right of the tee and a third lake in front of the green. Ryder Cup player, Sam Torrance, has described the 18th as 'possibly the strongest and most exciting in the world'.
18 holes, 6325metres, Par 73, SSS 73, Course record 69.
Club membership 260.
Visitors Mon-Sun & BHs. Booking required. Dress code.
Societies booking required. **Green Fees** not confirmed. **Prof** John Kelly **Course Designer** Craddock/Ruddy **Facilities** ⓦ ⓘ ⓛ ⌂ ⍩ ⚴ ⚓ ⚇ ⛳ ✦ **Location** 9km N of city centre off R122

Stackstown Kellystown Rd, Rathfarnham
☎ 01 4942338 & 4941993 📠 01 4933934
e-mail: stackstowngc@eircom.net
web: stackstowngolfclub.com
Pleasant course in the foothills of the Dublin mountains, affording breathtaking views of Dublin city and bay. Mature woodland borders every hole and premium is placed on accuracy off the tee. In 1999 the course was remodelled and the mountain streams which run through the course were harnessed to bring them into play and provide attractive on-course water features.
18 holes, 5625mtrs, Par 72, SSS 72, Course record 68.
Club membership 1092.
Visitors Mon-Sun & BHs. Booking required. **Societies** Booking required **Green Fees** €35 (€45 Sun). ⊛ **Prof** Michael Kavanagh **Course Designer** Shaftrey **Facilities** ⓦ ⓘ ⓛ ⌂ ⍩ ⚑ ⚓ ⚴ ⛳ ✦ **Conf** facs Corporate Hospitality Days **Location** 9km S of city centre. M50 junct 13, signs for Rathfarnham, 3rd lights left for Leopardstown, next lights follow road under M50, club 300 metres
Hotel ★★★ 74% HL Jurys Montrose Hotel, Stillorgan Rd, DUBLIN ☎ 01 2693311 178 en suite

DUN LAOGHAIRE   MAP 01 D4

Dun Laoghaire Eglinton Park, Tivoli Rd
☎ 01 2803916 📠 01 2804868
e-mail: dlgc@iol.ie
web: www.dunlaoghairegolfclub.ie
18 holes, 5313mtrs, Par 69, SSS 68, Course record 63.
Course Designer Harry Colt **Location** 1.2km from town centre port
Telephone for further details

HOWTH   MAP 01 D4

Deer Park Hotel, Golf & Spa D13
☎ 01 8322624 📠 01 8392405
e-mail: sales@deerpark.iol.ie
web: www.deerpark-hotel.ie

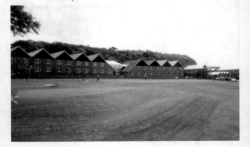

St Fintans: 9 holes, 3084metres, Par 37.
Deer Park: 18 holes, 6245metres, Par 72.
Grace O'Malley: 9 holes, 2862metres, Par 35. Short
Course: 12 holes, 1655metres, Par 36.
Course Designer Fred Hawtree **Location** "14.5km NE of city centre, off coast road 0.8km before Howth Harbour"
Telephone for further details
Hotel ★★★ 72% HL Deer Park Hotel, Golf & Spa, HOWTH ☎ 01 8322624 80 en suite

See advert on page 431

Ireland

CHAMPIONSHIP COURSE
CO DUBLIN — PORTMARNOCK

THE LINKS

Map 01 D4

Strand Road, Portmarnock
☎ 01 8462968 📄 01 8462601
e-mail: **emer@portmarnockgolfclub.ie**
web: **www.portmarnockgolfclub.ie**
Old Course: 18 holes, 6567metres, Par 72, SSS 73.
New Course: 9 holes, 3082metres, Par 37.
Club membership 1100.
Visitors booking required. Handicap certificate. Dress code. **Societies** booking required.
Green Fees Phone. **Prof** Joey Purcell
Course Designer W Pickeman **Facilities** ⑪
🍴 by prior arrangement 🏠 🖥 🍷 ⚒ 🏖 🏪 ♿ ✂
🚗 ✂ **Location** S of town off R106

Universally acknowledged as one of the truly great links courses, The Links has hosted many great events from the British Amateur Championships of 1949 and the Canada Cup in 1960, to 12 stagings of the revised Irish Open. Founded in 1894, the serpentine championship course offers a classic challenge: surrounded by water on three sides, no two successive holes play in the same direction. Unlike many courses that play nine out and nine home, The Links demands a continual awareness of wind direction. Extraordinary holes include the 14th, which Henry Cotton regarded as the best hole in golf; the 15th, which Arnold Palmer regards as the best Par 3 in the world; and the 5th, regarded as the best on the course by the late Harry Bradshaw. Bradshaw was for 40 years The Link's golf professional and runner-up to AD Locke in the 1949 British Open, playing his ball from an empty bottle of stout.

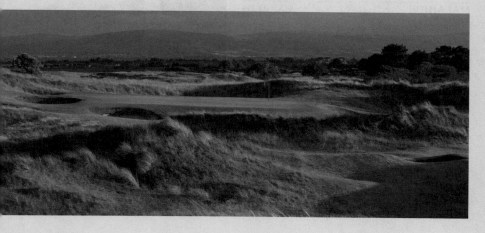

KILLINEY   MAP 01 D4

Killiney Ballinclea Rd
☎ 01 2852823 📄 01 2852861
e-mail: killineygolfclub@eircom.net
9 holes, 5655mtrs, Par 70, SSS 70.
Telephone for further details
Hotel ★★★★ 72% HL Fitzpatrick Castle Hotel, KILLINEY ☎ 01 2305400
113 en suite

LUCAN   MAP 01 D4

Hermitage Ballydowd
☎ 01 6268491 📄 01 6238881
e-mail: hermitagegolf@eircom.net
web: www.hermitagegolf.ie
Part level, part undulating course bordered by the River Liffey and
offering some surprises.
18 holes, 6034mtrs, Par 71, SSS 71.
Club membership 1100.
Visitors Mon, Thu & Fri. Booking required. Handicap certificate. Dress code.
Societies Booking required. **Green Fees** €80 per round. **Prof** Simon
Byrne **Course Designer** J McKenna **Facilities** ⑪ ⑩ 🐛 ⌨ 🏐 🏌 🛒 🍴 🏌
🏌 **Conf** Corporate Hospitality Days **Location** On N4
Hotel ★★★ 74% HL Finnstown Country House Hotel, Newcastle Rd,
Lucan, DUBLIN ☎ 01 6010700 25 en suite 28 annexe en suite

Lucan Celbridge Rd
☎ 01 6282106 📄 01 6282929
e-mail: luncangolf@eircom.net
web: lucangolfclub.ie
Founded in 1897 as a nine-hole course and extended to 18 holes
in 1988, Lucan involves playing over a lane which bisects the 1st
and 7th holes. The front nine is undulating while the back nine is flatter
and features water hazards and a 531-metre Par 5 18th hole.
18 holes, 5958mtrs, Par 71, SSS 71, Course record 67.
Club membership 920.
Visitors Mon, Tue & Fri. Dress code. **Societies** Booking required. **Green
Fees** €45 per round. **Course Designer** Eddie Hackett **Facilities** ⑪ ⑩ 🐛
⌨ 🏐 🏌 🍴 🏌 **Location** W of town towards Celbridge
Hotel ★★★ 67% HL Lucan Spa Hotel, LUCAN ☎ 01 6280494 71 rms
(61 en suite)

MALAHIDE   MAP 01 D4

Malahide Beechwood, The Grange
☎ 01 8461611 📄 01 8461270
e-mail: manager@malahidegolfclub.ie
web: www.malahidegolfclub.ie

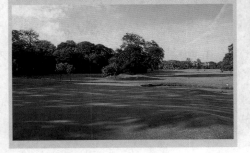

PORTMARNOCK   MAP 01 D4

Portmarnock see page 435
Hotel ★★★★ HL Portmarnock Hotel & Golf Links, Strand Rd,
PORTMARNOCK ☎ 01 8460611 98 en suite

Portmarnock Hotel & Golf Links Strand Rd
☎ 01 8460611 📄 01 8462442
e-mail: golfres@portmarnock.com
web: www.portmarnock.com
This links course makes full use of the dunes and natural terrain to
provide an authentic links layout. The elevated tees and greens, blind
approaches and doglegs - not to mention sea breezes, will keep
the golfer thinking through every round. Gently undulating fairways
leading to large fast greens must be negotiated through 98 strategically
placed bunkers, while hillocks, wild grasses and gorse await wayward
shots.
18 holes, 5992metres, Par 71, SSS 72, Course record 67.
Visitors Mon-Sun & BHs. Dress code. **Societies** booking required. **Green
Fees** not confirmed. **Course Designer** Bernhard Langer **Facilities** ⑪
⑩ 🐛 ⌨ 🏐 🏌 🛒 🏌 🏌 **Leisure** sauna, gymnasium. **Conf** facs
Corporate Hospitality Days
Hotel ★★★★ HL Portmarnock Hotel & Golf Links, Strand Rd,
PORTMARNOCK ☎ 01 8460611 98 en suite

RATHCOOLE   MAP 01 D4

Beech Park Johnstown
☎ 01 4580522 📄 01 4588365
e-mail: info@beechpark.ie
web: www.beechpark.ie
Undulating flat parkland course with heavily wooded fairways. Famous
for its Amen Corner (holes 10 to 13).

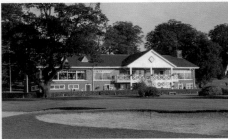

18 holes, 5753metres, Par 72, SSS 70, Course record 67.
Club membership 1038.
Visitors Mon & Thu-Fri. Booking required. Dress code. **Societies** booking
required. **Green Fees** not confirmed. **Prof** Zak Rouiller **Course Designer**
Eddie Hackett **Facilities** ⑪ ⑩ 🐛 ⌨ 🏐 🏌 🛒 🏌 🏌 **Conf** Corporate

Continued

Hospitality Days **Location** From N7, take exit signed Rathcoole North. Follow local signs.
Hotel ★★★ 74% HL Finnstown Country House Hotel, Newcastle Rd, Lucan, DUBLIN ☎ 01 6010700 25 en suite 28 annexe en suite

RUSH   MAP 01 D4

Rush

☎ 01 8438177 (Office) & 8437548
📄 01 8438177
e-mail: info@rushgolfclub.com
Seaside borders three fairways on this links course. There are 28 bunkers and undulating fairways to add to the challenge of the variable and strong winds that blow at all times and change with the tides. There are no easy lies.
9 holes, 5598mtrs, Par 70, SSS 69. Club membership 500.
Visitors Mon-Fri. Booking required. Dress code. **Societies** Booking required. **Green Fees** €32 per 18 holes. ⊛ **Facilities** ⒤ ⦿ ⓛ ⏛ ⏛ ⚷
⚷ **Location** SW of town

SAGGART   MAP 01 D4

City West Hotel & Golf Resort

☎ 01 4010500 & 4010878 (shop) 📄 01 4588565
e-mail: info@citywest-hotel.iol.ie
web: citywesthotel.com
Championship: 18 holes, 5774metres, Par 70, SSS 70, Course record 65.
Executive: 18 holes, 4713metres, Par 65, SSS 69.
Course Designer Christy O'Connor Jnr **Location** Off N7 S to village
Telephone for further details
Hotel ★★★ 69% HL Bewleys Hotel Newlands Cross, Newlands Cross, Naas Rd, DUBLIN 22 ☎ 01 4640140 & 4123301 📄 01 4640900 299 en suite

SKERRIES   MAP 01 D4

Skerries Hacketstown

☎ 01 8491567 📄 01 8491591
e-mail: admin@skerriesgolfclub.ie
web: www.skerriesgolfclub.ie
Tree-lined parkland course on gently rolling countryside, with sea views from some holes. The 1st and 18th are particularly challenging.
18 holes, 6081mtrs, Par 73, SSS 72, Course record 67.
Club membership 1200.
Visitors Mon-Sun & BHs. Booking required Tue, Wed, Sat, Sun & BHs. Handicap certificate. Dress code. **Societies** Booking required **Green Fees** €50 per round. **Prof** Bobby Kinsella **Facilities** ⒤ ⦿ ⓛ ⏛ ⏛ ⚷ ⚷
Location S of town off R127
Hotel ★★★ 70% HL Boyne Valley Hotel & Country Club, Stameen, Dublin Rd, DROGHEDA ☎ 041 983 7737 73 en suite

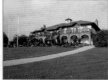

Malahide Golf Club

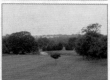

Golfers visiting this 27-hole parkland course will find a scenically beautiful course, consistently maintained to the highest standards.

The motto of the club is "A light heart and a cheerful spirit", also reflected in the warmth of our welcome both to individuals and Societies, which sees many returning year after year.

For beginner or established players, our friendly Golf Professional John Murray is on hand to offer advice or lessons to improve your game.

From the Clubhouse there are breath-taking views of Howth Head and the Wicklow Mountains, matched by the hospitality cuisine found in out Restaurant and bar.

Beechwood, The Grange, Malahide, Co. Dublin
For bookings please contact Mark Gannon, General Manager
Email: manager@malahidegolfclub.ie
Tel: +353 (01) 846-1611   Fax: +353 (01) 846-1270
Website: www.malahidegoldclub.ie

SWORDS   MAP 01 D4

Swords Open Golf Course Balheary Av, Swords

☎ 01 8409819 & 8901030 📄 01 8409819
e-mail: info@swordsopengolfcourse.com
web: www.swordsopengolfcourse.com
Parkland beside the River Broadmeadow, in countryside 16km from Dublin.
18 holes, 5612metres, Par 70, SSS 70, Course record 73.
Club membership 475.
Visitors Mon-Sun & BHs. Booking required. Dress code. **Societies** booking required. **Green Fees** not confirmed. ⊛ **Course Designer** T Halpin
Facilities ⏛ ⏛ ⚷ ⚷ **Location** N of town centre

TALLAGHT   MAP 01 D4

Dublin City Ballinascorney

☎ 01 4516430 📄 01 4598445
e-mail: info@dublincitygolf.com
web: www.dublincitygolf.com
Set in the valley of Glenasmole, this very scenic course offers a variety of terrain, where every hole is different, many would be considered feature holes.
18 holes, 5061metres, Par 69, SSS 67, Course record 63.
Club membership 500.
Visitors Mon-Sun & BHs. Booking required. Dress code. **Societies** booking required. **Green Fees** not confirmed. **Course Designer** Eddie Hackett
Facilities ⒤ ⦿ ⓛ ⏛ ⏛ ⚷ ⚷ ⚷ ⚷ **Conf** facs **Location** 12km SW of city centre on R114
Hotel ★★★ 74% HL Lynch Green Isle Hotel, Naas Rd, Newlands Cross, Naas Rd, DUBLIN 22 ☎ 01 4593406 240 en suite

Ireland

CO GALWAY

BALLINASLOE
MAP 01 B4

Ballinasloe Rosglos
☎ 090 9642126 🖹 090 9642538
e-mail: ballinasloegolfclub@eircom.net
web: ballinasloegolfclub.com

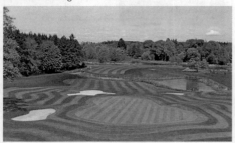

18 holes, 5865mtrs, Par 72, SSS 70, Course record 69.
Course Designer E Hackett/E Connaughton **Location** 3km S on R355
Telephone for further details

BALLYCONNEELY
MAP 01 A4

Connemara
☎ 095 23502 & 23602 🖹 095 23662
e-mail: links@iol.ie
web: www.connemaragolflinks.com
This championship links course has a spectacular setting by the
Atlantic Ocean, with the Twelve Bens Mountains in the background.
Established in 1973, it is a tough challenge, due in no small part
to its exposed location, with the back nine the equal of any in the
world. The last six holes are exceptionally long and offer a great
challenge to golfers of all abilities. When the wind blows, club
selection is crucial. Notable holes are the 13th (200yd Par 3), the
long Par 5 14th, the 15th with a green nestling in the hills, the 16th
guarded by water and the 17th and 18th, both Par 5s over 500yds
long.

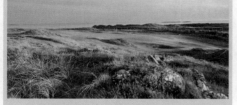

Championship: 18 holes, 6095mtrs, Par 72, SSS 73,
Course record 64.
New: 9 holes, 2754mtrs, Par 35. Club membership 970.
Visitors Mon-Sun & BHs. **Societies** Booking required. **Green Fees** €60
per round (€70 Fri-Sun). **Prof** Hugh O'Neill **Course Designer** Eddie
Hackett **Facilities** ⑪ 🍴 🛒 ♨ 🎱 ⚒ ⛳ ✔ 🏌 ✦ 🏴 **Conf** Corporate
Hospitality Days **Location** W of village off R342
Hotel ★★★★ 77% HL Abbeyglen Castle Hotel, Sky Rd, CLIFDEN
☎ 095 21201 45 en suite

BEARNA
MAP 01 B3

Bearna Golf and Country Club Corboley
☎ 091 592677 🖹 091 592674
e-mail: info@bearnagolfclub.com
web: www.bearnagolfclub.com
Set amid the beautiful landscape of the west of Ireland and enjoying
commanding views of Galway Bay, the course covers more than 100
hectares. This has resulted in generously proportioned fairways,
many elevated tees and some splendid carries. Water comes into
play at thirteen holes and the final four holes provide a memorable
finish. Lakes on 6th, 7th and 10th holes.

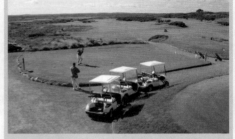

18 holes, 5746metres, Par 72, SSS 72, Course record 68.
Club membership 600.
Visitors Mon-Sun & BHs. Dress code. **Societies** welcome. **Green
Fees** not confirmed. **Prof** Declan Cunningham **Course Designer**
Robert J Brown **Facilities** ⑪ 🍴 🛒 ♨ 🎱 ⚒ ⛳ 🏌 ✦ **Conf** facs
Location 3.5km N of Bearna, off R336
Hotel ★★★★ 76% HL Galway Bay Hotel Conference & Leisure Centre,
The Promenade, Salthill, GALWAY ☎ 091 520520 153 en suite

GALWAY
MAP 01 B4

Galway Blackrock, Salthill
☎ 091 522033 🖹 091 529783
e-mail: galwaygolf@eircom.net
web: galwaygolf.com
Designed by Dr A McKenzie, this course is inland by nature,
although some of the fairways run close to the ocean. The terrain
is of gently sloping hillocks with plenty of trees and furze bushes
to catch out the unwary. Although not a long course it continues to
delight visiting golfers.
18 holes, 5995metres, Par 70, SSS 71, Course record 67.
Club membership 1238.
Visitors Mon, Wed-Sat & BHs. Booking required. Handicap certificate.
Dress code. **Societies** booking required. **Green Fees** not confirmed.
Prof Don Wallace **Course Designer** McKenzie **Facilities** ⑪ 🍴 🛒 ♨
🎱 ⚒ ⛳ 🏌 ✦ 🏌 ✦ **Conf** Corporate Hospitality Days **Location** 3km
W in Salthill

GORT
MAP 01 B3

Gort Castlequarter
☎ 091 632244 🖹 091 632387
e-mail: info@gortgolf.com
web: www.gortgolf.com
Set in 65 hectares of picturesque parkland. The 515-metre 9th and
the 472-metre 17th are played into a prevailing wind and the Par 4
dog-leg 7th will test the best.   *Continued*

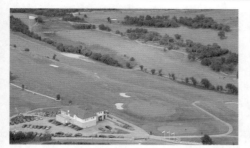

Gort

18 holes, 5705mtrs, Par 71, SSS 69, Course record 67.
Club membership 1060.
Visitors Mon-Sun & BHs. Booking required. Dress code. **Societies** Booking required. **Green Fees** €25 per day (€30 Sat & Sun). **Course Designer** Christy O'Connor Jnr **Facilities** ⑪ ⑩ ⓘ ☶ ☷ ⅄ ☖ ☗ ⅃ ✎ ✐

LOUGHREA   MAP 01 B3

Loughrea Bullaun Rd, Graigue
☎ 091 841049 📄 091 847472
e-mail: loughreagolfclub@eircom.net
An excellent parkland course with good greens and extended in 1992 to 18-holes. The course has an unusual feature in that it incorporates a historic souterrain (underground shelter/food store).
18 holes, 5825mtrs, Par 71, SSS 70, Course record 68.
Club membership 700.
Visitors Mon-Sat & BHs. Booking required Wed, Sat & BHs. Dress code. **Societies** Booking required. **Green Fees** €25 per day. **Course Designer** Eddie Hackett **Facilities** ⑪ ☶ ☷ ☖ ⅄ ✎ ✐ **Location** Follow signs from bypass for Mountbellew/New Inn. 1.5m N of town.

MOUNTBELLEW   MAP 01 B4

Mountbellew Ballinasloe
☎ 0905 79259 📄 0905 79274
9 holes, 5143mtrs, Par 69, SSS 66, Course record 63.
Location Off N63
Telephone for further details

ORANMORE   MAP 01 B3

Athenry Palmerstown
☎ 091 794466 📄 091 794971
e-mail: athenrygc@eircom.net
web: athenrygolfclub.net
A mixture of parkland and heathland built on a limestone base against the backdrop of a large pine forest. The Par 3 holes are notable with a feature hole at the 12th - from an elevated tee played between beech and pine trees.
18 holes, 5687metres, Par 70, SSS 70, Course record 67.
Club membership 1000.
Visitors Mon-Sat & BHs. Booking required Wed, Fri-Sat & BHs. Dress code. **Societies** booking required. **Green Fees** not confirmed. **Prof** Raymond Ryan **Course Designer** Eddie Hackett **Facilities** ⑪ ⑩ ☶ ☷ ☖ ⅄ ☗ ✎ ☖ ✐ ⅃ **Conf** Corporate Hospitality Days **Location** 6km E on R348

Galway Bay Golf Resort Renville
☎ 091 790711 📄 091 792510
e-mail: info@galwaybaygolfresort.com
web: www.galwaybaygolfresort.com
A championship golf course surrounded on three sides by the Atlantic Ocean and featuring water hazards on a number of holes. Each hole has its own characteristics made more obvious by the everchanging seaside winds. The design of the course highlights and preserves the ancient historic features of the Renville Peninsula. The spectacular setting and distractingly beautiful and cleverly designed mix of holes presents a real golfing challenge, demanding total concentration.
18 holes, 6533metres, Par 72, SSS 73, Course record 68.
Club membership 280.
Visitors contact club for details. **Societies** booking required. **Green Fees** not confirmed. **Prof** Eugene O'Connor **Course Designer** Christy O'Connor Jnr **Facilities** ⑪ ⑩ ☶ ☷ ☖ ⅄ ☗ ✐ ✎ ⅃ **Leisure** sauna **Conf** Corporate Hospitality Days **Location** 5km SW of village

PORTUMNA   MAP 01 B3

Portumna
☎ 090 9741059 📄 090 9741798
e-mail: info@portumnagolfclub.ie
web: www.portumnagolfclub.ie
18 holes, 6225mtrs, Par 72, SSS 72.
Course Designer E Connaughton **Location** 4km W of town on R352
Telephone for further details

RENVYLE   MAP 01 A4

Renvyle House Hotel
☎ 095 43511 📄 43515
e-mail: renvyle@iol.ie
web: www.renvyle.com
Pebble Beach: 9 holes, 3200metres, Par 36,
Course record 34.
Location "Renvyle 6km off N59, course NW of village"
Telephone for further details
Hotel ★★★ 74% HL Renvyle House Hotel, RENVYLE ☎ 095 43511 68 en suite

TUAM   MAP 01 B4

Tuam Barnacurragh
☎ 093 28993 📄 093 26003
18 holes, 5513mtrs, Par 72, SSS 69.
Course Designer Eddie Hackett **Location** 1km S of town on R347
Telephone for further details

CO KERRY (CIARRAÍ)

BALLYBUNION   MAP 01 A3

Ballybunion see page 441

Ireland

BALLYFERRITER
(BAILE AN FHEIRTEARAIGH)
MAP 01 A2

Dingle Links
☎ 066 9156255 📠 066 9156409
e-mail: dinglegc@iol.ie
web: www.dinglelinks.com
This most westerly course in Europe has a magnificent scenic location. It is a traditional links course with beautiful turf, many bunkers, a stream that comes into play on 14 holes and, usually, a prevailing wind.

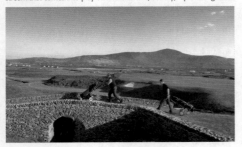

18 holes, 6126metres, Par 72, SSS 71, Course record 72. Club membership 432.
Visitors Mon-Sun & BHs. Booking required. Handicap certificate. Dress code. **Societies** booking required. **Green Fees** not confirmed. **Course Designer** Hackett/O'Connor Jnr **Facilities** ⑪ ⑩ ⓛ ⓑ ⓠ ⓨ ⓓ 🏌 🏌 **Leisure** buggies for hire May-Oct. **Location** 2.5km NW of village off R559

CASTLEGREGORY
MAP 01 A2

Castlegregory Stradbally
☎ 066 7139444 📠 066 7139958
e-mail: castlegregorygolf@oceanfree.net
web: www.castlegregorygolflinks.com
A links course sandwiched between the sea and a freshwater lake and mountains on two sides. The 3rd hole is visually superb with a 234-metre drive into the wind.
9 holes, 2569mtrs, Par 68, SSS 68, Course record 67. Club membership 426.
Visitors Mon-Sun & BHs. Booking required Sat & Sun & BHs. Dress code. **Societies** Booking required. **Green Fees** €32 per 18 holes, €20 per 9 holes. 🏌 **Course Designer** Dr Arthur Spring **Facilities** ⓠ ⓨ ⓨ **Leisure** fishing. **Location** 3km W of town near Stradbally
Hotel ★★★ 72% HL Abbey Gate Hotel, Maine St, TRALEE ☎ 066 7129888 100 en suite

GLENBEIGH
MAP 01 A2

Dooks
☎ 066 9768205 📠 066 9768476
e-mail: office@dooks.com
web: dooks.com
Long-established course on the shore between the Kerry mountains and Dingle Bay. Sand dunes are a feature (the name Dooks is a derivation of the Gaelic word for sand bank) and the course offers a fine challenge in a superb Ring of Kerry location. Redesigned by Martin Hantree.
18 holes, 5944mtrs, Par 71, SSS 70, Course record 73. Club membership 1000.

Visitors Mon-Sat & BHs. Booking required. Dress code. **Societies** Booking required. **Green Fees** €80 per 18 holes. **Course Designer** Martin Hawtree **Facilities** ⑪ ⑩ ⓛ ⓑ ⓠ ⓨ ⓓ 🏌 🏌 🏌 **Conf** Corporate Hospitality Days **Location** NE of village off on N70
Hotel ★★★ 74% HL Gleneagle Hotel, Muckross Rd, KILLARNEY ☎ 064 36000 250 en suite

KENMARE
MAP 01 B2

Ring of Kerry Golf & Country Club Templenoe
☎ 064 42000 📠 064 42533
e-mail: reservations@ringofkerrygolf.com
web: www.ringofkerrygolf.com
A world class golf facility with spectacular views across Kenmare Bay. Opened in 1998, the club has gone from strength to strength and is fast becoming a must-play course for golfers visiting the area. Every hole is memorable.

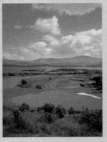

18 holes, 6236mtrs, Par 72, SSS 73, Course record 68. Club membership 260.
Visitors Mon-Sun & BHs. Booking required Sat & Sun. Handicap certificate. Dress code. **Societies** Booking required. **Green Fees** €80 per round, €120 per 36 holes (€90/€130 Sat & Sun). **Prof** Adrian Whitehead **Course Designer** Eddie Hackett **Facilities** ⑪ ⑩ ⓛ ⓠ ⓨ ⓓ 🏌 🏌 🏌 **Conf** facs Corporate Hospitality Days **Location** 6.5km W of Kenmare
Hotel ★★★★ CHH Sheen Falls Lodge, KENMARE ☎ 064 41600 66 en suite

KILLARNEY
MAP 01 B2

Beaufort Golf Resort Churchtown, Beaufort
☎ 064 44440 📠 064 44752
e-mail: beaufortgc@eircom.net
web: www.beaufortgolfclub.com

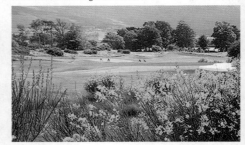

A championship-standard parkland course designed by Dr Arthur Spring. This course is in the centre of south-west Ireland's golfing

Continued

BALLYBUNION

Map 01 A3

Sandhill Rd
☎ 068 27146 📠 068 27387
e-mail: bbgolfgc@ioe.ie
web: www.ballybuniongolfclub.ie
Old Course: 18 holes, 6083mtrs, Par 71, SSS 72, Course record 67.
Cashen: 18 holes, Par 72, SSS 71, Course record 69.
Club membership 1500.
Visitors Mon-Sat. Booking required. Handicap certificate. Dress code. **Societies** Booking required. **Green Fees** Old Course: €165 per round, Cashen Course: €110 per round, Both courses: €240. **Prof** Brian O'Callaghan
Course Designer Simpson **Facilities** ⑪ ⑩
🛏 ⌨📱 🍴 🏌 📷 🛎 ⛳ 🚗 ⛳ ⛳ **Leisure** sauna
Location 2km S of town

Having excellent links, Ballybunion is recognised for its fine development of the natural terrain. Mr Murphy built the Old Course in 1906. With large sand dunes and an Atlantic backdrop, Ballybunion offers the golfer an exciting round of golf in a scenic location. But be warned, the Old course is difficult to play in the wind. President Clinton played Ballybunion on his historic visit to Ireland in 1998. Although overshadowed by the Old Course, the Cashen Course designed by Robert Trent Jones is also world class, characterised by narrow fairways, small greens and large dunes.

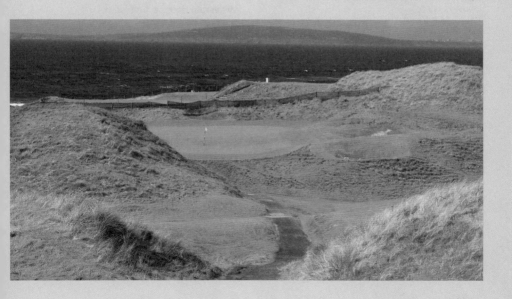

mecca. Ruins of a medieval castle dominate the back nine and the whole course is overlooked by the MacGillycuddy Reeks. The Par 3 8th and Par 4 11th are two of the most memorable holes.

18 holes, 6035mtrs, Par 71, SSS 72, Course record 68. Club membership 350.

Visitors Mon-Sun & BHs. Booking required Fri-Sun & BHs. Dress code. **Societies** Booking required. **Green Fees** €50 per round (€60 weekends). **Prof** Keith Coveney **Course Designer** Arthur Spring **Facilities** ⊕ ⑩ ﹦ ⌷ ⑂ ⚲ 📠 🏊 🍴 ✦ **Conf** Corporate Hospitality Days **Location** 11km W of Killarney off N72

Hotel ★★★ 71% HL Castlerosse Hotel, KILLARNEY ☎ 064 31144 121 en suite

Castlerosse Hotel
☎ 064 31144 🖹 064 31031
e-mail: res@castlerosse.ie
web: www.castlerosse.com

Set in mature parkland, the course commands stunning views and has fully irrigated USGA standard greens plus a practice green.

9 holes, 2761metres, Par 36. Club membership 70.

Visitors Mon-Sun & BHs. Handicap certificate. **Societies** booking required. **Green Fees** not confirmed. **Course Designer** H Wallace **Facilities** ⑩ ﹦ ⌷ ⑂ ⚲ 📠 🍴 ✦ **Leisure** hard tennis courts, heated indoor swimming pool, sauna, gymnasium. **Conf** facs

Hotel ★★★ 71% HL Castlerosse Hotel, KILLARNEY ☎ 064 31144 121 en suite

Killarney Golf & Fishing Club Mahony's Point
☎ 064 31034 🖹 064 33065
e-mail: reservations@killarney-golf.com
web: www.killarney-golf.com

The three courses are lakeside with tree-lined fairways; many bunkers and small lakes provide no mean challenge. Mahoney's Point Course has a particularly testing Par 5, 4, 3 finish and the courses call for great skill from the tee. Killarney has been the venue for many important events and is a favourite of many famous golfers.

Mahony's Point: 18 holes, 5826mtrs, Par 72, SSS 72, Course record 64.
Killeen: 18 holes, 6047mtrs, Par 72, SSS 72, Course record 68.
Lackabane: 18 holes, 6011mtrs, Par 72, SSS 72, Course record 64. Club membership 1600.

Visitors Mon-Sun & BHs. Booking required. Handicap certificate. Dress code. **Societies** Booking required. **Green Fees** per 18 holes, Mahony's Point: €100, Killeen: €120, Lackabane: €80. **Prof** Tony Coveney **Course Designer** H Longhurst/Sir Guy Campbell **Facilities** ⊕ ⑩ ﹦ ⌷ ⑂ ✦ ✦ **Conf** Corporate Hospitality Days **Location** 3.5km W on N72

Hotel ★★★★★ HL Aghadoe Heights Hotel & Spa, KILLARNEY ☎ 064 31766 74 en suite

Killorglin Stealroe
☎ 066 9761979 🖹 066 9761437
e-mail: kilgolf@iol.ie
web: killorglingolf.ie

A parkland course designed by Eddie Hackett as a challenging but fair test of golf, surrounded by magnificent views.

18 holes, 5941metres, Par 72, SSS 71, Course record 68. Club membership 510.

Visitors Mon-Sun & BHs **Societies** Booking required. **Green Fees** not confirmed. **Prof** Hugh Duggan **Course Designer** Eddie Hackett **Facilities** ⊕ ⑩ ﹦ ⌷ ⑂ ⚲ 📠 🍴 ✦ 🍴 ✦ **Leisure** fishing. **Location** 3km NE on N70

Parknasilla
☎ 064 45122 🖹 064 45323
9 holes, 5400mtrs, Par 70, SSS 69.
Course Designer Arthur Spring **Location** Near village off N70
Telephone for further details
Hotel ★★★★ 81% HL Parknasilla Hotel, PARKNASILLA ☎ 064 45122 24 en suite 59 annexe en suite

Tralee West Barrow
☎ 066 7136379 🖹 066 7136008
e-mail: info@traleegolfclub.com
web: www.traleegolfclub.com

The first Arnold Palmer designed course in Europe, this magnificent 18-hole links is set in spectacular scenery on the Barrow peninsula, surrounded on three sides by the sea. Perhaps the most memorable hole is the Par 4 17th which plays from a high tee, across a deep gorge to a green perched high against a backdrop of mountains. The back nine is very difficult and challenging. Not suitable for beginners.

18 holes, 5970mtrs, Par 71, SSS 71, Course record 66. Club membership 1306.

Visitors Mon-Sat. Booking required. Handicap certificate. Dress code. **Green Fees** €170 per round. **Prof** David Power **Course Designer** Arnold Palmer **Facilities** ⊕ ⑩ ﹦ ⌷ ⑂ ⚲ 📠 ✦ ✦ **Location** 13km NW of Tralee off R558

Hotel ★★★★ 76% HL Meadowlands Hotel, Oakpark, TRALEE ☎ 066 7180444 57 en suite

Waterville House & Golf Links
☎ 066 9474102 🖹 066 9474482
e-mail: wvgolf@iol.ie
web: www.watervillegolflink.ie

On the western tip of the Ring of Kerry, this course is highly regarded by many top golfers. The feature holes are the Par 5 11th, which runs along a rugged valley between towering dunes, and the Par 3 17th, which features an exceptionally elevated tee. Needless to say, the surroundings are beautiful.

18 holes, 6202mtrs, Par 72, SSS 72, Course record 65.

Visitors Mon-Sun & BHs. Booking required. Handicap certificate. Dress code. **Societies** Booking required **Green Fees** €165 per round (€115 before 8am & after 4pm Mon-Thur). **Prof** Liam Higgins **Course Designer** Eddie Hackett/Tom Fazio **Facilities** ⊕ ⑩ ﹦ ⌷ ⑂ ⚲ 📠 ✦ ✦ **Leisure** fishing, sauna, short game area. **Location** 0.5km from Waterville on N70

Hotel ★★★ 69% HL Derrynane Hotel, CAHERDANIEL ☎ 066 9475136 70 en suite

CHAMPIONSHIP COURSE

CO KILDARE — STRAFFAN

THE K CLUB

Map 01 D4

☎ 01 6017300 🖹 01 6017399
e-mail: golf@kclub.ie
web: www.kclub.ie
Palmer Course: 18 holes, 6526mtrs, Par 74, SSS 72, Course record 65.
Smurfit Course: 18 holes, 6636mtrs, Par 72, SSS 72.
Club membership 540.
Visitors booking required. **Societies** booking required. **Green Fees** Palmer £350, Smurfit £130. Reduced winter rates. **Prof** John McHenry/Peter O'Hagan
Course Designer Arnold Palmer **Facilities** ⑨
🍴 🛏 🖵 🍺 🧍 🖨 ⛳ ◇ 🏌 🛒 ⚒ 🏹
Leisure heated indoor swimming pool, fishing, sauna, solarium, gymnasium.
Conf facs Corporate Hospitality Days
Location W of village off R403

The K Club was the Ryder Cup's venue in 2006, the first time that Ireland has hosted the event. The course reflects the personality of its architect, Arnold Palmer, covering 220 acres of Kildare woodland, with 14 man-made lakes and the River Liffey providing the water hazards. From the instant you arrive at the 1st tee, you are enveloped by a unique atmosphere: the courses are both cavalier and charismatic. The Palmer Course is one of Europe's most spectacular courses, charming, enticing, and invariably bringing out the very best in your game. The best way to describe the Smurfit Course is that of an inland links. It has many dramatic landscapes with dunes moulding throughout, while some 14 acres of water have been worked in to the design, especially through the holes 13-18. The course is entirely different from the Palmer Course located just across the River Liffey.

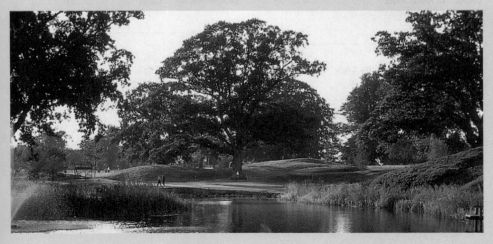

CO KILDARE

ATHY
MAP 01 C3

Athy Geraldine
☎ 059 8631729 📠 059 8634710
e-mail: info@athygolfclub.com
web: www.athygolfclub.com
18 holes, 5921metres, Par 72, SSS 71.
Course Designer Jeff Howes **Location** 1.6km NE of town on N78
Telephone for further details
Hotel Ⓣ Clanard Court Hotel, Dublin Rd, ATHY ☎ 059 864 0666
38 en suite

CARBURY
MAP 01 C4

Highfield Highfield House
☎ 046 9731021 📠 046 9731021
e-mail: highfieldgolf@eircom.ie
web: www.highfield-golf.ie
Relatively flat parkland with interesting undulations, enhanced by the fast stream that runs through many holes. The 4th dog-legs over the lake, the 7th is a great Par 5 with a challenging green, the 10th Par 3 is over rushes onto a plateau green (out of bounds on left). The 1st tee is situated on top of the cedar log clubhouse, which provides a spectacular starting point.
18 holes, 5493mtrs, Par 70, SSS 69. Club membership 500.
Visitors Mon-Sun & BHs. Booking required. **Societies** Booking required.
Green Fees €25-€35 per day (€35-€45 Sat & Sun). **Prof** Conor Devery
Course Designer Alan Duggan **Facilities** ⑪ 🍴🍽 🍺 🖳 🛅 🏖 🛄 🏌🛈
🏊 🍴🛈 **Conf** facs Corporate Hospitality Days **Location** 4.5km NW of village off R402
Hotel ★★★★ 74% HL Keadeen Hotel, NEWBRIDGE ☎ 045 431666
75 en suite

CASTLEDERMOT
MAP 01 C3

Kilkea Castle
☎ 0599 9145156
web: www.kilkeacastle.ie
18 holes, 6200mtrs, Par 71, SSS 71.
Telephone for further details
Hotel ★★★ 75% HL Seven Oaks Hotel, Athy Rd, CARLOW ☎ 059 9131308
89 en suite

DONADEA
MAP 01 C4

Knockanally Golf & Country Club
☎ 045 869322 📠 045 869322
e-mail: golf@knockanally.com
web: www.knockanally.com
Home of the Irish International Professional Matchplay championship, this parkland course is set in a former estate, with a Palladian-style clubhouse.
18 holes, 5930mtrs, Par 72, SSS 72, Course record 66. Club membership 500.
Visitors Mon-Sun & BHs. Booking required Wed, Fri-Sun & BHs. Dress code.
Societies Booking required. **Green Fees** €35 per round (€50 Sat & Sun).
Prof Martin Darcy **Course Designer** Noel Lyons **Facilities** ⑪ 🍴🍽 🍺 🖳

🖳 🛅 🏖 🍴 🍴 🍴 🏌 **Leisure** fishing. **Conf** Corporate Hospitality Days
Location 6km NW of village off M4
Hotel ★★★ 70% HL The Hamlet Court Hotel, Johnstownbridge, ENFIELD
☎ 046 9541200 30 en suite

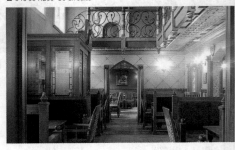

See advert on page 452

KILDARE
MAP 01 C3

Cill Dara Cill Dara, Little Curragh
☎ 045 521295 & 521433
e-mail: cilldaragolfclub@ireland.com
9 holes, 5852mtrs, Par 71, SSS 70, Course record 64.
Location 1.6km E of town
Telephone for further details
Hotel ★★★★ 74% HL Keadeen Hotel, NEWBRIDGE ☎ 045 431666
75 en suite

The Curragh Curragh
☎ 045 441238 & 441714 📠 045 442476
e-mail: curraghgolf@eircom.net
web: www.curraghgolf.com
A particularly challenging course, well wooded and with lovely scenery all around.
18 holes, 6035mtrs, Par 72, SSS 71, Course record 63. Club membership 1040.
Visitors Mon & Wed-Fri. Booking required. Dress code. **Societies** Booking required. **Green Fees** €32 per 18 holes. 🏌 **Prof** Gerry Burke **Facilities** ⑪
🍴🍽 🖳 🍴🛈 🛅 🏖 🍴🛈 🏌 **Location** E of town off R413
Hotel ★★★★ 74% HL Keadeen Hotel, NEWBRIDGE ☎ 045 431666
75 en suite

KILL
MAP 01 D4

Killeen
☎ 045 866003 📠 045 875881
e-mail: admin@killeengc.ie
18 holes, 5561mtrs, Par 71, SSS 71, Course record 70.
Course Designer Pat Ruddy/M Kelly **Location** Signed off N7 at Kill
Telephone for further details
Hotel Ⓣ Barberstown Castle, STRAFFAN ☎ 01 6288157 59 en suite

MAYNOOTH   MAP 01 D4

Carton House

☎ 01 5052000 📠 01 6286555
e-mail: reservations@cartonhouse.com
web: www.cartonhouse.com
The O'Meara is a parkland course surrounded by the ancient specimen trees of this fine estate. Feature holes include the 14th, 15th and 16th - a pair of Par 3s wrapped around a Par 5 crossing the loops of the river Rye. The Montgomerie plays like a links course with bunker hazards and a prevailing wind. The fairways run firm and fast and the bunker complexes demand strategic and shot making excellence and the ground game is always in play.
O'Meara: 18 holes, 6042metres, Par 72, SSS 72.
Montgomerie: 18 holes, 6237metres, Par 72, SSS 73,
Course record 68. Club membership 600.
Visitors Mon-Sun & BHs. Booking required. Handicap certificate. Dress code. **Societies** booking required. **Green Fees** not confirmed. **Prof** Francis Howley **Course Designer** O'Meara/Lobb & Montgomerie/Edy **Facilities** ⊕ ⊙ ⬥ 🖳 ☰ ✻ 🏌 **Leisure** fishing, sauna, solarium, gymnasium. **Conf** facs Corporate Hospitality Days **Location** N4 W from Dublin, exit Leixlip West, signed

---

NAAS   MAP 01 D4

Craddockstown Blessington Rd

☎ 045 897610 📠 045 896968
e-mail: enquires@craddockstown.com
web: www.craddockstown.com
A parkland course with easy walking. A major redevelopment was completed in 2004 with new tee boxes, 2 new greens, many water features, fairway improvements and the redevelopment of all greenside bunkers.
18 holes, 5748mtrs, Par 72, SSS 72, Course record 66.
Club membership 800.
Visitors Mon, Tue, Thu, Fri & Sun. Booking required. Dress code. **Societies** Booking required. **Green Fees** €40 (€45 Fri, €50 Sat &Sun & BHs).
Course Designer A Spring & R Jones **Facilities** ⊕ ⊙ 🖳 🖳 ⬥ ✻ 🏌 **Conf** facs Corporate Hospitality Days **Location** SE of town off R410

Naas Kerdiffstown

☎ 045 897509 & 874644 📠 045 896109
e-mail: info@naasgolfclub.com
web: naasgolfclub.com
This course is a truly unique challenge with water hazards, bunkers and sand-based greens. The Par 3 17th hole is now one of the most challenging tee shots where a round of golf can be won or lost.
18 holes, 5663mtrs, Par 71, SSS 69, Course record 65.
Club membership 1200.
Visitors Mon, Wed, Fri, Sat & BHs. Booking required. Dress code. **Societies** booking required. **Green Fees** €40 (€45 Sat & BHs). **Prof** Gavin Lunny **Course Designer** E Hackett/A Spring/J Howes **Facilities** ⊕ ⊙ 🖳 🖳 ⬥ 🏌 **Location** NE of town, off N7 onto Johnstown-Sallins road

---

STRAFFAN   MAP 01 D4

Castlewarden

☎ 01 4589254 & 4589838 📠 01 4588972
e-mail: info@castlewardengolfclub.com
web: www.castlewardengolfclub.com
18 holes, 5940metres, Par 72, SSS 70.
Course Designer Tommy Halpin **Location** 6km S of village off N7
Telephone for further details

The K Club see page 443

Hotel ★★★★★ CHH The K Club, STRAFFAN ☎ 01 6017200 69 en suite 10 annexe en suite

CALLAN   MAP 01 C3

Callan Geraldine

☎ 056 25136 & 25949 📠 056 55155
e-mail: info@callangolfclub.com
web: www.callangolfclub.com
18 holes, 5872metres, Par 72, SSS 70, Course record 66.
Course Designer B Moore/J Power **Location** 1.6km SE of village on R699
Telephone for further details
Hotel ★★★★ 70% HL Newpark Hotel, KILKENNY ☎ 056 7760500 129 en suite

---

KILKENNY   MAP 01 C3

Kilkenny Glendine

☎ 056 7765400 📠 056 7723593
e-mail: enquiries@kilkennygolfclub.com
web: www.kilkennygolfclub.com
One of Ireland's most pleasant inland courses, noted for its tricky finishing holes and its Par 3s. Features of the course are its long 11th and 13th holes and the challenge increases year by year as thousands of trees planted over the last 30 years or so are maturing. As host of the Kilkenny Scratch Cup annually, the course is permanently maintained in championship condition.
18 holes, 5925mtrs, Par 71, SSS 70, Course record 68.
Club membership 1368.
Visitors Mon-Sat & BHs. Booking required Fri, Sat & BHs. Dress code. **Societies** Booking required. **Green Fees** €35 per 18 holes (€40 Sat & BHs). **Prof** Jimmy Bolger **Facilities** ⊕ ⊙ 🖳 🖳 ⬥ ✻ 🏌 **Leisure** snooker & pool. **Conf** Corporate Hospitality Days **Location** 1.6km N of town on N77
Hotel ★★★ 69% HL The Kilkenny Inn Hotel, 15/15 Vicar St, KILKENNY ☎ 056 7772828 30 en suite

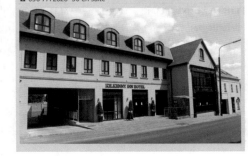

THOMASTOWN MAP 01 C3

Mount Juliet Hotel & Golf Club see page 447

Hotel ★★★★ CHH Mount Juliet Conrad Hotel, THOMASTOWN
☎ 056 7773000 32 en suite 27 annexe en suite

Hotel ★★★★ 78% HL Kilkenny River Court Hotel, The Bridge, John St,
KILKENNY ☎ 056 7723388 Fax 056 7723389 90 en suite

Hotel ★★★★ 70% HL Newpark Hotel, KILKENNY ☎ 056 7760500
Fax 056 7760555 129 en suite

Hotel ★★★ 70% HL Langtons Hotel, 69 John St, KILKENNY
☎ 056 776 5133 552 1728 Fax 056 776 3693 14 en suite 16 annexe
en suite

CO LAOIS

ABBEYLEIX MAP 01 C3

Abbeyleix Rathmoyle
☎ 057 8731450
e-mail: info@abbeyleixgolfclub.ie
web: www.abbeyleixgolfclub.ie
A pleasant, parkland 18-hole course. Undulating with water features
at five holes.
18 holes, 5557mtrs, Par 72, SSS 70. Club membership 470.
Visitors Mon-Sun. Booking required Sat-Sun. Dress code. **Societies**
Booking required. **Green Fees** €25 per round (€30 Sat & Sun).
Course Designer Mel Flanagan **Facilities** ⮕ **Location** 0.6km from Abbeyleix on Ballyroan road
Hotel ★★★★ 70% HL Newpark Hotel, KILKENNY ☎ 056 7760500
129 en suite

MOUNTRATH MAP 01 C3

Mountrath Knockanina
☎ 057 8732558 📠 057 8732643
e-mail: mountrathgc@eircom.net
web: www.mountrathgolfclub.ie
A picturesque course at the foot of the Slieve Bloom Mountains in
central Ireland. The 18-hole course has fine fairways and well-bunkered
greens, the River Nore flows through the course.
18 holes, 5732mtrs, Par 71, SSS 70, Course record 68.
Club membership 600.
Visitors Mon-Sun & BHs. Booking required Sat-Sun & BHs. Dress code.
Societies Booking required. **Green Fees** €25 per round (€30 Sat, Sun
& BHs). **Facilities** ⮕ **Conf** facs Corporate
Hospitality Days **Location** 2.5km SW of town off N7
Hotel ★★★★ 74% HL Keadeen Hotel, NEWBRIDGE ☎ 045 431666
75 en suite

PORTARLINGTON MAP 01 C3

Portarlington Garryhinch
☎ 057 8623115 📠 057 8623044
e-mail: portalingtongc@eircom.net
web: www.portalingtongolf.com
Lovely parkland course designed around a pine forest with flat terrain.
It is bounded on the 16th and 17th by the River Barrow which makes
the back 9 very challenging.
18 holes, 5723mtrs, Par 71, SSS 70, Course record 66.
Club membership 900.
Visitors Mon-Wed & Fri-Sun except BHs. Booking required Sat & Sun
Societies Booking required. **Green Fees** €35 per round (€40 Sat & Sun).

Course Designer Eddie Hackett **Facilities** ⮕ **Conf** facs Corporate Hospitality Days **Location** 6.5km SW of town on R423
Hotel ★★★★ 74% HL Keadeen Hotel, NEWBRIDGE ☎ 045 431666
75 en suite

PORTLAOISE MAP 01 C3

The Heath
☎ 057 8646533 📠 057 8646866
e-mail: info@theheathgc.ie
web: www.theheathgc.ie
Course noted for its rough heather and gorze furze and scenic views of
the rolling hills of Co Laois. Remarkably dry conditions all year round.
18 holes, 5857mtrs, Par 71, SSS 70, Course record 67.
Club membership 950.
Visitors Mon-Sat. Booking required. **Societies** Booking required. **Green
Fees** €20 per round (€30 Sat). **Prof** Mark O'Boyle **Course Designer** Jeff
Howes **Facilities** ⮕ **Location** 6.5km
N on N7
Hotel ★★★★ 74% HL Keadeen Hotel, NEWBRIDGE ☎ 045 431666
75 en suite

RATHDOWNEY MAP 01 C3

Rathdowney
☎ 0505 46170 📠 0505 46065
e-mail: rathdowneygolf@eircom.net
web: rathdowneygolfclub.com
An 18-hole parkland course, with undulating terrain. The 17th hole is a
tricky Par 3, 12th and 15th are particularly tough Par 4s and the 6th is a
challenging Par 5 (503 metres) into the prevailing wind. A good test for
golfers of all abilities.
18 holes, 5894metres, Par 71, SSS 70, Course record 67.
Club membership 500.
Visitors Mon-Sun & BHs. Booking required Fri-Sun & BHs. Dress code.
Societies booking required. **Green Fees** not confirmed. **Course
Designer** Eddie Hackett **Facilities** ⮕ **Conf** Corporate
Hospitality Days **Location** 0.8km SE, Johnstown signs from town square
Hotel ★★★★ 70% HL Newpark Hotel, KILKENNY ☎ 056 7760500
129 en suite

CO LEITRIM

BALLINAMORE MAP 01 C4

Ballinamore
☎ 071 9644346
A very dry and very testing nine-hole parkland course along the
Ballinamore-Ballyconnell Canal. Not busy on weekdays which makes
it ideal for high handicap golfers, while at the same time it tests the
ability of even a scratch golfer.
9 holes, 5194mtrs, Par 70, SSS 68, Course record 66.
Club membership 300.
Visitors Mon-Sun & BHs. Booking required Sat-Sun & BHs. Handicap
certificate. Dress code. **Societies** Booking Required **Green Fees** €20 per
day. **Course Designer** A Spring **Facilities** ⮕ **Leisure**
fishing. **Location** 3km W of town along Shannon-Erne canal
Hotel ★★★★ 76% HL Slieve Russell Hotel Golf and Country Club,
BALLYCONNELL ☎ 049 9526444 219 en suite

CHAMPIONSHIP COURSE

CO KILKENNY — THOMASTOWN

MOUNT JULIET HOTEL

Map 01 C3

☎ 056 7773064 🖶 056 7773078
e-mail: golfinfo@mountjuliet.ie
web: www.mountjuliet.com
18 holes, 6639metres, Par 72, SSS 75,
Course record 62.
Club membership 500.
Visitors Mon-Sun & BHs. Booking required Sat-Sun. Dress code. **Societies** booking required.
Green Fees from £75 in winter to £160
weekend summer. **Prof** Sean Cotter
Course Designer Jack Nicklaus **Facilities** ⑪
🍽 🍸 💻 🎱 🏌 🛒 ◇ 🏌 🛺 🏌 🦯
Leisure hard tennis courts, heated indoor
swimming pool, fishing, sauna, solarium,
gymnasium, Archery/clay shooting/equestrian.
Conf facs   Corporate Hospitality Days
Location 4km S of town off N9

Venue for the American Express
Championship in 2002 and 2004, Mount
Juliet's superb 18-hole course was designed
by Jack Nicklaus. It has also hosted many
prestigious events including the Irish
Open on three occasions. The course has a
cleverly concealed drainage and irrigation
system, perfect even when inclement
weather would otherwise halt play. It takes
advantage of the estate's mature landscape
to provide a world-class 72-Par challenge
for professionals and high-handicap
golfers alike. A unique three-hole golfing
academy has been added to allow novice
and experienced players ample opportunity
to improve their game, while a new 18-hole
putting course provides an extra dimension
of golfing pleasure and is the venue for the
National Putting Championship.

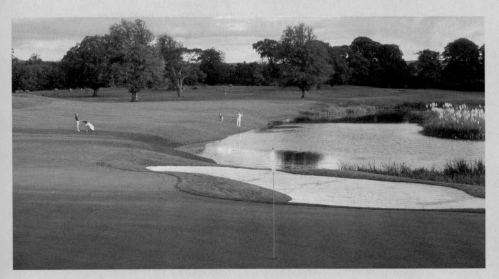

CARRICK-ON-SHANNON — MAP 01 C4

Carrick-on-Shannon Woodbrook
☎ 071 9667015 📠 071 9667015
e-mail: ckgc@eircom.net
web: www.carrickgolfclub.ie
An 18 hole course with a delightful diversity of scenery. Recently extended from 9 holes on preserved marshland that sweeps down to a lake and the Boyle river. The original 9 holes are set in mature parkland and under the new layout will constitute the first 5 and last 4 holes of the course. Two spectacular holes are the 8th where the tee is surrounded by water which requires a carry over the river and the 13th, a frightening Par 3.
18 holes, 5728mtrs, Par 70, SSS 68. Club membership 400.
Visitors Mon-Sun & BHs. Booking required. Dress code. **Societies** Booking required **Green Fees** €35 per 18 holes (€25 Tue, €40 Fri-Sun). **Course Designer** Eddie Hackett, Marc Westenborg **Facilities** ⑪ ⑩ ℔ ♀ ⑪ ♨ ❀ ➴ ✦ **Location** 6.5km W of town on N4
Hotel ★★★★ 76% HL Slieve Russell Hotel Golf and Country Club, BALLYCONNELL ☎ 049 9526444 219 en suite

CO LIMERICK

ADARE — MAP 01 B3

Adare Manor
☎ 061 396204 📠 061 396800
e-mail: info@adaremanorgolfclub.com
web: www.adaremanorgolfclub.com
An 18-hole parkland course surrounding the ruins of a 13th-century castle and a 15th-century abbey.
18 holes, 5304mtrs, Par 69, SSS 69, Course record 63. Club membership 750.
Visitors Mon-Fri. Booking required. Handicap certificate. Dress code. **Societies** Booking required **Green Fees** €40 per round. **Course Designer** Ben Sayers/Eddie Hackett **Facilities** ⑪ ⑩ ℔ ♀ ⑪ ♨ ❀ ✦ **Location** NE of town off N21
Hotel ★★★★ 80% HL Dunraven Arms Hotel, ADARE ☎ 061 396633 86 en suite

LIMERICK — MAP 01 B3

Castletroy Castletroy
☎ 061 335753 & 335261 📠 061 335373
e-mail: cgc@iol.ie
web: www.castletroygolfclub.com
Mature, parkland course extensively redeveloped in recent years. Out of bounds left of the first two holes and well maintained fairways demand accuracy off the tee. The long Par 5 6th hole is set into water. The Par 3 14th hole features a panoramic view from the tee with the green surrounded by water while the picturesque 18th is a stern test to finish with the green guarded by bunkers on both sides.
18 holes, 6284mtrs, Par 72, SSS 73, Course record 65. Club membership 1062.
Visitors Mon, Wed, Fri, Sat & BHs. Booking required. Handicap certificate. Dress code. **Societies** Booking required **Green Fees** €50 per 18 holes (€60 Fri-Sun & BHs). **Course Designer** Eddie Connaughton **Facilities** ⑪ ⑩ ℔ ♀ ⑪ ♨ ❀ ➴ ✦ ❀ ✦ **Conf** Corporate Hospitality Days **Location** 5km E of city centre
Hotel ★★★★ 78% HL Castletroy Park Hotel, Dublin Rd, LIMERICK ☎ 061 335566 107 en suite

Limerick Ballyclough
☎ 061 415146 📠 061 319219
e-mail: pat.murray@limerickgc.com
web: www.limerickgc.com
Tree-lined parkland course. The club is the only Irish winner of the European Cup Winners Team Championship.
18 holes, 5938mtrs, Par 72, SSS 71, Course record 63. Club membership 1500.
Visitors Mon-Sun & BHs. Booking required. Handicap certificate. Dress code. **Societies** Booking required. **Green Fees** €50 per round (€70 Fri-Sun &BHs). **Prof** Lee Harrington/Denise Mullew **Course Designer** A McKenzie **Facilities** ⑪ ⑩ ℔ ♀ ⑪ ♨ ❀ ➴ ✦ ❀ ✦ **Conf** facs **Location** 5km S on R511

Limerick County Golf & Country Club Ballyneety
☎ 061 351881 📠 061 351384
e-mail: lcgolf@ioi.ie
web: www.limerickcounty.com
Limerick County was designed by Des Smyth and presents beautifully because of the strategic location of the main features. It stretches over undulating terrain with one elevated section providing views of the surrounding countryside. It features over 70 bunkers with six lakes and several unique design features.
18 holes, 5686mtrs, Par 71, SSS 70, Course record 70. Club membership 800.
Visitors Mon-Sun & BHs. Booking required. Dress code. **Societies** Booking required. **Green Fees** €40 per round (€50 Sat, Sun). **Prof** Donal McSweeney **Course Designer** Des Smyth **Facilities** ⑪ ⑩ ℔ ♀ ⑪ ♨ ❀ ➴ ✦ ❀ ✦ **Conf** facs Corporate Hospitality Days **Location** 8km SE of city on R512
Hotel ★★★ 70% HL Hotel Greenhills, Caherdavin, LIMERICK ☎ 061 453033 18 rms (13 en suite)

NEWCASTLE WEST — MAP 01 B3

Killeline Cork Rd
☎ 069 61600 📠 069 77428
e-mail: killeline@eircom.net
web: www.killeline.com
18 holes, 6100metres, Par 72, SSS 68.
Location 0.4km off N21
Telephone for further details
Hotel ★★★★ 80% HL Dunraven Arms Hotel, ADARE ☎ 061 396633 86 en suite

Newcastle West Ardagh
☎ 069 76500 📠 069 76511
e-mail: info@newcastlewestgolf.com
web: www.newcastlewestgolf.com
Course set in 160 acres of countryside, built to the highest standards on sandy free draining soil. A practice ground and driving range are included. Hazards on the course include lakes, bunkers, streams and trees. A signature hole is the Par 3 6th playing 185yds over a lake.

Continued

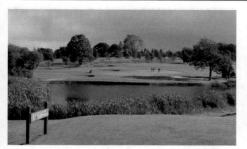

Newcastle West

18 holes, 5615mtrs, Par 71, SSS 72, Course record 67. Club membership 1019.
Visitors Mon-Sat & BHs. Booking required Sat. Dress code. **Societies** Booking required **Green Fees** Phone. **Prof** Conor McCormick **Course Designer** Dr Arthur Spring **Facilities** ⑪ ⑩ᐣ ⅃ ▯ ⑬ ⌗ ⚲ 🛪 ᔿ ⚐ 🏌 **Conf** facs Corporate Hospitality Days **Location** 3.5km off N21
Hotel ★★★★ 80% HL Dunraven Arms Hotel, ADARE ☎ 061 396633 86 en suite

CO LONGFORD

LONGFORD
MAP 01 C4

County Longford Glack, Dublin Rd
☎ 043 46310 📄 043 47082
e-mail: colonggolf@eircom.net
A lovely 18-hole parkland course with lots of trees.
18 holes, 5766metres, Par 72, Course record 71. Club membership 819.
Visitors Mon-Sun & BHs. Booking required. **Societies** booking required.
Green Fees not confirmed. ⊛ **Course Designer** Irish Golf Design
Facilities ⑪ ⅃ ▯ ⑬ ⌗ ⚲ ᔿ ⚐ 🏌 **Location** E of town
Hotel ★★★ 75% HL Abbey Hotel, Galway Rd, ROSCOMMON
☎ 090 6626240 50 en suite

CO LOUTH

ARDEE
MAP 01 D4

Ardee Townparks
☎ 041 6853227 📄 041 6856137
e-mail: ardeegolfclub@eircom.net
web: www.ardeegolfclub.com
Pleasant parkland with mature trees and natural water features.
The 13th hole, a Par 3 over water, is the main feature of the course.
18 holes, 5934mtrs, Par 71, SSS 72, Course record 64. Club membership 680.
Visitors Mon-Sat & BHs. Booking required Wed, Sat & BHs. Dress code.
Societies Welcome. **Green Fees** €35 per 18 holes (€50 Sat). **Prof** Scott Kirkpatrick **Course Designer** Eddie Hackett & Declan Branigan **Facilities** ⑪ ⑩ᐣ ⅃ ▯ ⑬ ⚲ ᔿ ᔿ ⚐ 🏌 **Conf** Corporate Hospitality Days **Location** N33 to Ardee, 400 metres from Fair Green
Hotel ★★★★ 77% HL Ballymascanlon House Hotel, DUNDALK
☎ 042 9358200 90 en suite

BALTRAY
MAP 01 D4

County Louth
☎ 041 9881530 📄 041 9881531
e-mail: reservations@countylouthgolfclub.com
web: www.countylouthgolfclub.com
Generally held to have the best greens in Ireland, this links course was designed by Tom Simpson to have well-guarded and attractive greens without being overly dependant on bunkers. It provides a good test for the modern champion, notably as the annual venue for the East of Ireland Amateur Open.
18 holes, 6141mtrs, Par 72, SSS 72, Course record 64. Club membership 1342.
Visitors Mon & Thu-Sat. Booking required. Handicap certificate. Dress code. **Societies** Booking required **Green Fees** €115 per round (€135 Sat). **Prof** Paddy McGuirk **Course Designer** Tom Simpson **Facilities** ⑪ ⑩ᐣ ⅃ ▯ ⑬ ⚲ ᔿ ⚲ 🛪 ᔿ ⚐ 🏌 **Leisure** hard tennis courts.
Location 8km NE of Drogheda

DUNDALK
MAP 01 D4

Ballymascanlon House Hotel
☎ 042 9358200 📄 042 9371598
e-mail: info@ballymascanlon.com
web: www.ballymascanlon.com
A testing 18-hole parkland course with numerous water hazards and two difficult holes through woodland, this very scenic course is set at the edge of the Cooley Mountains.

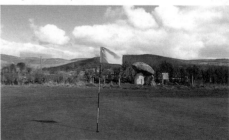

18 holes, 5073mtrs, Par 68, SSS 66.
Visitors Mon-Sun & BHs. Booking required Fri-Sun & BHs. Dress code.
Societies Booking required. **Green Fees** Phone. **Course Designer** Craddock/Ruddy **Facilities** ⑪ ⑩ᐣ ⅃ ▯ ⑬ ⚲ ᔿ ⚲ 🛪 ᔿ ⚐ 🏌 **Leisure** hard tennis courts, heated indoor swimming pool, sauna, gymnasium. **Conf** facs Corporate Hospitality Days **Location** 5km NE of town on R173
Hotel ★★★★ 77% HL Ballymascanlon House Hotel, DUNDALK
☎ 042 9358200 90 en suite

Dundalk Blackrock
☎ 042 9321731 📄 042 9322022
e-mail: manager@dundalkgolfclub.ie
web: www.dundalkgolfclub.ie
18 holes, 6028mtrs, Par 72, SSS 71.
Location 4km S of town on R172 coast road
Telephone for further details
Hotel ★★★★ 77% HL Ballymascanlon House Hotel, DUNDALK
☎ 042 9358200 90 en suite

eland

Killin Park Killin Park
☎ 042 9339303 📄 042 9320848
e-mail: johnfmcann@eircom.net
Opened in 1991 and designed by Eddie Hackett, this undulating 18-hole parkland course has mature woodland and river features. It provides challenging golf and breathtaking scenery. Bordered on the north side by Killin Wood and on the south by the Castletown River.
18 holes, 4840metres, Par 69, SSS 65, Course record 65.
Club membership 300.
Visitors Mon-Sun & BHs. Booking required Sat-Sun & BHs. Dress code.
Societies booking required. **Green Fees** not confirmed. ⊕ **Prof** Stephen Hoey **Course Designer** Eddie Hackett **Facilities** 🍴 by prior arrangement 🍺 ⬛🏷️ ⚲ 🏌️ ✦ ✦ **Location** 4.5km NW of village off N53
Hotel ★★★★ 77% HL Ballymascanlon House Hotel, DUNDALK
☎ 042 9358200 90 en suite

GREENORE   MAP 01 D4

Greenore
☎ 042 9373212 & 9373678 📄 042 9383898
e-mail: greenoregolfclub@eircom.net
web: www.greenoregolfclub.com
Situated amid beautiful scenery on the shores of Carlingford Lough, with views of the Mourne Mountains. The pine trees here are an unusual feature on a part-links course. There are quite a number of water facilities, tight fairways and very good greens.
18 holes, 6078mtrs, Par 71, SSS 73, Course record 69.
Club membership 1035.
Visitors Mon-Sun & BHs. Booking required. Dress code. **Societies** Welcome. **Green Fees** €35 per round (€50 weekends & bank holidays).
Prof Mr Robert Giles **Course Designer** Eddie Hackett **Facilities** ⊕ 🍴 🍺 ⬛🏷️ ⚲ 🏌️ ✦ ✦ **Leisure** Golf lessons available on request but must be pre booked. **Conf** Corporate Hospitality Days **Location** Near village off R175
Hotel ★★★★ 77% HL Ballymascanlon House Hotel, DUNDALK
☎ 042 9358200 90 en suite

TERMONFECKIN   MAP 01 D4

Seapoint
☎ 041 9822333 📄 041 9822331
e-mail: golflinks@seepoint.ie
web: seapointgolfclub.com
18 holes, 6470mtrs, Par 72, SSS 74.
Course Designer Des Smyth **Location** 6.5km NE of Drogheda
Telephone for further details
Hotel ★★★ 70% HL Boyne Valley Hotel & Country Club, Stameen, Dublin Rd, DROGHEDA ☎ 041 983 7737 73 en suite

---

CO MAYO (MAIGH EO)

BALLINA   MAP 01 B4

Ballina Mossgrove, Shanaghy
☎ 096 21050 📄 096 21718
e-mail: ballinagc@eircom.net
web: ballinagolfclub.com
Undulating but mostly flat inland course.
18 holes, 5581metres, Par 71, SSS 69, Course record 69.
Club membership 520.
Visitors Mon-Sun & BHs. Booking required. Handicap certificate. Dress code. **Societies** booking required. **Green Fees** not confirmed. **Prof** Eddie Tracey **Course Designer** E Hackett **Facilities** 🍺 ⬛🏷️ ⚲ 🏌️ ✦ 🛒 ✦ **Location** 1.5km W of town on R294
Hotel ★★★ 74% HL Teach Iorrais Hotel, Geesala, BALLINA ☎ 097 86888
31 en suite

BALLINROBE   MAP 01 B4

Ballinrobe Cloonacastle
☎ 094 9541118 📄 094 9541889
e-mail: info@ballinrobegolfclub.com
web: ballinrobegolfclub.com
A championship parkland 18-hole course, set in the mature woodlands of a historic estate at Cloonacastle. The layout of the course incorporates seven man-made lakes with the River Robe flowing at the back of the 3rd and 5th greens. Ballinrobe is full of character, typified by the 19th-century residence now used as the clubhouse.
18 holes, 6334metres, Par 73, SSS 72, Course record 67.
Club membership 650.
Visitors Mon-Sat & BHs. Booking required. Dress code. **Societies** booking required. **Green Fees** not confirmed. **Prof** Courtney Cougar **Course Designer** Eddie Hackett **Facilities** ⊕ 🍴 🍺 ⬛🏷️ ⚲ 🏌️ ✦ ✦ **Conf** facs Corporate Hospitality Days **Location** NE of town on R331
Hotel ★★★★★ 85% HL Ashford Castle, CONG ☎ 094 9546003
83 en suite

BALLYHAUNIS   MAP 01 B4

Ballyhaunis Coolnaha
☎ 094 9630014
e-mail: tmack@tinet.ie
9 holes, 5413mtrs, Par 70, SSS 68, Course record 68.
Location 5km N on N83
Telephone for further details
Hotel ★★★ 69% HL Knock House Hotel, Ballyhaunis Rd, KNOCK
☎ 094 9388088 68 en suite

BELMULLET
(BÉAL AN MHUIRTHEAD)

MAP 01 A5

Carne Carne
☎ 097 82292 📠 097 81477
e-mail: carngolf@iol.ie
web: www.carnegolflinks.com

A wild tumultuous roller-coaster landscape, which has been shaped into an inspirational links course by Eddie Hackett.

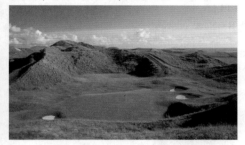

18 holes, 6119mtrs, Par 72, SSS 72, Course record 66.
Club membership 460.
Visitors Mon-Sun & BHs. Booking required. Dress code. **Societies** Booking advisable. **Green Fees** €60 per day (€60 per round Sat & Sun). **Course Designer** Eddie Hackett **Facilities** ⑪ ⒩ ⓛ ⓓ ⒯⓵ ⓟ ⓐ ⓔ ⓟ ⓥ ⓜ ⒡
Location 3km W of town off R313
Hotel ★★★ 74% HL Teach Iorrais Hotel, Geesala, BALLINA ☎ 097 86888 31 en suite

CASTLEBAR

MAP 01 B4

Castlebar Hawthorn Av, Rocklands
☎ 094 21649 📠 094 26088
e-mail: info@castlebargolfclub.ie
web: www.castlebargolfclub.ie

Course opened September 2000. Fast greens with severe borrows. Accuracy is essential from the tee on most holes. Long difficult course from blue (championship) tees.

18 holes, 5698metres, Par 71, SSS 70.
Club membership 650.
Visitors Mon-Sat & BHs. Booking required. Dress code. **Societies** booking required. **Green Fees** not confirmed. **Prof** David McQuillan **Course Designer** Peter McEvoy **Facilities** ⓛ ⓓ ⒯⓵ ⓐ ⓔ ⒡ ⓜ ⒡
Location 1.6km SE of town off N84
Hotel ★★ 64% HL Welcome Inn Hotel, CASTLEBAR ☎ 094 9022288 & 9022054 📠 094 9021766 40 en suite

CLAREMORRIS

MAP 01 B4

Claremorris Castlemacgarrett
☎ 094 9371527 📠 094 9372919
e-mail: info@claremorrisgolfclub.com
web: www.claremorrisgolfclub.com

A 18-hole parkland course designed by Tom Craddock, designer of Druids Glen. It consists of many eye-catching water features, bunkers, trees and wooded backgrounds. The feature hole is the short Par 4 14th with its island green.

18 holes, 6600mtrs, Par 73, SSS 70, Course record 68.
Club membership 600.

Visitors Mon-Sat & BHs. Booking required Thu, Sat & BHs. Dress code. **Societies** Booking required. **Green Fees** Oct-Mar €26/€32 per round; Apr-Sep €32/€40. **Course Designer** Tom Craddock **Facilities** ⑪ ⒩ ⓛ ⓓ ⒯⓵ ⓐ ⓔ ⓜ ⒡ **Location** 2km S of town on N17
Hotel ★★★ 67% HL Belmont Hotel, KNOCK ☎ 094 9388122 63 en suite

KEEL

MAP 01 A4

Achill Achill Island, Westport
☎ 098 43456 📠 098 43456
e-mail: achillgolfclub@eircom.net
web: www.achillgolfclub.com

Seaside links in a scenic location by the Atlantic Ocean.

9 holes, 5416mtrs, Par 70, SSS 66, Course record 69.
Club membership 240.
Visitors Mon-Sun & BHs. Booking required. **Societies** Booking required.
Green Fees Phone. ⊛ **Course Designer** Paddy Skirrit **Facilities** ⓓ ⓐ ⒡
Location E of Keel on R319
Hotel ★★★ 82% HL Hotel Westport Leisure, Spa & Conference, Newport Rd, WESTPORT ☎ 098 25122 129 en suite

SWINFORD

MAP 01 B4

Swinford Brabazon Park
☎ 094 9251378 📠 094 9251378
e-mail: sheetsjj@eircom.net
web: www.swinfordgolf.com

Pleasant parkland with good views of the beautiful surrounding countryside. Tough Par 3s.

9 holes, 5542metres, Par 70, SSS 68. Club membership 300.
Visitors Mon-Sun & BHs. **Societies** booking required. **Green Fees** not confirmed. ⊛ **Facilities** ⒯⓵ ⓐ ⒡ **Location** S of town on R320
Hotel ★★ 64% HL Welcome Inn Hotel, CASTLEBAR ☎ 094 9022288 & 9022054 📠 094 9021766 40 en suite

WESTPORT

MAP 01 B4

Westport Carrowholly
☎ 098 28262 & 27070 📠 098 27217
e-mail: info@westportgolfclub.com
web: www.westportgolfclub.com

This is a beautiful course with wonderful views of Clew Bay, with its 365 islands, and the holy mountain called Croagh Patrick, famous for the annual pilgrimage to its summit. Golfers indulge in a different kind of penance on this challenging course with many memorable holes. Perhaps the most exciting is the Par 5 15th, 580yds long and featuring a long carry from the tee over an inlet of Clew Bay.

18 holes, 6148mtrs, Par 73, SSS 71, Course record 61.
Club membership 600.
Visitors Mon-Sun & BHs. Booking required Fri-Sun & BHs. Dress code. **Societies** Booking required. **Green Fees** €38/€45 per round (€42/€55 Sat & Sun). **Prof** Alex Mealia **Course Designer** Fred Hawtree **Facilities** ⑪ ⒩ ⓛ ⓓ ⒯⓵ ⓐ ⓔ ⒡ ⓜ ⒡ ⒡ **Conf** Corporate Hospitality Days **Location** 4km from town off N59
Hotel ★★★ 82% HL Hotel Westport Leisure, Spa & Conference, Newport Rd, WESTPORT ☎ 098 25122 129 en suite

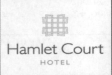

CO MEATH

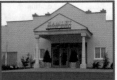

Hamlet Court
HOTEL

Johnstownbridge, Enfield, Co. Meath
Tel: 00 353 469541200   Fax: 00 353 469541704
email: info@thehamlet.ie   web: www.thehamlet.ie

The Hamlet Court Hotel is situated in the village of Johnstown bridge, just one mile from Enfield and twenty minutes from Dublin on the new M4. Centrally located and accessible to all mainline rail and bus links The Hamlet Court Hotel offers a luxurious and elegant setting in the heart of Ireland. And while you're here our friendly and attentive start will ensure that you want for nothing. Our award winning team of Chefs, draw upon fresh local produce wherever possible to create inspirational and sumptuous dishes. The Hamlet Court Hotel encompasses Pub, foyer, restaurant, free car parking, conference, banqueting & wedding facilities, nightclub, live music, dinner dances, babysitting, golf & equestrian packages, wheelchair accessible, TV, telephone, modem/data port connection, ensuite, laundry, executive rooms, suites & numerous local attractions. Whether your visit is for business or pleasure you can always unwind at our family owned and run hotel.

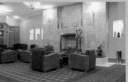

Whether you are staying with us on a golfing trip or you would just like an enjoyable game of golf, there is a wide variety of Golf Courses within travelling distance of The Hamlet Court Hotel to choose from. Also you can check out our special golf packages at www.thehamlet.ie

BETTYSTOWN
MAP 01 D4

Laytown & Bettystown
☎ 041 9827170 📠 041 9828506
e-mail: links@landb.ie
web: www.landb.ie
A very competitive and trying links course.
18 holes, 5652mtrs, Par 71, SSS 70, Course record 65.
Club membership 950.
Visitors Mon-Sun & BHs. Booking required. Handicap certificate. Dress code. **Societies** Booking required. **Green Fees** €60 per 18 holes (€75 Sat, Sun & BHs). **Prof** Robert J Browne **Facilities** ⑪ ⑩ ℔ ⌁ ⍾ ⚐ ⚏ ⚑ ⚐ **Leisure** hard tennis courts. **Location** N of village on R150

DUNSHAUGHLIN
MAP 01 D4

Black Bush Thomastown
☎ 01 8250021 📠 01 8250400
e-mail: info@blackbushgolfclub.ie
web: www.blackbushgolfclub.ie
Three 9-hole courses, giving three possible 18-hole combinations, set in lovely parkland, with a lake providing a hazard at the 1st. Creeks, trees and bunkers make for challenging and accurate shot-making.
Black Bush: 18 holes, 6337metres, Par 73, SSS 72.
Agore: 18 holes, 6033metres, Par 71, SSS 69.

Thomastown: 18 holes, 5882metres, Par 70, SSS 68.
Club membership 950.
Visitors contact club for details. **Societies** welcome. **Green Fees** not confirmed. **Prof** Shane O'Grady **Course Designer** Bobby Browne **Facilities** ⑪ ⑩ ℔ ⌁ ⍾ ⚐ ⚏ ⚑ ⚐ **Location** 2.5km E of village on R125
Hotel ★★★ 74% HL Finnstown Country House Hotel, Newcastle Rd, Lucan, DUBLIN ☎ 01 6010700 25 en suite 28 annexe en suite

KELLS
MAP 01 C4

Headfort
☎ 046 9240146 📠 046 9249282
e-mail: info@headfortgolfclub.ie
web: www.headfortgolfclub.ie
Headfort Old Course is a delightful parkland course which is regarded as one of the best of its kind in Ireland. There are ample opportunities for birdies, but even if these are not achieved, provides a challenging test. The New Course is a modern course which criss-crosses the Blackwater river, making use of two islands.

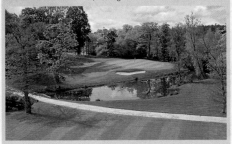

Old Course: 18 holes, 5973mtrs, Par 72, SSS 71.
New Course: 18 holes, 6164metres, Par 72, SSS 74.
Club membership 1700.
Visitors Mon-Sun & BHs. Booking required. Dress code. **Societies** Booking required. **Green Fees** Old Course: €50 per round (€55 Fri-Sun). New Course; €65 per round (€70 Fri-Sun). **Prof** Brendan McGovern **Course Designer** Christy O'Connor jnr **Facilities** ⑪ ⑩ ℔ ⌁ ⍾ ⚐ ⚏ ⚑ ⚐ **Location** 0.8km E of village on N3

See advert on opposite page

KILCOCK
MAP 01 C4

Kilcock Gallow
☎ 01 6287592 📠 01 6287283
e-mail: kilcockgolfclub@eircom.net
web: www.kilcockgolfclub.com
A parkland course with generous fairways, manicured greens and light rough only.
18 holes, 5775mtrs, Par 72, SSS 70, Course record 69.
Club membership 700.
Visitors Mon-Fri. Booking required. Dress code. **Societies** Booking required. **Green Fees** €25 per 18 holes (€32 Fri). **Course Designer** Eddie Hackett **Facilities** ⑪ ⑩ ℔ ⌁ ⍾ ⚐ ⚏ ⚑ **Location** "M4 exit Kilcock, course 3km "
Hotel ★★★ 67% HL Lucan Spa Hotel, LUCAN ☎ 01 6280494 71 rms (61 en suite)

Ireland

Headfort Golf Club

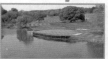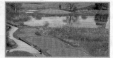

So you want to play on one of Ireland's Top 25 Courses (2005 Golf Digest Readers' Survey)?

You want to visit a 36-hole complex rated as potentially the best member's facility in Ireland and one of the country's top 10 parkland courses by the world-renowned golfing writer Dermot Gilleece?

If the answer is Yes then you want to play Headfort in

Co. Meath, the progressive and welcoming golf club in North Leinster that is home to two of the most natural parkland courses in Ireland.

The New Course, designed by Christy O'Connor Jnr. meanders around the river Blackwater and 13 of the holes feature a water challenge on a layout with that 'wow' factor.

Visitors are always welcome any day.
Because of our two Courses, we can guarantee golf to visitors 7 days a week.
For more information and details of 'Special Offers',
visit us at www.headfortgolfclub.ie

Headfort Golf Club, Navan Road, Kells,
County Meath, Ireland
Telephone: +353469240146
Timesheets: +353469282001
Fax: +353469249282
Email: info@headfortgolfclub.ie • Web site:
www.headfortgolfclub.ie
Adm. Secretary: Nora Murphy
Professional: Brendan McGovern PGA Pro

NAVAN   MAP 01 C4

Royal Tara Bellinter
☎ 046 25508 & 25244 📠 046 25508
e-mail: info@royaltaragolfclub.com
web: royaltaragolfclub.com
Pleasant parkland course offering plenty of variety. Situated close to the Hill of Tara, the ancient seat of the Kings of Ireland.
New Course: 18 holes, 5757mtrs, Par 71, SSS 70.
Bellinter Nine: 9 holes, 2911mtrs, Par 35, SSS 35.
Club membership 1000.
Visitors Mon-Sun & BHs. Booking required. Dress code. **Societies** Booking required **Green Fees** €45 per 18 holes (€55 weekends). **Prof** John Byrne **Course Designer** Des Smyth **Facilities** ⑪ ⑩ ⬛ ⬛ ⬛ ⬛ ⬛ ⬛ ⬛ **Conf** facs Corporate Hospitality Days **Location** 20km from Navan on N3

TRIM   MAP 01 C4

County Meath Newtownmoynagh
☎ 046 31463 📠 046 37554
web: trimgolf.net
18 holes, 6720mtrs, Par 73, SSS 72, Course record 68.
Course Designer Eddie Hackett/Tom Craddock **Location** 5km SW of town on R160
Telephone for further details

CO MONAGHAN

CARRICKMACROSS   MAP 01 C4

Mannan Castle Donaghmoyne
☎ 042 9663308 📠 042 9663308
e-mail: mannancastlegc@eircom.net
18 holes, 5944metres, Par 70, SSS 69.
Course Designer F Ainsworth **Location** 6.5km N of town
Telephone for further details
Hotel ★★★★ 77% HL Ballymascanlon House Hotel, DUNDALK
☎ 042 9358200   90 en suite

Nuremore
☎ 042 9671368 📠 042 9661853
e-mail: nuremore@eircom.net
web: www.nuremore-hotel.ie

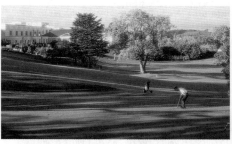

18 holes, 6400yds, Par 71, SSS 69, Course record 64.
Course Designer Eddie Hackett **Location** 1.6km SE of town on N2
Telephone for further details
Hotel ★★★★ 79% HL Nuremore Hotel, CARRICKMACROSS
☎ 042 9661438   72 en suite

CASTLEBLAYNEY   MAP 01 C4

Castleblayney Onomy
☎ 042 9740451 📠 042 9740451
e-mail: rayker@eircom.com
9 holes, 4918metres, Par 68, SSS 66, Course record 65.
Course Designer Bobby Browne **Location** In town on Hope Castle Estate
Telephone for further details
Hotel ★★★★ 77% HL Ballymascanlon House Hotel, DUNDALK
☎ 042 9358200   90 en suite

CLONES   MAP 01 C5

Clones Hilton Park
☎ 047 56017 & 56913 📠 047 56913
e-mail: clonesgolfclub@eircom.net
web: clonesgolf.com
A parkland course set in drumlin country and renowned for the quality of the greens and the wildlife. Due to a limestone belt, the course is very dry and playable all year.
18 holes, 5549mtrs, Par 70, SSS 69, Course record 62.
Club membership 450.
Visitors Mon-Sun & BHs. Booking required Sat, Sun & BHs. Dress code
Societies Booking required **Green Fees** €30 per round. **Course**

Continued

Designer Dr Arthur Spring **Facilities** ⊕ ⍥ 🏌 ⌸ ⌹ 🏊 ✐ 🛒 ✐ ⚑ **Conf**
Corporate Hospitality Days **Location** 5km S of town on R212
Hotel ⅬⅡ Hillgrove Hotel, Old Armagh Rd, MONAGHAN ☎ 047 4781288
44 en suite

MONAGHAN   MAP 01 C5

Rossmore Rossmore Park, Cootehill Rd
☎ 047 71222
e-mail: golffees@hotmail.com
An undulating, 18-hole parkland course in beautiful countryside.
18 holes, 5590mtrs, Par 70, SSS 69, Course record 68.
Club membership 650.
Visitors Mon-Sun & BHs. Booking required Thu, Sat-Sun & BHs. Dress code.
Societies Booking required. **Green Fees** €30 per round (€40 Sat, Sun &
BHs). **Prof** Ciaran Smyth **Course Designer** Des Smyth **Facilities** ⊕ ⍥ 🏌
⌸ ⌹ 🏊 ⚐ ✐ 🛒 ✐ ⚑ **Leisure** snooker. **Conf** Corporate Hospitality
Days **Location** 3km S of town on R188
Hotel ⅬⅡ Hillgrove Hotel, Old Armagh Rd, MONAGHAN ☎ 047 4781288
44 en suite

CO OFFALY

BIRR   MAP 01 C3

Birr The Glenns
☎ 0509 20082 🖷 0509 22155
e-mail: birrgolfclub@eircom.net
web: www.globalgolf.com
18 holes, 5700mtrs, Par 70, SSS 70, Course record 62.
Course Designer Eddie Connaughton **Location** 3km N of town on R439
Telephone for further details

DAINGEAN   MAP 01 C4

Castle Barna
☎ 057 9353384 🖷 057 9353077
e-mail: info@castlebarna.ie
web: www.castlebarna.ie
Parkland beside the Grand Canal. Many mature trees, natural streams
and the naturally undulating landscape provide a great challenge for
golfers of all abilities.
18 holes, 5798mtrs, Par 72, SSS 71, Course record 68.
Club membership 600.
Visitors Mon-Sun & BHs. Booking required Sat-Sun & BHs. Dress code.
Societies Booking required. **Green Fees** €22 per round (€35 Sat, Sun
& BHs). **Course Designer** Alan Duggan/Kieran Monahan **Facilities** ⊕
by prior arrangement ⍥ by prior arrangement 🏌 ⌸ ⌹ 🏊 ⚐ ✐ 🛒 ✐
Conf Corporate Hospitality Days **Location** 11km off N6 Dublin-Galway
road at Tyrellspass

EDENDERRY   MAP 01 C4

Edenderry
☎ 046 9731072 🖷 046 9733911
e-mail: enquiries@edenderrygolfclub.com
web: www.edenderrygolfclub.com
A most friendly club which offers a relaxing game in pleasant
surroundings. In 1992 the course was extended to 18 holes.
18 holes, 6029metres, Par 72, SSS 72, Course record 66.
Club membership 900.

Visitors Mon-Wed & Fri. Booking required. Dress code. **Societies** booking
required. **Green Fees** not confirmed. **Course Designer** Havers/Hackett
Facilities ⊕ ⍥ 🏌 ⌸ ⌹ 🛒 ✐ **Conf** facs Corporate Hospitality Days
Location 1.2km outside Edenderry on Dublin route

TULLAMORE   MAP 01 C4

Esker Hills
☎ 057 9355999 🖷 057 9355021
e-mail: info@eskerhillsgolf.com
web: www.eskerhillsgolf.com
Esker Hills is built on a landscape of plateaus, sweeping valleys and
natural lakes created by the retreating glaciers the ice age 10,000
years ago. In a unique setting with 18 challenging holes, no two of
which are remotely alike. A parkland course with a links feel and
sand based greens.
18 holes, 6051mtrs, Par 71, SSS 71, Course record 65.
Club membership 280.
Visitors Mon-Sun & BHs. Booking required. **Societies** Booking
required. **Green Fees** €35 per round (€48 Sat, Sun & BHs).
Course Designer Christy O'Connor jnr **Facilities** ⊕ ⍥ 🏌 ⌸ ⌹ 🏊
⚐ ⚑ ✐ 🛒 ✐ **Location** 3m from Tullamore off N80 Tullamore to
Clara road

Tullamore Brookfield
☎ 057 9321439 🖷 057 9341806
e-mail: tullamoregolfclub@eircom.net
web: www.tullamoregolfclub.ie
Course set in mature parkland of oak, beech and chestnut. The original
design was by James Braid and this has been radically altered to meet
the highest standards of the modern game, with new sand-based
undulating greens, lakes, bunkering, mounding and more trees.
18 holes, 5666mtrs, Par 70, SSS 71, Course record 68.
Club membership 1200.
Visitors Mon-Sat. Booking required. Dress code **Societies** Booking required
Green Fees €37 per 18 holes (€48 Sat). **Prof** Donagh McArdle **Course
Designer** James Braid/Paddy Merrigam **Facilities** ⊕ ⍥ 🏌 ⌸ ⌹ 🏊 ⚐ ⚑
🛒 ✐ **Location** 4km SW of town on R421
Hotel ★★★★ 74% HL Hodson Bay Hotel, Hodson Bay, ATHLONE
☎ 090 6442000 133 en suite

CO ROSCOMMON

ATHLONE   MAP 01 C4

Athlone Hodson Bay
☎ 090 6492073 🖷 090 6494080
e-mail: athlonegolfclub@eircom.net
web: www.athlonegolfclub.ie
A picturesque course with a panoramic view of Lough Ree. Overall, it
is a tight, difficult course with some outstanding holes and is noted for
its magnificent greens. All greens and tees have been rebuilt to sand
based, including a new Par 3 6th hole. Three new water features.
18 holes, 5854mtrs, Par 71, SSS 71, Course record 66.
Club membership 1250.
Visitors Mon-Sat (except BHs). Booking required. Handicap certificate.
Dress code. **Societies** Welcome. **Green Fees** €35 per round (€40 Sat).
Prof Kevin Grealy **Course Designer** J McAllister **Facilities** ⊕ ⍥ 🏌 ⌸ ⌹
🏊 ⚐ ⚑ ✐ 🛒 ✐ **Location** 6.5km from town beside Lough Ree off N61

Hotel ★★★★ 74% HL Hodson Bay Hotel, Hodson Bay, ATHLONE
☎ 090 6442000   133 en suite

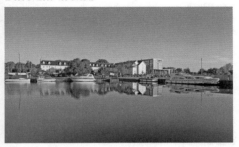

BALLAGHADERREEN
MAP 01 B4

Ballaghaderreen
☎ 094 9860295

Mature nine-hole course with an abundance of trees. Accuracy off the tee is vital for a good score. Small protected greens require a good short-iron plan. The Par 3, 5th hole at 178yds has ruined many a good score.

9 holes, 5237metres, Par 70, SSS 67, Course record 68. Club membership 400.

Visitors Mon-Sun & BHs. **Societies** booking required. **Green Fees** not confirmed. ☻ **Course Designer** Paddy Skerritt **Facilities** ☒ ♂
Location 3.5km S of town

BOYLE
MAP 01 B4

Boyle Roscommon Rd
☎ 071 9662594

Situated on a low hill and surrounded by beautiful scenery, this is an undemanding course where, due to the generous fairways and semi-rough, the leisure golfer is likely to finish the round with the same golf ball.

9 holes, 5324mtrs, Par 68, SSS 66, Course record 65. Club membership 621.

Visitors Mon-Sun & BHs. **Societies** Booking required. **Green Fees** €15 per day. ☻ **Course Designer** E Hackett **Facilities** ⊕ by prior arrangement ⦿ by prior arrangement ⧫ ⧠ ⧢ ☒ **Location** 3km S off N61
Hotel ★★★★ 66% HL The Landmark Hotel, CARRICK-ON-SHANNON
☎ 071 962 2222   50 en suite

CASTLEREA
MAP 01 B4

Castlerea Clonalis
☎ 094 9620068

9 holes, 4974mtrs, Par 68, SSS 66, Course record 62.
Location Near town centre on N60
Telephone for further details
Hotel ★★★ 75% HL Abbey Hotel, Galway Rd, ROSCOMMON
☎ 090 6626240   50 en suite

ROSCOMMON
MAP 01 B4

Roscommon Mote Park
☎ 090 6626382 📄 090 6626043
e-mail: rosegolfclub@eircom.net
web: www.golfclubireland.com/roscommon
Located on the rolling pastures of the Mote Park estate. Numerous water hazards, notably on the tricky 13th, multi-tiered greens and an excellent irrigation to give an all-weather surface.

18 holes, 6290mtrs, Par 72, SSS 70. Club membership 700.
Visitors Mon-Sun & BHs. Booking required Sun. Handicap certificate. Dress code. **Societies** Booking required. **Green Fees** €30 per round (€35 Sat & Sun). ☻ **Course Designer** E Connaughton **Facilities** ⊕ ⦿ ⧫ ⧠ ⧢ ☒
⧤ ♂ **Location** 0.8km S of town
Hotel ★★★ 75% HL Abbey Hotel, Galway Rd, ROSCOMMON
☎ 090 6626240   50 en suite

STROKESTOWN
MAP 01 C4

Strokestown Bumlin
☎ 071 9633528

Picturesque nine-hole course set in parkland with fine views.

9 holes, 2615mtrs, Par 68. Club membership 250.
Visitors Mon-Sat & BHs. Booking required Sat, Sun & BHs. Dress code.
Societies Booking required. **Green Fees** €15 per 18 holes. ☻ **Course Designer** Mel Flanagan **Facilities** ☒ **Location** 2.5km SW of village off R368
Hotel ★★★ 75% HL Abbey Hotel, Galway Rd, ROSCOMMON
☎ 090 6626240   50 en suite

CO SLIGO

BALLYMOTE
MAP 01 B4

Ballymote Ballinascarrow
☎ 071 9183089 📄 071 9183089
e-mail: john.mccarrick@gmail.com
web: www.ballymotegolfclub.com
Although Ballymote was founded in 1940, the course dates from 1993 and has matured well into a parkland with ample fairways and large greens. The feature Par 4 7th hole has been redesigned with the green surrounded by water and Ballinascarrow Lake in the background. A challenging course set in breathtaking scenery.

9 holes, 5302mtrs, Par 70, SSS 68, Course record 63. Club membership 250.
Visitors Mon-Sun & BHs. Booking required Sat, Sun & BHs **Societies** Booking required. **Green Fees** €20 per day. ☻ **Course Designer** Eddie Hacket/Mel Flanagan **Facilities** ⊕ by prior arrangement ⦿ by prior arrangement ⧫ by prior arrangement ⧠ by prior arrangement ☒ ⧫ ♂
Leisure fishing. **Location** 1.5km from Ballymote centre
Hotel ★★★ 76% HL Sligo Park Hotel, Pearse Rd, SLIGO ☎ 071 9190400
137 en suite

INISHCRONE — MAP 01 B5

Enniscrone
☎ 096 36297 📠 096 36657
e-mail: enniscronegolf@eircom.net
web: www.enniscronegolf.com
27 holes, 6125metres, Par 73, SSS 72, Course record 70.
Course Designer E Hackett/Donald Steel **Location** 0.8km S of village
Telephone for further details
Hotel ★★★ 74% HL Teach Iorrais Hotel, Geesala, BALLINA
☎ 097 86888 31 en suite

SLIGO — MAP 01 B5

County Sligo Rosses Point
☎ 071 9177134 & 9177186 📠 071 9177460
e-mail: teresa@countysligogolfclub.ie
web: countysligogolfclub.ie
Now considered to be one of the top links courses in Ireland, County Sligo is host to a number of competitions, including the West of Ireland championships and internationals. Set in an elevated position on cliffs above three large beaches, the prevailing winds provide an additional challenge. Tom Watson described it as 'a magnificent links, particularly the stretch of holes from the 14th to the 17th'.
18 holes, 6136mtrs, Par 71, SSS 72, Course record 67.
Bomore: 9 holes, 2785mtrs, Par 35, SSS 69.
Club membership 1250.
Visitors Mon-Sun & BHs. Booking required. Handicap certificate. Dress code. **Societies** Booking required. **Green Fees** Championship Course: €75 per 18 holes (€90 Fri-Sun & BHs), Bowmore: €25 9 holes €40 18 holes. **Prof** Jim Robinson **Course Designer** Harry Colt **Facilities** ⑪ 🍴 🏌 ☕ 🏠 🛍 🚗 ⛳ 🏌 ✂ **Conf** facs Corporate Hospitality Days **Location** N of town off N15

Strandhill Strandhill
☎ 071 9168188 📠 037191 68811
e-mail: strandhillgc.eircom.net
This scenic course is situated between Knocknarea Mountain and the Atlantic, offering golf in its most natural form amid the sand dunes of the West of Ireland. The 1st, 16th and 18th are Par 4 holes over 364 metres; the 2nd and 17th are testing Par 3s which vary according to the prevailing wind; the Par 4 13th is a testing dogleg right. This is a course where accuracy will be rewarded.
18 holes, 5516mtrs, Par 69, SSS 68. Club membership 450.
Visitors Mon-Sun & BHs. Booking required. Handicap certificate. Dress code. **Societies** Booking required. **Green Fees** Phone. **Prof** Anthony Gray **Facilities** ⑪ 🍴 🏌 ☕ 🏠 🛍 🚗 ✂ 🏌 ✂ **Location** 8km W of town off R292
Hotel ★★★ 76% HL Sligo Park Hotel, Pearse Rd, SLIGO ☎ 071 9190400 137 en suite

TOBERCURRY — MAP 01 B4

Tobercurry
☎ 071 85849 📠 071 9185888
e-mail: contact@tubbercurrygolfclub.com
web: www.tubbercurrygolfclub.com
A nine-hole parkland course designed by Edward Hackett. The 8th hole, a Par 3, is regarded as being one of the most testing in the west of Ireland. An exceptionally dry course, playable all year round.
9 holes, 5490mtrs, Par 70, SSS 69, Course record 65.
Club membership 350.
Visitors Mon-Sun & BHs. Booking required Sun. **Societies** Booking required **Green Fees** €20 per day/round. ⊕ **Course Designer** Eddie Hackett **Facilities** ⑪ 🍴 🏌 ☕ 🏠 🚗 ⛳ ✂ **Conf** Corporate Hospitality Days **Location** 0.4km from town centre

CO TIPPERARY

CAHIR — MAP 01 C3

Cahir Park Kilcommon
☎ 052 41474 📠 052 42717
e-mail: management@cahirparkgolfclub.com
web: www.cahirparkgolfclub.com
Parkland dissected by the River Suir, which adds a challenge to the Par 4 8th and Par 3 16th. Water in play on seven holes.
18 holes, 5806metres, Par 71, SSS 71, Course record 66.
Club membership 750.
Visitors Mon-Fri. Contact club for details. Dress code. **Societies** booking required. **Green Fees** not confirmed. ⊕ **Course Designer** Eddie Hackett **Facilities** ⑪ 🍴 🏌 ☕ 🏠 🚗 🛍 🍴 ✂ 🏌 **Location** 1.6km SW of town centre on R668

CARRICK-ON-SUIR — MAP 01 C2

Carrick-on-Suir Garvonne
☎ 051 640047 📠 051 640558
e-mail: cosgc@eircom.net
18 holes, 6061mtrs, Par 72, SSS 71, Course record 69.
Course Designer Eddie Hackett **Location** 3km SW of town
Telephone for further details
Hotel ★★★ 76% HL Hotel Minella, CLONMEL ☎ 052 22388 70 en suite

CLONMEL — MAP 01 C2

Clonmel Lyreanearla, Mountain Rd
☎ 052 24050 📠 052 83349
e-mail: cgc@indigo.ie
web: clonmelgolfclub.com
Set in the scenic, wooded slopes of the Comeragh Mountains, this is a testing course with lots of open space and plenty of interesting features. It provides an enjoyable round in exceptionally tranquil surroundings.
18 holes, 5804metres, Par 72, SSS 71.
Club membership 850.
Visitors Mon-Sun & BHs. Booking required Wed, Sat & Sun. Handicap certificate. Dress code. **Societies** booking required. **Green Fees** not confirmed. **Prof** Robert Hayes **Course Designer** Eddie Hackett **Facilities** ⑪ by prior arrangement 🏌 ☕ 🏠 🚗 🛍 🍴 ✂ **Location** 5km from Clonmel off N24
Hotel ★★★ 76% HL Hotel Minella, CLONMEL ☎ 052 22388 70 en suite

MONARD
MAP 01 B3

Ramada Hotel Ballykisteen, Limerick Junction
☎ 062 33333 📠 062 31555
web: www.ramadaireland.com
Ballykisteen is set in emerald green countryside just two miles
from Tipperary. The course, with landscaped surroundings against
a backdrop of mountains, lakes and streams, offers an excellent
challenge for the champion golfer. The use of forward tees provide a
course that is playable and enjoyable for the average golfer.
18 holes, 6186metres, Par 72, SSS 72.
Club membership 350.
Visitors Mon-Sun & BHs. Booking required. Dress code. **Societies** booking
required. **Green Fees** not confirmed. **Prof** James Harris **Course Designer**
Des Smith **Facilities** ⑪ ⓧ ⒧ ⒬ ⒭ ⒱ ⒯ ⒳ ⒴ ⒵ **Leisure**
tennis courts, indoor swimming pool, sauna, gymnasium. **Conf** facs
Location 1.6km SE of village on N24 towards Tipperary

NENAGH
MAP 01 B3

Nenagh Beechwood
☎ 067 31476 📠 067 34808
e-mail: nenaghgolfclub@eircom.net
web: www.nenaghgolfclub.com
The sand-based greens guarded by intimidating bunkers are a
challenge for even the most fastidious putters. Excellent drainage and
firm surfaces allow play all year round.
18 holes, 6029mtrs, Par 72, SSS 72, Course record 68.
Club membership 1100.
Visitors Mon-Sun & BHs. Booking required. Handicap certificate. Dress
code. **Societies** Booking required. **Green Fees** €30 per 18 holes. **Prof**
Robert Kelly **Course Designer** Patrick Merrigan **Facilities** ⑪ by prior
arrangement ⓧ by prior arrangement ⒧ ⒬ ⒭ ⒱ ⒯ ⒳ ⒴ ⒵
Location 5km NE of town on R491

ROSCREA
MAP 01 C3

Roscrea Golf Club Derryvale
☎ 0505 21130 📠 0505 23410
e-mail: roscreagolf@eircom.net
Course situated on the eastern side of Roscrea in the shadows of the
Slieve Bloom Mountains. A special feature of the course is the variety
of the Par 3 holes, most noteworthy of which is the 165-metre 4th,
which is played almost entirely over a lake. It is widely recognised that
the finishing six holes will prove a worthy challenge to even the best
players. The most famous hole on the course in the 5th, referred to
locally as the Burma Road, a Par 5 of over 457 metres with the fairway
lined with trees and out of bounds on the left side.
18 holes, 5809mtrs, Par 71, SSS 70, Course record 66.
Club membership 600.
Visitors Mon-Sun & BHs. Booking required Sat-Sun & BH's. Dress code.
Societies Booking required. **Green Fees** €30 (€35 Sat & Sun). **Course
Designer** A Spring **Facilities** ⑪ ⓧ ⒧ ⒬ ⒭ ⒱ ⒯ **Conf** Corporate
Hospitality Days **Location** E of town on N7

TEMPLEMORE
MAP 01 C3

Templemore Manna South
☎ 0504 31400 & 32923
Parkland with many mature and some newly planted trees, which
provide a pleasant test without being too difficult.
9 holes, 5780mtrs, Par 71, SSS 71, Course record 68.
Club membership 330.
Visitors Mon-Sun & BHs. Booking required. **Societies** Booking requested.
Green Fees €15 per day (€20 Sat & Sun). ⊛ **Facilities** ⑪ ⓧ ⒧ ⒬ ⒯
⒮ **Leisure** hard tennis courts. **Location** 0.8km S of town on N62

THURLES
MAP 01 C3

Thurles Turtulla
☎ 0504 21983 & 24599 📠 0504 24647
18 holes, 5904mtrs, Par 72, SSS 71, Course record 67.
Course Designer Mr J McMlister **Location** 1.6km S of town on N62
Telephone for further details

TIPPERARY
MAP 01 C3

County Tipperary Golf & Country Club Dundrum
House Hotel, Dundrum
☎ 062 71717 📠 062 71718
e-mail: dundrumh@id.ie
web: www.dundrumhousehotel.com
18 holes, 6447metres, Par 72, SSS 72, Course record 70.
Course Designer Philip Walton **Location** 12km NE of town on R505
Telephone for further details

Tipperary Rathanny
☎ 062 51119 📠 062 51119
e-mail: tipperarygolfclub@eircom.net
18 holes, 5761mtrs, Par 71, SSS 71, Course record 66.
Location 1.6km S of town on R664
Telephone for further details

CO WATERFORD

DUNGARVAN
MAP 01 C2

Dungarvan Knocknagranagh
☎ 058 41605 & 43310 📠 058 44113
e-mail: dungarvangc@eircom.net
web: www.dungarvangolfclub.com
A championship-standard course beside Dungarvan Bay, with seven
lakes and hazards placed to challenge all levels of golfer. The greens
are considered to be among the best in Ireland.
18 holes, 5998metres, Par 72, SSS 71, Course record 66.
Club membership 900.
Visitors contact club for details. **Societies** welcome. **Green Fees** not
confirmed. **Prof** David Hayes **Course Designer** Moss Fives **Facilities** ⒧
⒬ ⒯ ⒮ ⒱ **Leisure** snooker. **Location** Off N25
Hotel ★★★ 63% HL Lawlors Hotel, DUNGARVAN ☎ 058 41122 & 41056
📠 058 41000 89 en suite

Ireland

Gold Coast Golf & Leisure Ballinacourty
☎ 058 44055 ▤ 058 44055
e-mail: goldcoastgolf@cablesurf.com
web: www.goldcoastclub.com
Parkland beside the Atlantic Ocean with unrivalled views of Dungarvan Bay. The mature tree-lined fairways of the old course are tastefully integrated with the long and challenging newer holes to create a superb course.
18 holes, 6171mtrs, Par 72, SSS 72, Course record 70. Club membership 600.
Visitors Mon-Sun & BHs. Booking required Fri-Sun & BHs. Dress code. **Societies** Booking required. **Green Fees** €35 per 18 holes (€45 Sat & Sun). **Course Designer** Maurice Fives **Facilities** ⊕ ⏍ ⌚ 🍴 🔽 🚴 🏊 ☀ ♦ ✦ 🛄 ✦ **Leisure** hard tennis courts, heated indoor swimming pool, sauna, gymnasium. **Conf** facs Corporate Hospitality Days **Location** 3km N of town off N25
Hotel ★★★ 63% HL Lawlors Hotel, DUNGARVAN ☎ 058 41122 & 41056 ▤ 058 41000 89 en suite

West Waterford Golf & Country Club
☎ 058 43216 & 41475 ▤ 058 44343
e-mail: info@westwaterfordgolf.com
web: www.westwaterfordgolf.com
Designed by Eddie Hackett, the course is on 150 acres of rolling parkland by the Brickey River with a backdrop of the Comeragh Mountains, Knockmealdowns and Drum Hills. The first nine holes are laid out on a large plateau featuring a stream which comes into play at the 3rd and 4th holes. The river at the southern boundary affects several later holes.
18 holes, 6137mtrs, Par 72, SSS 72, Course record 70. Club membership 525.
Visitors Mon-Sun & BHs. Booking required. Dress code. **Societies** Booking required. **Green Fees** €33 per 18 holes (€44 weekends and bank holidays). **Course Designer** Eddie Hackett **Facilities** ⊕ ⏍ ⌚ 🔽 🍴 🚴 🏊 ☀ ✦ 🛄 ✦ **Leisure** hard tennis courts. **Conf** Corporate Hospitality Days **Location** 5km W of town off N25
Hotel ★★★ 63% HL Lawlors Hotel, DUNGARVAN ☎ 058 41122 & 41056 ▤ 058 41000 89 en suite

DUNMORE EAST   MAP 01 C2

Dunmore East
☎ 051 383151 ▤ 051 383151
e-mail: info@dunmoreeastgolfclub.ie
web: www.dunmoreeastgolfclub.ie
Overlooking the village, bay and the Hook peninsula, this course features a number of holes with cliff top trees and greens, promising challenging golf for the high or low handicap golfer.

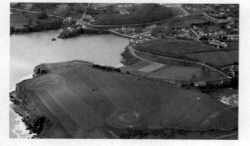

18 holes, 5400mtrs, Par 72, SSS 69, Course record 65. Club membership 500.
Visitors Mon-Sun & BHs. Booking required Sat, Sun & BHs. Dress code. **Societies** Booking required. **Green Fees** Apr-Oct: €30, Nov-Mar: €25 per 18 holes (€35/€30). **Course Designer** W H Jones **Facilities** ⊕ ⏍ ⌚ 🔽 🍴 🚴 🏊 ☀ ♦ 🛄 ✦ **Location** Into Dunmore East, left after fuel station, left at Strand Inn right
Hotel ★★★ 69% HL Majestic Hotel, TRAMORE ☎ 051 381761 60 en suite

LISMORE   MAP 01 C2

Lismore Ballyin
☎ 058 54026 ▤ 058 53338
e-mail: lismoregolf@eircom.net
web: www.lismoregolf.org
Picturesque, tree-dotted, sloping, nine-hole parkland course on the banks of the Blackwater River.
9 holes, 2748mtrs, Par 69, SSS 68. Club membership 400.
Visitors Mon-Sun & BHs. Booking required Wed, Sat, Sun & BHs. Dress code. **Societies** Booking required. **Green Fees** €20 per 18 holes. ⊕ **Prof** T. W. Murphy **Course Designer** Eddie Hackett **Facilities** 🔽 🍴 🚴 ☀ ✦ 🛄 ✦ 🛄 **Location** 1.6km W of town on R666
Hotel ★★★ 63% HL Lawlors Hotel, DUNGARVAN ☎ 058 41122 & 41056 ▤ 058 41000 89 en suite

TRAMORE   MAP 01 C2

Tramore Newtown Hill
☎ 051 386170 ▤ 051 390961
e-mail: tragolf@iol.ie
web: www.tramoregolfclub.com
This course has matured nicely over the years to become a true championship test and has been chosen as the venue for the Irish Professional Matchplay Championship and the Irish Amateur Championship. Most of the fairways are lined by evergreen trees, calling for accurate placing of shots, and the course is continuing to develop.
18 holes, 5923mtrs, Par 72, SSS 72, Course record 66. Club membership 1200.
Visitors Mon-Sat except BHs. Booking required. Dress code. **Societies** Booking required. **Green Fees** May-Sep: €45, Apr-Oct: €35, Nov-Mar: €30 (€60/€45/€35 Fri-Sat). **Prof** John Byrne **Course Designer** Capt H C Tippet **Facilities** ⊕ ⏍ 🔽 🍴 🚴 🏊 ☀ ✦ 🛄 ✦ **Conf** Corporate Hospitality Days **Location** 0.8km W of town on R675 coast road
Hotel ★★★ 69% HL Majestic Hotel, TRAMORE ☎ 051 381761 60 en suite

WATERFORD   MAP 01 C2

Faithlegg Faithlegg
☎ 051 382000 ▤ 051 382010
e-mail: golf@faithlegg.com
web: www.faithlegg.com
Set on the banks of the River Suir, the course has been integrated into a landscape textured with mature trees, flowing parkland and five lakes. Length is not the main defence, rather the greens provide a test for all levels making a good score a true reflection of good golf. Long Par 3's and tricky to mange Par 4's provide a challenge while reachable Par 5's may allow you to reclaim a shot or two.
18 holes, 6629yds, Par 72, SSS 72, Course record 69. Club membership 620.

Continued

Visitors Mon-Sun & BHs. Booking required Fri-Sun & BHs. Handicap certificate. Dress code. **Societies** booking required. **Green Fees** not confirmed. **Prof** Darragh Tighe & Ryan Hault **Course Designer** Patrick Merrigan **Facilities** ⊕ ⌕ ⌂ ⌱ ♨ ⌱ ♨ ⌂ ♨ ◌ ♪ ⌂ ♪ **Leisure** hard tennis courts, heated indoor swimming pool, fishing, sauna, solarium, gymnasium, full P.G.A. club repair & custom fitting service available, coaching specialists. **Conf** facs **Location** 9km E of town off R684 towards Cheekpoint

Waterford Newrath
☎ 051 876748 📄 051 853405
e-mail: info@waterfordgolfclub.com
web: www.waterfordgolfclub.com
One of the finest inland courses in Ireland. This is exemplified by the spectacular closing stretch, in particular the downhill 18th with its elevated tee, a wonderful viewpoint and a narrow gorse lined fairway demanding a very accurate tee shot.
18 holes, 5722mtrs, Par 71, SSS 70, Course record 64.
Club membership 1102.
Visitors Mon-Sun & BHs. Booking required. Dress code. **Societies** Booking required **Green Fees** Phone. **Prof** Harry Ewing **Course Designer** W Park/J Braid **Facilities** ⊕ ⌕ ⌂ ⌱ ♨ ⌂ ♨ ◌ ♪ **Location** 1.6km N of town on N77

Waterford Castle The Island, Ballinakill
☎ 051 871633 📄 051 871634
e-mail: golf@waterfordcastle.com
web: www.waterfordcastle.com/golf
A unique 130-hectare island course in the River Suir and accessed by private ferry. The course has four water features on the 2nd, 3rd, 4th and 16th holes with a Swilken Bridge on the 3rd hole. Two of the more challenging holes are the Par 4s at the 9th and 12th, the 9th being a 379-metre uphill, dog-leg right. The 417-metre 12th is a fine test of accuracy and distance. The views from the course are superb.
18 holes, 6231mtrs, Par 72, SSS 71, Course record 65.
Club membership 770.
Visitors Mon-Sat & BHs. Booking required. Dress code.
Societies Booking required. **Green Fees** Winter €48-€52; Summer €52-€62. **Course Designer** Des Smyth **Facilities** ⊕ ⌕ ⌂ ⌱ ♨ ◌ ♪ ⌂ ♪ **Leisure** hard tennis courts. **Conf** facs Corporate Hospitality Days **Location** 3km E of town via private ferry
Hotel ★★★★ HL Waterford Castle Hotel, The Island, WATERFORD
☎ 051 878203 19 en suite

CO WESTMEATH

ATHLONE   MAP 01 C4

Glasson Golf Hotel Glasson
☎ 090 6485120 📄 090 6485444
e-mail: info@glassongolf.ie
web: www.glassongolf.ie
Opened in 1993, the course has a reputation for being one of the most challenging and scenic courses in Ireland. Designed by Christy O'Connor Jnr it is reputedly his best yet. Surrounded on three sides by Lough Ree the views from everywhere on the course are breathtaking.
18 holes, 6251mtrs, Par 74, SSS 74, Course record 65.
Club membership 220.
Visitors Mon-Sun & BHs. Booking required. Dress code. **Societies** booking required. **Green Fees** €60 (€65 Fri & Sun, €75 Sat). **Course Designer** Christy O'Connor Jnr **Facilities** ⊕ ⌕ ⌂ ⌱ ♨ ⌂ ♨ ◌ ♪ ⌂ ♪

Leisure sauna, gymnasium, chipping green, hot tub, steam room. **Conf** facs Corporate Hospitality Days **Location** 10km N of town on N55
Hotel ★★★★ 74% HL Hodson Bay Hotel, Hodson Bay, ATHLONE
☎ 090 6442000 133 en suite

DELVIN   MAP 01 C4

Delvin Castle Clonyn
☎ 044 64315 & 64671 📄 044 64315
18 holes, 5800mtrs, Par 70, SSS 68.
Course Designer John Day **Location** On N52
Telephone for further details

MOATE   MAP 01 C4

Moate
☎ 090 6481271 📄 090 6482645
web: www.moategolfclub.ie
18 holes, 5742mtrs, Par 72, SSS 70, Course record 67.
Course Designer B Browne **Location** 1.6km N of town
Telephone for further details
Hotel ★★★★ 74% HL Hodson Bay Hotel, Hodson Bay, ATHLONE
☎ 090 6442000 133 en suite

Mount Temple Mount Temple Village
☎ 090 6481841 6481957 📄 0902 81957
e-mail: mttemple@iol.ie
web: www.mounttemplegolfclub.com
A traditionally built, championship course with unique links-type greens and natural undulating fairways. A challenge for all levels of golfers and all year golfing available.
18 holes, 6020metres, Par 72, SSS 72, Course record 71.
Club membership 250.
Visitors Mon-Sun & BHs. Booking required Sat-Sun & BHs. Dress code. **Societies** booking required. **Green Fees** not confirmed. **Prof** David Keenan **Course Designer** Michael Dolan **Facilities** ⊕ ⌕ ⌂ ⌱ ♨ ◌ ♪ ⌂ ♪ **Conf** Corporate Hospitality Days **Location** 5km NW of town to Temple Mount
Hotel ★★★★ 74% HL Hodson Bay Hotel, Hodson Bay, ATHLONE
☎ 090 6442000 133 en suite

MULLINGAR   MAP 01 C4

Mullingar ☎ 044 48366 📄 044 41499
18 holes, 5858metres, Par 72, SSS 71, Course record 63.
Course Designer James Braid **Location** 5km S of town on N52
Telephone for further details
Hotel ★★★★ 73% HL Mullingar Park Hotel, Dublin Rd, MULLINGAR
☎ 044 44446 & 37500 📄 044 35937 95 en suite

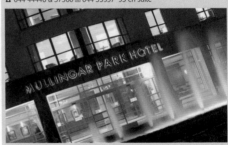

CO WEXFORD

ENNISCORTHY   MAP 01 D3

Enniscorthy Knockmarshall
☎ 053 9233191
e-mail: info@enniscorthygc.ie
web: www.enniscorthygc.ie
A pleasant course suitable for all levels of ability.
18 holes, 6115mtrs, Par 72, SSS 72. Club membership 900.
Visitors Mon-Sun & BHs. Booking required. Handicap certificate. Dress code. **Societies** Booking required **Green Fees** €30 per round (€40 Fri-Sun & BHs). **Prof** Martin Sludds **Course Designer** Eddie Hackett **Facilities** ⑪ ⑩ ⓛ ⌷ 孔 ⚒ ✿ 🍴 ✎ ⚒ ⌀ **Conf** Corporate Hospitality Days **Location** 1.6km W of town on N30

GOREY   MAP 01 D3

Courtown Kiltennel
☎ 055 25166 📠 055 25553
e-mail: courtown@iol.ie
web: www.courtowngolfclub.com
18 holes, 5898mtrs, Par 71, SSS 71, Course record 65.
Course Designer Harris & Associates **Location** 5km SE of town off R742 **Telephone for further details**
Hotel ★★★★ 73% HL Ashdown Park Hotel, The Coach Rd, GOREY TOWN ☎ 053 9480500 79 en suite

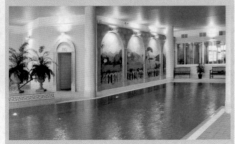

NEW ROSS   MAP 01 C3

New Ross Tinneranny
☎ 051 421433 📠 051 420098
18 holes, 5259metres, Par 70, SSS 70.
Course Designer Des Smith **Location** 5km from town **Telephone for further details**

ROSSLARE   MAP 01 D2

Rosslare Rosslare Strand
☎ 053 9132203 📠 053 9132263
e-mail: office@rosslaregolf.com
web: www.rosslaregolf.com
This traditional links course is within minutes of the ferry terminal at Rosslare. Many of the greens are sunken and are always in beautiful condition, but the semi-blind approaches are among features of this course which provide a healthy challenge. Celebrated 100 years of golf in 2005.
Old Course: 18 holes, 6042mtrs, Par 72, SSS 72, Course record 66.

Burrow: 12 holes, 3617metres, Par 46. Club membership 1000.
Visitors Mon-Sun & BHs. Booking required. Dress code. **Societies** Booking required. **Green Fees** Phone. **Prof** Johnny Young **Course Designer** Hawtree/Taylor **Facilities** ⑪ ⑩ ⓛ ⌷ 孔 ⌀ ⚒ ✿ 🍴 🞿 ✎ **Leisure** sauna. **Conf** Corporate Hospitality Days **Location** N of Rosslare village
Hotel ★★★★ HL Kelly's Resort Hotel & Spa, ROSSLARE ☎ 053 32114 118 annexe en suite

St Helen's Bay Golf & Country Club St Helens, Kilrane
☎ 053 9133234 📠 053 9133803
e-mail: info@sthelensbay.com
web: www.sthelensbay.com
Eighteen hole championship course with an additional 9 holes opened in 2003. Overlooking beach with accommodation on site.
27 holes, 5894mtrs, Par 72, SSS 72, Course record 69. Club membership 700.
Visitors Mon-Sun & BHs. Dress code. **Societies** Booking details **Green Fees** Nov-Mar: €25 per 18 holes, Apr-Oct: €40. (€30/€50 Sat & Sun). €25 all year per 9 holes **Course Designer** Philip Walton **Facilities** ⑪ ⑩ ⓛ ⌷ 孔 ⚒ ✿ 🍴 🞿 ✎ **Leisure** hard tennis courts, golf academy and tuition area. **Location** SE of Rosslare Harbour off N25
Hotel ★★★★ 78% HL Ferrycarrig Hotel, Ferrycarrig Bridge, WEXFORD ☎ 053 9120999 102 en suite

WEXFORD   MAP 01 D3

Wexford Mulgannon
☎ 053 42238 📠 053 42243
e-mail: info@wexfordgolfclub.ie
web: www.wexfordgolfclub.ie
Parkland with panoramic view of the Wexford coastline and mountains.
18 holes, 5578mtrs, Par 72, SSS 70. Club membership 800.
Visitors Mon-Sat & BHs. Booking required Thu & Sat. Dress code. **Societies** Booking required. **Green Fees** €32 per 18 holes, €27 winter (€38 Sat, Sun & BHs). **Prof** Liam Bowler **Facilities** ⑪ ⑩ ⓛ ⌷ 孔 ⚒ ✿ 🍴 🞿 ✎ **Hotel** ★★★ 78% HL Talbot Hotel Conference & Leisure Centre, The Quay, WEXFORD ☎ 053 22566 & 55559 📠 053 23377 109 en suite

CO WICKLOW

ARKLOW   MAP 01 D3

Arklow Abbeylands
☎ 0402 32492 📠 0402 91604
e-mail: arklowgolflinks@eircom.net
Scenic links course.
18 holes, 5802mtrs, Par 69, SSS 68, Course record 64. Club membership 780.
Visitors Tue-Sat. Booking required. Handicap certificate. Dress code. **Societies** Booking required. **Green Fees** €40 per round (€50 Fri-Sat). **Course Designer** Hawtree & Taylor **Facilities** ⑪ ⑩ ⓛ ⌷ 孔 ⚒ ✿ 🍴 **Location** 0.8km E of town centre
Hotel ★★★ CHH Marlfield House Hotel, GOREY ☎ 053 94 21124 20 en suite

BALTINGLASS

MAP 01 D3

Baltinglass Dublin Rd
☎ 059 6481350 🖹 059 6481842
e-mail: baltinglassgc@eircom.net
web: baltinglassgc.com
An 18-hole course overlooking Baltinglass town with breathtaking views of the Wicklow Mountains. Abundant mature trees make this course a good test of golf for all levels of handicap.
18 holes, 5912mtrs, Par 71, SSS 71, Course record 68.
Club membership 600.
Visitors Mon-Sun & BHs. Booking required **Societies** Booking required **Green Fees** Phone. ☏ **Course Designer** Eddie Connaughton **Facilities** ⓣ ⓘ ⓛ ⯑ ⓣ 🖧 ⎠ ♪ ⛴ ♪ **Location** 500 metres N of village
Hotel ★★★ 75% HL Seven Oaks Hotel, Athy Rd, CARLOW ☎ 059 9131308 89 en suite

BLAINROE

MAP 01 D3

Blainroe
☎ 0404 68168 🖹 0404 69369
e-mail: blainroegolfclub@eircom.net
web: www.blainroe.com
18 holes, 6175mtrs, Par 72, SSS 72, Course record 71.
Course Designer Fred Hawtree **Location** 5km SE of Wicklow on R750 coast road
Telephone for further details

BLESSINGTON

MAP 01 D3

Tulfarris Hotel & Golf Resort
☎ 045 867644 & 867600 🖹 045 867000
e-mail: info@tulfarris.com
web: www.tulfarris.com
Designed by Paddy Merrigan, this course is on the Blessington lakeshore with the Wicklow Mountains as a backdrop. The use of the natural landscape is evident throughout the whole course, the variety of trees guarding fairways and green approaches.
18 holes, 6507metres, Par 72, SSS 74, Course record 68.
Club membership 255.
Visitors Booking required Sat-Sun. **Societies** booking required. **Green Fees** not confirmed. **Prof** Stephen Brown **Course Designer** Patrick Merrigan **Facilities** ⓣ ⓘ ⓛ ⯑ ⓣ 🖧 ⎠ ♪ ◇ ♪ 🖧 ♪ **Leisure** hard tennis courts, fishing, gymnasium. **Conf** facs Corporate Hospitality Days **Location** 3.5km from village off N81

BRAY

MAP 01 D4

Bray Greystones Rd
☎ 01 2763200 🖹 01 2763262
e-mail: info@braygolfclub.com
web: www.braygolfclub.com
A USGA standard parkland course of nearly 81 hectares, combining stunning scenery with a classic layout. The 11th Par 4 signature hole provides a fine view of the coastline.
18 holes, 5990mtrs, Par 71, SSS 72, Course record 66.
Club membership 812.
Visitors Mon, Thu-Sat. Booking required. Dress code. **Societies** Booking required. **Green Fees** €25 before 9:30am, €40 before noon, €50 after noon (€70 Sat). **Prof** Ciaran Carroll **Course Designer** Smyth/Brannigan **Facilities** ⓣ ⓘ ⓛ ⯑ ⓣ 🖧 ⎠ ♪ 🖧 ♪ **Conf** facs Corporate Hospitality Days **Location** Near town off R761

Hotel ★★★ 68% HL Royal Hotel & Leisure Centre, Main St, BRAY
☎ 01 2862935 98 en suite

Old Conna Ferndale Rd
☎ 01 2826055 & 2826766 🖹 01 2825611
e-mail: info@oldconna.com
Parkland course set in wooded terrain with panoramic views of the Irish Sea and the Wicklow mountains.
18 holes, 5989mtres, Par 72, SSS 72, Course record 68.
Club membership 1000.
Visitors Mon-Fri. Booking required. Dress code. **Societies** booking required. **Green Fees** not confirmed. **Prof** Michael Langford **Course Designer** Eddie Hackett **Facilities** ⓣ ⓘ ⓛ ⯑ ⓣ 🖧 ⎠ ♪ 🖧 ♪ **Conf** facs Corporate Hospitality Days **Location** 3.5km from town centre
Hotel ★★★ 68% HL Royal Hotel & Leisure Centre, Main St, BRAY
☎ 01 2862935 98 en suite

Woodbrook Dublin Rd
☎ 01 2824799 🖹 01 2821950
e-mail: golf@woodbrook.ie
web: www.woodbrook.ie
Perched on top of 30-metre seacliffs, the course has recently been redesigned with 18 new sand-based, bent-grass greens of varying sculpture and built to USGA specification. Cunning placement of fairway and greenside bunkers call for shot making virtuosity of the highest calibre.
18 holes, 6017metres, Par 72, SSS 71, Course record 65.
Club membership 1200.
Visitors Mon, Thu-Fri. Booking required. Handicap certificate. Dress code. **Societies** booking required. **Green Fees** not confirmed. **Prof** Billy Kinsella **Course Designer** Peter McEvoy **Facilities** ⯑ ⓣ ⎠ ♪ 🖧 ♪ 🖧 ♪ **Location** On N11
Hotel ★★★ 68% HL Royal Hotel & Leisure Centre, Main St, BRAY
☎ 01 2862935 98 en suite

BRITTAS BAY

MAP 01 D3

The European Club
☎ 0404 47415 🖹 0404 47449
e-mail: info@europeanclub.com
web: www.theeuropeanclub.com
A links course that runs through a large dunes system. Since it was opened in 1992 it is rapidly gaining recognition as one of Irelands best courses. Notable holes include the 7th, 13th and 14th.
20 holes, 6737metres, Par 71, SSS 73, Course record 67.
Club membership 100.
Visitors Mon-Sun & BHs. Booking required. Dress code. **Societies** welcome. **Green Fees** not confirmed. **Course Designer** Pat Ruddy **Facilities** ⓣ ⓘ ⓛ ⯑ ⓣ 🖧 ♪ 🖧 ♪ **Conf** Corporate Hospitality Days **Location** 1.6km from Brittas Bay

DELGANY

MAP 01 D3

Delgany
☎ 01 2874536 🖹 01 2873977
e-mail: delganygolf@eircom.net
web: www.delganygolfclub.com
18 holes, 5473mtrs, Par 69, SSS 68.
Course Designer H Vardon **Location** 1.2km from village off N11
Telephone for further details
Hotel ★★★★ 69% HL Glenview Hotel, Glen O' the Downs, DELGANY
☎ 01 2873399 70 en suite

Glen of the Downs Coolnaskeagh

☎ 01 2876240 📠 01 2870063
e-mail: info@glenofthedowns.com
web: www.glenofthedowns.com
A parkland course that plays much like a links course with sand-based greens and tees. Among its features is a five-tier double green, which is shared by the 8th and 10th holes. Sandwiched in between is a fine Par 5, the 9th, which measures 457 metres off the back.
18 holes, 5980yds, Par 71, SSS 70, Course record 68.
Club membership 650.
Visitors may play Mon-Sun & BHs. Advance booking required. Dress code. **Societies** advance booking required. **Green Fees** not confirmed. **Course Designer** Peter McEvoy **Facilities** ⑪ 🍴 🍺 ♻ 🎲 ⅃ 🛍 ☂ ✦ 🏌 ⚴ **Conf** facs Corporate Hospitality Days **Location** off N11 southbound, 4m from Bray
Hotel ★★★★ 69% HL Glenview Hotel, Glen O' the Downs, DELGANY
☎ 01 2873399 70 en suite

DUNLAVIN MAP 01 D3

Rathsallagh

☎ 045 403316 📠 045 403295
e-mail: info@rathsallagh.com
web: www.rathsallagh.com
Designed by Peter McEvoy and Christy O'Connor Jnr, this is a spectacular course which will test the pro's without intimidating the club golfer. Set in 525 acres of lush parkland with thousands of mature trees, natural water hazards and gently rolling landscape. The greens are of high quality, in design, construction and condition.
18 holes, 6324mtrs, Par 72, SSS 74, Course record 68.
Club membership 410.
Visitors Mon-Sun & BHs. Booking required. Dress code. **Societies** Booking required. **Green Fees** €60 per round (€80 Fri-Sat & BHs). **Prof** Brendan McDaid **Course Designer** McEvoy/O'Connor **Facilities** ⑪ 🍴 🍺 ♻ 🎲 ⅃ 🛍 ☂ ✦ ⚴ 🏌 🍴 **Leisure** hard tennis courts, sauna, private jacuzzi/steam room, croquet lawn, walled garden. **Conf** facs Corporate Hospitality Days **Location** SW of village off N9

GREYSTONES MAP 01 D3

Charlesland Golf & Country Club Hotel

☎ 01 2874350 & 2878200 📠 01 2874360
e-mail: teetimes@charlesland.com
web: www.charlesland.com
Championship length, Par 72 course with a double dog-leg at the 9th and 18th. Water hazards at the 3rd and 11th.
18 holes, 5963mtrs, Par 72, SSS 72, Course record 68.
Visitors Mon-Sun & BHs. Booking required. Dress code. **Societies** Booking required. **Green Fees** €32 per round (€45 Fri-Sun). **Prof** Peter Duignan **Course Designer** Eddie Hackett **Facilities** ⑪ 🍴 🍺 ♻ 🎲 ⅃ 🛍 ☂ ✦ ⚴ 🏌 **Conf** facs Corporate Hospitality Days **Location** 1.6km S of town on R762
Hotel ★★★★ 69% HL Glenview Hotel, Glen O' the Downs, DELGANY
☎ 01 2873399 70 en suite

Greystones

☎ 01 2874136 📠 01 2873749
e-mail: secretary@greystonesgc.com
web: www.greystonesgc.com
18 holes, 5322mtrs, Par 69, SSS 68.
Course Designer P Merrigan
Telephone for further details
Hotel ★★★★ 69% HL Glenview Hotel, Glen O' the Downs, DELGANY
☎ 01 2873399 70 en suite

KILCOOLE MAP 01 D3

Druids Glen Golf Club see page 463

Hotel ★★★★★ 73% HL Marriott Druids Glen Hotel & Country Club, NEWTOWNMOUNTKENNEDY ☎ 01 2870800 145 en suite
Hotel ★★★ 72% HL Hunter's Hotel, RATHNEW ☎ 0404 40106 Fax 0404 40338 16 en suite
Hotel ★★★★ 69% HL Glenview Hotel, Glen O' the Downs, DELGANY
☎ 01 2873399 Fax 01 2877511 70 en suite

Kilcoole

☎ 01 2872066 📠 01 2010497
e-mail: adminkg@eircom.net
web: www.kilcoolegolfclub.com
Beautifully manicured nine holes with water features on five holes. The course is dry and flat with sand based greens and the Sugarloaf Mountain in the background provides a pleasing view. Near the sea but well protected by tree lined fairways.
9 holes, 5506mtrs, Par 70, SSS 69, Course record 66.
Club membership 600.
Visitors Mon-Sun & BHs. Booking required. Dress code. **Societies** Booking required. **Green Fees** Phone. **Facilities** ⑪ 🍴 🍺 ♻ 🎲 ⅃ 🛍 ☂ ✦ **Conf** facs Corporate Hospitality Days **Location** S of village on R761
Hotel ★★★★ 69% HL Glenview Hotel, Glen O' the Downs, DELGANY
☎ 01 2873399 70 en suite

RATHDRUM MAP 01 D3

Glenmalure Greenane

☎ 0404 46679 📠 0404 46783
e-mail: golf@glenmalure-golf.ie
web: www.glenmalure-golf.ie
18 holes, 4846metres, Par 71, SSS 67, Course record 71.
Course Designer P Suttle **Location** 3km W of town
Telephone for further details
Hotel ★★★ 70% HL Woodenbridge Hotel, WOODEN BRIDGE
☎ 0402 35146 23 en suite

CHAMPIONSHIP COURSE

CO WICKLOW — KILCOOLE

DRUIDS GLEN GOLF CLUB

Map 01 D3

Newtownmountkennedy
☎ 01 2873600 📠 01 2873699
e-mail: info@druidsglen.ie
web: www.druidsglen.ie
18 holes, 5987metres, Par 71, SSS 73,
Course record 62.
Club membership 219.
Visitors advance booking essential.
Societies advance booking essential
Green Fees Phone. **Prof** George Henry
Course Designer Tom Craddock/Pat Ruddy
Facilities ⑪ 🍽 🛒 ▭🍴 ⚒ 🏠 ⛳◇ 🏌 🚚
🏊 🏋 **Leisure** heated indoor swimming pool,
sauna, gymnasium. **Location** S of village on
R761

Druids Glen from the 1st tee to the 18th green
creates an exceptional golfing experience, with
its distinguished surroundings and spectacular
views. It is the culmination of years of
preparation, creating a unique inland course
that challenges and satisfies in equal parts.
Special features include an island green on
the 17th hole and a Celtic Cross on the 12th.
Druids Glen hosted the Murphy's Irish Open
in 1996, 1997, 1998 and for an unprecedented
fourth time in 1999. In 2000 Druids Glen
won the title of European Golf Course of the
Year and in 2002 it hosted the Seve trophy.
The world's top professionals and club golfers
alike, continue to enjoy the challenge here.
A variety of teeing positions are available
and there is a practice area, including three
full-length academy holes. Individual and
corporate members enjoy generous reserved
tee times; visitors are very welcome.

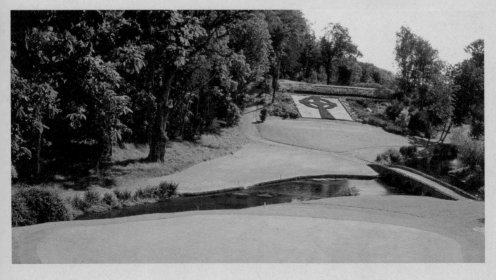

ROUNDWOOD

MAP 01 D3

Roundwood Newtown, Mountkennedy
☎ 01 2818488 & 2802555 ▤ 01 2843642
e-mail: rwood@indigo.ie
Heathland and parkland course with forest and lakes set in beautiful countryside with views of the coast and the Wicklow Mountains.
18 holes, 6113mtrs, Par 72, SSS 72, Course record 70.
Club membership 220.
Visitors Mon-Sun & BHs. Booking required. Dress code. **Societies** Booking required **Green Fees** €40 per round (€58 Sat, Sun & BHs). **Prof** Seamus Clinton **Facilities** ⑪ ⑩ ⓛ ⌷ ⅋ ⌲ ⛳ ♣ ♪ **Conf** Corporate Hospitality Days **Location** 4km NE of village on R765
Hotel ★★★ 66% HL The Glendalough Hotel, GLENDALOUGH
☎ 0404 45135 44 en suite

SHILLELAGH

MAP 01 D3

Coollattin Coollattin
☎ 053 9429125 ▤ 053 9429930
e-mail: coollattingolfclub@eircom.net
web: www.coollattingolfclub.com
Plenty of trees provide features on this 18-hole parkland course.
18 holes, 5622mtrs, Par 70, SSS 68, Course record 70.
Club membership 1115.
Visitors Mon-Sun & BHs. Booking required. Dress code. **Societies** Booking required **Green Fees** €30 per round (€45 Sat, Sun & BHs). **Prof** Peter Jones **Course Designer** Peter McEvoy **Facilities** ⑪ ⑩ ⓛ ⌷ ⅋ ⌲ ♣ ♪ ♣ ♪ **Conf** Corporate Hospitality Days
Hotel ★★★ CHH Marlfield House Hotel, GOREY ☎ 053 94 21124
20 en suite

WICKLOW

MAP 01 D3

Wicklow Dunbur Rd
☎ 0404 67379 ▤ 0404 64756
e-mail: info@wicklowgolfclub.ie
web: www.wicklowgolfclub.ie
Situated on the cliffs overlooking Wicklow Bay, this course provides a challenging test of golf, each hole having individual features. Spectacular views of the coastline from every hole.

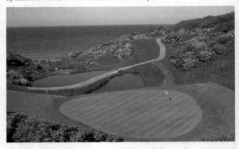

18 holes, 5437mtrs, Par 71, SSS 70. Club membership 700.
Visitors Mon-Sun & BHs. Booking required. Dress code. **Societies** Booking required **Green Fees** €40 per round (€45 Sat, Sun & BHs). **Prof** E McLoughlin, D McLoughlin **Course Designer** Craddock & Ruddy
Facilities ⑪ ⑩ ⓛ ⌷ ⅋ ⌲ ♣ ♪ ♣ ♪ **Location** SE of town centre

WOODENBRIDGE

MAP 01 D3

Woodenbridge Woodenbridge, Arklow
☎ 0402 35202 ▤ 0402 35754
e-mail: wgc@eircom.net
web: www.woodenbridgegolfclub.com
18 holes, 5852metres, Par 71, SSS 70, Course record 71.
Course Designer Patrick Merrigan **Location** N of village
Telephone for further details
Hotel ★★★ 70% HL Woodenbridge Hotel, WOODEN BRIDGE
☎ 0402 35146 23 en suite

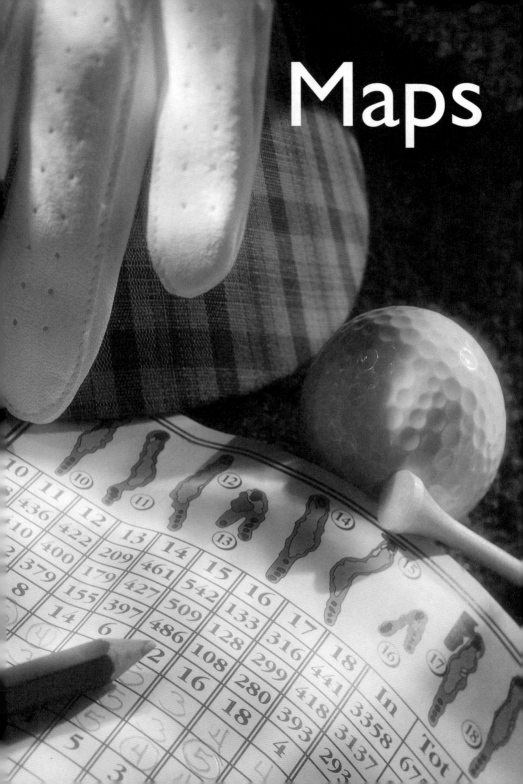

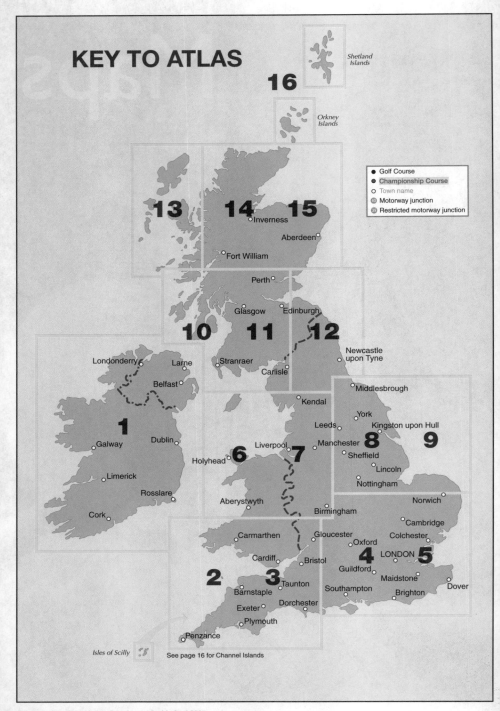

KEY TO ATLAS

Shetland Islands

16

Orkney Islands

- ● Golf Course
- ● Championship Course
- ○ Town name
- Ⓜ Motorway junction
- Ⓡ Restricted motorway junction

13 **14** **15**

Inverness

Aberdeen

Fort William

Perth

Glasgow   Edinburgh

10 **11** **12**

Newcastle upon Tyne

Londonderry   Larne   Stranraer

Belfast   Carlisle

Middlesbrough

Kendal

York

Leeds   Kingston upon Hull

1   Dublin   Liverpool   Manchester   **8**   **9**

Galway   Holyhead   **6**   **7**   Sheffield

Limerick   Lincoln

Rosslare   Nottingham

Aberystwyth   Norwich

Cork   Birmingham   Cambridge

Carmarthen   Gloucester   Colchester

Cardiff   Oxford

2   **3**   Bristol   **4** LONDON **5**

Taunton   Guildford   Maidstone

Barnstaple   Southampton   Brighton   Dover

Exeter   Dorchester

Plymouth

Penzance

Isles of Scilly   See page 16 for Channel Islands

© Automobile Association Developments Limited 2007

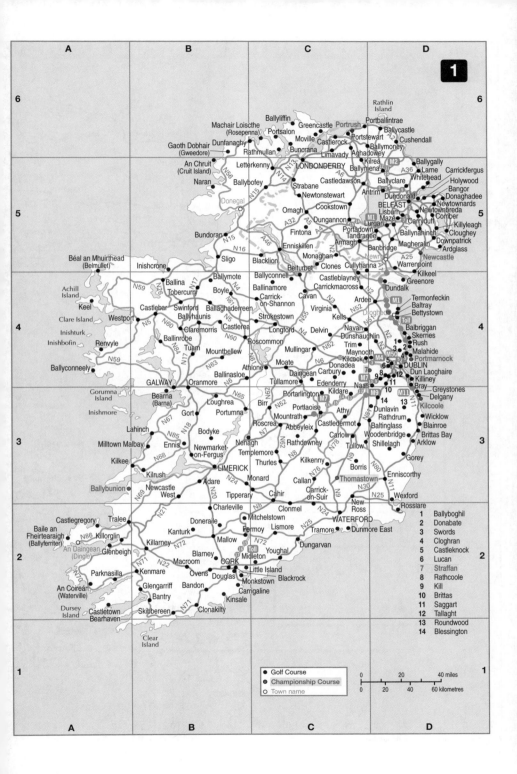

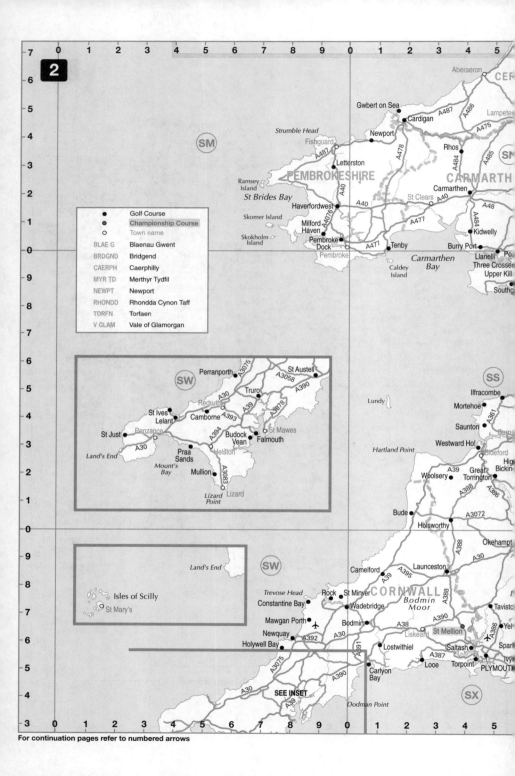

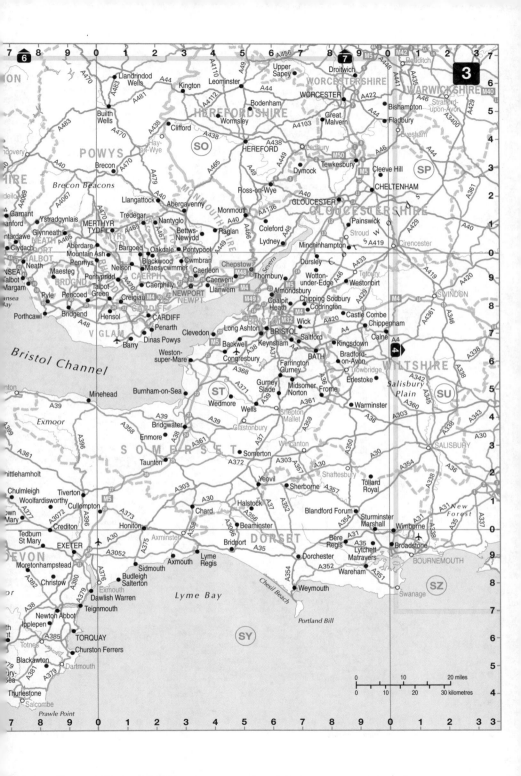

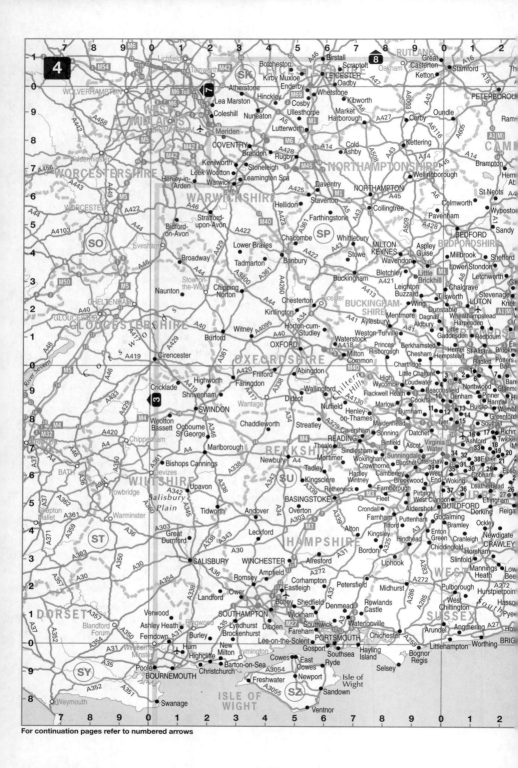

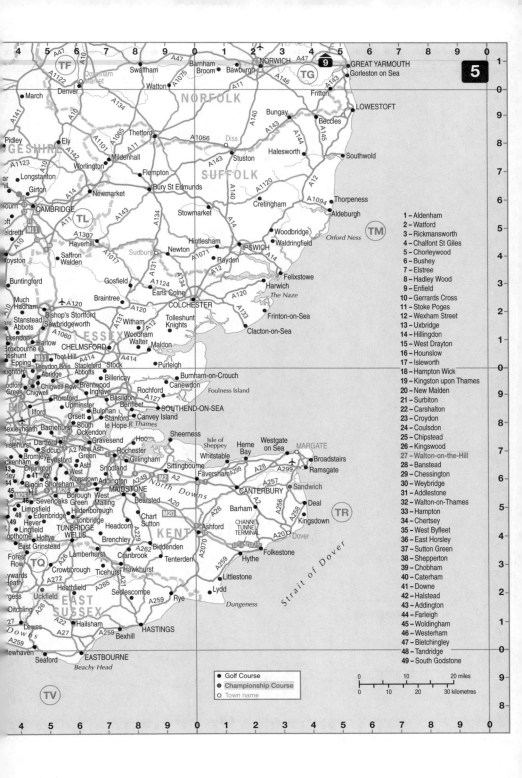

5

1 – Aldenham
2 – Watford
3 – Rickmansworth
4 – Chalfont St Giles
5 – Chorleywood
6 – Bushey
7 – Elstree
8 – Hadley Wood
9 – Enfield
10 – Gerrards Cross
11 – Stoke Poges
12 – Wexham Street
13 – Uxbridge
14 – Hillingdon
15 – West Drayton
16 – Hounslow
17 – Isleworth
18 – Hampton Wick
19 – Kingston upon Thames
20 – New Malden
21 – Surbiton
22 – Carshalton
23 – Croydon
24 – Coulsdon
25 – Chipstead
26 – Kingswood
27 – Walton-on-the-Hill
28 – Banstead
29 – Chessington
30 – Weybridge
31 – Addlestone
32 – Walton-on-Thames
33 – Hampton
34 – Chertsey
35 – West Byfleet
36 – East Horsley
37 – Sutton Green
38 – Shepperton
39 – Chobham
40 – Caterham
41 – Downe
42 – Halstead
43 – Addington
44 – Farleigh
45 – Woldingham
46 – Westerham
47 – Bletchingley
48 – Tandridge
49 – South Godstone

● Golf Course
● Championship Course
○ Town name

0   10   20 miles
0   10   20   30 kilometres

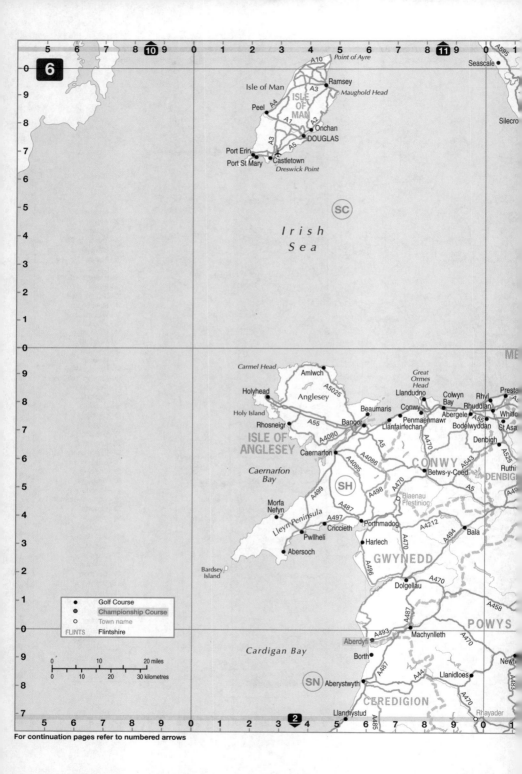

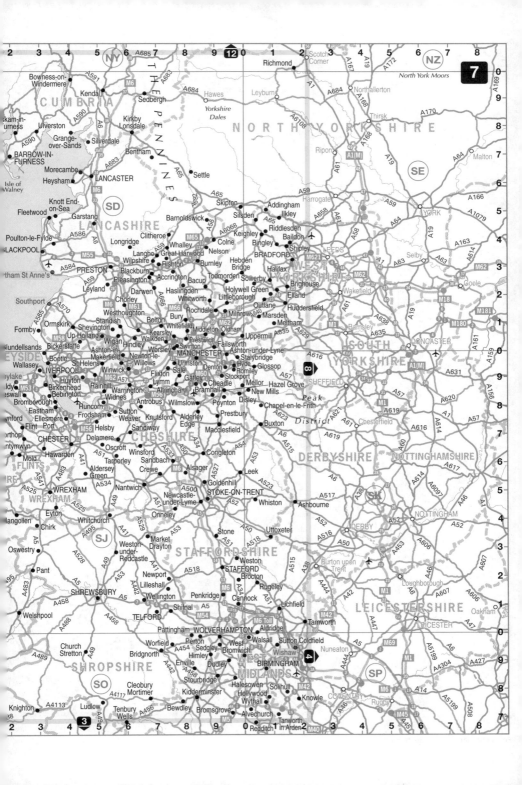

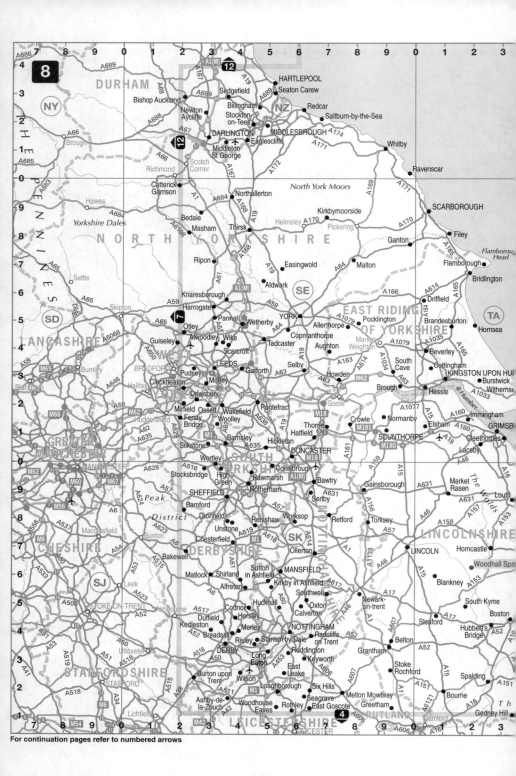

For continuation pages refer to numbered arrows

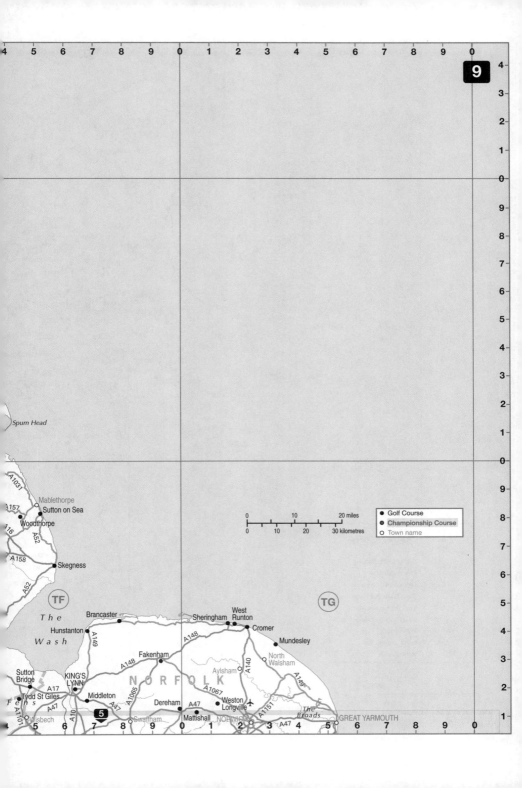

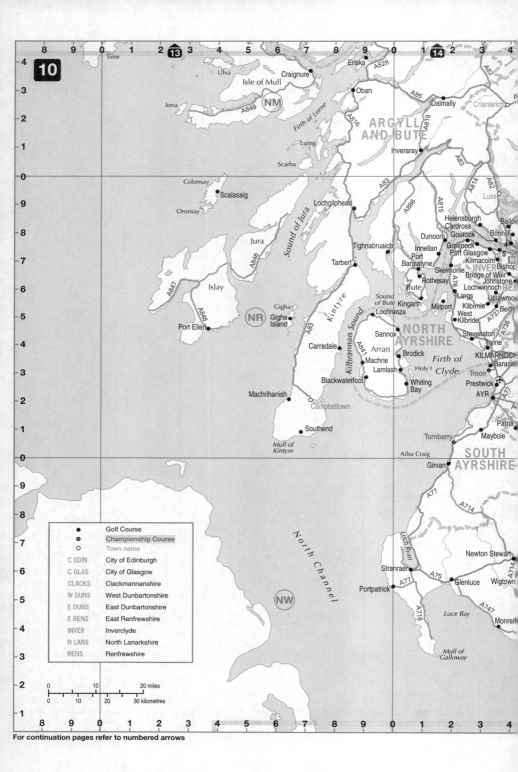

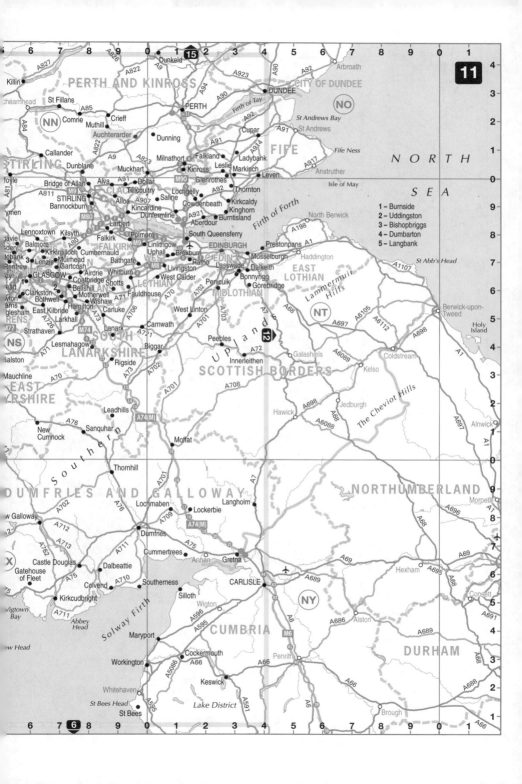

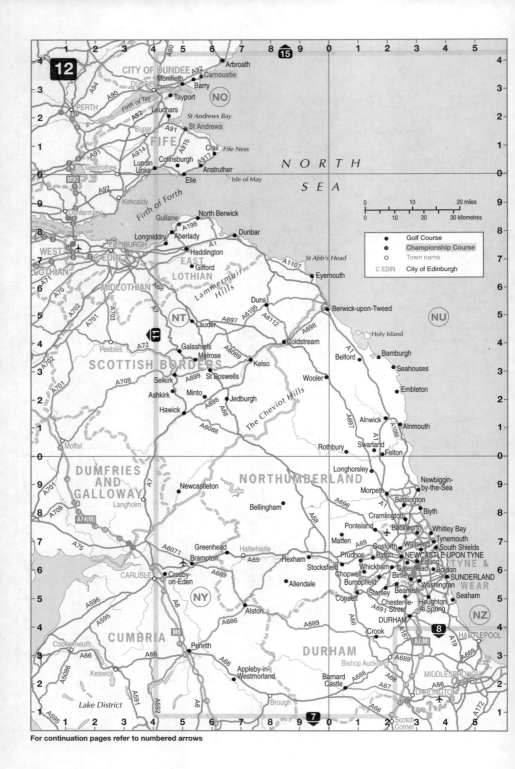

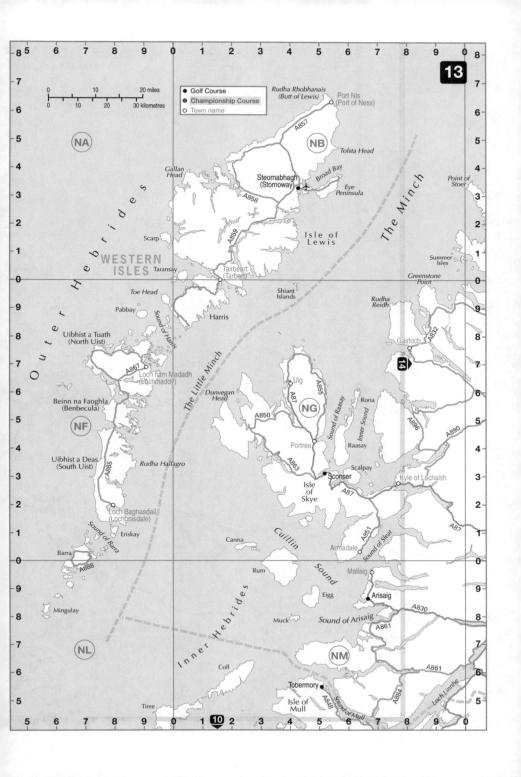

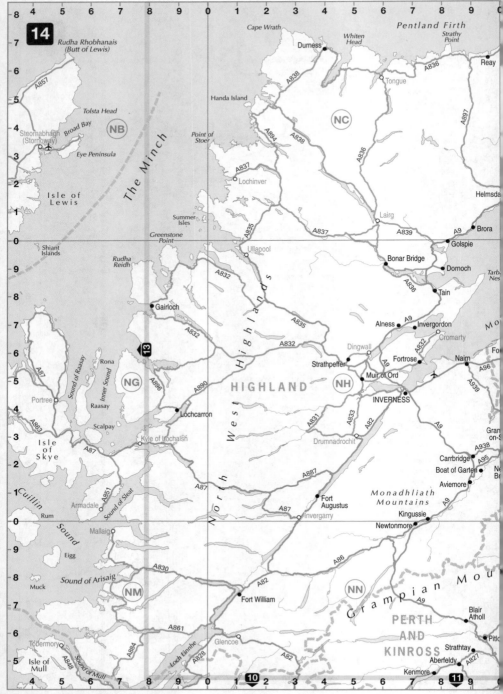

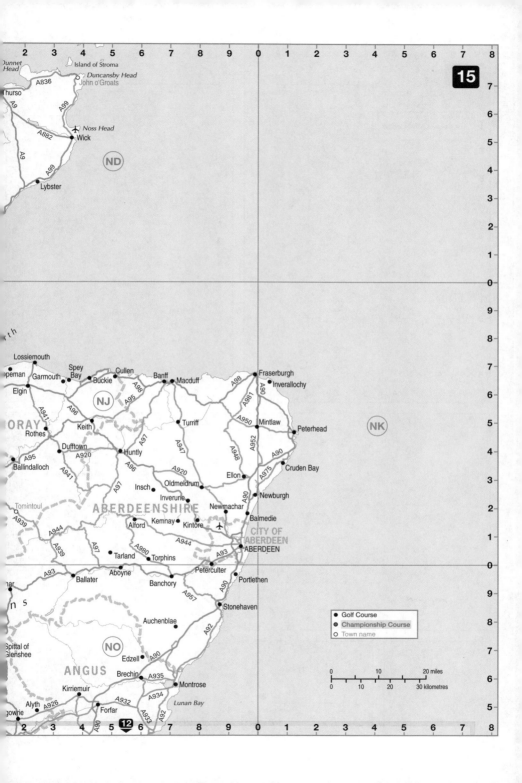

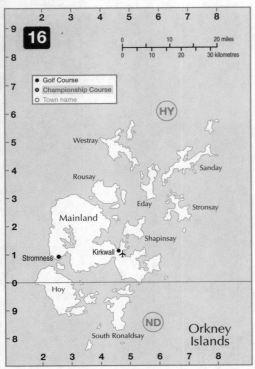

● Golf Course
● Championship Course
○ Town name

HY

20 miles
0 — 10 — 20 miles
0 — 10 — 20 — 30 kilometres

Westray

Rousay

Sanday

Eday

Stronsay

Mainland

Shapinsay

Stromness   Kirkwall ✈

Hoy

ND

South Ronaldsay

Orkney
Islands

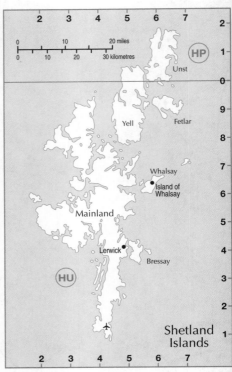

HP

Unst

0 — 10 — 20 miles
0 — 10 — 20 — 30 kilometres

Yell

Fetlar

Whalsay
● Island of
Whalsay

Mainland

Lerwick ●

Bressay

HU

✈

Shetland
Islands

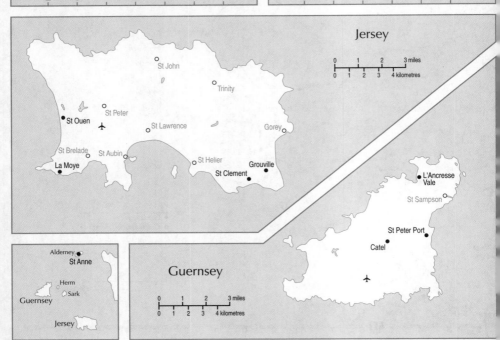

Jersey

St John

Trinity

0 — 1 — 2 — 3 miles
0 — 1 — 2 — 3 — 4 kilometres

St Peter

● St Ouen

St Lawrence

Gorey ○

St Brelade   St Aubin

St Helier

Grouville

La Moye ●

St Clement ●

● L'Ancresse
Vale

St Sampson ○

● St Peter Port

Catel ●

Alderney ○●
St Anne

Herm

Sark

Guernsey

Guernsey

Jersey

0 — 1 — 2 — 3 miles
0 — 1 — 2 — 3 — 4 kilometres

✈

Driving Ranges

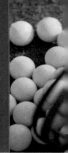

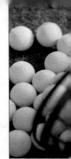

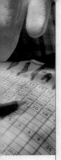

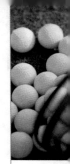

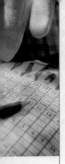

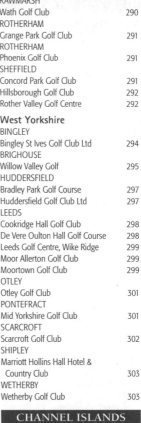

CHANNEL ISLANDS

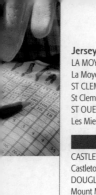

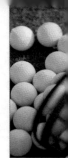

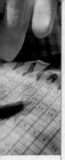

Location Index

Golf Course Index

Golf Course Index

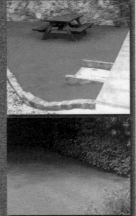
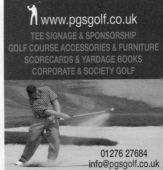
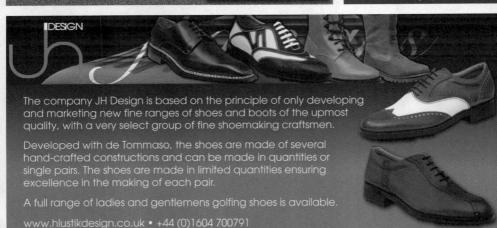
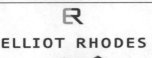
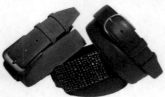
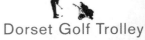
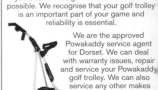